AVOIDING ERRORS IN THE EMERGENCY DEPARTMENT

THIRD EDITION

MICHAEL E. WINTERS, MD, MBA
Professor of Emergency Medicine and Medicine
Vice Chair for Clinical and Administrative Affairs
Department of Emergency Medicine
University of Maryland School of Medicine
Baltimore, Maryland

DALE P. WOOLRIDGE, MD, PHD
Professor of Emergency Medicine and Pediatrics
Department of Emergency Medicine and Pediatrics
University of Arizona College of Medicine
Tucson, Arizona

EVIE MARCOLINI, MD, MBE
Associate Professor of Emergency Medicine and Neurology
Vice Chair of Faculty Affairs, Department of Emergency Medicine
Geisel School of Medicine at Dartmouth
Hanover, New Hampshire

MIMI LU, MD
Clinical Professor of Emergency Medicine
Division of Pediatric Emergency Medicine
Department of Emergency Medicine
University of California, San Francisco School of Medicine
San Francisco, California

SARAH B. DUBBS, MD
Associate Professor of Emergency Medicine
Residency Program Director
Department of Emergency Medicine
University of Maryland School of Medicine
Baltimore, Maryland

Wolters Kluwer

Philadelphia · Baltimore · New York · London
Buenos Aires · Hong Kong · Sydney · Tokyo

Acquisitions Editor: James Sherman
Senior Development Editor: Ashley Fischer
Editorial Coordinator: Priyanka Alagar
Marketing Manager: Kirsten Watrud
Senior Production Project Manager: Catherine Ott
Managers, Graphic Arts & Design: Stephen Druding, Leslie Caruso
Manufacturing Coordinator: Lisa Bowling
Prepress Vendor: S4Carlisle Publishing Services

Third Edition

Copyright © 2025 Wolters Kluwer.

Copyright © 2017 Wolters Kluwer. Copyright © 2010 Lippincott Williams & Wilkins, a Wolters Kluwer business. All rights reserved. This book is protected by copyright. No part of this book may be reproduced or transmitted in any form or by any means, including as photocopies or scanned-in or other electronic copies, or utilized by any information storage and retrieval system without written permission from the copyright owner, except for brief quotations embodied in critical articles and reviews. Materials appearing in this book prepared by individuals as part of their official duties as U.S. government employees are not covered by the above-mentioned copyright. To request permission, please contact Wolters Kluwer at Two Commerce Square, 2001 Market Street, Philadelphia, PA 19103, via email at permissions@lww.com, or via our website at shop.lww.com (products and services).

9 8 7 6 5 4 3 2 1

Printed in Mexico

Library of Congress Cataloging-in-Publication Data
ISBN-13: 978-1-975211-86-8
Library of Congress Control Number: 2024914371

This work is provided "as is," and the publisher disclaims any and all warranties, express or implied, including any warranties as to accuracy, comprehensiveness, or currency of the content of this work.

This work is no substitute for individual patient assessment based upon healthcare professionals' examination of each patient and consideration of, among other things, age, weight, gender, current or prior medical conditions, medication history, laboratory data and other factors unique to the patient. The publisher does not provide medical advice or guidance and this work is merely a reference tool. Healthcare professionals, and not the publisher, are solely responsible for the use of this work including all medical judgments and for any resulting diagnosis and treatments.

Given continuous, rapid advances in medical science and health information, independent professional verification of medical diagnoses, indications, appropriate pharmaceutical selections and dosages, and treatment options should be made and healthcare professionals should consult a variety of sources. When prescribing medication, healthcare professionals are advised to consult the product information sheet (the manufacturer's package insert) accompanying each drug to verify, among other things, conditions of use, warnings and side effects and identify any changes in dosage schedule or contraindications, particularly if the medication to be administered is new, infrequently used or has a narrow therapeutic range. To the maximum extent permitted under applicable law, no responsibility is assumed by the publisher for any injury and/or damage to persons or property, as a matter of products liability, negligence law or otherwise, or from any reference to or use by any person of this work.

shop.lww.com

Associate Editors

MICHAEL ABRAHAM, MD, MS
Associate Professor
Department of Emergency Medicine
University of Maryland School of Medicine
Baltimore, Maryland

MICHAEL G. ALLISON, MD
Chief, Critical Care Medicine
Department of Medicine
University of Maryland St. Joseph Medical Center
Towson, Maryland

PATRICIA RUTH ATCHINSON, DO
Assistant Professor
Staff Physician
Department of Emergency Medicine and Critical Care
Dartmouth Hitchcock Medical Center
Lebanon, New Hampshire

LAURA J. BONTEMPO, MD, MEd
Associate Professor
Department of Emergency Medicine
University of Maryland School of Medicine
Baltimore, Maryland

JOELLE BORHART, MD
Program Director
Associate Professor of Emergency Medicine
Department of Emergency Medicine
Georgetown University Hospital
Washington Hospital Center
Washington, District of Columbia

WILLIAM J. BRADY, MD
Professor of Emergency Medicine and Medicine
Vice Chair of Emergency Medicine
The David A. Harrison Distinguished Educator
University of Virginia School of Medicine
Operational Medical Director
Albemarle County Fire Rescue
Charlottesville, Virginia

VINCENT J. CALLEO, MD
Medical Director, Upstate NY Polson Center
Department of Emergency Medicine
SUNY Upstate Medical University
Syracuse, New York

JOSHUA EASTER, MD, MS
Associate Professor
Department of Emergency Medicine
University of Virginia School of Medicine
Charlottesville, Virginia

LILLIAN LIANG EMLET, MD, MS
Professor
Department of Critical Care Medicine and Emergency Medicine
University of Pittsburgh School of Medicine
University of Pittsburgh Medical Center
Pittsburgh, Pennsylvania

KAYLA T. ENRIQUEZ, MD, MPH
Associate Professor
Department of Emergency Medicine
University of California, San Francisco School of Medicine
San Francisco, California

Associate Editors

Molly K. Estes, MD, FACEP, FAAEM
Associate Professor
Department of Emergency Medicine
Loma Linda University School of Medicine
Loma Linda, California

J. David Gatz, MD
Assistant Professor
Department of Emergency Medicine
University of Maryland School of Medicine
Baltimore, Maryland

Daniel B. Gingold, MD, MPH
Associate Professor
Department of Emergency Medicine
University of Maryland School of Medicine
Baltimore, Maryland

Joshua Glasser, MD, FAAP
Assistant Professor
Department of Emergency Medicine and Pediatrics
Penn State Health
Hershey, Pennsylvania

Kami M. Hu, MD
Assistant Professor
Department of Emergency Medicine
Department of Internal Medicine
University of Maryland School of Medicine
Baltimore, Maryland

Stephen Y. Liang, MD, MPHS
Associate Professor of Medicine
Department of Emergency Medicine
Division of Infectious Diseases
Department of Medicine
Washington University School of Medicine
St. Louis, Missouri

Phillip D. Magidson, MD, MPH
Assistant Professor
Division of Geriatric Medicine and Gerontology
Department of Emergency Medicine
The Johns Hopkins University School of Medicine
Baltimore, Maryland

Heather Murphy-Lavoie, MD
Director of Faculty Development
Department of Emergency Medicine
Louisiana State University School of Medicine
New Orleans, Louisiana

Adedamola Ogunniyi, MD
Associate Director, Residency Training Program
Department of Emergency Medicine
Harbor-UCLA Medical Center
Torrance, California

Ryan Raam, MD
Associate Professor of Clinical Emergency Medicine
Department of Emergency Medicine
Los Angeles General Medical Center
Los Angeles, California

Priti Rawani-Patel, MD, MA
Assistant Professor
Department of Emergency Medicine
University of Arizona College of Medicine
Tucson, Arizona

Jennifer Repanshek, MD
Adjunct Associate Professor of Clinical Emergency Medicine
Lewis Katz School of Medicine at Temple University
Temple University Hospital
Philadelphia, Pennsylvania

Scott W. Rodi, MD, MPH
Chair
Department of Emergency Medicine
Dartmouth Hitchcock Medical Center
Lebanon, New Hampshire

Manpreet Singh, MD, MBE, FACEP, AEMUS-FDP
Director, Undergraduate Medical Education
Department of Emergency Medicine
Harbor-UCLA Medical Center
Torrance, California

ANGELA D. SMEDLEY, MD
Assistant Professor
Medical Director
Department of Emergency Medicine
University of Maryland School of Medicine
Baltimore, Maryland

RYAN SPANGLER, MD
Assistant Professor
Department of Emergency Medicine
University of Maryland Medical Center
University of Maryland School of Medicine
Baltimore, Maryland

RAMIN TABATABAI, MD, MACM
Physician
Department of Emergency Medicine
Los Angeles General Medical Center
Los Angeles, California

JULIE T. VIETH, MD
Associate Professor
Department of Emergency Medicine
Larner College of Medicine at University of Vermont
Burlington, Vermont

HEIDI WERNER, MD, MSHPEd
Associate Clinical Professor
Departments of Emergency Medicine and Pediatrics
University of California, San Francisco School of Medicine
San Francisco, California

R. GENTRY WILKERSON, MD
Associate Professor
Department of Emergency Medicine
University of Maryland School of Medicine
Baltimore, Maryland

CHRISTOPHER G. WILLIAMS, MD, FAWM
Associate Professor
Department of Emergency Medicine
University of Arizona College of Medicine
Tucson, Arizona

GEORGE C. WILLIS, MD, FAAEM, FACEP
Vice Chair of Faculty Affairs
Department of Emergency Medicine
UT Health Science Center at San Antonio
San Antonio, Texas

BRIAN J. WRIGHT, MD, MPH
Clinical Associate Professor
Department of Emergency Medicine
Renaissance School of Medicine
Stony Brook, New York

Contributors

Beza Abebe, MD, MPH
Physician
Department of Emergency Medicine
Los Angeles General Medical Center
Los Angeles, California

Michael Abraham, MD, MS
Associate Professor
Department of Emergency Medicine
University of Maryland School of Medicine
Baltimore, Maryland

Jose Acosta, MD
Resident
Department of Emergency Medicine
Highland Hospital
Alameda Health System
Oakland, California

Surriya Ahmad, MD
Clinical Instructor
Ronald O. Perelman Department of Emergency Medicine
NYU Grossman School of Medicine
Attending Emergency Medicine
Department of Emergency Medicine
Bellevue Hospital/NYC Health and Hospitals
New York, New York

Peter Aiello, PharmD, MBA
Pediatric Clinical Pharmacy Specialist
Department of Pharmacy
SUNY Upstate Medical University
Syracuse, New York

Aslam Abbasi Akhtar, MD, PhD
Physician
Department of Emergency Medicine
Los Angeles County Harbor UCLA
Torrance, California

Nour Al Jalbout, MD
Assistant Fellowship Director
Harvard Emergency Ultrasound
Department of Emergency Medicine
Massachusetts General Hospital
Boston, Massachusetts

Irina Aleshinskaya, DO, MS
Physician
Department of Emergency Medicine
Staten Island University Hospital
Staten Island, New York

Rasheed Alhadi, MD
Resident
Department of Emergency Medicine
University of California, San Francisco School of Medicine
San Francisco, California

Afrah A. Ali, MBBS
Assistant Professor
Department of Emergency Medicine
University of Maryland School of Medicine
Baltimore, Maryland

Aaron Alindogan, MD
Physician
Department of Emergency Medicine
UT Health Science Center at San Antonio
San Antonio, Texas

Jack Allan, MD
Physician
Department of Emergency Medicine
Temple University Hospital
Philadelphia, Pennsylvania

Ashley Rebekah Allen, BSN, MD
Physician
Department of Emergency Medicine
LA General Medical Center
Los Angeles, California

Dennis Allin, MD, FAAEM, FAEMS, FACEP
EMS Medical Director
Event Medicine Medical Director
Professor
Department of Emergency Medicine
University of Kansas Health System
Kansas City, Kansas

Michael G. Allison, MD
Chief, Critical Care Medicine
Department of Medicine
University of Maryland St. Joseph Medical Center
Towson, Maryland

Ahmed Alsakha, MBBS, FRCPC, FAAEM, FACEP
Fellow
Department of Emergency Medicine
SUNY Upstate Medical University
Syracuse, New York

Andrea Alvarado, MD
Physician
Department of Critical Care Medicine
University of Pittsburgh Medical Center
Pittsburgh, Pennsylvania

Chance Anderson, MD, MS
Physician
Department of Emergency Medicine
Los Angeles General Medical Center
Los Angeles, California

Robert Anderson, MD
Physician
Department of Emergency Medicine
Maine Medical Center
Portland, Maine

Nicholas Andrew, MD
Clinical Instructor
Department of Emergency Medicine
Loma Linda University School of Medicine
Loma Linda, California

Matthew E. Anton, MD, MPH
Resident
Department of General Surgery
Dartmouth Hitchcock Medical Center
Lebanon, New Hampshire

Joseph H. Ash, MD
Resident
Department of Emergency Medicine
Penn State Health Milton S. Hershey Medical Center
Hershey, Pennsylvania

Carmen Avendano, MD
Physician
Department of Emergency Medicine
St. Francis Hospital
University of Minnesota Masonic Children's Hospital
Minneapolis, Minnesota

Ani Aydin, MD
Associate Professor
Department of Emergency Medicine
Yale School of Medicine
New Haven, Connecticut

Keith Azevedo, MD
Physician
Departments of Emergency Medicine and Internal Medicine
University of New Mexico School of Medicine
Albuquerque, New Mexico

Melissa Bacci, MD, MS
Fellow
Department of Critical Care Medicine
University of Pittsburgh Medical Center
Pittsburgh, Pennsylvania

Sarah Badin, MD
Fellow
Department of Emergency Medicine
Massachusetts General Hospital
Boston, Massachusetts

Nicola Baker, MD
Clinical Assistant Professor
Department of Emergency Medicine
Banner University Medical Center
Tucson, Arizona

LEKHA BAPU, DO
Resident
Department of Emergency Medicine
Medical University of South Carolina
Charleston, South Carolina

ALEXANDRA BARBOSA, MD
Resident
Departments of Emergency Medicine and Pediatrics
University of Arizona College of Medicine
Tucson, Arizona

AARON BARKSDALE, MD
Vice Chair of Research
Department of Emergency Medicine
University of Nebraska Medical Center
Omaha, Nebraska

ADAM BARNATHAN, DO
Physician
Department of Emergency Medicine
St. Anthony's Hospital
Tampa, Florida

ANDREW BARNETT, MD
Assistant Professor
Department of Emergency Medicine
University of Nebraska Medical Center
Omaha, Nebraska

RYAN BARNICLE, MD, MSED
Director of Emergency Critical Care
Department of Emergency Medicine
Brown Emergency Physicians
Providence, Rhode Island

DAVID BASILE, MD
Physician
Department of Emergency Medicine
Penn State Health Milton S. Hershey Medical Center
Hershey, Pennsylvania

LISA BELL, MD
Resident
Department of Emergency Medicine
Harbor-UCLA Medical Center
Torrance, California

ANDREW BELUS, PA-C, MPAS
Physician Assistant
Department of Emergency Medicine
Banner University Medical Center
Tucson, Arizona

AUBREY BETHEL, MD
Simulation Director
Department of Emergency Medicine
Dignity Health East Valley
Chandler, Arizona

RYAN BIERLE, DMSC, PA
Assistant Professor of Emergency Medicine and Medicine/Clinical
Department of Emergency Medicine
UT Health Science Center at San Antonio
San Antonio, Texas

MICHAEL BILLET, MD
Assistant Professor
Department of Emergency Medicine
University of Maryland School of Medicine
Baltimore, Maryland

STEVEN S. BIN, MD
Health Sciences Clinical Professor
Department of Emergency Medicine
University of California, San Francisco School of Medicine
San Francisco, California

AARON M. BLACKSHAW, MD
Physician
Department of Emergency Medicine
Novant Health Mint Hill Medical Center
Charlotte, North Carolina

JAMES BOHAN, MD
Chair of Emergency Medicine
Department of Emergency Medicine
Arnot Health
Elmira, New York

MICHAEL C. BOND, MD
Professor
Department of Emergency Medicine
University of Maryland School of Medicine
Baltimore, Maryland

MATTHEW P. BORLOZ, MD
Associate Professor
Department of Emergency Medicine
Virginia Tech Carilion School of Medicine
Roanoke, Virginia

B. BARRIE BOSTICK, MD
Pediatric Director, EM Residency
AdventHealth East Orlando
Department of Emergency Medicine
AdventHealth Orlando
Orlando, Florida

KIMBERLY BOSWELL, MD
Assistant Professor of Emergency Medicine
Department of Emergency Medicine
University of Maryland School of Medicine
Baltimore, Maryland

KAYLA BOURGEOIS, PHARMD
Fellow
Department of Emergency Medicine
SUNY Upstate Medical University Hospital
Syracuse, New York

MARINA BOUSHRA, MD
Assistant Professor
Physician
Emergency Services Institute
Respiratory Institute
Cleveland Clinic Foundation
Cleveland, Ohio

ALEXANDER BRACEY, MD
Assistant Professor
Department of Emergency Medicine
Albany Medical Center
Albany, New York

LAUREN E. R. BRADY, MD
Resident
Department of Emergency Medicine
Trident Medical Center
Charleston, South Carolina

WILLIAM J. BRADY, MD
Professor of Emergency Medicine and Medicine
Vice Chair of Emergency Medicine
The David A. Harrison Distinguished Educator
University of Virginia School of Medicine
Operational Medical Director
Albemarle County Fire Rescue
Charlottesville, Virginia

CAROLINE BRANDON, MD
Assistant Professor of Clinical Emergency Medicine
Department of Emergency Medicine
Lewis Katz School of Medicine at Temple University
Philadelphia, Pennsylvania

GRAHAM BRANT-ZAWADZKI, MD, MA
Associate Professor
Department of Emergency Medicine
University of Utah School of Medicine
Salt Lake City, Utah

ALLYSON M. BRIGGS, MD
Assistant Professor
Department of Emergency Medicine
The University of Kansas Medical Center
Kansas City, Kansas

TIMOTHY J. BRIGHT, MD, FAAP
Medical Director, Pediatric Emergency Department
Department of Pediatric Emergency Medicine
Tucson Medical Center
Tucson, Arizona

JOHN BROWN, MD, MPA
Medical Director
Department of Emergency Medical Services Agency
Department of Public Health
San Francisco, California

JOSEPH BROWN, MD
Assistant Professor
Department of Emergency Medicine
University of Colorado School of Medicine
Aurora, Colorado

CAROLINE BURKE, MD
Resident
Department of Emergency Medicine
University of California, San Francisco School of Medicine
San Francisco, California

CAROLINE W. BURMON, MD
Assistant Professor
Emergency Department
Mount Sinai Beth Israel
New York, New York

ADDIE BURTLE, MD
Physician
Department of Emergency Medicine
Washington University
St. Louis, Missouri

KYLE BURTON, MD, MPP
Resident
Department of Emergency Medicine
The Johns Hopkins Hospital
Baltimore, Maryland

MANZY BYRD, DO, MS
Resident
Department of Emergency Medicine
Arnot Ogden Medical Center
Elmira, New York

NIKKI CALI, MD
Attending Physician
Department of Emergency Medicine
University of Maryland Baltimore Washington Medical Center
Glen Burnie, Maryland

DANIEL CALICK, MD
Resident
Emergency Department
Virginia Tech Carilion School of Medicine
Carilion Clinic
Roanoke, Virginia

VINCENT J. CALLEO, MD
Medical Director, Upstate NY Polson Center
Department of Emergency Medicine
SUNY Upstate Medical University
Syracuse, New York

BRIAN CAMERON, MD
Assistant Professor
Department of Emergency Medicine
UT MD Anderson Cancer Center
Houston, Texas

LAUREN CAMERON-COMASCO, MD
Director of Geriatric Emergency Medicine
Department of Emergency Medicine
Corewell Health William Beaumont University Hospital
Royal Oak, Michigan

WILLIAM CAPUTO, MD
Residency Director, Associate Chair of Training and Education
Department of Emergency Medicine
Staten Island University Hospital—Northwell Health
Staten Island, New York

GUSTAVO CARMEN LOPEZ, MD
Resident
Department of Emergency Medicine
University of Virginia School of Medicine
Charlottesville, Virginia

CASEY CARR, MD
Assistant Professor
Division of Critical Care Medicine
Department of Emergency Medicine
University of Florida College of Medicine
Gainesville, Florida

JANET CARROLL, RN
Nurse Manager
Department of Forensic Nursing Program
Dartmouth Hitchcock Medical Center
Lebanon, New Hampshire

GLENNETTE CASTILLO, MD
Resident
Department of Emergency Medicine
MedStar Washington Hospital Center
Washington, District of Columbia

CALEB CHAN, MD, MPH
Assistant Professor
Department of Emergency Medicine and Internal Medicine
University of Maryland School of Medicine
Baltimore, Maryland

ANDREW K. CHANG, MD, MS
Professor and Vice Chair of Research and Academic Affairs
Department of Emergency Medicine
Albany Medical Center
Albany, New York

WAN-TSU W. CHANG, MD
Associate Professor
Departments of Emergency Medicine, Neurology, and Program in Trauma
University of Maryland School of Medicine
Baltimore, Maryland

DREW CHARLES, DO
Fellow
Department of Internal Medicine
University of Maryland Medical Center
Baltimore, Maryland

MONICA CHARPENTIER, MD, PHD
Fellow
Department of Emergency Medicine
University of California, San Francisco School of Medicine
San Francisco, California

SUMMER CHAVEZ, DO, MPH, MPM
Clinical Assistant Professor
Department of Health Systems and Population Health Sciences
University of Houston Tilman J. Fertitta Family College of Medicine
Houston, Texas

MARY CHEFFERS, MD
Clinical Faculty
Department of Emergency Medicine
Keck School of Medicine of USC
Los Angeles General Medical Center
Los Angeles, California

CAROL C. CHEN, MD, MPH
Associate Professor
Department of Emergency Medicine
University of California, San Francisco School of Medicine
San Francisco, California

ANDREW E. CHERTOFF, MD
Associate Professor
Department of Emergency Medicine
Albert Einstein College of Medicine
Bronx, New York

JOAN CHOU, MD
Resident
Department of Emergency Medicine
SUNY Upstate Medical University
Syracuse, New York

GAVIN K. CLARK, MS, MD
Resident
Department of Emergency Medicine
Dartmouth Hitchcock Medical Center
Hanover, New Hampshire

KATEY S. COHEN, MD, MSED
Resident
Department of Emergency Medicine
Temple University Hospital
Philadelphia, Pennsylvania

ALESSANDRA CONFORTO, MD
Clinical Associate Professor of Emergency Medicine (Clinician Educator)
Department of Emergency Medicine
Keck School of Medicine of USC
Los Angeles, California

MATTHEW W. CONNELLY, MD
Physician
Department of Emergency Medicine
Indiana University
Indianapolis, Indiana

TARA COPPER, MD, MS
Assistant Professor of Pediatrics
Department of Pediatrics
Washington University School of Medicine
St. Louis, Missouri

BENJAMIN CORNWELL, MD
Resident
Department of Emergency Medicine
University of Maryland Medical Center
Baltimore, Maryland

AMANDA CORREIA, DO, MS
Fellow
Department of Critical Care Medicine
Dartmouth Hitchcock Medical Center
Lebanon, New Hampshire

JONATHAN P. COSS, MD
Physician
Departments of Emergency Medicine and Pediatrics
Banner University Medical Center
University of Arizona College of Medicine
Tucson, Arizona

RYAN F. COUGHLIN, MD
Assistant Professor
Department of Emergency Medicine
Yale School of Medicine
New Haven, Connecticut

JEFF COVITZ, MA, NRP, FP-C
Paramedic Captain
San Francisco Fire Department
San Francisco, California

MATTHEW CRAVENS, MD
Fellow
Department of Critical Care Medicine
Maine Medical Center
Portland, Maine

JOSEPH CRUZ, DO
Assistant Medical Director
Emergency Department
Novant Rowan Medical Center
Mid-Atlantic Emergency Medicine Associates (MEMA)
Charlotte, North Carolina

LIA C. CRUZ, DO
Assistant Professor
Departments of Emergency Medicine and Pediatrics
Atrium Health Levine Children's Hospital
Charlotte, North Carolina

ERIKA DANELSKI, DO
Resident
Department of Emergency Medicine
Advocate Christ Medical Center
Oak Lawn, Illinois

ANNA DARBY, MD, MPH, MS
Clinical Assistant Professor
Assistant Program Director
Department of Emergency Medicine
Keck School of Medicine of USC
Los Angeles General Hospital
Los Angeles, California

NEIL K. DASGUPTA, MD
Clinical Associate Professor
Department of Emergency Medicine
New York Institute of Technology College of Osteopathic Medicine
Vice Chair
Department of Emergency Medicine
Nassau University Medical Center
East Meadow, New York

SUPRIYA J. DAVIS, MD
Resident
Department of Emergency Medicine
Washington Hospital Center
Washington, District of Columbia

LINDSEY DEGEORGE, MD
Attending Physician
Department of Emergency Medicine
MedStar Southern Maryland Hospital
Clinton, Maryland

JESSICA DEITRICK, DO
Resident
Department of Emergency Medicine
Penn State Health Milton S. Hershey Medical Center
Hershey, Pennsylvania

ELISHA PAUL DEKONING, MD, MS
Residency Program Director
Department of Emergency Medicine
Dartmouth Hitchcock Medical Center
Lebanon, New Hampshire

MATTHEW C. DELANEY, MD
Associate Professor
Department of Emergency Medicine
UAB Heersink School of Medicine
Birmingham, Alabama

MATTHEW ALAN DEMAREST, MD
Resident
Department of Emergency Medicine
Los Angeles General Medical Center
Los Angeles, California

IAN J. DEMPSEY, MD
Assistant Professor
Department of Orthopaedic Surgery
Virginia Tech Carilion School of Medicine
Carilion Clinic
Roanoke, Virginia

SEAN DENNY, MD
Resident
Department of Emergency Medicine
Harbor-UCLA Medical Center
Torrance, California

CURTIS DICKEY, DO
Fellow
Department of Critical Care Medicine
University of Pittsburgh Medical Center
Pittsburgh, Pennsylvania

HAEDAN DOTY, DO
Resident
Department of Emergency Medicine
University of Arizona College of Medicine
Tucson, Arizona

SARAH B. DUBBS, MD
Associate Professor of Emergency Medicine
Residency Program Director
Department of Emergency Medicine
University of Maryland School of Medicine
Baltimore, Maryland

JEFFREY DUBIN, MD, MBA
Senior Vice President, Medical Affairs and Chief Medical Officer
Professor of Clinical Emergency Medicine
Georgetown University School of Medicine
Department of Medical Affairs
MedStar Washington Hospital Center
Washington, District of Columbia

KAYLA DUELAND-KUHN, MD
Assistant Professor
Departments of Emergency Medicine and Pediatrics
SUNY Upstate University Hospital
Syracuse, New York

JOSHUA EASTER, MD, MS
Associate Professor
Department of Emergency Medicine
University of Virginia School of Medicine
Charlottesville, Virginia

WILLIAM EGGLESTON, PHARMD
Assistant Professor
Department of Pharmacy Practice
Binghamton University School of Pharmacy and Pharmaceutical Sciences
Binghamton, New York

MICHAEL R. EHMANN, MD, MPH, MS
Assistant Professor
Department of Emergency Medicine
The Johns Hopkins University School of Medicine
Baltimore, Maryland

ERICK A. EITING, MD, MPH, MMM
Vice Chair
Department of Emergency Medicine
Mount Sinai Beth Israel
New York, New York

KAYLA T. ENRIQUEZ, MD, MPH
Associate Professor
Department of Emergency Medicine
University of California, San Francisco School of Medicine
San Francisco, California

LANE EPPS, MD
Resident
Department of Emergency Medicine
University of California, San Francisco School of Medicine
San Francisco, California

DAN ERASO, MD
Assistant Professor
Department of Emergency Medicine
University of Florida College of
 Medicine—Jacksonville
Jacksonville, Florida

MOLLY K. ESTES, MD, FACEP, FAAEM
Associate Professor
Department of Emergency Medicine
Loma Linda University School of
 Medicine
Loma Linda, California

BRIAN EUERLE, MD
Associate Professor
Department of Emergency Medicine
University of Maryland School of
 Medicine
Baltimore, Maryland

CHEYENNE FALAT, MD
Assistant Professor
Department of Emergency Medicine
University of Maryland School of
 Medicine
Baltimore, Maryland

TIFFANY FAN, MD
Resident
Department of Emergency Medicine
Harbor-UCLA Medical Center
Torrance, California

JOSHUA D. FARKAS, MD, MS
Associate Professor
Department of Pulmonary and Critical Care
Larner College of Medicine at University
 of Vermont
Burlington, Vermont

ISAAC J. FARRELL, MD
Assistant Professor
Department of Emergency Medicine
University of Arizona College of Medicine
Tucson, Arizona

NAILLID FELIPE, MD, MPH
Clinical Instructor
Department of Emergency Medicine
New York University Langone Health
New York, New York

PATRICIA FERMIN, MD
Attending Physician
Department of Emergency Medicine
VA Greater Los Angeles Medical Center
Los Angeles, California

ALBERT FIORELLO, MD
Associate Professor of Emergency
 Medicine
Residency Program Director
Department of Emergency Medicine
University of Arizona College of Medicine
Tucson, Arizona

KYLE FISCHER, MD, MPH
Clinical Assistant Professor
Department of Emergency Medicine
University of Maryland School of
 Medicine
Baltimore, Maryland

DELANEY FISHER, DO
Resident
Departments of Emergency Medicine and
 Pediatrics
University of Arizona College of Medicine
Tucson, Arizona

KALLE J. FJELD, MD
Resident
Department of Emergency Medicine
Dartmouth Hitchcock Medical Center
Lebanon, New Hampshire

KEVIN J. FLANAGAN, DO, FPD-AEMUS
Assistant Professor
Department of Emergency Medicine
University of Maryland Medical Center
Baltimore, Maryland

HARRY V. FLASTER, MD
Resident
Department of Emergency Medicine
The Johns Hopkins University School of
 Medicine
Baltimore, Maryland

TIFFANY C. FONG, MD
Attending Physician
Department of Emergency Medicine
The Johns Hopkins University School of
 Medicine
Baltimore, Maryland

Eric R. Friedman, MD
Core Faculty, Trident Emergency Medicine Residency
Department of Emergency Medicine
Trident Medical Center
Charleston, South Carolina

Brian M. Fuller, MD, MSCI
Physician
Departments of Anesthesiology and Emergency Medicine
Washington University in St. Louis School of Medicine
St. Louis, Missouri

Brian L. Fuquay, DO
Resident
Department of Emergency Medicine
Carilion Clinic
Roanoke, Virginia

Emma R. Furlano, MD
Assistant Professor
Department of Emergency Medicine
Albany Medical College
Albany, New York

Gregory Gafni-Pappas, DO
Physician
Department of Emergency Medicine
Chelsea Hospital (Part of Trinity Health)
Chelsea, Michigan

J. David Gatz, MD
Assistant Professor
Department of Emergency Medicine
University of Maryland School of Medicine
Baltimore, Maryland

Curtis Geier, PharmD
Associate Clinical Professor
Emergency Medicine Clinical Pharmacist
Department of Emergency Medicine
San Francisco General Hospital
San Francisco, California

Cameron J. Gettel, MD, MHS
Assistant Professor
Department of Emergency Medicine
Yale School of Medicine
New Haven, Connecticut

Daniella Giardina, MD
Resident
Department of Emergency Medicine
SUNY Upstate Medical University
Syracuse, New York

Ryan C. Gibbons, MD
Associate Professor
Department of Emergency Medicine
Lewis Katz School of Medicine at Temple University
Philadelphia, Pennsylvania

Sarah Ring Gibbs, MD
Resident
Department of Emergency Medicine
Mount Sinai Icahn School of Medicine
New York, New York

Daniel B. Gingold, MD, MPH
Associate Professor
Department of Emergency Medicine
University of Maryland School of Medicine
Baltimore, Maryland

Zoe Glick, MD
Resident
Department of Emergency Medicine
University of Maryland School of Medicine
Baltimore, Maryland

Nicholas Goodmanson, MD
Program Director, Adult Critical Care Medicine Fellowship
Division of Critical Care Medicine
Advocate Lutheran General Hospital and Advocate Christ Medical Center
Chicago, Illinois

Rachel Gorodetsky, PharmD
Associate Professor
Department of Pharmacy Practice
D'Youville University School of Pharmacy
Buffalo, New York

Michael Gottlieb, MD, RDMS, FAAEM, FACEP
Ultrasound Division Director
Clinical Ultrasound Fellowship Director
Associate Professor of Emergency Medicine
Department of Emergency Medicine
Rush University Medical Center
Chicago, Illinois

Madeline Grade, MD, MSc
Physician
Department of Emergency Medicine
University of California, San Francisco School of Medicine
San Francisco, California

Sally Graglia, MD, MPH
Assistant Clinical Professor
Department of Emergency Medicine
University of California, San Francisco School of Medicine
San Francisco, California

Matthew J. Grant, MD
Assistant Professor
Department of Pediatrics
University of Maryland School of Medicine
Baltimore, Maryland

John C. Greenwood, MD, MS
Assistant Professor
Department of Emergency Medicine
Department of Anesthesiology and Critical Care
Perelman School of Medicine at the University of Pennsylvania
Philadelphia, Pennsylvania

David Alexander Gregor, MD
Resident
Department of Emergency Medicine
Keck School of Medicine of USC
Los Angeles General Medical Center
Los Angeles, California

Jennifer Guyther, MD
Assistant Professor
Departments of Emergency Medicine and Pediatrics
University of Maryland School of Medicine
Baltimore, Maryland

Andrés Guzmán, MD
Assistant Professor
Division of Emergency Medicine
Schulich School of Medicine and Dentistry
Western University Ontario
London, Ontario, Canada

Ruben Guzman, MD
Resident
Department of Emergency Medicine
Los Angeles General Medical Center
Los Angeles, California

Hania Habeeb, MD, MS, FACEP
Associate Chair
Department of Emergency Medicine
MedStar Harbor Hospital
Baltimore, Maryland

Kaytlin E. Hack, MD
Assistant Professor
Department of Emergency Medicine
MedStar Georgetown University Hospital
Washington, District of Columbia

Jon Halling, MD, MBA
Program Director
Department of Anesthesiology Residency
Grand Strand Medical Center
Myrtle Beach, South Carolina

Bachar Hamade, MD, MSc
Associate Staff
Department of Intensive Care and Resuscitation, Center for Emergency Medicine
Cleveland Clinic Foundation
Cleveland, Ohio

Jin H. Han, MD, MSc
Professor
Department of Geriatric Research, Education, and Clinical Center
Tennessee Valley Healthcare Center
Nashville, Tennessee

Gregory Hand, MD
Physician
Department of Pediatrics
University of Texas at Austin Dell Medical School
Austin, Texas

Kevin Hanley, MD
Associate Physician
Department of Emergency Medicine
University of California, San Francisco School of Medicine
San Francisco, California

Jonathan Hansen, MD, MBA
Assistant Professor
Department of Emergency Medicine
The Johns Hopkins University School of Medicine
Baltimore, Maryland

Samuel Harris, MD
Resident
Department of Emergency Medicine
Tampa General Hospital
University of South Florida Morsani College of Medicine
Tampa, Florida

Shorok Hassan, DO
Physician
Department of Emergency Medicine
Staten Island University Hospital
Staten Island, New York

Colman Hatton, MD
Physician
Department of Emergency Medicine
Maine Medical Center
Portland, Maine

Chen He, MD
Residency Program Director and Assistant Professor
Department of Emergency Medicine
Mount Sinai Morningside West
New York, New York

Sean Heavey, MD
Fellow
Department of Emergency Medicine
UC Davis School of Medicine
Sacramento, California

Madeleine Heller, MD
Resident
Department of Emergency Medicine
Los Angeles General Medical Center
Los Angeles, California

John Herrick, DO, FACEP
Associate Program Director
Department of CHRISTUS Health/Texas A&M Emergency Medicine Residency
CHRISTUS Spohn Shoreline
Corpus Christi, Texas

Harry E. Heverling, DO
Assistant Professor
Department of Emergency Medicine
The Johns Hopkins University School of Medicine
Baltimore, Maryland

Marvin Heyboer III, MD, FUHM, FACCWS
Professor
Department of Emergency Medicine
SUNY Upstate Medical University
Syracuse, New York

Guyon J. Hill, MD
Director of Emergency Ultrasound
Department of Pediatric Emergency Medicine
Dell Children's Medical Center
University of Texas at Austin Dell Medical School
Austin, Texas

Michael Hodgman, MD, FACMT, FAACT
Clinical Assistant Professor of Emergency Medicine
Department of Emergency Medicine
SUNY Upstate Medical University
Medical Toxicologist
Upstate New York Poison Center
Syracuse, New York

Akilesh Honasoge, MD, MA
Fellow
Department of Cardiology
Rush University Medical Center
Chicago, Illinois

Jaime Hope, MD
Medical Director
Assistant Professor
Department of Emergency Medicine
Beaumont Corewell Health
Royal Oak, Michigan

SAMANTHA HUNT, MD
Resident
Emergency Department
Dartmouth Hitchcock Medical Center
Lebanon, New Hampshire

LAUREN M. HUNTER, MSN
Nurse Practitioner
Department of Emergency Medicine
Novant Health Mint Hill Medical Center
Charlotte, North Carolina

NICHOLAS B. HURST, MD, MS, FAAEM, FACEP
Assistant Professor of Emergency Medicine
Department of Emergency Medicine
University of Arizona College of Medicine
Tucson, Arizona

ABBAS HUSAIN, MD
Associate Program Director
Department of Emergency Medicine
Staten Island University Hospital
Staten Island, New York

CHINEZIMUZO IHENATU, MD
Physician
Department of Emergency Medicine
Hospital of the University of Pennsylvania
Philadelphia, Pennsylvania

DAN IM, MD
Resident
Department of Emergency Medicine
Harbor-UCLA Medical Center
Torrance, California

ERRETT JACKS, MD
Physician
Department of Emergency Medicine
Grand Strand Medical Center
Myrtle Beach, South Carolina

LAURA JANNECK, MD, MPH
Assistant Professor
Department of Emergency Medicine
University of Oklahoma School of Community Medicine
Tulsa, Oklahoma

GREGORY JASANI, MD
Assistant Professor of Emergency Medicine
Department of Emergency Medicine
University of Maryland School of Medicine
Baltimore, Maryland

NATHAN JASPERSE, MD
Resident
Department of Emergency Medicine
Harbor-UCLA Medical Center
Torrance, California

LEE JOHNSON, MD
Resident
Department of Emergency Medicine
Denver Health
Denver, Colorado

NICHOLAS J. JOHNSON, MD
Associate Professor and Section Head of Critical Care
Department of Emergency Medicine
Division of Pulmonary, Critical Care, and Sleep Medicine
Department of Medicine
University of Washington
Seattle, Washington

MELISSA JOSEPH, MD
Assistant Professor
Department of Emergency Medicine
Yale School of Medicine
New Haven, Connecticut

AMANDA L. JOY, MS, PA-C
Associate Medical Director
MedStar Health Urgent Care
MedStar Health
Columbia, Maryland

JORDAN A. JUSTICE, MD, FACEP, FAAP
Director of Pediatric Emergency Education
Departments of Emergency Medicine and Pediatrics
Santa Barbara Cottage Hospital
Santa Barbara, California

ANNAHIETA KALANTARI, DO, MED
Vice Chair of Education
Department of Emergency Medicine
Penn State Health Milton S. Hershey Medical Center
Hershey, Pennsylvania

SHRUTI KANT, MBBS
Associate Professor
Departments of Emergency Medicine and Pediatrics
University of California, San Francisco School of Medicine
San Francisco, California

SAM KAPLAN, MD
Resident
Department of Emergency Medicine
University of Arizona College of Medicine
Tucson, Arizona

ELIZABETH KARAGOSIAN, MD
Physician
Emergency Department
Southern New Hampshire Medical Center
Nashua, New Hampshire

ALYSSA KARL, MD
Assistant Professor of Clinical Emergency Medicine
Department of Emergency Medicine
Lewis Katz School of Medicine at Temple University
Philadelphia, Pennsylvania

NEENA KASHYAP, MD
Resident
Department of Emergency Medicine
Temple University Hospital
Philadelphia, Pennsylvania

MICHAEL KEENAN, MD
Clinical Instructor
Department of Emergency Medicine
SUNY Upstate Medical University
Syracuse, New York

RICHARD E. KENNEDY, MD, PhD
Associate Professor
Department of Medicine
UAB Heersink School of Medicine
Birmingham, Alabama

DANYA KHOUJAH, MBBS, MEHP
Attending Physician
Department of Emergency Medicine
AdventHealth Tampa
Tampa, Florida

VANESSA KHOURY, MD
Physician
Department of Emergency Medicine
University of Virginia School of Medicine
Charlottesville, Virginia

EUNHYE (GRACE) KIM, MD
Physician
Department of Emergency Medicine
Loma Linda University School of Medicine
Loma Linda, California

MICHAEL KIM, MD
Resident
Department of Emergency Medicine
Washington University School of Medicine
St. Louis, Missouri

BRENT KING, MD, MMM
Professor and Vice Chair for Quality, Safety, and Innovation
Department of Emergency Medicine
University of Maryland School of Medicine
Baltimore, Maryland

SAMANTHA A. KING, MD
Assistant Professor
Department of Emergency Medicine
University of Maryland School of Medicine
Baltimore, Maryland

KELLIE KITAMURA, MD
Physician
Department of Emergency Medicine
UCLA Ronald Reagan–Olive View Medical Center
Los Angeles, California

KEVIN M. KLAUER, DO, EJD
Chief Medical Officer
Department of Administration
HCA Florida Ocala and West Marion Hospitals
Ocala, Florida

BRIANNA KLUCHER, MD
Resident
Department of Emergency Medicine
University of Maryland Medical Center
Baltimore, Maryland

ALEX Y. KOO, MD, FACEP
Assistant Professor of Emergency
  Medicine
Department of Emergency Medicine
Georgetown University and Washington
  Hospital Center
Washington, District of Columbia

OLENA KOSTYUK, MD
Fellow
Department of Pediatric Emergency
  Medicine
Oklahoma Children's Hospital
Oklahoma City, Oklahoma

ERIK J. KRAMER, MD
Physician
Department of Emergency Medicine
University of California, San Francisco
  School of Medicine
San Francisco, California

JESSICA KUXHAUSE, MD
Physician
Department of Emergency Medicine
Beaumont Hospital
Royal Oak, Michigan

AARON R. KUZEL, DO, MBA
Assistant Professor of Emergency
  Medicine
Department of Emergency Medicine
University of Louisville School of
  Medicine
Louisville, Kentucky

JUSTIN LACKEY, MD
Resident Physician
Department of Emergency Medicine
Carilion Clinic
Roanoke, Virginia

JEREMY LACOCQUE, DO
Assistant Professor of Emergency Medicine
Department of Emergency Medicine
University of California, San Francisco
  School of Medicine
San Francisco, California

DIANA LADKANY, MD
Physician
Department of Emergency Medicine
Georgetown University School of Medicine
Washington, District of Columbia

STEVEN LAI, MD
Assistant Clinical Professor
Department of Emergency Medicine
David Geffen School of Medicine at UCLA
Los Angeles, California

DANIELLE LANGAN, DO
Physician
Department of Emergency Medicine
Staten Island University Hospital
Staten Island, New York

CORNELIA LATRONICA, MD
Associate Professor
Division of Pediatric Emergency Medicine
Department of Emergency Medicine
University of California, San Francisco
  School of Medicine
San Francisco, California

ERIK LAURIN, MD
Professor of Emergency Medicine
Department of Emergency Medicine
UC Davis School of Medicine
Sacramento, California

IAN H. LAW, BSE, MD
Professor
Department of Pediatrics
University of Iowa Stead Family
  Department of Pediatrics
Iowa City, Iowa

**MARIA MAGDALENA
LAWRYNOWICZ, MD, MS**
Assistant Professor
Assistant Program Director
Department of Emergency Medicine
Georgetown University School of Medicine
Georgetown University Hospital
MedStar Washington Hospital Center
Washington, District of Columbia

KERRI LAYMAN, MD
Chief
Department of Emergency Medicine
MedStar Georgetown University Hospital
Washington, District of Columbia

KARLY LEBHERZ, MD
Physician
Department of Emergency Medicine
Ochsner Medical Center
New Orleans, Louisiana

J. Austin Lee, MD, MPH
Adjunct Clinical Assistant Professor
Department of Emergency Medicine
Indiana University School of Medicine
Bloomington, Indiana

Kenneth Lee, MD
Resident
Department of Emergency Medicine
Harbor-UCLA Medical Center
Torrance, California

Ryan Lee, MD
Chief Fellow
Department of Critical Care Medicine
University of Maryland Medical Center
Baltimore, Maryland

Sarah Lee, MD
Faculty Physician
Clinical Instructor
Department of Emergency Medicine
University of Maryland School of Medicine
Baltimore, Maryland

Tracy Leigh LeGros, MD, PhD
Full Professor
Director of Faculty Development
Regional One Trauma Center
University of Tennessee Health Sciences Center
Memphis, Tennessee

Evan Leibner, MD, PhD
Assistant Professor of Emergency Medicine
Departments of Emergency Medicine and Cardiology
Institute for Critical Care Medicine
The Mount Sinai Hospital
New York, New York

Miguel Lemus, MD
Physician
Department of Emergency Medicine
West Los Angeles Veterans Affairs Medical Center
Los Angeles, California

Kathy LeSaint, MD
Associate Professor
Department of Emergency Medicine
University of California, San Francisco School of Medicine
San Francisco, California

Matthew J. Levy, MD
Associate Professor
Department of Emergency Medicine
The Johns Hopkins University School of Medicine
Baltimore, Maryland

Kelly Lew, MD
Resident
Department of Emergency Medicine
MedStar Washington Hospital Center/ Georgetown University Hospital
Washington, District of Columbia

Philana H. Liang, PA-C, MPH, MSHS
Physician Assistant
Division of Infectious Diseases
Department of Medicine
Washington University School of Medicine
St. Louis, Missouri

Stephen Y. Liang, MD, MPHS
Associate Professor of Medicine
Department of Emergency Medicine
Division of Infectious Diseases
Department of Medicine
Washington University School of Medicine
St. Louis, Missouri

Megan M. Lieb, DO
Fellow
Department of Emergency Medicine
Albany Medical Center
Albany, New York

Margaret Lin-Martore, MD
Associate Clinical Professor
Departments of Emergency Medicine and Pediatrics
University of California, San Francisco School of Medicine
San Francisco, California

Mei-Ling Liu, MD
Assistant Professor
Department of Emergency Medicine
Hospital of the University of Pennsylvania
Philadelphia, Pennsylvania

SHAN W. LIU, MD, SD
Associate Professor of Emergency
  Medicine
Department of Emergency Medicine
Massachusetts General Hospital
Boston, Massachusetts

KRISTI LIZYNESS, DO
Physician
Department of Emergency Medicine
Hartford Healthcare
Hartford, Connecticut

JOSEPHINE LO BELLO, MD
Resident
Department of Emergency Medicine
The Johns Hopkins University School of
  Medicine
Baltimore, Maryland

DAVID LOCKE, MD
Physician
Department of Emergency Medicine
Penn State Health
Hershey, Pennsylvania

BRIT LONG, MD
Associate Professor of Military and
  Emergency Medicine
Attending, Emergency Physician
Department of Emergency Medicine
Brooke Army Medical Center
Fort Sam Houston, Texas

HEATHER LOUNSBURY, MD
Assistant Professor
Department of Emergency Medicine
University of Virginia School of Medicine
Charlottesville, Virginia

SPENCER LOVEGROVE, MD
Attending Physician
Department of Emergency Medicine
University of Maryland Baltimore
  Washington Medical Center
Glen Burnie, Maryland

BOBBI-JO LOWIE, MD
Clinical Instructor
Department of Emergency Medicine
University of Maryland School of
  Medicine
Baltimore, Maryland

JONATHAN SCOTT LOWRY, MD
Associate Professor
Department of Emergency Medicine
Banner University Medical Center
Tucson, Arizona

CHRISTINA LU, MD
Associate Professor
Department of Emergency Medicine
Hartford Hospital
Hartford, Connecticut

MIMI LU, MD
Clinical Professor of Emergency
  Medicine
Division of Pediatric Emergency
  Medicine
Department of Emergency Medicine
University of California, San Francisco
  School of Medicine
San Francisco, California

CHASE LUTHER, MD
Physician
Department of Emergency Medicine
Kern Medical
Bakersfield, California

NHI Y. LUU, DO
Fellow
Department of Emergency Medicine/
  Anesthesia
University of Florida College of
  Medicine
Gainesville, Florida

NICHOLAS MACALUSO, MD
Physician
Department of Emergency Medicine
Harbor-UCLA Medical Center
Torrance, California

PHILLIP D. MAGIDSON, MD, MPH
Assistant Professor
Division of Geriatric Medicine and
  Gerontology
Department of Emergency Medicine
The Johns Hopkins University School of
  Medicine
Baltimore, Maryland

Christyn Magill, MD
Assistant Professor, Pediatric Emergency Medicine
Department of Emergency Medicine
Atrium Health Carolinas Medical Center
Levine Children's Hospital
Charlotte, North Carolina

Sarah Mahonski, MD
Assistant Professor of Emergency Medicine
Department of Emergency Medicine
SUNY Upstate Medical University
Syracuse, New York

Darcy James Mainville, MD
Assistant Professor, Emergency Medicine
Physician, Critical Care Intensivist
Department of Emergency Medicine
Loma Linda University Health
Loma Linda University School of Medicine
Loma Linda, California

Trent R. Malcolm, MD, MS
Physician
Department of Emergency Medicine
Jefferson Health New Jersey
Sewell, New Jersey

Elizabeth Malik, MD
Physician
Department of Emergency Medicine
Dartmouth Hitchcock Medical Center
Lebanon, New Hampshire

Sara Manning, MD
Assistant Professor of Emergency Medicine
Department of Emergency Medicine
Indiana University School of Medicine
Indianapolis, Indiana

Mustfa Khalid Manzur, MD, MPH, MS
Resident
Department of Emergency Medicine
Montefiore Medical Center
Jacobi Medical Center
Bronx, New York

Catherine A. Marco, MD
Physician
Department of Emergency Medicine
Penn State Health
Hershey, Pennsylvania

Jeanna M. Marraffa, PharmD, MPH
Clinical Director, Upstate NY Poison Center
Clinical Professor
Department of Emergency Medicine
SUNY Upstate Medical University
Syracuse, New York

Alison Marshall, MD
Assistant Professor
Department of Emergency Medicine
Dartmouth Hitchcock Medical Center
Lebanon, New Hampshire

Kenneth D. Marshall, MD, MA
Associate Professor
Department of Emergency Medicine
University of Kansas Medical Center
Kansas City, Kansas

John W. Martel, MD, PhD
Assistant Professor, Emergency Medicine
Department of Emergency Medicine
Tufts University School of Medicine
Boston, Massachusetts
Physician
Maine Medical Center
Portland, Maine

Victoria J. Martin, MD
Assistant Professor
Department of Emergency Medicine
Dartmouth Hitchcock Medical Center
Lebanon, New Hampshire

Ashley N. Martinelli, PharmD
Clinical Pharmacy Specialist, Emergency Medicine
Department of Pharmacy
University of Maryland Medical Center
Baltimore, Maryland

DEREK MARTINEZ, DO
Resident
Department of Emergency Medicine
University of Oklahoma School of
  Community Medicine
Tulsa, Oklahoma

NICHOLAS MAXWELL, MD
Resident
Department of Emergency Medicine
Washington University School of
  Medicine
St. Louis, Missouri

MARYANN MAZER-AMIRSHAHI, PHARMD, MD, MPH, PHD
Professor of Emergency Medicine
Department of Emergency Medicine
Georgetown University School of Medicine
Washington, District of Columbia

KAITLYN MCBRIDE, MD
Resident
Department of Emergency Medicine
Carilion Clinic
Roanoke, Virginia

TAYLOR MCCORMICK, MD, MSC
Director, Pediatric Emergency Department
  and Urgent Care
Department of Emergency Medicine
Denver Health
Denver, Colorado

JACK MCGEACHY, MD
Attending Physician
Department of Emergency Medicine
Tampa General Hospital
Tampa, Florida

JENNIFER MCGOWAN, MD
Assistant Professor of Emergency Medicine
Department of Emergency Medicine
University of Louisville School of
  Medicine
Louisville, Kentucky

MICHAEL P. MCGREGOR, MD
Assistant Residency Program Director
Attending Physician
Department of Emergency Medicine
Montefiore Medical Center
Bronx, New York

NORA MCNULTY, MD
Resident
Department of Emergency Medicine
Montefiore Medical Center
Jacobi Medical Center
Bronx, New York

CHELSEY MILLER, MD, MPH
Resident
Department of Emergency Medicine
Yale New Haven Health
New Haven, Connecticut

EMILY MILLER, MD
Resident
Department of Emergency Medicine
UT Health Science Center at San Antonio
San Antonio, Texas

GABRIELLA MILLER, MD
Resident
Department of Emergency Medicine
University of Maryland Medical Center
Baltimore, Maryland

TAYLOR MILLER, MD, MPHIL
Physician
Department of Emergency Medicine
University of Maryland Medical Center
Baltimore, Maryland

JOSEPH M. MINICHIELLO, MD
Physician
Department of Emergency Medicine
Maine Medical Center
Portland, Maine

KELLIE A. MITCHELL, MD
Fellow
Department of Emergency Medicine
University of Virginia Health System
Charlottesville, Virginia

JOSEPH J. MOELLMAN, MD
Professor of Emergency Medicine
Department of Emergency Medicine
University of Cincinnati College of Medicine
Cincinnati, Ohio

MUKUND MOHAN, MD
Resident
Department of Emergency Medicine
Staten Island University Hospital–
  Northwell Health
Staten Island, New York

CONTRIBUTORS

LAURA HEMKER MOLES, MD, MS
Physician
Department of Emergency Medicine
Los Angeles General Medical Center
Los Angeles, California

ELISE MOLNAR, MD
Resident
Department of Emergency Medicine
Harbor-UCLA Medical Center
Torrance, California

KEVIN MOLYNEUX, MD
Emergency Physician
Department of Emergency Medicine
Columbia University College of Physicians and Surgeons
New York, New York

LUIS A. AGUILAR MONTALVAN, MD
Resident
Department of Emergency Medicine
Jacobi Medical Center
Montefiore Medical Center
Albert Einstein Medical Center
Bronx, New York

RENE MONZON, MD
Physician
Department of Emergency Medicine
University of California, San Francisco School of Medicine
San Francisco, California

ANDREW B. MOORE, MD, MCR
Assistant Professor
Department of Emergency Medicine
Virginia Tech Carilion School of Medicine
Carilion Clinic
Roanoke, Virginia

JESSICA MOORE, MD
Assistant Professor of Clinical Emergency Medicine
Department of Emergency Medicine
Lewis Katz School of Medicine at Temple University
Philadelphia, Pennsylvania

LAUREN MOORE, MD
Fellow
Department of Critical Care Medicine
Cleveland Clinic Foundation
Cleveland, Ohio

FINNELLA MORGAN, PHARMD
Clinical Pharmacy Specialist
Department of Emergency Medicine
Johns Hopkins Bayview Medical Center
Baltimore, Maryland

TODD D. MORRELL, MD
Assistant Professor
Department of Emergency Medicine
Geisel School of Medicine at Dartmouth
Hanover, New Hampshire

NATHAN J. MORRISON, DO, MENG
Physician
Department of Emergency Medicine
Penn State Health Milton S. Hershey Medical Center
Hershey, Pennsylvania

HILLARY CAROLINE MOSS, MD
Assistant Professor of Emergency Medicine
Attending Physician
Department of Emergency Medicine
Montefiore Medical Center
Albert Einstein College of Medicine
Bronx, New York

MEGHIN MOYNIHAN, PHARMD, BCEMP
Emergency Medicine Clinical Pharmacy Specialist
Department of Emergency Medicine
The Johns Hopkins Hospital
Baltimore, Maryland

KELLY-ANN MUNGROO, DO
Resident
Department of Emergency Medicine
Zucker School of Medicine at Hofstra
Staten Island University Hospital–Northwell Health
Staten Island, New York

JESSICA MUÑOZ, MD
Resident
Department of Emergency Medicine
Loma Linda University School of Medicine
Loma Linda, California

FREDERICK R. MURPHY JR, MPT, MPH
Geriatric Clinical Specialist
Department of Rehabilitation Services
Johns Hopkins Bayview Medical Center
Baltimore, Maryland

PAUL I. MUSEY JR, MD, MS
Associate Professor of Emergency Medicine; Vice Chair, Research and Innovation
Department of Emergency Medicine
Indiana University School of Medicine
Indianapolis, Indiana

M. KATHRYN MUTTER, MD, MPH
Associate Professor
Department of Emergency Medicine
University of Virginia School of Medicine
Charlottesville, Virginia

BENNETT A. MYERS, MD
Assistant Professor
Department of Emergency Medicine
University of Maryland School of Medicine
Baltimore, Maryland

ARSAM NADEEM, MD
Resident
Department of Emergency Medicine
Jefferson Health New Jersey
Stratford, New Jersey

ARUN NAGDEV, MD
Director, Emergency Ultrasound
Department of Emergency Medicine
Highland Hospital
Alameda Health System
Oakland, California

ARUN NAIR, MD, MPH
Physician
Department of Emergency Medicine
St. David's Medical Center
Austin, Texas

DEANNA BRIDGE NAJERA, MPAS, MS, PA-C
Physician Assistant
Department of Emergency Medicine
MedStar Montgomery Medical Center
Olney, Maryland

ANTHONY J. NASTASI, MD, MHS
Resident
Department of Emergency Medicine
Perelman School of Medicine at the University of Pennsylvania
Philadelphia, Pennsylvania

JOSEPH A. NELSON MD, MBA
Assistant Professor
Department of Emergency Medicine/Critical Care Medicine
University of Maryland/Shock Trauma Center
Baltimore, Maryland

VIVIENNE NG, MD, MPH
Assistant Professor
Department of Emergency Medicine
University of Arizona College of Medicine
Tucson, Arizona

JOSHUA (JOSH) NICHOLS, MD
Physician
Department of Emergency Medicine
Virginia Tech Carilion School of Medicine
Carilion Clinic
Roanoke, Virginia

CHRISTOPHER P. NICKSON, BSc (HONS), BHB, MBChB, MCLINEPID (CLINTOX)
Senior Intensivist
Department of Intensive Care Unit
Alfred Health
Melbourne, Victoria, Australia

MAHNOOSH NIK-AHD, MD, MPH
Assistant Clinical Professor
Division of Pediatric Emergency Medicine
Department of Emergency Medicine
University of California, San Francisco School of Medicine
San Francisco, California

ROBERT OLYMPIA, MD
Professor
Attending Physician
Departments of Emergency Medicine and Pediatrics
Penn State College of Medicine
Penn State Health Milton S. Hershey Medical Center
Penn State Children's Hospital
Hershey, Pennsylvania

HILARY ONG, MD
Assistant Professor of Pediatrics, Emergency Medicine
Department of Emergency Medicine
University of California, San Francisco School of Medicine
San Francisco, California

JESSICA LANGE OSTERMAN, MS, MD
Associate Professor of Clinical Emergency Medicine
Department of Emergency Medicine
Keck School of Medicine of USC
Los Angeles, California

JAKOB OTTENHOFF, DO
Assistant Professor
Department of Emergency Medicine
University of Virginia School of Medicine
Charlottesville, Virginia

GARRETT S. PACHECO, MD
Assistant Professor
Departments of Emergency Medicine and Pediatrics
University of Arizona College of Medicine
Tucson, Arizona

JOSEPH PALTER, MD
Associate Medical Director
Department of Emergency Medicine
Stroger Hospital of Cook County
Chicago, Illinois

NIKITA PARIPATI, MD
Resident
Department of Emergency Medicine
Hospital of the University of Pennsylvania
Philadelphia, Pennsylvania

TENNESSEE PARK, MD
Physician
Department of Emergency Medicine
University of Virginia
Charlottesville, Virginia

BRIAN PARKER, MD, MS
Assistant Professor
Department of Emergency Medicine
UT Health Science Center at San Antonio
San Antonio, Texas

M. KAITLIN PARKS, DO
Attending Physician, Core Faculty
Department of Emergency Medicine
Norman Regional Health System
Norman, Oklahoma

DEVANG PATEL, MD
Associate Professor
Department of Medicine
University of Maryland School of Medicine
Baltimore, Maryland

SIMA PATEL, MD
Associate Professor
Department of Emergency Medicine
University of California, San Francisco School of Medicine
San Francisco, California

KYRA PATICOFF, OMS IV
Medical Student
Department of Emergency Medicine
Staten Island University Hospital
Staten Island, New York

EMILY PEARCE, MD
Resident
Department of Emergency Medicine
University of New Mexico School of Medicine
Albuquerque, New Mexico

LEE PLANTMASON, MD, MPH
Physician
Department of Emergency Medicine
Sharp Memorial Hospital
San Diego, California

STEVEN POLEVOI, MD
Clinical Professor of Emergency Medicine
Attending Physician
Department of Emergency Medicine
University of California, San Francisco School of Medicine
San Francisco, California

ELIZABETH PONTIUS, MD
Associate Professor of Emergency Medicine
Department of Emergency Medicine
Georgetown University School of Medicine
Washington, District of Columbia

NICHOLAS D. POOLE, MD
Resident
Department of Emergency Medicine
Dartmouth Hitchcock Medical Center
Lebanon, New Hampshire

ARTHUR J. POPE, MD, PHD
Assistant Professor of Clinical Emergency Medicine
Department of Emergency Medicine
Perelman School of Medicine at the University of Pennsylvania
Philadelphia, Pennsylvania

JENNIFER V. POPE, MD
Assistant Professor of Emergency Medicine
Department of Emergency Medicine
Dartmouth Hitchcock Medical Center
Lebanon, New Hampshire

MATTHEW POREMBA, PHARMD
Clinical Pharmacist, Emergency Medicine
Department of Pharmacy
University of Maryland Medical Center
Baltimore, Maryland

BO QIN, MD
Resident
Department of Emergency Medicine
Perelman School of Medicine at the University of Pennsylvania
Philadelphia, Pennsylvania

RYAN RAAM, MD
Associate Professor of Clinical Emergency Medicine
Department of Emergency Medicine
Los Angeles General Medical Center
Los Angeles, California

AMIR ROMBOD RAHIMIAN, MD, MPH
Physician
Department of Emergency Medicine
University of Arizona College of Medicine
Tucson, Arizona

PRITI RAWANI-PATEL, MD, MA
Assistant Professor
Department of Emergency Medicine
University of Arizona College of Medicine
Tucson, Arizona

NEIL A. RAY, MD
Clinical Assistant Professor of Emergency Medicine
Department of Emergency Medicine
Perelman School of Medicine at the University of Pennsylvania
Philadelphia, Pennsylvania

CHLOE RENSHAW, MD
Clinical Educator
Department of Emergency Medicine
University of Maryland School of Medicine
Baltimore, Maryland

JENNIFER REPANSHEK, MD
Adjunct Associate Professor of Clinical Emergency Medicine
Lewis Katz School of Medicine at Temple University
Temple University Hospital
Philadelphia, Pennsylvania

ZACHARY REPANSHEK, MD
Associate Professor
Department of Emergency Medicine
Lewis Katz School of Medicine at Temple University
Philadelphia, Pennsylvania

RANDALL T. RHYNE, MD
Assistant Professor
Department of Emergency Medicine
The Johns Hopkins University School of Medicine
Baltimore, Maryland

DIANE RIMPLE, MD
Interim Chair
Department of Emergency Medicine
University of New Mexico School of Medicine
Albuquerque, New Mexico

LINDSAY RITTER, MD
Intensivist
Department of Critical Care
MedStar Washington Hospital Center
Washington, District of Columbia

MEGAN RIVERA, MD
Resident
Department of Emergency Medicine
University of Florida College of Medicine
Gainesville, Florida

EMILY C. Z. ROBEN, MD, MS
Associate Professor of Pediatric Emergency Medicine
Department of Emergency Medicine
UCSF Benioff Children's Hospital
University of California, San Francisco School of Medicine
San Francisco, California

KELLI ROBINSON, MD
Physician
Department of Emergency Medicine
University of Maryland Medical Center
Baltimore, Maryland

CLARE ROEPKE, MD
Assistant Professor
Department of Emergency Medicine
Lewis Katz School of Medicine at Temple University
Philadelphia, Pennsylvania

ANTHONY ROGGIO, MD
Assistant Professor
Department of Emergency Medicine
University of Maryland School of Medicine
Baltimore, Maryland

MATTHEW A. ROGINSKI, MD, MPH
Assistant Professor of Emergency Medicine and Medicine
Department of Emergency Medicine
Dartmouth Hitchcock Medical Center
Lebanon, New Hampshire

KEVIN ROLNICK, MD
Resident
Department of Emergency Medicine
University of California, San Francisco School of Medicine
San Francisco General Hospital
San Francisco, California

CALIXTO ROMERO, MD
Physician and Fellow
Departments of Emergency Medicine and Critical Care Medicine
Dartmouth Hitchcock Medical Center
Lebanon, New Hampshire

ANNIE ROMINGER, MD, MPH, MSU
Associate Professor
Department of Emergency Medicine
Atrium Health Carolinas Medical Center
Wake Forest University School of Medicine
Charlotte, North Carolina

EMILY ROSE, MD
Associate Professor of Clinical Emergency Medicine
Department of Emergency Medicine
Keck School of Medicine of USC
Los Angeles, California

TINA GODINHO ROSENBAUM, MD, MPH
Attending Physician
Department of Emergency Medicine
MedStar Washington Hospital Center
Washington, District of Columbia

EFRAT ROSENTHAL, MD
Assistant Professor of Emergency Medicine
Department of Emergency Medicine
University of California, San Francisco School of Medicine
San Francisco, California

AMIR A. ROUHANI, MD
Associate Clinical Professor
Department of Emergency Medicine/Internal Medicine
UCLA–Olive View Medical Center
Sylmar, California

STEVEN ROUMPF, MD, MBA
Medical Director
Department of Emergency Medicine
Indiana University Health and Indiana University School of Medicine
Indianapolis, Indiana

CATHERINE ROWBOTTOM, DO, MS
Resident
Department of Emergency Medicine
Case Western Reserve University School of Medicine
The MetroHealth System
Cleveland Clinic Foundation
Cleveland, Ohio

THOMAS H. ROZEN, MBBS, FCICM, FRACP
Director of Paediatric Intensive Care
Department of Paediatric Intensive Care Unit
Royal Children's Hospital
Melbourne, Victoria, Australia

RAWAN SAFA, MD
Resident
Department of Emergency Medicine
Washington University School of Medicine
Barnes Jewish Hospital
St. Louis, Missouri

CHRISTINA SAJAK, MD
Resident
Department of Emergency Medicine
University of Maryland Medical Center
Baltimore, Maryland

NICHOLAS SANTAVICCA, MD
Assistant Professor
Department of Emergency Medicine
Montefiore Medical Center
Bronx, New York

EMILY SCHAEFFER, DO
Resident
Department of Emergency Medicine
Virginia Tech Carilion School of Medicine
Roanoke, Virginia

VERENA SCHANDERA, MD
Associate Professor
Department of Emergency Medicine
UC Davis School of Medicine
Sacramento, California

JORDAN B. SCHOOLER, MD, PhD
Assistant Professor
Department of Emergency Medicine
Heart and Vascular Institute CCU
Penn State Health
Hershey, Pennsylvania

JOSEPH SCHRAMSKI, DO
Program Director, Emergency Medicine
Department of Emergency Medicine
Corewell Health
Trenton, Michigan

KRAFTIN E. SCHREYER, MD, MBA
Associate Professor of Emergency Medicine
Department of Emergency Medicine
Temple University Hospital
Philadelphia, Pennsylvania

ROBERT W. SEABURY, PharmD
Clinical Staff Pharmacist
Department of Pharmacy
SUNY Upstate University Hospital
Syracuse, New York

JUSTIN SEMPSROTT, MD
Director
International Drowning Researchers' Alliance
Kuna, Idaho

JORGE SERRANO, MD
Resident
Department of Emergency Medicine
Los Angeles General Medical Center
Los Angeles, California

RICCARDO SERRO, MD
Resident
Department of Neurosurgery
University of Maryland School of Medicine
Baltimore, Maryland

KINJAL SETHURAMAN, MD, MPH
Associate Professor
Department of Emergency Medicine
University of Maryland School of Medicine
Baltimore, Maryland

Aalap Shah, MD
Assistant Professor
Department of Emergency Medicine
Medical University of South Carolina
Charleston, South Carolina

Aesha Shah, MD
Resident
Department of Emergency Medicine
Penn State Health Milton S. Hershey Medical Center
Hershey, Pennsylvania

Michael Shamoon, MD
Clinical Assistant Professor of Emergency Medicine
Assistant Program Director, LA General/USC Emergency Medicine Residency
Department of Emergency Medicine
Keck School of Medicine of USC
Los Angeles, California

Tori Shank, DO
Resident
Department of Emergency Medicine
Trident Medical Center
Charleston, South Carolina

Daniel Sheets, MD, MPH
Clinical Instructor
Department of Emergency Medicine
Regions Hospital
Saint Paul, Minnesota

Christina L. Shenvi, MD, PhD, MBA
Associate Professor of Emergency Medicine
Department of Emergency Medicine
University of North Carolina School of Medicine
Chapel Hill, North Carolina

Guy Shochat, MD
Professor of Emergency Medicine
Department of Emergency Medicine
University of California, San Francisco School of Medicine
San Francisco, California

Ashley Shreves, MD
Physician
Department of Emergency Medicine
Department of Palliative Care
Ochsner Medical Center
New Orleans, Louisiana

Richard Sinert, DO
Professor of Emergency Medicine
Department of Emergency Medicine
NYC Health + Hospitals/Kings County
SUNY Downstate Health Sciences University
Brooklyn, New York

Manpreet Singh, MD, MBE, FACEP, AEMUS-FDP
Director, Undergraduate Medical Education
Department of Emergency Medicine
Harbor-UCLA Medical Center
Torrance, California

Lucas Sjeklocha, MD
Assistant Professor
Department of Emergency Medicine
University of Maryland School of Medicine
Baltimore, Maryland

Rachel M. Skains, MD, MSPH
Assistant Professor
Department of Emergency Medicine
UAB Heersink School of Medicine
Birmingham, Alabama

Janet Anne Smereck, MD
Associate Professor
Department of Emergency Medicine
Georgetown University School of Medicine
Washington, District of Columbia

Moira Smith, MD, MPH
Clinical Informatics Fellow
Department of Emergency Medicine
University of Virginia Health System
Charlottesville, Virginia

SARAH SOMMERKAMP, MD
Assistant Professor
Department of Emergency Medicine
University of Maryland School of
  Medicine
Baltimore, Maryland

PRATHAP SOORIYAKUMARAN, MD
Assistant Clinical Professor
Department of Emergency Medicine
Zuckerberg San Francisco General
  Hospital
University of California, San Francisco
  School of Medicine
San Francisco, California

ANNALISE SORRENTINO, MD
Professor of Pediatrics
Division of Emergency Medicine
Department of Pediatrics
UAB Heersink School of Medicine
Birmingham, Alabama

CECILY KOPPUZHA SOTOMAYOR, MD
Attending Physician
Department of Emergency
  Medicine
University of California, San Francisco
  School of Medicine
San Francisco, California

RYAN SPANGLER, MD
Assistant Professor
Department of Emergency Medicine
University of Maryland Medical Center
University of Maryland School of
  Medicine
Baltimore, Maryland

RORY SPIEGEL, MD
Assistant Professor
Department of Emergency Medicine and
  Critical Care
MedStar Washington Hospital Center
Washington, District of Columbia

SARAH BETH SPIEGEL, MD
Resident
Department of Emergency Medicine
NYU Bellevue
New York, New York

JEREMY ST. THOMAS, MD
Resident
Departments of Emergency Medicine and
  Pediatrics
University of Maryland Medical Center
Baltimore, Maryland

DARREN STAPLETON, MD
Resident
Department of Emergency Medicine
University of Arizona College of
  Medicine
Tucson, Arizona

KATHLEEN STEPHANOS, MD
Assistant Professor
Departments of Emergency Medicine and
  Pediatrics
University of Maryland School of
  Medicine
Baltimore, Maryland

ROBERT J. STEPHENS, MD, MSCI
Resident
Department of Emergency
  Medicine
Washington University School of
  Medicine
Saint Louis, Missouri

KELLY STEWART, MD
Physician
Department of Emergency Medicine
Denver Health
Denver, Colorado

KATRINA STIME, MD
Chief Resident
Department of Emergency
  Medicine
University of California, San Francisco
  School of Medicine
San Francisco, California

JOHN STOCKTON, MD, MPH
Fellow
Department of Emergency Medicine
Harbor-UCLA Medical Center
Torrance, California

Christine M. Stork, PharmD, MPH, DABAT, FAACT
Co-Pharmacology Thread Leader, Norton College of Medicine
Toxicologist, Upstate NY Poison Center
Professor
Departments of Pharmacology and Emergency Medicine
SUNY Upstate Medical University
Syracuse, New York

Steven Straube, MD, MBA
Assistant Professor
Department of Emergency Medicine
University of California, San Francisco School of Medicine
San Francisco, California

Jonathan Stuart, DO
Physician
Department of Emergency Medicine
University of Washington School of Medicine
Seattle, Washington

Salvador J. Suau, MD
Residency Program Director
Department of Emergency Medicine
Ochsner Clinic Foundation
New Orleans, Louisiana

Michael D. Sullivan, MD
Resident
Department of Emergency Medicine
University of Maryland Medical Center
Baltimore, Maryland

Mark Sutherland, MD
Assistant Professor
Department of Emergency Medicine
University of Maryland School of Medicine
Baltimore, Maryland

Danielle Sutton, MD
Attending Physician
Department of Pediatric Emergency Medicine
Atrium Health Levine Children's Hospital
Charlotte, North Carolina

Stuart Swadron, MD
Adjunct Professor of Clinical Emergency Medicine and Medical Education
Department of Emergency Medicine
Keck School of Medicine of USC
Los Angeles, California

Anand K. Swaminathan, MD, MPH
Assistant Professor of Emergency Medicine
Department of Emergency Medicine
Staten Island University Hospital–Northwell Health
Staten Island, New York

Eric R. Swanson, MD
Professor
Department of Emergency Medicine
University of Utah School of Medicine
Salt Lake City, Utah

Ramin Tabatabai, MD, MACM
Physician
Department of Emergency Medicine
Los Angeles General Medical Center
Los Angeles, California

William F. Taber, MD
Resident
Department of Emergency Medicine
Virginia Tech Carilion School of Medicine
Carilion Clinic
Roanoke, Virginia

Sierra Tackett, MD
Resident
Department of Emergency Medicine
Indiana University School of Medicine
Indianapolis, Indiana

Farid K. Tadros, MD
Emergency Medicine Resident
Department of Emergency Medicine
Los Angeles General Medical Center
Los Angeles, California

Tianyu Tang, MD
Resident
Department of Emergency Medicine
University of California, San Francisco School of Medicine
San Francisco, California

LLOYD TANNENBAUM, MD
Physician
Department of Emergency Medicine
Brooke Army Medical Center
San Antonio, Texas

MATTHEW TANZI, MD
Clinical Assistant Professor
Department of Emergency Medicine
Stony Brook University Hospital
Stony Brook, New York

ISAAC TAWIL, MD
Professor
Department of Emergency Medicine
University of New Mexico School of Medicine
Albuquerque, New Mexico

HEIDI MARIA TEAGUE, MD, MS
Assistant Professor
Department of Emergency Medicine
University of Maryland School of Medicine
Baltimore, Maryland

NATALIE J. TEDFORD, MD
Clinical Instructor
Research Fellow
Division of Pediatric Emergency Medicine
Department of Pediatrics
University of Utah School of Medicine
Salt Lake City, Utah

LISA TENORIO, MD
Physician
Department of Emergency Medicine
St. Joseph's Medical Center
Stockton, California

RONALD B. TESORIERO, MD
Associate Professor of Surgery
Department of Surgery
University of California, San Francisco School of Medicine
San Francisco, California

CHRISTOPHER THOM, MD
Associate Professor of Emergency Medicine
Department of Emergency Medicine
University of Virginia Health System
Charlottesville, Virginia

J. JEREMY THOMAS, MD, MBA
Professor and Endowed Chair
Department of Emergency Medicine
University of Louisville, School of Medicine
Louisville, Kentucky

C. NICOLE THOMPSON, MD, MBA
Assistant Professor of Emergency Medicine
Division of Emergency Medicine
Department of Surgery
Texas Tech University Health Sciences Center
Lubbock, Texas

HALLIE TIBURZI, BSc
Patient and Customer Experience Liaison
Department of Emergency Medicine
Staten Island University Hospital
Staten Island, New York

DANIEL TIRADO, MD, MS
Resident
Department of Emergency Medicine
SUNY Upstate University Hospital
Syracuse, New York

NICOLE TITZE, MD
Physician
Department of Emergency Medicine
Harbor-UCLA Medical Center
Torrance, California

MICHAEL TOM, MD
Attending Physician
Department of Emergency Medicine
St. Francis Hospital
Federal Way, Washington
Clinician
Department of Hyperbaric Medicine
Department of Emergency Medicine
Hospital of the University of Pennsylvania
Philadelphia, Pennsylvania

NAM TRINH, MD
Resident
Department of Emergency Medicine
MedStar Georgetown University
Washington, District of Columbia

Rachel E. Tsolinas, MD
Resident
Department of Emergency Medicine
University of California, San Francisco School of Medicine
San Francisco, California

Richard Diego Gonzales y Tucker, MD
Assistant Professor
Department of Emergency Medicine
University of California, San Francisco School of Medicine
San Francisco, California

Katren Tyler, MD
Clinical Professor of Emergency Medicine
Department of Emergency Medicine
UC Davis School of Medicine
Sacramento, California

Nicolas A. Ulloa, MD
Attending Physician and Core Faculty
Department of Emergency Medicine
Mount Sinai Medical Center
Miami Beach, Florida

Jeffrey Uribe, MD
Assistant Clinical Professor
Department of Emergency Medicine
Georgetown University School of Medicine
Attending Physician
Department of Emergency Medicine
MedStar Health
Washington, District of Columbia

Raizada Vaid, MD
Fellow
Division of Pediatric Emergency Medicine
Department of Emergency Medicine
SUNY Upstate University Hospital
Syracuse, New York

Julie Y. Valenzuela, MD
Assistant Professor of Surgery
Division of Trauma, Burns, and Surgical Critical Care
Department of Surgery
University of Miami Leonard M. Miller School of Medicine
Miami, Florida

Rolando G. Valenzuela, MD, DTMH
Clinical Assistant Professor
Department of Emergency Medicine
University of Miami Jackson Memorial
Miami, Florida

Kristina van de Goor, MD
Physician
Department of Emergency Medicine
Los Angeles General Medical Center
Los Angeles, California

James Vandenberg, MD, MSc
Assistant Professor of Clinical Emergency Medicine
Department of Emergency Medicine
Lewis Katz School of Medicine at Temple University
Philadelphia, Pennsylvania

Alvin Varghese, MD
Physician
Emergency Department
University of Maryland Medical Center
Baltimore, Maryland

Balakrishna Vemula, MD
Fellow
Department of Emergency Medicine
The Johns Hopkins Hospital
Baltimore, Maryland

Haley Vertelney, MD
Emergency Physician
Department of Emergency Medicine
University of California, San Francisco School of Medicine
San Francisco, California

Hurnan Vongsachang, MD, MPH
Fellow
Department of National Clinical Scholars Program at UCLA
David Geffen School of Medicine at UCLA
Los Angeles, California

JOYCE WAHBA, MD
Physician
Department of Emergency Medicine
Harbor-UCLA Medical Center
Torrance, California

SHABANA WALIA, MD, MPH, FACEP
Assistant Professor
Department of Emergency Medicine
McGovern Medical School
UTHealth Houston
Houston, Texas

ANNE WALKER, MD
Physician
Department of Emergency Medicine
St. Joseph's Medical Center
Stockton, California

DAVID JOHN WALLACE, MD, MPH
Adjunct Associate Professor
Critical Care Medicine
University of Pittsburgh
Pittsburgh, Pennsylvania

JORDAN WARCHOL, MD, MPH
Assistant Professor
Department of Emergency Medicine
University of Nebraska Medical Center
Omaha, Nebraska

DILLON WARR, MD
Resident
Department of Emergency Medicine
Temple University Hospital
Philadelphia, Pennsylvania

ANNA L. WATERBROOK, MD
Professor, Emergency and Sports Medicine
Department of Emergency Medicine
University of Arizona College of Medicine
Tucson, Arizona

MONICA KATHLEEN WATTANA, MD
Associate Professor
Department of Emergency Medicine
UT MD Anderson Cancer Center
Houston, Texas

LEIGH-ANN J. WEBB, MD, MBA
Assistant Professor of Emergency Medicine
Department of Emergency Medicine
University of Virginia Health System
Charlottesville, Virginia

MITCHELL WEEMAN, MD
Physician
Department of Emergency Medicine
University of Louisville School of Medicine
Louisville, Kentucky

MATTHEW WELLES, MD
Fellow
Department of Critical Care Medicine
University of Pittsburgh School of Medicine
Pittsburgh, Pennsylvania

SARAH K. WENDEL, MD, MBA
Assistant Professor
Department of Emergency Medicine
University of Virginia School of Medicine
Charlottesville, Virginia

HEIDI WERNER, MD, MSHPEd
Associate Clinical Professor
Departments of Emergency Medicine and Pediatrics
University of California, San Francisco School of Medicine
San Francisco, California

R. GENTRY WILKERSON, MD
Associate Professor
Department of Emergency Medicine
University of Maryland School of Medicine
Baltimore, Maryland

CHRISTOPHER G. WILLIAMS, MD, FAWM
Associate Professor
Department of Emergency Medicine
University of Arizona College of Medicine
Tucson, Arizona

KELLY WILLIAMSON, MD
Associate Professor
Department of Emergency Medicine
Northwestern University, Feinberg School of Medicine
Chicago, Illinois

GEORGE C. WILLIS, MD, FAAEM, FACEP
Vice Chair of Faculty Affairs
Department of Emergency Medicine
UT Health Science Center at San Antonio
San Antonio, Texas

CASEY LEE WILSON, MD
Residency Program Director
Department of Emergency Medicine
Grand Strand Medical Center
Myrtle Beach, South Carolina

RACHEL WILTJER, DO
Clinical Instructor
Departments of Emergency Medicine and Pediatrics
University of Maryland School of Medicine
Baltimore, Maryland

T. ANDREW WINDSOR, MD
Assistant Professor
Department of Emergency Medicine
University of Maryland School of Medicine
Baltimore, Maryland

MAIA WINKEL, MD, MS
Resident
Department of Emergency Medicine
Jacobi Medical Center
Montefiore Medical Center
Bronx, New York

MATTHEW L. WONG, MD, MPH
Associate Professor of Clinical Emergency Medicine
Department of Emergency Medicine
Lewis Katz School of Medicine at Temple University
Philadelphia, Pennsylvania

SHAHRZAD WOODBRIDGE, DO
Physician
Department of Emergency Medicine
University of Utah School of Medicine
Salt Lake City, Utah

WILLIAM WOODS, MD
Associate Professor of Emergency Medicine
Department of Emergency Medicine
University of Virginia Health System
Charlottesville, Virginia

WINSTON WU, MD
Resident
Department of Emergency Medicine
University of Virginia School of Medicine
Charlottesville, Virginia

SAMANTHA J. YARMIS, MD
Physician
Department of Emergency Medicine
University of Maryland Medical Center
Baltimore, Maryland

TYLER YATES, MD
Physician
Department of Emergency Medicine
Northwell at Staten Island University Hospital
New York, New York

JULIANNE YEARY, PharmD, BCCCP, BCEMP
Clinical Pharmacy Specialist, Emergency Medicine
Department of Pharmacy
Barnes Jewish Hospital
St. Louis, Missouri

MICHAEL J. YOO, MD
Core Faculty
Assistant Professor of Military and Emergency Medicine
San Antonio Uniformed Services Health Education Consortium
Fort Sam Houston, Texas

CONOR YOUNG, MD
Fellow and Physician
Department of Emergency Medicine
SUNY Upstate Medical University
Syracuse, New York

KRISTA YOUNG, MD
Fellow
Department of Pediatrics
University of Iowa Hospitals and Clinics
Iowa City, Iowa

JENNIFER YU, MD
Assistant Chair
Department of Critical Care Medicine
MedStar Washington Hospital Center
Washington, District of Columbia

VIAN ZADA, MD
Resident
Department of Emergency Medicine
Los Angeles General Medicine Center
Los Angeles, California

WESLEY ZEGER, DO
Professor
Department of Emergency Medicine
University of Nebraska Medical Center
Omaha, Nebraska

LARA ZEKAR, MD
Chief Emergency Medicine Resident
Emergency Department
UC Davis Medical Center
Sacramento, California

ALEXANDER ZIRULNIK, MD, MPH
Resident
Emergency Department
Massachusetts General Hospital
Brigham and Women's Hospital
Boston, Massachusetts

MELISSA E. ZUKOWSKI, MD, MPH
Medical Director
Department of Emergency Medicine
Banner University Medical Center
University of Arizona College of Medicine
Tucson, Arizona

SARAH ZYZANSKI, MD
Physician
Department of Emergency Medicine
Harbor-UCLA Medical Center
Torrance, California

PREFACE

Emergency medicine (EM) is a high-risk specialty, where emergency care providers must quickly evaluate and treat unfamiliar patients in an overcrowded and often underresourced environment. Conditions in our emergency departments with respect to inpatient boarding, staffing shortages, and extended wait times seem to have only increased as we emerge from the COVID-19 pandemic. The great challenge in EM is to be able to quickly, efficiently, and safely evaluate each patient to find and treat those with deadly, time-sensitive conditions. Given the myriad of patients with non-life-threatening conditions, emergency care providers can be easily lulled into a false sense of security that the patient before them has a benign condition. With the need to rapidly diagnose time-sensitive conditions, efficiently deliver high-quality care, quickly and effectively communicate with patients, and discharge patients with proper instructions, errors in EM are inevitable. This textbook was created to help the emergency care provider minimize those errors by discussing common mistakes and pitfalls that may occur in the daily practice of EM.

As with prior editions, we have included 365 chapters in this textbook and strongly encourage readers to simply read one chapter per day over the course of a year. Chapters have been organized into various organ systems (eg, cardiovascular, gastrointestinal, neurologic), key EM categories (eg, resuscitation, airway management, critical care, trauma, pediatrics, pain management), as well as key nonclinical aspects of EM (eg, clinical practice). The majority of this third edition contains new content written by new authors. Chapters previously contained in the second edition have been updated with the most recent evidence-based information. The result is that this text reads more like a third volume rather than a third edition. We anticipate that readers will continue to benefit from the outstanding content in the first and second editions even as they read this third edition.

We would like to thank the authors and associate editors of this textbook for the significant time and effort that they have devoted to making their chapters cutting-edge, evidence-based, and practical. We would also like to thank Dr Amal Mattu, for providing us with the opportunity to create what we believe is an outstanding text and contribution to EM. Our sincere thanks also to the publisher, managing editors, and staff at Wolters Kluwer for their dedication and support to this textbook. Finally, we would like to thank our families and colleagues for their support and for providing the inspiration for us to complete this textbook.

We hope that you find this text usable, practical, and informative about common errors in EM. Best wishes to you and your patients!

MICHAEL E. WINTERS, MD, MBA
DALE P. WOOLRIDGE, MD, PHD
EVIE MARCOLINI, MD, MBE
MIMI LU, MD
SARAH B. DUBBS, MD

Acknowledgments

I would like to thank my wife, Erika, and my wonderful children, Hayden, Emma, Taylor, and Olivia, for their selfless love, support, and encouragement. You are my world. A special thanks also to Dr Mattu for all of the amazing educational opportunities that he has provided to many of us, including the opportunity for this third edition! You are a wonderful colleague, inspirational mentor, and dear friend. Finally, thank you to the faculty and residents in the Department of Emergency Medicine at the University of Maryland. It is humbling to work with such amazing physicians each and every day in our department.

—**Michael E. Winters, MD, MBA**

I would like to thank my long-time mentor, Dr Marc Tischler, who not only inspired me but more importantly believed in me. His influence and friendship have made me a better person. Marc will forever be missed.

—**Dale P. Woolridge, MD, PhD**

Thank you Paul, for your unwavering support, your inspiration, and for teaching me how to teach. Thank you Dr Mattu, for your mentorship, your role model, and the opportunities to bring education to Emergency Medicine in so many ways. It is a privilege to work with this team—thank you Mike Winters for leading us. And finally, my heartful thank you to all the Emergency Medicine clinicians who bring excellent care to all patients every day.

—**Evie Marcolini, MD, MBE**

Never enough thank-yous to express... *My Family:* Our wild, wacky, and wonderful ways have shaped who I am, and inspire me to live my fullest life. *My Dearest Popo:* Not a day goes by in which I don't miss you and remember you. *Dr. Mattu:* You shared your love and gift of education with me and so many others. *My Coeditors:* Your friendship and support was immense. *My UMEM and UCSF Fellow Warriors:* I love being in the trenches with you.

—**Mimi Lu, MD**

Matthew, Emily, and Abigail—I love you so much and am thankful every day for our family. Amal, remember when you asked me what my 10-year plan was, and I said, "I just want to teach"? Thank you for the endless opportunities over the years, you have been an incredible mentor and sponsor. To my coeditors—we made it—I am privileged to have taken this journey with you. To my residents and colleagues at UMEM—you inspire me every day! AEIOU.

—**Sarah B. Dubbs, MD**

Contents

ASSOCIATE EDITORS iii
CONTRIBUTORS vi
PREFACE xxxix
ACKNOWLEDGMENTS xl
ABBREVIATIONS lxii

SECTION I RESUSCITATION
Book Editor: Michael E. Winters
Associate Editors: Kami M. Hu and Michael G. Allison

1. Highest Quality CPR   *Luis A. Aguilar Montalvan and Andrew E. Chertoff* 1
2. Properly Position Those Pads!   *Samantha J. Yarmis and Caleb Chan* 3
3. Are Epinephrine, Calcium, or Bicarbonate Beneficial in Cardiac Arrest?   *Catherine Rowbottom and Bachar Hamade* 6
4. Resuscitating Refractory Ventricular Tachycardia and Ventricular Fibrillation   *Akilesh Honasoge and Caleb Chan* 8
5. Know the Indications for Initiating ECMO in the ED   *Nhi Y. Luu and Casey Carr* 11
6. Optimize Oxygenation and Ventilation in Your Patient Who Has Experienced a Cardiac Arrest   *Zoe Glick and Lindsay Ritter* 14
7. What MAP Should You Target in the Postarrest Patient?   *Ryan Lee and Wan-Tsu W. Chang* 16
8. When to Activate the Cardiac Cath Team Following Sudden Cardiac Arrest—Don't Be Afraid to Call   *Matthew J. Levy* 18
9. Has Enthusiasm for TTM Cooled Off?   *Catherine Rowbottom and Bachar Hamade* 20
10. Making a Difference in Undifferentiated Shock   *Daniel Sheets and Randall T. Rhyne* 22
11. POCUS Pearls for Undifferentiated Shock   *Samantha A. King and T. Andrew Windsor* 25
12. Should You Administer Balanced Fluids or Normal Saline?   *Nam Trinh and Rory Spiegel* 28

13 Don't Make These Peripheral Pressor Pitfalls *Joseph A. Nelson and Mark Sutherland* 30

14 Massive Transfusion or Massive Confusion? *Mustfa Khalid Manzur and Hillary Caroline Moss* 32

15 Should You Ever Perform an ED Thoracotomy? *Harry V. Flaster and Michael R. Ehmann* 34

16 Know the Indications for REBOA Placement in the ED *Casey Lee Wilson and Errett Jacks*...36

17 Recognize and Resuscitate Cardiac Tamponade Before Your Patient Crashes *Nora McNulty and Nicholas Santavicca* 38

18 Know How to Mend a Broken Heart *Michael G. Allison* 41

19 CPAP, BiPAP, and HFNC—OH MY! *Bo Qin and John C. Greenwood* 44

20 Interpreting the Post-ROSC ECG *Maia Winkel and Michael P. McGregor* 47

21 Pearls for the Patient With Pulmonary Hypertension *Taylor Miller and Lucas Sjeklocha* 49

22 When Should I Give Lytics for PE? *Nour Al Jalbout and Sarah Badin* 52

23 Know How to Resuscitate the Crashing Tox Patient *Tiffany C. Fong and Harry E. Heverling* 54

SECTION II AIRWAY MANAGEMENT
Book Editor: Michael E. Winters
Associate Editors: Kayla T. Enriquez

24 Properly Performing BVM Ventilation *Lara Zekar, Verena Schandera, and Erik Laurin* 61

25 Resuscitate Before You Intubate! *Rene Monzon and Kayla T. Enriquez* 63

26 Know Your RSI Meds *Lee Johnson and Joseph Brown*...................66

27 What Is Your Plan B, C, D? *Lara Zekar and Erik Laurin* 68

28 Don't Make These Mistakes in Intubating the Patient Who Is Obese *Katrina Stime and Guy Shochat* 70

29 Pitfalls in Intubating the Crashing Asthmatic *Lara Zekar and Verena Schandera* 73

30 Avoid the Clean Kill—Intubating the Patient With Acidosis *Madeline Grade and Guy Shochat* 76

31 What to Do When You Lose Your View *Jeremy Lacocque and Erik J. Kramer* 78

32	Know How to Perform a Bougie-Assisted Cricothyroidotomy *Lee Johnson and Joseph Brown* 81
33	Baby on Board—Intubating the Pregnant Patient *Haley Vertelney and Cecily Koppuzha Sotomayor* 84

SECTION III CRITICAL CARE

Book Editor: Evie Marcolini
Associate Editors: Brian J. Wright

34	Know Your Initial Vent Settings *Ryan Barnicle and Chelsey Miller* 89
35	Don't Forget Post-Intubation Analgesia and Sedation *Matthew Tanzi* 93
36	Phenobarbital for Alcohol Withdrawal Syndrome *Kevin Rolnick and Rory Spiegel* 96
37	Monitoring Ventilator Pressures Is a Must *Christina Lu and Kristi Lizyness* 99
38	Know How to Interpret Ventilator Waveforms *Nicolas A. Ulloa and Dan Eraso* 103
39	What's Up With Alternative Modes of Mechanical Ventilation? *Alexander Bracey and Megan M. Lieb* 108
40	Know How to Evaluate and Manage the Intubated Patient With Refractory Hypoxemia *Thomas H. Rozen and Christopher P. Nickson* 111
41	Think Before You Hang Those Fluids! Consider a Tailored Fluid Strategy for Critically Ill Patients *Michael G. Allison* 114
42	Who Needs RRT in the ED? *Sarah Ring Gibbs and Evan Leibner* 116
43	Know How to Care for the ICU Boarder in Your ED *Joshua D. Farkas* 120
44	Push-Dose Pressor Pitfalls *C. Nicole Thompson* 122
45	Perform the Simple Interventions That Make a Big Difference in Preventing Ventilator-Associated Pneumonia *Jonathan Stuart and Nicholas J. Johnson* 125
46	ECMO in the Emergency Department *David John Wallace and Nicolas A. Ulloa* 128
47	Be Ready to Discuss and Deliver End-of-Life Care in the Emergency Department *Ashley Shreves* 130

SECTION IV CARDIOLOGY
Book Editor: Mimi Lu
Associate Editors: William J. Brady and Joshua Easter

48. Beyond Chest Pain: Recognizing Acute Coronary Syndrome in Diverse Patient Populations   *Leigh-Ann J. Webb* 135
49. Don't Miss ACS in Older Adults   *M. Kathryn Mutter and Moira Smith* 137
50. Proceed With Caution! Diagnosing Anxiety in the Patient With Chest Pain   *J. Austin Lee and Paul I. Musey Jr* 139
51. Do Not Rely on a Single ECG to Evaluate Chest Pain in the ED in Patients With High Clinical Suspicion for Acute Coronary Syndrome   *William J. Brady* 141
52. Know the Differential for ST Segment Elevation: It's More Than Just Acute Coronary Syndrome   *Lloyd Tannenbaum and Brit Long* 144
53. Be Able to Recognize Lead Misplacement   *Summer Chavez* 148
54. Can You Diagnose Stemi in RBBB?   *William J. Brady* 151
55. High-Sensitivity Troponins—High Yield or High Risk   *Wesley Zeger and Andrew Barnett* 153
56. Do Not Forget the Non-ACS Causes of Chest Pain   *Jennifer McGowan and J. Jeremy Thomas* 155
57. Pitfalls in Adults With Congenital Heart Disease   *Sarah K. Wendel and William Woods* 158
58. Occlusion Myocardial Infarction: Time to Move Past the STEMI Paradigm   *Christopher Thom* 160
59. Is a Recent Stress Test Helpful in the ED Patient With Chest Pain?   *Jordan Warchol and Aaron Barksdale* 162
60. Know the Mimics of Ventricular Tachycardia   *Mitchell Weeman and J. Jeremy Thomas* 164
61. Management of Ventricular Storm   *Jakob Ottenhoff and Winston Wu* 167
62. In Pace of Emergency   *Moira Smith and M. Kathryn Mutter* 169
63. Management of Atrial Fibrillation: Rate Control Versus Rhythm Conversion   *Aaron R. Kuzel and J. Jeremy Thomas* 172
64. Mismanagement of Atrial Fibrillation in Wolff-Parkinson-White Syndrome   *Kellie A. Mitchell and William J. Brady* 174
65. Pitfalls in Hypertensive Emergencies   *Lauren M. Hunter and Aaron M. Blackshaw* 177

66	Chest Pain Plus ... Don't Miss Aortic Dissection *J. David Gatz*	180
67	Don't Overlook Atypical Risk Factors for ACS *Michael J. Yoo and Brit Long*	182
68	Be Aggressive With Nitroglycerin in Acute Cardiogenic Pulmonary Edema *Jakob Ottenhoff and Gustavo Carmen Lopez*	187
69	When Good VADs Go Bad *William J. Brady*	189
70	The Myocarditis Masquerade *Tennessee Park and Joshua Easter*	191
71	One Syncope Rule to Rule Them All? *Vanessa Khoury and Heather Lounsbury*	195

Section V Gastroenterology

Book Editor: Michael E. Winters
Associate Editors: Jennifer Repanshek

72	Can Appendicitis Be Treated With Antibiotics Alone? *Clare Roepke*	199
73	Don't Underestimate an Acute Variceal Hemorrhage! *Lee Plantmason*	201
74	High Risk: Acute Mesenteric Ischemia *Kalle J. Fjeld and Alison Marshall*	203
75	When Should You Image Patients With Acute Pancreatitis? *Kalle J. Fjeld and Alison Marshall*	205
76	When Should You Image Patients With Inflammatory Bowel Disease? *Jack Allan*	207
77	Can You Discharge That Patient With Acute Diverticulitis? *Ryan C. Gibbons*	209
78	Pitfalls in Esophageal Perforation *James Vandenberg*	212
79	What Are the Priorities in Patients With Acute Liver Failure? *Matthew L. Wong*	214
80	Know When to Administer Antibiotics for Severe Acute Pancreatitis *Alyssa Karl*	217
81	Acalculous Cholecystitis: No Stones, No Problems? *Clare Roepke*	219
82	Who Needs an Emergent EGD in the ED? *Jessica Moore*	221
83	Know How to Deal With the Displaced PEG Tube *Julie Y. Valenzuela and Rolando G. Valenzuela*	223
84	Biliary POCUS Pitfalls *Ryan C. Gibbons*	225

85	Ticking Time Bomb: The Gastric Bypass Patient With Abdominal Pain *Dillon Warr and Zachary Repanshek* 235
86	Don't Miss Aortoenteric Fistula: A Rare But Life-Threatening Cause of Gastrointestinal Bleeding! *Neena Kashyap and Zachary Repanshek* 238
87	Don't Miss the Patient With Perforated Peptic Ulcer *Katey S. Cohen and Zachary Repanshek* 240
88	Don't Be Fooled by a Subtle Presentation—SBP Can Be Deadly! *Alessandra Conforto* 243
89	Acute Cholangitis aka Biliary Sepsis *Prathap Sooriyakumaran* 245
90	Beware of the Patient With Painless Jaundice *Rolando G. Valenzuela and Andrés Guzmán* 247
91	Twist and Shout! The Patient With Volvulus *Kraftin E. Schreyer* 249
92	Don't Be Afraid to Order a CT on a Pregnant Patient If They Really Need It *Jennifer Repanshek* 251

SECTION VI CUTANEOUS
Book Editor: Michael E. Winters
Associate Editors: Heather Murphy-Lavoie

93	Is This Necrotizing Fasciitis? *Tracy Leigh LeGros* 255
94	Cutaneous Bullous Pemphigoid vs Pemphigus Vulgaris *Tracy Leigh LeGros* 258
95	Common Cellulitis Mimics *Shabana Walia* 261
96	Know When Should You Prescribe Antibiotics After I&D of an Abscess *Chance Anderson and Emily Rose* 263
97	Chickenpox or Mpox? How Do I Tell the Difference? *Emily Rose and Kristina van de Goor* 265
98	Don't Miss Systemic Illnesses That Present With Cutaneous Signs and Symptoms *Annalise Sorrentino* 267
99	Staphylococcal Toxic Shock Syndrome *Hurnan Vongsachang and Emily Rose* 270
100	Should You I&D That Abscess in the Patient With Hidradenitis? *Matthew Alan Demarest and Emily Rose* 272

SECTION VII ENDOCRINE/METABOLIC
Book Editor: Dale P. Woolridge
Associate Editors: George C. Willis

| 101 | A Normal Bicarbonate Value Does Not Exclude an Acid-Base Disturbance   *Emily Miller and George C. Willis* .... 275 |

102	Pitfalls in the Management of Adults with DKA *Anthony Roggio* 277
103	Do Not Rely on Orthostatic Vital Signs to Diagnose Volume Depletion *Mukund Mohan and Anand K. Swaminathan*............. 280
104	Hyperglycemic Hyperosmolar State: When High Sugar Gets You Down *Jaime Hope* 282
105	VBG Wizardry: The Down and Dirty on Interpreting the VBG *Joshua (Josh) Nichols and William F. Taber* 284
106	Bicarbonate Useless? Current Indications for the Use of Bicarbonate Therapy *Kimberly Boswell*....................................... 286
107	Pass the Steroids: Don't Miss Adrenal Insufficiency *William Caputo and Sarah Lee*.. 289
108	The Crashing Infant: Don't Miss Inborn Errors of Metabolism *Kyra Paticoff and Danielle Langan* 291
109	Fever and Altered Mental Status: Don't Forget Thyroid Storm *Shorok Hassan and Hallie Tiburzi* 293
110	Know How to Recognize and Treat Myxedema Coma *Kevin Molyneux and Chen He*.. 296
111	Know Causes of Ketoacidosis in the Patient Without Diabetes *Tyler Yates and Irina Aleshinskaya*.............................. 298
112	Pitfalls in Hyperkalemia *Steven Polevoi* 300
113	Pitfalls in the Management of Hyponatremia *Kelly-Ann Mungroo and Abbas Husain*... 304

SECTION VIII ENVIRONMENTAL
Book Editor: Sarah B. Dubbs
Associate Editors: Christopher G. Williams

114	Acclimatize, Descend, or Die! *Kevin Hanley* 307
115	Smoke Inhalation: Commonly Overtreated and Undertreated Aspects *Dennis Allin*... 310
116	Exercise-Associated Hyponatremia: Drinking Yourself to Death (With Water) *Emily Pearce*.. 312
117	A Deep Dive on Decompression Illness *Michael Tom*.................. 314
118	Dry Drowning Is Not a Thing, So Stop Blowing Smoke! *Justin Sempsrott* 317
119	Pitfalls in Heat Stroke Management *Christopher G. Williams*...... 319
120	When, How, and Why to Call Your Friendly Neighborhood Hyperbaric Doc *Michael Tom*... 322
121	Accidental Hypothermic Cardiac Arrest *Graham Brant-Zawadzki* 325

| 122 | Don't Be Bitten by the Bite *Nicholas B. Hurst* .... 327 |

SECTION IX HEAD, EARS, EYES, NOSE, AND THROAT (HEENT)
Book Editor: Mimi Lu
Associate Editors: Laura J. Bontempo

123	Recognizing Zoster Ophthalmicus and How to Treat It *Kelli Robinson* 331
124	Killer Sore Throats: Epiglottitis *Diane Rimple* 333
125	Consider a Deep Neck Space Infection in a Child With Fever and Neck Pain or Torticollis *Natalie J. Tedford* 335
126	Now Hear This: First Do No Harm When Treating Tympanic Membrane Perforation *John Herrick* 337
127	Know the Can't Miss Causes of a Red Eye *Gregory Jasani* 339
128	Eyeing the Causes of Acute Atraumatic Vision Loss *Gregory Gafni-Pappas* 342
129	Digging for Gold: Some Nuggets About Epistaxis *Shahrzad Woodbridge and Eric R. Swanson* 345
130	Properly Treating Dental Infections *Kinjal Sethuraman* 347
131	Fishing for Foreign Bodies *Eunhye (Grace) Kim and Molly K. Estes* 349
132	Don't Miss the Tracheoinnominate Fistula *Sierra Tackett and Sara Manning* 352
133	How to Successfully Replace a Dislodged Trach *Melissa Bacci* 354
134	Know How to Perform a Lateral Canthotomy With Cantholysis *Michael D. Sullivan and Cheyenne Falat* 356
135	Beware of the Post-Tonsillectomy Bleed *Lia C. Cruz and Joseph Cruz* 359
136	Expertly Manage Dental Trauma *Elizabeth Pontius* 361
137	POCUS Pearls for the Eye *Brianna Klucher and Samantha A. King* 364

SECTION X HEMATOLOGY/ONCOLOGY
Book Editor: Sarah B. Dubbs
Associate Editors: Molly K. Estes

| 138 | Thrombotic Thrombocytopenic Purpura and Hemolytic Uremic Syndrome: Bloody Zebras With a Bad Bite *Naillid Felipe* .... 367 |
| 139 | High Temps and Low Counts: Treat Patients With Febrile Neutropenia With Early and Appropriate Antibiotics *Matthew W. Connelly, Steven Roumpf, and Molly K. Estes* .... 370 |

140	My Chest! My Back! My Sickle Cell Attack! *Karly Lebherz and Salvador J. Suau* 372
141	Emergent Anticoagulant Reversal: A^2—Appropriately Aggressive *Keith Azevedo and Isaac Tawil* 375
142	Know How to Evaluate and Manage the CAR-T Patient *Monica Kathleen Wattana and Brian Cameron* 378
143	All Aboard! Don't Miss TRALI and TACO *Darcy James Mainville and Jessica Muñoz* 381
144	When Should You Transfuse Blood Products and Factors? *Nicholas Andrew and Matthew P. Borloz* 383
145	Know This Clinical Presentation of Leukemia in the Pediatric Patient *B. Barrie Bostick* 386

SECTION XI IMMUNOLOGY
Book Editor: Dale P. Woolridge
Associate Editors: Joshua Glasser

146	There Are *No* Absolute Contraindications for Epinephrine in Anaphylaxis *Joseph H. Ash and Robert Olympia* 391
147	Second-Line Medications in Anaphylaxis Are Just That—Second Line! *Lekha Bapu and Aalap Shah* 393
148	Avoid These Pitfalls in the Management of ACE-Inhibitor Angioedema *Aalap Shah and Joseph J. Moellman* 395
149	Know How to Identify Immune-Based Therapy Toxicities *David Locke and Catherine A. Marco* 399
150	Dazed and Confused: Immune-Mediated Encephalitides *Aesha Shah and Jessica Deitrick* 401
151	How Should You Evaluate Shortness of Breath in a Patient Post Lung Transplant? *Nathan J. Morrison and Jordan B. Schooler* 405
152	What Do You Need to Know About the Sick Liver Transplant Patient? *David Basile and Annahieta Kalantari* 407

SECTION XII INFECTIOUS DISEASE
Book Editor: Dale P. Woolridge
Associate Editors: Adedamola Ogunniyi

153	Don't Miss Acute Retroviral Syndrome *Sally Graglia* 411
154	Understand When and How to Initiate HIV Post-Exposure Prophylaxis in the Emergency Department *Philana H. Liang and Stephen Y. Liang* 413
155	Toxic Shock Syndrome: Do Not Hesitate—Resuscitate *Olena Kostyuk* 416

156	Meningitis Doesn't Have to Be a Pain in the Neck! *Nicholas Macaluso* 418
157	Avoid These Common Pitfalls in Influenza Treatment *Maryann Mazer-Amirshahi* 421
158	Treating Pneumonia in COPD *Diana Ladkany and Jeffrey Dubin* 423
159	Know When to Immunize for Mpox *Dan Im* 425
160	Diagnostic Delays in the Diagnosis of Osteomyelitis *Kenneth Lee* 427
161	Don't Forget These Conditions in the Febrile Traveler *Richard Diego Gonzales y Tucker and Nathan Jasperse* 429
162	Syphilis Is Back! Or Was It Ever Gone? *Elise Molnar* 432
163	By Land, by Sea, by Air: Know These Best-Practice Strategies to Prevent Infectious Spread *Lisa Bell* 436
164	Antibiotic Timing in Sepsis: What Really Matters? *Sean Denny* 438
165	Timely Source Control in Sepsis *John Stockton* 439

Section XIII Musculoskeletal (Nontrauma)
Book Editor: Michael E. Winters
Associate Editors: Priti Rawani-Patel

166	Ugh! Another Repeat Visit for Back Pain?! Keep Epidural Abscess on the Differential! *Aubrey Bethel and Haedan Doty* 443
167	Under Pressure: Rapidly Diagnosing and Treating Acute Compartment Syndrome of the Extremities *Darren Stapleton and Anna L. Waterbrook* 445
168	Don't Get Broken Up About Muscle Breakdown— Rhabdomyolysis *Amir Rombod Rahimian and Isaac J. Farrell* 447
169	When Back Pain Is an Emergency *James Bohan and Manzy Byrd* 450
170	What Works for MSK Low Back Pain? Steroids, Muscle Relaxers, Opioids? *Jonathan P. Coss and Priti Rawani-Patel* 452
171	Knee Pain? Don't Forget to Check the Hip! *Alexandra Barbosa* 454
172	Avoid These Pitfalls in the Diagnosis of Septic Joint *Delaney Fisher and Priti Rawani-Patel* 456
173	Don't Miss (Infectious) Flexor Tenosynovitis *Sam Kaplan and Nicola Baker* 458

SECTION XIV NEUROLOGY
Book Editor: Evie Marcolini
Associate Editors: Ramin Tabatabai and Ryan Raam

- **174** Diagnosing Cervical Artery Dissection in the ED: A Real Pain in the Neck! *Amir A. Rouhani, Kellie Kitamura, and Steven Lai* 461
- **175** Understand the Utility and Limitations of Diagnostic Imaging in Nontraumatic Subarachnoid Hemorrhage *Miguel Lemus* 464
- **176** Leave It Alone: Blood Pressure Measurement in Ischemic Stroke *Amir A. Rouhani, Steven Lai, and Kellie Kitamura* 466
- **177** Cerebral Venous Sinus Thrombosis: A Rare Diagnosis With a Common Chief Complaint *Steven Lai, Kellie Kitamura, and Amir A. Rouhani*.. 468
- **178** Blood Pressure in the Patient With Intracerebral Hemorrhage *Kellie Kitamura, Amir A. Rouhani, and Steven Lai* 471
- **179** How to Disposition the Patient With Suspected TIA *Patricia Fermin*.. 473
- **180** Know When to Use, and NOT to Use, the HINTS Examination *Laura Hemker Moles and Ryan Raam* 475
- **181** Stop Asking Your Patient What They Mean by "Dizzy" *Beza Abebe and Ryan Raam* 477
- **182** Know How to Properly Perform the Dix-Hallpike and Epley Maneuvers *Madeleine Heller and Mary Cheffers*......................... 480
- **183** Don't Underdose Your Antiseizure Medications *Farid K. Tadros and Caroline Brandon* 484
- **184** Know the Can't Miss Causes of Headache *Jorge Serrano and Ryan Raam* 487
- **185** Don't Miss the Myasthenic *Ashley Rebekah Allen and Anna Darby*... 490
- **186** What Do I Do With Wake-Up Stroke? *David Alexander Gregor and Michael Shamoon*............................. 492
- **187** It's Not All in My Head! Evaluation of the Patient With Suspected Psychogenic Nonepileptiform Seizures *Vian Zada and Ramin Tabatabai*... 495
- **188** Can't Miss Moves in the Patient With TBI *Chase Luther and Ryan Raam* 497

SECTION XV OBSTETRICS/GYNECOLOGY
Book Editor: Sarah B. Dubbs
Associate Editors: Joelle Borhart and Julie T. Vieth

- **189** Pitfalls in the Pursuit of Ovarian Torsion *Matthew C. DeLaney* .. 501

#		
190	Seizing Young Female? Think Eclampsia. Thinking Eclampsia? Think Again *Kenneth D. Marshall and Allyson M. Briggs*	503
191	Time's a Wastin': Perimortem Cesarean Delivery *Vivienne Ng*	505
192	Dyspnea in Pregnancy *Tina Godinho Rosenbaum and Nam Trinh*	507
193	Peripartum Cardiomyopathy Pearls *Glennette Castillo and Diana Ladkany*	509
194	Know These Postabortion Complications *Maria Magdalena Lawrynowicz and Jeffrey Uribe*	513
195	Evaluating the Pregnant Patient After a Motor Vehicle Crash *Kaytlin E. Hack and Jennifer Yu*	516
196	Do You Need to Do a Pelvic Exam in the ED Anymore? *Amanda L. Joy and Alex Y. Koo*	518
197	Caring for the Sexual Assault Survivor *Deanna Bridge Najera and Maryann Mazer-Amirshahi*	520
198	Hyperemesis Gravidarum *Lindsey DeGeorge and Kelly Lew*	523
199	Critical Considerations in Postmenopausal Bleeding *Sarah B. Dubbs and Mimi Lu*	526
200	Pitfalls in the Care of Patients Who Have Had IVF *Diana Ladkany and Hania Habeeb*	528
201	How Do I Evaluate a Breast Mass in the Emergency Department? *Janet Anne Smereck and Gavin K. Clark*	530
202	Errors in Ectopic Pregnancy Evaluation and Management *Supriya J. Davis and Kerri Layman*	533

Section XVI   Psychology

Book Editor: Evie Marcolini
Associate Editors: Daniel B. Gingold

#		
203	Differentiating Dementia Versus Delirium *Casey Carr and Megan Rivera*	537
204	Ask About Suicide Risk *Arsam Nadeem and Trent R. Malcolm*	540
205	Anxiety in the Emergency Department *Afrah A. Ali*	542
206	Substance Use Disorders in the Emergency Department *Laura Janneck and Derek Martinez*	545
207	Mastering Management of the Acutely Agitated Patient *Kyle Fischer and Rachel Wiltjer*	549
208	Droperidol Is BACK *Ashley N. Martinelli and Daniel B. Gingold*	551
209	Do Not Forget About Me: The Psych Boarder in Your ED *Kelli Robinson*	554

210	Do You Have the Capacity to Assess Capacity? *Bobbi-Jo Lowie and Christina Sajak*	556
211	Do You Really Need Those Labs for Medical Clearance? *Spencer Lovegrove and Gabriella Miller*	559

SECTION XVII GENITOURINARY
Book Editor: Sarah B. Dubbs
Associate Editors: Ryan Spangler

212	Caring for the Patient Who Has Had Gender Affirming Surgery *Matthew J. Grant*	563
213	Fournier Gangrene: A Lethal Infection You Can't Sit On! *Bobbi-Jo Lowie*	566
214	Testicular Torsion Trickery *Jeremy St. Thomas and Kathleen Stephanos*	568
215	Pyelonephritis: When It's Complicated Urine Trouble *Devang Patel and Drew Charles*	570
216	What Goes Up Must Come Down *Jessica Lange Osterman*	571
217	The Bleeding Dialysis Fistula *Christina Sajak*	573
218	What Are We Doing With Stones These Days? *Alvin Varghese and Ryan Spangler*	575
219	Don't Get Left Behind: New STI Treatment Guidelines *Bobbi-Jo Lowie and Matthew Poremba*	577
220	Pitfalls in Prostatitis *Meghin Moynihan and Ryan Spangler*	580
221	Chronic Catheters—Do I Treat That UA? *Arthur J. Pope and Chinezimuzo Ihenatu*	583

SECTION XVIII THORACIC
Book Editor: Sarah B. Dubbs
Associate Editors: Lillian Liang Emlet

222	Properly Risk Stratify the Patient With Suspected Pulmonary Embolism *Kelly Williamson*	585
223	Know the Management of Hemoptysis *Daniel Calick and Matthew P. Borloz*	588
224	Use High-Flow Nasal Cannula in Patients With Mild-to-Moderate Respiratory Distress From Hypoxemia *Matthew Welles and Neil K. Dasgupta*	591
225	Know Which Patients With Submassive Pulmonary Embolism May Benefit From Thrombolytic Therapy *Curtis Dickey and Joseph Schramski*	593
226	Know How to Manage Pneumomediastinum *Ani Aydin*	597

227	Does Magnesium Work in Acute Asthma Exacerbation? *Marina Boushra and Lauren Moore* 600
228	Be Careful With Fluids in Pulmonary Hypertension *Andrea Alvarado* 602
229	Know the Causes of Shortness of Breath—It's Not All in the Lungs *Chloe Renshaw* 605
230	Ventilator Management for the Boarded ED Patient *Erika Danelski and Nicholas Goodmanson* 608

SECTION XIX TOXICOLOGY
Book Editor: Dale P. Woolridge
Associate Editors: Vincent J. Calleo

231	Alcohol Intoxication and Withdrawal *Kevin Hanley and Kevin Rolnick* 611
232	Acetaminophen Toxicity: Getting Reacquainted With Matthew and Rumack *Peter Aiello and Vincent J. Calleo* 613
233	Toxic Alcohols *Sarah Mahonski* 616
234	Salicylate Poisoning: The Malicious Mimic *Robert W. Seabury* 618
235	Managing the Hot and Bothered: Sympathomimetic Overdoses *Arun Nair* 620
236	Emerging Substances of Use: What's Old Is New Again *Conor Young and Kayla Dueland-Kuhn* 623
237	Don't Forget Carbon Monoxide Toxicity in the Differential of HA *Joan Chou and Marvin Heyboer III* 625
238	Don't Forget Serotonin Toxicity in Your Patient With Agitation *Ahmed Alsakha and Christine M. Stork* 628
239	Be Sure to Ask About Herbal Remedies *Daniella Giardina and Jeanna M. Marraffa* 630
240	Dude, Don't Make These Marijuana Mistakes *Raizada Vaid and Michael Hodgman* 633
241	Know the Differences Between Calcium Channel and Beta-Blocker Overdoses *Curtis Geier and Kathy LeSaint* 636
242	Don't Stumble on the Dialyzable Toxins *Daniel Tirado and Vincent J. Calleo* 638
243	TCA Toxicities Still Happen *Rachel Gorodetsky* 640
244	Deadly in Small Doses *Timothy J. Bright and Vincent J. Calleo* 643
245	Know the Indications for High-Dose Insulin Therapy *Kayla Bourgeois and William Eggleston* 645
246	What's the Latest on Decontamination? *Michael Keenan* 647

Section XX Trauma
Book Editor: Evie Marcolini
Associate Editors: Patricia Ruth Atchinson

247	Managing Penetrating Neck Injuries: Hard or Soft, Superficial or Deep? *Melissa Joseph and Ryan F. Coughlin*	651
248	Save a Limb! Vascular Injury in Penetrating Extremity Trauma *Taylor McCormick and Kelly Stewart*	654
249	Judicious Abdominal Imaging in Trauma *Caroline W. Burmon and Erick A. Eiting*	656
250	When to Suspect Blunt Cerebrovascular Injury *Steven Straube and Ronald B. Tesoriero*	659
251	Closing the Book: Using a Bedsheet to Stabilize Pelvic Fractures *Michael Gottlieb and Stuart Swadron*	661
252	Spinal Immobilization or Spinal Motion Restriction: Which Is Better? *Joseph Palter*	664
253	The ABCs of Major Burns *Mary Cheffers, Ruben Guzman, and Stuart Swadron*	666
254	OR Versus IR, Where Should Your Trauma Patient Go? *Matthew Cravens and Colman Hatton*	669
255	Getting It Right in Globe Rupture *Amanda Correia*	672
256	Traumatic Cardiac Arrest *Matthew E. Anton and Matthew A. Roginski*	674
257	Know When to Drain a Pericardial Effusion in Trauma *Calixto Romero*	677
258	Anticoagulant and Antiplatelet Reversal in Trauma *Elizabeth Malik and Samantha Hunt*	679
259	Fluids, PRBCs, or Whole Blood for Trauma? *Alison Marshall and Kalle J. Fjeld*	681

Section XXI Orthopedics
Book Editor: Evie Marcolini
Associate Editors: Michael Abraham

260	Admit Displaced Supracondylar Fractures for Neurovascular Checks *Danielle Sutton*	685
261	Know the Difference Between Jones and Pseudo-Jones Fractures *Kaitlyn McBride and Andrew B. Moore*	688
262	Always Search for Other Injuries in Patients With Scapula Fracture *John W. Martel and Joseph M. Minichiello*	690
263	Don't Miss the Proximal Fibula Fracture in Patients With Ankle Fracture *Danielle Sutton*	692

264	Check for Snuffbox Tenderness and Don't Miss a Scaphoid Fracture *Danielle Sutton*	694
265	Calcaneal Fracture? Don't Miss a Spinal Injury! *Michael Abraham*	697
266	Beware of Benign-Appearing High-Pressure Injection Injuries *Andrew B. Moore and Emily Schaeffer*	698
267	Lisfranc Injury: Danger in the Midfoot *Brian L. Fuquay*	700
268	Tibial Plateau Fractures Can Be Subtle *Lauren E.R. Brady and Eric R. Friedman*	703
269	Can I Reduce the Shoulder Dislocation With a Fracture? *Justin Lackey and Ian J. Dempsey*	707
270	Leaving It All up to Chance *Tori Shank and Eric R. Friedman*	711

Section XXII Procedures/Skills

Book Editor: Sarah B. Dubbs
Associate Editors: J. David Gatz

271	Sedation Pearls and Pitfalls: Procedural Sedation in the Emergency Department *Benjamin Cornwell and J. David Gatz*	713
272	Arthrocentesis Tips *Benjamin Cornwell and J. David Gatz*	717
273	Lumbar Puncture and the Champagne Tap *Kevin Hanley*	719
274	Tapping the Belly: Paracentesis in the Emergency Department *Ryan Bierle and Brian Parker*	722
275	What Nerve! Ultrasound-Guided Regional Nerve Blocks *Casey Lee Wilson and Jon Halling*	724
276	A Needling Issue: Decompressing Tension Pneumothorax *Arun Nair*	727
277	Is Ultrasound Sufficient for Line Confirmation? *Samantha A. King and Brian Euerle*	729
278	Nasopharyngoscopy in the ED *Michael Billet*	731
279	Foley Catheter Follies *Arthur J. Pope and Chinezimuzo Ihenatu*	733
280	Mind the Pressure! Balloon Tamponade for UGIB *Aaron Alindogan and Brian Parker*	736
281	Pearls for Proper Splint Placements *Tianyu Tang and Steven Straube*	738
282	Chest Tube Placement in the Patients Who Are Obese *Neil A. Ray and Anthony J. Nastasi*	742
283	Pitfalls in US-Guided IV Placement *Kevin J. Flanagan and Sarah Sommerkamp*	745

284	Lifesaving Procedures in an Austere Environment *Anne Walker and Lisa Tenorio*	748
285	Shunt Tap: Tricks of the Trade *Riccardo Serro and Wan-Tsu W. Chang*	750
286	Tips and Tricks for the Bedside Hip Reduction in the Emergency Room *Nikita Paripati and Mei Ling Liu*	753

Section XXIII Pediatrics

Book Editor: Mimi Lu
Associate Editors: Heidi Werner

287	Recognize Child Abuse Early *Carol C. Chen*	757
288	Keep the Baby Warm! And Other Steps in Neonatal Resuscitation *Caroline Burke and Heidi Werner*	759
289	The Pediatric Airway: Learn It, Live It, Control It! *Alexandra Barbosa and Garrett S. Pacheco*	761
290	All That Barks Is Not Croup *Steven S. Bin*	764
291	Pediatric Procedural Sedation in the ED: Dealer's Choice *Jordan A. Justice*	766
292	Urinary Tract Infection in Young Children *Cornelia Latronica*	768
293	Beware Pediatric Appendicitis *Christyn Magill*	771
294	Diagnoses Not to Miss in the Acutely Limping Child *Gregory Hand and Guyon J. Hill*	774
295	Back Pain in Kids Is Never Normal *Rachel E. Tsolinas and Emily C. Z. Roben*	776
296	Kid ECGs Are Not Just Little Adult ECGs *Krista Young and Ian H. Law*	778
297	What's New in Managing Pediatric Diabetic Ketoacidosis *Hilary Ong and Mimi Lu*	781
298	Make PALS Your Pal *Rasheed Alhadi and Efrat Rosenthal*	783
299	Is Procalcitonin Helpful in Young Infants? *Monica Charpentier and Sima Patel*	786
300	The Hard Truth of Constipation—Don't Miss the Potentially Serious Causes of Constipation *Jennifer Guyther and Carmen Avendano*	789
301	Mishaps in Pediatric Myocarditis *Madeline Grade and Margaret Lin-Martore*	791
302	The Kitchen Sink—Pediatric Status Asthmaticus *Mahnoosh Nik-Ahd*	793

303	Overscanning the Pediatric Patient With Trauma *Jennifer Guyther and Mimi Lu* 796
304	Pediatric Status Epilepticus: Pearls and Pitfalls of Emergency Management *Lane Epps and Shruti Kant* 798
305	Easy Does It: Be Cautious With the Pediatric Patient With Cyanosis Who Has Undergone Cardiac Surgery *Christyn Magill* 801

Section XXIV Geriatrics

Book Editor: Mimi Lu
Associate Editors: Phillip D. Magidson

306	Do Not Underestimate the Potential Morbidity of Abdominal Pain in Older Adults *Christina L. Shenvi* 805
307	Rib, Hip, and Vertebral Compression Fractures *Sean Heavey and Katren Tyler* 807
308	The Geriatric Patient With Trauma Is Sicker Than You Realize *Sarah Beth Spiegel and Surriya Ahmad* 810
309	Respecting Thy Elders: Defining, Detecting, and Reporting of Geriatric Abuse *Alexander Zirulnik and Shan W. Liu* 812
310	Pain Medications and Procedural Sedation in Older Adults *Jessica Kuxhause and Lauren Cameron-Comasco* 815
311	Overdiagnosing and Overtreating UTIs in the Older Person *Robert Anderson* 817
312	Be Attentive to Inattention: Delirium Management Pearls in the ED *Brianna Klucher and Danya Khoujah* 819
313	Evaluating the Asymptomatic Patient With Dementia *Surriya Ahmad and Richard Sinert* 822
314	Defining Goals of Care in Your Geriatric ED Patient *Josephine Lo Bello and Balakrishna Vemula* 824
315	Know How to Cognitively Screen Your Geriatric Patient *Rachel M. Skains, Jin H. Han, and Richard E. Kennedy* 826
316	Safely Discharging Your Older Patient to Home *Kyle Burton and Cameron J. Gettel* 828
317	Perform Mobility Testing in Your Older Patient With a Ground Level Fall *Frederick R. Murphy Jr and Phillip D. Magidson* 830
318	Too Much of a Good Thing: Polypharmacy in Older Adults *Finnella Morgan and Jonathan Hansen* 832

Section XXV Wound Care
Book Editor: Sarah B. Dubbs
Associate Editors: Manpreet Singh

319 Sutures: What, When, Why, and Why Not? *Bobbi-Jo Lowie*........ 835
320 Pitfalls in Emergency Department Abscess Incision and Drainage *Annie Rominger* 837
321 Plantar Puncture Wound Pearls and Pitfalls *R. Gentry Wilkerson*.. 839
322 Do Not Believe the Adage That Epinephrine Cannot Be Used for Digital Blocks *Bennett A. Myers and Michael C. Bond* 842
323 When Are Prophylactic Antibiotics Indicated for Wounds? *Annie Rominger*.. 844
324 Eyelid Lacerations: When to Repair and When to Refer *Annie Rominger*.. 846
325 Ear Injuries and Lacerations *Sarah B. Dubbs*............................... 849
326 Just Under the Surface: Tendon and Nerve Injuries *Sarah B. Dubbs*.. 851
327 What Do I Do With Road Rash? *Joyce Wahba and Manpreet Singh* 853
328 What's New in the Care of Minor Burns *Aslam Abbasi Akhtar*.... 855
329 Do Not Miss a Foreign Body in a Wound *Tiffany Fan* 858
330 Fingernail Faux Pas *Sarah Zyzanski*.. 860
331 Scalp Wounds *Nicole Titze* 862

Section XXVI Covid-19
Book Editor: Dale P. Woolridge
Associate Editors: Stephen Y. Liang

332 Know the Varying Clinical Presentations of COVID-19 *Rawan Safa and Stephen Y. Liang*.. 865
333 Don't Miss MIS-C *M. Kaitlin Parks and Tara Copper*................ 867
334 In It for the Long Haul: Long COVID *Michael Kim and Stephen Y. Liang*.. 869
335 How Accurate Are the COVID-19 Tests *Addie Burtle*.................. 872
336 What Pharmacologic Management Matters in COVID-19 *Julianne Yeary and Stephen Y. Liang*.. 875
337 Mechanical Ventilation in the Patient With COVID-19 *Robert J. Stephens and Brian M. Fuller*.. 878

338	Beating the Beast: Evolution of COVID-19 Vaccines *Nicholas Maxwell and Stephen Y. Liang* 881
339	Complications and Myths in COVID-19 Vaccinations *Olena Kostyuk* 883

SECTION XXVII CLINICAL PRACTICE
Book Editor: Dale P. Woolridge
Associate Editors: Angela D. Smedley and Scott W. Rodi

340	Improving Patient Trust: Tips for Patient Satisfaction *Todd D. Morrell* 887
341	Your Patient Has Died: How to Deliver Bad News to Family Members *Heidi Maria Teague* 889
342	Discharge Documentation: Keep It Clear, Concise, Yet Complete *Albert Fiorello* 891
343	Advanced Practice Provider Supervision in the Emergency Setting *Melissa E. Zukowski and Andrew Belus* 893
344	What to Do With So Many? Strategies for Reducing Emergency Department Overcrowding *Jonathan Scott Lowry* 896
345	It's Not My Fault! Hospital Issues Leading to ED Boarding and How to Fix Them *Jonathan Scott Lowry* 898
346	Your Deposition *Kevin M. Klauer* 900
347	Say What? How to Maximize the Transfer of Care With Your EMS Providers *John Brown and Jeff Covitz* 902
348	I'm Out of Here! Pitfalls in the AMA Process *Christina Sajak* 904
349	I've Been Served! What Do I Do Now? *Christina Sajak and Gregory Jasani* 906
350	See No Evil: Mandatory Reporting Obligations *Gregory Jasani and Rachel Wiltjer* 908
351	Material Injury: Simple Steps to Preserve Forensic Evidence *Janet Carroll and Elizabeth Karagosian* 910
352	Caring for the Intimate Partner Violence Victim *Victoria J. Martin* 913
353	Identifying Victims of Human Trafficking *Janet Carroll and Elisha Paul DeKoning* 915
354	Pearls for the Safer Sign-Out *Brent King* 918
355	Collaborating With Difficult Consultants *Nikki Cali* 920
356	Caring for the Inpatient Boarder *Nicholas D. Poole and Jennifer V. Pope* 922

Section XXVIII Pain Management
Book Editor: Evie Marcolini
Associate Editors: R. Gentry Wilkerson

357	Ketamine for Procedural Sedation and Pain Management in the Emergency Department *R. Gentry Wilkerson*	925
358	Pitfalls in Ultrasound-Guided Nerve Blocks *Jose Acosta and Arun Nagdev*	928
359	Trama-Don't: Reasons to Avoid Using Tramadol *Jack McGeachy*	930
360	NSAIDs in Older Adults *Andrew K. Chang and Emma R. Furlano*	932
361	Dose Your Opioids Correctly *T. Andrew Windsor and Meghin Moynihan*	935
362	Awesome Analgesic Adjuncts *Adam Barnathan and Samuel Harris*	937
363	Time Matters! Effective Pain Management in Your Sickle Cell Patient *Annie Rominger*	940
364	Effective Strategies for the Treatment of Patients With Opioid Dependency *Kathy LeSaint and Curtis Geier*	942
365	Management of Acute Pain in Patients on Buprenorphine *R. Gentry Wilkerson*	945

Index 949

Abbreviations

4AT	4 As test	ACS-COT	American College of Surgeons Committee on Trauma
A4C	apical four chamber		
AAA	abdominal aortic aneurysm		
AAEM	American Academy of Emergency Medicine	AD	Alzheimer disease
		AD	aortic dissection
AAP	American Academy of Pediatrics	ADA	American Diabetes Association
		ADAPT	Accelerated Diagnostic Protocol for Chest Pain
AAST	American Association for the Surgery of Trauma	ADEM	acute disseminated encephalomyelitis
ABC	absolute band count		
ABC	airway, breathing, and circulation	ADH	alcohol dehydrogenase
		ADH	antidiuretic hormone
ABC	assessment of blood consumption	ADHF	acute decompensated heart failure
ABCD	airway, breathing, circulation, disability	ADL	activities of daily living
		ADP	adenosine diphosphate
ABEM	American Board of Emergency Medicine	AEF	aortoenteric fistula
		AEM	*Academic Emergency Medicine*
ABG	arterial blood gas	AER	annual event rates
ABI	ankle-brachial index	AES	American Epilepsy Society
ABP	acute bacterial prostatitis	AF	atrial fibrillation
AC	activated charcoal	AFE	amniotic fluid embolism
AC	assist/control	AG	anion gap
ACC	American College of Cardiology	AGE	arterial gas embolism
ACC	aorta cross-clamping	AGS	American Geriatrics Society
ACCP	anti-cyclic citrullinated peptide	AHA	American Heart Association
ACE	angiotensin-converting enzyme	AHA/ASA	American Heart Association and American Stroke Association
ACE2	angiotensin-converting enzyme 2	AHCA	accidental hypothermic cardiac arrest
ACE-II	angiotensin-converting enzyme II	AHL	anterior humeral line
ACE-inh	angiotensin-converting enzyme inhibitors	*aHUS*	atypical hemolytic uremic syndrome
ACEP	American College of Emergency Physicians	AIDS	acquired immunodeficiency syndrome
AChEI	acetylcholine esterase inhibitor	AIN	anterior interosseous nerve
ACL	anterior collateral ligament	AIR	Appendicitis Inflammatory Response score
ACLE	acute cutaneous lupus erythematosus	AIS	acute ischemic stroke
ACLS	advanced cardiac life support	AIVR	accelerated idioventricular rhythm
ACOG	American College of Obstetricians and Gynecologists	AKI	acute kidney injury
ACS	acute coronary syndrome		

AL	anterolateral	ATACH-2	Antihypertensive Treatment of Acute Cerebral Hemorrhage 2
ALDH	aldehyde dehydrogenase		
ALF	acute liver failure	ATLS	advanced trauma life support
ALI	acute lung injury	ATP	adenosine triphosphate
ALOC	altered level of consciousness	AV	atrioventricular
ALS	advanced life support	AVAPS	average volume-assured pressure support
ALT	alanine transaminase		
AMA	against medical advice	AVB	atrioventricular block
AMA	American Medical Association	AVH	acute variceal hemorrhage
AMI	acute mesenteric ischemia	AVOID Study	Air Verses Oxygen In myocarDial infarction study
AMI	acute myocardial infarction		
AMP	adenosine monophosphate	AVP	arginine vasopressin
AMPA	alpha-amino-3-hydroxy-5-methyl-4-isoxazolepropionic acid receptor	AVRT	atrioventricular reentrant tachycardia
		AVS	acute vestibular syndrome
AMS	altered mental status	AWS	alcohol withdrawal syndrome
AMT	Abbreviated Mental Test	AXR	abdominal x-ray
AMT-4	Abbreviated Mental Test	BAS	Brief Alzheimer Screen
ANA	antinuclear antibody	BASE	Brief Abuse Screen for the Elderly
ANC	absolute neutrophil count		
Anti-TNF	antitumor necrosis factor	BASICS	Balanced Solutions in Intensive Care Study
ANUG	acute necrotizing ulcerative gingivitis		
		BATiC	blunt abdominal trauma in children
AP	acute pancreatitis		
AP	anteroposterior	BB	beta-blocker
APAP	acetaminophen	BBB	bundle branch block
aPCC	activated prothrombin complex concentrate	bCAM	Brief Confusion Assessment Method
APHL	Association of Public Health Laboratories	BCVI	blunt cerebrovascular injury
		BER	benign early repolarization
API	arterial pressure index	beta-HCG	beta-human chorionic gonadotropin
APP	advanced practice provider		
APRV	airway pressure release ventilation	BID	twice daily
		BiPAP	bilevel positive airway pressure
ARB	angiotensin receptor blocker	BiVAD	biventricular assist device
ARDS	acute respiratory distress syndrome	BMI	body mass index
		BMP	basic metabolic panel
ARF	acute renal failure	BNP	brain natriuretic peptide
ARN	acute retinal necrosis	BNP	B-type natriuretic peptide
ARS	acute retroviral syndrome	BOX trial	Blood Pressure and Oxygenation Targets in Postresuscitation Care trial
ART	assisted reproductive technology		
ASA	acetylsalicylic acid		
ASA	American Society of Anesthesiologists	BP	blood pressure
		bpm	beats per minute
ASA	American Stroke Association	BPPV	benign paroxysmal positional vertigo
ASAP	as soon as possible		
ASD	acute stress disorder	BTD	balloon tamponade device
ASH	American Society of Hematology	BTF	Brain Trauma Foundation
		BUC	buccal
ASM	antiseizure medication	BUN	blood urea nitrogen
AST	aspartate transaminase	BVM	bag valve mask

B-W	Burch-Wartofsky	CK	creatine kinase
BZ	benzodiazepine	CKD	chronic kidney disease
CA-ASB	catheter-associated asymptomatic bacteriuria	CLABSI	central-line associated bloodstream infections
CAB	circulation, airway, breathing	CLE	cutaneous lupus erythematosus
CAD	cervical artery dissection	CLOVERS trial	Crystalloid Liberal or Vasopressors Early Resuscitation in Sepsis trial
CAD	coronary artery disease		
CAG	coronary angiography		
CAM	Confusion Assessment Method	CMP	complete metabolic panel
CAPD	Cornell Assessment for Pediatric Delirium	CMP	comprehensive metabolic panel
CAR-T	chimeric antigen receptor T cell	CMS	Centers for Medicare and Medicaid Services
CAS	Clinical Anxiety Scale		
CAUTIs	catheter-associated urinary tract infections	CMV	cytomegalovirus
		CN	cranial nerve
CBC	complete blood count	CNS	central nervous system
CBD	cannabidiol	CO	carbon monoxide
CBD	common bile duct	CO	cardiac output
CBP	chronic bacterial prostatitis	COHb	carboxyhemoglobin
CBT	cognitive-based therapy	COMACARE trial	Carbon dioxide, Oxygen and Mean arterial pressure After Cardiac Arrest and Resuscitation trial
CCB	calcium channel blocker		
CCF	chest compression fraction		
CCTA	coronary computed tomography angiography		
		COPD	chronic obstructive pulmonary disease
CD	Crohn disease		
CDC	Centers for Disease Control and Prevention	COVID	coronavirus disease
		COWS	Clinical Opiate Withdrawal Scale
CDT	catheter-directed therapy		
CDT	catheter-directed thrombolysis	COX	cyclooxygenase
CES	cauda equina syndrome	CP	chest pain
CF	cystic fibrosis	CP/CPPS	chronic prostatitis/chronic pelvic pain syndrome
CHA2DS2-VASc	CHADS plus vascular disease, age 65-74, sex (ie, female)		
		CPAP	continuous positive airway pressure
CHADS2	congestive heart failure, hypertension, age >75, diabetes, prior stroke		
		CPC	Cerebral Performance Category score
CHD	congenital heart disease		
CHEST	American College of Chest Physicians	CPP	cerebral perfusion pressure
		CPP	coronary perfusion pressure
CHF	congestive heart failure	CPR	cardiopulmonary resuscitation
CHS	cannabinoid hyperemesis syndrome	CPS	Child Protective Service
		CRAO	central retinal artery occlusion
CI	cognitive impairment	CRASH-2	Clinical Randomization of an Antifibrinolytic in Significant Hemorrhage 2
CICO	can't intubate, can't oxygenate		
CIWA	Clinical Institute Withdrawal Assessment		
		CRE	carbapenem-resistant Enterobacteriaceae
CIWA	Clinical Institute Withdrawal Assessment for Alcohol		
		CRP	C-reactive protein
CIWA-Ar	Clinical Institute Withdrawal Assessment for Alcohol-Revised	CRRT	continuous renal replacement therapy
		CRS	cytokine release syndrome

CSF	cerebrospinal fluid	DKA	diabetic ketoacidosis
CSRS	Canadian Syncope Risk Score	DL	direct laryngoscopy
C-SSRS	Columbia Suicide Severity Rating Scale	DM	diabetes mellitus
		DNS	delayed neurologic sequelae
CT	computed tomography	DOAC	direct oral anticoagulant
CTA	computed tomography angiography	DOACs	direct-acting oral anticoagulants
		DOREMI	dobutamine compared with milrinone
CTV	computed tomographic venography	DRE	digital rectal examination
		DRESS	drug reaction with eosinophilia and systemic symptom
CV	cardiovascular		
CVA	cardiovascular accident	DSA	digital subtraction angiography
CVA	costovertebral angle	dsDNA	double-stranded deoxyribonucleic antibodies
CVC	central venous catheter		
CVD	cardiovascular disease	DSED	double sequential external defibrillation
CVP	central venous pressure		
CVST	cavernous sinus thrombosis	DSI	delayed sequence intubation
CVST	cerebral venous sinus thrombosis	DTI	direct thrombin inhibitors
		DTs	delirium tremens
CVT	cerebral vascular thrombosis	DTS	Delirium Triage Screen
CVT	cerebral venous thrombosis	DVT	deep vein thrombosis
CVVH	continuous veno-venous hemofiltration	DVT	deep venous thrombosis
		DWI	diffusion-weighted imaging
CWI	cold water immersion	EAH	exercise-associated hyponatremia
CXR	chest radiography		
CXR	chest x-ray	EASI	Elder Abuse Suspicion Index
D&E	dilation and evacuation	EAST	Eastern Association for the Surgery of Trauma
DAN	Divers Alert Network		
DAWN	DWI or CTP Assessment with Clinical Mismatch in the Triage of Wake-Up and Late Presenting Strokes Undergoing Neurointervention with Trevo	EBV	Epstein-Barr virus
		ECASS	European Cooperative Acute Stroke Study
		ECG	electrocardiogram
		ECG	electrocardiography
DBP	diastolic blood pressure	Echo	echocardiography
DBZD	designer benzodiazepine	ECLS	extracorporeal life support
DC	direct current	ECMO	extracorporeal membrane oxygenation
DCI	decompression illness		
DCS	decompression sickness	ECPR	extracorporeal cardiopulmonary resuscitation
DDAVP	desmopressin acetate		
DEA	Drug Enforcement Administration	ECTR	extracorporeal treatments
		ED Senior AID	ED Senior Abuse Identification
DEET	diethyltoluamide		
DEFUSE	Endovascular Therapy Following Imaging Evaluation for Ischemic Stroke	ED	emergency department
		EDACS	Emergency Department Assessment of Chest Pain Score
DF	disoproxil fumarate		
DI	distensibility index	EDT	emergency department thoracotomy
DIC	disseminated intravascular coagulation		
		EEG	electroencephalogram
DIHS	drug-induced hypersensitivity symptom	EF	ejection fraction
		EGD	esophagogastroduodenoscopy
DIP	distal-interphalangeal		

EJ	external jugular	FICB	fascia iliaca compartment block
EKG	electrocardiogram	FIO_2	fraction of inspired oxygen
ELISA	enzyme-linked immunosorbent assay	FLAIR	fluid-attenuated inversion recovery
ELM	external laryngeal manipulation	FM	facemask
ELSO	Extracorporeal Life Support Organization	FNA	fine-needle aspiration
		FNB	femoral nerve block
EM	emergency medicine	FNP	family nurse practitioners
EMPs	emergency medicine providers	FOOSH	fall on an outstretched hand
EMRs	electronic medical records	FRC	functional residual capacity
EMS	emergency medical service	FT	finger thoracostomy
EMT	Emergency Medical Technician	FTA-ABS	fluorescent treponemal antibody absorption
EN	erythema nodosum		
ENT	ear, nose, and throat	GABA	gamma aminobutyric acid
ENT	otolaryngology	GAD	generalized anxiety disorder
EOL	end of life	GAS	gender-affirming surgeries
EP	emergency physician	GBS	Guillain-Barré syndrome
EP	emergency provider	GCA	giant cell arteritis
EPAP	expiratory positive airway pressure	GCS	Glasgow Coma Scale
		GCSE	generalized convulsive status epilepticus
Epi	epinephrine		
EPS	extrapyramidal side effects	GDMT	goal-directed medical therapies
ERCP	endoscopic retrograde cholangiopancreatography	GEAR	Geriatric Emergency care Applied Research
ESBL	extended-spectrum beta-lactamase	GFR	glomerular filtration rate
		GGT	Gamma-glutamyl transferase
ESC	European Society of Cardiology	GI	gastrointestinal
ESETT	Established Status Epilepticus Treatment Trial	GIB	gastrointestinal bleeding
		GJ	Gastrojejunal
ESI	Emergency Severity Index	GLF	ground-level fall
ESR	erythrocyte sedimentation rate	GPC	gram-positive cocci
ESRD	end-stage renal disease	GRACE	Guideline for Recurrent Low-Risk Chest Pain
ET	endotracheal		
ETCO$_2$	end-tidal carbon dioxide	GSW	gunshot wound
ETI	endotracheal intubation	gtt	continuous infusion
ETOH	ethanol	GU	genitourinary
ETT	endotracheal tube	GYN	gynecology
EUA	Emergency Use Authorization	HA	headache
EUS	endoscopic ultrasound	HACA	hypothermia after cardiac arrest
EVS	episodic vestibular syndrome	HADS-A	Hospital Anxiety Depression Scale-Anxiety
EVT	endovascular thrombectomy		
FAST	focused assessment with sonography in trauma	HAE	hereditary angioedema
		HAPE	high-altitude pulmonary edema
FBA	foreign body aspiration	HAV	hepatitis A virus
FBs	foreign bodies	HBO	hyperbaric oxygen
FDA	Food and Drug Administration	HBOT	hyperbaric oxygen therapy
FEIBA	factor eight inhibitor bypassing activity	HbS	sickle hemoglobin
		HBV	hepatitis B virus
FFP	fresh frozen plasma	HC	hydrocephalus
FFS	facial feminization surgery	hCG	human chorionic gonadotropin
FG	Fournier gangrene	HDI	high-dose insulin

HDN	high-dose nitroglycerin	ICAD	internal carotid artery dissection
HEART	history, electrocardiogram, age, risk factors, and troponin	ICANS	immune effector cell-associated neurotoxicity syndrome
HELLP	hemolysis with a microangiopathic blood smear, elevated liver enzymes, and a low platelet count	ICD	implantable cardioverter defibrillator
		ICE	immune effector cell-associated encephalopathy
HF	heart failure	ICH	intracerebral hemorrhage
HF	hydrofluoric	ICP	intracerebral pressure
HFNC	high-flow nasal cannula	ICP	intracranial pressure
HFNO	high-flow nasal oxygen	ICS	intercostal space
HG	hyperemesis gravidarum	ICU	intensive care unit
HHS	hyperglycemic hyperosmolar state	ID	infectious disease
		IDDM	insulin-dependent diabetes mellitus
HIEs	health information exchanges		
HIET	high-dose insulin-euglycemia therapy	IDSA	Infectious Disease Society of America
HI-MAP	Heart, IVC-Morison pouch, Aorta, Pulmonary	IEM	inborn errors of metabolism
		IFE	intravenous fat emulsion
HINTS	Head Impulse, Nystagmus, Test of Skew	IgG	immunoglobulin G
		IgM	immunoglobulin M
HIT	heparin-induced thrombocytopenia	IHD	intermittent hemodialysis
		IJ	internal jugular
HIV	human immunodeficiency virus	IL-6	interleukin 6
hpf	high-power field	ILCOR	International Liaison Committee on Resuscitation
HPV	human papillomavirus		
HQ-CPR	high-quality cardiopulmonary resuscitation	ILD	interstitial lung disease
		IM	intramuscular
HR	heart rate	IMC	Intermediate Care Unit
HS	heart stroke	IMV	invasive mechanical ventilation
HS	hidradenitis suppurativa	IN	intranasal
hs-Tn	high-sensitivity troponins	iNO	inhaled nitric oxide
hsTrop	high-sensitivity troponin	iNPH	idiopathic normal pressure hydrocephalus
HSV	herpes simplex virus		
HT	human trafficking	INR	international normalized ratio
HTN	hypertension	INTERACT2	Intensive Blood Pressure Reduction in Acute Cerebral Hemorrhage Trial
HTS	hypertonic saline		
HUS	hemolytic uremic syndrome		
HZO	herpes zoster ophthalmicus	IO	intraosseous
I STUMBLED/NH	isopropyl alcohol; salicylates; theophylline, tenormin (atenolol); uremia, methanol, metformin; barbiturates; lithium; ethylene glycol; dabigatran, depakote	IOP	intraocular pressure
		IPAP	inspiratory positive airway pressure
		IPV	intimate partner violence
		IR	interventional radiology
		ISAR	Identification of Seniors At Risk
		ITP	intrathoracic pressure
I&D	incision and drainage	IUD	intrauterine device
I:E	inspiration-to-expiration	IUP	intrauterine pregnancy
IABP	intra-aortic balloon pumps	IV	intravenous
IBD	inflammatory bowel disease	IVC	inferior vena cava
IBW	ideal body weight	IVFs	intravenous fluids

IVH	in vitro fertilization	LWOT	left without treatment
IVIG	intravenous immunoglobulin	mAb	monoclonal antibodies
IVS	intercostal space	MAC	Macintosh
JAK	Janus kinase	MACE	major adverse cardiac event
JJ	jejunojejunal	MAD	mucosal atomization device
JVD	jugular venous distention	MAHA	microangiopathic hemolytic anemia
KOR	kappa-opioid receptor		
KUB	kidney, ureter, and bladder	MAKE30	major adverse kidney events in 30 days
LA	left arm		
LAST	local anesthetic systemic toxicity	MAP	mean airway pressure
LBBB	left bundle branch block	MAP	mean arterial pressure
LCP	Leg-Calvé-Perthes	MASH	Movement, Air Entry, Symmetry, Heard breath sounds
LD	loop drainage		
LDH	lactate dehydrogenase	MAT	medical-assisted therapy
LE	leukocyte esterase	MC	myxedema coma
LE	lower extremity	MC	myxedema crisis
LE	lupus erythematosus	MCP	metacarpophalangeal
LES	lower esophageal sphincter	MCS	mechanical circulatory support
LET	lidocaine-epinephrine-tetracaine	MDMA	3,4-methylenedioxymethamphetamine
LFT	liver function test		
LIJ	left internal jugular	MDRO	multidrug resistant organism
LKWT	last known well time	MET	medical expulsive therapy
LL	left leg	MG	myasthenia gravis
LMA	laryngeal mask airway	MI	myocardial infarction
LMWH	low-molecular-weight heparin	MIP	maximal inspiratory pressure
LNT	Linton-Nachlas tube	MIS	multisystem inflammatory syndrome
LOD	limit of detection		
LOV-ED	Lung-Protective Ventilation Initiated in the Emergency Department	MIS-A	multisystem inflammatory syndrome in adult
		MIS-C	multisystem inflammatory syndrome in children
LP	lumbar puncture		
LPM	liters per minute	MMSE	Mini-Mental State Examination
LPS	lipopolysaccharide	MOA	mechanism of action
LPV	lung-protective ventilation	MOR	mu-opioid receptor
LR	lactated Ringer	MPHR	maximum predicted heart rate
LR	likelihood ratio	MPI	myocardial perfusion imaging
LRINEC	Laboratory Risk Indicator for Necrotizing Fasciitis	MR	magnetic resonance
		MRA	magnetic resonance angiography
LRMs	lung recruitment maneuvers		
LSD	lysergic acid diethylamide	MRCP	magnetic resonance cholangiopancreatography
LT	lactated Ringer		
LUQ	left upper quadrant	MRI	magnetic resonance imaging
LV	left ventricle	MRN	medical record number
LV	left ventricular	mRNA	messenger RNA
LVAD	left ventricular assist device	mRS	modified Rankin scale
LVEDV	left ventricular end-diastolic volume	MRSA	methicillin-resistant *Staphylococcus aureus*
LVEF	left ventricular ejection fraction	mRSI	modified rapid sequence intubation
LVH	left ventricular hypertrophy		
LVO	large vessel occlusion	MRV	magnetic resonance venography
LVOT	left ventricular outflow tract	MSK	musculoskeletal

MSM	men who have sex with men	NPA	nasopharyngeal airways
MSSA	methicillin-susceptible *Staphylococcus aureus*	nPEPE	nonoccupational postexposure prophylaxis
MSUD	maple syrup urine disease	NPO	no prior preparation
MT	massive transfusion	NPO	nothing by mouth
mTOR	mammalian target of rapamycin	NPPV	noninvasive positive pressure ventilation
MV	mechanical ventilation		
MV	minute ventilation	NPV	negative predictive value
MVCs	motor vehicle crashes	NRB	non-rebreather
	N$_2$O nitrous oxide	NS	normal saline
NAAT	nucleic acid amplification test	NSAID	nonsteroidal anti-inflammatory drug
NAC	*N*-acetylcysteine		
NAD	nicotinamide adenine dinucleotide	NSTE	non–ST-segment elevation
		NSTEMI	non–ST-segment elevation myocardial infarction
NADH	reduced form of NAD+		
NAEMSP	National Associated of Emergency Medical Services Physicians	NSTI	necrotizing soft tissue infection
		NT	needle thoracostomy
NAPQI	*N*-acetyl-*p*-benzoquinone imine	NT-proBNP	N-terminal pro-brain natriuretic peptide
NASPGHAN	North American Society of Pediatric Gastroenterology, Hepatology and Nutrition	O3DY	Ottawa 3DY
		OB/GYN	obstetrician/gynecologist
		OCP	oral contraceptive pill
NAT	non-accidental trauma	OCS	ocular compartment syndrome
NC	nasal cannula	ODS	osmotic demyelination syndrome
NCCTH	noncontrast computed tomography of the head		
		OH	orthostatic hypotension
NEDOCS	National Emergency Department Overcrowding Study	OHCA	out-of-hospital cardiac arrest
		OHSS	ovarian hyperstimulation syndrome
NF	necrotizing fasciitis		
NGL	nasogastric lavage	OIs	opportunistic infections
NIAID/FAAN	National Institute of Allergy and Infectious Diseases/Food Allergy and Anaphylaxis Network	OM	otitis media
		OMI	occlusion myocardial infarction
		OPA	oropharyngeal airway
		OR	odds ratio
NICU	Neonatal Intensive Care Unit	OR	operating room
NIF	negative inspiratory force	OT	occupational therapy
NIH	National Institutes of Health	OUD	opioid use disorder
NIPPV	noninvasive positive pressure ventilation	PA	physical assistant
		PA	posterior-anterior
NIV	noninvasive ventilation	PAH	pulmonary arterial hypertension
NMB	neuromuscular blocking		
NMDA	*N*-methyl-D-aspartate	PALabS	Pediatric Appendicitis Laboratory Score
NMS	neuroleptic malignant syndrome		
		PALS	pediatric advanced life support
NOMI	non-occlusion myocardial infarction		
		pARC	Pediatric Appendicitis Risk Calculator
NOTR	no objective testing rule		
NP	nurse practitioner	PAS	Pediatric Appendicitis Score
		PAT	pediatric assessment triangle

PATCH	Platelet transfusion versus standard care after acute stroke due to spontaneous cerebral hemorrhage associated with antiplatelet therapy	PIOPED	Prospective Investigation of Pulmonary Embolism Diagnosis
PAWSS	Prediction of Alcohol Withdrawal Severity Scale	PIP	peak inspiratory pressure
		PIP	proximal interphalangeal
PBC	primary biliary cholangitis	PIV	peripheral intravenous
PBW	predicted body weight	PLASMIC	*p*latelet count, *h*emolysis markers (LDH, bilirubin), *a*bsolute reticulocyte count, *s*erum creatinine, *m*arkers of organ involvement, *i*nternational normalized ratio, and *c*omplement levels
pCAM	Pediatric Confusion Assessment Method		
PCC	prothrombin complex concentrates		
PCI	percutaneous coronary intervention	PLUS	Plasma-Lyte 148 versus Saline
		PLWD	persons living with dementia
PCL	posterior collateral ligament	PMCD	perimortem cesarean delivery
PCP	phencyclidine	PML	progressive multifocal leukoencephalopathy
PCP	potent compound phencyclidine		
PCP	primary care provider	PMN	polymorphonuclear leukocytes
PCR	polymerase chain reaction	PNES	psychogenic nonepileptiform seizures
PCT	procalcitonin		
PD	panic disorder	PNI	penetrating neck injury
PDE	phosphodiesterase	PNP	pediatric nurse practitioners
PDP	push-dose pressors	PNS	peripheral nervous system
PE	phenytoin sodium equivalents	PO	by mouth
PE	pulmonary embolism	PO	orally
PEA	pulseless electrical activity	POC	point-of-care
PECARN	Pediatric Emergency Care Applied Research Network	POCUS	point-of-care ultrasound
		POCUS	point-of-care ultrasonography
PEEP	positive end expiratory pressure	POLST	Physician Orders for Life-Sustaining Treatment
PEG	percutaneous endoscopic gastrostomy	PORN	progressive outer retinal necrosis
PEG	polyethylene glycol	PPAs	parapharyngeal abscesses
PEP	postexposure prophylaxis	PPCM	peripartum cardiomyopathy
PERC	pulmonary embolism rule-out criteria	PPD	purified protein derivative
		PPE	personal protective equipment
PESI	Pulmonary Embolism Severity Index	PPI	proton pump inhibitor
		Pplat	plateau pressure
PET	positron emission tomography	PPV	positive predictive value
PET-CT	positron emission tomography-computed tomography	PPV	positive pressure ventilation
		PR	per rectum
PF4	platelet factor 4	PRBC	packed red blood cell
PH	pulmonary hypertension	PrEP	preexposure prophylaxis
PICA	post (or peri)-intubation cardiac arrest	PRIS	propofol-related infusion syndrome
PICU	pediatric intensive care unit	PRN	as needed
PID	pelvic inflammatory disease	PROPPR	The Pragmatic, Randomized Optimal Platelet and Plasma Ratios trial
PIMs	potentially inappropriate medications		

PRVC	pressure-regulated volume control	ROSC	return of spontaneous circulation
PS	pressure support	ROX	ratio of oxygen saturation
PSC	primary sclerosing cholangitis	RPAs	retropharyngeal abscesses
PSL	parasternal long	RPOC	retained products of conception
PSS	parasternal short	RPR	rapid plasma regain
PSV	pressure support ventilation	RR	respiratory rate
PSVT	paroxysmal supraventricular tachycardia	RRT	renal replacement therapy
PT	physical therapy	RSI	rapid sequence intubation
PT	prothrombin time	RSV	respiratory syncytial virus
PT/INR	prothrombin time/international normalized ratio	RT	resuscitative thoracotomy
PT/PTT	prothrombin time and partial thromboplastin time	RT-PCR	reverse transcription-polymerase chain reaction
PTC	percutaneous transhepatic cholangiography	RUE	right upper extremity
		RUQ	right upper quadrant
PTH	parathyroid hormone	RUSH	Rapid Ultrasound for Shock and Hypotension
PTSD	posttraumatic stress disorder	RV	right ventricle
PTT	activated partial thromboplastin time	RVAD	right ventricular assist device
		RVR	rapid ventricular rate
PTX	pneumothorax	RWMA	regional wall motion abnormalities
PUD	peptic ulcer disease		
pUF	peritoneal ultrafiltration	RYGB	Roux-en-Y gastric bypass
PUL	pregnancy of unknown location	SA	sinoatrial
		SAFE	sexual assault forensic examination
PVC	premature ventricular contractions	SAFE	sexual assault forensic examiner
PVR	pulmonary vascular resistance	SAFE-T	Suicide Assessment Five-Step Evaluation and Triage
QTc	corrected QT interval		
RA	rheumatoid arthritis	SAH	subarachnoid hemorrhage
RA	right arm	SALAD	Suction Assisted Laryngoscopy and Airway Decontamination
RA	right atrial		
RAFT	Rapid Appraisal for Trafficking	SALT-ED	Saline Against Lactated Ringer's or Plasma-Lyte in the Emergency Department
RASS	Richmond Agitation Sedation Scale		
		SANE	Sexual Assault Nurse Examiner
RAT	rapid antigen testing	SAPB	serratus anterior plane block
RBBB	right bundle branch block	SARS	severe acute respiratory syndrome
RBC	red blood cell		
RCA	right coronary artery	SBI	serious bacterial infection
RCT	randomized controlled trial	SBP	spontaneous bacterial peritonitis
REBOA	resuscitative endovascular balloon occlusion of the aorta	SBP	systolic blood pressure
		SBT	Sengstaken-Blakemore tube
RF	rheumatoid factor	SBT	Short Blessed Test
RIJ	right internal jugular	SCA	sudden cardiac arrest
RL	right leg	SCAPE	sympathetic crashing acute pulmonary edema
RNS	reactive nitrogen species		
RNs	registered nurses	SCD	sickle cell disease
ROS	reactive oxygen species	SCFE	slipped capital femoral epiphysis
ROS	review of systems		

SCOT	succinyl-CoA: 3-ketoacid CoA transferase	SSRI	selective serotonin reuptake inhibitor
SCRAs	synthetic cannabinoid receptor agonists	SSTIs	skin and soft tissue infections
		ST	serotonin toxicity
SCUF	Slow continuous ultrafiltration	START	screening tool to alert doctors to the right treatment
SDD	selective digestive decontamination	STDs	sexually transmitted diseases
SEA	spinal epidural abscess	STE	ST elevation
SEP-1	severe sepsis and septic shock early management bundle	STEADI	Stopping Elderly Accidents, Deaths & Injuries
SFSR	San Francisco Syncope rule	STEC	Shiga toxin-producing *Escherichia coli*
SGA	supraglottic airway		
SGLT2	sodium-glucose transport protein 2	STEMI	ST-segment elevation myocardial infarction
SHoC	Sonography in Hypotension and Cardiac	STI	sexually transmitted infections
SI	shock index	STOPP	Screening Tool of Older Persons Prescriptions
SIADH	syndrome of inappropriate antidiuretic hormone secretion	STSE	ST-segment elevation
SIMV	synchronized intermittent mandatory ventilation	STSS	Staphylococcal toxic shock syndrome
SIRS	systemic inflammatory response syndrome	SV	stroke volume
		SVC	superior vena cava
SIS	six-item screener	SVR	systemic vascular resistance
SJS/TEN	Stevens-Johnson syndrome/ toxic epidermal necrolysis	SVT	supraventricular tachycardia
		T2DM	type 2 diabetes, also known as non–insulin-dependent diabetes
SLE	systemic lupus erythematosus		
SLED	sustained low-efficiency dialysis		
		TACO	transfusion-associated circulatory overload
SMA	superior mesenteric artery		
SMART	Isotonic Solutions and Major Adverse Renal Events trial	TAD	thoracic aortic dissection
		TAPSE	tricuspid annular plane systolic excursion
SNAC	scaphoid nonunion advanced collapse		
		TAPSE: PASP	tricuspid annular plane systolic excursion:pulmonary artery systolic pressure
SNRIs	serotonin/norepinephrine reuptake inhibitors		
SOAP	sepsis occurrence in acutely ill patients	TB	tuberculosis
		TBI	traumatic brain injury
SOGI	sexual orientation & gender identity	TBSA	total body surface area
		TCA	traumatic cardiac arrest
SPA	suprapubic aspiration	TCA	tricyclic antidepressant
SPECT	single photon emission computed tomography	TCP	transcutaneous cardiac pacing
		TcP	transcutaneous pacing
SPGB	sphenopalatine ganglion block	TdP	Torsades de Pointes
SPLIT0.9%	*Saline* vs *Plasma-Lyte* 148 for *ICU* Fluid *Therapy*	TEE	transesophageal echocardiogram
SPMSQ	Short Portable Mental Status Questionnaire	TEE	transesophageal echocardiography
SS	serotonin syndrome	TEG	thromboelastogram
SSD	silver sulfadiazine	TEG	thromboelastography

THAWS	thrombolysis for acute wake-up and unclear-onset strokes with alteplase at ≤4.5 hours after symptom time	UGNB	ultrasound-guided nerve block
		UGRA	ultrasound-guided regional anesthesia
THC	tetrahydrocannabinol	UHMS	Undersea and Hyperbaric Medical Society
TIA	transient ischemic attack		
TIC	trauma-induced coagulopathy	UPT	urine pregnancy test
TIC	trauma-informed care	URI	upper respiratory illness
TID	three times daily	URI	upper respiratory infection
TIFs	tracheo-innominate artery fistulas	URL	upper reference limit
		US	ultrasonography
		US	ultrasound
TIMI	thrombolysis in myocardial infarction	USGPIV	ultrasound-guided peripheral IV
TIPS	transjugular intrahepatic portosystemic shunt	UTI	urinary tract infection
		V̇/Q̇	ventilation/perfusion
TiTrATE	*ti*ming, *tr*iggers, *a*nd *t*argeted bedside eye *e*xaminations	VA ECMO	venoarterial ECMO
		VA	venoarterial
TLS	tumor lysis syndrome	VAD	ventricular assist device
TM	tympanic membrane	VAD	vertebral artery dissection
TMP-SMX	trimethoprim-sulfamethoxazole	VAERS	Vaccine Adverse Events Reporting System
TMT	tarsometatarsal	VAP	ventilator-associated pneumonia
tPA	tissue plasminogen activator	VAT	video-assisted thoracostomy
TPX	tension pneumothorax	VATS	video-assisted thoracic surgery
TRALI	transfusion-related acute lung injury	VBG	venous blood gas
		VC	vector change
TS	transient synovitis	VC	vital capacity
TSH	thyroid-stimulating hormone	VCF	vertebral compression fractures
TSLO	thoracic-lumbar sacral orthosis	V_d	volume of distribution
TSS	toxic shock syndrome	VDRL	Venereal Disease Research Laboratory
TSST	toxic shock syndrome toxin		
TSST-1	toxic shock syndrome toxin-1	VE	vaccine efficacy
TTE	transthoracic echo	VEGF	vascular endothelial growth factor
TTI	transthoracic impedance		
TTM	targeted temperature management	VF	ventricular fibrillation
		VILI	ventilator-induced lung injury
TTP	thrombotic thrombocytopenic purpura	VIT	velocity-time integral
		VITT	vaccine induced thrombotic thrombocytopenia
TUG	timed up and go		
TV	tidal volume	VKA	vitamin K antagonists
TvP	transvenous pacing	VL	video laryngoscopy
TVUS	transvaginal ultrasound	VOC	vaso-occlusive crisis
TWI	T-wave inversion	VOE	vaso-occlusive episode
TXA	tranexamic acid	VP	ventriculoperitoneal
UA	urinalysis	VRE	vancomycin-resistant enterococci
UC	ulcerative colitis		
UDS	urine drug screen	VRE	vancomycin-resistant *Enterococcus*
UFH	unfractionated heparin		
UGIB	upper gastrointestinal bleeding		
UGIS	upper gastrointestinal series	VS	ventricular storm

VT	ventricular tachycardia	WBC	white blood cell
VTE	venous thromboembolism	WCT	wide complex tachycardia
VV ECMO	venovenous ECMO	WE	Wernicke encephalopathy
		WES	wall echo shadow
VV	venovenous	WFWB	warm fresh whole blood
VZV	varicella zoster virus	WHO	World Health Organization
WAKE-UP	Efficacy and Safety of MRI-Based Thrombolysis in Wake-Up Stroke	WPW	Wolff-Parkinson-White
		XR	x-ray

SECTION I
RESUSCITATION

1

HIGHEST QUALITY CPR

LUIS A. AGUILAR MONTALVAN AND ANDREW E. CHERTOFF

HQ-CPR is the most important aspect of cardiac arrest management. While there is a lack of strong data to support some of its elements, endeavors by the ILCOR, AHA, and others are growing our shared knowledge on this subject. Here is what we know to be the components of HQ-CPR:

- A CCF of at least 80%. Interruptions for any reason should be minimized and maintained no longer than 10 seconds at a time.
- A compression rate maintained at 100 to 120 bpm
- A compression depth of 5 to 6 cm (2-2.5 inches) for adults, 5 cm (2 inches) for children, and 4 cm (1.5 inches) for infants, with full chest recoil between each compression
- Compressors changed every 2 minutes or sooner if needed
- A compression-to-breath ratio of 30:2 in patients without an advanced airway (15:2 if pediatric and single rescuer), with each breath delivered to achieve chest rise
- Continuous compressions with 1 breath every 6 to 8 seconds given over 1 second in patients with an advanced airway (1 breath every 2-3 seconds for pediatric patients)

CCF, the ratio of time spent performing compressions to the entire duration of the resuscitation, improves the likelihood of ROSC when maintained above 60%, with the aim being 80% or higher. Compressors should switch out after 2 minutes or sooner if the compressor is feeling fatigued, to avoid decay in chest compression depth and rate. Pauses in CPR should be minimized and kept to less than 10 seconds to prevent avoidable nadirs in CPP, as a CPP of greater than 15 mm Hg is generally accepted as necessary to achieve ROSC. Decreased "hands-off" time can be facilitated by steps such as having an ultrasound or Doppler in place for cardiac or pulse evaluation prior to a pause in compressions.

Hand position during CPR should be over the lower half of the sternum, just below the nipple line. If a shock is required, then compressions should persist while another member charges the defibrillator, and once the shock is delivered, compressions should be immediately resumed without pausing to check for a pulse. If available, ultrasonography should be used rather than manual pulse checks for earlier pulse detection. POCUS for other purposes risks prolonging compression pauses and should only be incorporated if the team can ensure maintenance of a high CCF. A successful strategy to include cardiac POCUS during resuscitations utilizes a team member assigned to this role, with instructions to place the phased array transducer in an easily accessible view prior to pausing CPR.

There are three recommended methods of airway management: BVM, SGA placement, and ETI. BVM is widely available and SGAs can be placed relatively easily with minimal setup, while ETI is the airway of choice after ROSC. Some studies have found that ETI is associated with ROSC, survival to hospital admission, and discharge with good neurologic outcomes. After several subsequent head-to-head comparisons failed to consistently demonstrate superiority, recommendations regarding method, use of an advanced airway, and timing of placement are dependent on specific patient and situational characteristics, while still optimizing compression quality. The 2020 AHA guidelines recommend earlier prioritization of oxygenation and definitive airway for pregnant patients in cardiac arrest, cardiac arrests secondary to primary respiratory etiology, and in pediatric arrests, which most commonly occur due to respiratory issues.

Mechanical chest compression devices can lower personnel demand and, when applied correctly, may eliminate human variation in location, rate, compression depth, and chest recoil. Studies have yet to establish superiority to manual compressions with regard to clinically relevant patient outcomes. Potential advantages of such a device may come at the cost of prolonged hands-off time during device application and ineffective compressions if malpositioned. The advantages of such a device must always be weighed against the swiftness and familiarity with which it can be applied.

Real-time feedback monitoring is essential for HQ-CPR, as observer-only feedback overestimates compression performance. The heterogeneity of existing real-time feedback devices limits the ability to comparatively interpret existing data, but the overall consensus is that some sort of nondisruptive feedback system is needed. The use of devices that rest on the chest and assess mechanical CPR quality (depth, recoil, rate) has been associated with improved ROSC and short-time survival in patients with cardiac arrest. Adjuncts like $ETCO_2$ monitoring provide CPR quality feedback and have some prognostic value; higher $ETCO_2$ readings indicate better perfusion, with $ETCO_2$ readings of at least 10 mm Hg and ideally greater than 20 mm Hg correlating with the delivery of 25% or more of cardiac output, which is the aim of CPR. Persistent $ETCO_2$ readings less than 10 mm Hg despite good CPR at the 20-minute mark are associated with a 0.5% likelihood of ROSC.

Additional considerations include minimization of aortocaval compression in pregnant patients at or beyond 20 weeks gestation. Manual left uterine displacement allows appropriate CPR performance while optimizing venous return and is recommended by the AHA over lateral tilt or wedge. While pediatric cardiac arrests with HQ-CPR are generally associated with higher rates of ROSC than those adults, depth of compressions in infants and neonates is frequently suboptimal and efforts should be made to specifically monitor this parameter during resuscitations.

PEARLS

- Higher CCFs are associated with ROSC, with a goal CCF 80% or more.
- CPR monitoring must be intentional to ensure the highest quality, using real-time feedback devices and avoiding prolonged interruptions (>10 seconds) that compromise the achieved CPP.
- The ventilation rate for pediatric patients with an advanced airway is now 20 to 30 breaths/min.

- $ETCO_2$ monitoring during CPR has both feedback value and prognostic value at the 20-minute mark.
- Manual left uterine displacement is recommended over lateral tilt or wedge during cardiac arrest in pregnant patients with gestation of 20 weeks or more.

Suggested Readings

Paiva EF, Paxton JH, O'Neil BJ. The use of end-tidal carbon dioxide ($ETCO_2$) measurement to guide management of cardiac arrest: a systematic review. *Resuscitation*. 2018;123:1-7.

Tang Y, Sun M, Zhu A. Outcome of cardiopulmonary resuscitation with different ventilation modes in adults: a meta-analysis. *Am J Emerg Med*. 2022;57:60-69.

Wang PL, Brooks SC. Mechanical versus manual chest compressions for cardiac arrest. *Cochrane Database Syst Rev*. 2018;8(8):CD007260.

Wyckoff MH, Singletary EM, Soar J, et al. 2021 International Consensus on Cardiopulmonary Resuscitation and Emergency Cardiovascular Care Science With Treatment Recommendations: Summary From the Basic Life Support; Advanced Life Support; Neonatal Life Support; Education, Implementation, and Teams; First Aid Task Forces; and the COVID-19 Working Group. *Resuscitation*. 2021;169:229-311.

2

Properly Position Those Pads!

Samantha J. Yarmis and Caleb Chan

Defibrillator pads are commonly used in the ED, whether for cardioversion of uncontrolled arrhythmias, defibrillation of shockable rhythms in cardiac arrest, or TCP in symptomatic bradycardia or heart block. For these procedures to be successful, a critical mass of the involved cardiac muscle must be depolarized. Factors that affect TTI, that is, the resistance to flow of current through the thorax, determine the success of cardioversion/defibrillation attempts. These factors include the distance between electrodes and the amount of energy delivered, both of which are affected by pad placement, as is the portion of heart muscle receiving the current.

Defibrillator pads can be placed in either an AL or AP position (**Figures 2.1** and **2.2**). Most pads come with a pictorial guide, but proper AL positioning involves one pad just to the right of the right upper sternal border below the right clavicle, with the other centered in the left midaxillary line, while in AP orientation, one pad is in the front either at the right midsternal border or just below the left nipple, with the other just below the scapula on the patient's back. Breast tissue may need to be lifted or laterally displaced to position the anterior pad. Optimal pad placement includes the absence of contact with other items such as electrodes or piercings and full skin contact with minimal body hair, although shaving is not always feasible in emergent situations. Topical medications or patches must be removed before pad placement to avoid burns as well as to optimize skin contact.

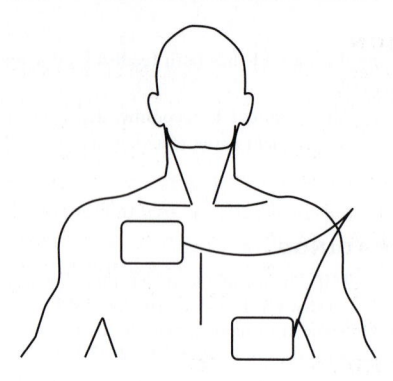

FIGURE 2.1 Anterolateral pad placement.

DEFIBRILLATION

AL pad placement is often used during cardiac arrest due to ease of placement; it does not require rolling or turning the patient to place the pads and avoids interrupting CPR efforts. This convenience can minimize hands-off time and may decrease time to shock delivery, but the optimal initial pad orientation for successful defibrillation in cardiac arrest has not been determined.

Up to half of patients in cardiac arrest due to pulseless VT or VF are refractory to defibrillation. Based on the results of the DOSE-VF trial, discussed in more detail in Chapter 4, the addition of a second set of pads in the opposite orientation with rapid sequential shock delivery (DSED) should be attempted if possible due to its association with an increased chance of VF termination, ROSC, and neurologically intact survival to hospital discharge. If DSED is not possible, then transition to the other pad orientation (VC defibrillation) should be pursued, as it was associated with increased odds of VF termination and survival to discharge in the study.

Existing data do not support one over the other, AL or AP, in terms of initial pad orientation and defibrillation success, and current AHA guidelines note that either is reasonable.

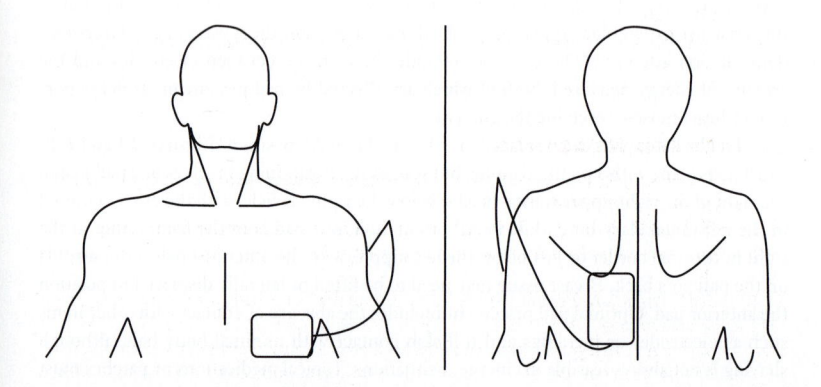

FIGURE 2.2 Anteroposterior pad placement.

CARDIOVERSION

AP pad placement has been traditionally considered to be superior to AL for the termination of atrial arrhythmias, such as atrial fibrillation and flutter, with data supporting the superiority of AP positioning in decreasing TTI and restoring sinus rhythm using monophasic defibrillators. Studies evaluating pad placement with biphasic defibrillators have had mixed results, with either no difference or AL performing better. Subgroup analysis of a more recent study demonstrating no significant benefit to either orientation did note a trend toward increased success when using AL pad placement in older patients, in patients who are obese, and in patients with a longer duration of atrial fibrillation. Larger studies and meta-analyses have not shown a significant difference in the success of cardioversion between the two.

TRANSCUTANEOUS PACING

There is only small-study electrophysiology lab data regarding pad placement in TCP, but it supports AP over AL pad positioning in terms of success of capture and the decreased energy required to do so.

CONCLUSION

Optimal pad placement for cardioversion, defibrillation, and pacing is not yet definitively known. For patients who are unstable, the choice of pad placement should be guided primarily by speed with which pads can be appropriately positioned with good skin contact and the familiarity of the medical staff. For relatively stable patients, AL positioning may be considered over AP for atrial cardioversions, and AP over AL for transcutaneous pacing.

PEARLS

- Early defibrillation improves survival in cardiac arrest due to VT or VF. Fast and effective pad placement matters more than the specific location of pads, and all medical staff should be familiar with both AP and AL orientations.
- For patients in VT/VF refractory to initial shocks, VC or DSED may increase the success of terminating the dysrhythmia.
- AL pad placement may improve success in terminating atrial dysrhythmias, particularly in patients who are obese or older, or those with prolonged dysrhythmia duration.
- AP pad placement may improve capture for successful transcutaneous pacing.

SUGGESTED READINGS

Cheskes S, Verbeek PR, Drennan IR, et al. Defibrillation strategies for refractory ventricular fibrillation. *N Engl J Med*. 2022;387:1947-1956.

Moayedi S, Patel P, Brady N, Witting M, Dickfeld TL. Anteroposterior pacer pad position is better than anterolateral for transcutaneous cardiac pacing. *Resuscitation*. 2022;181: 140-146.

Steinberg MF, Olsen J-A, Persse D, et al. Efficacy of defibrillator pads placement during ventricular arrhythmias, a before and after analysis. *Resuscitation*. 2022;174:16-19.

Virk SA, Rubenis I, Brieger D, Raju H. Anteroposterior versus anterolateral electrode position for direct current cardioversion of atrial fibrillation: a meta-analysis of randomised controlled trials. *Heart Lung Circ*. 2022;31:1640-1648.

3

ARE EPINEPHRINE, CALCIUM, OR BICARBONATE BENEFICIAL IN CARDIAC ARREST?

CATHERINE ROWBOTTOM AND BACHAR HAMADE

The AHA recommendations for OHCA are modified with each guideline update, using the latest literature to provide recommendations that may increase patients' chances of survival. Nearly 90% of patients with OHCA do not survive to hospital discharge, and of those that do survive, just over 60% of patients live 10 years after their initial cardiac arrest. Though medications are only one piece of the chain of survival, many resources are allocated to the provision of pharmacologic support during cardiac arrest. This chapter reviews the most commonly used medications for OHCA.

EPINEPHRINE

Epinephrine has continued to be an integral part of ACLS algorithms in OHCA with a recommended dose of 1 mg (1:10,000 concentration) every 3 to 5 minutes. Several studies have shown benefits to the use of epinephrine. A randomized control trial in 2011 found that epinephrine improved rates of ROSC and survival to admission; however, the trial was terminated early and could not explain any differences in long-term survival or effects on neurologic outcomes. Another randomized control trial performed in 2018 on patients with OHCA showed an improved 30-day survival rate with administration of epinephrine when compared to placebo. In 2019, the AHA continued to advocate for epinephrine based on data from a meta-analysis of two randomized control trials that compared epinephrine to placebo in patient who had cardiac arrest. The meta-analysis found that there was an increase in survival to hospital discharge in patients receiving epinephrine, regardless of their presenting cardiac rhythm.

SODIUM BICARBONATE

Sodium bicarbonate administration during cardiac arrest has remained a controversial topic. Bolus administration of a hypertonic bicarbonate solution has a variety of detrimental physiologic effects. By reducing systemic vascular resistance, sodium bicarbonate can compromise cerebral perfusion pressure. It may also create extracellular alkalosis, shifting the oxyhemoglobin saturation curve to the left, thereby inhibiting oxygen release to the tissues. In addition, by producing excess carbon dioxide, it can paradoxically contribute to intracellular acidosis. Two meta-analyses, performed in 2020 and 2021, support the decision to omit sodium bicarbonate from the current AHA guidelines. Treatment with sodium bicarbonate did not show a statistically significant increase in survival to discharge or ROSC. However, the 2020 AHA guidelines state that there are clinical scenarios where sodium bicarbonate treatment is a beneficial adjunct to other standard-of-care treatments, as in patients with severe hyperkalemia or overdose of medications causing sodium channel blockade (such as tricyclic antidepressant medications).

CALCIUM

In 1970, the AHA recommended the use of calcium for patients presenting with cardiac arrest. Between 1980 and 1983, multiple trials challenged this recommendation, and the AHA guidelines stopped recommending the routine use of calcium in patients who had cardiac arrest. A randomized control trial in 2021 redemonstrated the lack of benefit of calcium in OHCA. In 2022, a systematic review not only showed lack of benefit with calcium administration but also demonstrated potential harm in this patient population.

There are a few specific circumstances where the administration of calcium can be considered. Calcium can be used in patients with significant hyperkalemia to stabilize the myocardial cell membrane, as an adjunct in patients who had cardiac arrest when hypermagnesemia is suspected, and in patients with suspected beta-blocker or calcium channel blocker toxicity who are in refractory shock.

AMIODARONE AND LIDOCAINE

A randomized, double-blinded trial published in 2016 compared amiodarone, lidocaine, and saline in addition to standard of care in cardiac arrest with shock-refractory pulseless VT or VF. The study found an increased rate of survival to admission but did not find a statistically significant increase in rate of survival to hospital discharge or survival with improved neurologic outcomes. Interestingly, administration of amiodarone and lidocaine did show an improved rate of survival in bystander-witnessed cardiac arrest compared to placebo, possibly indicating a time-dependent benefit of treatment with antiarrhythmics. The current 2020 AHA guidelines recommend amiodarone or lidocaine for shock-resistant VF and pulseless VT through either intravenous or intraosseous routes. The current ACLS algorithm recommends initial administration of 300 mg of amiodarone with a subsequent dose of 150 mg or initial administration of 1 to 1.5 mg/kg of lidocaine with a second dose of 0.5 to 0.75 mg/kg.

MAGNESIUM SULFATE

The 2020 AHA guidelines do not recommend the routine use of magnesium for patients who had cardiac arrest. Magnesium may be considered for special situations in cardiac arrest, such as in patients with torsades de pointes (polymorphic VT due to a long QT interval).

VASOPRESSIN

The 2020 AHA guidelines state that vasopressin can be considered for use in patients who had cardiac arrest, either administered alone or in conjunction with epinephrine. However, this is not a strong recommendation. In a recent systematic review, vasopressin use, either alone or when combined with epinephrine, did not improve outcomes when compared to epinephrine administration alone. The studies were underpowered, which is why the weak recommendation for vasopressin persists in the guidelines.

PEARLS

- Early use of epinephrine may increase the chance of ROSC and survival to hospital discharge.
- Sodium bicarbonate is recommended for severe hyperkalemia and overdose with sodium channel blocking agents such as tricyclic antidepressants.
- Calcium can be considered in hyperkalemia, hypermagnesemia, and beta-blocker or calcium channel blocker toxicity.

- Amiodarone or lidocaine may be used in cardiac arrest with VT or VF refractory to defibrillation.
- Magnesium is recommended for polymorphic VT.
- Vasopressin may be considered in cardiac arrest; the current literature has not shown it to outperform epinephrine in trials that have been mostly underpowered.

Suggested Readings

Amacher SA, Bohren C, Blatter R, et al. Long-term survival after out-of-hospital cardiac arrest: a systematic review and meta-analysis. *JAMA Cardiol*. 2022;7(6):633-643.

Holmberg MJ, Issa MS, Moskowitz A, et al; International Liaison Committee on Resuscitation Advanced Life Support Task Force Collaborators. Vasopressors during adult cardiac arrest: a systematic review and meta-analysis. *Resuscitation*. 2019;139:106-121.

Kudenchuk PJ, Brown SP, Daya M, et al; Resuscitation Outcomes Consortium Investigators. Amiodarone, lidocaine, or placebo in out-of-hospital cardiac arrest. *N Engl J Med*. 2016; 374(18):1711-1722.

Vallentin MF, Granfeldt A, Meilandt C, et al. Effect of intravenous or intraosseous calcium vs. saline on return of spontaneous circulation in adults with out-of-hospital cardiac arrest. *JAMA*. 2021;326(22):2268-2276.

4

Resuscitating Refractory Ventricular Tachycardia and Ventricular Fibrillation

Akilesh Honasoge and Caleb Chan

Sustained ventricular arrhythmias are common in ED resuscitations, accounting for approximately half of all out-of-hospital cardiac arrests. Initial treatment is reliant on whether the patient is in arrest or has hemodynamic instability as a result of the tachycardia. ACLS guidelines for abnormal ventricular arrhythmias recommend sedation with cardioversion/defibrillation or a variety of medications such as amiodarone, procainamide, lidocaine, and adenosine to assist in these resuscitations. However, when initial attempts at ventricular arrhythmia correction fail or when the arrhythmia becomes recurrent despite medical treatment, the guidelines are less instructive on which subsequent therapies to consider.

Defining Electrical Storm

Recurrent or refractory VT and VF are often classified as "electrical storm." This entity is defined as three or more episodes of sustained VT, VF, or appropriate defibrillator shocks within a 24-hour period. Sustained VT is further defined as either more than 30 seconds or any length of VT requiring termination due to hemodynamic compromise. In the absence of a known fascicular VT, outflow tract VT, or prolonged QT, first-line medical treatment of ventricular arrhythmias should remain either amiodarone, procainamide, or lidocaine. The single best first-line medication remains widely debated. However, when these medications alone are ineffective, knowledge of the pathophysiologic mechanisms of VT may provide clues to the appropriate treatment modality for refractory cases.

Monomorphic Ventricular Arrhythmias

Reentrant ventricular arrhythmias are more common in patients with a history of prior myocardial infarction, structural/congenital heart disease, or infiltrative diseases such as sarcoidosis. A specifically timed depolarization can loop through a reentrant circuit and often leads to monomorphic VT. These reentrant circuits are often difficult to manage with antiarrhythmic drugs and frequently require an ablation procedure.

TdP

Spontaneous fluctuations in the membrane potential can trigger PVCs. If these PVCs occur before complete repolarization of the myocytes, it can cause a form of polymorphic VT called TdP. This can be exacerbated by delayed repolarization in conditions such as a prolonged QT interval. Magnesium administration for TdP predominantly works to prevent these early PVCs. rather than affect the QT interval; thus, it is not possible to use the QT interval changes to guide magnesium dosage. If magnesium alone is not adequate, isoproterenol or overdrive pacing should be used to shorten the QT interval. Isoproterenol is a nonselective beta-1 and beta-2 agonist that induces a high sympathetic tone and sinus tachycardia. Termination of an offending agent that prolongs the QT is an important focus after initial resuscitation.

Other Polymorphic Ventricular Arrhythmias

Spontaneous PVCs that are triggered during a fully repolarized state can also lead to multiple types of ventricular arrhythmia, including monomorphic or polymorphic VT. These are often caused by abnormal levels of intracellular calcium, such as caused by a high catecholaminergic state, electrolyte abnormalities, digoxin toxicity, or ischemic tissue during a myocardial infarction. Thus, treatment is focused on the reversal of these states. Given the catecholaminergic causes of VT, aggressive sedation is often recommended for refractory cases, including consideration of intubation and the initiation of medications such as propofol. When sedation alone is inadequate to treat the sympathetic storm, a percutaneous stellate ganglion block can be performed.

Use of Beta-Blockers

Given the high rates of refractory ventricular arrhythmias exacerbated by high catecholaminergic states, there has been recent interest in the use of beta-blockers during resuscitations. Though there are numerous case reports on the use of esmolol for refractory cases, only three very small retrospective trials exist. Although all trials had a trend toward higher rates of ROSC in patients who received esmolol, only one trial reached statistical significance, and no trial had significant differences in neurologic or survival outcomes. Some historical data suggest that an electrical storm due to acute myocardial infarction may respond better to sympathetic blockade. Selection of beta-blockers may be important, as some studies suggest that propranolol may be superior to metoprolol, especially when combined with amiodarone. Overall, there is no clear recommendation or evidence that broad use of beta-blockers is helpful during all electrical storm resuscitations, but it may be effective in some difficult-to-control circumstances.

Defibrillation Troubleshooting

Finally, if defibrillation attempts do not have any appreciable effect on the ventricular rhythm, the first step must be to troubleshoot the defibrillator setup. If synchronization is required, ensure the appropriate mode with maximum energy has been selected and that the QRS complex and not another wave have been synchronized by the machine. If not correct, consider changing the lead setting on the device to find the lead with the clearest QRS complex. Carefully consider adequate adhesion of the pads to the chest wall, especially if hair or sweat is present. If adhesion issues are suspected, hands-on defibrillation with external pressure on the anterior pad with a gloved hand has been used. However, the data have not consistently shown the safety of this practice with a potential for harm to the provider. Furthermore, traditional hands-off defibrillation has historically been very effective when there are minimal delays in hands-off time. Although widely debated, the appropriate positioning of the defibrillator pads (anterior-posterior vs anterior-lateral) is not clear. If initial attempts at defibrillation are not successful, consider switching to a different pad position.

Dual Sequential Defibrillation

If the patient remains in VT/VF despite three defibrillation attempts, consider DSED. Several case reports demonstrate the potential successes of transitioning to DSED in refractory cases. However, a meta-analysis of 10 different randomized control trials on DSED versus standard defibrillation comprising 1,347 patients showed statistically insignificant differences between the groups regarding termination of refractory VF. The 2022 DOSE-VF randomized control trial found significant benefit to DSED in patients with refractory VF after three conventional defibrillation attempts, resulting in a greater percentage of patients surviving to hospital discharge with a good neurologic outcome.

PEARLS

- VT and VF have heterogeneous causes and mechanisms.
- Consider the underlying cause of the refractory arrhythmia before selecting treatment options.
- Refractory monomorphic reentrant VT or VF is unlikely to be effectively managed with medications alone.
- Beta-blockers may worsen refractory TdP; beta-blockers may also improve refractory VT/VF due to high sympathetic activity or acute myocardial infarction.
- If repeat defibrillation attempts are unsuccessful, add an additional pad for DSED.

Suggested Readings

Al-Khatib SM, Stevenson WG, Ackerman MJ, et al. 2017 AHA/ACC/HRS guideline for management of patients with ventricular arrhythmias and the prevention of sudden cardiac death: a report of the American College of Cardiology/American Heart Association Task Force on clinical practice guidelines and the heart rhythm society. *Heart Rhythm*. 2018;15(10):e73-e189.

Cheskes S, Verbeek PR, Drennan IR, et al. Defibrillation strategies for refractory ventricular fibrillation. *N Engl J Med*. 2022;387(21):1947-1956.

Lee YH, Lee KJ, Min YH, et al. Refractory ventricular fibrillation treated with esmolol. *Resuscitation*. 2016;107:150-155.

Lemkin DL, Witting MD, Allison MG, Farzad A, Bond MC, Lemkin MA. Electrical exposure risk associated with hands-on defibrillation. *Resuscitation*. 2014;85(10):1330-1336.

Li Y, He X, Li Z, Li D, Yuan X, Yang J. Double sequential external defibrillation versus standard defibrillation in refractory ventricular fibrillation: a systematic review and meta-analysis. *Front Cardiovasc Med*. 2022;9:1017935.

Neumann T, Gruenewald M, Lauenstein C, Drews T, Iden T, Meybohm P. Hands-on defibrillation has the potential to improve the quality of cardiopulmonary resuscitation and is safe for rescuers-a preclinical study. *J Am Heart Assoc*. 2012;1(5):e001313.

Zeppenfeld K, Tfelt-Hansen J, de Riva M, et al. 2022 ESC guidelines for the management of patients with ventricular arrhythmias and the prevention of sudden cardiac death: developed by the task force for the management of patients with ventricular arrhythmias and the prevention of sudden cardiac death of the European Society of Cardiology (ESC) Endorsed by the Association for European Paediatric and Congenital Cardiology (AEPC). *Eur Heart J*. 2022;43(40):3997-4126.

5

KNOW THE INDICATIONS FOR INITIATING ECMO IN THE ED

NHI Y. LUU AND CASEY CARR

ECMO is a modified cardiopulmonary bypass, increasingly utilized to oxygenate the blood and provide hemodynamic support in patients with critical heart or lung pathology who are failing conventional maneuvers. ECMO provides additional time to treat underlying illnesses and can serve as a temporary bridge to transplantation. When used for the management of cardiac arrest, the use of ECMO is termed *extracorporeal cardiopulmonary resuscitation*.

BASIC CONFIGURATION

The two basic types of ECMO are VV and VA (**Figure 5.1**). VV-ECMO accesses and returns blood via the venous system and provides extrapulmonary gas exchange, and is thereby used solely for respiratory support. VA-ECMO accesses the venous system and provides oxygenated blood to the arterial system, and is used for hemodynamic instability with or without respiratory failure.

The configuration of ECMO is highly variable, and several pump drive and pumpless systems exist. The basic configuration consists of a specialized cannula, circuit tubing, a centrifugal pump, heat exchanger, bladder reservoir, and a membrane that oxygenates blood and removes carbon dioxide. The tubing runs to and from the patient, and blood is driven through the oxygenation membrane by the centrifugal pump head, warmed to an appropriate degree, and returned to the patient. This is typically done under systemic anticoagulation, in which unfractionated heparin is commonly used.

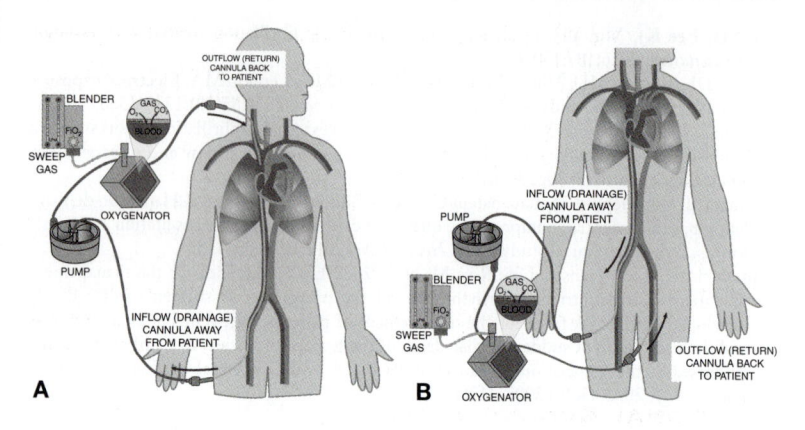

FIGURE 5.1 Veno-venous and veno-arterial extracorporeal membrane oxygenation. **(A)** VV-ECMO dual-site cannulation. The drainage cannula is inserted into the right femoral vein and the return cannula is inserted into the right jugular vein. **(B)** VA-ECMO dual-site cannulation, with drainage cannula inserted into the right femoral vein, and the return cannula in the left femoral artery. (Courtesy of Catherine Cichon, MD, MPH. Illum B, Odish M, Minokadeh A, et al. Evaluation, treatment, and impact of neurologic injury in adult patients on extracorporeal membrane oxygenation: a review. *Curr Treat Options Neurol.* 2021;23(5):15. Figure 2.)

VV-ECMO may be performed in a variety of ways. Typically, deoxygenated blood is removed via a cannula in the right femoral vein, with oxygenated blood returned via the right internal jugular vein. VA-ECMO cannulation is typically performed at the bilateral femoral sites, with a venous catheter inserted into one femoral vein and an arterial catheter in the contralateral femoral artery.

INDICATIONS FOR ECMO IN THE ED

- **Acute PE**—Massive PE or high risk of imminent mortality by the PESI score (≥Class IV) or Bova score (>4) are clear indications for potential ECMO, to serve as a bridge to endovascular or catheter-based interventions. For patients who are hemodynamically stable or at only intermediate risk (PESI Class III or Bova score 3-4), acceptable patient factors for cannulation are likely to vary depending on the individual institution but consultation should be considered.
- **Refractory cardiogenic shock**—Whether due to myocarditis, refractory malignant arrhythmias, or toxic overdose (eg, calcium-channel blocker), VA-ECMO ensures organ perfusion and decreases vasoactive requirements.
- **Refractory cardiac arrest with reversible cause**—VA-ECMO serves as a bridge to reversal of the inciting cause of arrest, such as acute STEMI, refractory malignant arrhythmias, accidental hypothermia, and massive PE. The data comparing ECPR to conventional CPR in terms of optimizing survival and neurologic outcomes after arrest are mixed. ECPR is most successful when performed in a highly selective subset of patients, including those with witnessed arrest, minimal downtime (<5 minutes)

and bystander CPR, shockable rhythms, and with short duration of time between arrest and initiation of ECMO flow. The ELSO suggests an age limit of 70 years and recommends establishing adequate ECMO flow within 60 minutes of arrest, but institutions vary in their internal criteria and may defer cannulation with more stringent criteria. An exception is cardiac arrest due to accidental hypothermia, where patients can do well despite prolonged downtimes (on the order of hours).
- **Respiratory failure with refractory hypoxia**—VV-ECMO is the usual mode of choice for acute respiratory failure failing standard rescue therapies and is also used as a bridge to lung transplant for acute or chronic respiratory failure in patients already on the transplant list. Initiation of VV-ECMO in the ED is likely to be a rare event but should be considered for those patients with refractory hypoxia despite optimal ventilator settings and rescue therapies, and in any patient known to be listed for lung transplant.

ADDITIONAL CONSIDERATIONS

Risks inherent to the use of ECMO include arterial occlusion leading to limb ischemia, hemorrhage secondary to anticoagulation, thrombosis and embolization from the centrifugal pump, heparin-induced thrombocytopenia, and potential air embolism if the tubing is not primed appropriately.

ECMO is a costly and time- and manpower-intensive resource, leading to strict selection criteria for its use. Suggested exclusion criteria for initiation of ECMO include history of severe neurologic dysfunction, intracranial hemorrhage, terminal malignancy, uncontrolled bleeding, and severe peripheral vascular disease.

PEARLS

- ECMO is a temporary rescue therapy providing cardiopulmonary support to critically ill patients undergoing treatment for a reversible pathology. VV-ECMO provides gas exchange for patients with respiratory failure while VA-ECMO provides circulatory support in addition to gas exchange.
- Potential considerations for ECMO include acute respiratory failure with refractory hypoxia failing conventional rescue therapies, refractory cardiogenic shock, refractory cardiac arrest, cardiotoxic ingestions, and massive PE.
- Indications and optimal factors for ECPR outcomes include reversible etiology of arrest, witnessed arrest, downtime less than 5 minutes and bystander CPR, short time to cannulation (<60 minutes), and shockable rhythms, *without* other terminal comorbidities.

SUGGESTED READINGS

Richardson AC, Tonna JE, Nanjayya V, et al. Extracorporeal cardiopulmonary resuscitation in adults. Interim guideline consensus statement from the extracorporeal life support organization. *ASAIO J*. 2021;67(3):221-228.

Tramm R, Ilic D, Davies AR, Pellegrino VA, Romero L, Hodgson C. Extracorporeal membrane oxygenation for critically ill adults. *Cochrane Database Syst Rev*. 2015;1(1):CD010381.

Wengenmayer T, Tigges E, Staudacher DL. Extracorporeal cardiopulmonary resuscitation in 2023. *Intensive Care Med Exp*. 2023;11(1):74.

6

OPTIMIZE OXYGENATION AND VENTILATION IN YOUR PATIENT WHO HAS EXPERIENCED A CARDIAC ARREST

ZOE GLICK AND LINDSAY RITTER

Optimizing both oxygenation and ventilation in patients who have experienced cardiac arrest is important. Patients who have experienced cardiac arrest should continue to receive airway and ventilatory support even after they achieve ROSC. Those who remain comatose, if they did not previously have their airway secured, should undergo endotracheal intubation and mechanical ventilation. Optimizing oxygenation and ventilation in patients who have experienced cardiac arrest by preventing hypoxia is essential in minimizing multiorgan system injury and irreversible damage.

Although advancements have been made in resuscitative measures in critically ill patients, the prognosis after ROSC has improved little since the first large multicenter report on patients who have experienced cardiac arrest was published in the 1950s. Mechanisms driving cardiac arrest are complex and a secondary postarrest resuscitation begins even after ROSC is achieved. Now called "post–cardiac arrest syndrome," this phenomenon is the physiologic response to whole-body ischemia and reperfusion. This is further complicated by baseline comorbidities and the underlying cause of cardiac arrest. Post–cardiac arrest syndrome is a unique pathophysiologic process that involves postarrest brain and cardiac injury in addition to systemic ischemia and reperfusion response. Optimal oxygenation and ventilation strategies in patients who have experienced arrest can help ameliorate the effects of postarrest syndrome and improve morbidity and mortality. This is achieved by monitoring and adjusting levels of oxygen and carbon dioxide in the blood to goal levels.

During cardiac arrest, the ILCOR suggests using the highest possible inspired oxygen concentration. Most studies define hypoxia as arterial partial pressure of oxygen (PaO_2) less than 60 mm Hg and hyperoxia as PaO_2 greater than 300 mm Hg. The AHA guidelines define hypoxia as SaO_2 less than 94%. According to ILCOR, care should be taken to avoid hypoxemia as well as hyperoxia following ROSC.

While hypoxia can lead to organ damage via insufficient brain oxygen delivery and is consistently linked with worse neurologic outcomes, hyperoxia can conversely cause a secondary brain injury via generated injurious reactive free radical oxygen species from the increased amount of dissolved oxygen in the blood. Although some literature has shown an association with PaO_2 greater than 300 mm Hg and increased in-hospital mortality after OHCA, results from hyperoxia are not consistent across all studies. Despite conflicting results, unnecessary administration of oxygen leading to a PaO_2 greater than 300 mm Hg should not be targeted as no obvious benefit has been elucidated.

Postarrest, current guidelines advise that 100% inspired oxygen should be administered with the goal of titrating to an arterial oxygen saturation of 94% to 98% or PaO_2 of 75 to 100 mm Hg. Of note, peripheral vasoconstriction after ROSC can make pulse oximetry levels unreliable. Obtaining an arterial blood gas is useful in measuring oxyhemoglobin saturation and can be used before titrating FiO_2. Keep in mind that patients who are hypothermic or undergoing targeted temperature management should use a temperature-corrected approach to measuring blood gases. Laboratory values for Pa_{CO_2} can be higher than the patient's true carbon dioxide level when their temperature is below normal.

AHA guidelines recommend normocarbia, with an end-tidal CO_2 of 30 to 40 mm Hg or arterial pressure of carbon dioxide (Pa_{CO_2}) of 35 to 45 mm Hg. Arterial blood gases and end-tidal CO_2 should also be used to carefully monitor ventilation in patients who have experienced arrest. Observational studies have shown worse neurologic outcomes associated with hypocarbia, defined as Pa_{CO_2} less than 30 mm Hg. One observational study found hypocarbia to be independently associated with worse neurologic function, as it causes cerebral vasoconstriction, decreasing cardiac output to the brain, thereby increasing the risk of anoxic brain injury and poor neurologic recovery. Although hyperventilation can be used as a temporizing measure in cases of acute cerebral edema, this should be balanced with the subsequent increased risk of brain injury. While hypocarbia has been associated with worse neurologic outcomes, outcomes associated with hypercarbia are inconsistent.

Utilizing protective ventilatory settings in the patient who has experienced ROSC can help prevent further damage. Low-tidal volumes of 6 to 8 cm^3/kg IBW are generally used in patients who have experienced ROSC; however, there are no clear guidelines or evidenced-based recommendations for this patient population. Instead, ventilation settings are usually adapted from those in patients with lung injury. Keeping Pplat less than 30 cm H_2O can also reduce ventilatory-associated lung injury. Given the decreased cardiac output and cerebral perfusion associated with hyperventilation, starting with 10 to 12 breaths per minute and titrating to achieve the target carbon dioxide levels, as previously mentioned, is suggested. There are a variety of methods used to monitor and optimize oxygenation and ventilation in post–ROSC cardiac arrest (see **Figure 6.1**). Generally, it is recommended to maintain normocarbia and normoxemia; however, an individualized approach should be used for special populations when appropriate.

Special consideration should be given to patients whose cause of cardiac arrest is related to COPD or asthma exacerbation, ARDS, or patients who have experienced arrest who subsequently develop ARDS. Due to existing lung injury, targeting a Pa_{CO_2} of 35 to 45 mm Hg

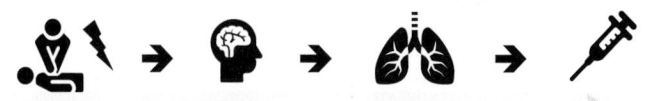

Emergency Department to Intensive Care Unit

Cardiac Arrest Management	Preserve Brain Oxygenation	Ventilator Management	Blood Gas
• Achieve return of spontaneous circulation	• Target normoxia • Avoid hyperventilation	• 6-8 cc/kg IBW tidal volume • Goal Pplat <30 cm H_2O	• Obtain post intubation • Goal Pa_{O_2} 75-100 mm Hg • Goal Pa_{CO_2} 35-55 mm Hg

FIGURE 6.1 Suggested clinical management of oxygenation and ventilation in the cardiac arrest patient who has achieved return of spontaneous circulation.

may not be feasible, as permissive hypercarbia may be necessary to prevent further lung injury. The clinician must balance the risk of hypercarbia and acidosis with the need to use protective lung ventilation, keeping the Pplat less than 30, and preventing hypoxia. In general, targeting a pH greater than 7.2 with a hypercapnic acidosis is recommended.

PEARLS

- Regulation of oxygenation and ventilation is important in the management of patients who have experienced arrest.
- Arterial blood gas measurements, when available, can be helpful in obtaining desired oxygen and carbon dioxide levels.
- It is reasonable to aim for an end-tidal CO_2 of 30 to 40 mm Hg or Pa_{CO_2} of 35 to 45 mm Hg.
- Oxygen should be administered with the goal of titrating to an arterial oxygen saturation of 94% to 98% or Pa_{O_2} of 75 to 100 mm Hg.

SUGGESTED READINGS

Callaway CW, Donnino MW, Fink EL, et al. Part 8: post–cardiac arrest care. *Circulation.* 2015;132(18 suppl 2):S465-S482.

Hickling KG, Walsh J, Hendersons S, Jackson R. Low mortality rate in adult respiratory distress syndrome using low-volume, pressure limited ventilation with permissive hypercapnia: a prospective study. *Crit Care Med.* 1994;22:1568-1578.

Kilgannon JH, Jones AE, Shapiro NI, et al. Emergency Medicine Shock Research Network (EMShockNet) Investigators. Association between arterial hyperoxia following resuscitation from cardiac arrest and in-hospital mortality. *JAMA.* 2010;303(21):2165-2171.

Morrison LJ, Deakin CD, Morley PT, et al. Part 8: advanced life support: 2010 international consensus on cardiopulmonary resuscitation and emergency cardiovascular care science with treatment recommendations. *Circulation.* 2010;122(16 suppl 2):S345-421.

Nolan JP, Sandroni C, Böttiger BW, et al. European Resuscitation Council and European Society of Intensive Care Medicine guidelines 2021: post-resuscitation care. *Intensive Care Med.* 2021;47(4):369-421.

7

WHAT MAP SHOULD YOU TARGET IN THE POSTARREST PATIENT?

RYAN LEE AND WAN-TSU W. CHANG

Maintaining end-organ perfusion following ROSC is paramount in postcardiac arrest patients. MAP is the critical hemodynamic marker used by clinicians to ensure they are maintaining adequate perfusion. Low MAP may cause inadequate blood flow to vital organs, leading to ischemia and cell death; however, elevated MAP may contribute to increased oxygen demand and stress on the heart. MAP is normally tightly regulated by a variety of homeostatic mechanisms but varies widely as a part of postcardiac arrest syndrome. Further, while cerebral perfusion pressure, a product of MAP minus intracranial pressure, is autoregulated in healthy individuals, this process is disrupted in the time following cardiac arrest. Therefore, patients with hypoxic-ischemic brain injury following cardiac arrest may be more dependent on an adequate MAP to maintain cerebral perfusion.

CLINICAL TRIALS OF POSTARREST BLOOD PRESSURE GOALS

Observational studies have associated a higher MAP with improved neurologic outcomes. Two recent trials compared lower versus higher MAP targets in postcardiac arrest patients. The COMACARE Trial, published in 2018, randomized 120 patients with OHCA and ventricular fibrillation or tachycardia to a MAP of 65 to 75 mm Hg or 80 to 100 mm Hg. The study failed to show any difference in neuron-specific enolase level as a surrogate marker of neurologic injury at 48 hours. In 2019, the NEUROPROTECT Trial randomized 112 patients with OHCA of any initial rhythm to a MAP target of 65 mm Hg or 85 to 100 mm Hg. There was no significant difference in brain injury as measured by diffusion-weighted MRI at day 5. Neither of these trials were powered to detect patient-oriented outcomes.

Most recently, the BOX Trial was designed specifically to address this question and powered to detect mortality difference. About 802 patients with OHCA were randomized to either a low or high MAP target of 63 mm Hg or 77 mm Hg, respectively. Baseline characteristics and other postarrest care were similar between groups. No significant difference was seen in the composite primary outcome of death from any cause or severe disability as defined by CPC score of 3 or 4 at 90 days. No difference was seen across any secondary outcomes, rate of adverse events, or between prespecified subgroups.

GUIDELINE RECOMMENDATIONS

The 2020 AHA guidelines offer a level 2a recommendation of avoiding hypotension by maintaining a systolic blood pressure of at least 90 mm Hg and a MAP of at least 65 mm Hg in the postresuscitation period. Utilizing dynamic indices to assess volume status and guide fluid administration is reasonable, while administering norepinephrine to treat postarrest hypotension was associated with lower mortality when compared to epinephrine in a large retrospective study and has been recommended as a first-line vasopressor. In light of the most recent evidence, any benefit of higher MAP targets remains unproven. Optimal postarrest MAP targets may need to be individualized and warrant further evaluation.

PEARLS

- Postarrest hemodynamic instability is common, and maintaining end-organ perfusion is a paramount goal in resuscitation.
- Maintaining an adequate MAP has been proposed as one intervention to mitigate neurologic injury following ROSC.
- Guidelines and recent evidence support maintaining a MAP of at least 65 mm Hg and a systolic blood pressure of at least 90 mm Hg.
- While higher MAP has been associated with better neurologic outcomes, the most recent prospective studies failed to show any benefit.
- Norepinephrine is a reasonable first-line vasopressor for postarrest hypotension.

Suggested Readings

Ameloot K, De Deyne C, Eertmans W, et al. Early goal-directed haemodynamic optimization of cerebral oxygenation in comatose survivors after cardiac arrest: the Neuroprotect post-cardiac arrest trial. *Eur Heart J.* 2019;40:1804-1814.

Beylin ME, Perman SM, Abella BS, et al. Higher mean arterial pressure with or without vasoactive agents is associated with increased survival and better neurological outcomes in comatose survivors of cardiac arrest. *Intensive Care Med.* 2013;39(11):1981-1988.

Bougouin W, Slimani K, Renaudier M, et al. Epinephrine versus norepinephrine in cardiac arrest patients with post-resuscitation shock. *Intensive Care Med.* 2022;48(3):300-310.

Jakkula P, Pettila V, Skrifvars MB, et al. Targeting low-normal or high-normal mean arterial pressure after cardiac arrest and resuscitation: a randomised pilot trial. *Intensive Care Med.* 2018;44:2091-2101.

Kjaergaard J, Møller JE, Schmidt H, et al. Blood-pressure targets in comatose survivors of cardiac arrest. *N Engl J Med.* 2022;387(16):1456-1466.

Neumar RW, Nolan JP, Adrie C, et al. Post-cardiac arrest syndrome: epidemiology, pathophysiology, treatment, and prognostication. A consensus statement from the International Liaison Committee on Resuscitation (American Heart Association, Australian and New Zealand Council on Resuscitation, European Resuscitation Council, Heart and Stroke Foundation of Canada, InterAmerican Heart Foundation, Resuscitation Council of Asia, and the Resuscitation Council of Southern Africa); the American Heart Association Emergency Cardiovascular Care Committee; the Council on Cardiovascular Surgery and Anesthesia; the Council on Cardiopulmonary, Perioperative, and Critical Care; the Council on Clinical Cardiology; and the Stroke Council. *Circulation.* 2008;118(23):2452-2483.

8

When to Activate the Cardiac Cath Team Following Sudden Cardiac Arrest—Don't Be Afraid to Call

Matthew J. Levy

Emergent CAG and subsequent PCI are mainstays of modern emergency medical care. It is well established that emergent CAG should be promptly performed in patients experiencing acute STEMIs. The benefits of emergent CAG have had a profound effect in the form of decreased mortality and morbidity for those patients with an acute "culprit" obstructing coronary artery lesion and a very low complication rate. The role and indications for emergent CAG in patients who have experienced a SCA, especially OHCA with ROSC, continues to be an area of ongoing discovery and discussion. These patients are classically stratified based on factors that include the presence of an initial shockable rhythm and the presence of ST-segment elevation on postarrest ECG.

ECG Stratification

A subset of ROSC patients will not demonstrate a STEMI on ECG but still have an acutely obstructing coronary artery lesion. Thus, the subsequent challenge is identifying which ROSC patients without ST-segment elevations on their ECG will benefit from coronary angiography. It has been noted that SCA may not be accompanied by antecedent symptoms or classic ECG manifestations of STEMI following ROSC. Further, many original studies examining emergent PCI in patients with STEMI excluded cardiac arrest.

Guideline Recommendations

The ILCOR published a systematic review on this topic in 2021 and updated it in 2022. This review stratified patients after ROSC into the following key categories and their abbreviated key findings:

1) Without ST-elevation and *all* initial rhythms: Two small RCTs were identified, and no significant difference was found between early, late, or no CAG.
2) Without ST-elevation and initial *shockable* rhythms: Two RCTs and two other observational studies showed low or very low certainty evidence for favorable neurologic outcomes associated with early CAG.
3) With ST-elevation: One observational study was identified with very low certainty evidence that found no effect on survival or favorable neurologic outcome with early CAG compared with late or no CAG.

The 2022 ILCOR guidelines primarily reference the 2021 guidelines and make the following treatment recommendations: For comatose postarrest ROSC patients without ST-segment elevation, either an early or a delayed approach for CAG is reasonable (weak recommendation, low-certainty evidence). However, the 2021 guidelines also say, "There may be subgroups of patients without ST-segment elevation with high-risk features who would benefit from earlier CAG." The ILCOR guidelines stop short of describing what high-risk features may support an earlier CAG; however, 2015 AHA guidelines suggest considering hemodynamic instability, electrical instability, comorbid conditions, and ongoing cardiac ischemia. Don't be afraid to call the interventional cardiologist, discuss the case, and arrive at a plan that's best for that patient.

The guidelines are unequivocal in their support for early CAG in ROSC patients with STEMI.

PEARLS

- Early PCI should be performed in patients with ECG findings of ST-segment elevation.
- An early or delayed approach for CAG is reasonable for postarrest patients without ECG findings of ST-segment elevation.
- Consider hemodynamic instability, electrical instability, and ongoing ischemia when deciding whether PCI may be indicated in a postarrest patient without STEMI.
- When in doubt, call and discuss the case with the interventional cardiologist.

Suggested Readings

Singh M, Holmes DR Jr, Dehmer GJ, et al. Percutaneous coronary intervention at centers with and without on-site surgery: a meta-analysis. *JAMA*. 2011;306:2487-2494.

Wyckoff MH, Greif R, Morley PT, et al. 2022 International Consensus on Cardiopulmonary Resuscitation and Emergency Cardiovascular Care Science With Treatment Recommendations: Summary From the Basic Life Support; Advanced Life Support; Pediatric Life

Support; Neonatal Life Support; Education, Implementation, and Teams; and First Aid Task Forces. *Circulation.* 2022;146(25):e483-e557.

Wyckoff MH, Singletary EM, Soar J, et al. 2021 International Consensus on Cardiopulmonary Resuscitation and Emergency Cardiovascular Care Science With Treatment Recommendations: Summary From the Basic Life Support; Advanced Life Support; Neonatal Life Support; Education, Implementation, and Teams; First Aid Task Forces; and the COVID-19 Working Group. *Resuscitation.* 2021;169:229-311.

9

HAS ENTHUSIASM FOR TTM COOLED OFF?

CATHERINE ROWBOTTOM AND BACHAR HAMADE

PATHOPHYSIOLOGIC RATIONALE AND TARGETED OUTCOMES OF TTM

Resuscitated cardiac arrest is associated with global hypoxia and ischemia with the potential for reperfusion injury and excitotoxicity, increasing the risk of poor neurologic outcomes. Hypothermia decreases the metabolic rate and accumulation of waste products, decreases excitatory neurotransmitter and free radical production, and modulates inflammatory processes responsible for neuronal cell damage and cerebral injury. Hypothermia also improves cardiac performance indices in postcardiac arrest patients. These possible benefits of hypothermia are countered by adverse effects including coagulopathy, arrhythmias, hyperglycemia, and infection. Contraindications include patient responsiveness, bleeding, coagulopathy, or cardiac arrest resulting from trauma, sepsis, or hemorrhagic shock.

BACKGROUND OF THERAPEUTIC HYPOTHERMIA

The 2005 AHA guidelines for cardiopulmonary resuscitation and emergency cardiovascular care first introduced "therapeutic hypothermia" for comatose patients following successful ROSC. Two trials published in 2002 studied the effects of therapeutic hypothermia in patients with ROSC after cardiac arrest due to shockable rhythms and prompted this major change from the 2000 AHA guidelines.

The trial by Bernard et al. randomized comatose survivors of OHCA to treatment with hypothermia at 33 °C or normothermia at 37 °C. The HACA study by Holzer et al. compared the effects of therapeutic hypothermia at 32 °C to 34 °C and normothermia at 37 °C. Both studies showed favorable neurologic outcomes in patients who underwent therapeutic hypothermia.

The 2010 AHA guidelines reinforced the use of therapeutic hypothermia for patients with cardiac arrest due to shockable rhythms. Recommendations included cooling of comatose adult patients with ROSC after OHCA due to pulseless ventricular tachycardia or fibrillation at 32 °C to 34 °C for 12 to 24 hours and consideration of hypothermia for other comatose adult patients with ROSC with any associated rhythm.

A 2013 RCT performed by Nielsen et al. compared neurologic outcomes of patients at either 33 °C or 36 °C after OHCA regardless of initial rhythm. Patients were maintained at target temperatures for 28 hours with subsequent rewarming to 37 °C and aggressive prevention of hyperthermia. Results showed no significant differences in mortality or neurologic outcomes. Therefore, the 2015 AHA guidelines recommended a temperature of 32 °C to 36 °C for all comatose patients with ROSC for at least 24 hours followed by avoidance of hyperthermia. The terminology for cooling patients after resuscitated cardiac arrest changed from "therapeutic hypothermia" to the term TTM, encompassing different strategies including prevention of fever, maintenance of normothermia, or induction of mild hypothermia.

Guidelines for Use of TTM in Cardiac Arrest Patients

Multiple studies have been performed since the 2015 AHA guidelines, most including patients presenting with a shockable rhythm. The "Hypothermia After Cardiac Arrest With Nonshockable Rhythm" trial is the only RCT comparing therapeutic hypothermia and normothermia in patients presenting with a nonshockable rhythm. This trial compared therapeutic hypothermia at 33 °C with maintenance of normothermia at 37 °C and showed improved neurologic outcomes at 3 months in the hypothermia group.

The 2019 trial, "Targeted Normothermia After Out-of-Hospital Cardiac Arrest" (TTM2 trial), compared the effects of therapeutic hypothermia at 33 °C and targeted normothermia at less than 37.8 °C in postcardiac arrest patients after ROSC. This trial excluded patients with an unwitnessed cardiac arrest, an initial rhythm of asystole, or an admission temperature of below 30 °C. Results did not show improvement in the 6-month mortality rate or neurologic outcomes between the groups.

A 2021 systematic review and meta-analysis evaluated patients with ROSC after OHCA due to any rhythm and demonstrated that TTM at 32 °C to 34 °C showed no improvement in survival rates or favorable neurologic outcomes when compared to normothermia. Additionally, a 2021 meta-analysis of 10 RCTs did not find improved survival rates or functional outcomes in patients undergoing any level of hypothermia compared to maintenance of normothermia. However, it demonstrated the possible adverse effects caused by hypothermia, including the development of arrhythmias.

Based on the literature over the past 20 years, therapeutic hypothermia has not been found to improve outcomes when compared to maintenance of normothermia in postcardiac arrest patients, except potentially in patients who present with a nonshockable rhythm. Despite this, the 2020 AHA guidelines continue to recommend TTM for comatose adults achieving ROSC in both OHCA and in-hospital cardiac arrest from shockable and nonshockable rhythms. The guidelines also recommend temperature maintenance between 32 °C and 36 °C and maintenance of TTM for at least 24 hours with a goal of preventing hyperthermia. It seems likely that AHA will move to update their next guidelines with new recommendations for TTM based on initial presenting rhythm.

PEARLS

- Two landmark trials in 2002 showed neurologic benefit from therapeutic hypothermia.
- AHA adopted therapeutic hypothermia in 2005.
- A large 2013 trial showed no difference in neurologic outcome between targeted temperatures of 33 °C and 36 °C.

- The 2019 TTM2 trial did not show a difference in outcomes of postcardiac arrest patients maintained at 33 °C or avoiding fever at less than 37.8 °C.
- The 2020 AHA updates recommend TTM between 32 °C and 36 °C for 24 hours post ROSC.
- Fever should be avoided as part of TTM.

Suggested Readings

Bernard SA, Gray TW, Buist MD, et al. Treatment of comatose survivors of out-of-hospital cardiac arrest with induced hypothermia. *N Engl J Med*. 2002;346(8):557-563.

Holzer M, et al. Mild Therapeutic Hypothermia to Improve the Neurologic Outcome After Cardiac Arrest. *N Engl J Med*. 2002; 346(8):549-556.

Hypothermia after Cardiac Arrest Study Group. Mild therapeutic hypothermia to improve the neurologic outcome after cardiac arrest. *N Engl J Med*. 2002;346(8):549-556.

Lascarrou JB, Merdii H, Le Gouge A, et al. Targeted temperature management for cardiac arrest with nonshockable rhythm. *N Engl J Med*. 2019;381(24):2327-2337.

Neumar RW, Shuster M, Callaway CW, et al. Part 1: Executive summary: 2015 American Heart Association Guidelines update for cardiopulmonary resuscitation and emergency cardiovascular care. *Circulation*. 2015;132(18 suppl 2):S315-S367.

Nielsen N, Wetterslev J, Cronberg T, et al. Targeted temperature management at 33 degrees C versus 36 degrees C after cardiac arrest. *N Engl J Med*. 2013;369(23):2197-2206.

Peberdy MA, Callaway CW, Neumar RW, et al. Part 9: Post-cardiac arrest care: 2010 American Heart Association guidelines for cardiopulmonary resuscitation and emergency cardiovascular care. *Circulation*. 2010;122(18 suppl 3):S768-S786.

10

Making a Difference in Undifferentiated Shock

Daniel Sheets and Randall T. Rhyne

The patient in undifferentiated shock presents a unique challenge, as the emergency physician must perform a time-critical resuscitation with limited diagnostic information. In addition to a focused assessment of the ABCs, special attention should be paid to "the pump," "the tank," and "the pipes" for a systematic approach to the patient with hypotension. Early recognition and treatment of the underlying etiology are crucial, as sustained hypotension is a strong predictor of subsequent organ failure and mortality.

Shock is defined as an imbalance in tissue oxygen supply and demand. This imbalance results in cellular injury with toxic increases in intracellular calcium, anaerobic respiration, lactate production, cellular death, and the release of systemic proinflammatory cytokines, a cascade ultimately resulting in end-organ damage and possibly multiple organ dysfunction syndrome and death. The four broad classifications of shock are:

1) **Hypovolemic**: due to depleted intravascular blood volume (eg, hemorrhage, fluid losses, third spacing)
2) **Cardiogenic**: due to decreased cardiac output from an intrinsic cardiac pathology (eg, myocardial infarction, valvular dysfunction, decompensated heart failure)
3) **Obstructive**: due to mechanical obstruction that reduces cardiac output (eg, cardiac tamponade, massive pulmonary embolism, tension pneumothorax)
4) **Distributive**: due to excessive vasodilation (eg, sepsis, anaphylaxis, adrenal crisis, neurogenic shock)

The initial step in the management of undifferentiated shock includes obtaining peripheral venous access and ensuring adequate ventilation and oxygenation. This may require noninvasive or even invasive mechanical ventilation, and it is important to ensure appropriate circulatory support has been provided, as the associated decrease in venous return with positive pressure may trigger circulatory decompensation. A trial bolus of crystalloid solution should be considered with careful monitoring of clinical response. If anaphylaxis is suspected based on history and physical exam, administration of epinephrine during initial resuscitation is key.

Early evaluation includes patient history, exam, bloodwork, ECG, and imaging, including bedside ultrasound. An early focus on "the pump" helps discriminate between the four classifications of shock and decreases time to lifesaving interventions. An ECG should be performed early to assess for STEMI, complete heart block, right heart strain suggesting massive pulmonary embolism, or electrical alternans suggesting cardiac tamponade. Bedside ultrasound can quickly reveal pericardial effusion and provide an assessment of cardiac contractility as well as filling. A large pericardial effusion with right-sided diastolic collapse suggests cardiac tamponade causing obstructive shock. A hypokinetic heart with dilated cardiac chambers suggests cardiogenic shock potentially necessitating inotropic support. A dilated RV with intraventricular septal bowing and decreased LV filling suggests RV failure, possibly due to pulmonary embolism. A hyperdynamic heart (ie, higher than normal ejection fraction) with underfilled chambers suggests distributive or hypovolemic shock.

Following evaluation of "the pump," an assessment of "the tank" helps determine intravascular volume status. Physical exam findings such as elevated jugular venous pressure, bilateral rales on lung auscultation, or lower extremity edema suggest whole-body fluid overload, although they may not be entirely representative of intravascular volume. A passive leg raise can be performed to see if increasing venous return improves cardiac output, indicating fluid responsiveness. Bedside ultrasound may also detect intra-abdominal free fluid indicating possible hemorrhage and helps provide further assessment of intravascular status. An IVC diameter less than 2 cm, as measured 2 to 3 cm distal to the right atrial junction, with inspiratory collapse of over 50% in spontaneously breathing patients not on PPV, suggests the patient is intravascularly depleted. PPV and elevated right heart pressures make interpretation of the dilated IVC less reliable, while a small IVC with respiratory variation remains suggestive of hypovolemia. IVC visualization can also clarify cardiac findings: for example, a small or collapsing IVC in the presence of pericardial effusion makes tamponade unlikely. Ultrasound can also be used to reassess intravascular status after fluid resuscitation. Vasopressors are often necessary to manage continued hypotension despite adequate fluid repletion, and some physicians opt to start them early while fluid resuscitation is ongoing.

Evaluation of "the pipes" completes shock assessment. Cool extremities with sluggish cap refill hint at peripheral vasoconstriction and possibility of a cardiogenic

TABLE 10.1	ULTRASOUND AND EXAM FINDINGS OF THE FOUR CLASSIFICATIONS OF SHOCK			
CLASSIFICATION	**THE PUMP**	**THE TANK**	**THE PIPES**
Hypovolemic	Any contractility, although hyperdynamic is most suggestive. Small cardiac chambers	IVC <2 cm >50% collapsibility (spontaneously breathing patients)	Normal or vasoconstricted (increased SVR) Intra-abdominal free fluid, possible AAA
Distributive	Any contractility, although hyperdynamic is most suggestive. Small- or normal-sized cardiac chambers	IVC <2 cm >50% collapsibility (spontaneously breathing patients)	Vasodilated (decreased SVR)
Cardiogenic	Decreased contractility Large cardiac chambers Large RV with small LV in RV failure	Dilated (>2 cm) IVC <50% collapsibility	Vasoconstricted
Obstructive	Tamponade: pericardial effusion, right-sided diastolic collapse, hyperdynamic, underfilled cardiac chambers PE: dilated RV, septal bowing, small LV, potential clot in transit Tension PTX: lateral shift of cardiac windows, small cardiac chambers, absence of lung sliding	Dilated (>2 cm) IVC <50% collapsibility	Vasoconstricted Lower extremity DVT

DVT, deep venous thrombosis; IVC, inferior vena cava; LV, left ventricle; PTX, pneumothorax; RV, right ventricle; SVR, systemic vascular resistance.

component or profound hypovolemia, while warm extremities may be indicative of distributive shock. Physical exam may reveal a pulsatile abdominal mass suggestive of AAA, which may also be detected with ultrasound. Exam findings or ultrasound suggestive of DVT may indicate massive pulmonary embolism as the source of obstructive shock.

A systematic evaluation of "the pump," "the tank," and "the pipes" can aid in the prompt recognition of the etiology of undifferentiated shock (**Table 10.1**) and help guide ongoing resuscitation to improve outcomes.

PEARLS

- Use a systematic approach to "the pump," "the tank," and "the pipes" to determine classification of shock.
- Integrate the use of bedside ultrasound into resuscitation of patients with undifferentiated shock to help make the diagnosis and guide interventions.

Suggested Readings

Atkinson P, Bowra J, Milne J, et al. International Federation for Emergency Medicine Consensus Statement: sonography in hypotension and cardiac arrest (SHoC): an international consensus on the use of point of care ultrasound for undifferentiated hypotension and during cardiac arrest. *CJEM*. 2017;19(6):459-470.
Goldberg SA, Liu P. Undifferentiated shock. *Crit Decis Emerg Med*. 2015;29(3):9-19.
Jones AE, Aborn LS, Kline J. Severity of emergency department hypotension predicts adverse hospital outcome. *Shock*. 2004;22(5):410-414.
Perera P, Mailhot T, Riley D, et al. The RUSH exam: rapid ultrasound in shock in the evaluation of the critically ill. *Emerg Med Clin North Am*. 2010;28:29-56.
Vincent J, De Backer D. Circulatory shock. *N Engl J Med*. 2013;368(18):1726-1734.

11

POCUS Pearls for Undifferentiated Shock

Samantha A. King and T. Andrew Windsor

POCUS has a wide variety of applications in the acute care setting, and multiple protocols have been developed for its utilization in the care of patients who have undifferentiated hypotension. These protocols improve diagnostic accuracy and impact additional diagnostic and treatment decisions in the initial phases of resuscitation.

POCUS is generally more helpful to rule in pathology than to rule it out. One would hope that the introduction of POCUS-guided targeted resuscitative strategies would improve outcomes, but recent literature has not uniformly supported this conclusion. Research into long-term outcomes is limited, and studies have mostly shown the impact of ultrasound on initial management and diagnostic uncertainty.

RUSH Examination

Initial approaches to ultrasound in patients who have undifferentiated hypotension involve quick multiorgan assessment, with the most predominant protocol being the RUSH examination. The RUSH components can be remembered using the mnemonic HI-MAP (**Figure 11.1A**). Another conceptualization is to consider the components of the examination as an evaluation of the "pump," the "tank," and the "pipes."

The goal of this examination is to quickly assess clinically oriented questions: How is the heart contracting? Are there signs of right heart strain or obstructive shock? Is the IVC plethoric, normal, or collapsed? Is there free fluid in the abdomen? Does the aorta have an obvious dissection or aneurysm? Is there a pneumothorax? Initial reports of the examination showed the ability to complete the entirety of the examination within 2 minutes. Critics of this protocol note that some of the portions of the examination, such as the search for intraabdominal free fluid and abdominal aortic aneurysm evaluation, are of low yield in undifferentiated shock, while supporters argue that such findings are must-not-miss.

RUSH Exam: HIMAP versus Pump/Tank/Pipes Protocolization

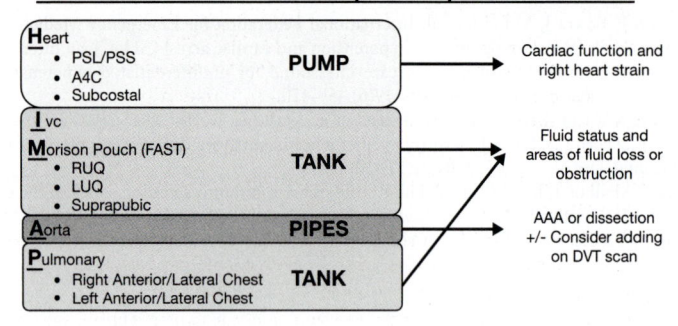

Heart — PSL/PSS, A4C, Subcostal — **PUMP** → Cardiac function and right heart strain

Ivc
Morison Pouch (FAST) — RUQ, LUQ, Suprapubic — **TANK** → Fluid status and areas of fluid loss or obstruction

Aorta — **PIPES** → AAA or dissection +/- Consider adding on DVT scan

Pulmonary — Right Anterior/Lateral Chest, Left Anterior/Lateral Chest — **TANK**

A

SHoC Protocol: Hierarchical Scanning

Hierarchy	Views	Goals
Addtl. Views	DVT, FAST, and AAA exams	Thrombosis and sources of blood loss
Supplementary Views	Cardiac—Additional views	Additional cardiac information
Core Views	Cardiac—Subxiphoid and parasternal views, lung, IVC	Pericardial effusion, cardiac form and function, pleural fluid, and filling status

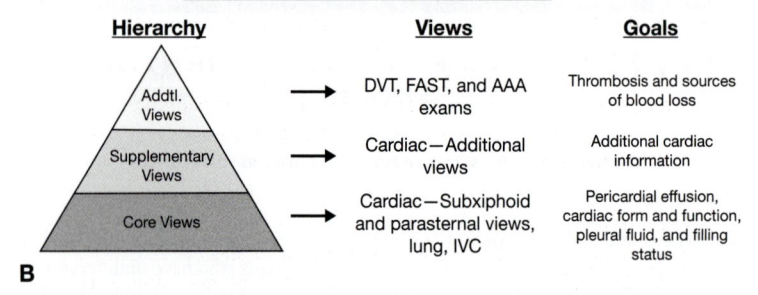

B

FIGURE 11.1 RUSH (A) and SHoC (B) protocols for evaluation of the patient who has undifferentiated hypotension. AAA, abdominal aortic aneurysm; A4C, apical four chamber; DVT, deep vein thrombosis; FAST, Focused Assessment with Sonography in Trauma; IVC, inferior vena cava; LUQ, left upper quadrant; PSL, parasternal long; PSS, parasternal short; RUQ, right upper quadrant.

SHoC Undifferentiated Hypotension Protocol

SHoC investigators created a more tiered approach (**Figure 11.1B**) based on the probability of identifying abnormal findings. The focus for each scan in the protocol is evaluation for fluid, form, function, and filling. This protocol recommends "core" views be performed on all patients; these include evaluation of the IVC and cardiac function and filling, as well as assessment for tamponade and signs of volume overload in the lungs. "Supplementary" cardiac views are indicated for patients where further information may be obtained without limiting further resuscitation, whereas "Additional" views searching for pathology such as intraabdominal free fluid or aortic aneurysm are only recommended based on individual patient circumstances.

Fluid Management

In addition to evaluation for shock etiology, POCUS can also assist in the fluid management of patients in shock. Both the RUSH and SHoC protocols include the evaluation of the IVC for volume assessment. A collapsed or nearly collapsed IVC is likely to predict a patient who is intravascularly depleted and therefore likely volume responsive.

Otherwise, IVC evaluation is less reliable in assessing the volume responsiveness of a patient without incorporating clinical context. For instance, although a plethoric IVC can be indicative of hypervolemia, the plethoric IVC in patients with cardiac tamponade or tension pneumothorax is not necessarily reflective of their volume status, and they may be volume depleted. Similarly, respiratory variation requirements depend on whether the patient is breathing spontaneously or undergoing positive pressure ventilation. In general, inspiratory IVC collapse of 50% or more indicates volume responsiveness in a spontaneously breathing patient, while for patients undergoing mechanical ventilation, evidence supports use of the IVC-DI over IVC distension alone in determining volume responsiveness. [IVC-DI = (change in IVC diameter/ minimum IVC diameter) × 100%] with an IVC-DI greater than 18% indicating volume responsiveness in patients who are passively breathing on the ventilator. Thus, IVC evaluation should be interpreted in the context of the patient's entire status rather than in isolation.

Given the limitations of IVC measurement, alternative strategies have been proposed to evaluate fluid responsiveness. Measurement of stroke volume variation using the LVOT-VTI can provide information about the potential volume responsiveness of the patient, with an increase in the VTI by 10% to 15% after a passive leg raise suggesting fluid responsiveness. There is ongoing research into other potential markers, including carotid flow time, IVC versus carotid measurements, and venous congestion evaluation, but these measurements are not quite ready for widespread use.

TEE

Finally, TEE can be considered for patients who have unstable hypotension. TEE allows for visualization of the heart without the obstruction of lungs, lines, or other monitoring devices. In the ED, TEE can be a consideration in patients who are intubated who have limited evaluation by TTE or need continuous, ongoing visualization of the heart. TEE requires both further training and equipment, however, limiting widespread implementation.

PEARLS

- Ultrasound can reduce diagnostic uncertainty and impact initial management decisions in undifferentiated shock, with a focus on the heart, lungs, and IVC, maximizing diagnostic yield.
- Inspiratory collapse of the IVC 50% or greater is suggestive of volume responsiveness in a spontaneously breathing patient, while an IVC-DI greater than 18% indicates fluid responsiveness in patients who are passively breathing and intubated.
- The LVOT-VTI with passive leg raise is a better assessment of volume responsiveness and should be used if the IVC is without marked respiratory variation.
- TEE plays a role in the resuscitation in patients who have limited transthoracic views or require continuous monitoring.

Suggested Readings

Barbier C, Loubières Y, Schmit C, et al. Respiratory changes in inferior vena cava diameter are helpful in predicting fluid responsiveness in ventilated septic patients. *Intensive Care Med.* 2004;30(9):1740-1746.

Milne J, Atkinson P, Lewis D, et al. Sonography in Hypotension and Cardiac Arrest (SHoC): rates of abnormal findings in undifferentiated hypotension and during cardiac arrest as a basis for consensus on a hierarchical point of care ultrasound protocol. *Cureus*. 2016;8(4):e564.

Shokoohi H, Boniface KS, Pourmand A, et al. Bedside ultrasound reduces diagnostic uncertainty and guides resuscitation in patients with undifferentiated hypotension. *Crit Care Med*. 2015;43(12):2562-2569.

Stolz LA, Shah A. Rapid Ultrasound for Shock and Hypotension (RUSH): hypotension evaluation. Sonoguide: Ultrasound Guide for Emergency Physicians. Published November 10, 2021. Accessed January 12, 2023. https://www.acep.org/sonoguide/advanced/rush/

12

Should You Administer Balanced Fluids or Normal Saline?

Nam Trinh and Rory Spiegel

The use of IV fluid administration in critically ill patients has been a topic of controversy since Alexis Hartmann first added sodium and bicarbonate to water. Most recently, a number of studies comparing the use of NS to "balanced" alternatives have advanced our understanding of this century-old debate. Early studies examining 0.9% sodium chloride solutions described an association between their use and hyperchloremic acidosis. The concern was that supraphysiologic concentrations of chloride would lead to or worsen hyperchloremia and metabolic acidosis. This can result in renal vasoconstriction, decreased GFR, and delayed time to first micturition. Experts feared that such disturbances in renal homeostasis could then lead to AKI, the need for invasive RRT, and even death.

Evidence

A recent barrage of RCTs examining this question has given us a far better understanding of the topic in question. In 2015, the SPLIT trial was published in *JAMA*, where the authors enrolled 2,278 patients in a cluster-randomized fashion to receive NS or buffered crystalloid. In this trial, balanced fluids did not decrease the risk of AKI, need for RRT, or mortality. Unfortunately, this trial suffered from several limitations. More than 70% of patients came from the operating room, and the majority of patients only received 1 to 2 L of NS. Given these limitations, it is unclear if this trial was capable of identifying the harms of NS in large volume resuscitation in critically ill patients.

In 2018, the SALT-ED trial and the SMART trial were published in concert in the *NEJM*. The SALT-ED, a single-center, unblinded RCT, showed no difference in hospital-free days in noncritically ill ED patients. The SMART, a non-blinded, cluster-randomized study with multiple crossovers, compared saline to balanced crystalloids in critically ill adults with sepsis. It found that patients randomized to the balanced fluids group experienced a 1.1% decrease in MAKE30. Unfortunately, this study was not blinded and the physicians could change fluid choice if they thought it was clinically appropriate. Moreover, SMART enrolled over 15,000 patients only finding a 1.1% difference in a composite outcome, which included death from any cause, new renal-replacement therapy, or persistent renal dysfunction. None of the individual components were found to be statistically significant, and most importantly the difference in the rate of persistent renal failure did not differ between the two groups, calling into question the validity of the underlying physiologic concern and thus the composite outcome used to demonstrate harm.

In August 2021, Zampieri et al published a large RCT examining the use of balanced solutions in the critically ill. The BASICS trial enrolled critically ill patients from 75 ICUs in Brazil requiring fluid resuscitation. The authors compared balanced solutions to 0.9% saline and found no difference in all-cause mortality at 90 days. The trial addressed many of the concerns of the previous trials examining this topic. It was a large, multicenter, blinded RCT. The patients received relatively high volumes of IV crystalloid: greater than 3 L over 72 hours. Despite enrolling critically ill patients who received aggressive fluid resuscitation strategies, the authors were unable to identify harm associated with the use of NS. In the same year, Finfer et al published the PLUS trial, another large-scale multicenter, double-blinded RCT including 53 ICUs in Australia and New Zealand. The authors enrolled 5,037 patients and like BASICS before it, they found no statistically significant difference in all-cause mortality at 90 days or evidence of AKI.

Conclusion

While it is well-documented that resuscitation using saline solutions will lead to a hyperchloremic acidosis, the current literature suggests its use does not affect clinically relevant outcomes such as hospital-free days, ICU-free days, need for RRT, and mortality. If there are no differences in those outcomes, when choosing the correct fluid, simple factors such as cost, availability, and physician comfort should play the major role. Ultimately, the initial choice of fluids does not appear to matter, especially when given judiciously. Rather, our focus should be on the volume of fluid administered, with the goal of restoring circulatory blood volume, while limiting the known harms associated with overaggressive fluid administration.

PEARLS

- NS administration can cause or worsen hyperchloremic acidosis.
- Multiple RCTs have found no difference in the incidence of AKI, need for RRT, or mortality, whether balanced fluids or NS is administered.
- Rather than focusing on fluid type, our primary concern should be to identify the appropriate volume of fluid to administer and avoid over-resuscitation.

Suggested Readings

Finfer S, Micallef S, Hammond N, et al. Balanced multielectrolyte solution versus saline in critically ill adults. *N Engl J Med*. 2022;386:815-826.

Self WH, Semler MW, Wanderer JP, et al. Balanced crystalloids versus saline in noncritically ill adults. *N Engl J Med*. 2018;378(9):819-828.

Young P, Bailey M, Beasley R, et al. Effect of a buffered crystalloid solution vs saline on acute kidney injury among patients in the intensive care unit: the SPLIT randomized clinical trial. *JAMA*. 2015;314(16):1701–1710.

Zampieri FG, Machado FR, Biondi RS, et al. Effect of intravenous fluid treatment with a balanced solution vs 0.9% saline solution on mortality in critically ill patients: the BaSICS randomized clinical trial. *JAMA*. 2021;326(9):818-829.

13

DON'T MAKE THESE PERIPHERAL PRESSOR PITFALLS

JOSEPH A. NELSON AND MARK SUTHERLAND

The administration of vasopressors through a peripheral IV catheter when central venous access is not immediately available has become a widely accepted practice. Historically, peripheral administration of vasopressors was contraindicated, given concerns for extravasation, limb ischemia, and tissue necrosis; however, delaying vasopressor administration until central venous access can be obtained can put patients at risk of decompensation. Recent analyses of critically ill patients observed a 2% increase in mortality for each hour vasopressor initiation was delayed. In this setting, the Surviving Sepsis Campaign guideline now recommends the prioritization of peripheral vasopressors to reverse systemic shock and prevent end-organ hypoperfusion if central access is not readily available. Peripheral vasopressor infusions can expedite appropriate management in critically ill patients and in some patients, obviate the need for central venous access altogether.

RISKS OF PERIPHERAL VASOPRESSOR ADMINISTRATION

A systematic review has estimated the risk of vasopressor extravasation at 1.8% in adults and 3.3% in children. These percentages are comparable to the risks associated with central venous access, such as pneumothorax, central line–associated deep vein thrombosis, and central line–associated blood stream infection. Serious complications related to peripheral vasopressors are infrequently documented. Most recently, an analysis of 1,300 patients did not find any adverse events of limb ischemia or tissue necrosis.

SELECTION OF AN IV SITE FOR PERIPHERAL VASOPRESSORS

Loubani et al. performed a systematic review demonstrating that the risk of extravasation was higher in lines placed distal to the antecubital fossa. This is corroborated by a prospective study conducted in 55 ED patients who received vasopressors for various forms of shock. Of these patients, two suffered extravasation injuries, one in the hand and the other in the antecubital fossa. Despite these complications, none were serious nor did they require further intervention. In addition to attaining proximal access, the utilization of a large-bore catheter is predicted to decrease the risk of infiltration. NYU Langone Medical Center conducted a chart review that found an increased risk of complications in smaller gauge IVs, as 75% of the complications were associated with a 20-gauge IV or smaller. Thus, it would prove beneficial to use larger proximal vessels with larger bore peripheral IVs for vasopressor administration.

USING A DILUTE CONCENTRATION OF VASOPRESSOR

Dilute concentrations of vasopressors may improve the safety of peripheral administration. A retrospective cohort study analyzed 14,385 perioperative patients receiving peripheral norepinephrine infusions and found an estimated risk of 0 to 2 events per 10,000 patients. One of the metrics that informed their low rate of adverse events was the use of a dilute norepinephrine infusion (20 mcg/mL). At present, no studies have compared the risk of complications in various concentrations of peripheral infusions. Until there is a better understanding of the safety profiles of higher concentration infusions, it is advisable to use lower concentrations of vasopressors peripherally to minimize the risk of complications.

Evaluate the Peripheral Vasopressor Infusion Site

The attention given to peripheral vasopressor infusions is highly variable among providers. To decrease the risk of complications, some studies propose an interdisciplinary protocol to increase awareness of peripheral infusions across pharmacy, physicians, and nursing to ensure frequent monitoring and create contingency plans for complications. Some examples include implementing monitoring or documentation guidelines or limiting the duration of infusion at each site. Long Island Jewish Medical Center protocolized vasopressor administration by ensuring peripheral infusions were initiated with ultrasound-guided access, in a vein larger than 4 mm, frequent assessments of the access site, and with a maximum duration of 72 hours per infusion site. With this protocol, there was a 2% risk of PIV infiltration and no patients developed long-standing tissue injury. Other centers have observed an increased risk of infiltration with infusions beyond 24 hours. Given these findings, it may be beneficial to limit peripheral vasopressor infusions to less than 24 hours or switch access points beyond this time frame. If complications should occur, be aware that peripheral vasopressor infusions more often resulted in severe hypotension in comparison to central catheters. This may occur in the setting of suboptimal vasopressor absorption systemically and delays with transitioning the medication to an alternate site. To mitigate the risk of hypotension, maintaining at least two working access sites at all times could ensure a quick transition of the infusion to an alternate access point.

There are many trade-offs associated with central vasopressor infusions versus peripheral vasopressor administration. With a low incidence of minor complications, the preponderance of evidence suggests that vasopressors can be safely administered peripherally and may improve mortality by allowing quicker initiation of therapy. Implementing safety measures following peripheral vasopressor initiation and maintenance will minimize the risks of extravasation.

PEARLS

- Mortality is increased for each hour delay in vasopressor administration, and the Surviving Sepsis Campaign guidelines recommend the prioritization of peripheral vasopressors to treat hypotension if central access is not readily available.
- Large-gauge IVs (>20 gauge) in proximal arm locations have lower risks of extravasation.
- Dilute vasopressor infusions may reduce the complications from an extravasation event.
- Establish a process or protocol to evaluate the sites of peripheral vasopressor infusions to reduce the chance of extravasation injury.

Suggested Readings

Cardenas-Garcia J, Schaub KF, Belchikov YG, Narasimhan M, Koenig SJ, Mayo PH. Safety of peripheral intravenous administration of vasoactive medication. *J Hosp Med.* 2015;10(9):581-585.

Lewis T, Merchan C, Altshuler D, Papadopoulos J. Safety of the peripheral administration of vasopressor agents. *J Intensive Care Med.* 2019;34(1):26-33.

Loubani OM, Green RS. A systematic review of extravasation and local tissue injury from administration of vasopressors through peripheral intravenous catheters and central venous catheters. *J Crit Care.* 2015;30(3):653.e9-653.e6.53E17.

Marti K, Hartley C, Sweeney E, Mah J, Pugliese N. Evaluation of the safety of a novel peripheral vasopressor pilot program and the impact on central line placement in medical and surgical intensive care units. *Am J Health Syst Pharm.* 2022;79(suppl 3):S79-S85.

Medlej K, Kazzi AA, El Hajj Chehade A, et al. Complications from administration of vasopressors through peripheral venous catheters: an observational study. *J Emerg Med.* 2018;54(1):47-53.

Owen VS, Rosgen BK, Cherak SJ, et al. Adverse events associated with administration of vasopressor medications through a peripheral intravenous catheter: a systematic review and meta-analysis. *Crit Care.* 2021;25(1):146.

Pancaro C, Shah N, Pasma W, et al. Risk of major complications after perioperative norepinephrine infusion through peripheral intravenous lines in a multicenter study. *Anesth Analg.* 2020;131(4):1060-1065.

Tian DH, Smyth C, Keijzers G, et al. Safety of peripheral administration of vasopressor medications: a systematic review. *Emerg Med Australas.* 2020;32(2):220-227.

Tran QK, Mester G, Bzhilyanskaya V, et al. Complication of vasopressor infusion through peripheral venous catheter: a systematic review and meta-analysis. *Am J Emerg Med.* 2020;38(11):2434-2443.

14

Massive Transfusion or Massive Confusion?

Mustfa Khalid Manzur and Hillary Caroline Moss

MT is typically defined as an infusion of 4 units of blood within an hour, 50% of blood volume replacement within 3 hours, or 10 units of blood within 24 hours. The exact definitions and protocols defining MT vary widely because they are developed and implemented at an institutional level. MT is particularly important in the management of hemorrhagic shock, where the keys to effective management are tripartite: restore oxygenation, maintain volume, and prevent additional losses of blood by correcting coagulopathies and establishing control of bleeding.

Selection of patients for MT has been inconsistent. Purely relying on gestalt is a poor predictor of actual need for MT. The most widely used approach partners gestalt with the prospectively validated ABC scoring system. ABC assigns one point each for a heart rate above 120 bpm, systolic blood pressure below 90 mm Hg, a penetrating trauma mechanism, and a positive FAST examination. A score greater than 2 indicates that the patient will likely need MT. This is an imperfect approach because tachycardia above 120 bpm may be stymied by beta-blocker or calcium channel blocker therapy, for example. Thus, most clinicians partner the ABC score with other factors to activate an MT protocol: clinical instability, the presence of active bleeding, and multiple transfusions in the ED.

Historically, the first step in resuscitation was to immediately restore intravascular volume with a crystalloid infusion. This approach has come into question recently due to crystalloid infusion's unintended consequences—acidosis and hemodilution—leading secondarily to coagulopathy already present in many critically ill patients. Large bolus administration of crystalloid is associated with dilutional coagulopathy, compartment syndrome, acute respiratory distress syndrome, multiple organ dysfunction syndrome, and hypoxemia. Even small volumes of crystalloid have been associated with increased mortality in traumatic patients with hypotension. A shift away from crystalloid infusion to both earlier transfusion of blood products and early infusion of plasma has now come into vogue. Early resuscitation with plasma is associated with improved likelihood of survival.

The 2015 PROPPR study was the landmark study that evaluated the ideal ratio of blood product transfusion (plasma:platelets:RBCs). This randomized control trial found that patients who received a 1:1:1 ratio of these blood products, as compared to a 1:1:2 ratio, had no significant difference in mortality, but did have lower rates of exsanguination and higher rates of hemostasis. There was no difference in complication rates between the two groups. Based on this trial, utilization of a 1:1:1 ratio for plasma, platelets, and RBCs is recommended in the setting of MT protocol.

Additionally, TXA is a common agent available for use in the ED to help curb blood loss in an acutely hemorrhaging patient. TXA is an antifibrinolytic agent that inhibits the activation of plasminogen to plasmin. Plasmin, in turn, is responsible for the breakdown of fibrin, which plays a crucial role in the lattice structure of blood clots. Notably, the role of TXA in the hemorrhaging trauma patient was investigated in the CRASH-2 study, an international, randomized, controlled trial of over 20,000 trauma patients with or at risk for significant bleeding. TXA, given intravenously as a bolus of 1 g over 10 minutes followed by 1 g over 8 hours, significantly reduced all-cause mortality and death due to bleeding as compared to placebo, without any increase in vasoocclusive events or deaths. In order to optimize its benefits, TXA should be given within the first 3 hours after trauma.

TEG may be used to curb the overall amount of blood product during MT. TEG is a laboratory test that comprehensively profiles the function of platelets in a sample, including fibrin formation, time to achieve sufficient clot strength, and amount of fibrinolysis. Each aspect of a TEG profile from a sample of blood can be specifically addressed by fresh frozen plasma, cryoprecipitate, platelets, desmopressin, or TXA. If TEG is not available at your institution, fibrinogen level may be a viable alternative.

Risks of MT are not insignificant. Besides the usual risk of transfusion reactions and transmission of blood-borne diseases, patients undergoing MT are at risk for volume overload, hypocalcemia (due to the presence of citrate preservative in blood products that precipitates calcium), hyperkalemia, acidosis, and hypothermia. Physical trauma to tissue and acute renal failure secondary to hypoxia drive the development of hyperkalemia and must be monitored for and corrected to the extent possible to prevent dysrhythmia. Calcium levels should be monitored during MT or alternatively calcium should be empirically dosed to overcome the effect of citrate.

PEARLS

- Plasma should be the first line for initial volume replacement in the setting of hemorrhagic shock; crystalloid administration should be avoided.
- Blood product transfusion ratio during MT is optimized when provided in a 1:1:1 ratio for plasma, platelets, and packed RBCs.
- Calcium level should be monitored during MT and, if not possible, calcium should be empirically dosed to overcome the effect of citrate, which is a blood product preservative that precipitates calcium.
- TEG should be utilized when possible to curb the overall amount of blood product during MT. If TEG is not available at your institution, fibrinogen level may be a viable alternative.

SUGGESTED READINGS

Chang R, Holcomb JB. Optimal fluid therapy for traumatic hemorrhagic shock. *Crit Care Clin.* 2017;33(1):15-36.

D'Amore K, Swaminathan A. Massive gastrointestinal hemorrhage. *Emerg Med Clin North Am.* 2020;38(4):871-889.

Elmer J, Wilcox SR, Raja AS. Massive transfusion in traumatic shock. *J Emerg Med.* 2013;44(4):829-838.

Holcomb JB, Tilley BC, Baraniuk S, et al. Transfusion of plasma, platelets, and red blood cells in a 1:1:1 vs. a 1:1:2 ratio and mortality in patients with severe trauma: the PROPPR randomized clinical trial. *JAMA.* 2015;313(5):471-482.

Pham HP, Shaz BH. Update on massive transfusions. *Br J Anaesth.* 2013;111(suppl 1):i71-i82.

Pommerening MJ, Goodman MD, Holcomb JB, et al. Clinical gestalt and the prediction of massive transfusion after trauma. *Injury.* 2015;46(5):807-813.

Shakur H, Roberts I, Bautista R, et al. Effects of tranexamic acid on death, vascular occlusive events, and blood transfusion in trauma patients with significant haemorrhage (CRASH-2): a randomised, placebo-controlled trial. *Lancet.* 2010;376(9734):23-32.

15

SHOULD YOU EVER PERFORM AN ED THORACOTOMY?

HARRY V. FLASTER AND MICHAEL R. EHMANN

Resuscitative thoracotomy (RT), also termed ED thoracotomy, is perhaps the most dramatic—and certainly the most invasive—procedure in the emergency physician's armamentarium. It is also among the most controversial, but when performed correctly on the appropriate patient for the appropriate indications, RT can be associated with significantly improved survival for a moribund patient.

RT is a temporizing measure and should not be performed in the absence of rapid access to an operating room with an appropriately trained surgeon. RT is indicated for patients who have suffered a penetrating thoracic injury and are observed by health care personnel (either prehospital or ED) to have objective signs of life prior to cardiopulmonary arrest and loss of vital signs. Objective signs of life include pupillary response, spontaneous ventilation, carotid pulse, measurable or palpable blood pressure, spontaneous movement, cardiac motion on ultrasound, or cardiac electrical activity. The procedure may be considered in patients sustaining penetrating nonthoracic injury, though the likelihood of survival is lower than for penetrating thoracic injury. Due to the very low rate of post-thoracotomy survival in patients who have suffered blunt traumatic injury, RT may be considered only very rarely for survivors of blunt trauma with vital signs in the ED who subsequently suffer cardiopulmonary arrest witnessed by ED personnel. RT in patients with blunt injury without signs of life on presentation is not recommended because of dismal neurologically intact survival (0.1%) and the inherent risk of the procedure to health care personnel.

Successful RT requires choreographed resuscitation of the patient with many simultaneous actions occurring in parallel. All patients undergoing RT require a definitive airway, right-sided chest tube or finger thoracostomy, adequate vascular access, and blood products available for hemodynamic support. Throughout this high-intensity procedure, coordination is of the utmost importance to ensure the safety of the entire treatment team, as the procedure places clinicians at high risk for blood-borne pathogen exposure.

Available equipment, including a thoracotomy tray, chest tubes, stapler, a suction device, internal defibrillator paddles, and ACLS medications, should be readied. While preparing for the procedure, CPR should be continued with personnel performing external chest compressions on the patient's right side to avoid interfering with thoracotomy setup on the patient's left. The clinician performing the RT should be familiar with the indications for the procedure and the steps required to perform RT. Patients who regain vital signs following resuscitative efforts and completion of the RT must be transferred immediately to the operating room for definitive management of their injuries.

Common complications of RT include phrenic nerve injury, coronary artery injury, postprocedure infection, and injury or disease transmission to health care workers. While the RT has been practiced for over half a century, investigation of novel techniques in the management of cardiopulmonary arrest secondary to trauma is ongoing. New tools—such as REBOA—may augment or replace resuscitative thoracotomy, depending on the location of the injury (see Chapter 16).

PEARLS

- RT is indicated for penetrating thoracic injury with observed signs of life prior to cardiopulmonary arrest.
- RT may be considered for penetrating nonthoracic injury though rates of survival are low.
- Survival and neurologic recovery following RT are the highest for patients with witnessed signs of life, penetrating thoracic injury, stab wounds, and cardiac injury.
- Correct placement of the rib spreader with the crossbar located laterally and the handle and ratchet bar oriented parallel to the floor to allow the operator to extend the left anterolateral thoracotomy incision to a clamshell incision, if necessary.
- RT should be undertaken only if the treating facility has resources to provide definitive care for the patient and if the safety of all treatment team members can be assured.

Suggested Readings

Burlew CC, Moore EE, Moore FA, et al. Western trauma association critical decisions in trauma: resuscitative thoracotomy. *J Trauma Acute Care Surg*. 2012;73(6):1359-1363.

DuBose J, Fabian T, Bee T, et al. Contemporary utilization of resuscitative thoracotomy: results from the AAST Aortic Occlusion for Resuscitation in Trauma and Acute Care Surgery (AORTA) multicenter registry. *Shock*. 2018;50(4):414-420.

Liu A, Nguyen J, Ehrlich H, et al. Emergency resuscitative thoracotomy for civilian thoracic trauma in the field and emergency department settings: a systematic review and meta-analysis. *J Surg Res*. 2022;273:44-55.

Seamon MJ, Haut ER, Van Arendonk K, et al. An evidence-based approach to patient selection for emergency department thoracotomy: a practice management guideline from the Eastern Association for the Surgery of Trauma. *J Trauma Acute Care Surg*. 2015;79(1):159-173.

Slessor D, Hunter S. To be blunt: are we wasting our time? Emergency department thoracotomy following blunt trauma: a systematic review and meta-analysis. *Ann Emerg Med*. 2015;65(3):297-307.e16.

16

Know the Indications for REBOA Placement in the ED

Casey Lee Wilson and Errett Jacks

ED RT with ACC remains the most common procedure for hemorrhage control in patients with penetrating trauma and witnessed loss of vital signs. Unfortunately, current survival rates for RT remain a dismal 15%. ED RT also incurs significant potential risks to the providers who perform them. REBOA has been developed as an adjunct for hemorrhage control and to sustain vital perfusion until definitive hemostasis can be achieved. REBOA has seen more frequent use since the introduction of a catheter specifically adapted for ED use. The primary indication for REBOA is abdominopelvic trauma noncompressible hemorrhage that is suspected to be below the diaphragm. Multiple meta-analyses demonstrate that REBOA may result in a lower mortality rate compared to RT with ACC in patients with penetrating trauma.

REBOA Zones and Appropriate Placement

REBOA can be quickly placed when performed according to a protocol. Placement within the aorta occurs via the common femoral artery, and the depth of placement is guided by the level of trauma, which is approximated via an external measurement. Zone I is the supradiaphragmatic location within the thoracic aorta and allows for control of lower torso, abdominal, or lower extremity bleeding; this location is relevant for hemorrhagic abdominal trauma. Zone I placement is measured externally from the femoral insertion site to the xiphoid process (~46 cm). Zone II placement is extremely variable and should be avoided, as it is associated with vascular complications from celiac and renal artery disruption. Zone III is considered the least complicated and is inferior to the renal arteries and proximal to the iliac bifurcation. Zone III placement is intended to control bleeding in the pelvis and lower extremities. Zone III placement is measured externally from the femoral insertion site to the level of the umbilicus (~27 cm). Bedside aortic ultrasound can be utilized to obtain the appropriate level of occlusion when fluoroscopy is not readily available.

Noncompressible torso hemorrhage has a mortality rate that approaches 50%. Animal studies that have compared REBOA to RT demonstrated improved physiologic parameters and improved survival with REBOA. REBOA can serve as a salvage method of circulatory support until definitive hemostasis is obtained in patients with end-stage hypovolemic shock. Inflation of the balloon allows for increased mean arterial pressure and improved afterload support. Shorter times of balloon inflation lower the risk of ischemic insult and result in greater patient survival. Zone III inflation is generally 60 to 90 minutes compared to the shorter time of 30 to 60 minutes for Zone I inflation.

Previous studies in the vascular and cardiothoracic surgery literature have demonstrated poor outcomes with ACC. Spinal cord injury and paralysis are the most devastating complications and occur in up to 23% of patients. The beneficial hemodynamic effect of REBOA must be balanced by the potential untoward metabolic sequelae from ischemia-reperfusion injury. Critical care facilities and anticipated organ support are essential in any environment where REBOA is used.

REBOA in Pediatric Patients

REBOA has been used in pediatric patients, with research demonstrating a significant increase in systolic blood pressure following balloon deployment with no reported REBOA-related complications. As in adult patients, proper selection of pediatric patients that would most benefit from REBOA remains an area of investigation.

REBOA is an emerging alternative to RT or laparotomy for the rapid control of exsanguinating noncompressible torso and abdominopelvic trauma. It is ideal in military and resource-poor settings, where damage control resuscitation is critical. In addition, REBOA has demonstrated promise in the prehospital setting where mortality remains high because of hemorrhagic shock. To sustain broad utilization of REBOA, further investigation and the eventual protocolization of patient selection and intervention timing are critical. As techniques and technology advance, physicians will need to carefully consider the available evidence and resources to determine its applicability in their respective practice settings. REBOA continues to remain an exciting area of investigation for the proactive management of noncompressible truncal hemorrhage, and future adaptations may also show a role in nontraumatic cardiac arrest.

PEARLS

- RT with open ACC and internal cardiac massage remain the current treatment for traumatic circulatory arrest.
- Ongoing REBOA studies suggest that procedure-related deaths and major complications are minimal, and REBOA holds promise as an alternative treatment for noncompressible torso hemorrhage.
- REBOA may be a "future consideration" in terms of widespread use by emergency physicians as an alternative to ED RT.
- No high-quality data currently exist to support the widespread use of REBOA; however, meta-analyses suggest decreased mortality.
- Further research, as well as institution-dependent resources and expertise, will need to be conducted prior to pervasive use of REBOA.

SUGGESTED READINGS

Khalid S, Khatri M, Siddiqui MS, Ahmed J. Resuscitative endovascular balloon occlusion of aorta versus aortic cross-clamping by thoracotomy for noncompressible torso hemorrhage: a meta-analysis. *J Surg Res.* 2021;270:252-260.

Moore LJ, Brenner M, Kozar RA, et al. Implementation of resuscitative endovascular balloon occlusion of the aorta as an alternative to resuscitative thoracotomy for noncompressible truncal hemorrhage. *J Trauma Acute Care Surg.* 2015;79(4):523-532.

Morrison JJ, Ross JD, Markov NP, et al. The inflammatory sequelae of aortic balloon occlusion in hemorrhagic shock. *J Surg Res.* 2014;191:423-431.

Samuels JM, Sun K, Moore EE, et al. Resuscitative endovascular balloon occlusion of the aorta—interest is widespread but need for training persists. *J Trauma Acute Care Surg.* 2020;89(4):e112-e116.

17

RECOGNIZE AND RESUSCITATE CARDIAC TAMPONADE BEFORE YOUR PATIENT CRASHES

NORA MCNULTY AND NICHOLAS SANTAVICCA

Pericardial effusions are common and may be infectious or noninfectious in etiology. Cardiac tamponade, however, is relatively rare and occurs when the pressure of the accumulated pericardial fluid restricts diastolic filling of the ventricles, thereby decreasing venous return and cardiac output. The pericardium is relatively stiff and the rate of fluid accumulation impacts its ability to accommodate higher volumes. Sudden ventricular free wall rupture, for example, will cause rapid pericardial fluid expansion with dramatic pressure increases even with volumes as small as 50 mL, while subacute or chronic effusions give the pericardium time to stretch, accommodating as much as 2 to 3 L of fluid.

CLINICAL PRESENTATION

Patient presentations may vary considerably, from relatively asymptomatic to critically ill. The most common presenting symptom is dyspnea, which occurs in the majority of cases. Other symptoms include palpitations, chest pain, and lethargy. The classically described Beck triad (muffled heart sounds, jugular venous distension, and hypotension) is infrequently seen and is neither sensitive nor specific. As a result, it is important for emergency clinicians to maintain a high clinical suspicion for this entity.

EVALUATION

After history and physical, ECG and US are the two main modalities for the detection of cardiac tamponade. ECG findings are neither sensitive nor specific but may demonstrate:

- Sinus tachycardia or arrhythmia
- Low QRS voltage (see **Figure 17.1**)
    - Electrical alternans (alternation of the height of QRS complexes as the heart "swings" within the fluid-filled pericardium)

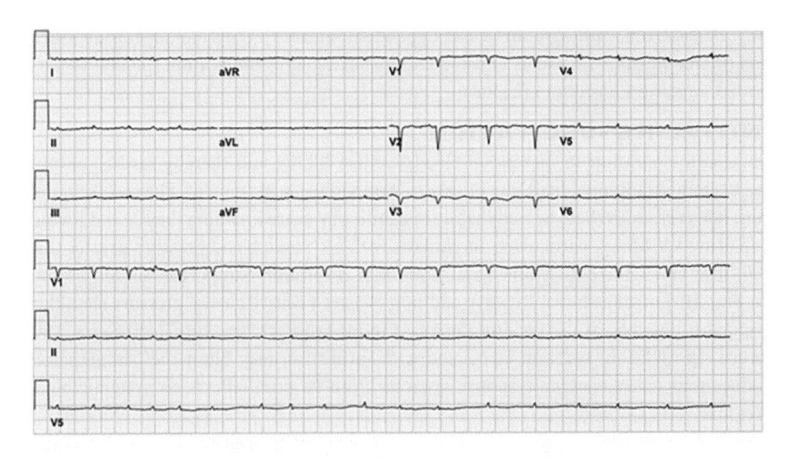

FIGURE 17.1 ECG with sinus tachycardia and low QRS voltage in the setting of cardiac tamponade. (Courtesy of Jason Lupow, MD and Molly Moseley, MD, Montefiore Medical Center.)

Bedside echocardiography will typically reveal hypoechoic fluid surrounding the heart, with various findings suggesting obstructed cardiac filling due to tamponade:

- RA systolic collapse; earliest sign, highly sensitive
- Diastolic RV collapse (see **Figure 17.2**); highly specific
- IVC dilation without respiratory variation (see **Figure 17.2**); sensitive
    - Exaggerated inspiratory variation in mitral valve (25% decrease) and tricuspid valve (40% increase) in-flow velocities, with pulse-wave Doppler placed at the tips of the valves on apical four-chamber view; "ultrasonographic pulsus paradoxus," relatively sensitive

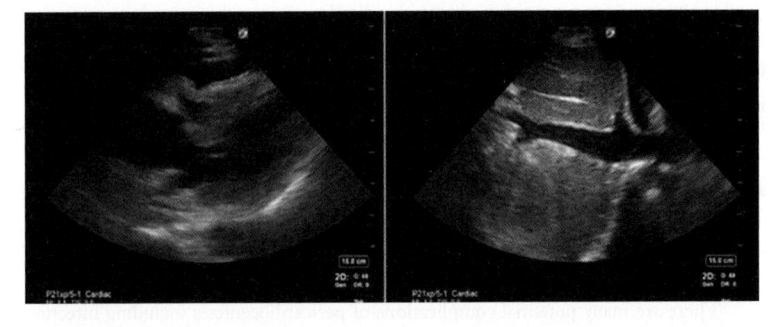

FIGURE 17.2 Parasternal long cardiac view showing hypoechoic region anteriorly suggestive of effusion with left right ventricular collapse (**left**) and IVC dilation with minimal respiratory variation in the setting of cardiac tamponade (**right**). (Courtesy of Taylor Burden, MD, Jacobi Medical Center.)

Bedside echocardiography is user dependent; notable pitfalls include misidentification of an epicardial fat pad as effusion and mistaking effusion location (pleural vs pericardial, missing a posterior effusion).

Initial Resuscitation

Fluid administration to increase preload, cardiac filling, and thereby cardiac output, has been the traditional mainstay of cardiac tamponade management. Overresuscitation may, however, exacerbate hemodynamic instability by overdistending the RV and further impairing LV filling, particularly in patients with a systolic blood pressure greater than 100 mm Hg. Utilize high-flow nasal cannula if respiratory support is needed beyond the standard nasal cannula. Invasive and noninvasive positive airway pressure should be avoided if possible, as the resulting increase in intrathoracic pressure decreases venous return. In addition, sedation associated with intubation may blunt the compensatory endogenous catecholamine response separate from its usual effects on systemic blood pressure.

Vasoactive use in cardiac tamponade has historically been unhelpful. The body's endogenous surge of catecholamines during tamponade increases chronotropy and inotropy of the heart in an attempt to maintain systemic perfusion, and additional exogenous catecholamines provide minimal additional effect. If the patient does not have tachycardia on presentation, however, norepinephrine or epinephrine infusions *may* be considered to increase the heart rate and mean arterial pressure, avoiding overcorrection of afterload and worsening of obstructive shock. Systemic vasodilators such as dobutamine and milrinone are not recommended.

Definitive Management

The definitive management of cardiac tamponade involves pericardial drainage. In the ED, stabilization is best achieved by needle pericardiocentesis, except in cases of tamponade requiring emergent surgical intervention, such as that secondary to trauma, myocardial free wall rupture, and aortic dissection.

While various approaches have been described, the subxiphoid approach using ultrasound guidance is the simplest. While patients in cardiac arrest will be supine, patients with a pulse should be positioned with their head of bed slightly elevated to help decrease respiratory distress and bring the pericardium closer to the chest wall. Ultrasound identification of the largest effusion diameter beforehand maximizes pericardiocentesis success rate, while direct visualization during the procedure minimizes inappropriate intracardiac drainage and allows clues into potential clotted hemopericardium if blood cannot be immediately aspirated.

- Under as sterile a technique as possible depending on patient stability, insert a long 18-gauge pericardiocentesis or spinal needle through the skin at a 30° to 45° angle.
- Aspirate with a syringe while advancing the needle in line with the transducer's view, toward the left shoulder, until there is fluid return.
  - The required amount of drainage and overall success of the pericardiocentesis are determined by hemodynamic improvement.

There are many potential complications of pericardiocentesis including infection, injury to neighboring intraabdominal and intrathoracic structures, and others. Patients with cardiac tamponade require specialist consultation and close monitoring in an ICU setting after ED stabilization.

PEARLS

- Beck triad is insensitive. Maintain a high level of suspicion for cardiac tamponade in patients presenting with dyspnea, especially without pulmonary findings.
- Echocardiography remains the best modality to identify cardiac tamponade. The absence of RA systolic collapse and a dilated IVC without respiratory variation have high sensitivities, while RV diastolic collapse and the presence of more than 25% mitral valve in-flow respiratory variation are quite specific.
- Initial hemodynamic stabilization may involve fluid administration, but overresuscitation can worsen hemodynamics. Vasoactives are generally unhelpful.
- The definitive treatment for most cases of tamponade is pericardiocentesis, except for those requiring surgery in which pericardiocentesis is contraindicated.

SUGGESTED READINGS

Alerhand S, Carter JM. What echocardiographic findings suggest a pericardial effusion is causing tamponade? *Am J Emerg Med*. 2019;37(2):321-326.

Alerhand S, Adrian RJ, Long B, Avila J. Pericardial tamponade: a comprehensive emergency medicine and echocardiography review. *Am J Emerg Med*. 2022;58:159-174.

Flint N, Siegel RJ. Echo-guided pericardiocentesis: when and how should it be performed? *Curr Cardiol Rep*. 2020;22(8):71.

Kearns MJ, Walley KR. Tamponade: hemodynamic and echocardiographic diagnosis. *Chest*. 2018;153(5):1266-1275.

Synovitz CK, Brown EJ. Pericardiocentesis. *In:* Cline DM, Ma O, Cydulka RK, Meckler GD, Handel DA, Thomas SH, eds. *Tintinalli's Emergency Medicine: A Comprehensive Study Guide*. 7th ed. The McGraw-Hill Companies, Inc.; 2011:250-257.

18

KNOW HOW TO MEND A BROKEN HEART

MICHAEL G. ALLISON

Cardiogenic shock is a condition of inadequate organ perfusion due to cardiac dysfunction and has an inpatient mortality rate of over 50%. Patients present in varying degrees of extremis and are usually described as being "cold" on the classic warm/cold dichotomy used to describe patients with heart failure. Patients can present with a variety of etiologies for cardiac dysfunction, such as myocardial infarction, valvular disorders, arrhythmias, and even toxicologic causes. Cardiogenic shock is defined by a constellation of hemodynamic alterations leading to decreased organ perfusion. There are varying societal definitions and clinical trial inclusion criteria, but nearly all include some component of hypotension (usually SBP <90 mm Hg) and organ hypoperfusion (manifested on clinical examinations, labs, or urinary output). Cardiogenic shock has an incidence of about 6%, and outcomes for patients who are diagnosed with shock have improved, mainly as a result of early reperfusion therapies provided to patients with acute myocardial infarction. Hemodynamic support of the patient in shock is essential to get patients to definitive therapy and to support organ dysfunction until cardiac function improves.

Pharmacologic Support

Inotropic support is the mainstay of immediate therapy for patients with cardiogenic shock. Inotropes act by increasing cardiac contractility. Guidelines do not recommend one particular agent over another, due to the general paucity of consistent data from randomized, controlled trials to direct a preferred agent. Choices include inopressors such as norepinephrine and epinephrine, and inodilators such as dobutamine and milrinone. Norepinephrine and epinephrine are catecholamines that act through alpha- and beta-receptor agonism, whereas dobutamine is a catecholamine that acts primarily through beta-2 receptor agonism. Milrinone is a phosphodiesterase inhibitor that acts through induction of increased cyclic AMP. Dopamine is another inopressor with alpha- and beta-activities but has demonstrated increased tachydysrhythmias and increased mortality when used in patients with cardiogenic shock when compared with norepinephrine. Dopamine has widely fallen out of favor since the publication of the SOAP II trial in 2010. Norepinephrine has become the default first-line inopressor for many types of shock, including cardiogenic shock. A study in 2018 (OptimaCC) looked at the comparison between norepinephrine and epinephrine in patients with acute myocardial infarction. Though just 57 patients were enrolled, epinephrine had a statistically significant increase in refractory shock. Other adverse events did not reach statistical significance, perhaps due to the small sample size. The 2022 DOREMI trial compared dobutamine with milrinone in the treatment of 192 patients with cardiogenic shock and found no difference in the primary outcome of a composite endpoint that included death, arrest, need for mechanical support, stroke, or renal failure. The pragmatic approach suggested in the 2017 AHA cardiogenic shock guidelines represents a reasonable starting point for hemodynamic management. In classic cases of cardiogenic shock, use of norepinephrine plus either dobutamine or milrinone represents a reasonable starting point, adjusting therapy once the etiology of cardiogenic shock is better delineated.

Other considerations for initial management include withholding antihypertensives and negative inotropic agents. This includes avoiding the continuation of home beta-blockers and not initiating any intravenous beta-blockade for tachydysrhythmias. For patients with suspected ischemia, a P2Y12 inhibitor (such as clopidogrel, prasugrel, or ticagrelor) should not be initiated before coronary imaging. This practice allows for the safe planning of cardiac surgery for patients in need of urgent or emergent invasive revascularization or valvular intervention based upon the results of subsequent cardiac studies.

Intravenous Fluids

The administration of intravenous fluids is generally avoided in patients with cardiogenic shock, as these patients are often on the flat portion of the Frank-Starling curve and will not improve their cardiac output with volume loading. Two scenarios in which fluids may be indicated—in small aliquots with close monitoring—include patients who develop cold and dry heart failure with shock due to rapid titration of diuretics and GDMT and patients with right ventricular failure due to infarction. GDMT therapies (beta-blockers, aldosterone receptor blockers, angiotensin-converting enzyme inhibitors, and neprilysin inhibitors) are the mainstay of outpatient medical therapy for heart failure but may cause volume depletion, kidney injury, and negative inotropic effects on cardiovascular function. Diuretics should be held in patients who appear "cold and dry." A low ejection fraction does not preclude the use of small volumes of fluid for hypovolemia. Similarly, patients with right ventricular dysfunction may see initial benefit from the use of intravascular volume expansion with crystalloids.

Temporary MCS

MCS is added on for patients who fail to improve their cardiac index and organ perfusion despite the addition of inotropes and vasopressors. These devices work by mechanically pumping blood, making it more efficient for the heart itself to pump blood. IABP have traditionally been used to increase coronary perfusion pressure during acute coronary syndromes. IABPs inflate and deflate in the descending aorta, creating a vacuum through which cardiac output increases (by ~0.5 L/min) and systemic vascular resistance decreases. The cardiac output is rather modest compared with other support devices like the Impella, a percutaneous transvalvular left ventricular assist device. This device uses an impellor motor within the device to suction blood from the left ventricle and pump it into the ascending aorta. Depending on the device inserted, the Impella can improve cardiac output by 1 to 5 L/min. Venoarterial ECMO can provide complete circulatory support and is used in cases where there is biventricular cardiac failure as a bridge to recovery or definitive therapy.

PEARLS

- Patients in cardiogenic shock have a very high mortality rate. Finding and correcting the underlying cause can improve patient outcomes.
- Dopamine should be avoided in patients with cardiogenic shock due to increased incidence of tachydysrhythmias and increased mortality.
- Norepinephrine is a reasonable first-line agent for patients in shock, and an inodilator such as dobutamine or milrinone can be added to augment cardiac output.
- Avoid giving patients in cardiogenic shock beta-blockers.
- Consider early referral to a center capable of providing MCS for cases refractory to initial therapy.

Suggested Readings

Combes A, Price S, Slutsky AS, Brodie D. Temporary circulatory support for cardiogenic shock. *Lancet*. 2020;396(10245):199-212.

De Backer D, Biston P, Devriendt J, et al. Comparison of dopamine and norepinephrine in the treatment of shock. *N Engl J Med*. 2010;362(9):779-789.

Mathew R, Di Santo P, Jung RG, et al. Milrinone as compared with dobutamine in the treatment of cardiogenic shock. *N Engl J Med*. 2021;385(6):516-525.

van Diepen S, Katz JN, Albert NM, et al. Contemporary management of cardiogenic shock: a scientific statement from the American Heart Association. *Circulation*. 2017; 136(16):e232-e268.

19

CPAP, BiPAP, AND HFNC—OH MY!

BO QIN AND JOHN C. GREENWOOD

Resuscitation of patients in acute respiratory distress is a core component of emergency medicine, where prompt interventions are critical to avoid serious complications and death. Noninvasive modalities of respiratory support, specifically CPAP, BiPAP, and HFNC, have demonstrated significant utility in the management of respiratory failure from a variety of conditions in the ED.

NPPV

The two forms of NPPV are CPAP and BiPAP. CPAP delivers a constant amount of pressure throughout the entire respiratory cycle. BiPAP delivers a distinct pressure during inspiration and expiration. The inspiratory positive airway pressure is abbreviated IPAP and the expiratory positive airway pressure is abbreviated EPAP. The EPAP component of BiPAP is equivalent to the PEEP prescribed with CPAP and improves oxygenation by recruiting collapsed alveoli, redistributing pulmonary fluid, and diminishing ventilation-perfusion mismatch. BiPAP additionally improves ventilation by generating a pressure gradient between the inspiratory phase and expiratory phase, increasing ventilatory support in patients with hypercapnic respiratory failure (**Figure 19.1**).

HFNC

HFNC delivers heated, humidified oxygen at flow rates up to 60 LPM. This supports oxygenation by matching or exceeding the patient's inspiratory flow demands, thereby reducing oxygen dilution from the entrainment of room air. The prescribed flow rate may provide a low level of dynamic positive airway pressure, as well as support ventilation through carbon dioxide washout and reducing dead space. In general, it should be assumed that HFNC provides negligible ventilation support and only addresses hypoxia.

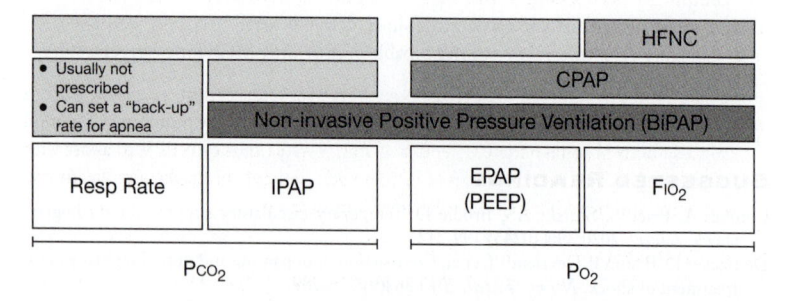

FIGURE 19.1 Modes of noninvasive respiratory support and how they affect specific targets of respiratory failure. BiPAP, bilevel positive airway pressure; CPAP, continuous positive airway pressure; EPAP, expiratory positive airway pressure; FiO_2, fraction of inspired oxygen; HFNC, high-flow nasal cannula; IPAP, inspiratory positive airway pressure; PEEP, positive end-expiratory pressure.

Patient Selection

Primary contraindications for NPPV and HFNC include hemodynamic instability, inability to protect the airway, upper airway obstruction, and facial trauma. NPPV or HFNC should be initiated as soon as possible in patients who exhibit significant work of breathing or hypoxia refractory to standard nasal cannula therapy to prevent worsening respiratory decompensation.

When placing a patient on NPPV, the initial step is to select the appropriate mask. The oronasal mask is most commonly used. After the patient is correctly fitted, the NPPV mode and pressure settings are selected. It is best to start with lower inspiratory pressure(s) to allow the patient to adapt to the mask and ventilator. Oxygenation can be improved by increasing the FIO_2 or by increasing the PEEP (or EPAP in BiPAP mode). Ventilation can be increased on BiPAP by increasing the difference (delta) between IPAP and EPAP, thus increasing ventilatory driving pressure. Beware of prescribing an IPAP greater than 20 cm H_2O, as this has been associated with an increased risk of gastric insufflation and aspiration. High inspiratory pressures may additionally result in significant mask leaking, which can impact the ability to provide long-standing NPPV therapy.

For a patient requiring HFNC, the initial step is to set the FIO_2 and oxygen flow rate. The FIO_2 can be titrated to the patient's oxygen saturation goal, while the flow can be titrated based on the patient's respiratory status and comfort. Patients with greater respiratory distress may require higher flow to reduce entrainment of room air.

After initiation of NPPV or HFNC, patients should be closely monitored to ensure an appropriate response to the intervention. The key components of reevaluation include vital signs, mental status, cardiopulmonary exam, and blood gas values. NPPV can be challenging for patients to tolerate, but can be alleviated with verbal guidance, changes in pressure settings, or pharmacologic agents such as short-acting opioids, benzodiazepines, low-dose ketamine, haloperidol, or dexmedetomidine.

Indications

CHF and COPD

There is robust evidence to support NPPV as a first-line respiratory support in patients with respiratory failure from exacerbations of CHF and COPD. In this patient population, NPPV has been shown to decrease the need for intubation, shorten hospital and ICU stay, and improve mortality.

Asthma Exacerbation

While data on the use of NPPV in patients with asthma exacerbation are mixed when it comes to reduction in intubation and mortality, NPPV may improve pulmonary function and decrease both hospital and ICU length of stay. A short trial of NPPV to assist with ventilatory fatigue is a reasonable choice in asthmatic patients, given the significant risk of barotrauma and hyperinflation associated with intubation.

Primary Hypoxemic Respiratory Failure

The optimal oxygenation strategy in patients with primary hypoxemic respiratory failure, most commonly pneumonia or exacerbation of interstitial lung diseases, remains controversial. A recent meta-analysis showed a reduction in mortality with NPPV and a reduction in the rate of intubation with both NPPV and HFNC. In a large 2015 randomized controlled trial, the use of HFNC resulted in lower mortality compared with both NPPV and standard oxygen. While further studies are needed, a trial of HFNC or NPPV is usually warranted in the patient with primary hypoxemic respiratory failure.

High Risk of Failure	Moderate Risk	Low Risk of Failure
ROX Index ≤ 3	ROX Index 3-5	ROX Index > 5

FIGURE 19.2 Clinical approach to using the ROX index for identifying patients at risk for HFNC failure. Dark gray indicates high risk for HFNC failure, light gray indicates moderate risk, and white indicates low risk.

The ROX index, defined as ($[SpO_2/FIO_2]$/respiratory rate), is a simple clinical tool that can help predict the need for intubation for patients on HFNC. In a prospective cohort study, a ROX index greater than or equal to 4.88 at 2, 6, and 12 hours was associated with a lower risk of requiring intubation, while an index less than 2.85, 3.47, and 3.85 at 2, 6, and 12 hours, respectively, was associated with increased risk (**Figure 19.2**).

Preoxygenation Prior to Intubation

Patients who require intubation are typically preoxygenated with 100% oxygen delivered by nasal cannula and nonrebreather in order to prevent desaturation during the apneic period. There are times when this method may not be sufficient to provide adequate preoxygenation. The literature suggests that patients who are preoxygenated with NPPV tend to have fewer desaturations during intubation compared to patients receiving either standard oxygen or HFNC.

PEARLS

- HFNC should generally be used in patients with pure hypoxemic respiratory insufficiency.
- NPPV has the highest level of evidence for benefit in patients with acute exacerbations of COPD and CHF.
- A short trial of NPPV or HFNC is appropriate for alert patients with hypoxemic or hypercapnic respiratory insufficiency.
- HFNC should generally be avoided in patients with hypercapnic respiratory failure, as it provides negligible ventilatory support.
- Increasing EPAP/PEEP/CPAP improves oxygenation while increasing IPAP improves ventilation.
- Patients on NPPV or HFNC require frequent reevaluation. Worsening clinical status or lack of improvement is an indication to escalate to endotracheal intubation.

SUGGESTED READINGS

Cabrini L, Landoni G, Oriani A, et al. Non-invasive ventilation and survival in acute care settings: a comprehensive systematic review and meta-analysis of randomized controlled trails. *Crit Care Med*. 2015;43(4):880-888.

Ferreyro BL, Angriman F, Munshi L, et al. Association of non-invasive oxygenation strategies with all-cause mortality in adults with acute hypoxemic respiratory failure: a systematic review and meta-analysis. *JAMA*. 2020;324:1-12.

Fong KM, Au SY, Ng GWY. Preoxygenation before intubation in adult patients with acute hypoxemic respiratory failure: a network meta-analysis of randomized trials. *Crit Care*. 2019; 23:319.

Frat JP, Thille AW, Mercat A, et al. High-flow oxygen through nasal cannula in acute hypoxemic respiratory failure. *N Engl J Med*. 2015;372:2185-2196.

Martin J, Hall RV. Non-invasive ventilation. *Crit Decis Emerg Med*. 2015;29(2):11-18.

Nava S, Hill N. Non-invasive ventilation in acute respiratory failure. *Lancet*. 2009;374:250-259.

Ozyilmaz E, Ugurlu AO, Nava S. Timing of non-invasive ventilation failure: causes, risk factors, and potential remedies. *BMC Pulm Med*. 2014;13:14-19.

Roca O, Caralt B, Messika J, et al. An index combining respiratory rate and oxygenation to predict outcome of nasal high-flow therapy. *Am J Respir Crit Care Med*. 2019;199(11):1368-1376.

Vital FM, Ladeira MT, Atallah AN. Non-invasive positive pressure ventilation (CPAP or bilevel NPPV) for cardiogenic pulmonary oedema. *Cochrane Database Syst Rev*. 2013;(5): CD00531.

20

Interpreting the Post-ROSC ECG

Maia Winkel and Michael P. McGregor

A 12-lead ECG should be performed following ROSC in a patient resuscitated from cardiac arrest. An early postarrest ECG is critical to determine the presence of STEMI or STEMI equivalent. ECG patterns suggestive of STEMI or STEMI equivalents include the following:

1) Classic STEMI criteria
   ST segment elevations greater than 1 mm in two or more contiguous leads with two exceptions:
   a) In V2 and V3, ST-segment elevation should be 1.5 mm or more in female patients, 2.0 mm or more in male patients who are 40 years or above, and 2.5 mm or more in male patients below 40 years
   b) ST-segment depression in V1-V3 instead of elevation (indicative of posterior MI)
2) Modified Sgarbossa criteria in the setting of a left-bundle branch block or paced rhythm
   a) Concordant ST-segment elevation 1 mm or more in any lead with a positive QRS complex
   b) Concordant ST-segment depression 1 mm or more in V1, V2, or V3
   c) Excessive discordant ST elevation as 25% or more of the depth of the preceding S wave
3) Left main equivalent disease
   a) Greater than or equal to 70% stenosis of the proximal left anterior descending coronary artery and proximal left circumflex artery with less than or equal to 50% stenosis of the left main coronary artery
   b) Associated ECG findings include ST-segment elevations in aVR greater than or equal to V1 in the presence of diffuse ST-segment depressions in leads I, II, and V4-V6
4) Diffuse ST-segment depressions

If the ECG demonstrates any of these findings, the next step in postcardiac arrest care is emergent cardiac catheterization with potential PCI. Recent literature has questioned the need for immediate coronary angiography in the absence of STEMI on a post-ROSC ECG.

A Push for Delayed Post-ROSC ECGs

Standard postcardiac arrest care entailed obtaining a post-ROSC ECG as soon as possible. This practice has been called into question based on a 2021 study that demonstrated post-ROSC ECGs obtained within the first 7 minutes after ROSC were often falsely positive for a STEMI (18.5%). These ECGs suggested an ischemic cause of arrest, however, did not correlate with findings at the time of catheterization. ECGs performed between 8 and 33 minutes had fewer false positives (7.2%). If the initial post-ROSC ECG is obtained within the first few minutes following ROSC, the emergency physician should consider repeating the ECG after a few more minutes to more accurately evaluate for the presence of a STEMI or STEMI equivalents.

It is essential to remember two main points:

1) STE is not always initially present during the most acute phase of coronary occlusion (or occlusive presentations, such as left main equivalents or multivessel disease).
2) A decreased flow state during and immediately after cardiac arrest can cause global or regional coronary ischemia leading to nonocclusive STE. This "demand" ischemia and associated ECG findings should improve with IV fluids and vasopressors as appropriate.

Multiple trials have demonstrated that there is no benefit to immediate angiography for patients with ROSC and no evidence of STE on ECG when compared with delayed angiography. It can be helpful to consider this evidence when deciding how emergently a post-ROSC patient should be taken for cardiac catheterization.

A Push for Immediate Post-ROSC ECGs

A common belief is that the severe metabolic derangements present in the immediate post-ROSC period may prevent accurate analysis of the post-ROSC ECG, resulting in erroneous decisions to proceed with angiography. However, a 2020 study demonstrated that the initial post-ROSC ECG and follow-up ECG interpretations were similarly able to predict angiographically and clinically significant acute coronary occlusions in out-of-hospital cardiac arrest when read by experienced clinicians.

Considerations

The primary objective of obtaining an accurate interpretation of the post-ROSC ECG is to appropriately direct the resources necessary to stabilize the patient. If the underlying cause is coronary occlusion, the patient will need emergent catheterization with reperfusion. If the cause is not cardiac, performing catheterization may delay resuscitation and other diagnostic studies to find the cause of arrest.

PEARLS

- If an immediate post-ROSC ECG is obtained, order another at least 8 minutes afterward to ensure that the ECG findings persist.
- Hypoperfusion can produce STE on the ECG that is due to nonocclusive demand ischemia.

- If there is any doubt, consult cardiology for possible catheterization lab activation; acute culprit lesions can be the cause of cardiac arrest without necessarily producing STEs.

Suggested Readings

Baldi E, Schnaubelt S, Caputo ML, et al. Association of timing of electrocardiogram acquisition after return of spontaneous circulation with coronary angiography findings in patients with out-of-hospital cardiac arrest. *JAMA Netw Open*. 2021;4(1):e2032875.

Brown MA, Klusewitz S, Elefteriades J, Prescher L. The current state of coronary revascularization: percutaneous coronary intervention versus coronary artery bypass graft surgery. *Int J Angiol*. 2021;30(3):228-242.

Desch S, Freund A, Akin I, et al. Angiography after out-of-hospital cardiac arrest without ST-segment elevation. *N Engl J Med*. 2021;385:2544-2553.

Fasolino A, Compagnoni S, Baldi E, et al. Updates on post-resuscitation care. After the return of spontaneous circulation beyond the 2021 guidelines. *Rev Cardiovasc Med*. 2022;23(11):373.

Lemkes JS, Janssens GN, van der Hoeven NW, et al. CAG after cardiac arrest without ST-segment elevation. *N Engl J Med*. 2019;380:1397-1407.

Sharma A, Miranda DF, Rodin H, Bart BA, Smith SW, Shroff GR. Do not disregard the initial 12 lead ECG after out-of-hospital cardiac arrest: it predicts angiographic culprit despite metabolic abnormalities. *Resusc Plus*. 2020;4:100032.

Sharma A, Miranda DF, Rodin H, Bart BA, Smith SW, Shroff GR. Interobserver variability among experienced electrocardiogram readers to diagnose acute thrombotic coronary occlusion in patients with out of hospital cardiac arrest: impact of metabolic milieu and angiographic culprit. *Resuscitation*. 2022;172:24-31.

21

Pearls for the Patient With Pulmonary Hypertension

Taylor Miller and Lucas Sjeklocha

PH is a broad and underappreciated diagnosis that has increased in prevalence. Symptoms of PH are often nonspecific, and the diagnosis can be delayed by years. PH was recently redefined as a mean pulmonary artery pressure of above 20 mm Hg (from over 25 mm Hg). Numerous other indicators that reflect high pulmonary pressures with an elevated workload on the RV can be obtained by less invasive diagnostic methods. PH is currently classified into five groups (**Table 21.1**).

PH and RV Failure

The RV is a thin-walled, crescent-shaped, low-pressure pump that supplies the usually compliant pulmonary arteries. As such, it is afterload sensitive, and disturbances in volume status, medication compliance, oxygenation, ventilation, acid-base status, and poor

Table 21.1 Classification of PH

WHO Classification	Mechanism	Management
Group 1	Primary PAH that may or may not be associated with other systemic diseases	Specialty input on PAH-specific therapy
Group 2	Elevated pulmonary pressure due to left heart failure	Treatment of underlying disorder
Group 3	Elevated pulmonary pressure associated with lung disease or chronic hypoxia	Treatment of underlying disorder
Group 4	Chronic thromboembolic PH or other obstructive processes	Treatment of underlying disorder
Group 5	Unknown mechanisms including systemic disorders such as sarcoidosis or hematologic disorders	Treatment of underlying disorder

PAH, pulmonary arterial hypertension; PH, pulmonary hypertension; WHO, World Health Organization.

systemic perfusion can trigger a vicious cycle of pulmonary vasoconstriction and RV failure that can be difficult to reverse. Several aspects of RV and pulmonary physiology contribute to this feedback loop:

- Increased RV afterload impedes flow, leading to RV overdistension, decreased pump function, and tricuspid regurgitation.
- RV overload leading to increased RV pressures and poor LV filling causes interventricular septal bowing, further impinging on LV preload and reducing cardiac output.
- As cardiac output decreases and right-sided pressures rise relative to systemic blood pressure, RV perfusion decreases, worsening RV ischemia and function and exacerbating RV overload.

Decompensated PH and RV dysfunction are often not considered by clinicians despite clinical signs. Patients often present with volume overload—a lack of pulmonary edema despite other signs of peripheral edema or cardiogenic shock may suggest RV failure. These patients experience congestion in the abdominal circulation as well, so gastrointestinal symptoms should also prompt consideration of RV dysfunction. Common resuscitative maneuvers such as intubation or fluid boluses may cause further deterioration if instituted before the RV is supported. Because of this, PH should be considered in patients with seemingly paradoxical responses to these initial therapies.

Early assessment with bedside ultrasound is crucial in critically ill patients. Echocardiographic signs of PH or RV dysfunction include an elevated RV to LV ratio, echocardiographic "D sign," and decreased TAPSE.

RESUSCITATE THE RV TO AVOID DETERIORATION

Systemic hypotension can be catastrophic, leading to poor RV perfusion and the vicious cycle noted earlier. Aggressively defend the MAP with early vasopressors; norepinephrine is an appropriate general first-line vasopressor. Vasopressin is a second-line vasopressor and has desirable effects in advanced PH. Avoid pure alpha agonists like phenylephrine in patients with PH. Inotropes may be needed in those with cardiogenic shock, with preference for dobutamine, although low-dose epinephrine or milrinone can also be used. Fluid administration should be judicious, if fluids are given at all, with small aliquots and frequent reassessment. Indeed, in patients with decompensation due to volume overload, initiation of diuresis after institution of vasopressor and/or inotropic support may be needed.

Cardiac arrhythmias, including atrial fibrillation, are common in PH and may trigger decompensation. Prompt rhythm control is desirable, avoiding negative inotropes such as beta-blockers and calcium channel blockers in decompensated RV failure; early cardioversion may be needed. Support oxygenation and ventilation, as hypoxia and hypercarbia cause pulmonary vasoconstriction that worsens PH and RV afterload. Avoidance of positive pressure ventilation is ideal given its effects on RV preload, but if needed, lower PEEP strategies should be implemented after appropriate hemodynamic support. In critically ill patients, inhaled pulmonary vasodilators (eg, nitric oxide), prostacyclins (eg, epoprostenol), or milrinone can be administered via either HFNC or mechanical ventilator to reduce RV afterload. It is important that these medications are given via inhaled route rather than IV to avoid systemic vasodilatation and ventilation-perfusion mismatch that can induce RV collapse. Critically ill patients may also be candidates for mechanical circulatory support or transplant, and early referral to specialized centers should be made in consultation with a PH specialist or intensivist, if possible.

Optimize the Intubation That Can't Be Avoided

In general, intubation should be avoided in severe PH with RV failure, given the well-recognized risk of hemodynamic collapse. It may, however, be necessary while treating the underlying cause of PH, especially in Group 2 or Group 3 patients. If intubation is necessary, every effort should be made to perform a hemodynamically neutral procedure with minimization of sedation, use of more hemodynamically stable sedatives, effective preoxygenation, and peri-procedure administration of vasopressors and/or inotropes. Strongly consider a continuous vasopressor infusion initiated prior to intubation and consider awake intubation in suitable patients.

Continue PAH Medications in the ED

Abrupt discontinuation of home PH medications can trigger rapid cardiovascular collapse. Common oral medications include riociguat, PDE-5 inhibitors (eg, sildenafil, tadalafil), and endothelin receptor antagonists (eg, bosentan, ambrisentan). Prostacyclin agonists can be given via the oral (selexipag), inhaled (treprostinil), or infusion (epoprostenol, treprostinil) routes. Ensure access to home medications during the ED visit, and consider early specialty consultation if the patient encounters any disruptions in supply.

PEARLS

- Ensure home PH medication continuation in the ED.
- Assess RV function and fluid status with bedside ultrasound in patients with known PH.
- Avoid intubation, if possible, but support the RV and optimize hemodynamics if intubation is required.
- Discuss with a PH specialist or intensivist, and consider early referral to a specialty center.

SUGGESTED READINGS

Konstam MA, Kiernan MS, Bernstein D, et al. Evaluation and management of right-sided heart failure. *Circulation*. 2018;137:e578–e622.
Simon E, Bridwell RE, Montrief T, et al. Evaluation and management of pulmonary hypertension in the emergency department setting. *Am J Emerg Med*. 2020;38(6):1237–1244.
Taichman DB. Pulmonary arterial hypertension. *N Engl J Med*. 2021;385:2361-2376.
Wilcox SR, Kabrhel C, Channick RN. Pulmonary hypertension and right ventricular failure in emergency medicine. *Ann Em Med*. 2015;66(6):619-628.

22

WHEN SHOULD I GIVE LYTICS FOR PE?

NOUR AL JALBOUT AND SARAH BADIN

Acute PE affects as many as 900,000 Americans and is responsible for more than 100,000 annual deaths in the United States. It is associated with long-term morbidity, risk of recurrence, and high medical costs. The workup of acute PE is aided by signs and symptoms, risk factor analysis, and the support of decision rules. Symptoms include chest pain, dyspnea, cough, hemoptysis, syncope, or symptoms of DVT. Signs of PE include tachycardia, tachypnea, fever, hypoxia, hypotension, severe bradycardia, altered mental status, or signs of DVT. Risk factors include a variety of hypercoagulable states, such as pregnancy, active malignancy, coagulation disorders, recent surgery, major trauma, lower extremity fractures, immobilization, and oral contraceptives or hormone replacement therapy. Prior venous thromboembolism is a significant risk factor for PE. Decision rules such as Wells criteria, Geneva score, and PERC have been developed to help clinicians in the workup of suspected PE, given the multiple signs, symptoms, and clinical presentations. The most common diagnostic test employed for PE is a CT pulmonary angiography.

STRATIFICATION OF PE

Once a PE is diagnosed, the next step in management is to classify the type of PE. Risk stratification is essential for guiding subsequent management. High-risk (massive) PE, or hemodynamically unstable PE, is defined as a PE with sustained hypotension (a systolic blood pressure <90 mm Hg or a drop of ≥40 mm Hg from baseline for at least 15 minutes); hypotension requiring inotropic support that is not explained by other causes; or persistent profound bradycardia (heart rate <40 bpm) with signs or symptoms of shock. The term massive PE is sometimes used interchangeably with high-risk PE, and it refers to the presence of hemodynamic compromise rather than the size of the PE. Patients with hemodynamically unstable PE are more likely to die from severe RV dysfunction and obstructive shock, especially in the first 2 hours. Tools such as the PESI and Bova scores are used to stratify hemodynamically stable patients into intermediate (submassive) or low risk based on their risk of developing complications. While the PESI takes into account patient characteristics, medical history, vital signs, and clinical status, and is used alongside other imaging and biomarker (pro-BNP and troponin) results, the Bova score incorporates BP, HR, troponin levels, and signs of RV dysfunction on echocardiography or CT.

MANAGEMENT OF ACUTE PE

The initial management of patients presenting with PE is centered on optimizing their oxygenation and hemodynamics. In hemodynamically unstable PE, the priority is restoring adequate circulation and initiating definitive therapy promptly. In both hemodynamically stable and unstable PE, point-of-care echocardiography is extremely useful for ruling in signs of RV dysfunction, identifying alternative diagnoses for shock, and guiding further resuscitation. Anticoagulation is the mainstay of therapy for all patients without major contraindications. Initial treatment regimens may include UFH for high-risk PE and LMWH or fondaparinux for intermediate- and low-risk PE.

WHO SHOULD RECEIVE THROMBOLYSIS?

The decision to administer thrombolytic agents depends on an individualized assessment and must incorporate patient wishes, life expectancy, comorbidities, and risk of bleeding.

Systemic thrombolysis is recommended in patients with high-risk PE as it decreases all-cause mortality, decreases PE recurrence, and leads to stabilization of respiratory and cardiovascular function (low evidence) at the expense of increasing both major (moderate evidence) and minor hemorrhagic events (low evidence). These recommendations are supported by society guidelines from the ACC, the CHEST, and the ESC. While there is a strong indication for thrombolysis in patients with high-risk/massive PE, those with low-risk PE should not receive thrombolytics.

The decision to administer thrombolytics is more difficult for patients classified as having intermediate-risk PE. Some institutions have formed PE response teams, and this team should be consulted for guidance, if available. The ACC recommends that patients who are at intermediate risk by PESI score and have evidence of RV dysfunction should be considered for systemic thrombolysis or CDT. The rationale for thrombolysis is based on the observation that severe RV dysfunction is associated with a worse prognosis. Patients who decompensate despite initial anticoagulation should be considered for rescue thrombolytic therapy as supported by multiple guidelines. Patients with absolute contraindications to thrombolysis or other high risk for bleeding should not receive this therapy. Instead, assessment for CDT is warranted.

CHOICE AND ADMINISTRATION OF THROMBOLYTIC

Thrombolytic therapy is typically administered via a peripheral intravenous catheter as an infusion. Alteplase and tenecteplase are available in the United States, whereas streptokinase and urokinase are available as additional treatment options in other countries. Alteplase is administered at 100 mg dose as a continuous infusion over 2 hours (for lower rates of bleeding) while withholding anticoagulation during the infusion period. Tenecteplase is dosed based on the patient's weight. In cases of cardiac arrest, alteplase can be administered as a bolus or as an infusion over 15 minutes.

PEARLS

- Patients with hemodynamic instability due to acute PE should receive thrombolytic therapy unless there is an absolute contraindication.
- Bedside ultrasound can be used to determine the presence of RV dysfunction and aid in the risk stratification of patients with acute PE.

- Patients with intermediate-risk PE should have an individualized approach to the administration of thrombolytics.
- Patients with low-risk PE should not receive thrombolysis.

SUGGESTED READINGS

Giri J, Sista AK, Weinberg I, et al. Interventional therapies for acute pulmonary embolism: current status and principles for the development of novel evidence: a scientific statement from the American Heart Association. *Circulation.* 2019;140(20):e774–e801.

Jaff MR, McMurtry MS, Archer SL, et al. Management of massive and submassive pulmonary embolism, iliofemoral deep vein thrombosis, and chronic thromboembolic pulmonary hypertension: a scientific statement from the American Heart Association. *Circulation.* 2011;123(16):1788-1830.

Konstantinides SV, Meyer G, Becattini C, et al. 2019 ESC guidelines for the diagnosis and management of acute pulmonary embolism developed in collaboration with the European Respiratory Society (Ers). *Eur Heart J.* 2020;41(4):543-603.

Stevens SM, Woller SC, Kreuziger LB, et al. Antithrombotic therapy for VTE disease. *Chest.* 2021;160(6):e545-e608.

Zuo Z, Yue J, Dong BR, Wu T, Liu GJ, Hao Q. Thrombolytic therapy for pulmonary embolism. *Cochrane Database Syst Rev.* 2021;2021(4):CD004437.

23

KNOW HOW TO RESUSCITATE THE CRASHING TOX PATIENT

TIFFANY C. FONG AND HARRY E. HEVERLING

Resuscitation of the critically ill poisoned patient requires careful consideration to avoid exacerbating the underlying toxicologic pathophysiology, yet usually occurs with incomplete or erroneous information. Obtaining a reliable history from the patient is challenging, and offending agents and dosages are rarely identified. For this reason, an understanding of typical toxidromes (**Table 23.1**) is essential, although presentations may still vary due to patient-specific factors and potential confounding by polysubstance ingestions.

EVALUATION OF THE POISONED PATIENT

Initial focus on the "ABCs", or "CABs", takes priority, with an added "D-E" for immediate external decontamination and enhanced elimination if indicated. Evaluation of the patient's vital signs and perfusion while obtaining IV access and a 12-lead ECG and placing the patient on telemetry and pulse oximetry monitoring are crucial first steps for all poisoned patients. Continuous end-tidal CO_2 monitoring may be appropriate for early detection of hypercarbia and respiratory failure. Assessment of the patient's neurologic status overlaps with the patient's hemodynamic and respiratory evaluation but remains

TABLE 23.1 COMMON TOXIDROMES

	MENTAL STATUS	T	BP	HR	RR	PUPILS	SKIN	OTHER	EXAMPLES OF TOXIC AGENTS
Sympathomimetic	Agitated, hypervigilant, paranoid, hallucinating	↑	↑	↑	↑	Dilated	Diaphoretic	Tremor, seizures	Cocaine, amphetamines, synthetic cathinones ("bath salts"), pseudoephedrine
Ethanol or sedative-hypnotic withdrawal	Restless, anxious, agitated, disoriented, hallucinating	↑	↑	↑	↑	Dilated	Diaphoretic	Tremor, seizures	
Serotonin syndrome	Normal to confused or agitated delirium	↔/↑	↑	↑	↔/↑	Dilated or normal	Diaphoretic or normal	Tremor, hyperreflexia, clonus, seizures, diarrhea	SSRI, SNRI, MAOI, TCA, meperidine, dextromethorphan
Opioid withdrawal	Normal to anxious, dysphoric, or agitated	↔	↑	↑	↔	Dilated	Diaphoretic	Vomiting, diarrhea, rhinorrhea, piloerection, yawning	
Anticholinergic	Delirious, hallucinating, mumbling speech	↑	↔/↑	↑	↔/↑	Dilated	Dry and flushed	Dry mucous membranes, urinary retention	Antihistamines, prochlorperazine, cyclobenzaprine, TCA, atropine
Hallucinogen	Hallucinating, perceptual distortion, to delirious or agitated	↔/↑	↔/↑	↔/↑	↔/↑	Usually dilated	Variable	Nystagmus in some	MDMA ("ecstasy"), PCP, ketamine, LSD, psilocybin, mescaline

(continued)

TABLE 23.1 COMMON TOXIDROMES (CONTINUED)

	MENTAL STATUS	T	BP	HR	RR	PUPILS	SKIN	OTHER	EXAMPLES OF TOXIC AGENTS
Cholinergic	Normal to depressed	↔	↔/↓	↓	↑/↓	Constricted	Diaphoretic	"SLUDGE" (salivation, lacrimation, urination, diarrhea, GI cramping, emesis) "Killer Bs" (bradycardia, bronchorrhea, bronchospasm), seizures, fasciculations, paralysis	Organophosphate and carbamate insecticides, nerve agents (sarin, soman, VX, tabun, Novichok), nicotine, physostigmine, edrophonium
Sedative-hypnotic	Sedated, confused, comatose	↔/↓	↓	↓	↓	Variable	Variable	Nystagmus, hyporeflexia, ataxia, respiratory depression	Benzodiazepines, barbiturates, ethanol and other alcohols, gabapentin, zolpidem
Opioid	Sedated, comatose	↓	↓	↓	↓	Constricted	Variable	Hyporeflexia	Opioids (heroin, fentanyl morphine, oxycodone, hydromorphone, methadone), loperamide

↑, increases; ↓, decreases; ↔, unchanged; BP, blood pressure; HR, heart rate; GI, gastrointestinal; LSD, lysergic acid diethylamide; MAOI, monoamine oxidase inhibitor; MDMA, 3,4-methylenedioxymethamphetamine; PCP, phencyclidine; RR, respiratory rate; SNRI, serotonin-norepinephrine reuptake inhibitor; SSRI, selective serotonin reuptake inhibitor; T, temperature; TCA, tricyclic antidepressant; VX, venomous agent X.

a key part of the poisoning primary survey, with depressed mentation, agitation, and/or seizures potentially requiring immediate intervention and, in conjunction with pupillary findings, providing clues as to offending agents.

After primary evaluation and stabilization of emergent hemodynamic, respiratory, or neurologic issues, a comprehensive secondary survey must be performed. Potentially life-threatening extremes of temperature must be identified and managed, notably severe hyperthermia (core temperature >106 °F or 41.1 °C), which requires aggressive cooling to below 101.5 °F (38.7 °C) within 30 minutes. Medications may be indicated in specific circumstances, such as dantrolene for malignant hyperthermia caused by inhalational anesthetics and rarely by succinylcholine. A thorough head-to-toe examination should be performed to rule out the presence of medication patches as well as trauma, as intoxicated patients are at higher risk of traumatic injury.

Circulation

Unstable dysrhythmias result from direct effects on cardiac myocytes and the autonomic nervous system and are exacerbated by hypoxia, acidemia, and electrolyte abnormalities. WCT can result from several classes of drugs that block sodium channels, including Type IA antidysrhythmics (eg, procainamide, lidocaine, flecainide, quinidine), local anesthetics, antihistamines, bupropion, carbamazepine, topiramate, TCAs, and cocaine. Bradycardia can manifest as the end-stage of several poisonings but is classically seen with beta-blockers, calcium channel blockers, and digoxin. Hypo- or hypertension may occur depending on the drug's effects on cardiac function, vascular smooth muscle, and patient volume status. POCUS should be performed, evaluating volume status and cardiac function, to help guide resuscitation, and vasopressors or inotropes started if needed. Antidotes directed at the specific causative agent are definitive treatment, but initial stabilization can require additional treatment considerations (**Table 23.2**).

Airway and Breathing

Sedatives and other depressants may cause respiratory compromise if no immediate antidote (eg, naloxone, dextrose) is available. Stabilization can range from airway repositioning or nasal cannula to endotracheal intubation, which is generally indicated for airway protection with a GCS score of 8 or less, even without hypoxia. Hypercarbia can be present before oxygen saturation is affected; end-tidal CO_2 monitoring and/or blood gas sampling helps identify early respiratory failure. For bradypnea or respiratory arrest due to suspected opiate overdose, a trial of IV or IN naloxone provides both diagnostic and potential therapeutic benefits.

Neurotoxicity

Depressed mentation can occur as a direct or indirect effect of the offending agent. Agitation may be caused by drug intoxication or withdrawal, traumatic brain injury, or psychosis. If medication is needed, benzodiazepines are the preferred agents, especially midazolam (rapid intramuscular absorption) and diazepam due to rapid onset and time-to-peak effect. Antipsychotic agents such as haloperidol and droperidol should be used with caution as they may impair heat dissipation, lower seizure threshold, cause QTc prolongation, and are contraindicated in serotonin syndrome and NMS. Seizures may be precipitated by numerous agents, whether due to intoxication or withdrawal. They tend to be less responsive to standard antiepileptic drugs, and benzodiazepines are the mainstay of treatment due to their efficacy and ability to avoid worsening the underlying toxicity. Refractory or recurrent seizures can occur in some poisonings if the underlying

TABLE 23.2	EXAMPLES OF TOXIN-DEPENDENT STABILIZATION CONSIDERATIONS	
	PRESENTATION	STABILIZING THERAPY
Sodium-channel blocker	Unstable, wide complex tachycardia	Sodium bicarbonate: 1-2 mEq/kg IV bolus every 3-5 min until QRS <100 ms, followed by an infusion at double the maintenance rate with goal serum pH 7.50-7.55
	Unstable bradycardia	1. Atropine: 0.5-1.0 mg IV every 2-3 min to a maximum dose of 3 mg 2. Epinephrine: 2-10 mcg/min IV titrated to heart rate
Calcium channel beta blocker digoxin		3. Temporary transcutaneous or transvenous cardiac pacing for medication—refractory bradycardia
	Cardiogenic shock	1. Concentrated regular insulin: 1 unit/kg/h, IV with concomitant dextrose bolus and infusion 2. ECMO consultation for treatment-refractory shock
Long-acting opiate	Recurrent bradypnea, hypercarbic hypoxic respiratory failure, respiratory arrest	Naloxone IV infusion: initial rate two-thirds effective awakening dose, titrated to respiratory rate >12 breaths/min
Isoniazid	Refractory/recurrent seizures	Pyridoxine: 1 g IV per gram of ingested isoniazid, or 5 g if amount of isoniazid is unknown.

ECMO, extracorporeal membrane oxygenation; g, gram; IV, intravenous; kg, kilogram; mEq, milliequivalents; mg, milligram.

etiology is not addressed, such as with sodium-channel blockers, carbon monoxide, isoniazid, and hypoglycemic agents.

Decontamination

External decontamination may be crucial in poisonings due to dermal exposure, but GI decontamination is *not* part of the initial resuscitation of a poisoned patient. Historically considered in patients presenting within 1 hour after ingestion, large overdoses, or overdoses without antidote, methods such as gastric lavage, whole bowel irrigation, and use of emetics (eg, syrup of ipecac) have attendant risk, are not supported by evidence, and are rarely—if ever—indicated. Activated charcoal may be considered in cooperative patients with preserved mental status and a stable airway who have had ingested large dosages, sustained-release products, substances that form concretions or bezoars, or those that undergo enterohepatic or enteroenteric recirculation.

Enhanced Elimination

ECTR like hemodialysis and hemoperfusion may enhance the elimination of certain absorbed poisons. ECTR may be considered in patients with serious illness that is nonresponsive to supportive care or impairment of the physiologic means of elimination (renal or liver). This strategy is used infrequently because many toxins cannot be extracorporeally removed; it is most commonly applied in severe poisoning from salicylates, lithium, and toxic alcohols.

Urinary alkalinization with sodium bicarbonate infusion may enhance the excretion of some drugs, such as salicylates, phenobarbital, and other renally excreted weak acids.

Poison Control Consultation

Consultation with the Poison Control Center (1-800-222-1222) or a local toxicologist will provide vital input into the ongoing care of the poisoned patient.

PEARLS

- Obtain collateral information from EMS providers, family, friends, and medical/pharmacy records.
- Toxidromes serve as a framework to approach the undifferentiated patient, but presentations may vary depending on patient comorbidities, timing and dosage of agents, and coingestants.
- WCT in the undifferentiated poisoned patient require sodium bicarbonate therapy.
- Benzodiazepines are the treatment of choice for both seizure and agitation management.
- In most cases, meticulous supportive care is more important than an antidote.

Suggested Readings

Farkas, J. Approach to the critically ill poisoned patient. *The Internet Book of Critical Care*. Accessed May 10, 2021. https://emcrit.org/ibcc/tox/

Skolnik A, Monas J. The crashing toxicology patient. *Emerg Med Clin North Am*. 2020;38(4):841-856.

Upchurch C, Blumenberg A, Brodie D, et al. Extracorporeal membrane oxygenation use in poisoning: a narrative review with clinical recommendations. *Clin Toxicol (Phila)*. 2021;59(10):877-887.

SECTION II
AIRWAY MANAGEMENT

24

Properly Performing BVM Ventilation

Lara Zekar, Verena Schandera, and Erik Laurin

Effective BVM ventilation is an essential component of airway management. The operator has to be aware of the intricacies of proper BVM techniques that significantly affect the efficacy of BVM ventilation.

Equipment

The standard BVM is composed of a self-inflating, manually compressible bag attached to a patient connector, which comprises a unidirectional valve, exhalation port, and patient connection port that attaches to either a FM, SGA, or ETT. On the other end, the bag is attached to an oxygen reservoir with tubing attached to an oxygen source.

In theory, with an effective FM seal, the BVM can deliver 100% oxygen to the patient at a flow rate of 15 L/min. It is crucial to provide enough oxygen flow to keep the reservoir inflated; otherwise, the delivered FIO_2 can precipitously drop by entraining room air through a rescue valve within the BVM instead of 100% oxygen from the reservoir.

The BVM is primarily used as a positive-pressure ventilation device and does not supply passive blow-by oxygen in the same manner as a nonrebreather mask or nasal cannula. If a BVM is used for oxygenation in a spontaneously breathing patient (without bag compression), oxygen delivery is driven only by the patient's own negative inspiratory force. This can be problematic in patients with reduced respiratory effort. To avoid inadequate oxygenation, it is beneficial to apply positive-pressure ventilation coordinated with the patient's own respiration in a spontaneously breathing patient via manually squeezing the compressible bag.

The exhalation port is another area of the BVM that requires attention. Most modern BVMs have a one-way disk valve on the exhalation port, which allows exhaled gas to escape but closes if the patient has any negative inspiratory force with a spontaneous breath. It is important to note that if this exhalation valve is not present, room air will enter through the exhalation port with negative pressure inspiration, causing a significant drop in FIO_2.

Many adult and pediatric BVMs have a positive-pressure relief valve ("pop-off valve") to prevent delivery of excessive pressure (above 20-45 cm H_2O). This positive-pressure relief valve can be disabled if higher pressures are needed to achieve adequate ventilation.

Some manufacturers produce BVMs with extra features that may enhance safety, such as in-line manometer, LED light, PEEP valve, and CO_2 waveform capnography. The manometer measures the pressure in the bowl of the mask, so the operator can prevent airway pressures above 20 to 30 cm H_2O, which would exceed the lower esophageal opening pressure, causing gastric insufflation and subsequent regurgitation. Some BVMs have an integrated LED light that illuminates every 6 seconds to prevent overventilation. Integral PEEP valve allows improved oxygenation. Lastly, in-line CO_2 waveform capnographs can provide objective evidence of gas exchange by the presence of a waveform. This is especially important with faulty or inaccurate pulse oximeters, such as during cardiopulmonary resuscitation.

Mask Seal

An important element of good BVM ventilation is an adequate mask seal. Masks come in a variety of sizes and should be chosen appropriately. Both under- and overinflation of the mask cushion may disrupt the seal.

Providers can achieve good mask seals with several one-handed and two-handed techniques.

In single operator BVM ventilation, a conventional teaching is the C-E technique, with a thumb and index finger forming a "C" encircling and stabilizing the mask over the nose and mouth, while the middle, ring, and little fingers are in "E" formation along the mandible, providing a jaw thrust.

There are two generally accepted two-handed techniques, when a second operator is available to compress the bag: a two-handed C-E technique, positioning both hands on either side of the mask as described earlier, and the V-E technique, often called the thenar grip. In the thenar grip, the thumb and thenar eminence of both hands are positioned in parallel on either side of the bag connector on the mask, with four fingers on each hand providing an anterior jaw thrust on each side of the mandible. Compared to the double C-E grip, the thenar grip is superior and results in greater peak pressures and higher tidal volumes due to a tighter seal.

When discussing mask seal, the edentulous patient warrants special consideration. Repositioning the mask such that the caudal edge rests above the lower lip (ie, moving the mask up the face so the bottom sinks into the mouth) may improve ventilation by opening the airway and allowing a better jaw thrust. If dentures are available, they should be placed in the patient's mouth. Alternatively, rolled gauze pads can be placed between the gums and the cheeks bilaterally to provide support for the lateral aspect of the mask to form the seal.

Ventilation

A common acronym for proper BVM ventilation technique is JAWS:

- Jaw thrust
- Airway placement (oropharyngeal or nasopharyngeal)
- Work together
- Small and slow squeeze

Optimal manual compression of the BVM bag should deliver 6 to 7 mL/kg of ideal body weight per breath over 1 to 2 seconds and not exceed a rate of 12 breaths/min. Lower rates (6-8 breaths/min) may be appropriate in patients with severe obstructive pulmonary disease to prevent air-trapping. Typical adult BVM bags are around 1.5 L, which means that manual compression of one-third of the bag will deliver a 500-mL tidal volume; additional compression will likely deliver unnecessarily large volumes. Paying close attention to rate and volume is critical since common issues with BVM ventilation are hyperventilation and inappropriate tidal volumes.

PEARLS

- Training in BVM should be continually refreshed.
- Ensure a high-flow oxygen source (15 L/min) and inflate reservoir.
- Optimize mask seal and airway patency with a thenar grip, good jaw thrust, and oral/nasal airway placement.
- Pay close attention to rate, volume, and pressures when ventilating a patient.
- Provide synchronized assist breaths when using BVM to oxygenate a spontaneously breathing patient.
- Use CO_2 waveform capnography, pressure manometry, and PEEP valves for optimal BVM use.

Suggested Readings

Hart D, Reardon R, Ward C, et al. Face mask ventilation: a comparison of three techniques. *J Emerg Med.* 2013;44(5):1028-1033.

Joffe AM, Hetzel S, Liew EC. A two-handed jaw-thrust technique is superior to the one-handed "EC-clamp" technique for mask ventilation in the apneic unconscious person. *Anesthesiology.* 2010;113(4):873-879.

Kheterpal S, Han R, Tremper KK, et al. Incidence and predictors of difficult and impossible mask ventilation. *Anesthesiology.* 2006;105:885-891.

Neumar RW, Otto CW, Link MS, et al. Part 8: adult advanced cardiovascular life support: 2010 American Heart Association Guidelines for Cardiopulmonary Resuscitation and Emergency Cardiovascular Care. *Circulation.* 2010;122(Suppl 3):S729-S767.

Racine SX, Solis A, Hamou NA, et al. Face mask ventilation in edentulous patients: a comparison of mandibular groove and lower lip placement. *Anesthesiology.* 2010;112(5): 1190-1193.

25

Resuscitate Before You Intubate!

Rene Monzon and Kayla T. Enriquez

ETI of the critically ill patient is a hallmark emergency medicine procedure. Securing an endotracheal tube is inherently risky and comes with life-threatening complications that can be avoided if proper measures are taken to resuscitate the patient before intubating. Arrhythmias, failed intubation, hypotension, hypoxemia, and even post-intubation cardiac arrest are all common obstacles, well documented in airway literature. By understanding the hemodynamic effects of intubation shared in this chapter, you will feel more comfortable foreseeing potential pitfalls and have a higher chance of safe and successful intubation.

Hemodynamic Effects of Intubation

During spontaneous inspiration, there is a decrease in ITP secondary to the diaphragm contracting and increasing the size of thoracic space. The decrease in ITP is associated with a decrease in right atrial pressure and a concomitant increase in venous return and preload. Conversely, during a mechanically ventilated breath, with high tidal volume or high PEEP, there is an increase in ITP and right atrial pressure, which results in a decrease in venous return and preload. If the patient is not prophylactically resuscitated, the decrease in preload with mechanical ventilation can worsen hypotension in an already hypovolemic patient. Of note, the increase in right atrial pressure increases the risk of PVC and other life-threatening arrhythmias.

Intubation also causes significant changes in plasma concentration of noradrenaline, which may result in tachycardia and hypertension. While the mechanism of this reflex sympathetic response is not completely understood, it may involve provocation of the baroreceptor system by stimulation of the epipharynx and laryngopharynx during intubation.

"Induction induced sympatholysis" is often a neglected cause of hypotension. This is the phenomenon wherein fully sedating a patient in partially compensated shock inevitably blunts the adrenergic drive and impairs the compensatory response. This hemodynamic effect has been seen with every major induction agent.

Who Is at Risk for Decompensation? How Do You Predict Potential Pitfalls?

If hemodynamics are not closely monitored throughout RSI, serious life-threatening complications may arise such as PICA. The risk of decompensation and cardiac arrest can be decreased with the useful tool of the SI. The SI is the heart rate divided by the systolic blood pressure (eg, for a heart rate of 80, and an SBP of 120, the SI would be 0.67). A pre-RSI SI of 0.9 or more has been associated with cardiac arrest. Several studies have shown that decompensation is increased for patients with the following:

- Pre-intubation hypotension (SBP <90 mm Hg)
- Pre-intubation hypoxemia (SpO_2 <90%)
- Pre-intubation SI (≥0.9)

Heffner et al found that the prevalence of PICA was approximately 4% in ED intubations, and that increasing SI was associated with increasing risk of PICA, with the odds of cardiac arrest increasing 1.16 times for every 0.1 increase in SI.

Fluid resuscitation and vasopressors can be utilized prior to intubation to prevent hypotension, and thus PICA. While there is no specific SI or SBP that makes ETI completely benign, an effort should be made to correct an SI of 1.0 or an SBP of less than 90 mm Hg. Furthermore, hypoxemia should be corrected to the extent possible, and preoxygenation should be a standard part of every ETI.

Pre-intubation Resuscitation

To overcome pre-intubation hypotension, physicians should rely on administering intravenous fluids or blood (depending on the clinical scenario). Administration of 1 to 2 L of intravenous fluids (plasmalyte or normal saline) unless otherwise contraindicated (ie, congestive heart failure, chronic kidney disease, etc) is recommended for patients who are hypovolemic or septic. Blood administration is the preferred treatment for acute bleeding. If this initial resuscitation does not improve SBP above the 90 mm Hg threshold, vasopressors can be given. Examples include the following:

- Push dose Epi: 9 mL of NS + 1 mL Epi (100 mcg/mL) = 10 mcg/mL—0.5 to 2 mL every 2 to 5 minutes
- Norepinephrine infusion: 0.02 to 1.0 mcg/kg/min
- Vasopressin infusion: 0.01 to 0.04 units/min

Correcting pre-intubation hypoxemia is covered in more detail in a separate chapter but briefly: Preoxygenation may be accomplished via a nonrebreather mask, NIPPV, or BVM devices. Head elevation, jaw thrust, OPA, and NPA are all airway adjuncts for maximal effect during preoxygenation. In the event of an unsuccessful first pass, augmenting preoxygenation with passive (apneic) oxygenation between intubation attempts is strongly recommended.

Induction medications should be carefully considered when resuscitating a hypotensive patient. Ketamine (0.5-2 mg/kg) causes sympathetic stimulation and is among the most hemodynamically stable induction agents when dealing with pre-intubation hypotension. Etomidate (0.3 mg/kg), although shown to have very few cardiovascular effects, can cause sympatholysis and hypotension, thus a reduced dose should be considered if using this agent. Benzodiazepines, such as midazolam, are often used as induction agents but have been associated with moderate hypotension and therefore would not be the first-line induction agent in a hypotensive patient. Lastly, propofol has been shown to inhibit the sympathetic nervous system and cause significant hypotension, and therefore less attractive for intubating hypotensive patients.

In addition to correcting hypovolemia and hypoxemia, it is important to identify and be aware of preexisting pathologies that may complicate intubation. For example, in a trauma patient, needle decompression of a suspected PTX should be performed prior to intubation to prevent worsening of the PTX, tension physiology, or hypotension due to decreased venous return. In a patient with a suspected spinal cord injury, cervical spine precautions and neck stabilization should be implemented and airway adjuncts brought to the bedside. These airway adjuncts include bougie device, D-blade, LMA, and surgical airway equipment.

PEARLS

- Intubation greatly affects a patient's hemodynamics.
- The SI can be helpful to predict life-threatening complications such as PICA.
- Patients at greatest risk for decompensation are those who have not adequately been resuscitated (hypotensive, hypoxemic, SI [≥ 0.9]).
- Resuscitate with fluids, blood, pressors, and adequate preoxygenation.
- Consider induction medications and their physiologic effects carefully.

Suggested Readings

Bruder N, Ortega D, Granthil C. Consequences and prevention methods of hemodynamic changes during laryngoscopy and intratracheal intubation. *Ann Fr Anesth Reanim.* 1992;11(1):57-71.

Heffner AC, Swords DS, Neale MN, Jones AE. Incidence and factors associated with cardiac arrest complicating emergency airway management. *Resuscitation.* 2013;84(11):1500-1504.

List JI. Peri-intubation cardiac arrest: new insights into an uncommon and potentially preventable cause of mortality in critically ill patients. Critical Care Medicine, American College of Emergency Physicians; 2018.

Park YC, Ryu HH, Baik SW, Chung KS, Choi IC. The hemodynamic changes following tracheal intubation with special reference to age. *Korean J Anesthesiol.* 1991;24(6):1138-1146.

26

Know Your RSI Meds

Lee Johnson and Joseph Brown

RSI is a technique commonly used by physicians to manage emergency airways. This technique uses induction agents to bring about an unconscious state followed quickly by paralytic agents to aid in the rapid and safe intubation of an airway. Strictly, RSI is performed without ventilation after medications are given; however, in practice many patients receive bag-valve-mask ventilation until an intubation attempt. It is critical to have a structured approach to RSI and know the medications used in this process. This chapter focuses only on RSI medications and does not address other aspects of the intubation process.

Premedication, induction, and paralysis are the steps involving medications in RSI. Awake patients should be adequately sedated before being paralyzed. This can be done by having your induction agent pushed intravenously, followed immediately by your paralytic agent. There is evidence that a small number of ED patients experience awareness of paralysis during and immediately after RSI. Understanding the duration of action of your medications is crucial to preventing this complication.

Premedication

Premedication is the use of agents such as fentanyl or lidocaine to blunt the physiologic response to intubation. The practice of pretreatment has largely fallen out of favor, as available evidence has not shown a benefit to this practice. Two notable exceptions include fentanyl in patients with intracranial hemorrhage and atropine in pediatric intubations. While distinct from historical pretreatment regimens, medications may be utilized prior to RSI to facilitate preoxygenation and improve hemodynamics as part of a "resuscitate before you intubate" algorithm.

Sedation

Sedation can be achieved by many routes. Etomidate, ketamine, and propofol are three commonly utilized medications, each with distinct advantages and drawbacks. Etomidate (0.3 mg/kg/IV) has a quick onset of action and a short duration making it favorable as an induction agent. It is blood pressure neutral and lowers intracranial pressure. It has been suggested that etomidate causes adrenal insufficiency in patients with septic shock; however, current evidence evaluating the use of a single dose of etomidate has not demonstrated any mortality effects.

Ketamine (1-2 mg/kg/IV) is associated with less respiratory depression and generally will support or increase blood pressure. Ketamine is a good alternative in septic shock patients. Despite the suggestions that ketamine may increase intracranial pressure in patients with traumatic brain injury, the literature has not born this out and the lack of associated hypotension may be beneficial in this patient population.

Propofol (0.5 mg/kg/IV) is a great anticonvulsant and has the shortest duration of action of the three induction agents listed but is relatively contraindicated in hypotensive patients due to its vasodilatory and negative inotropic effects.

Paralysis

Deciding on the best paralytic is similar to sedatives in that there are advantages and drawbacks to available drugs. The most commonly used paralytics are depolarizing and nondepolarizing agents, with succinylcholine and rocuronium being the most common in each class, respectively.

Succinylcholine (1-1.5 mg/kg/IV) has a faster onset and shorter duration of action (approximately 10 minutes) than any nondepolarizing agent. Contraindications include burns, crush injuries, and denervation injuries occurring greater than 72 hours prior to induction. Instances when a rise in serum potassium would not be tolerable and neuromuscular diseases are also contraindications.

Rocuronium (0.6-1.5 mg/kg/IV) is the other most common paralytic. When dosed appropriately, rocuronium has a similar onset of action and produces similar intubating conditions to succinylcholine. Its duration of action is significantly longer at approximately 45 minutes. If utilizing rocuronium, you must pay meticulous attention to postintubation sedation to prevent awareness with paralysis.

PEARLS

- Induction and paralysis are the key steps involving medications in RSI.
- Etomidate, ketamine, and propofol are three commonly used drugs for sedation.
- Etomidate (0.3 mg/kg/IV) has a quick onset of action and a short duration, is blood pressure neutral, and lowers ICP. Ketamine (1-2 mg/kg) is relatively contraindicated in hypertensive patients, is as effective as etomidate, and can be used in sepsis. Propofol (0.5 mg/kg) is contraindicated in hypotensive patients and can be used as an anticonvulsant.
- Succinylcholine (1.5 mg/kg/IV) is a depolarizing agent, has a rapid onset of action and short duration, but is contraindicated in patients at risk for denervation or hyperkalemia. Rocuronium (1.0-1.5 mg/kg/IV) is a nondepolarizing agent and has a longer duration of effect compared to succinylcholine.

Suggested Readings

April MD, Arana A, Pallin DJ, et al. Emergency department intubation success with succinylcholine versus rocuronium: a National Emergency Airway Registry study. *Ann Emerg Med.* 2018;72(6):645-653.

April MD, Arana A, Schauer SG, et al. Ketamine versus etomidate and peri-intubation hypotension: a National Emergency Airway Registry study. *Acad Emerg Med.* 2020;27(11): 1106-1115.

Brown CA III, Walls RM. Rapid sequence intubation. In: Brown CA III, Sakles JC, Mick NW, eds. *The Walls Manual of Emergency Airway Management*. 5th ed. Wolters Kluwer; 2018:235.

Bruder EA, Ball IM, Ridi S, Pickett W, Hohl C. Single induction dose of etomidate versus other induction agents for endotracheal intubation in critically ill patients. *Cochrane Database Syst Rev.* 2015;(1):CD010225.

Cohen L, Athaide V, Wickham ME, Doyle-Waters MM, Rose NG, Hohl CM. The effect of ketamine on intracranial and cerebral perfusion pressure and health outcomes: a systematic review. *Ann Emerg Med.* 2015;65(1):43-51.e2.

Driver BE, Prekker ME, Wagner E, et al. Recall of awareness during paralysis among ED patients undergoing tracheal intubation. *Chest.* 2023;163(2):313-323.

Fuller BM, Pappal RD, Mohr NM, et al. Awareness with paralysis among critically ill emergency department patients: a prospective cohort study. *Crit Care Med.* 2022;50(10):1449-1460.

Leede E, Kempema J, Wilson C, et al. A multicenter investigation of the hemodynamic effects of induction agents for trauma rapid sequence intubation. *J Trauma Acute Care Surg.* 2021;90(6):1009-1013.

Mallon WK, Keim SM, Shoenberger JM, et al. Rocuronium vs succinylcholine in the emergency department: a critical appraisal. *J Emerg Med.* 2009;37(2):183-188.

27

What Is Your Plan B, C, D?

Lara Zekar and Erik Laurin

Emergency airway management is a lifesaving intervention for patients and one of the most high-risk procedures that the emergency physician will perform. The cognitive burden of airway management is high, so a standardized plan for intubation is vital. Closed-loop communication, avoiding repeated attempts with the same technique, prompt recognition of failure, and transitioning to the next step requires practice and will maximize success in difficult airway management. Before beginning, make sure to have all the tools necessary for airway management in close reach. Anticipate failure and have backup devices ready at the bedside. The popular SOAP ME mnemonic outlines the minimum equipment necessary:

- **S:** Suctioning device capable of clearing airway debris. Historically, Yankauer suction catheters have been used, but improved suction devices such as the DuCanto suction catheter can be lifesaving if particulates or large-volume debris must be cleared. Ensure suction tubing is long enough to reach the patient, with the suction device attached and tucked under the patient's shoulder or mattress. Put it on the right side, in a consistent position, so it can be grabbed without taking your eyes off the airway. In soiled airways, lead with the suction device ahead of the laryngoscope blade (SALAD technique, see Chapter 31).
- **O:** Oxygen attached to devices and turned on. A BVM will be needed after intubation and should be connected to continuous waveform CO_2 capnography. For optimal preoxygenation, use a nonrebreather face mask at high-flow rate (>30 L/min oxygen),

NIPPV, or HFNC. For apneic oxygenation, use a standard nasal cannula at 15 L/min oxygen flow or HFNC, if rapid desaturation is anticipated.
- **A:** Airway equipment should include several sizes of laryngoscopes (ideally videolaryngoscopy), ETTs, SGAs, a cricothyrotomy kit, and a bougie.
- **P:** Pharmaceuticals. Medications for induction, paralysis, intravenous fluids, and vasopressors if hypotension is expected. Verbalize the plan for induction, paralysis, and post-intubation sedation. Pharmacists are extremely valuable when using high-risk medications during a resuscitation, so involve them whenever possible.
- **M:** Monitors. Have the patient on a cardiac monitor. Turning on the audible pulse oximetry tone allows the intubator to be continuously aware of the patient's oxygen saturation. Waveform end-tidal CO_2 capnography will give confirmation of correct ETT placement and help manage ventilator settings in the post-intubation period. Blood pressure should be set to cycle every 3 to 5 minutes.
- **E:** Emergency equipment, including defibrillator and invasive airway equipment.

Approach

One of the first decision points in the approach to intubation is whether the patient is appropriate for RSI, or is it safer to keep the patient spontaneously breathing and use an awake approach with topical anesthesia. Although the factors that determine this decision are beyond the scope of this chapter, the vast majority of emergency intubations are performed with RSI. Since RSI renders a patient apneic and oxygen desaturation frequently occurs with multiple intubation attempts, it is paramount to have a predetermined plan for subsequent oxygenation and intubation attempts if the first-pass fails.

The initial attempt at intubation is often the best attempt because subsequent attempts result in operator fatigue as well as airway trauma, secretions, blood, and swelling. Therefore, the first attempt should be performed with optimal patient positioning, the best devices available, suction, bougie, ELM, and appropriate RSI medication dosing. If the first attempt fails, then the next step depends on the oxygen saturation—this is Plan B. If the saturation is normal, which is more likely if apneic oxygenation has been used, then another intubation attempt can be performed with close attention to anything that can be *improved* for the next attempt. Another attempt with the same device and operator and no change in the approach will likely result in an unsuccessful second attempt. Therefore, to succeed, change the device, reposition the patient, improve ELM technique, use a bougie, or change the operator. If the patient has desaturated to less than 93%, Plan B should focus on reoxygenation.

Reoxygenation can occur with either a BVM or SGA. The decision on which device to use is determined by the operator's assessment of intubation success on the next attempt. For instance, if the operator feels that something can be changed and a second attempt will likely be successful, then BVM reoxygenation is appropriate. Special attention should be paid to peak pressures and volumes delivered to minimize gastric insufflation and regurgitation. It is then easy to remove the BVM and allow a second intubation attempt.

However, if the operator feels that intubation success is unlikely on a second attempt, then reoxygenation should occur with an SGA, specifically one made as a conduit for intubation. These intubating SGAs are excellent at rescue oxygenation and ventilation and have a very high success rate of intubation through them, especially if a flexible endoscope is used. Reoxygenation and then intubation can proceed through the SGA.

Failure of reoxygenation is vital to recognize early since desaturation occurs rapidly. Plan C would then include rescue BVM, maximizing technique with a thenar grip, oropharyngeal and nasopharyngeal airways, and two operators. If an SGA has not yet been tried for reoxygenation, it should be attempted.

At the same time, preparation for Plan D—a surgical airway—should begin. The neck anatomy needs to be palpated to identify the thyroid cartilage and cricothyroid membrane. The cricothyrotomy can begin when the operator feels that reoxygenation is impossible, which is known as a CICO situation. The cricothyrotomy should be done with a bougie-aided, scalpel technique.

PEARLS

- Be methodical when setting up for emergency intubation and have backup equipment immediately available.
- The first intubation attempt is often the best, so optimize it for first-pass success.
- Reoxygenate with a BVM or convert to an intubating SGA early.
- Surgical airway needs to be performed quickly when a CICO situation occurs.

SUGGESTED READINGS

Henderson JJ, Popat MT, Latto IP, Pearce AC, Difficult Airway Society. Difficult Airway Society guidelines for management of the unanticipated difficult intubation. *Anaesthesia.* 2004;59(7):675-694.

Levitan RM, Heitz JW, Sweeney M, Cooper RM. The complexities of tracheal intubation with direct laryngoscopy and alternative intubation devices. *Ann Emerg Med.* 2011; 57(3):240-247.

Nelson JG, Wewerka SS, Woster CM, et al. Evaluation of the Storz CMAC®, Glidescope® GVL, AirTraq®, King LTS-D™, and direct laryngoscopy in a simulated difficult airway. *Am J Emerg Med.* 2013;31(3):589-592.

Sagarin MJ, Barton ED, Chng YM, Walls RM, National Emergency Airway Registry Investigators. Airway management by US and Canadian emergency medicine residents: a multicenter analysis of more than 6,000 endotracheal intubation attempts. *Ann Emerg Med.* 2005;46(4):328-336.

28

DON'T MAKE THESE MISTAKES IN INTUBATING THE PATIENT WHO IS OBESE

KATRINA STIME AND GUY SHOCHAT

Obesity causes physiologic changes that can complicate airway management, including decreased respiratory reserve due to decreased FRC and increased airway pressures due to heavier chest walls and abdominal girth. Given these physiologic changes, there are important considerations for preoxygenation, positioning, medication dosing, laryngoscopy, cricothyroidotomy, and initiating mechanical ventilation in patients who are obese.

Preoxygenation is essential to increase safe apnea time; however, it is less effective in patients who are obese due to abdominal girth, which pushes up the diaphragm and reduces FRC. To improve preoxygenation, patients who are obese should be placed in an upright or semi-upright position, which decreases pressure on the chest wall and improves alveolar recruitment. Preoxygenation can usually be accomplished using an NRB mask for spontaneously breathing patients or a BVM for unconscious patients for 3 to 5 minutes. BVM ventilation is often more difficult in patients who are obese due to redundant soft tissue in the upper airway causing pharyngeal collapse. The two-person thenar grip technique is recommended in this patient population (see **Figure 28.1**). Nasopharyngeal or oropharyngeal airways may also be used if the patient is obtunded. End-tidal CO_2 monitoring can be used to evaluate the effectiveness of preoxygenation. If the patient is persistently hypoxemic, NIPPV can help reduce intrapulmonary shunting due to atelectasis.

Proper positioning is essential for successful laryngoscopy and intubation in patients who are obese. All patients should be placed with the head of bed at 30° to reduce upward pressure on the diaphragm. If not in cervical spine precautions, the patient should be ramped using the bed, blankets, or commercially available ramps to align the external auditory meatus with the sternal notch. It is the authors' preference to use the hospital bed itself to position the patient (see **Figure 28.2**). The ramped position has been shown to be superior to the sniffing position in patients who are obese.

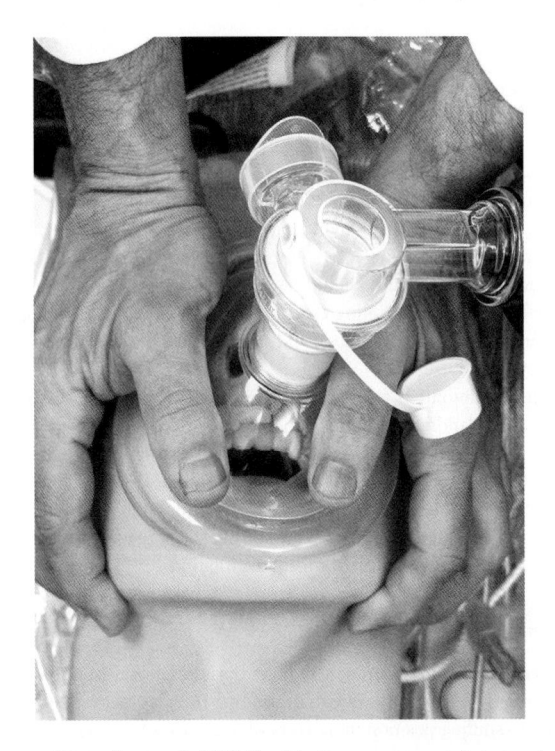

Figure 28.1 Bag valve mask (BVM) with the two-person thenar grip technique.

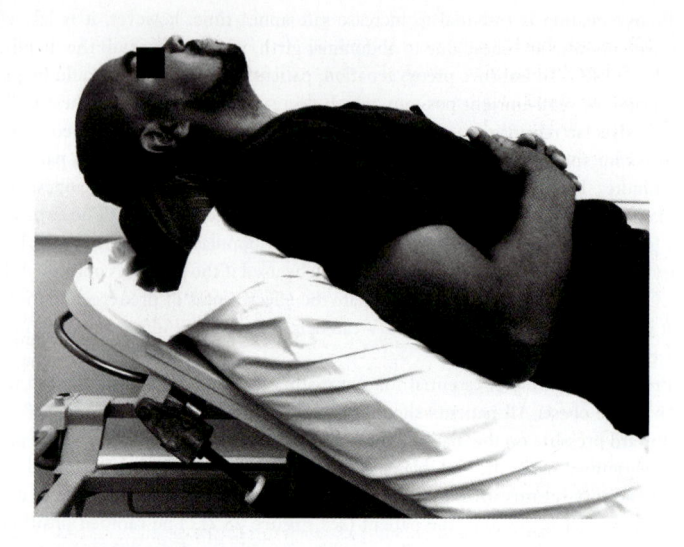

FIGURE 28.2 Ramping using the bed to align the external auditory meatus with the sternal notch.

There are important dosing adjustments for RSI medications in patients who are obese. NMB agents, which are not lipophilic, can be dosed by IBW or slightly more than IBW to rapidly achieve optimal intubating conditions. Induction agents, which are somewhat lipophilic, should be dosed using adjusted body weight. This can be estimated by IBW + 0.5 (actual body weight − IBW).

Rapid oxygen desaturation is more common in patients who are obese due to decreased oxygen reserve and increased oxygen consumption. Given this physiologic change, laryngoscopy techniques should be optimized for speed. Larger laryngoscope blades may be helpful for controlling excess soft tissue. Video laryngoscopy may be superior to DL in patients who are obese, and it is possible to take a first DL look with a MAC video laryngoscope blade.

If a cricothyroidotomy is needed to secure the airway, excess neck tissue can make it difficult to identify landmarks. In this patient population, it is recommended to make a generous vertical incision and then use the "scalpel-finger-bougie" technique.

When initiating mechanical ventilation, tidal volumes should be calculated based on IBW, as obesity does not affect lung volumes. Ramping the patient and using higher levels of positive end-expiratory pressure may be necessary to reduce atelectasis, improve $\dot{V}/\dot{Q}$ mismatch, and improve oxygenation and ventilation.

PEARLS

- Preoxygenate patients who are obese in an upright or semi-upright position.
- Ramp patient to align the external auditory meatus with the sternal notch (superior to sniffing position in patients who are obese).

- NMB agents should be dosed based on slightly more than IBW; induction agents should be dosed based on adjusted body weight (approximately halfway between actual body weight and IBW).
- Choose a reliable intubation technique such as video laryngoscopy.
- Calculate tidal volumes using IBW.

Suggested Readings

Altermatt FR, Muñoz HR, Delfino AE, Cortínez LI. Pre-oxygenation in the obese patient: effects of position on tolerance to apnoea. *Br J Anaesth*. 2005;95(5):706-709. PMID: 16143575.

Collins JS, Lemmens HJ, Brodsky JB, Brock-Utne JG, Levitan RM. Laryngoscopy and morbid obesity: a comparison of the "sniff" and "ramped" positions. *Obes Surg*. 2004;14(9): 1171-1175. PMID: 15527629.

De Jong A, Wrigge H, Hedenstierna G, et al. How to ventilate obese patients in the ICU. *Intensive Care Med*. 2020;46(12):2423-2435. PMID: 33095284.

Parker BK, Manning S, Winters ME. The crashing obese patient. *West J Emerg Med*. 2019;20(2):323-330. PMID: 30881553.

Zhi G, Xin W, Ying W, Guohong X, Shuying L. "Obesity paradox" in acute respiratory distress syndrome: asystematic review and meta-analysis. *PLoS One*. 2016;11(9):e0163677.

29

Pitfalls in Intubating the Crashing Asthmatic

Lara Zekar and Verena Schandera

More than 25 million Americans carry the diagnosis of asthma, representing more than 8% of the US population. It is the most common chronic medical condition among pediatric patients. Approximately 2% of patients with an asthma exacerbation who present to the ED are intubated. Acute severe asthma necessitates immediate recognition and aggressive management, as it is associated with significant morbidity and mortality.

The underlying pathology of asthma exacerbation consists of bronchospasm, airway inflammation with increased vascular permeability, and increased secretions, causing obstruction. It leads to dynamic hyperinflation, gas trapping, intrinsic auto-PEEP, and hypoventilation. If not recognized and reversed, it ultimately leads to respiratory arrest and hemodynamic compromise due to increased intrathoracic pressures and the inability to oxygenate and ventilate. The mainstays of therapies focus on bronchodilation and inflammation reduction, and include inhaled short-acting beta-2 agonists, inhaled anticholinergics, and systemic corticosteroids. Systemic bronchodilation in the form of IV magnesium sulfate can serve as an adjunct in acute severe asthma. Systemic beta-agonist therapy with subcutaneous terbutaline or IM epinephrine can be administered in patients not responding to the therapies mentioned earlier. For patients with profound hypotension or symptoms refractory to IM epinephrine, IV epinephrine is another option.

NIPPV

If a patient is refractory to first-line medical management and has worsening hypercarbia, refractory hypoxia, worsening mental status, fatigue, and bradypnea/apnea, it is necessary to pursue more aggressive treatment modalities such as NIPPV or mechanical ventilation.

The benefit of NIPPV in severe acute asthma remains inconclusive according to a 2012 Cochrane review. Several studies suggest promising results, such as reduced need for intubation, decreased work of breathing, improved ventilation-perfusion mismatch, and shorter hospital stays. BIPAP specifically has additional inspiratory pressure, supporting air movement, and improving beta-adrenergic aerosol delivery to smaller airways. In-line inhaled medications should be continued while the patient is on NIPPV.

HFNC has shown some benefit in the pediatric population but is based on limited evidence. Its role is still unclear in the adult population, but it can be attempted as an alternative to NIPPV in patients with contraindications or relative contraindications.

Altered mental status is a relative contraindication for NIPPV; however, patients with asthma often achieve rapid improvement in cognitive function shortly after being placed on NIPPV. The patient should be closely monitored until improvement is seen, and airway management equipment should be readily available. If the patient needs NIPPV but is unable to tolerate the face mask, the physician can attempt DSI.

DSI is a relatively new concept with limited data in patients with asthma, however, can help optimize preoxygenation prior to intubation. Ketamine (1-2 mg/kg) or dexmedetomidine (1 mcg/kg over 10 minutes) can provide sedation with preserved respiratory drive, can improve oxygenation and ventilation achieved with NIPPV, and allow for proper preoxygenation before intubation. As mentioned earlier, airway equipment should be readily available, as there are reports of low-dose ketamine causing apnea in critically ill patients. If respiratory distress continues despite cooperation with maximal noninvasive therapy, then a paralytic (with or without more induction agent, depending on the degree of consciousness) can be given and the patient can be intubated having had optimized preoxygenation. DSI should be thought of as "procedural sedation for the procedure of preoxygenation." Preoxygenation is vital to avoid peri-intubation complications and cardiac arrest; therefore, every attempt should be made for maximal preoxygenation in the patient with hypoxemic asthma given these patients have little cardiopulmonary reserve.

Endotracheal Intubation

Endotracheal intubation in the asthmatic is associated with significant morbidity and mortality, and should be avoided if possible.

Preoxygenation is important to minimize the risk of hypoxemia and extend the duration of safe apnea. As mentioned earlier, NIPPV used with DSI can serve as a bridge to intubation by improving oxygenation in a patient not tolerating NIPPV alone. Maintenance of oxygenation during the time from early paralysis to intubation is extremely important as these patients desaturate rapidly that can result in a respiratory arrest. If NIPPV is used for preoxygenation, then using a backup respiratory rate on the NIPPV machine will preserve oxygenation and ventilation during induction, until the patient is fully paralyzed. If NIPPV is not used, HFNC or a standard NC at 15 L/min oxygen flow can be used for apneic oxygenation.

Either ketamine or etomidate is considered a reasonable induction agent. Ketamine is a historically recommended induction agent for intubation due to its bronchodilatory effect. Some authors suggest pretreatment with an anticholinergic agent (glycopyrrolate or atropine) to reduce post-intubation secretions associated with ketamine. Most studies show similar first-pass success rates comparing ketamine and etomidate, and it is unlikely that the bronchodilatory effects of ketamine have effects beyond the aggressive treatment regimens already used prior to intubation.

Despite the distress and anxiety of patients prior to intubation, pretreatment with sedatives should be avoided due to possible respiratory depression. Rocuronium or succinylcholine can both be used for paralysis, and both are dosed at 1.0 to 1.5 mg/kg to shorten the time of onset, as rapid paralysis is desired for patients at risk for rapid desaturation. If possible, larger endotracheal tubes (8.0 mm) are recommended due to their decreased effects on airway resistance.

Once intubated, it is important to reduce the patient's minute ventilation. Start at a tidal volume of 6 mL/kg of ideal body weight (lower if plateau pressures are >30 cm H_2O) and respiratory rate of 6 to 10 breaths/min. The inspiratory to expiratory ratio should be reduced to 1:4 or less, allowing patients to fully exhale prior to receiving another breath. At times, manual assistance to help these patients exhale by disconnecting them from a ventilator and squeezing their chests is required. Permissive hypercarbia is recommended to prevent hyperinflation and barotrauma.

Post-intubation hypotension is common, likely due to insensible fluid loss, effects of sedation, severe lung hyperdistention (increased intrathoracic pressure), and positive pressure ventilation, which can cause hemodynamic compromise. Pre-intubation administration of IV fluids is recommended to increase preload. If needed, epinephrine or phenylephrine should be readily available and can be used to improve hypotension, after reversible causes have been identified.

PEARLS

- Avoid intubation if possible as it has been shown to increase morbidity and mortality.
- Maximize oxygenation and medication delivery with NIPPV when not contraindicated.
- Physiologically optimize the patient prior to intubation.
- Remember DSI for uncooperative hypoxemic patients.
- Ketamine or etomidate is recommended as induction agent.
- Avoid high respiratory rates (follow recommended 6-10 breaths/min) to avoid breath stacking and barotrauma.

Suggested Readings

Agnihotri NT, Saltoun C. Acute severe asthma (status asthmaticus). *Allergy Asthma Proc.* 2019;40(6):406-409.

Brenner B, Corbridge T, Kazzi A. Intubation and mechanical ventilation of the asthmatic patient in respiratory failure. *Proc Am Thorac Soc.* 2009;6:371-379.

Godwin HT, Fix ML, Baker O, Madsen T, Walls RM, Brown 3rd CA. Emergency department airway management for status asthmaticus with respiratory failure. *Respir Care.* 2020;65(12):1904-1907.

Lim WJ, Akram RM, Carson KV, et al. Non-invasive positive pressure ventilation for treatment of respiratory failure due to severe acute exacerbations of asthma. *Cochrane Database Syst Rev.* 2012;(12):CD004360.

Long B, Lentz S, Koyfman A, Gottlieb M. Evaluation and management of the critically ill adult asthmatic in the emergency department setting. *Am J Emerg Med.* 2021;44:441-451.

Mannam P, Siegel MD. Analytic review: management of life-threatening asthma in adults. *J Intensive Care Med.* 2010;25(1):3-15.

30

AVOID THE CLEAN KILL—INTUBATING THE PATIENT WITH ACIDOSIS

MADELINE GRADE AND GUY SHOCHAT

In most cases, intubating a patient in respiratory distress is a life saving procedure. However, intubating a patient with severe acidosis can result in disastrous outcomes if not expertly managed. Patients with severe acidosis exist in a perilous balance, in which their respiratory drive is the very mechanism preventing their pH from falling into potentially fatal levels of acidosis. Any decrease in minute ventilation in these patients, let alone complete cessation of respiratory effort with paralysis, can be catastrophic. Thus, it is critical to maintain minute ventilation as much as possible and to properly prepare for any adverse events should there be a decrease in minute ventilation.

In general, a pH below 6.8 is considered incompatible with life. At present, a clearly defined pH threshold below which should raise concern for adverse outcomes from intubation has not been well defined. Often, it depends in large part on how quickly the patient has arrived at their state of acidosis (eg, a patient with diabetic ketoacidosis who has been declining over several days vs a sudden severe lactic acidosis without respiratory compensation). Notwithstanding, a pH below 7.1 is very serious if considering intubation, and most clinicians would agree that deterioration may occur rapidly and unpredictably at pH values below 7.0.

The best way to manage the airway in a patient with acidosis is to prevent decompensation and avoid intubation altogether. Even if your patient's initial P_{CO_2} is perfectly within the expected range of respiratory compensation, it is important not to become complacent. While some patients can sustain this compensatory effort for extended periods of time, others may not. As patients fatigue, they decrease their minute ventilation, which can lead to hypercarbia, worsened mental status, concurrent respiratory acidosis, rapid decreases in pH, and eventually dysrhythmias and cardiovascular collapse. Obtain serial blood gases, take note of respiratory effort and mental status over time, and attempt to treat the primary cause of acidosis. The administration of sodium bicarbonate therapy for severe acidosis remains controversial and debated. Many clinicians opt to administer bicarbonate for extremely low pH, due to concern for myocyte dysfunction, especially at the first signs of hypotension or bradycardia. Theoretically, it may sequester enough hydrogen ions to provide a temporary buffer against a drop in pH if used immediately prior to intubation. However, evidence for this practice is lacking, and if your patient with acidosis is already maximizing their rate of bicarbonate conversion and CO_2 exhalation, extra bicarbonate may contribute to an excess of CO_2 and lead to respiratory acidosis.

NIPPV can be useful in the management of severe metabolic acidosis by reducing inspiratory work of breathing and boosting alveolar minute ventilation, especially as patients begin to tire. It also can be helpful to measure a patient's pre-intubation tidal volume and respiratory rate in order to determine their required minute ventilation post-intubation. Patients with very high requirements may need spontaneous breathing ventilator modes to match this level of compensation post-intubation. NIPPV should be utilized in lieu of intubation for as long as possible, provided there are no contraindications to its use (ie, decreased mental status, concern for airway protection).

If a definitive airway must be established, it is important to proceed swiftly but thoughtfully. The most critical component to airway management of the patient with acidosis is to minimize apnea time. Patients in severe acidosis teeter on a precarious inflection point at which even minor increases in carbon dioxide can cause precipitous drops in pH and lead to cardiovascular collapse. Intubation in these circumstances should be performed by a highly experienced clinician to maximize the chance of first-pass success.

Awake intubation should be considered in many high-risk anatomic and physiologic situations, where paralysis can limit ventilation or cause soft tissue relaxation that obstructs the airway. Critical acidosis is a classic indication for awake intubation, as it allows maintenance of minute ventilation. Awake nasal intubation can be challenging and slow even in expert hands, but awake laryngoscopy is a skill every emergency physician can master. The more cooperative the patient, the more one can use topical agents alone instead of systemic medications. If IV sedation is required, ketamine is an ideal choice to keep respiratory drive intact. The authors prefer a simplified approach using nebulized lidocaine 4% or 2% (5 mL in a standard neb unit is fast and very effective) followed by ketamine 1 mg/kg (less if obtunded) given by slow IV push (as rapid push can result in laryngospasm and apnea). Topical lidocaine can also be administered nasally via atomization or orally via viscous solution. A Macintosh blade video laryngoscope is preferred, as the rigid stylet used with hyperangulated blades is challenging in the patient with spontaneous respiratory effort. Size down, lubricate the endotracheal tube, and be ready with additional IV sedation the moment the tube passes the vocal cords.

If RSI is unavoidable, it is advisable to continue to administer a few slow controlled breaths (10-12/min) through continued positive pressure ventilation or a BVM while your paralytic and sedative take effect. A very elegant option is to place a LMA after topicalization and sedation or RSI, thus continuing to ventilate the patient while subsequently transitioning to an endotracheal tube. This is an excellent time for an emergency physician to use a fiber-optic scope, as intubating with a scope via an LMA is far easier to master than nasal intubation. Some LMA brands are designed to allow an endotracheal tube to pass over a scope directly through the LMA itself, and with the aid of a bronchoscopy adapter you can ventilate the patient while doing so. Alternatively, you can also pass a disposable scope through any supraglottic airway, then cut the scope at its base with shears once you are past the cords, remove the LMA over the scope remnant, and use that scope as a bougie to guide your endotracheal tube.

Once you have successfully intubated the patient, confirmed placement, and transitioned to mechanical ventilation, your airway management is not yet complete. It is critically important to set the appropriate ventilator settings after the period of reduced ventilation during intubation. Immediately increase the tidal volume (eg, 8 mL/kg) and respiratory rate (eg, 30 breaths/min) and ensure your patient is well sedated to tolerate these settings, or choose a pressure support mode that allows the patient to set their own minute ventilation. Keep a close initial eye on the ventilator tracing and adjust settings to match the minute ventilation requirement without air trapping.

PEARLS

- Reassess your patients with metabolic acidosis and trend blood gas to identify signs of decompensation as early as possible. Don't forget to treat the underlying cause.
- Don't just pre-oxygenate, pre-ventilate. Buy time, improve minute ventilation, and in some cases avoid intubation by providing positive pressure when able.
- Minimize apnea time. Acidosis will sharply worsen as intubation time increases.
- Consider awake intubation with ketamine and/or topical analgesia in patients with other difficult airway characteristics that make paralysis too risky. You aren't done once the tube is in. Don't forget to customize your ventilator settings (higher tidal volume and respiratory rate) and give adequate sedation.

Suggested Readings

Kornas RL, Owyang CG, Sakles JC, Foley LJ, Mosier JM, Society for Airway Management's Special Projects Committee. Evaluation and management of the physiologically difficult airway: consensus recommendations from society for airway management. *Anesth Analg.* 2021;132(2):395-405.

Moiser JM, Joshi R, Hypes C, Pacheco G, Valenzuela T, Sakles JC. The physiologically difficult airway. *West J Emerg Med.* 2015;16(7):1109-1117.

Weingart S, Swaminathan A. Critical care mailbag: intubating with severe acidosis. EM:RAP. Accessed January 5, 2023. https://www.emrap.org/episode/emrap20213/criticalcare.

31

What to Do When You Lose Your View

Jeremy Lacocque and Erik J. Kramer

The initial assessment of every critically ill ED patient begins with an evaluation of the airway. In the following chapter, the authors discuss strategies for approaching the deteriorating airway and what to do when you cannot obtain a view of the vocal cords or if you lose your view.

First-Pass Options

Knowing your tools and anatomy is key to navigating a difficult airway. The following are common tools used to successfully intubate the patient.

- VL: Generally, the default tool for intubation, as it can accommodate standard geometry blades and hyperangulated blades for anterior and difficult airways.

- DL: The authors recommend DL be used when VL is obscured by fluid, blood, or condensation. The Miller style blade is used by scooping the epiglottis up and out of view; because of this we recommend its use with DL as a first choice in cases of epiglottitis, pharyngeal masses, and is considered ideal in pediatric cases given the "floppier" epiglottis.
- Hyperangulated blades: Recommended for patients in cervical collars and in patients with poor neck mobility, short necks, or a small thyromental distance (less than two finger breadths). Be sure you use a rigid stylet to accommodate the hyperangulation, as a more pliable stylet will lose shape.
- Fiber-optic scope: Should be considered as a first-pass tool in known narrow airways, such as known stenosis, airway neoplasms, or surgically altered airways. It may also be considered for usage with nasotracheal intubation in cases of severe oral or tongue swelling or in cases of oral trauma. In additional, it can help intubate through certain laryngeal mask airways. Generally, fiber-optic use takes more time and is not recommended for the crashing patient.
- Suction: One to two suction catheters should be available at the head of the bed and used when inserting any blade or fiber-optic scope into the patient's naso- or oropharynx to ensure maximal visibility. In situations where the airway has large amounts of secretions, food particulate or fluid (blood, vomit), large bore suction should be used if available. If unavailable, taking the suction catheter off the tubing and inserting the tubing directly into the mouth can be helpful.

Rescue Approaches

When there is difficulty obtaining a definitive airway either via nasopharyngeal or oropharyngeal intubation, it is important to continue to oxygenate and ventilate the patient.

- BVM: Every "can't intubate, can't ventilate" situation deserves an attempt with BVM. The authors recommend that patients receive BVM ventilation for preoxygenation and in between multiple attempts at intubation to prevent hypoxia and hypercarbia. While not a definitive airway, patients with difficult anatomy but who are not at high risk of further airway obstruction or aspiration can receive BVM indefinitely until an airway can be secured either via intubation or surgical airway.
- Bougie: The bougie can be used to easily pass through the vocal cords under direct visualization or blindly in instances of airway obstruction from fluid. Use of the bougie when unable to obtain a good view of the vocal cords is done by feeling a "clicking" sensation as the coudé tip passes through the tracheal rings. The bougie can also be rotated right or left after passing the cords to selectively intubate the right or left mainstem in cases of massive hemoptysis.
- SGA: The SGA is often used as a temporizing rescue approach, as they can be inserted blindly and by a broader range of providers. While there is a higher risk of aspiration, they can be effective until a definitive airway is established.
- Cricothyrotomy: This is the last resort for securing the difficult airway. When patients can't be intubated or oxygenated/ventilated, cricothyrotomy is indicated. Needle cricothyrotomy should be performed on patients less than 8 years old and can be considered in older pediatric or adult patients as a temporizing measure to provide oxygenation. Note that minimal ventilation is provided by needle cricothyrotomy. For patients who can be oxygenated and ventilated, all other options should be exhausted before considering a cricothyrotomy.

Troubleshooting

When you are unable to pass the ETT, the solution depends on the problem.

Anatomy

If you're in the mouth and can't see the cords, are you using the right equipment? If you see mostly tongue, you may need to increase the size of your blade. If you see mostly mucosal tissue and the esophagus, you need to slowly retract your blade or use a smaller blade. Is the tube unable to advance? Try a smaller tube or bend your stylet to mirror the angle at which you are approaching the vocal cords. Try using a bougie to improve your chances of success. If the cords are anterior, will external pharyngeal manipulation help? Will a hyperangulated blade with a rigid stylet improve your view? Understanding these simple concepts and troubleshooting through them will help improve your view.

Obstruction

If the liquid is blocking your view and routine suctioning isn't effective, consider using DL instead of VL, as the VL camera can often become blurry and obstructed. Using the SALAD technique is helpful in obtaining a better view of the vocal cords. This technique is as follows:

1) Enter the mouth with the suction catheter followed by your DL or VL blade.
2) Once the oropharynx is suctioned thoroughly, the suction catheter is placed to the left of the blade where it continues to decontaminate the airway during intubation attempt on the right side of the blade.
3) In addition, placing the catheter in the esophagus will help to continuously suction emesis and improve your view.
4) In instances where this method is still not effective, an ETT can be placed in the esophagus as a tamponade for secretions and moved to the left of the blade while an attempt at securing the airway to the right of the blade is made.
5) If using a large bore catheter that accommodates bougie insertion and all of the techniques mentioned earlier fail due to profuse amounts of fluid obstructing your view, place the tip of the catheter through the vocal cords, disconnect the suction, place a bougie through the catheter, and exchange the suction catheter for an ETT over the bougie.
6) If the airway is obstructed by large particulates (ie, food, bone, tissue) and you are unable to suction or your suction becomes clogged, consider using McGill Forceps to improve your view. Once you are able to visualize the cords, attempt to pass your ETT.

Takeaway Message

It is important to know your limits. An airway attempt should not typically exceed 30 seconds. Minimize the chances for hypoxemia by applying apneic oxygenation with a nasal cannula at flush rate.

When you make a second attempt, make sure you've changed something between the first and second attempts. Don't expect a different outcome if you try the same thing twice. Do you need a different blade? Have you optimized the patient's positioning? Are the patient's three axes lined up?

Finally, reevaluate the patient's need for endotracheal intubation. If the patient can be well ventilated via BVM or SGA, use that in the meantime. You can put a patient on a ventilator with an SGA. Then, when the patient is otherwise stabilized, consider another attempt, involving a consultant or even intubating the patient through the SGA using a tube exchanger or fiberscope.

PEARLS

- Stay humble. If your attempt isn't successful within 30 seconds, go back to BVM and change something on your second attempt. Your goal is to oxygenate and ventilate the patient.
- Planning is just as important as execution. Set up your equipment and position your patient for success on the first attempt.
- Ensure you have easy access to tools for rescue approaches such as a bougie, SGA, suction, McGills, fiber-optic scope, and cricothyroidotomy equipment.
- Use the SALAD technique to clear the obstruction and help improve your view.
- When all else fails, perform a cricothyrotomy (or needle cricothyrotomy in patients <8 years old).

Suggested Readings

Intubating the Critically Ill Patient: A Step-by-Step Guide for Success in the ED and ICU. (2020). Germany: Springer International Publishing.
Root, Christopher W., et al. "Suction Assisted Laryngoscopy and Airway Decontamination (SALAD): A technique for improved emergency airway management." *Resuscitation Plus* 1 (2020): 100005.

32

Know How to Perform a Bougie-Assisted Cricothyroidotomy

Lee Johnson and Joseph Brown

A cricothyrotomy is indicated when attempts to oxygenate and ventilate have failed, when attempts to intubate have failed, or when attempts to intubate are not plausible (significant facial trauma or distorted facial anatomy).

The greatest pitfall in performing a cricothyrotomy is the delay in performing the procedure. This is often due to repeated failed attempts at nonsurgical efforts to establish an airway as a result of provider discomfort in performing a surgical airway.

Unfortunately, there are numerous studies that have revealed that most patients were already bradycardic or in cardiac arrest before cricothyrotomy. Oftentimes, the failure linked to cricothyrotomy is the result of a delay in performing the procedure rather than the failure in the procedure itself. Equally important is the preparation for the procedure as the end point of all intubation attempts. By doing so, in cases where there is an inability to establish a definitive airway, there will be clarity in moving to a surgical airway as the expected next step.

CONTRAINDICATIONS

In a life-threatening airway emergency, there are no absolute contraindications to a cricothyrotomy.

Relative contraindications to consider include prior neck surgery, obesity, neck pathology, prior radiation therapy to the area, potential distal airway obstruction, coagulopathy, trauma/burns, hematoma, or any features that distort anatomic landmarks. With these, it is important to anticipate difficulties, prepare accordingly, and consider consulting surgery, anesthesiology, or otolaryngology (ENT) prior to the procedure.

Surgical cricothyroidotomy is generally not recommended in children under the age of 8 as the small size of the cricothyroid membrane makes accessing this space difficult. In these children, transtracheal jet ventilation is preferred, unless a physician comfortable performing a tracheostomy in this age group is available.

PREPARATION

Prior to the procedure, obtain a cuffed 4.0 or 5.0 tracheostomy tube or a 6.0 endotracheal tube, a bougie, and a number 11 scalpel. Antiseptic swabs, suction, lighting, 4 × 4 gauze, and a tracheal hook may be beneficial if time allows. Prior to any expected difficult intubation, mark the cricothyroid membrane with a marking pen, both to familiarize yourself with the patient's anatomy and to prepare your team for the possibility of proceeding to a cricothyrotomy if necessary. In cases where a surgical airway is likely, such as in severe facial trauma, and time permits, consider injecting the skin overlying the cricothyroid membrane with lidocaine with epinephrine to assist with hemostasis.

PROCEDURE

Once the decision is made to perform a cricothyrotomy, position yourself on the same side of the patient as your dominant hand. Perform a "laryngeal handshake" with your nondominant hand, centering the larynx between your thumb and middle finger, and sweeping the chin cranially to expose the cricothyroid membrane. With your dominant hand, palpate up from the sternal notch. The most caudal bony prominence is the cricoid cartilage, followed cranially by the thyroid cartilage. The cricothyroid membrane will then be the depression noted between the thyroid and cricoid cartilages. The cricothyroid membrane is a dense fibroelastic sheet between the thyroid and cricoid cartilages with an average height and width of 10 mm (index finger width).

While maintaining control of the larynx, center the cricothyroid membrane between your thumb and middle finger of the nondominant hand and palpate the membrane with your first finger of the nondominant hand. This creates your crosshairs with the cricothyroid membrane centered between your thumb and middle finger and your first finger directly palpating the membrane.

Once identified, sterilize the area. Hold the trachea with your nondominant hand and make a 2- to 3-cm midline vertical incision through the skin with the scalpel in your dominant hand. In patients with a very large neck, a larger incision may be necessary. Once identified, make a 1- to 2-cm transverse stab incision through the cricothyroid membrane. Insert your little finger into the incision and through the cricoid membrane and feel the inside of the trachea; if you feel ridges, you are in the right place. Slide your bougie along your finger into the trachea, and reconfirm your location by feeling for tracheal rings. Insert your tube over the bougie and advance until the cuff is within the airway. Inflate the cuff, auscultate for breath sounds, and use end title CO_2 for confirmation of airway placement. Secure by suturing in place and/or with a twill tie or a commercial tube holder. Given this is a shorter airway, extra caution should be exercised when securing the airway.

POST CRICOTHYROTOMY

After securing the airway, one needs to be wary of the complications of performing a cricothyrotomy and appropriately document. Commonly cited complications include aspiration, mediastinal emphysema, hemorrhage, creation of false passage into the tissue, esophageal/tracheal laceration, or vocal cord injury.

A cricothyrotomy can be a stressful situation, however, and can also serve as a great learning opportunity. Debriefing after a cricothyrotomy allows for concerns to be heard and for everyone in the room to understand the procedure and decision making that was performed. It can also identify areas of improvement for future cannot intubate, cannot oxygenate scenarios.

As with any high-frequency, low-occurrence procedure, preparation starts well before the patient arrival. Periodically, reviewing and rehearsing this time-sensitive procedure is imperative.

PEARLS

- Do not delay cricothyrotomy; a delay could result in a worse outcome.
- At a minimum, you need a No. 11 scalpel, a bougie, and a cuffed 6.0 endotracheal tube.
- Once one has entered the cricothyroid membrane, make sure to always have either a surgical device, scalpel, or your finger in the opening at all times until the tube is placed.
- Make time for debriefing; this can be a stressful experience for all involved.

SUGGESTED READINGS

DeVore EK, Redmann A, Howell R, Khosla S. Best practices for emergency surgical airway: a systematic review. *Laryngoscope Investig Otolaryngol*. 2019;4(6):602-608.

Frerk C, Mitchell VS, McNarry AF, et al. Difficult Airway Society 2015 guidelines for management of unanticipated difficult intubation in adults. *Br J Anaesth*. 2015;115(6):827-848.

George, N, Consunji, G, Storkersen, J, et al. Comparison of emergency airway management techniques in the performance of emergent Cricothyrotomy. *Int J Emerg Med*. 2022;15(1):24.

Greenland KB, Acott C, Segal R, Goulding G, Riley RH, Merry AF. Emergency surgical airway in life-threatening acute airway emergencies—why are we so reluctant to do it? *Anaesth Intensive Care*. 2011;39(4):578-584.

Heidegger, T. Management of the difficult airway. *N Engl J Med*. 2021;384(19):1836-1847.

Langvad S, Hyldmo PK, Nakstad AR, Vist GE, Sandberg M. Emergency cricothyrotomy—a systematic review. *Scand J Trauma Resusc Emerg Med*. 2013;21:43.

Moroco AE, Armen SB, Goldenberg D. Emergency cricothyrotomy: a 10-year single institution experience. *Am Surg*. 2023;89(4):1243-1246.

Paix BR, Griggs WM. Emergency surgical cricothyroidotomy: 24 successful cases leading to a simple 'scalpel-finger-tube' method. *Emerg Med Australas*. 2012;24(1):23-30.

33

Baby on Board—Intubating the Pregnant Patient

Haley Vertelney and Cecily Koppuzha Sotomayor

Respiratory depression is a rare complication that occurs in approximately 0.2% of pregnancies; however, it carries a high morbidity of up to 30% of maternal deaths in the United States. Definitive airway management in this population poses unique challenges to the physician and requires additional training and consideration. Misunderstanding of the specific anatomic and physiologic characteristics of the pregnant patient can lead to poor maternal and fetal outcomes.

The high rate of complications is likely multifactorial. There are several conditions that can lead to respiratory distress in the gravid patient (**Table 33.1**). In general, there is less research on pregnant patients as they are frequently excluded from medical trials, including those that study respiratory failure. In addition, as with most low-frequency and high-acuity presentations, an emergency physician may be less comfortable managing respiratory distress in the pregnant patient simply from infrequency of exposure to the event. Physiologic and anatomic changes that occur during pregnancy also complicate management of respiratory depression in these patients. Consequently, the rate of failed intubation in this population is up to 10 times higher than in nonpregnant patients.

TABLE 33.1	CONDITIONS THAT CONTRIBUTE TO RESPIRATORY DEPRESSION IN THE GRAVID PATIENT
Pregnancy-specific	Preeclampsia/eclampsia
	Obstetric sepsis
	Peripartum cardiomyopathy
	Pulmonary edema secondary to tocolytics
	Increased fluid retention
	Pregnancy-induced weight gain
	Amniotic fluid embolism
Increased risk in pregnancy	Thromboembolism
	Aspiration
	Asthma
	Heart failure
	Pulmonary infection
	Urinary tract infection
	Transfusion associated lung injury
	Placental abruption
	Chorioamnionitis
	Obstetric hemorrhage
	Endometritis
Common in general population	Non-obstetric sepsis
	Aspiration pneumonia
	Atelectasis
	Trauma
	Drugs/toxins
	Underlying chronic conditions NOS
	Obesity

Several anatomic changes happen during pregnancy that increase the risk of respiratory depression during airway management. Weight gain and increased breast size can make optimizing head and chest positioning more difficult during intubation. Human placental growth hormone increases blood flow to the upper airways, which makes the vocal cords swollen and more friable. Furthermore, gravid patients are generally edematous due to low serum protein, high blood volume, and the antidiuretic effect of oxytocin. These edematous changes can make visualization difficult during laryngoscopy. In later pregnancy, the gravid uterus can compress the IVC, which predisposes a pregnant patient to peri-intubation hypotension due to decreased venous return to the heart, particularly if the patient is not positioned in a left-lateral tilt. Similarly, compression of the aorta can reduce uterine blood flow, which can lead to maternal hypotension. The FRC decreases up to 20% due to the expanded uterus pressing up against the diaphragm. FRC can decrease even further in patients who are supine or obese. Pressure from abdominal contents can compress lungs and lead to small-airway closure particularly when the patient is lying flat, which leads to worsening hypoxemia. The abdomen also presses up on the diaphragm, decreasing the tone of the gastroesophageal sphincter and predisposing the patient to aspiration of gastric contents.

The physiologic changes of pregnancy also complicate the management of respiratory depression in these patients. Fetal demand normally increases maternal oxygen consumption by up to 50%. Small variations in pH can significantly affect fetal physiology and lead to poor fetal outcomes. Hypocarbic status due to hyperventilation can cause ureteroplacental vasoconstriction and lead to fetal hypoxia. This process is normally regulated by maternal alkalosis, which regulates the transfer of acidic carbon dioxide from fetus to mother via elimination from maternal lungs. Hypoxia can develop quickly in response to hypoventilation or apnea. The immune system is downregulated during pregnancy to allow maternal tolerance of fetal tissue, but this can predispose pregnant patients to develop pneumonia and subsequent respiratory failure. Given these risks, it is imperative to be optimally prepared for intubation of the gravid patient (**Table 33.2**).

TABLE 33.2 PREPARATION FOR ESTABLISHING A DEFINITIVE AIRWAY FOR THE GRAVID PATIENT

Team meeting	■ Assign clear roles to entire team ■ Clarify plan including adjuncts, contingencies, and medications
Preoxygenation	■ Give 100% oxygen to prolong time to desaturation during apnea ■ Head of bed at least 30° during preoxygenation to increase functional residual capacity
Positioning	■ Ramped, sniffing position ■ Anticipate left uterine displacement with at least 15° of tilt to minimize aortocaval compression ■ Head of bed at least 30° to minimize aspiration risk
Equipment	■ Recommend video laryngoscopy. Consider short laryngoscope (for possibly decreased oropharyngeal diameter) ■ Consider awake tracheal intubation, as oxygenation and manual ventilation may be difficult due to upper airway collapse ■ Have backup supraglottic airway available (but avoid primary use as aspiration risk increases, particularly beyond second trimester) ■ Surgical airway kit at bedside ■ Backup smaller ETTs available ■ Materials and staff available for potential neonatal resuscitation in case of emergent delivery

This preparation includes a team meeting to assign roles and clarify plans, appropriate preoxygenation, and patient positioning to optimize venous return and decrease the risk of aspiration, as well as all appropriate intubation equipment needed for uncomplicated and complicated airways.

The medications for RSI for a pregnant patient should be the same as those used in nonpregnant patients. Ketamine should be carefully considered in patients with preeclampsia or eclampsia as it can exacerbate hypertension. Notably, all induction agents will cross the placenta; however, a definitive airway for a pregnant patient in respiratory distress is imperative; the risks of fetal hypoxia outweigh the risks of fetal exposure to induction medications. Paralytic agents are ionized, so they will not cross the placenta and will not affect the fetus.

PEARLS

- Airway management in a gravid patient is challenging due to anatomic and physiologic changes in pregnancy.
- The risk of failed airway is higher in pregnant patients with respiratory depression than in nonpregnant patients.
- Medications for induction agents and neuromuscular blocking agents should be used in pregnant patients for intubation.
- It is important to have a clear plan for intubation of the pregnant patient and several contingencies ready.

Suggested Readings

Hood D, Dewan D. Anesthetic and obstetric outcome in morbidly obese parturients. *Anesthesiology.* 1993;79(6):1210-1218.

Jenkins TM, Troiano NH, Graves CR, Baird SM, Boehm FH. Mechanical ventilation in an obstetric population: characteristics and delivery rates. *Am J Obstet Gynecol.* 2003;188(2):549-552.

Kinsella SM, Winton AL, Mushambi MC, et al. Failed tracheal intubation during obstetric general anaesthesia: a literature review. *Int J Obstet Anesth.* 2015;24:356-374.

Lapinsky SE. Cardiopulmonary complications of pregnancy. *Crit Care Med.* 2005;33: 1616-1622.

Lapinsky SE, Kruczynski K, Slutsky AS. Critical care in the pregnant patient. *Am J Respir Crit Care Med.* 1995;152(2):427-455.

LoMauro A, Aliverti A. Respiratory physiology of pregnancy. *Breathe (Sheff).* 2015; 11(4): 297-301.

Marina B. Respiratory failure and airway management in the pregnant patient. REBEL EM blog. Accessed December 31, 2020. https://rebelem.com/respiratory-failure-and-airway-management-in-the-pregnant-patient/

McDonnell NJ, Paech MJ, Clavisi OM, Scott KL; ANZCA Trials Group. Difficult and failed intubation in obstetric anaesthesia: an observational study of airway management and complications associated with general anaesthesia for caesarean section. *Int J Obstet Anesth.* 2008;17:292-297.

McKeen DM, George RB, O'Connell CM, et al. Difficult and failed intubation: incident rates and maternal, obstetrical, and anesthetic predictors. *Can J Anaesth.* 2011;58(6): 514-524.

Murphy VE, Gibson P, Talbot PI, Clifton VL. Severe asthma exacerbations during pregnancy. *Obstet Gynecol.* 2005; 106: 1046-1054.

Namazy JA, Schatz M. Pregnancy and asthma: recent developments. *Curr Opin Pulm Med*. 2005;11:56-60.

Rodrigues J, Neiderman MS. Pneumonia complicating pregnancy. *Clin Chest Med*. 1992; 13:679–691.

Saracoglu K, Saracoglu G. Airway management during pregnancy and labor. In: Shallik NA, eds. *Special Conditions in Human Airway Management*. IntechOpen; 2021:1577-1578.

Sista P, Chukwulebe S. Intubating the pregnant patient in the ED. NUEM Blog. Expert Commentary by Patel S. January 18, 2021. Retrieved from http://www.nuemblog.com/blog/intubating-the-pregnant-patient.

SECTION III

CRITICAL CARE

34

KNOW YOUR INITIAL VENT SETTINGS

RYAN BARNICLE AND CHELSEY MILLER

Any patient placed on IMV in the ED is at risk for VILI. Improper IMV settings will potentially worsen injured lungs or introduce lung injury to otherwise healthy patients regardless of the indication for endotracheal intubation. Injury occurs via multiple mechanisms and can lead to harmful complications for patients. Emergency physicians must be conscientious about initial ventilator settings to mitigate these deleterious forces at the beginning of IMV by defaulting to a LPV protocol.

In the LOV-ED study from 2018, Fuller et al showed that intentional implementation of an ED-based LPV protocol (**Figure 34.1**) is feasible and was associated with a clinically meaningful reduction in the instances of ARDS and other ventilator-associated conditions developing later in the ICU (14.5%-7.4%). Ventilator-free days, hospital-free days, and ICU-free days were all increased. Mortality decreased from 34.1% to 19.6%. A more recent large retrospective study showed similar clinical benefits as well as a significant reduction in the overall cost of care.

Initial settings for LPV that can be empirically applied to most ED patients have been published by Weingart and Fuller and are summarized later. Specific adjustments for those with obstructive lung disease are included.

- *Mode*: Volume-AC is an ideal ventilator mode for patients in the ED. The patient is permitted to breathe over a set minimum RR, but the ventilator will deliver the same set volume regardless of whether the cycle is triggered by time or patient inhalation. The major advantage of volume-AC is full respiratory support for the work of breathing in the post-intubation phase when paralytics and potent sedation are being utilized. Additionally, this mode can help minimize the metabolic demand of breathing while the patient is experiencing the acute phase of the emergency mandating intubation. It is a straightforward mode that allows the selection of accurate tidal volume and reliable monitoring of inspiratory plateau pressures (P_{plat}), the two most essential elements of LPV.
- *Tidal volume (V_t)*: The core of LPV is based on the landmark ARDSNet ARMA study, which demonstrated the superiority of targeting lower tidal volumes and established the standard of 4 to 8 mL/kg tidal volumes, based on a patient's PBW. Limiting maximum tidal volumes is thought to be a key factor in preventing VILI by preventing overdistension and volutrauma. Starting at a V_t of 8 mL/kg PBW is safe and can be

Initiate ED Ventilator Protocol

Obtain accurate patient height
- After patient stabilizes, use tape measure for height measurement

Volutrauma

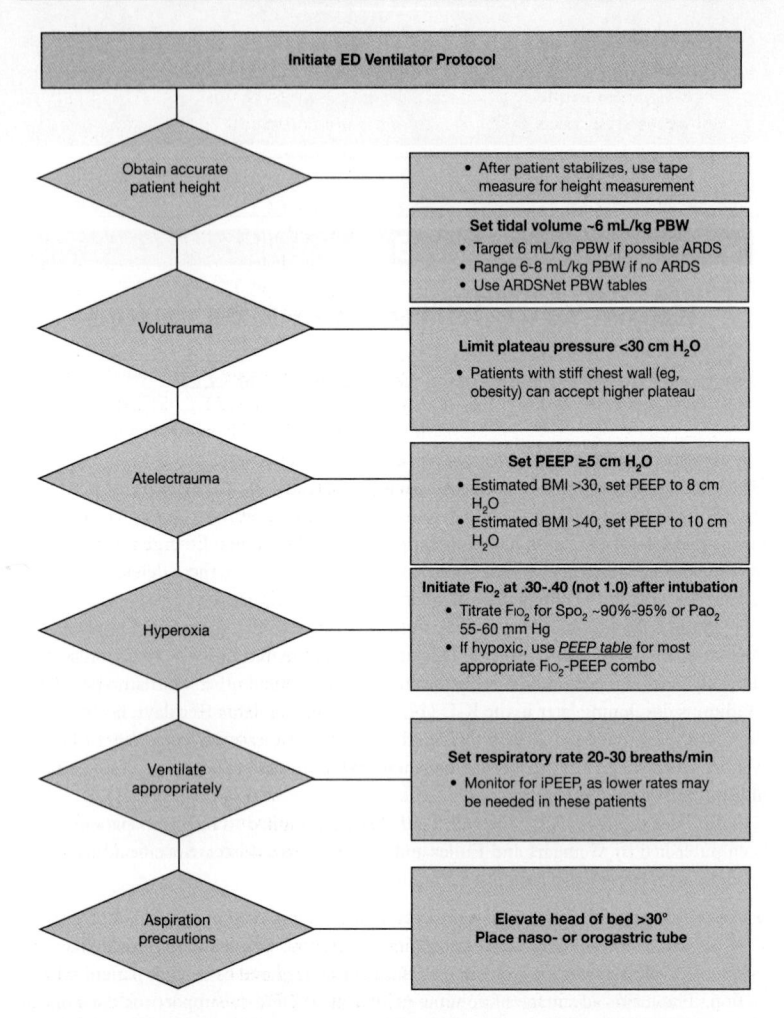

Set tidal volume ~6 mL/kg PBW
- Target 6 mL/kg PBW if possible ARDS
- Range 6-8 mL/kg PBW if no ARDS
- Use ARDSNet PBW tables

Limit plateau pressure <30 cm H₂O
- Patients with stiff chest wall (eg, obesity) can accept higher plateau

Atelectrauma

Set PEEP ≥5 cm H₂O
- Estimated BMI >30, set PEEP to 8 cm H₂O
- Estimated BMI >40, set PEEP to 10 cm H₂O

Hyperoxia

Initiate F$_{IO_2}$ at .30-.40 (not 1.0) after intubation
- Titrate F$_{IO_2}$ for S$_{pO_2}$ ~90%-95% or P$_{aO_2}$ 55-60 mm Hg
- If hypoxic, use _PEEP table_ for most appropriate F$_{IO_2}$-PEEP combo

Ventilate appropriately

Set respiratory rate 20-30 breaths/min
- Monitor for iPEEP, as lower rates may be needed in these patients

Aspiration precautions

Elevate head of bed >30°
Place naso- or orogastric tube

FIGURE 34.1 ED ventilator protocol. (Reprinted from Fuller BM, Ferguson IT, Mohr NM, et al. Lung-protective ventilation initiated in the emergency department (LOV-ED): a quasi-experimental, before-after trial. *Ann Emerg Med*. 2017; 70(3):406-418, with permission from Elsevier. Copyright © 2017 by the American College of Emergency Physicians.)

reduced further as needed if the patient is determined to have ARDS or high plateau pressures. Reducing V_t to as low as 4 mL/kg PBW may be necessary if plateau pressures continue to be elevated in patients with ARDS. Before setting the target tidal volume, a tape measure should be used to get an accurate patient height for the calculation of the correct PBW.

- *Inspiratory plateau pressure (P_{plat})*: Monitoring P_{plat}, or the static pressure at the level of the alveoli, is the best surrogate for estimating whether the current tidal volume will cause alveolar injury. Ideally, P_{plat} should be less than 30 cm H$_2$O. If pressures are elevated above this, the tidal volume can be reduced by 1 mL/kg at a time. P_{plat} is not equivalent to peak inspiratory pressure during volume-AC mode and needs to be measured by an inspiratory hold maneuver. Peak pressure is higher than P_{plat} and represents a combination of the pressure at the alveoli and the pressure needed to overcome airway resistance.

- *Inspiratory flow rate*: Patients who are spontaneously breathing expect large flow rates at the initiation of each breath and if the ventilator is set with a low inspiratory flow rate, significant ventilator dyssynchrony can develop due to patient discomfort. Starting with an initial inspiratory flow rate of 60 L/min is ideal, but patients with obstructive lung disease may need higher rates (ie. 80 L/min) to maximize exhalation time.
- *RR*: The exact goal Paco$_2$ will vary depending on the nature of the acute illness. The RR should be the first variable, and typically the only variable, that is manipulated based on Paco$_2$ levels. For most patients, set RR to 16 to 20 breaths/min and adjust as needed from 15 to 30 bpm based on subsequent end-tidal CO$_2$ and blood gas readings. Despite the risk of hypoventilation causing subsequent hypercapnia and respiratory acidosis, patients with obstructive lung disease should be started with a RR much lower than typical (around 10 bpm) to allow plenty of time for exhalation and avoid breath stacking and auto-PEEP.
- *PEEP and FIO$_2$*: Finally, oxygenation is managed via the settings for PEEP and FIO$_2$. Although FIO$_2$ should be kept at 100% for the intubation and subsequent transition to mechanical ventilation, FIO$_2$ should be reduced as low as possible to maintain adequate oxygen saturation and avoid ongoing oxygen toxicity. PEEP should be set to a minimum of 5 cm H$_2$O for most patients. A goal pulse oximetry (SpO$_2$) level of 88% to 95% can be targeted for most patients without brain injury or other contraindications such as acute cor pulmonale. Evidence suggests poor compliance with this fundamental oxygenation protocol in the ED, despite widely available PEEP-FIO$_2$ titration tables (**Table 34.1**) guiding titration. As more alveoli are recruited, SpO$_2$ may increase beyond 95%, and then down titration using the stepwise fashion can begin.

For patients with COPD or asthma, exhalation is inhibited by outflow obstruction. These patients are uniquely at risk for dynamic hyperinflation from progressive air entrapment. This can worsen VILI and lead to acute cardiovascular collapse. However, these patients still benefit from the same principles of LPV such as low tidal volumes. Ensuring adequate exhalation is the most important principle when patients on ventilation with obstructive lung disease. Modification to RR and inspiratory flow time as well as adequate sedation and analgesia is necessary. Physicians should monitor the flow waveform on the ventilator and ensure that the tracing of the expiratory limb returns to the baseline before the initiation of the next breath. Once the underlying pathophysiology has been adequately treated, such as acute bronchospasm in asthma, the RR and the necessary sedation may be more liberalized. In the meantime, hypercapnia and acidosis down to a pH of 7.2 can be well tolerated in most cases.

Overall compliance with LPV settings decreases with busy ED boarding, so protocolization of LPV as a standard of care is essential as the boarding crisis worsens internationally. The goal of mechanical ventilation is to maintain life-sustaining gas exchange and reduce the metabolic demands of breathing while avoiding VILI. **Table 34.2** summarizes LPV settings in the ED for convenient clinical reference.

TABLE 34.1 PEEP

FIO$_2$ (%)	PEEP (CM H$_2$O)
30	5
40	5
40	8
50	8
50	10
60	10
70	10
70	12
70	14
80	14
90	14
90	16
90	18
100	20
100	22
100	24

Adapted from Acute Respiratory Distress Syndrome Network, Brower RG, Matthay MA, et al. Ventilation with lower tidal volumes as compared with traditional tidal volumes for acute lung injury and the acute respiratory distress syndrome. *N Engl J Med*. 2000;342(18):1301-1308.

TABLE 34.2 SUMMARY TABLE FOR THE TWO VENTILATOR STRATEGIES

	LUNG PROTECTIVE STRATEGY	OBSTRUCTIVE STRATEGY
Mode	Volume assist control	Volume assist control
Tidal volume	Start at 8 mL/kg PBW; adjust for plateau pressure goal	8 mL/kg PBW
Inspiratory flow rate	Start at 60 L/min; adjust for comfort	60–80 L/min
RR	Start at 16 breaths/min; adjust for PaCO$_2$ goal	Start at 10 breaths/min; adjust to allow full expiration
PEEP	Start at 5 cm H$_2$O; adjust according to table	0 cm H$_2$O (some may treat patient with PEEP ≤5 cm H$_2$O)
FIO$_2$	Start at 40%; adjust according to table	Start at 40%; adjust for SpO$_2$ ≥88%
Check for safety	Measure plateau pressure. If ≥30 cm H$_2$O, decrease tidal volume by 1 mL/kg	Measure plateau pressure or observe flow time graph. If plateau pressure ≥30 cm H$_2$O or flow/time graph shows incomplete expiration, decrease RR

PBW, predicted body weight; RR, respiratory rate.

Reprinted from Weingart SD. Managing initial mechanical ventilation in the emergency department. *Ann Emerg Med*. 2016;68(5):614–617, with permission from Elsevier. Copyright © 2016 by the American College of Emergency Physicians.

PEARLS

- Patients in the ED requiring IMV should be placed in settings consistent with LPV (low V_t, higher PEEP, and minimal FIO$_2$).

- Use a tape measure to accurately measure a patient's height and then calculate the appropriate V_t based on PBW.
- Adjust the RR to manage minute ventilation when trying to target a specific $Paco_2$.
- All patients should be assessed for adequate exhalation and breath stacking, but patients with obstructive lung disease (ie, COPD, asthma) may need low RRs and high inspiratory flow rates to avoid this complication.
- During the acute post-intubation phase, ensure appropriate analgesia and sedation, so the patient can tolerate appropriate ventilator settings while other initial diagnostic and therapeutic tasks are completed.

Suggested Readings

Acute Respiratory Distress Syndrome Network, Brower RG, Matthay MA, et al. Ventilation with lower tidal volumes as compared with traditional tidal volumes for acute lung injury and the acute respiratory distress syndrome. *N Engl J Med*. 2000;342(18):1301-1308.

Fernando SM, Fan E, Rochwerg B, et al. Lung-protective ventilation and associated outcomes and costs among patients receiving invasive mechanical ventilation in the ED. *Chest*. 2021;159(2):606-618.

Fuller BM, Ferguson IT, Mohr NM, et al. Lung-Protective Ventilation Initiated in the Emergency Department (LOV-ED): a quasi-experimental, before-after trial. *Ann Emerg Med*. 2017;70(3):406-418.e4.

Lentz S, Roginski MA, Montrief T, Ramzy M, Gottlieb M, Long B. Initial emergency department mechanical ventilation strategies for COVID-19 hypoxemic respiratory failure and ARDS. *Am J Emerg Med*. 2020;38(10):2194-2202.

Mosier JM, Hypes CD. Mechanical ventilation strategies for the patient with severe obstructive lung disease. *Emerg Med Clin North Am*. 2019;37(3):445-458.

Owyang CG, Kim JL, Loo G, Ranginwala S, Mathews KS. The effect of emergency department crowding on lung-protective ventilation utilization for critically ill patients. *J Crit Care*. 2019;52:40-47.

Slutsky AS, Ranieri VM. Ventilator-induced lung injury. *N Engl J Med*. 2013;369(22):2126-2136.

Weingart SD. Managing initial mechanical ventilation in the emergency department. *Ann Emerg Med*. 2016;68(5):614-617.

Wilcox SR, Richards JB, Fisher DF, Sankoff J, Seigel TA. Initial mechanical ventilator settings and lung protective ventilation in the ED. *Am J Emerg Med*. 2016;34(8):1446-1451.

35

Don't Forget Post-Intubation Analgesia and Sedation

Matthew Tanzi

ETI is a vital resuscitative procedure performed by EP. Airway management is commonly performed via RSI using a variety of sedative and neuromuscular blockade medications. The immediate post-intubation period is critical for continued patient stabilization. Numerous adverse effects can occur if analgesia and sedation are not administered appropriately. These include, but are not limited to, self-extubation, catecholamine surge, hemodynamic instability, impaired psychological recovery, delirium, and ventilator dyssynchrony. Physicians must be especially diligent in recognizing the need for analgosedation for patients receiving long-acting paralytics. Recent studies have shown that EPs often neglect post-intubation analgesia and sedation. One retrospective study of ED intubated patients found that 33% had no anxiolytic, 53% had no analgesic, and 20% had neither anxiolytic nor analgesic in the peri-intubation period. The volume of critically ill patients presenting to the ED has increased rapidly without a proportional increase in ICU bed availability. Unfortunately, this has resulted in a nationwide boarding crisis and the requirement for prolonged care of intubated patients in the ED. Therefore, it is vital to understand how to appropriately implement post-intubation analgesia and sedation.

Fentanyl or Hydromorphone (Opioids)
Appropriate analgesia, with lower levels of sedation, results in decreased ICU length of stay and decreased time on mechanical ventilation. A potent opioid, typically fentanyl or hydromorphone, should be administered to transition the patient out of the induction phase. Fentanyl is simple to titrate and short acting. A dose of 1 mcg/kg typically results in a dose of 50 to 100 mcg. A fentanyl infusion can be started and titrated if a prolonged course is anticipated, yet with any infusion, the clinical effects can be prolonged. The sedative effect of hydromorphone is similar to fentanyl, but it is long acting. A standard dose of hydromorphone typically starts at 0.5 to 1 mg. Both fentanyl and hydromorphone can lead to a decrease in sympathetic tone causing hypotension.

Propofol
Analgesia alone may not adequately treat the acute undifferentiated intubated patient. Sedation is often necessary to facilitate further diagnostic workup and post-intubation comfort. Using an objective scale, such as the RASS, enables effective communication between physicians and nurses regarding patient arousability. After administration of a long-acting paralytic, it can be challenging to measure depth of sedation. After intubation, we aim for a deeper sedation goal. Once stabilized, it is not uncommon to fluctuate between RASS of −1 and −3. Propofol is a GABAergic medication that is highly lipophilic. It is a powerful anxiolytic and amnestic agent, but it provides no analgesia. Propofol is preferred for those presenting with status epilepticus or with other intracranial processes, as it is a powerful antiseizure medication and decreases cerebral oxygen consumption. It has a short half-life that enables physicians to facilitate awakening and frequent examination. The most common side effect of propofol is hypotension, and it is contraindicated in those with hypertriglyceridemia or those with an egg or soybean allergy. Of note, PRIS is a rare occurrence that has been observed in critically ill patients. It is characterized by severe unexplained metabolic acidosis, arrhythmias, ARF, rhabdomyolysis, hyperkalemia, and cardiovascular collapse. The standard dose of propofol is 5 to 10 mcg/kg/min with a typical ceiling of 50 mcg/kg/min, yet higher doses (60-80 mcg/kg/min) can be utilized.

Dexmedetomidine
Dexmedetomidine is a powerful alpha-2 agonist sedative with anxiolytic effects. Dexmedetomidine should not be bolused as hemodynamic collapse can occur, yet a continuous

infusion that is gradually uptitrated, typically 0.4 to 1.6 mcg/kg/h, can achieve sedation and agitation control without respiratory compromise. The peak effect is achieved around 45 minutes after initiation. Characteristic side effects include hypotension and bradycardia. In patients who require higher levels of sedation, other agents may be a better choice. Beneficially, a dexmedetomidine infusion can be continued post-extubation as it does not inhibit respiratory drive.

KETAMINE

Ketamine is a non-opiate, noncompetitive NMDA antagonist that provides both analgesia and sedation. It can be administered as an induction medication, a PRN agitation or analgesic medication, or a continuous infusion, starting at a rate of 0.5 to 2 mg/kg/h. The benefit of ketamine over propofol and dexmedetomidine is that it results in a catecholamine surge; thus, its sympathomimetic properties are hemodynamically friendly. However, because of this, we avoid ketamine in those with hypertensive and/or cardiovascular emergencies. Previous assumptions that ketamine increases intracranial pressure have been debunked and it is a powerful antiepileptic. Ketamine is a first-line medication for intubations related to respiratory disease as it directly prevents histamine-induced bronchoconstriction. Increased secretions and emergence reactions are the most likely side effects yet are not immediate concerns for intubated patients.

BENZODIAZEPINES

BZ should be avoided for sedation as better alternatives exist. BZ enhance inhibitory GABA mechanisms on postsynaptic neurons, thus limiting excitability. Midazolam and lorazepam (short- and intermediate-acting BZ, respectively) are the most frequently utilized. When BZ are contrasted against non-BZ, the latter was associated with decreased ICU length of stay and less time on mechanical ventilation. In addition, BZ are associated with high rates of delirium. However, BZ do possess a role, specifically for short-acting agitation control. BZ and/or phenobarbital (a long-acting barbiturate) are useful for status epilepticus or withdrawal syndromes (ie, ETOH withdrawal).

CONCLUSION

Post-intubation analgesia and sedation are of utmost importance with increasing rates of critically ill patients boarding in the ED. Intubation is a lifesaving procedure, yet it can create tremendous patient pain and anxiety in addition to the initial insult that requires the aforementioned intervention. An appropriate balance between analgesia and sedation can reduce ICU length of stay and time on mechanical ventilation, in addition to creating an improved patient experience.

PEARLS

- During setup for intubation, encourage staff to prepare post-intubation medications.
- Address analgesia first, then sedation.
- Keep the patient sedated; use fluid or vasopressors to support the MAP.
- Use RASS or other objective scale to assess pain and agitation and titrate medications (Table 35.1).
- Avoid benzodiazepines for sedation.

TABLE 35.1	RICHMOND AGITATION-SEDATION SCALE	
SCORE	TERM	DESCRIPTION
+4	Combative	Overtly combative, violent, immediate danger to staff
+3	Very agitated	Pulls or removes tube(s) or catheter(s); aggressive
+2	Agitated	Frequent nonpurposeful movement, fights ventilator
+1	Restless	Anxious but movements not aggressive vigorous
0	Alert and calm	
−1	Drowsy	Not fully alert, but has sustained awakening (eye opening/eye contact) to *voice* (≥10 seconds)
−2	Light sedation	Briefly awakens with eye contact to *voice* (<10 seconds)
−3	Moderate sedation	Movement or eye opening to *voice*
−4	Deep sedation	No response to voice, but movement or eye opening to *physical* stimulation
−5	Unarousable	No response to *voice* or *physical stimulation*

From Sessler CN, Gosnell M, Grap MJ, et al. The Richmond Agitation-Sedation Scale: validity and reliability in adult intensive care patients. *Am J Respir Crit Care Med.* 2002;166:1338-1344. Copyright © 1987-2024 American Thoracic Society, All Rights Reserved.

SUGGESTED READINGS

Bonomo JB, Butler AS, Lindsell CJ, Venkat A. Inadequate provision of postintubation anxiolysis and analgesia in the ED. *Am J Emerg Med.* 2008;26(4):469-472.

Lembersky O, Golz D, Kramer C, et al. Factors associated with post-intubation sedation after emergency department intubation: a report from The National Emergency Airway Registry. *Am J Emerg Med.* 2020;38(3):466-470.

Patel SB, Kress JP. Sedation and analgesia in the mechanically ventilated patient. *Am J Respir Crit Care Med.* 2012;185(5):486-497.

Sessler CN, Gosnell M, Grap MJ, et al. The Richmond Agitation-Sedation Scale: validity and reliability in adult intensive care patients. *Am J Respir Crit Care Med.* 2002; 166:1338-1344.

Wood S, Winters ME. Care of the intubated emergency department patient. *J Emerg Med.* 2011;40(4):419-427.

36

PHENOBARBITAL FOR ALCOHOL WITHDRAWAL SYNDROME

KEVIN ROLNICK AND RORY SPIEGEL

TRADITIONAL ALCOHOL WITHDRAWAL TREATMENT

AWS is a common ED presentation associated with significant morbidity and mortality. AWS occurs due to an imbalance in GABA and glutamate receptor activity. As a result of relative GABA inactivity and glutamate hyperactivity, AWS can present with dangerous clinical manifestations, including autonomic instability, agitation, delirium, and seizures. Benzodiazepines are usually effective in treating alcohol withdrawal as they act directly on

GABA receptors to amend this imbalance. While AWS is commonly treated with benzodiazepines such as lorazepam or diazepam, this treatment strategy is not without drawbacks. Phenobarbital is a useful alternative agent that has unique advantages over benzodiazepines.

When using benzodiazepines, it can be difficult to predict the total dose required for each patient early in their presentation. Evidence supports the use of a symptom-triggered benzodiazepine protocol rather than fixed-dose pathways. Given this, benzodiazepine-based strategies require frequent and time-intensive clinical reassessments to determine the need for re-dosing. Some benzodiazepines, such as lorazepam, have a relatively short half-life. This creates challenges, namely the potential for clinical deterioration after symptoms are initially controlled. In addition, benzodiazepines can precipitate paradoxical agitation and are associated with delirium.

Advantages of Phenobarbital for AWS

Phenobarbital is highly effective as a first-line agent for AWS and avoids many of the drawbacks of benzodiazepines. IV phenobarbital administration can be safely front-loaded as a 10 mg/kg dose. This strategy is associated with less need for mechanical ventilation and reduced sedative needs as compared to serial dosing of phenobarbital. In addition, the therapeutic phenobarbital levels that are used to treat AWS are far below the levels considered toxic. This allows clinicians to be aggressive with their initial loading dose without fear of inducing drug toxicity.

Another benefit of a phenobarbital is its protracted half-life (~140 hours), which effectively results in an "auto-taper" after a patient has been given a loading dose. As a result, patients who are treated with phenobarbital do not necessarily need benzodiazepine or oral phenobarbital tapers and experience similar duration of effects as patients that undergo a benzodiazepine taper.

Phenobarbital may also be effective in treating AWS that is refractory to benzodiazepines. Evidence suggests that patients who fail treatment with benzodiazepines respond to phenobarbital. There are two theories for the beneficial effects of phenobarbital versus benzodiazepines. First, phenobarbital acts independently on the GABA receptor and does not rely on endogenous GABA to be effective (unlike benzodiazepines). Second, in addition to its action on GABA receptors, phenobarbital also inhibits glutamate receptors. This can help to rectify the imbalance between competing neurotransmitters.

The evidence examining the use of phenobarbital for AWS suggests that protocols using phenobarbital result in decreased rates of ICU admission, decreased ICU and hospital length of stay, lower incidence of mechanical ventilation, and mitigate the need for adjunctive medications as compared to benzodiazepine-based protocols. In addition, the use of phenobarbital reduces the need for subsequent benzodiazepine infusions and the myriad associated complications and monitoring requirements. Importantly, phenobarbital for AWS is not associated with increased adverse outcomes such as intubation, seizures, or mortality.

Dosing

To administer phenobarbital through a loading dose strategy, start with 10 mg/kg IV phenobarbital infused over 30 minutes if the patient has not received significant benzodiazepines and does not have known severe liver disease. After the loading dose, reassess after 30 minutes and re-dose one to two additional 3 mg/kg doses of phenobarbital for ongoing withdrawal (**Figure 36.1**). An alternative effective dosing strategy is to give an initial dose of 260 mg, followed by clinical reassessment and serial doses of 130 mg as needed. While phenobarbital is effective and overall safe as compared to benzodiazepines, if it is being administered in conjunction with other sedating agents, be aware that its sedating

```
                    ┌─────────────────────┐
                    │   Suspected AWS     │
                    └─────────────────────┘
                              │
                    Has the Pt received >12 mg of Ativan in the
                    past 12 h or moderate liver disease
              No                              Yes
```

Initiate IV phenobarbital:
- 10 mg/kg load
- 3 mg/kg if still symptomatic
- Repeat 3 mg/kg if still symptomatic

Initiate IV phenobarbital:
- 6 mg/kg load
- 3 mg/kg if still symptomatic
- Repeat 3 mg/kg if still symptomatic

Disposition based on current symptoms and additional patient needs. Reference CIWA-ar dispo chart *, **

Disposition based on current symptoms and additional patient needs. Reference CIWA-ar dispo chart *, **

CIWA-ar Dispo Chart

Initial CIWA-Ar Score	Appropriate Level of Care
≥30	ICU level of care only
15-29	IMC/ICU level of care
<15 (& IV dosing options needed)	Med-Surg/IMC/ICU level of care (NOT behavioral health)
<15 (& NO IV dosing options needed)	ANY level of care (including behavioral health)

*Patients who have received full phenobarbital load and are otherwise appropriate for discharge should be discharged with strict instructions to hold alcohol use for the next 48 h.
** Patients who have received full phenobarbital loading dose and are still showing significant symptoms concerning for AWS, alternative diagnoses should be considered.

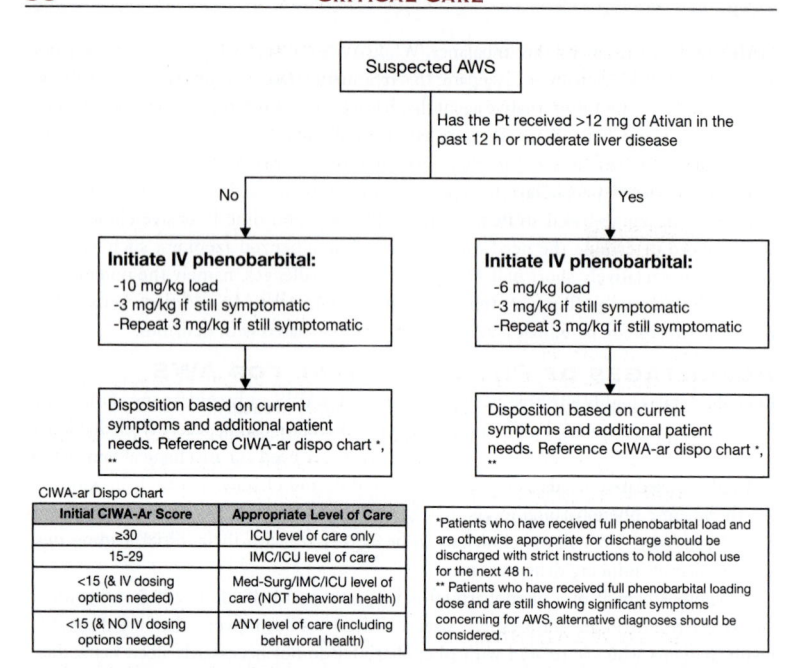

FIGURE 36.1 AWS, alcohol withdrawal syndrome; CIWA-Ar, clinical institute withdrawal assessment for alcohol - revised; ICU, intensive care unit; IMC, intermediate care unit; IV, intravenous.

effects may be amplified. This may include patients who have already received significant doses of benzodiazepines. If the patient has received significant benzodiazepines (eg, >12 mg of lorazepam-equivalents), consider adjusting the loading dose to 6 mg/kg. In addition, in patients with liver disease, care should be taken in treating AWS with phenobarbital as it is primarily hepatically metabolized. For patients who have undergone a full phenobarbital load plus approximately 15 mg/kg and are still exhibiting symptoms of AWS, consider alternative diagnoses that often mimic AWS. A serum phenobarbital level may be obtained. If the patient is still experiencing symptoms and has a therapeutic serum phenobarbital level, AWS is unlikely to be the cause of the patient's current clinical presentation.

DISPOSITION FOR AWS TREATED WITH PHENOBARBITAL

When patients present to the ED with AWS, it is important to understand the precipitating cause and determine any serious underlying etiology. Once a serious underlying cause for the patient's AWS has been ruled out and the patient has undergone a loading dose of phenobarbital, a decision can be made regarding disposition based on the patient's current clinical status. Patients who receive lower doses of phenobarbital (up to 10 mg/kg) for mild to moderate AWS with resolution of their symptoms may be discharged. This should occur after a period of observation and reassessment to ensure control of their symptoms and clinical stability. Discharge should only be considered in patients with sustained CIWA-ar lesser than 8 and without high-risk features such as a prior history of alcohol withdrawal seizures or delirium tremens, who have no other admission criteria, and preferably with a clear follow up plan in place. In patients with ongoing withdrawal, admission to the "Med/Surg" floor level of care is appropriate for more mild withdrawal (CIWA-ar <15). Consider admission to an IMC for patients with CIWA-ar 15 to 29 and ICU admission for patients with CIWA-ar greater than 30. IMC and ICU admission may be required for "mild" withdrawal patients with serious underlying pathologies (ie, cerebrovascular accidents, pancreatitis, pneumonia, etc).

PEARLS

- Phenobarbital is overall safe to use and not associated with significant negative sequelae (including the need for mechanical ventilation) in patients with AWS as compared to benzodiazepines.
- Phenobarbital dosing strategies include a 10 mg/kg loading dose or an initial dose of 260 mg with additional doses of 130 mg as needed.
- Be mindful of patients that have already received benzodiazepines or patients with severe liver failure, and consider reducing the dose to 6 mg/kg.
- Phenobarbital may effectively treat patients with AWS resistant to benzodiazepines—but be wary of oversedation given the potential for synergistic effects between the two drug classes.

SUGGESTED READINGS

Gold JA, Rimal B, Nolan A, Nelson LS. A strategy of escalating doses of benzodiazepines and phenobarbital administration reduces the need for mechanical ventilation in delirium tremens. *Crit Care Med*. 2007;35(3):724-730.

Hendey GW, Dery RA, Barnes RL, Snowden B, Mentler P. A prospective, randomized, trial of phenobarbital versus benzodiazepines for acute alcohol withdrawal. *Am J Emerg Med*. 2011;29(4):382-385.

Saitz R, Mayo-Smith MF, Roberts MS, Redmond HA, Bernard DR, Calkins DR. Individualized treatment for alcohol withdrawal. A randomized double-blind controlled trial. *JAMA*. 1994;272(7):519-523.

Shah P, Stegner-Smith KL, Rachid M, Hanif T, Dodd KW. Front-loaded versus low-intermittent phenobarbital dosing for benzodiazepine-resistant severe alcohol withdrawal syndrome. *J Med Toxicol*. 2022;18(3):198-204.

Young GP, Rores C, Murphy C, Dailey RH. Intravenous phenobarbital for alcohol withdrawal and convulsions. *Ann Emerg Med*. 1987;16(8):847-850.

37

MONITORING VENTILATOR PRESSURES IS A MUST

CHRISTINA LU AND KRISTI LIZYNESS

Ventilator management is a dynamic process that often requires reevaluation and manipulation of initial settings to mitigate VILI. Studies have shown that VILI results not only in a 12% increase in mortality but also in prolonged ICU stays with increased risk for infections and delirium. Understanding basic ventilator pressures including PIP, Pplat, and recognizing auto–PEEP can significantly improve patient outcomes by preventing barotrauma and volutrauma.

COMPLIANCE AND AIRWAY RESISTANCE

Fundamental to mechanical ventilation are the concepts of compliance and airway resistance. Compliance (C) describes the distensibility of alveoli and is defined as the amount of pressure (P) needed to achieve a certain lung volume (V).

$$C = \Delta V / \Delta P \qquad \text{Eq. 37.1}$$

Diseased lungs are often less compliant and require higher pressures to achieve desired tidal volumes. While compliance describes lung mechanics at an alveolar level; airway resistance describes the impedance of airflow through the airways and ET tubing. Resistance is heavily dependent on airway radius.

The amount of pressure needed to inflate the lungs is inversely proportional to lung compliance and directly proportional to airway resistance. Etiologies that decrease respiratory compliance or increase airway resistance will require increased airway pressures to provide adequate ventilation. Regardless of initial ventilation settings, diligent monitoring of the below pressures is essential to preventing VILI.

PEAK PRESSURE

PIP represents the maximum total pressure supplied by the ventilator during inspiration. Since most initial ventilator settings are volume-control assist-control, the PIP represents the pressure required to generate the desired tidal volume (V_t). The PIP is a summation of airway resistance plus alveolar pressure.

Normal PIPs range from 25 to 30 cm H_2O with goal pressures less than 40 cm H_2O. Pressures greater than 40 cm H_2O are associated with increased mortality. Lungs that are less compliant or have increased airway resistance will require higher peak pressures to maintain minute ventilation. Modern ventilators come equipped with peak pressure alarms generated from the pressure-time waveform displayed on the screen and will alarm when pressures approach approximately 40 cm H_2O. The PIP alarm can be adjusted on the ventilator in certain circumstances. Ventilation will cease after the PIP alarm is reached, which can lead to critical hypoventilation in some circumstances if not closely monitored.

INSPIRATORY PLATEAU PRESSURE

It is important to monitor Pplat in conjunction with PIP as both are required to determine the underlying etiology of the pressure alarm. The Pplat is measured by an end-inspiratory hold lasting approximately 0.5 to 1 second (**Figure 37.1**). During this time, there is no airflow through the circuit. Pressures equalize throughout the system resulting in a plateau pressure that is a surrogate marker for alveolar pressure. This maneuver is easy to perform; however, steps may vary slightly depending on the ventilator model. An important consideration is that the patient must be in synchrony with the ventilator when performing the maneuver. Inspiratory effort during the maneuver will give an inaccurate reading. As plateau pressures increase, the alveoli are at risk for over-distention and subsequent barotrauma. The goal is to keep Pplat less than 30 cm H_2O.

PEAK AND PLATEAU PRESSURE INTERPRETATION

To simplify, think of PIPs as the pressure required to overcome airway resistance and ET tubing, while plateau pressures are reflective of pressures inside the alveoli themselves. When troubleshooting the ventilator, there are two common scenarios:

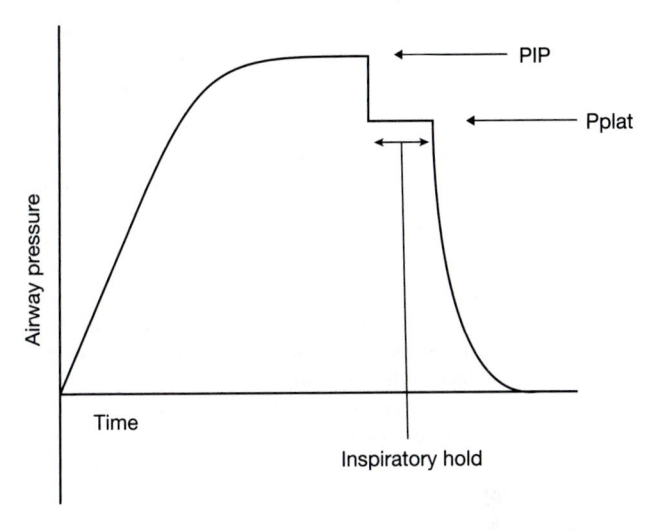

FIGURE 37.1 Peak inspiratory pressure (PIP) and inspiratory plateau pressure (Pplat).

1) High PIP and low/normal Pplat: The problem is airway resistance.
   - Kinking or blockage in the ETT or circuit
   - Biting the ETT
   - Ventilator dyssynchrony
   - Mucus plugging
   - Bronchospasm
   - Excessive gas flow rate

   Evaluate the tubing to ensure there is no kinking. Increasing sedation or applying a bite block may be required if the patient is biting on the tube or dyssynchronous with the ventilator. Consider suctioning for increased secretions or inhaled bronchodilators if the physical exam or ventilator waveform is consistent with bronchospasm. Adjust ventilator settings if the flow rate is too high.

2) High PIP and Pplat: The problem is at the alveolar level.
   - Mainstem intubation
   - Atelectasis
   - Pneumonia
   - Pulmonary edema
   - Pneumothorax
   - Pleural effusion or hemothorax
   - Excessive tidal volumes

   In these cases, the physical exam, a chest radiograph, and an ultrasound would greatly aid in the differential diagnosis. Once easily reversible etiologies are ruled out, good lung protective ventilator strategies must be employed. This involves down titration of the tidal volume to 4 to 6 mL/kg while maintaining plateau pressures less than 30 cm H_2O and allowing for permissive hypercapnia if there are no contraindications.

Auto-PEEP

Extrinsic PEEP is set by the physician to reduce alveolar collapse during expiration. This promotes alveolar recruitment and oxygenation by increasing the total surface area available for gas exchange. Intrinsic, or auto-PEEP, occurs when the minute ventilation or tidal volume is set too high and there is incomplete exhalation before initiation of the next breath. This results in hyperinflation and breath stacking. Patients with obstructive diseases such as COPD or asthma are at increased risk for developing this phenomenon. Auto-PEEP is important to monitor as excessive hyperinflation places the patient at increased risk for not only barotrauma and pneumothorax but also hemodynamic instability and circulatory collapse.

There are three separate ways to monitor for auto-PEEP. The first utilizes the end-expiratory hold, which is a pause maneuver done during exhalation. If pressure at the end of exhalation is greater than the ventilator set PEEP, the difference is the auto-PEEP. Observing an expiratory-flow curve that does not return to baseline before initiation of another breath also suggests this phenomenon (**Figure 37.2**). The final method involves the visual comparison of the inspiratory and expiratory volumes. An inspiratory volume significantly higher than the expiratory volume is concerning for auto-PEEP.

Management options to consider include prolonging expiration by decreasing respiratory rate, increasing inspiratory flow rate, or decreasing the *I:E* ratio. Decreasing the tidal volume also decreases the likelihood of auto-PEEP or breath stacking. If there is concern for auto-PEEP in the setting of hemodynamic instability, disconnect the patient from the ventilator to allow for complete exhalation.

Conclusion

VILI is a potentially life-threatening complication in mechanical ventilation. Patients with underlying lung disease such as COPD, asthma, or interstitial lung disease are at increased risk for this complication. Visibly apparent respiratory distress and hemodynamic instability are late sequelae of barotrauma. Monitoring ventilator pressures is a must.

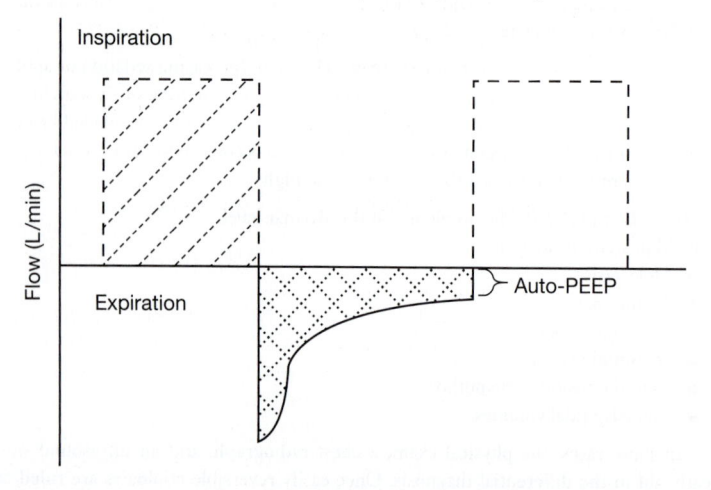

FIGURE 37.2 Auto-PEEP occurs when there is incomplete exhalation before the next breath.

PEARLS

- Monitoring ventilator pressures is important to prevent VILI and reduce mortality.
- Elevated PIP with low/normal Pplat indicates increased airway resistance.
- Elevated PIP with an elevated Pplat indicates the problem is at the alveolar level.
- Auto-PEEP can lead to breath stacking, dynamic hyperinflation, and ultimately hemodynamic instability.
- Auto-PEEP can be identified by an end-expiratory hold maneuver, observing the flow curve not returning to baseline, and comparing inspiratory and expiratory lung volumes.

Suggested Readings

Carlo WA, Ambalavanan N, Chatburn RL. Chapter 10—ventilator parameters. In: Donn SM, Sinha SK, eds. *Manual of Neonatal Respiratory Care.* 2nd ed. Mosby; 2006: 81-85, ISBN 9780323031769 (https://www.sciencedirect.com/science/article/pii/B9780323031769500155)

Diaz R, Heller D. Barotrauma and mechanical ventilation [Updated Aug 1, 2022]. In: *StatPearls [Internet]*. StatPearls Publishing; 2022. https://www.ncbi.nlm.nih.gov/books/NBK545226/

Marino PL, Sutin KM. *The ICU Book.* 3rd ed. Lippincott Williams & Wilkins; 2007.

Owens, W. *The Ventilator Book.* 3rd ed. First Draught Press; 2021.

Silva PL, Rocco PRM. The basics of respiratory mechanics: ventilator-derived parameters. *Ann Transl Med.* 2018;6(19):376. PMID: 30460250.

38

Know How to Interpret Ventilator Waveforms

Nicolas A. Ulloa and Dan Eraso

Ventilator Waveforms

Ventilator waveforms are graphical depictions of the flow of air or gas through the lungs during mechanical ventilation. Whereas the ventilator settings are the clinician's dictated parameters, the waveforms are a visual representation of the patient's physiologic response to those settings. The three most common and important waveforms are pressure, flow, and volume. These waveforms will vary slightly depending on whether a pressure or volume mode is selected. Optimal ventilator settings allow for the efficient exchange of gas while avoiding ventilator-induced lung injury. Suboptimal ventilator settings or pathophysiologic conditions can create ventilator asynchrony with resultant patient discomfort, ineffective gas exchange, and increased morbidity and mortality.

NORMAL WAVEFORMS

Pressure waveforms depict pressure on the y-axis over time on the x-axis. For a volume control setting, a normal pressure waveform will look like an upward ramp, as displayed in **Figure 38.1**, Part 1A. Initially, there is an abrupt increase in pressure as the ventilator delivers the breath with a steady increase in pressure until the entire breath is delivered. The peak of the graph is the PIP. During exhalation, there is a rapid drop in pressure until the exhalation is completed. At this point, the remaining pressure in the lungs is the PEEP. The graph can vary depending on the patient's lung compliance and airway resistance. An increase or decrease in PEEP will shift the entire waveform up and down, respectively.

Figure 38.1, Part 2A represents a normal pressure waveform for a pressure control setting. The appearance should resemble a box. During inhalation, the pressure will rapidly reach a set level based on the ventilator parameters. During exhalation, there is an abrupt decrease in pressure until it reaches the PEEP.

Flow waveforms measure the movement of gas in liters per minute plotted over time. To better conceptualize, the waveform should be split between inhalation and exhalation. For a volume control setting, the inspiratory portion will appear like a box with constant flow while the breath is given (**Figure 38.1**, Part 1B). The inhalation portion will be interpreted by the ventilator as a positive value above the x-axis. During exhalation, the waveform will have a negative value underneath the x-axis. The slope of the waveform will initially be sharp and then the flow will continue to decrease as the exhalation phase ends. The waveform should reach zero prior to the initiation of the next breath and the importance of this concept will be discussed later.

For pressure control, the concept is essentially the same, although the flow during inspiration may be variable. Typically, the flow rate is initially higher and then tapers off, which can be seen in **Figure 38.1**, Part 2B.

Finally, the volume waveform tends to be the most intuitive as seen in **Figure 38.1**, Part 1C and Part 2C. For a volume control setting, the waveform will show a triangle-shaped pattern demonstrating the changes in volume with inspiration and expiration. For pressure control, the waveform will look similar but less uniform as there may be breath-to-breath variation in volumes.

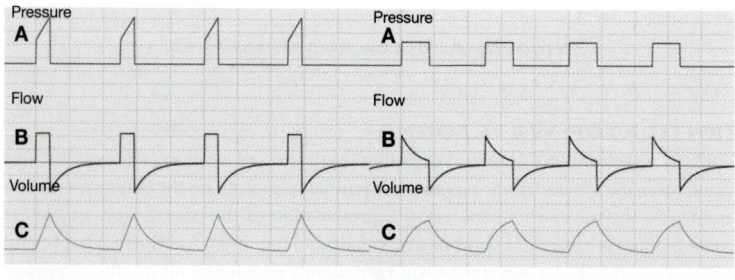

FIGURE 38.1 **Part 1, A-C.** Demonstrates a volume control setting which shows pressure, flow, and volume waveforms. **Part 2, A-C.** Demonstrates a pressure control setting which shows pressure, flow, and volume wave forms, respectively.

Patient-Ventilator Asynchrony

Patient-ventilator asynchrony is a very common problem among patients on mechanical ventilation. Asynchrony has been associated with discomfort, worse gas exchange, hypoxia, increased duration of mechanical ventilation, and mortality. The following will describe types of asynchronies and how to correct them. There may be a tendency to treat these patients with increased sedation. Although not always incorrect, patient-ventilator asynchrony deserves a more elegant approach to optimizing mechanical ventilation and avoiding excessive sedation.

Ineffective Triggering

Ineffective triggering occurs when the patient attempts to trigger a breath, but the ventilator fails to provide the mechanical breath. This can occur if the patient is overly sedated, too weak to trigger their own breath or there is a significant amount of auto–PEEP present. In additional, this can occur if the pressure sensor is too high to detect the patient's effort. **Figure 38.2** demonstrates the positive deflection on the flow and pressure waveforms, representing the patient's inspiratory effort without a subsequent mechanical breath. Treating causes of auto–PEEP, optimizing sedation to improve patient effort, or increasing the sensitivity of the pressure sensor can alleviate this issue.

Autotrigger

Autotrigger is the opposite of ineffective triggering. In autotriggering, the ventilator interprets pressure or flow changes from cardiac activity, cuff leaks, or oscillations from secretions in the ventilator circuit as the patient initiates a breath. The ventilator gives excessive ventilation. Management is directed at correcting the underlying cause and if that doesn't work adjusting the flow trigger sensitivity.

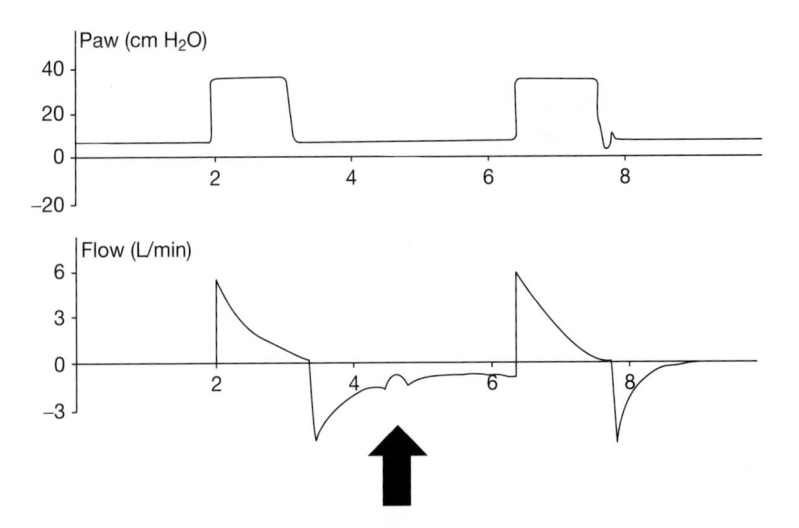

Figure 38.2 Ineffective triggering demonstrates the positive deflection during expiratory phase of the flow curve. This represents triggered breath without a delivered breath from the ventilator. (From Mellema MS. Ventilator waveforms. *Top Companion Anim Med.* 2013;28(3):112-123.)

Flow Asynchrony

Flow asynchrony occurs when the inspiratory flow of the ventilator does not match the inspiratory flow demands of the patient (as seen in **Figure 38.3**). "Flow hunger" or "flow starvation" is another term for this concept. For a volume control setting, the pressure waveform will show a negative dip which may imply the flow rate or tidal volumes are inadequate for the patient's comfort. In this scenario, the patient is essentially pulling flow from the circuit, leading to a dip in the pressure waveform. This issue can be corrected by increasing the flow rate or increasing the tidal volumes.

Double Triggering

Double triggering occurs when the patient receives a mechanical breath and before exhaling, triggers the ventilator again for an additional breath. Double triggering is usually due to premature termination of the mechanical breath. Occasionally with volume control settings, the tidal volume may be too low for the patient's comfort or the inspiratory time is too short. This leads to significant air hunger. The patient tries to compensate by breathing again prior to exhalation of the initial breath as demonstrated in **Figure 38.4**. The excess tidal volumes can cause elevated intrathoracic pressures and lung injury. Temporarily switching the ventilator to a pressure support mode (if the patient can tolerate it) can give the patient more control to reach their desired tidal volumes. The physician can note the tidal volumes that improve patient synchrony and then apply that tidal volume when switching back to volume control. This is a simple maneuver to "ask" the patient what tidal volumes they desire. In the event of double triggering, higher tidal volumes are permitted. For example, 8 cc/kg IBW is better than double triggering at 6 cc/kg IBW (effectively 12 cc/kg IBW). In additional, decreasing flow rates can also alleviate double triggering if the patient desires inspiratory time is longer than what the ventilator is providing.

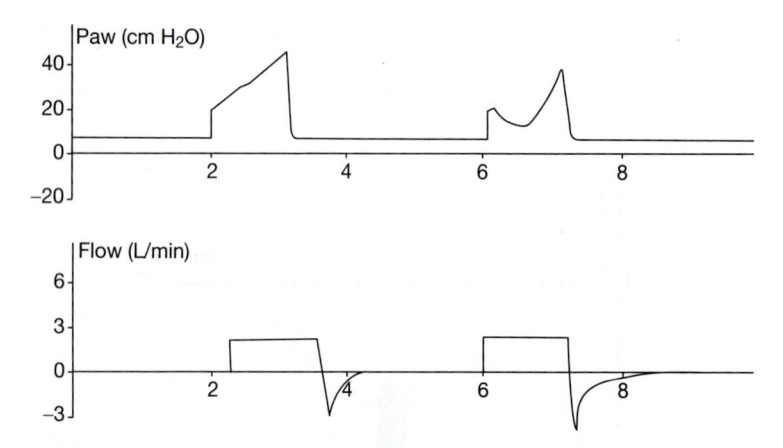

FIGURE 38.3 Flow asynchrony, which demonstrates the negative dip on the upslope of the pressure waveform. Here, the patient is pulling in extra flow from the ventilator leading to a mild drop in the pressure. This can be fixed by increasing the flow rates or tidal volumes. (Reprinted from Mellema MS. Ventilator waveforms. *Top Companion Anim Med*. 2013;28(3):112-123, with permission from Elsevier.)

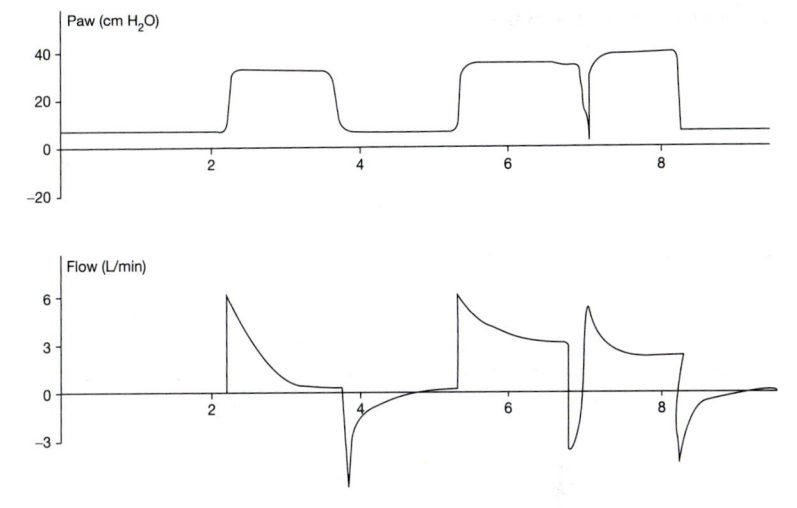

FIGURE 38.4 Double triggering, which demonstrates the additional breath prior to exhalation. Oftentimes, this happens when flow rates or tidal volumes are inadequate for the patient's demands. (Reprinted from Mellema MS. Ventilator waveforms. *Top Companion Anim Med*. 2013;28(3):112-123, with permission from Elsevier.)

AIR TRAPPING

Air trapping, also known as breath stacking, can occur in patients on mechanical ventilation who have underlying obstructive lung pathology such as COPD or asthma. This occurs when the patient does not have enough time to complete their exhalation before the ventilator delivers the next breath. In **Figure 38.5**, the flow waveform does not reach

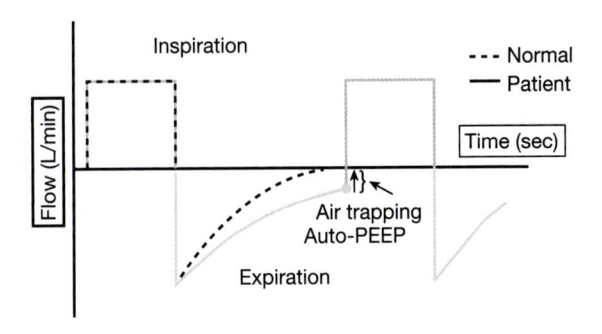

FIGURE 38.5 Air trapping/breath stacking, which demonstrates a failure to return to the baseline during expiratory phase of the flow waveform. This can be corrected by decreasing the respiratory rate or decreasing the *I:E* ratio to facilitate complete exhalation. (From Restrepo RD, Khusid F. Essentials of ventilatory graphics. *Ind J Resp Care*. 2014;3(1):396-404. Figure 4.)

zero before the upcoming breath. Over time this can lead to a significant increase in intrathoracic pressure that can impede venous return and lead to hemodynamic collapse. Decreasing the respiratory rate, increasing the flow, or increasing the expiratory time can allow for more time to facilitate expiration. Optimizing exhalation time may result in elevated pCO_2 levels. Increased sedation or even paralytics may be required if the clinician is having significant challenges maintaining an appropriately low respiratory rate.

PEARLS

- Monitoring the ventilator waveforms can provide critical information to optimize ventilation.
- The flow waveform often provides the most useful information when evaluating for asynchrony.
- Adjusting flow rates can help alleviate air hunger or flow hunger in flow asynchrony or double triggering.
- Breath stacking is observed when the flow curve does not return to zero prior to the initiation of another breath.
- Decrease the respiratory rate, increase the flow, or increase the *I:E* ratio to facilitate exhalation time.

SUGGESTED READINGS

Bailey JM. Management of patient-ventilator asynchrony. *Anesthesiology*. 2021;134(4): 629-636. PMID: 33592102.

Doerschug KC. Patient-ventilator synchrony. *Clin Chest Med*. 2022;43(3):511-518. PMID: 36116818.

Esperanza JA, Sarlabous L, de Haro C, Magrans R, Lopez-Aguilar J, Blanch L. Monitoring asynchrony during invasive mechanical ventilation. *Respir Care*. 2020;65(6):847-869. PMID: 32457175.

Leatherman J. Mechanical ventilation for severe asthma. *Chest*. 2015;147(6):1671-1680. PMID: 26033128.

39

WHAT'S UP WITH ALTERNATIVE MODES OF MECHANICAL VENTILATION?

ALEXANDER BRACEY AND MEGAN M. LIEB

Most patients in the ED will be started on a conventional mode of ventilation (eg, volume or pressure AC). However, a conventional mode may not be the optimal setting for a given patient or clinical scenario. Therefore, it is prudent for the emergency physician to be familiar with the alternate modes of ventilation to properly care for the patient on mechanical ventilation. Importantly, many of these alternative modes emphasize patient-initiated breaths. Such modes would be inappropriate for use in the patient with paralysis (eg, during the peri-intubation period).

PRVC

PRVC allows the operator to set a goal TV. This differs from volume AC as the ventilator in PRVC applies a PS to achieve the TV rather than setting a flow rate and volume limit as it does in volume AC. The ventilator in PRVC adjusts the PS on a breath-to-breath basis to maintain the goal TV.

The primary benefit of PRVC is that it ensures a MV using the minimal amount of PS necessary to achieve a given TV. This may have utility in ARDS. If a change in respiratory mechanics occurs (eg, compliance, patient effort) then the ventilator will adjust the PS to achieve the TV. Theoretically, as a patient on PRVC recovers from their illness, the ventilator will use incrementally less PS for a given TV, thereby allowing the patient to wean themselves from the ventilator.

This mode may fail if a patient has a high respiratory drive (eg, severe metabolic acidosis, respiratory distress, intubation for neurologic injury). In such instances, the patient's increased respiratory effort falsely indicates to the ventilator that *less* PS is required when the patient may actually need *more* PS. This can lead to respiratory muscle fatigue or patient discomfort and dyssynchrony.

SIMV

SIMV allows the operator to determine the rate of mandatory breaths to be given at a set TV. Patients may also spontaneously initiate breaths, which may be supported by a set PS. The patient's work of breathing will be inversely proportional to the amount of PS provided. The ventilator will attempt to synchronize the mandatory breaths with those taken by the patient by delaying a machine-delivered breath if the ventilator senses a patient-initiated breath, preventing a machine-delivered breath from occurring during exhalation.

Since SIMV allows for a patient to take spontaneous breaths with a set amount of support, it may have utility in weaning patients from IMV with less active titration by the operator compared to AC modes.

SIMV may fail if the patient is unable to maintain adequate TV and the mandatory breath rate or PS is too low. Also, SIMV may not adequately offset the work of breathing patients with high metabolic demands; therefore, conventional modes are usually preferred during the acute resuscitation period.

PSV

PSV allows for all the respiratory drive to be patient initiated without a mandatory RR. PS may be adjusted to achieve a target TV.

PSV is particularly useful for determining the appropriateness of extubation. Patients must initiate each breath and use their own respiratory mechanics to achieve ventilation. PS may be weaned until the patient is ready for a spontaneous breathing trial.

PSV may fail if the patient is not ready to perform the majority of the work of breathing (eg, respiratory muscle weakness, paralysis). Patients on PSV must be closely monitored for changes in RR, TV, and apnea. While modern ventilators have backup RR, they do not initiate until apnea ensues.

APRV

In APRV, most of the respiratory cycle is spent at continuously high pressure to increase MAP, thereby promoting recruitment and oxygenation. Intermittent releases in the pressure and spontaneous breathing over the set pressure achieve ventilation. Conceptually, APRV is CPAP with intermittent releases of pressure.

The benefits of APRV include $\dot{V}/\dot{Q}$ matching optimization, improved alveolar recruitment, and reduced barotrauma owing to lower peak and plateau pressures with higher MAP. Therefore, APRV is arguably the mode of choice in ARDS.

APRV may fail in several ways. Increased MAP results in higher intrathoracic pressure, which may cause hemodynamic instability. Furthermore, pressures set too aggressively may result in barotrauma or pneumothoraces. Additionally, spontaneous breathing is helpful for the successful application of APRV. Therefore, oversedation or chemical paralysis may result in suboptimal MV and potentially worsening hemodynamics, the latter owing to the loss of negative pressure inspiration from spontaneous breaths. Finally, as the settings in APRV are distinct from those set in other commonly used ventilator modes, the successful application of APRV requires familiarity with the settings and close patient monitoring.

AVAPS

AVAPS is a NIV mode conceptually similar to PRVC. It allows the operator to set a target TV that the ventilator then achieves by administering dynamic PS breaths until the goal TV is met. This contrasts with traditional NIV settings in which a PS is administered with volume as the variable. The dynamic change in PS breaths offers benefits over standard NIV settings as it can self-titrate to the set TV under dynamic clinical circumstances (eg, positional changes, increased patient wakefulness and effort).

AVAPS may be most useful in patients presenting with hypercapnic encephalopathy. In such cases, AVAPS has been demonstrated to have higher average TV and to normalize $Paco_2$ levels more rapidly, and resolve encephalopathy when compared to NIV with traditional settings. This may be particularly beneficial in busy EDs in which circumstances limit frequent NIV setting adjustments.

AVAPS can fail in the same ways that PRVC may (see earlier). In additional, increased PS risks aspiration if the PS overcomes the tone of the LES, with several studies suggesting 15 to 20 cm H_2O as the maximum. Close monitoring and weighing the benefits of increased ventilation versus the risks of aspiration is necessary for patients on AVAPS.

PEARLS

- EPs must be familiar with alternative modes of ventilation to optimally care for their patients on mechanical ventilation.
- Modes that emphasize patient-initiated breaths are inappropriate for the patient with paralysis.
- No single ventilator mode has been shown to be superior to another; rather, the correct ventilator mode should be tailored to the clinical scenario and operator familiarity.
- It is essential to have a knowledge of how each ventilator mode can be adjusted, and how they may fail to prevent adverse outcomes.

SUGGESTED READINGS

Briones Claudett KH, Briones Claudett M, Chung Sang Wong M. Noninvasive mechanical ventilation with average volume assured pressure support (AVAPS) in patients with chronic obstructive pulmonary disease and hypercapnic encephalopathy. *BMC Pulm Med.* 2013;13:12. PMID: 23497021.

Fredericks AS, Bunker MP, Gliga LA, et al. Airway pressure release ventilation: a review of the evidence, theoretical benefits, and alternative titration strategies. *Clin Med Insights Circ Respir Pulm Med.* 2020;14:1179548420903297. PMID: 32076372.

Isono S, Eikermann M, Odaka T. Facemask ventilation during induction of anesthesia: how "gentle" is "gentle" enough? *Anesthesiology.* 2014;120:263-265.

Owens W. *The Ventilator Book.* First Draught Press; 2018.

Singh G, Chien C, Patel S. Pressure regulated volume control (PRVC): set it and forget it? *Respir Med Case Rep.* 2019;29:100822. PMID: 32257782.

40

Know How to Evaluate and Manage the Intubated Patient With Refractory Hypoxemia

Thomas H. Rozen and Christopher P. Nickson

Refractory hypoxemia in an intubated patient is a time-critical emergency that demands a systematic approach. Assessment and management are performed concurrently, with life threats addressed in order of priority. The "DOPES" mnemonic helps guide initial actions, especially in the immediate post-intubation period (**Table 40.1**).

The first step in the management of the intubated patient with refractory hypoxemia is to disconnect the ventilator from the ETT. Once disconnected, look for signs of gas trapping (aka auto-PEEP or dynamic hyperinflation). If gas trapping is suspected, allow for prolonged expiration by adjusting the ventilator settings. This can be accomplished with a lower respiratory rate (eg, 6 breaths/min), increased inspiratory flow rate (eg, 100 L/min), prolonged expiratory time (eg, *I:E* ratio of <1:4), or decreased PEEP (eg, PEEP = 0 cm H_2O).

Once dynamic hyperinflation is excluded, connect a bag-valve-mask device to the ETT with 100% oxygen. If the patient is easy to ventilate and reoxygenate, then the culprit is either the ventilator or the circuit. If the patient is still difficult to ventilate, then there is a problem with the ETT or the patient. Importantly, never ventilate a patient with a tracheostomy before confirming tube position, due to the risk of causing catastrophic subcutaneous emphysema.

Table 40.1 The "DOPES" Mnemonic

Displaced ETT
Obstructed ETT
Patient disorders, such as pneumothorax
Equipment problems
"Stacked breaths" (dynamic hyperinflation)

Experts may avoid the step of disconnecting from the ventilator if they are confident that the ventilator and circuit are not malfunctioning and there is no dynamic hyperinflation. This avoids potential drawbacks of disconnection, such as lung de-recruitment and loss of diagnostic information provided by the ventilator.

Confirm ETT patency by passing a suction catheter and monitoring $ETCO_2$. Quantitative $ETCO_2$ monitoring is the gold standard for confirmation of endotracheal intubation and for detection of ETT malposition. Up to eight $ETCO_2$ waveforms over 30 seconds may be seen after esophageal intubation. If a bougie is used to confirm ETT position and patency, it should be passed gently to avoid tracheobronchial injury. "Hold up" of the bougie occurs at the carina (~30 cm) when the ETT is endotracheal. With esophageal ETT placement, the bougie will pass easily beyond 35 cm. Bronchoscopy or chest radiography can also be used to confirm ETT position; however, these modalities may take too long in a rapidly deteriorating patient.

Patients who are easy to ventilate with the bag-valve-mask device and yet remain hypoxemic may have a malpositioned ETT or a circuit leak (eg, cuff leak, disconnection, or a breach in the circuit). If in doubt, remove the ETT, continue bag-valve-mask ventilation, and prepare for reintubation.

If the etiologies mentioned earlier have been excluded and the patient remains hypoxemic, consider patient factors. To rapidly assess patient factors, use the "MASH" approach during bag-valve ventilation (**Table 40.2**). Asymmetric chest movement raises suspicion for unilateral endobronchial intubation, pneumothorax, pleural effusion, hemothorax, or lung collapse due to pneumonia. Other common patient causes of hypoxemia include pulmonary edema, bronchospasm, and pulmonary embolus.

Suspect ARDS in patients with bilateral pulmonary infiltrates on chest radiography. These patients (including those with coronavirus disease 2019) require protective lung ventilation with tidal volumes of 6 mL/kg predicted body weight, plateau pressures less than 30 cm H_2O, and an arterial pH above 7.15. Avoid excess fluid administration and perform head-up positioning to help preserve functional residual capacity. Useful therapies for refractory hypoxemia in ARDS are listed in **Table 40.3**.

Nonpulmonary causes of hypoxemia (eg, cyanotic heart disease or hemoglobinopathies) are rare but are worth considering in refractory cases. Finally, if the patient is easy to ventilate and the hypoxemia rapidly resolves, establish the immediate antecedents to hypoxemia. A simple disconnection of the ventilator/circuit or suctioning can lead to significant desaturation through de-recruitment and atelectasis (especially in small children).

For additional details, see Chapter 38.

TABLE 40.2 THE "MASH" APPROACH FOR RAPID PATIENT ASSESSMENT

- Movement of the chest
    - Movement bilateral, unilateral, or absent?
    - Is the chest hyper-expanded?
- Arterial saturation (SaO_2) and PaO_2
    - Obtain an arterial blood gas sample if time permits
- Skin color of the patient (turning blue or pinking up?)
    - Remember that the SpO_2 monitor lags behind the patient's true oxygen saturation
- Hemodynamic stability

Table 40.3	Therapies for Refractory Hypoxemia in Patients With ARDS

- Increase FIO_2 to 1.0 and titrate to acceptable SpO_2 target (eg, 88%-92%).
- Administer sedation and neuromuscular blockade, if required, to decrease oxygen consumption, improve chest wall compliance, and avoid patient-ventilator dyssynchrony.
- Provide suction, chest physiotherapy, and bronchoscopy to shift sputum plugs.
- Ventilator adjustments:
  - Optimize PEEP using the ARDSNet nomogram. Higher PEEP may be required for severe ARDS and for patients with obesity.
  - Increase the inspiratory time (and consequently the inspiratory-to-expiratory [I:E] ratio; eg, 1:1).
  - Inverse ratio ventilation or alternate ventilation modes, such as APRV, can be considered if the clinician has appropriate expertise. No particular strategy is proven to improve patient outcomes.
- Prone positioning can be performed in settings with teams trained in the procedure for patients with PaO_2/FIO_2 ratio <150 mm Hg. Prolonged proning (eg, >12 h/d) is associated with improved mortality.
- LRMs should not be performed routinely, but a simple approach is to apply 40 cm H_2O of positive pressure for 40s. LRMs have been found to improve oxygenation but not mortality. Stepwise recruitment maneuvers should be avoided.
- Pulmonary vasodilators, such as iNO, improve physiologic parameters but not mortality in patients with mechanically ventilated ARDS. Their routine use is not recommended; however, a trial of inhaled pulmonary vasodilator as a rescue therapy may be used in patients refractory to other therapies. The treatment should be tapered off if there is no rapid improvement in oxygenation. Venovenous ECMO is used for reversible respiratory disorders resulting in hypoxemia refractory to other measures.

PEARLS

- Use the "DOPES" mnemonic to remember the immediate life threats in the intubated patient with hypoxemia.
- Disconnection from the ventilator allows treatment of dynamic hyperinflation and excludes equipment causes.
- Quantitative $ETCO_2$ monitoring is the gold standard for confirming ETT positioning.
- The "MASH" approach allows rapid assessment of the patient while attempting to diagnose causes of hypoxemia.
- Numerous ventilatory and non-ventilatory strategies can help improve refractory hypoxemia in patients with ARDS.

Suggested Readings

Chiumello D, Brioni M. Severe hypoxemia: which strategy to choose. *Crit Care.* 2016; 20(1):132. PMID: 27255913. https://ccforum.biomedcentral.com/articles/10.1186/s13054-016-1304-7

Dragoi L, Siuba MT, Fan E. Lessons learned in mechanical ventilation/oxygen support in COVID19. *Clin Chest Med.* 2023;44(2):321-333.

Fan E, Del Sorbo L, Goligher EC, et al. An Official American Thoracic Society/European Society of Intensive Care Medicine/Society of Critical Care Medicine Clinical Practice Guideline: mechanical ventilation in adult patients with acute respiratory distress syndrome [published correction appears in *Am J Respir Crit Care Med*. 2017;195(11):1540]. *Am J Respir Crit Care Med*. 2017;195(9):1253-1263.

Nickson C. Post-intubation hypoxia. LITFL.com. 2015. Accessed January 12, 2023. https://litfl.com/post-intubation-hypoxia/

Thind A. Pros and pitfalls of disconnecting the ventilator during acute respiratory decompensation. Critical Care Now. Accessed January 12, 2023. https://criticalcarenow.com/pros-and-pitfalls-of-disconnecting-the-ventilator-during-acute-respiratory-decompensation/.

41

Think Before You Hang Those Fluids! Consider a Tailored Fluid Strategy for Critically Ill Patients

Michael G. Allison

Fluid resuscitation is one of the key therapies for ED patients with hypotension. Patients in shock are provided IVFs with the intent to increase stroke volume and improve organ perfusion. The optimal approach for administering IVFs in resuscitation is not well established due to limitations in the literature as well as the complexity and heterogeneity of critically ill patients. The fixed dose of IVFs (30 mL/kg) for sepsis recommended by the Surviving Sepsis Campaign and included in the SEP-1 measure by the Centers for Medicare & Medicaid Services is taken from decades-old research on early goal-directed therapy. The choice of 30 mL/kg was not based upon research evaluating the optimal fluid dose but has been carried on in subsequent randomized controlled trials in sepsis. Meanwhile, research highlighting the harms of providing large volume resuscitation has been mounting, especially as we understand that only 50% of critically ill patients with hypotension will respond to a fluid bolus. A thoughtful approach to providing fluids to patients in the ED should replace the indiscriminate use of liberal fluid resuscitation.

Benefits and Harms of Fluid Boluses

A variety of diseases and clinical syndromes can result in patients becoming hypotensive. Patients in cardiogenic or obstructive shock may be fluid intolerant. Patients can develop intravascular volume depletion due to a combination of poor intake, fluid losses, and/or increased capillary leak. Distributive shock can develop when a decrease in vasomotor tone leaves patients with dilated blood vessels and inadequate circulating volume. Multiple shock subtypes can be present in the same patient.

Provision of IVFs can increase venous return, augment stroke volume, and result in improved tissue perfusion in fluid responsive patients. Swift reversal of hypotension with fluids allows patients to avoid the potential need for invasive lines, the administration of vasopressors, and admission to a critical care setting.

Caution must be exercised when using large quantities of IVFs as volume resuscitation can be associated with a variety of complications. Patients with and without heart failure may develop pulmonary edema from fluid collecting in the interstitium of the lungs due to impaired capillary permeability and increased hydrostatic pressures.

Excessive fluids can make right heart failure syndromes worse. Renal injury may occur due to increased venous pressures, decreases in renal arterial blood flow, and interstitial edema causing tubular dysfunction. Mounting observational data has described a correlation between increased fluid resuscitation and worse outcomes—such as prolonged mechanical ventilation, acute kidney injury, and increased mortality. All of this data suggests that clinicians should be cautious with overzealous fluid administration.

Selecting an Initial Liberal Versus Restrictive Approach to Fluid Loading

Two general strategies exist for fluid resuscitation: liberal and restrictive. However, there is no consensus on what precisely defines each approach. Typically, a liberal strategy entails an initial bolus of at least 30 mL/kg of fluids, followed by additional fluids in response to persistent hypotension. In contrast, a restrictive approach also starts with 30 mL/kg of fluids but may use vasopressors simultaneously to improve blood pressure and increase venous return. In a restrictive approach, further intravenous volume resuscitation is not prompted by persistent hypotension unless there is compelling evidence of volume responsiveness or a significant clinical reason.

The CLOVERS trial, examining the effects of a liberal versus restrictive resuscitation practice in patients with septic shock, was published in 2023. Over 1,500 patients were randomized with the liberal fluid group receiving an additional 3.4 L after their initial resuscitation while the restrictive group received a median of 1.3 L. There were no notable differences in the primary outcome of death nor in secondary outcomes including days free from mechanical ventilation, days free from vasopressor uses, and days free from renal replacement therapy. Unfortunately, patients in the trial were enrolled only after initial fluid loading with a median amount of 2.0 L fluid, which equates to a 30 mL/kg load for a 67-kg patient.

Determining Volume Responsiveness After the Initial Fluid Strategy

Providing the precise amount of fluids tailored to a patient's individual need has been described as the holy grail in resuscitation. Deciding whether to continue IVFs based solely on noninvasive blood pressure measurements places patients at risk of overresuscitation while static markers of volume responsiveness, such as CVP measurements, are known to be unreliable tools. The adoption of dynamic methods of hemodynamic monitoring has shown promise in providing individualized fluid therapy based on an assessment of volume responsiveness. Volume responsiveness refers to the ability of a patient's stroke volume to increase by 10% to 15% after receiving a crystalloid or colloid fluid bolus. The promise of dynamic measures of volume responsiveness has been subsequently tempered by the lack of reliability and the consistent application to individual patients.

Techniques such as arterial waveform analysis, ultrasound evaluation of the inferior vena cava, echocardiographic assessments of stroke volume (via velocity-time integral), thoracic bioreactance, and impedance plethysmography have all been studied to help identify patients that may respond to further fluid loading. Selecting the correct technique for the hypotensive patient can be challenging. Spontaneously breathing patients are not able to use heart/lung interactions that inform the majority of arterial waveform analysis. Mechanically ventilated patients require high tidal volumes for many of these techniques to be predictive. A number of these techniques are not validated in patients with tachycardia and dysrhythmias or with right ventricular dysfunction.

Clinical training and local availability of devices significantly impact the ability to perform a volume responsiveness assessment in the ED. When available, these devices may not be perfectly predictive but can be better than best clinical estimate in assessing a patient's possible response to additional fluid loading. In the absence of experience, training, or devices that can estimate volume responsiveness or in challenging or unclear cases, consider a strategy of early vasopressor use with small bolus fluid challenges and assess and reassess response to treatment to ensure effectiveness of further fluid resuscitation.

PEARLS

- The use of initial boluses of 30 mL/kg of crystalloid fluids in patients with sepsis is not based on evidence but has emerged as a standard practice.
- There are many documented risks to providing large volume resuscitation including increased length of stay, increased renal injury, and increased mortality.
- A 2023 trial of early restrictive versus liberal fluid administration demonstrated no notable difference in patient outcomes.
- Performing dynamic measures of volume responsiveness in the ED can be challenging, given that their predictive ability is dependent upon clinical circumstances and can be influenced by patient-specific factors.
- Consider using vasopressors early in resuscitation and challenging patients with small additional fluid boluses to avoid overresuscitation.

Suggested Readings

Monnet X, Shi R, Teboul JL. Prediction of fluid responsiveness. What's new? *Ann Intensive Care*. 2022;12:46.

Nguyen HG, Jaehne AK, Jayaprakash N, et al. Early goal directed therapy in severe sepsis and septic shock: insights and comparisons to ProCESS, ProMISe and ARISE. *Crit Care*. 2016;20:160.

The National Heart, Lung, and Blood Institute Prevention and Early Treatment of Acute Lung Injury Clinical Trials Network. Early restrictive or liberal fluid management for sepsis-induced hypotension. *N Engl J Med*. 2023;388(6):499-510.

42

Who Needs RRT in the ED?

Sarah Ring Gibbs and Evan Leibner

RRT is used to substitute kidney function in cases of renal failure or to augment clearance of certain toxic ingestions. This is achieved by filtering blood from the patient and then using diffusion or convection across semipermeable membranes in a continuous or intermittent manner to extract solutes and/or water. There are several different modalities to choose from. The choice depends primarily on the patient's clinical status (specifically hemodynamic stability), preexisting access, purpose of RRT (solute or water removal), and availability.

INDICATIONS

RRT is indicated in the patient showing signs of renal failure complicated by volume overload, life-threatening and treatment-refractory hyperkalemia or metabolic acidosis, and/or significant uremia (ie, encephalopathy with obtundation, pericarditis, or neuropathy). Remember the mnemonic AEIOU (AEIOU: A—acidosis; E—electrolytes, principally hyperkalemia; I—ingestions or overdose of medications/drugs; O—overload of fluid causing heart failure; U—uremia). Likewise, RRT has been used in rhabdomyolysis for myoglobin clearance, though the benefits of this have not been fully established in the literature. For poisonings, RRT can be used independent of renal failure, depending on the volume of toxic exposure or the patient's clinical status. Not all toxins are suitable for removal with RRT. Those most amenable include ones that have a low-molecular weight, are primarily distributed in the blood as opposed to peripherally, have a low affinity for protein binding, and are excreted for clearance. Common dialyzable drugs/toxins include the following:

Aminoglycosides	Levetiracetam
Atenolol	Lithium
Barbiturates	Metformin
Dabigatran	Organophosphates
Dapsone	Procainamide
Deferoxamine	Salicylates
Diphenhydramine	Theophylline
Iron	Toxic alcohols
Isoniazid	Vancomycin

This list is not comprehensive, so in case of a large overdose it is worthwhile to check with your local poison control center or toxicology experts.

RISKS

As with any intervention, certain risks exist when initiating RRT in the ED. Inserting an appropriate catheter has risks, many of which are reduced with proper use of ultrasound. Risks include arterial or nerve puncture with the introducing needle, dilation of a major artery, hematoma formation, and pneumothorax. Additional risks exist specifically with subclavian access, such as an increased risk of proximal vein stenosis or thrombosis that can hinder future ability to create an arteriovenous fistula on the ipsilateral side. Likewise, given the location, hemopneumothorax is a higher risk with a subclavian entry site.

CLABSI are a risk with both the introduction of a catheter and recurrent use. Likewise, as the catheter is a retained foreign body, thrombosis and distal emboli are risks to maintaining access.

Finally, with the procedure of RRT, hemodynamic instability of the patient is a possibility given fluid and solute shifts. This can lead to hypotension, disequilibrium, cerebral edema, seizures, cardiac arrhythmias, and cardiovascular collapse. Though rare, equipment malfunction is also a possibility, leading to large-volume blood loss and electrolyte derangements.

Contraindications

There are relatively few in general and can be divided into contraindications for vascular catheter placement (if required) and to running RRT. Contraindications to vascular catheter placement include local infection at the site of insertion, thrombosis at the site of catheter placement that could cause an embolus, significant stenosis of the vessel as to cause damage with catheter manipulation, or abnormal anatomy that would preclude successful catheter placement. Bleeding can be a relative contraindication to both catheter placement (secondary to coagulopathy) or RRT due to inability to tolerate anticoagulation or to tolerate fluid shifts. Contraindications to running RRT largely include significant hemodynamic instability secondary to volume shifts or an uncooperative patient.

Access Site

When choosing an access site, order of preference should be RIJ, LIJ, either femoral vein, left subclavian, and then right subclavian. The RIJ is preferred as it is a direct line from catheter insertion to the caval-atrial junction. This will provide the highest blood flow for RRT. Furthermore, as it is direct, there are lower risks for catheter complications such as kinking or obstruction. The LIJ is the next preferred site if the RIJ is unavailable, however, because it is not direct, the patient could experience reduced flow during RRT. The next choice is the femoral vein. If selecting this site, care must be taken to use the longest catheter available to reach the distal IVC. Compared to IJ lines, femoral lines reduce patient mobility and have a higher rate of infection and thrombosis when left in for longer periods of time. The subclavian veins should be left as a last resort due to their tortuosity (often leading to reduced flow or difficulty with placement) and risk of causing proximal vein stenosis as mentioned before.

Location will also determine the length of catheter selected. Catheters vary widely in length depending on the manufacturer; however, each site has a suitable range of lengths. These include the following:

- RIJ: 12 to 15 cm
- LIJ: 15 to 20 cm
- Femoral vein: 20 to 24 cm
- Subclavian vein: approximately 15 cm

Modes of RRT

- iHD
  - Performed over shorter periods of time with a larger volume of blood dialyzed at a given time which could lead to increased risk of hemodynamic stability. It is less expensive, faster, has fewer bleeding/clotting complications, and does not often require anticoagulation. iHD is best for toxin removal. Can be performed with a fistula or a vascular catheter.
- CRRT
  - The most common modality used is CVVH. Generally, run over a 24-hour period and continuous anticoagulation is preferred. It is less likely to cause hypotension than iHD so is an alternative for the patient who is hemodynamically unstable. It can only be performed with a vascular catheter, and a fistula cannot be used. In additional, it is preferred with patients with brain injury as it has fewer fluid shifts that can affect the brain as well as for rhabdomyolysis. CRRT requires ICU level nursing with providers that are trained on its use, usually with a 1-to-1 ratio.
- SCUF

- A type of CRRT used to remove only excess fluid (not solute) from the bloodstream. Generally removes smaller volumes than CVVH when run over the same 24-hour time frame though it can be run for shorter time periods.
- Hybrid
  - SLED
    - Considered a hybrid therapy between iHD and CRRT, SLED is typically run over 6- to 12-hour sessions as compared to 3- to 4-hour sessions in iHD and 24-hour sessions in CRRT. Like CRRT is often used in patients who are more hemodynamically unstable as is less likely to cause hypotension. Can be performed with a fistula or a vascular catheter and no anticoagulation is required.
- pUF
  - Not frequently used in the ED unless the patient has a preexisting peritoneal catheter, and the ED has the capability to run it.

MODALITIES	ADVANTAGES	DISADVANTAGES	ADDITIONAL
iHD	Fastest (3-4 h sessions) Can use a fistula or vascular catheter Less expensive Anticoagulation not required Preferred for toxin removal	Increased risk for hemodynamic instability	
CRRT	Preferred in patients who are hemodynamically unstable Preferred in patients with brain injury (fewer fluid shifts) Rhabdomyolysis	Longer sessions than iHD (often 24 h/d) Continuous anticoagulation preferred Can only use a vascular catheter (cannot use fistula) Requires specific nursing training to run with 1:1 ratio	Includes modalities such as CVVH, CVVHD, and CVVHDF
SCUF	Preferred in patients who are hemodynamically unstable	Continuous anticoagulation preferred Longer sessions than iHD (variable though up to 24 h/d) Requires vascular catheter	A form of CRRT that removes excess fluid (not solute)
SLED	Preferred in patients who are hemodynamically unstable Can use a fistula or vascular catheter Anticoagulation not required	Longer sessions than iHD (6-12 h)	A hybrid between CRRT and iHD
pUF	Fewer side effects than iHD (nausea, vomiting, cramping) More convenient outpatient (can be performed at home and overnight)	Requires preexisting catheter (no emergent access) Facility may not have access to a pUF cycler	

PEARLS

- RRT is indicated in patients with specific toxic ingestions or renal failure complicated by volume overload, life-threatening and treatment-refractory hyperkalemia or metabolic acidosis, and/or significant uremia.
- Risks primarily involve injury to surrounding structures with placement of the dialysis catheter, infection, thrombosis with embolus, and hemodynamic instability while receiving RRT.
- When placing a temporary dialysis catheter, preference for location should be RIJ > LIJ > femoral veins > left subclavian vein > right subclavian vein.
- The choice between RRT modalities depends on the patient's hemodynamic status, access, purpose of RRT (solute or water removal), and facility availability.
- Hypotension does not preclude patients from receiving RRT; however, slower methods of filtration should be considered such as CRRT, SCUF, or SLED.

Suggested Readings

Antoun TA, Palevsky PM. Selection of modality of renal replacement therapy. *Semin Dial.* 2009;22:108-113.

Beecham GB, Narothama RA. Dialysis catheter. In: *StatPearls [Internet]*. NCBI Bookshelf; 2022.

Hechanova LA. Overview of renal replacement therapy—genitourinary disorders. *Merck Manuals Professional Edition.* 2022.

Mehta RL. Challenges and pitfalls when implementing renal replacement therapy in the ICU. *Crit Care.* 2015;19(Suppl 3)S9.

43

Know How to Care for the ICU Boarder in Your ED

Joshua D. Farkas

The number of critically ill patients presenting to the ED is rapidly growing. In addition to an increasing number, a prolonged length of stay can significantly impact the mortality of critically ill ED patients. The value of high-quality supportive care cannot be overstated, so this should be initiated in the ED while awaiting transfer to the ICU.

Avoid Excess Fluid Administration

Critically ill patients can gain approximately 1 L of fluid per day due to a myriad of sources. Multiple intravenous medications, continuous infusions, and repeated fluid boluses can lead to an excessively positive fluid balance. Over several days, this excess fluid may cause edema and lead to severe complications (including pulmonary edema, renal failure, abdominal compartment syndrome, and pressure ulceration).

Avoiding unnecessary fluid administration is critical. Reflexively giving fluid boluses to increase blood pressure or urine output should be avoided, unless the patient is truly volume depleted. Among patients with systemic inflammation (eg, sepsis, pancreatitis), fluid boluses may cause temporary improvement, but this fluid rapidly extravasates into the tissues. In addition to indiscriminate fluid boluses, "maintenance fluids" should also be avoided.

Avoid Unnecessary Blood Transfusion

Blood transfusion can cause several complications, including volume overload, immunosuppression, transfusion reactions, and transfusion-related acute lung injury. Non-bleeding ICU patients generally should not be transfused unless they have hemoglobin less than 7 mg/dL. Transfusing two units of blood at a time should also be avoided, as a patient's hemoglobin level may fluctuate over time. A landmark trial investigating upper gastrointestinal hemorrhage showed that a transfusion threshold of 9 mg/dL increased mortality compared to a transfusion threshold of 7 mg/dL. Importantly, this study excluded patients with exsanguinating hemorrhage or acute coronary syndrome.

Avoid Benzodiazepines

Traditionally, benzodiazepines were a mainstay for therapy of anxiety among critically ill patients. However, recent evidence shows that they increase the risk of delirium and duration of mechanical ventilation. Among intubated patients, a propofol or dexmedetomidine infusion is generally preferable (even if this requires a low-dose norepinephrine infusion to maintain hemodynamic stability). Other alternatives include antipsychotics such as haloperidol, droperidol, olanzapine, or quetiapine (which are *especially* preferred over benzodiazepines for the management of agitated delirium).

Avoid High-Dose Opioid Infusions

The ideal strategy for analgesia among critically ill patients is often multimodal analgesia. This utilizes moderate doses of several agents *synergistically*, with a goal of minimizing the toxicity due to any single agent. For example, a combination of scheduled acetaminophen (eg, 1 gram q6h), a pain-dose ketamine infusion (eg, 0.1-0.3 mg/kg/h), and as-needed boluses of opioid is often effective.

Higher-dose opioid infusions should be avoided if possible. A single dose of fentanyl has a short half-life, but if provided as a continuous infusion fentanyl accumulates in fat tissues with a prolonged duration of action. If opioid infusions are used without *organized* and *aggressive* efforts at weaning them, they may accumulate and delay extubation. Overutilization of opioids may also lead to tolerance and subsequent withdrawal among patients on mechanical ventilation for several days.

Avoid Nephrotoxic Medications

Renal failure is often the first organ failure to develop in the context of hypoperfusion. Consequently, nephrotoxins should be avoided among critically ill patients who are not chronically anuric and dialysis dependent.

NSAIDs in particular should be avoided. In addition to a risk of renal failure, NSAIDs increase the risk of gastric stress ulceration. ACE inhibitors and ARBs should generally be avoided, unless there is a strong indication for their use (eg, acute myocardial infarction).

Vancomycin may accumulate and cause renal failure over time, so ongoing use should be avoided if possible. As a general rule of thumb, vancomycin should usually be stopped within less than 48 hours if microbiologic data doesn't reveal methicillin-resistant *Staphylococcus aureus*. Also note that vancomycin isn't indicated for most community-acquired infections (eg, intra-abdominal or urinary tract infections).

Avoid DVT

Patients should receive DVT prophylaxis unless they are actively bleeding or have other contraindications. In renal failure, unfractionated heparin is the only option (eg, 5,000 IU every 8 hours). For most patients, low-molecular-weight heparin is preferred over unfractionated heparin since it carries a lower risk of heparin-induced thrombocytopenia (eg, enoxaparin 40 mg daily). Recall that heparin is *weight based*, so patients who are morbidly obese might benefit from proportionally higher doses (eg, 0.25 mg/kg enoxaparin every 12 hours).

PEARLS

- Avoid unnecessary maintenance fluids.
- Don't transfuse unless the patient is actively exsanguinating or the hemoglobin is less than 7 mg/dL.
- Utilize multimodal analgesia to achieve pain control while minimizing medication side effects.
- Avoid nephrotoxins if possible (eg, NSAIDs, ACE inhibitors, ARBs, vancomycin).
- Provide DVT prophylaxis unless contraindicated.

Suggested Readings

Devlin JW, Skrobik Y, Gelinas C, et al. Clinical Practice Guidelines for the prevention and management of pain, agitation/sedation, delirium, immobility, and sleep disruption in adult patients in the ICU. *Crit Care Med*. 2019;46(9):e825-e873.

Napolitano LM, Kurek S, Luchette FA, et al. Clinical Practice Guideline: red blood cell transfusion in adult trauma and critical care. *Crit Care Med*. 2009;37(12):3124-3157.

Villanueva C, Colomo A, Bosch A, et al. Transfusion strategies for acute upper gastrointestinal bleeding. *N Engl J Med*. 2013;368(1):11-21.

44

Push-Dose Pressor Pitfalls

C. Nicole Thompson

PDP, or bolus-dose vasopressors, have been adopted into the clinical practice of emergency medicine to temporarily treat hypotension. Although potentially lifesaving, administration can be challenging. To avoid common errors, clinicians should ensure proper patient selection, and ED stakeholders should develop system-based protocols to reduce human errors inherent to PDP.

Clinicians have used epinephrine and phenylephrine in the ED in bolus or push-dose formulations. Both have a short time to onset (<1 minute), short half-lives, and can be given via peripheral IV. Epinephrine acts as both inotrope and vasopressor with alpha- and beta-activity. This increases blood pressure and heart rate. Phenylephrine works as a pure vasopressor with only alpha-activity, and can improve MAP but carries a risk of reflex bradycardia. Phenylephrine can last 10 to 20 minutes, while epinephrine can last 5 to 10 minutes. The dosing of epinephrine is 5 to 20 mcg (or 1 mcg/kg in pediatrics) while the dosing of phenylephrine is 50 to 200 mcg (or 5-20 mcg/kg in pediatrics), or 10 times that of epinephrine.

	EPINEPHRINE	**PHENYLEPHRINE**
Mechanism	Alpha- and beta-1/2 agonist	Alpha-agonist
Action	Inotrope, chronotrope, and vasopressor	Pure vasopressor
Duration	5-10 min	10-20 min
Dose	5-20 mcg (1 mcg/kg in pediatrics)	50-200 mcg (5-20 mcg/kg in pediatrics)
Side effects	Tachydysrhythmias	Reflex bradycardia Variable effect on cardiac output

To prepare push-dose epinephrine, take a 10-mL syringe and draw up 9 mL of saline with 1 mL of 0.1 mg/mL epinephrine. This creates a 10 mcg/mL solution of epinephrine.

To prepare push-dose phenylephrine, inject 1 mL of 10 mg/mL phenylephrine into a 100-mL bag of normal saline. Then draw the solution into a syringe, creating a 100 mcg/mL of solution of phenylephrine.

PATIENT SELECTION

When utilizing PDP, clinicians must consider patient selection. For example, patients undergoing procedural sedation or rapid sequence induction for endotracheal intubation are classic candidates for PDP use. Post-intubation hypotension occurs in up to 25% of patients, and both epinephrine and phenylephrine can aid in managing this complication. A syringe of PDP should be immediately available at the start of induction, endotracheal intubation, and initiation of mechanical ventilation.

Patients with vasodilatory and distributive shock (including sepsis and anaphylaxis) are also appropriate candidates for PDP. If possible, patients should be adequately fluid resuscitated, but this can occur concurrently with PDP to temporize cardiac output and blood pressure while any necessary vasoactive infusions are prepared and initiated. The patient with neurotrauma may also be included in this category. Neurogenic shock patients benefit from the chronotropy and increased peripheral or systemic vascular resistance (SVR) of epinephrine, and patients with TBI benefit from the maintenance of MAP sufficient for adequate CPP. The risk of bradycardia or relative bradycardia (a normal heart rate in a shocked patient) makes phenylephrine a controversial, albeit historical, choice here.

In trauma or medical patients with suspected hemorrhagic shock receiving a massive transfusion, consider administration of push-dose vasopressin 1 to 4 units, as AVP levels decrease dramatically secondary to decreased pituitary secretion and loss of AVP in the shed blood. AVP deficiency results in venodilation and hypotension **resistant to catecholamines.**

Exercise caution with patients in undifferentiated shock. Perform a RUSH exam (see Chapter 11), at least concurrently with PDP, not only to rule out other treatable causes of hypotension (such as tension pneumothorax or pericardial tamponade) but also to monitor effects on cardiac function after the administration of the vasopressor. This will aid in the nuanced selection of agents for additional PDP or ongoing vasoactive infusions. For example, many patients, such as those with hyperdynamic or vasoplegic shock, will tolerate an increase in afterload caused by phenylephrine without a decrease in stroke volume. If, however, push-dose phenylephrine results in decreased cardiac function on bedside ultrasound, the clinician may opt for the inotropy of epinephrine for subsequent doses. Similarly, patients with bradycardia may benefit from the chronotropy of epinephrine over phenylephrine. However, in patients with hypertrophic obstructive cardiomyopathy physiology or with tachycardia or tachydysrhythmias, phenylephrine may be the better choice.

HUMAN ERROR

The use of PDP at bedside introduces the risk of human error. These medications require selection of appropriate dose calculation, dilution, and incremental administration in emergent high-risk and high-stress situations, often without the usual safety checks. Epinephrine is manufactured in multiple concentrations and forms, which can lead to overdosing errors. Asking for "code cart epinephrine" or just "epinephrine" may cause clinicians to select the 1:1,000 (1 mg/mL) epinephrine vials rather than the 1:10,000 (0.1 mg/mL) epinephrine ampule, resulting in a 10-fold overdose. Staff may interpret verbal orders of "push-dose epi" as "push a dose of epi," prompting a less experienced practitioner to give a full code dose of epinephrine (1 mg) and cause a significant overdose. Furthermore, dilutions of phenylephrine and epinephrine are performed differently, potentiating significant dosing errors if the procedures are mixed up. Finally, inadvertent overdose can occur due to a lack of proper labeling, leading to the inadvertent use of a PDP-containing syringe as a saline flush.

SYSTEMS-BASED PROTOCOLS

To reduce the risk of human errors, ED stakeholders should participate in the design of systems-based protocols. First, the department should agree on a uniform naming system. By agreeing on and educating the department of the name "push-dose epi," clinicians reduce the risk of administering a cardiac arrest dose or undiluted epinephrine. Second, the department should keep mixing instruction cards or placards readily accessible in the highest acuity situations to reduce dilution errors. Push-dose phenylephrine preparation has more steps, so stakeholders may consider accepting the additional cost of commercially available premixed syringes or choose to exclude phenylephrine as a push-dose option. Bedside-mixed syringes should be labeled after the medication is drawn up with an agreed-upon expiration time (typically 1 hour). Departments should educate nursing and pharmacy staff on a method to document doses administered. Finally, a nonpunitive system for adverse event reporting should be available to staff for ongoing quality improvement efforts.

PEARLS

- Epinephrine and phenylephrine are vasopressors commonly used in bolus-dose or push-dose formulations in the ED.

- A syringe of push-dose vasopressor should be available prior to high-risk procedures (RSI, sedation).
- Perform a RUSH exam to appropriately assess and treat causes of shock, but PDPs can help temporize cardiac output and maintain blood pressure.
- Involve and educate stakeholders on the design and execution of system-based protocols to reduce human errors.

Suggested Readings

Cole J, Knack S, Karl E, Horton G, Satpathy R, Driver B. Human errors and adverse hemodynamic events related to "push dose pressors" in the emergency department. *J Med Toxicol.* 2019; 15(4):276-286.

Kubena A, Weston S, Alvey H. Push-dose vasopressors in the emergency department: a narrative review. *J Emerg Crit Care Med.* 2022;6:22.

Sims CA, Holena D, Kim P, et al. Effect of low-dose supplementation of arginine vasopressin on need for blood product transfusions in patients with trauma and hemorrhagic shock: a randomized clinical trial. *JAMA Surg.* 2019;154(11):994-1003.

Tilton LJ, Eginger KH. Utility of push-dose vasopressors for temporary treatment of hypotension in the emergency department. *J Emerg Nurs.* 2016;42(3):279-281. PMID: 27156610.

Weingart S. Push-dose pressors for immediate blood pressure control. *Clin Exp Emerg Med.* 2015;2(2):131-132. PMID: 27752585.

45

Perform the Simple Interventions That Make a Big Difference in Preventing Ventilator-Associated Pneumonia

Jonathan Stuart and Nicholas J. Johnson

VAP is defined as pneumonia that arises in a mechanically ventilated patient more than 48 hours after endotracheal intubation. VAP occurs in 5% to 40% of all mechanically ventilated patients depending on country, hospital setting, and identification criteria. VAP has been associated with an all-cause mortality of up to 50%. Relevant for the emergency clinician, approximately half of all episodes of VAP occur within the first 4 days of mechanical ventilation. Increased ED length of stay has been shown to be a risk factor for the development of pneumonia in mechanically ventilated patients. A number of simple interventions have been demonstrated to reduce the risk of VAP. Many of these can easily be implemented in the ED.

The greatest risk factors for VAP are endotracheal intubation and mechanical ventilation. When it is possible and safe, avoiding intubation altogether is the best strategy for avoiding VAP. If tracheal intubation is required, the oral route is preferred. A similar principle applies to placement of gastric tubes. Orogastric is preferred over nasogastric as the nasal route has been associated with higher VAP and sinusitis risk. Noninvasive positive pressure ventilation should be considered in alert patients with respiratory failure due to chronic obstructive pulmonary disease, congestive heart failure, asthma, immunocompromised states, neuromuscular weakness, and may be used in selected patients with other conditions. Other noninvasive modalities, such as high-flow nasal cannula, may be considered in select patients with acute hypoxemic respiratory failure.

Semirecumbent positioning achieved by elevating a mechanically ventilated patient's head to greater than 30° to 45° is a simple intervention that likely reduces risk for VAP. Supine patient positioning has been demonstrated to facilitate aspiration in several studies. A 2016 *Cochrane* review confirmed the semirecumbent position is superior for prevention of clinically suspected VAP although there is a lack of evidence for microbiologically documented VAP. Mechanically ventilated patients in the ED should be placed in the semirecumbent position unless a contraindication, such as spinal immobilization, exists. If contraindications exist, reverse Trendelenburg position may suffice.

Colonization of the oropharynx has been identified as an independent risk factor for VAP. Oral decontamination with chlorhexidine has been routinely utilized to mitigate this risk. A 2013 Cochrane Review documented a 40% decrease in the likelihood of VAP among patients treated with oral chlorhexidine. However, recent studies have called the benefit of chlorhexidine into question, and a meta-analysis of prior randomized trials showed no association of chlorhexidine use with lower VAP rates. Nonetheless, the treatment remains routine but the optimal timing, and whether it must occur in the ED, is also unclear.

SDD with topical and/or systemic antibiotics has been associated with lower mortality rates, primarily in ICUs with low baseline antibiotic administration. A 2022 systematic review confirmed a reduced risk of mortality, VAP, and duration of mechanical ventilation, but this evidence was of low certainty. In contrast, a 2022 randomized clinical trial found no benefit to SDD. Fortunately, SDD was not associated with an increase in adverse events such as the development of *Clostridium difficile* infection or antimicrobial resistant organisms. However, the association with selective decontamination and the emergence of antimicrobial resistant organisms remains uncertain. Trauma patients and patients treated with targeted temperature management after out-of-hospital cardiac arrest are subpopulations who may benefit the most from SDD. Some randomized trials have reported lower VAP rates with administration of probiotics, but that signal is not present on subsequent meta-analysis.

Attention to endotracheal tube cuff pressure and shape may also aid in VAP prevention. Emergency clinicians should consider measuring endotracheal tube cuff pressure using a manometer after intubation. An endotracheal tube cuff pressure maintained at 20 to 30 cm H_2O can prevent leakage of bacterial pathogens around the cuff into the lower respiratory tract. Frequent pressure monitoring and devices designed to provide continuous control of endotracheal tube cuff pressure throughout the respiratory cycle have not been shown to consistently reduce the risk for VAP.

Endotracheal tubes with special features may also influence VAP prevention. Several meta-analyses have documented a decreased prevalence of VAP when endotracheal tubes with subglottic suctioning ports are used although recent studies have demonstrated no impact on time to extubation. Special features such as modified cuff shapes, materials, and/or antimicrobial coatings have not proven superior to conventional endotracheal

TABLE 45.1	MEASURES THAT MAY REDUCE RISK OF VAP

Avoidance of endotracheal intubation when possible
Noninvasive modalities for oxygenation and ventilation
Regular assessment for liberation from mechanical ventilation
Semirecumbent patient positioning
Orotracheal intubation as opposed to nasal
Orogastric tube placement and gastric decompression
SDD
Avoidance of unnecessary blood transfusion
Application of subglottic suction
Antimicrobial-coated endotracheal tubes
Endotracheal tube cuff pressure of 20-30 cm H_2O
Avoidance of unnecessary stress ulcer prophylaxis
Ventilator bundles

SDD, selective digestive decontamination; VAP, ventilator-associated pneumonia.

tubes. Silver-coated endotracheal tubes have been studied extensively and a Cochrane review confirmed a reduced risk of VAP but no decrease in ICU or hospital length of stay.

Many hospitals have adopted "ventilator bundles" based on the Institute for Healthcare Improvement's initiative to incorporate evidence-based practices into clinical care. The ventilator bundle includes five practices, three of which aim to prevent VAP: (1) elevation of the head of the bed to 30° to 45°, (2) daily "sedation vacation" and daily assessment of readiness to extubate, (3) peptic ulcer disease prophylaxis, (4) deep venous thrombosis prophylaxis, and (5) oral decontamination with chlorhexidine. The impact of these bundles is unclear as the results of implementation studies are mixed. A 2018 meta-analysis demonstrated a reduction of both overall mortality and VAP-related mortality with implementation of the ventilator bundle in the ICU setting. Ventilation bundles adapted for the ED setting including measures such as head-of-bed elevation, regular oral care, subglottic suctioning, sedation titration, spontaneous breathing trials, deep vein thrombosis prophylaxis, and stress ulcer prophylaxis have been shown to improve outcomes, but the role of these bundles in VAP prevention in the ED remains unclear (see also **Table 45.1**).

PEARLS

- The best way to avoid VAP is to avoid unnecessary intubation and mechanical ventilation and extubate as soon as possible.
- Simple measures such as elevating the head of the bed and SDD may reduce risk of VAP.
- Use of subglottic suctioning devices, antimicrobial-coated and/or modified endotracheal tubes, and attention to adequate endotracheal tube cuff pressure may prevent aspiration of oral secretions.
- SDD using topical or systemic antimicrobial agents may prevent VAP, but further investigation is needed.

Suggested Readings

Bhat R, Goyal M, Graf S, et al. Impact of post-intubation interventions on mortality in patients boarding in the emergency department. *West J Emerg Med*. 2014;15(6):708-711. PMID: 25247049.

DeLuca LA Jr, Walsh P, Davidson DD Jr, et al. Impact and feasibility of an emergency department-based ventilator-associated pneumonia bundle for patients intubated in an academic emergency department. *Am J Infect Control*. 2017;45(2):151-157. PMID: 27665031.

Hammond NE, Myburgh J, Seppelt I, et al. Association between selective decontamination of the digestive tract and in-hospital mortality in intensive care unit patients receiving mechanical ventilation: a systematic review and meta-analysis. *JAMA*. 2022;328(19):1922-1934. PMID: 36286098.

Klompas M, Li L, Kleinman K, et al. Associations between ventilator bundle components and outcomes. *JAMA Intern Med*. 2016;176(9):1277-1283. PMID: 27428482.

Klompas M, Speck K, Howell MD, et al. Reappraisal of routine oral care with chlorhexidine gluconate for patients receiving mechanical ventilation: systematic review and meta-analysis. *JAMA Intern Med*. 2014;174(5):751-761. PMID: 24663255.

46

ECMO in the Emergency Department

David John Wallace and Nicolas A. Ulloa

ECMO is used with increasing frequency in critically ill patients. The increase in use has resulted in earlier patient cannulation, often initiated in the ED. For the ED physician, knowing the indications for ECMO is paramount as recognition can lead to better outcomes for these time-sensitive conditions. Briefly, VV ECMO should be used primarily for severe lung pathology, and VA ECMO should be used for severe combined heart and lung pathology.

Application and Main Indications

With VV ECMO, the patient will have a large vascular cannula placed to access the venous circulation. The VV ECMO circuit will oxygenate the patient's venous blood and remove carbon dioxide. The circuit will then return the patient's blood into the venous circulation by a separate cannula (or channel if using a dual-lumen cannula). The objective is to protect vital organs from experiencing critical hypoxemia while allowing the lungs to recover. VV ECMO should be considered in patients who are persistently hypoxic or hypercapnic on optimal ventilator settings. The following are common indications for initiating VV ECMO in the ED:

- Severe acute respiratory distress syndrome, with refractory hypoxemia or hypercapnia
- Severe pneumonia, with refractory hypoxemia or hypercapnia
- Severe status asthmaticus, with refractory hypoxemia or hypercapnia

With VA ECMO, the patient will also have a large vascular cannula in place that removes venous blood. The VA ECMO circuit adds oxygen and removes carbon dioxide from the patient's venous blood. In addition, the VA ECMO circuit has a pump that propels the blood, which is returned to the patient's arterial circulation. The objective is to protect vital organs from experiencing critical hypoxemia or hypoperfusion, allowing the lungs and heart to recover. Typically, VA ECMO is used as a bridge to recovery, bridge to transplantation, or bridge to assist devices in the following examples:

- ED cardiac arrest
- Cardiogenic shock
- Right ventricular failure
- Refractory ventricular tachycardia or fibrillation

Other Indications

VA ECMO is used in severe cardioactive medication overdoses (ie, β-blockers and calcium channel blockers). VA ECMO provides hemodynamic support for patient's refractory to standard treatments, thus providing adequate perfusion to vital organs while the offending agent is metabolized over time.

In additional, accidental hypothermia is another instance in which ECMO should be considered. EMS recommendation for severe hypothermia (<28 °C) is to transport patients to hospitals with ECMO capabilities. The ECMO circuit, in addition to oxygenating, ventilating, and perfusing vital organs, will rewarm blood better than other passive and active rewarming techniques.

Exclusion Criteria

ECMO therapy requires significant resources, frequently over days to weeks; therefore, appropriate patient selection is essential. Although specific exclusion criteria may vary between institutions, the underlying rationale is to exclude patients from ECMO who are too sick to benefit, unable to tolerate the circuit itself, or are too healthy to benefit.

At one extreme of illness severity are patients who are too sick to benefit from ECMO. When a patient has severe acute multiorgan failure or severe organ failure in the setting of chronic end-stage disease, ECMO should not be initiated as it will not change the outcome for the patient. Many institutions use age thresholds for ECMO consideration, as a proxy for chronic disease burden and anticipated actuarial benefit. Although age cutoffs vary, older than 65 years is typically considered a relative contraindication. However, it is reasonable to discuss candidacy with the ECMO team on a case-by-case basis.

ECMO circuits typically require anticoagulation to prevent blood clotting in the conduit lines or other circuit elements. Patients with contraindications to anticoagulation are therefore generally excluded from ECMO consideration, though ECMO with minimal or no anticoagulation is performed in some centers and could be considered on a case-by-case basis in those settings.

Lastly, there are patients who are not sick enough to benefit from ECMO. For these patients, conventional therapy should result in a good outcome, so there is no room for ECMO to further improve morbidity or mortality. Although ECMO has become increasingly safe in the last decade, there are also therapy-associated risks that could result in a worse outcome for a lower severity of illness patients (ie, the patient is exposed to the risks of ECMO therapy but not the benefit, as they would have recovered without ECMO).

Implementing ED-Initiated ECMO

Successful use of ECMO requires special equipment and specific physician, nursing, perfusionist, and respiratory therapist expertise. ED ECMO is well-suited to clinical pathways that use a collaborative ECMO team for the early identification of patients and optimal initiation of therapy. Clinical pathways should be designed to facilitate the identification of candidate patients and facilitate communication between ED and in-patient ECMO team members. In EDs that do not have in-patient ECMO capability, clinical pathways can still facilitate coordination with an in-patient ECMO team at a referral center and specialized transport services. Finally, a multidisciplinary case review process should be implemented in all ED ECMO programs to track outcomes, case selection, and identify areas for system improvement.

PEARLS

- ECMO initiation is no longer limited to patients already in the intensive care unit or cardiac catheterization laboratory.
- Early consideration of ECMO for patients with severe respiratory or cardiovascular failure refractory to standard therapy can improve patient outcomes.
- The most common indication for ECMO is severe ARDS and cardiogenic shock.
- It is important to review inclusion and exclusion criteria as patient selection for ECMO is crucial to optimize outcome and resource utilization.

Suggested Readings

Brodie D, Bacchetta, M. Extracorporeal membrane oxygenation for ARDS in adults. *N Engl J Med.* 2011;365(20):1905-1914.
Guglin M, Zucker MJ, Bazan VM, et al. Venoarterial ECMO for adults: JACC Scientific Expert Panel. *J Am Coll Cardiol.* 2019;73(6):698-716. PMID: 30765037.
Harnisch L-O, Moerer O. Contraindications to the initiation of veno-venous ECMO for severe acute respiratory failure in adults: a systematic review and practical approach based on the current literature. *Membranes (Basel).* 2021;11(8):584.
Rao P, Khalpey Z, Smith R, Burkhoff D, Kociol RD. Venoarterial extracorporeal membrane oxygenation for cardiogenic shock and cardiac arrest. *Circ Heart Fail.* 2018;11(9):e004905. PMID: 30354364.
Tonna JE, Selzman CH, Mallin MP, et al. Development and implementation of a comprehensive, multidisciplinary emergency department extracorporeal membrane oxygenation program. *Ann Emerg Med.* 2017;70:32-40.

47

Be Ready to Discuss and Deliver End-of-Life Care in the Emergency Department

Ashley Shreves

Patients commonly visit the ED near the EOL. The needs of dying patients can easily overwhelm caregivers, even in the presence of hospice services. Palliative care consultative services are increasingly available but not able to meet the large demand generated by such patients in the ED. It is critical that emergency physicians be ready to discuss and deliver EOL care.

Most patients in the last hours to days of life lose decision-making capacity. For this reason, first steps in evaluating EOL patients often involve identifying an appropriate surrogate decision maker. The next of kin hierarchy varies by state but spouses are typically first, followed by adult children, parents, and then siblings. If the patient has legally identified a health care power of attorney or health care proxy, that person trumps all other "natural" surrogates. Next, in a patient without capacity, determining if advance directives exist is paramount. While the language of living wills is often vague and unhelpful, POLST forms are essentially portable EOL order sets that address specific medical interventions like intubation, artificial nutrition, and hydration frequently considered at the EOL. Most states now have a POLST program, and so it is important that emergency physicians understand how to interpret and apply these unique advance directives.

In the absence of clear advance directives, a discussion with patients and/or their surrogate decision makers regarding the goals of care should take place. These conversations work best when done systematically, with attention paid to specific words and language used. Broadly speaking, the physician should attempt to understand the patient's goals and values, assimilate that with information about the patient's prognosis, and then make a treatment recommendation, rather than simply asking the patient or surrogate what treatments they "want." Giving patients and families a menu of options is a common pitfall and can lead to medical decision making driven by poor health literacy and overwhelming fear, rather than a careful weighing of the risks and benefits of different pathways.

While many "Goals of care" roadmaps exist, most share the following common steps:

1) Preparation
2) Patient perception
3) Invitation/readiness
4) Knowledge exchange
5) Elicit values/goals
6) Medical recommendation

For step 1, it is important to have an accurate understanding of the clinical facts. This may necessitate a careful review of the electronic medical record and/or a discussion with the patient's primary care physician or specialist, like an oncologist. Sometimes it can be impossible to accurately prognosticate for a patient in the first minutes to hours of their ED stay based on the limited information and data points available. For step 2, the patient's perception of his or her illness is assessed. Patients and families cannot engage in EOL decision making and discussions until they have an accurate understanding of their condition. Large gaps between understanding and clinical reality must be bridged before high-quality decision making can take place. Phrases like "What have the doctors told you about your illness?" and "What's your sense of how things are going?" are useful. For step 3, the patient and family's readiness or willingness to proceed with what is likely to be an emotionally painful conversation should be assessed. Phrases like "I'm worried about you/her/him" and "I know you all are hoping for the best, but I'm wondering if we can also discuss and plan for the worst" can be helpful to gauge their willingness to move forward and consider care pathways not strictly focused on life prolongation.

Next, the physician should share his or her understanding of the clinical situation. Information should be delivered in small bites and medical jargon avoided, when possible. Phrases like "I think she's dying" and "time could be short" can better communicate how dire the situation is, rather than specific data points such as white blood cell counts and creatinine levels. Another helpful phrase is "At this point, I can't imagine how we could turn this situation around." Phrases like "I'm really worried" can be more effective at communicating a poor prognosis than statistics.

For step 5, what is most important to patients and their caregivers should be explored. Some will respond well to open-ended questions like "On hearing this news, what's most important to you?" and "Can you help me understand what is an acceptable quality of life to you?" Others will need more concrete guidance. For instance, "Some people in your situation would be willing to be put on life support and spend time in the ICU, even if there was only a small chance it would buy them more time or get them home with their family again. Other people would be unwilling to go through that and would prefer that we refocus on their comfort at this point. What kind of person are you?"

In step 6, the use of life-prolonging interventions should be discouraged if they are inconsistent with the patient's goals and/or not in the patient's best interest. For example, "I'm worried that using treatments like life support will only prolong her dying and add to her suffering" or "The best thing we can do right now is refocus all our efforts on her comfort and quality of life." Brief, direct statements like "In light of what we've discussed, it is in your loved one's best interest to have a natural death" and "When her heart stops, we will not interfere with that process" can address code status and are strongly preferred to questions like "Would she want to be resuscitated?" or "Is she full code?". Detailed descriptions of chest compressions and defibrillation are rarely necessary.

Clinicians should expect strong emotions in response to hearing bad news. Facing death can trigger feelings of grief, despair, anger, guilt, disappointment, shock, and more. This is normal and does not reflect poorly on the clinician's communication skills. Rather than saying "It's going to be ok" or walking back from the clinical reality, phrases like "I wish things were different" and "I can only imagine how disappointed you must be" are preferred to demonstrate empathy and communicate alignment.

PEARLS

- Emergency physicians must learn how to have EOL conversations.
- EOL conversations go best when done systematically.
- Patients at the EOL should never be given a menu of treatment options and be expected to choose wisely.
- Physicians should recommend treatments that meet patient goals.
- EOL conversations provoke strong emotional responses from patients and families. This is normal and does not reflect poorly on the clinician's communication skills.

Suggested Readings

Jesus JE, Geiderman JM, Venkat A, et al. Physician orders for life-sustaining treatment and emergency medicine: ethical considerations, legal issues, and emerging trends. *Ann Emerg Med*. 2014;64(2):140-144.

Lamas D, Rosenbaum L. Freedom from the tyranny of choice—teaching the end-of-life conversation. *N Engl J Med*. 2012;366(18):1655-1657.

Loffredo AL, Chan GK, Wang DH, et al. United States best practice guidelines for primary palliative care in the Emergency Department. *Ann Emerg Med*. 2021;78(5):658-669.

Ouchi K, Lawton AJ, Bowman J, Bernacki R, George N. Managing code status conversations for seriously ill older adults in respiratory failure. *Ann Emerg Med*. 2020;76(6):751-756.

Weissman DE. Decision making at a time of crisis near the end of life. *JAMA*. 2004;292(14):1738-1743.

SECTION IV
CARDIOLOGY

48

BEYOND CHEST PAIN: RECOGNIZING ACUTE CORONARY SYNDROME IN DIVERSE PATIENT POPULATIONS

Leigh-Ann J. Webb

Heart disease remains the leading cause of death in the United States. Recognizing ACS in a timely manner is crucial for the prompt initiation of appropriate treatment, which can help preserve heart function and improve morbidity and mortality. However, recognizing ACS can be challenging, especially in diverse populations. There are important considerations related to symptoms, risk factors, and diagnostic tests used to identify ACS in women, transgender patients, racial and ethnic minorities, and the older adults.

SEX DIFFERENTIATIONS

Both men and women share traditional population-based modifiable CV risk factors for CAD including hypertension, hyperlipidemia, diabetes mellitus, smoking, sedentary lifestyle, obesity, and poor diet. Non-modifiable risk factors such as family history, age, and gender also play a role. Smoking portends a higher relative risk for women. Estrogen is thought to have a protective effect in premenopausal women. Early menopause is associated with higher CV risk. Pregnancy complications such as gestational hypertension, preeclampsia, gestational diabetes, and preterm delivery portend higher CV risk for women both during pregnancy and in the postpartum period.

Classic presenting symptoms of ACS for both men and women include chest pain, diaphoresis, shortness of breath, arm pain, and nausea or vomiting. Women with ACS are more likely to present with pain between the shoulder blades, nausea or vomiting, and shortness of breath. The upper reference limits of hsTn assays are sex specific and formulated based on the population studied. Females have a lower upper threshold limit compared to males, but the clinical impact of this difference is unclear.

TRANSGENDER PATIENTS

Clinicians may experience unique challenges when it comes to interpreting hsTn results in transgender individuals. Although further research is needed, both sex at birth and gender-affirming hormone therapy, such as estrogen or testosterone, can affect hsTn levels and complicate the interpretation of the results, potentially leading to misdiagnosis of ACS.

Clinicians should inquire about biologic sex as well as the use of gender-affirming hormones and proceed with an individualized and patient-centered approach in transgender individuals with suspected ACS. One potential approach is to use the female reference intervals for patients whose biologic sex is female as well as for biologically male patients who are taking gender-affirming hormone therapy; consider obtaining a second (delta) hsTn if clinically appropriate.

RACE AND ETHNICITY CONSIDERATIONS

White, Black, and Hispanic populations are the racial and ethnic groups that have been most studied in the United States. There is a higher incidence of CVD among Black and Hispanic patients compared to non-Hispanic White patients. Black and Hispanic patients presenting with ACS are typically younger, female, and uninsured. The initial symptom presentation of ACS may vary. In some studies, Black patients with ACS reported more and higher severity of symptoms. At least one study suggests that Black patients experiencing chest pain with accompanying palpitations and unusual fatigue were more likely to have confirmed ACS than their White counterparts. Overall higher rates of CVD burden in Black patients are attributed to several social determinants of health leading to higher incidence of CV risk factors such as obesity, hypertension, hyperlipidemia, and diabetes. Black women have a higher rate of CVD compared to Black men. Hispanic patients also carry a higher burden of comorbidities compared to non–Hispanic White patients, including obesity, hypertension, and diabetes. However, they appear to have more favorable than expected CVD mortality, a phenomenon widely regarded as the *Hispanic Paradox*.

AGE DIFFERENCES

Older patients have the highest rates of CVD with high morbidity and mortality associated with ACS. Although the most common presenting symptom in all age groups is chest pain, older patients are more likely to present atypically which can lead to delays in diagnosis and treatment, and with significant impact on outcomes (see Chapter 49).

HEALTH DISPARITIES

Health disparities refer to differences in health outcomes that exist among different population groups. The factors contributing to these disparities are complex but can be influenced by a number of social determinants of health. Disparities have been well documented in patients with ACS, including negative impacts on quality of care and outcomes in women, the older adults, and Black patients compared to non-Hispanic White patients. These disparities can lead to significant consequences for affected individuals and communities. While potential strategies to advance health equity at the population level should be multidimensional and community needs driven, clinicians play a central role in the prompt recognition and management of ACS in individual patients and should strive to maintain a high level of patient-centered care, while keeping in mind the potential diagnostic challenges reviewed in this chapter. Clinicians should consider adopting a lower threshold to initiate further workup and evaluation for ACS in these patient populations.

PEARLS

- Women are more likely to present with atypical symptoms of ACS including pain between the shoulder blades, nausea and vomiting, and shortness of breath.

- hsTn tests should be interpreted with caution in transgender individuals. Consider using the female reference range for both biologic females and biologic males taking gender-affirming hormone therapy.
- Black and Hispanic populations presenting with ACS are more likely than White patients to be younger and female.
- Older patients with ACS are less likely to present with chest pain than younger age groups.

SUGGESTED READINGS

Bhatia PM, Daniels LB. High sensitive cardiac troponins: the evidence behind sex-specific cutoffs. *J Am Heart Assoc.* 2020;9(10):e015272.

Engberding N, Wenger NK. Acute coronary syndromes in the elderly. *F1000Res.* 2017;6:1791.

Graham G. Racial and ethnic differences in acute coronary syndrome and myocardial infarction within the United States: from demographics to outcomes. *Clin Cardiol.* 2016;39(5):299-306.

Gomez S, Blumer V, Rodriguez F. Unique cardiovascular disease risk factors in Hispanic individuals. *Curr Cardiovasc Risk Rep.* 2022;16:53-61.

Sandoval Y, Apple FS, Mahler SA. High-sensitivity cardiac troponin and the 2021 AHA/ACC/ASE/CHEST/SAEM/SCCT/SCMR guidelines for the evaluation and diagnosis of acute chest pain. *Circulation.* 2022;146(7):569-581.

Van Oosterhout R, de Boer AR, Maas A, Rutten FH, Bots ML, Peters S. Sex differences in symptom presentation in acute coronary syndromes: a systematic review and meta-analysis. *J Am Heart Assoc.* 2020;9(9):e014733.

49

DON'T MISS ACS IN OLDER ADULTS

M. KATHRYN MUTTER AND MOIRA SMITH

Timely recognition of ACS in older adults is complicated by age-related changes in symptom presentation and diagnostic test interpretation. Geriatric syndromes, such as multimorbidity, cognitive impairment, delirium, and functional decline, contribute to a more challenging history taking and diagnostic decision-making process.

SIGNS AND SYMPTOMS

Though chest pain is a common presenting sign of ACS, multiple other presenting complaints should prompt consideration of ACS in older adults. In the GRACE trial, 43% of patients greater than 75 years of age presented without chest pain, compared with 27% of patients 65 to 75 years of age and 29% of patients less than 65 years of age. Patients without chest pain were more likely to be female, diabetic, or have a history of hypertension or heart failure. The patients without chest pain were more likely to present with dyspnea (49%), diaphoresis (26%), and nausea and vomiting (24%). Though less common, delirium has additionally been recognized as a primary complaint with ACS in older adults.

Multimorbidity (>2 chronic conditions) occurs more frequently in the geriatric patient population, which can lead to confounding with presenting symptoms. For example, a patient with COPD and coronary artery disease may primarily present with dyspnea, but the underlying inciting illness is an MI. In the Framingham Study, unrecognized ACS, defined as previous MIs recognized by characteristic changes on a routine ECG, was found in 25% of all MIs, but in 60% of all MIs in men older than 75 years and 34% in women older than 75 years. Unrecognized MIs in this study included both "silent MIs," meaning no previous event could be discovered through the history, and misattributed symptoms.

Cognitive impairment is one of the most challenging geriatric syndromes for acute presentations, as it confounds symptomatology and increases the risk of delirium. In patients older than 85 years, altered mental status has been reported to be the presenting symptom of MI in up to 19% of cases. If there is lack of clarity or an acute change in cognition, maintaining a high index of suspicion by obtaining an ECG and troponin will help differentiate ACS from other presentations.

Age-related changes in cardiac structure and function predispose older patients to complications. Older patients with acute MI have a higher risk of arrhythmias, myocardial rupture, heart failure, renal failure, cardiogenic shock, and mortality. This association is likely multifactorial, not only related to changes in heart structure and function but also delays in presentation and diagnosis and multimorbidity. Congestive heart failure with STEMI also occurs significantly more often in the older patients. Therefore, when older patients present with signs or symptoms of acute decompensated heart failure, it is important to consider ACS.

Interpretation of the ECG

ECG abnormalities present at baseline in older adults can be a confounder in both STEMI and NSTEMI ACS presentations. Obtaining a prior ECG, as well as serial ECGs, is critical for comparison and may help differentiate concerning abnormalities from baseline changes. As with younger patients, for older patients with concerns for ACS and bundle branch block or ventricular pacing, utilization of decision tools such as the modified Sgarbossa Criteria will aid with differentiation.

Risk Stratification

hs-Tn has been helpful in its improved sensitivity for detecting myocardial injury, but it has reduced specificity, particularly in the presence of underlying chronic diseases. Chronic elevations of hs-Tn are found with fibrotic changes in heart structure, renal failure, age-related changes in body composition, hypertension, and heart failure, among other factors. In this case, a subsequent hs-Tn should be obtained, and if it rises this is concerning for acute injury. It can be challenging to differentiate Type 1 MI (plaque rupture) versus Type 2 MI (mismatch of myocardial oxygen supply due to other conditions, such as sepsis) in older adults as well, and will require attention to the ECG, rise of troponin levels, clinical presentation, and evaluation for other acute illnesses.

There are multiple decision rules that can aid in identification of patients suspected of ACS at low risk of 30-day major adverse cardiovascular events, including the HEART, EDACS, ADAPT (includes TIMI), NOTR, among others. The 2021 AHA guideline recommends the use of a clinical decision pathway using risk scores, particularly when conventional troponin assays are being used. There are limited studies to determine which risk score is most useful for correctly identifying low-risk older patients appropriate for outpatient management, but it is important to note that ADAPT places all patients older than 65 years in the intermediate category. Patients become not low risk above 75 years with EDACS and above 50 years with NOTR, regardless of other risk factors. A study by Ashburn et al, showed that the HEART pathway achieved high sensitivity (99%, 95% CI 97-100) for 30-day death or MI among adults older than 65 years. For patients without known CAD, in whom ACS is suspected and determined to be intermediate risk, the AHA guideline recommends CCTA for those below 65 years, but stress testing for those above 65 years.

PEARLS

- Patients above 65 years with ACS are more likely to present without chest pain.
- Cognitive and hearing impairment can lead to delays in presentation and diagnosis.
- Older patients are more likely to have underlying causes for chronically elevated troponin, so evaluating the pattern of rise or fall will be necessary.
- The HEART pathway is sensitive for identifying lower-risk older patients appropriate for outpatient management, but it may increase cardiac testing and may not reduce hospitalization rates.

SUGGESTED READINGS

Ashburn NP, Snavely AC, Paradee BE, et al. Age differences in the safety and effectiveness of the HEART pathway accelerated diagnostic protocol for acute chest pain. *J Am Geriatr Soc*. 2022;70(8):2245-2257.

Bayer AJ, Chadha JS, Farag RR, et al. Changing presentation of myocardial infarction with increasing old age. *J Am Geriatr Soc*. 1986;34:263-266.

Canto JG, Rogers WJ, Goldberg RJ, et al. Association of age and sex with myocardial infarction symptom presentation and in-hospital mortality. *JAMA*. 2012;307:813-822.

Damluji AD, Forman DE, Wang TY, et al. Management of acute coronary syndrome in the older adult population: a scientific statement from the American Heart Association. *Circulation*. 2023;147:e32-e62.

Gulati M, Levy PD, Mukherjee D, et al. 2021AHA/ACC/ASE/CHEST/SAEM/SCCT/SCMR guideline for the evaluation and diagnosis of chest pain. *J Am Coll Cardiol*. 2021;78(22):e187-e285.

50

PROCEED WITH CAUTION! DIAGNOSING ANXIETY IN THE PATIENT WITH CHEST PAIN

J. AUSTIN LEE AND PAUL I. MUSEY JR

Chest pain is one of the most frequent reasons for visits to the ED and can be the presenting symptom for many potentially life-threatening disorders. Most patients (80%-95%) presenting to the ED with chest pain are not found to have significant cardiac, pulmonary, or other emergent causes for their symptoms but uncertainty about the underlying etiology can produce marked stress and anxiety. Anxiety is a common problem contributing to patients seeking emergent evaluation of chest pain. Further complicating the issue is that while anxiety and panic can cause chest pain, a number of potentially dangerous causes of chest pain can also generate anxiety.

Symptoms of anxiety and panic disorders can include palpitations, tachycardia, dyspnea, chest pain, nausea, diaphoresis, and dizziness. These symptoms can overlap with symptoms of other emergent etiologies of chest pain, including MI or pulmonary embolism. In one study, anxiety was seen as a contributor to the symptoms of chest pain in 30% to 40% of patients who were determined to be at low risk for ACS.

Anxiety is highly prevalent after MI, but the association between anxiety and MI is not well established. Anxiety is more prevalent among patients with CVD than in the general population. Independent of depression, anxiety appears to be a risk factor for CVD. Theories about the association include increased incidence of risk factors for CVD including hypertension, alcohol and tobacco use, sedentary lifestyle, inflammatory responses, and reduced heart rate variability. Others hypothesize that the over-activation of the hypothalamic-pituitary-adrenal axis and the sympathetic nervous system, in concert with decreased sympathomimetic-vagal control, may increase the risk of CVD among anxious individuals.

Patients evaluated for chest pain in the ED with anxiety commonly have recurring and persistent symptoms and present a diagnostic and therapeutic challenge. In subjects with low-risk chest pain, the prevalence of abnormal anxiety symptoms was 47% and was associated with a high rate of repeat ED visits and a low rate of medical diagnoses. Panic and anxiety in patients with unexplained chest pain are often underrecognized and underdiagnosed by emergency medicine clinicians. Even when the clinician suspects a patient may have anxiety contributing to their symptoms, many emergency medicine clinicians do not discuss their concerns regarding anxiety with their patients, nor provide tools for patients to manage their symptoms. For patients with recurrent low-risk chest pain, screening for depression and anxiety and referral for treatment could reduce overall healthcare use and minimize return ED visits. Not addressing the role of anxiety and chest pain can impact patients' symptoms and thoughts about their ED care.

Current guidelines encourage clinicians to avoid reflexively ascribing symptoms of chest pain or dyspnea to anxiety. However, if no cardiopulmonary emergency is identified after a prudent evaluation (including a workup as outlined in local testing policies or as identified in the evidence-based GRACE *Guideline for Recurrent Low-Risk Chest Pain*), clinicians should then consider screening and referring such patients for evaluation of anxiety as a contributing or causative cause of symptoms. Tools to screen for anxiety in the ED include the validated GAD 7-item scale, the CAS, and the validated HADS-A subscale. When clinicians only rule out emergent causes of chest pain and then discharge patients home, anxiety can go undiagnosed and untreated. Interestingly, patients taking SSRIs do not have an increased risk of ACS; a meta-analysis showed that SSRIs taken for depression seem to reduce the risk of MI (though without mortality benefit). Diagnosing and treating anxiety is important to improve symptoms and may potentially reduce future ED visits for similar symptoms.

PEARLS

- Symptoms of anxiety can overlap with several emergent causes of chest pain, including MI. Avoid reflexively ascribing symptoms of chest pain or dyspnea to anxiety.

- Approximately 80% to 90% of patients who present to the ED for evaluation of chest pain will not have cardiac disease or a cardiopulmonary emergency.
- Patients with anxiety have high rates of healthcare utilization, and their anxiety is underdiagnosed and undertreated in the ED.
- Screening for anxiety in patients being discharged from the ED for chest pain after a prudent workup may be beneficial.

SUGGESTED READINGS

Almog R, Carasso S, Lavi I, Amir O. The risk for a first acute coronary syndrome in patients treated with different types of antidepressants: a population based nested case-control study. *Int J Cardiol.* 2018;267:28-34.

Fernandes N, Prada L, Rosa MM, et al. The impact of SSRIs on mortality and cardiovascular events in patients with coronary artery disease and depression: systematic review and meta-analysis. *Clin Res Cardiol.* 2021;110(2):183-193.

Karlsen HR, Matejschek F, Saksvik-Lehouillier I, Langvik E. Anxiety as a risk factor for cardiovascular disease independent of depression: a narrative review of current status and conflicting findings. *Health Psychol Open.* 2021;8(1):2055102920987462.

Musey PI, Patel R, Fry C, Jimenez G, Koene R, Kline JA. Anxiety associated with increased risk for emergency department recidivism in patients with low-risk chest pain. *Am J Cardiol.* 2018;122(7):1133-1141.

Tully PJ, Harrison NJ, Cheung P, Cosh S. Anxiety and cardiovascular disease risk: a review. *Curr Cardiol Rep.* 2016;18(12):120.

Wen Y, Yang Y, Shen J, Luo S. Anxiety and prognosis of patients with myocardial infarction: a meta-analysis. *Clin Cardiol.* 2021;44(6):761-770.

51

DO NOT RELY ON A SINGLE ECG TO EVALUATE CHEST PAIN IN THE ED IN PATIENTS WITH HIGH CLINICAL SUSPICION FOR ACUTE CORONARY SYNDROME

WILLIAM J. BRADY

Patients with chest pain or other presentations potentially consistent with ACS are evaluated with a focused history, physical examination, and 12-lead ECG; in selected cases, serum troponin values and other testing are also obtained. All three subtypes of ACS, unstable angina, NSTEMI, and STEMI, can demonstrate ST segment and/or T-wave abnormalities. Not all such ACS presentations, however, will initially demonstrate ECG abnormality. In fact, when considering AMI, including both NSTEMI and STEMI, approximately half of such patients will demonstrate significant ECG findings on initial presentation ... while the remaining 50% of patients will not demonstrate significant ECG abnormalities. Thus, patients with a high clinical concern for AMI and a nondiagnostic ECG can be monitored with serial ECGs.

The dynamic nature of the ECG ST segment and T-wave abnormalities results from the similarly dynamic nature of ACS event itself, which includes intracoronary plaque rupture followed by thrombus formation and vasospasm; coronary obstruction to flow and the resultant ACS can initially be intermittent and/or minimal in magnitude. If the ECG is performed during a period of sustained coronary flow in the early stages of active ACS, it will likely demonstrate a nondiagnostic ECG, an ECG lacking significant ST segment and/or T-wave findings. The performance of repeat, or serial, ECGs in such high clinical likelihood patients increases the possibility of detecting the ST segment and/or T-wave changes indicative of evolving ACS.

In patients ultimately found to have AMI, the initial, nondiagnostic ECG can range from entirely normal to minimally abnormal with nonspecific ST segment and/or T-wave abnormalities. The ECG can be entirely normal in 1% to 5% of individuals diagnosed with AMI in the subsequent 24 hours after ED presentation. Similarly, the initial ECG can demonstrate nonspecific ST segment and/or T-wave abnormalities; this classification is a "transition interpretation" between entirely normal and obviously abnormal, with ST-segment deviation and/or T-wave inversion. Nonspecific ST segment and/or T-wave abnormalities include ST-segment deviation, either elevation or depression, up to 1 mm in magnitude and/or T waves that are blunted, flattened, or biphasic. Nonspecific ST segment and/or T-wave abnormalities are encountered in 5% to 12% of patients found to have AMI in the subsequent 24 hours of presentation.

The remaining groups of ECG categories include those patients with significant ST-segment depression and/or dynamic T-wave changes as well as patients with confounding ECG patterns, such as LBBB or right ventricular paced rhythms (VPR) from an implanted pacemaker. ST-segment depression with or without dynamic T-wave changes can be seen in 10% to 25% of ED patients ultimately diagnosed with AMI. Confounding ECG patterns are seen in the remainder of patients without a diagnostically abnormal ECG.

While it is important to identify all forms of ACS as soon as clinically feasible, rapid detection of STEMI is of paramount importance and allows for consideration of urgent reperfusion therapy, including either fibrinolysis or percutaneous coronary intervention. In a patient with a convincing clinical description of ACS who demonstrates a nondiagnostic ECG, obtaining serial ECGs can demonstrate increases in the magnitude of the elevated ST segment and/or changes in the contour of the ST segment, both findings that can suggest an evolving AMI (**Figure 51.1A**). The evolution of other ECG presentations with the development of progressive ST segment and/or T-wave abnormalities also identifies patients at higher risk of ACS and adverse outcomes; earlier detection of these patients allows for prompt treatment.

In addition to the nondiagnostic ECG described earlier, serial ECGs can also be used in the various STEMI mimic presentations (**Figure 51.1B**), such as BER, acute myopericarditis, LBBB, left ventricular hypertrophy with strain pattern, and VPR. Such mimicking patterns demonstrate ST segment and/or T-wave abnormalities not related to ACS and can be difficult to distinguish from evolving ACS.

Serial ECGs significantly increased the diagnosis of STEMI in patients suspected of AMI who had initial nondiagnostic ECGs or confounding ECG patterns of LBBB. The sensitivity for AMI diagnosis of the single, initial ECG increased from 55% to 68% for serial ECGs with a similar increase in the number of patients who were candidates for urgent reperfusion therapy (48%–62%, respectively).

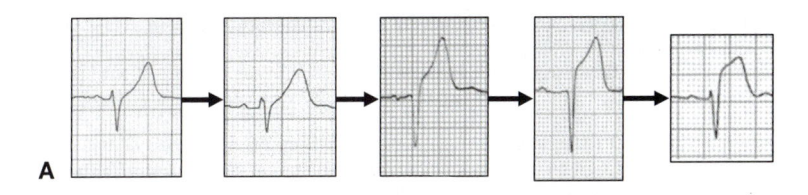

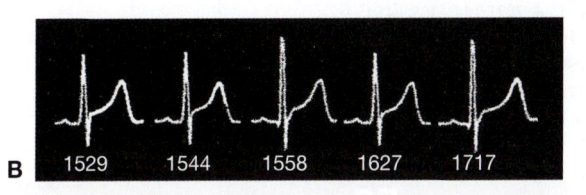

FIGURE 51.1 A. Serial ECGs demonstrating evolving anterior wall STEMI. Lead V$_3$ is shown from sequential 12-lead ECGs obtained over a 44-minute period from a patient with chest pain, dyspnea, and diaphoresis. At 0645 hours, no ST-segment elevation is noted and the contour of the ST segment is concave. Minimal change is noted on the next ECG at 0703 hours. From 0703 to 0715 hours, the ECG demonstrated a change in the ST segment with significant elevation appearing. Further ST-segment elevation is noted at 0721 hours and, eventually, a change in the contour of the elevated ST segment at 0729 hours. **B.** Serial ECGs demonstrating the absence of change in ST-segment elevation and the ST-segment contour in a patient ultimately found to have electrocardiographic benign early repolarization. (Lead III is shown.)

If clinically warranted, serial ECGs should be performed at time intervals appropriate for the diagnostic question being considered. The time intervals can range from very frequent, such as every 2 to 3 minutes in acutely ill patients with high clinical suspicion for AMI, to much less frequent, ranging from every 10 to 60 minutes. The timing for repeat ECG should be guided by the overall clinical status. In addition, resource availability will also impact the time interval of serial ECG performance.

PEARLS

- Serial ECGs can be helpful in the subset of patients who present with a high clinical suspicion for AMI and yet a nondiagnostic ECG.
- Serial ECGs are not appropriate for all patients with chest pain, only those individuals with a nondiagnostic ECG on initial presentation in whom the clinician is significantly concerned about AMI.

SUGGESTED READINGS

Berberian J, Brady WJ, Matt A, eds. *EMRA EKG Guide*. 2nd ed. Emergency Medicine Residents' Association/American College of Emergency Physicians; 2022.

Brady WJ, Truwit JD, eds. *Critical Decisions in Electrocardiography*. London, BMJ-Wiley-Blackwell Publishing Group, 2009.

Fesmire FM. ECG diagnosis of acute myocardial infarction in the presence of left bundle-branch block in patients undergoing continuous ECG monitoring. *Ann Emerg Med*. 1995;26:69-82.

Fesmire FM, Percy RF, Bardoner JB, Wharton DR, Calhoun FB. Usefulness of automated serial 12-lead ECG monitoring during the initial emergency department evaluation of patients with chest pain. *Ann Emerg Med*. 1998;31:3-11.

Gulati M, Levy PD, Mukherjee D, et al. 2021 AHA/ACC/ASE/CHEST/SAEM/SCCT/SCMR guideline for the evaluation and diagnosis of chest pain: a report of the American College of Cardiology/American Heart Association Joint Committee on Clinical Practice Guidelines. *Circulation*. 2021;144:e368-e454.

Mattu A, Tabas J, Brady WJ, eds. *Electrocardiography in Emergency Medicine*. American College of Emergency Physicians Publishing; 2019.

52

KNOW THE DIFFERENTIAL FOR ST SEGMENT ELEVATION: IT'S MORE THAN JUST ACUTE CORONARY SYNDROME

LLOYD TANNENBAUM AND BRIT LONG

While STSE on an ECG can be due to an acute MI related to acute coronary occlusion, other non-ACS entities can also cause STSE. Clinicians should maintain a broad differential regarding the various causes of ST segment. We recommend the mnemonic ELEVATIONS when approaching an ECG with STSE:

Electrolytes
LBBB and paced
Early repolarization
Ventricular hypertrophy
Aneurysmal left ventricle
Thrombotic occlusion (MI)
Inflammation (pericarditis)
Osborn (hypothermia)
Neurogenic
Sudden death (Brugada)

When attempting to differentiate STSE associated with acute coronary occlusion from other STEMI mimics, the history and examination must also be considered. Evaluating the entire ECG is essential, including ST-segment depressions, T-wave inversions, reciprocal changes, Q waves, and terminal QRS distortion.

ELECTROLYTES

Electrolyte abnormalities including hyperkalemia and hypercalcemia can result in STSE. Hyperkalemia may have STSE with peaked T waves, seen most prominently in V1 and

V2, but STSE is concave. Hypercalcemia may have STSE seen most prominently in the anterior leads but also a short QT interval.

LBBB AND VENTRICULAR-PACED RHYTHM

LBBB and ventricular-paced rhythms mimic an anterior STEMI, but the QRS complexes will be widened. Modified Sgarbossa Criteria should be utilized for diagnosis of acute coronary occlusion in the setting of LBBB or paced rhythm (discussed elsewhere) to assess for ECG evidence of acute MI.

EARLY REPOLARIZATION

Early repolarization can mimic STEMI, but the STSE is often diffuse, and there should be neither ST-segment depression nor hyperacute T waves (**Figure 52.1**).

Benign early repolarization is most commonly found in healthy patients below 50 years. The ECG typically demonstrates significant widespread J point elevation, with unique T-wave morphology. The J point demonstrates notching or slurring (fish hook pattern), and the initial half of the T wave is concavely curved upwards, followed by a sharp, downward second half. The ratio of STSE to T-wave height rate in V6 should be less than 0.25. There should also be no terminal QRS distortion and no reciprocal changes. Terminal QRS distortion is defined by the absence of an S wave and J wave in either of leads V2 or V3 and is often present in anterior STEMI.

VENTRICULAR HYPERTROPHY

LVH with strain pattern (ie, ST segment and T-wave abnormalities) is another STEMI mimic (**Figure 52.2**). There are several criteria for LVH diagnosis, including the Sokolov-Lyon criteria (S wave depth in V1 plus tallest R wave in V5-V6 is >35 mm). In LVH, there may be ST-segment depression and T-wave inversion in the left-sided leads, known as the strain pattern. The ECG may also demonstrate increased R wave peak time more than 50 ms in lead V5 and/or V6. Left axis deviation is common, and the STSE in leads V1 to V3 is discordant to the deep S waves. Unfortunately, voltage criteria alone are not definitive for LVH, and ECG changes are insensitive for diagnosis.

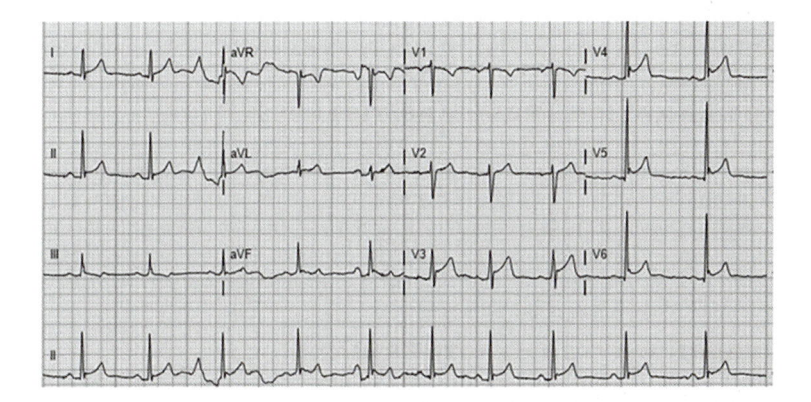

FIGURE 52.1 Benign early repolarization with diffuse ST-segment elevation and lack of ST-segment depression.

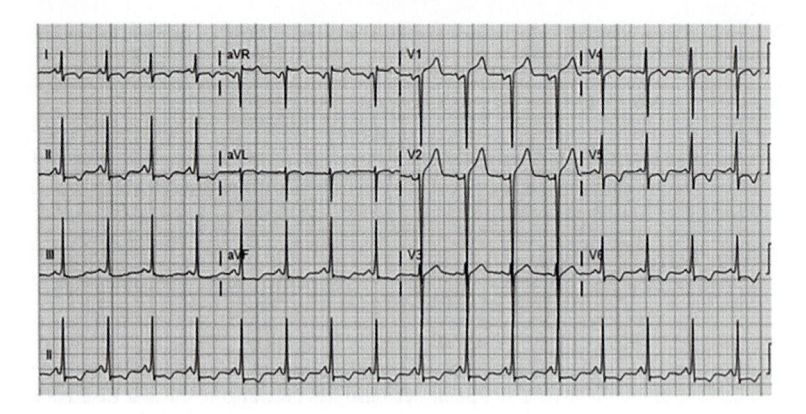

FIGURE 52.2 ECG demonstrating LVH with strain.

ANEURYSMAL LV

A LV aneurysm can cause persistent STSE after an MI, typically lasting longer than 2 weeks. STSE is most commonly present in anterior leads. The ECG may demonstrate concave or convex morphology with well-formed Q or QS waves. The T waves have relatively small amplitude when compared to the QRS complex in contrast to hyperacute T waves. There is an absence of reciprocal ST-segment depression or dynamic ECG changes, and well-formed Q waves. New ST changes, progressing or dynamic ECG changes, reciprocal ST-segment depression, and a toxic-appearing patient are suggestive of STEMI.

THROMBOTIC OCCLUSION (MI)

No differential diagnosis of STSE is complete without STEMI and acute coronary occlusion. Hyperacute T waves, prolonged QT, and reciprocal changes are concerning for acute coronary occlusion. The PAILS mnemonic can be used to evaluate reciprocal ST-segment depressions. PAILS stands for Posterior – Anterior – Inferior – Lateral – Septal. This mnemonic identifies the leads that most commonly result in reciprocal changes.

INFLAMMATION (PERICARDITIS)

The ECG may demonstrate diffuse STSE without ST-segment depressions, except in V1 and aVR. Whereas PR segment depression may be present, ST-segment depression should only be in leads V1 and aVR. ST-segment depression in other leads suggests acute coronary occlusion. STEMI due to acute coronary occlusion can be associated with convex ST segments with STSE greater in lead III compared to II. Pericarditis STSE is concave, diffuse, and greater in lead II compared to III. Spodick sign may be found in pericarditis (downsloping of the TP segment).

OSBORN WAVES (HYPOTHERMIA)

Osborn waves are most commonly associated with hypothermia but may also occur in hypercalcemia, takotsubo cardiomyopathy, neurologic conditions, myocarditis, and Brugada syndrome. This is a positive deflection at the J point in precordial and true limb leads, with typically reciprocal negative deflection in aVR and V1. The size of the Osborn waves is proportional to the degree of hypothermia. These patients are at risk of ventricular arrhythmia. Shiver artifact may also be present in hypothermic patients, most commonly in lead V1.

NEUROGENIC

Increased intracranial pressure can cause ECG changes. Common changes include STSE, ST-segment depression, and/or biphasic T waves seen in V2/V3 and the deeply inverted, symmetric T waves seen in V4 to V6. Patients may end up in the catheterization lab before neuroimaging is obtained for the diagnosis. History is essential, especially from bystanders or EMS in the altered patient.

SUDDEN DEATH (BRUGADA)

Brugada syndrome is a rare, inherited arrhythmic disorder with increased risk of syncope and sudden death. In Type 1 Brugada syndrome, the T waves in V1 and V2 have a "backslash" (\) morphology, and in Type 2 Brugada syndrome, the T wave in V2 has a "saddleback" morphology. Patients with syncope and Brugada syndrome discovered on ECG should receive cardiology consultation and likely admission. If this pattern is discovered incidentally in a patient without presyncope or syncope, follow-up with cardiology is recommended. Brugada pattern may also occur in patients with fever, infection, illicit drug use, and sodium channel-blocking agent use.

PEARLS

- Not all causes of STSE are due to ACS.
- The ELEVATIONS mnemonic can help differentiate between common causes of STSEs: Electrolytes, LBBB and paced, Early repolarization, Ventricular hypertrophy, Aneurysmal left ventricle, Thrombotic occlusion (MI), Inflammation (pericarditis), Osborn (hypothermia), Neurogenic, Sudden death (Brugada).

SUGGESTED READINGS

de Bliek EC. ST elevation: differential diagnosis and caveats. A comprehensive review to help distinguish ST elevation myocardial infarction from nonischemic etiologies of ST elevation. *Turk J Emerg Med*. 2018;18(1):1-10.

Hanna EB, Glancy DL. ST-segment elevation: differential diagnosis, caveats. *Cleve Clin J Med*. 2015;82(6):373-384.

Klein LR, Shroff GR, Beeman W, Smith SW. Electrocardiographic criteria to differentiate acute anterior ST-elevation myocardial infarction from left ventricular aneurysm. *Am J Emerg Med*. 2015;33(6):786-790.

Lee DH, Walsh B, Smith SW. Terminal QRS distortion is present in anterior myocardial infarction but absent in early repolarization. *Am J Emerg Med*. 2016;34(11):2182-2185.

Smith SW, Dodd KW, Henry TD, Dvorak DM, Pearce LA. Diagnosis of ST-elevation myocardial infarction in the presence of left bundle branch block with the ST-elevation to S-wave ratio in a modified Sgarbossa rule. *Ann Emerg Med*. 2012;60(6):766-776.

Tannenbaum L, Bridwell R, Inman B. *EKG Teaching Rounds*. Springer Nature; 2022.

Witting MD, Hu KM, Westreich AA, Tewelde S, Farzad A, Mattu A. Evaluation of Spodick's sign and other electrocardiographic findings as indicators of STEMI and pericarditis. *J Emerg Med*. 2020;58(4):562-569.

53

BE ABLE TO RECOGNIZE LEAD MISPLACEMENT

SUMMER CHAVEZ

Unrecognized ECG lead misplacement can have serious clinical consequences—misdiagnosis causing incorrect medical treatment and subsequent delay in appropriate treatment of the original underlying condition. However, certain identifiable patterns exist that can clue the physician into lead misplacement. Both the precordial (chest) and limb leads can be affected by lead reversal and misplacement. There are six precordial leads: V1 (right sternal margin at the 4th ICS), V2 (left sternal margin at the 4th ICS), V3 between V2 and V4 (5th ICS at the midclavicular line), V5 (anterior axillary line at the 5th ICS), V6 (midaxillary line at the 5th ICS). There are four limb electrodes (LA, RA, LL, RL). The augmented leads (aVF [RA & LA], aVL [RA & LL], and aVR [LA & LL]) are the averages of their corresponding leads and are designated with the "a" prefix. Discrepancies in the position and placement of the electrodes affect the leads (I, II, III, aVL, aVF, aVR), consequently changing the ECG patterns based on Einthoven triangle. Every lead has a vector composed of summing or subtracting voltages from the corresponding electrodes. In general, lead I should have a positive P wave and R wave while aVR will have negative P wave and R wave. R-wave progression, or the gradually increasing magnitude of the R wave, should be visualized in leads V1 to V4.

The most common error occurs when the limb leads are reversed (LA and RA). Lead I is totally inverted while leads II and III are switched with each other (**Figures 53.1**

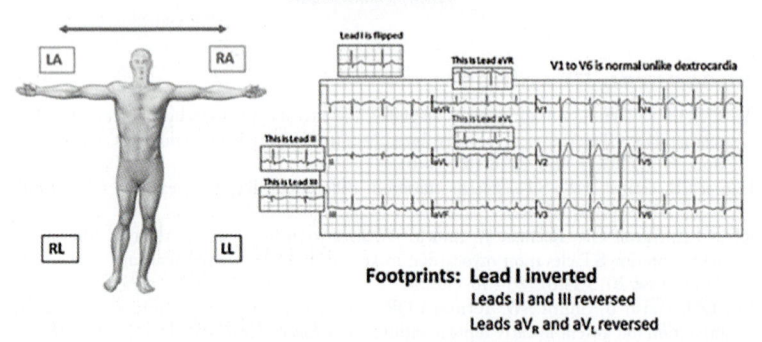

FIGURE 53.1 ECG features of limb lead reversal. (Reprinted from Mond HG, Garcia J, Visagathilagar T. Twisted leads: the footprints of malpositioned electrocardiographic leads. *Heart Lung Circ*. 2016;25(1):61-67, with permission from Elsevier. Copyright © 2015 Australian and New Zealand Society of Cardiac and Thoracic Surgeons (ANZSCTS) and the Cardiac Society of Australia and New Zealand (CSANZ). Published by Elsevier Ltd. All rights reserved.)

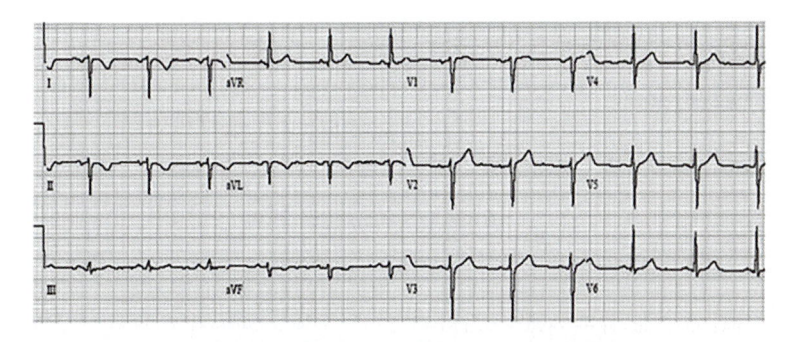

FIGURE 53.2 ECG features of limb lead reversal. (Reprinted from Harrigan RA, Chan TC, Brady WJ. Electrocardiographic electrode misplacement, misconnection, and artifact. *J Emerg Med.* 2012;43(6):1038-1044, with permission from Elsevier.)

and 53.2). In addition, leads aVL and aVR are also switched, while aVF is unchanged. There may be right axis deviation or lead aVR is positive. In patients with limb lead reversal, it may appear that the patient has dextrocardia; however, there will be normal R-wave progression. Clinicians may be tipped off to limb lead reversal as the negative P wave and QRS complexes in inverted lead I are atypical, especially if there is cardiac disease. Generally, the direction of the QRS complex in leads I and V6 should match each other.

Arm and leg electrodes, such as in the instance of the RA and RL electrodes (**Figure 53.3**), may also occur. In this instance, the main giveaway is the isoelectric voltage of lead II. Leads I and III switch with each other. A negative P wave in lead I may also be present. A more difficult pattern to identify is the reversal of LA and LL electrodes. This causes lead III to be inverted. Leads I and II switch as well as aVL and aVF with each

Reversed Right Arm-Right Leg

Footprints: Lead II isoelectric
Leads I and III mirror image
Leads I and aV$_L$ identical
Lead I inverted P wave

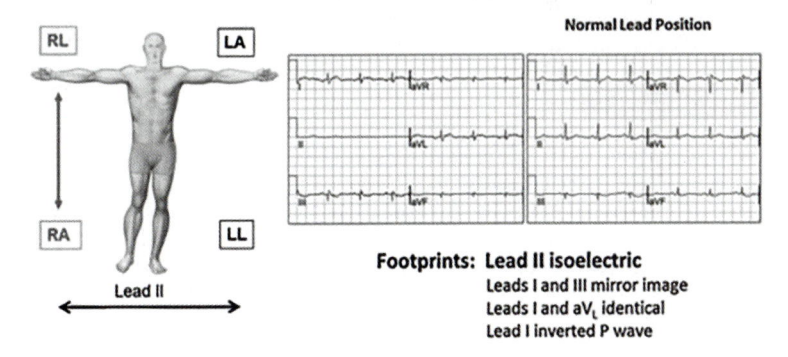

FIGURE 53.3 ECG features of RA/RL reversal. (Reprinted from Mond HG, Garcia J, Visagathilagar T. Twisted leads: the footprints of malpositioned electrocardiographic leads. *Heart Lung Circ.* 2016;25(1):61-67, with permission from Elsevier. Copyright © 2015 Australian and New Zealand Society of Cardiac and Thoracic Surgeons (ANZSCTS) and the Cardiac Society of Australia and New Zealand (CSANZ). Published by Elsevier Ltd. All rights reserved.)

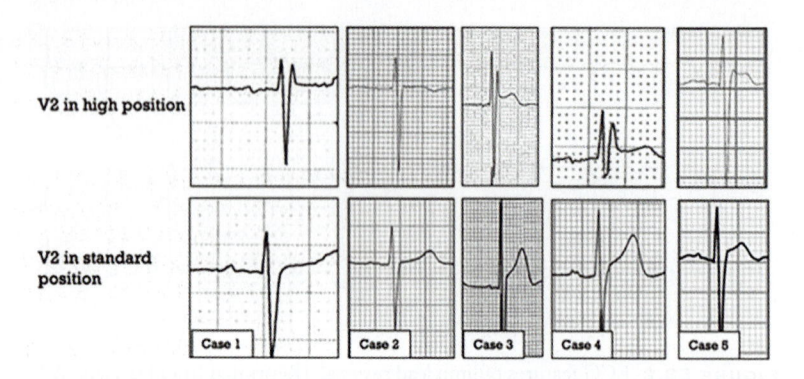

FIGURE 53.4 ECG features of superior lead placement of V1 and V2. (Reprinted from Walsh B. Misplacing V1 and V2 can have clinical consequences. *Am J Emerg Med*. 2018;36(5):865-870, with permission from Elsevier.)

other. aVR is unchanged. Aside from the inverted lead III, clinicians can be tipped off by a larger P wave in lead I than lead II, poor R-wave progression, and shifts in the QRS axis.

Precordial electrode misplacement, especially due to difficulties related to obesity and female anatomy, can also cause pathology mimics such as pseudoinfarction patterns. V1 and V2 can be placed too superiorly, leading to false patterns of incomplete RBBB, Brugada syndrome, anterior TWI, STEMI, Q waves concerning for a prior septal infarct, and poor R-wave progression (**Figure 53.4**). EM physicians should have a strong suspicion when the P wave in V1 is completely negative or in V2 is biphasic.

While other variations exist of lead misplacement, these are the most common ones. Ultimately, if the clinical picture and the ECG do not seem to correlate, physicians should take special care to repeat the ECG and consider the electrode placement. By having knowledge of proper ECG placement, recognition of the patterns generated by improper lead placement in combination with pretest probabilities, physicians can identify this scenario.

PEARLS

- Positive P wave and R wave in lead I, but negative in aVR. QRS complex direction in lead I and V6 should match.
- Limb lead reversal: Lead I inverted. Leads II and II switched. Right axis deviation.
- Arm/leg lead reversal: Isoelectric lead II or inverted lead III.
- Misplaced leads can cause pathology mimics.

SUGGESTED READINGS

Harrigan RA, Chan TC, Brady WJ. Electrocardiographic electrode misplacement, misconnection, and artifact. *J Emerg Med*. 2012;43(6):1038-1044.

Mond HG, Garcia J, Visagathilagar T. Twisted leads: the footprints of malpositioned electrocardiographic leads. *Heart Lung Circ*. 2016;25(1):61–67.

Walsh B. Misplacing V1 and V2 can have clinical consequences. *Am J Emerg Med*. 2018; 36(5):865–870.

CAN YOU DIAGNOSE STEMI IN RBBB?

WILLIAM J. BRADY

The prevalence of RBBB varies across populations. When present, it is most often pathologic, involving either age-related degeneration of the conduction system or the development of myocardial disease. The age-dependent occurrence of RBBB is quite striking with an increasing occurrence in older individuals, usually considered a manifestation of degeneration of the conduction system. RBBB is also seen more often in patients with diabetes mellitus and past anterior wall myocardial infarction. RBBB is considered a normal variant in approximately 1% of the population in patients with an otherwise normal heart. Patients with RBBB and no underlying heart disease have an excellent prognosis, while those with underlying cardiac illness have increased rates of morbidity and mortality. Conversely, the presence of LBBB, whether new-onset or preexisting, is most often a manifestation of significant underlying myocardial disease and a marker of the risk of adverse outcomes.

The diagnosis of AMI in the setting of bundle branch block is possible yet more challenging, whether it be LBBB or RBBB. As is commonly known, the presence of LBBB *confounds* the ECG's ability to demonstrate ECG changes related to AMI; in addition, the anticipated ECG abnormalities encountered in uncomplicated LBBB can mimic changes related to coronary ischemia or infarction when, in fact, they represent the expected repolarization findings of LBBB. Application of the modified Sgarbossa criteria can assist in this challenging situation. Conversely, RBBB does not confound the ECG diagnosis of AMI; clinicians unaware of the anticipated ECG findings in RBBB, however, will be less likely to note unexpected abnormalities (ie, those related to AMI). Importantly, the modified Sgarbossa has no applicability in RBBB considerations of AMI.

The traditional ECG criteria required for the diagnosis of RBBB include the following criteria (**Figure 54.1A**):

1) QRS complex width greater than 0.12 seconds
2) RsR' QRS complex in lead V1
3) Widened or "slurred" S wave in leads I and V6.

The appearance of the ST segment and, to a lesser extent, the T wave is changed by the altered repolarization patterns seen in RBBB. The basic, anticipated relationship of the QRS complex and ST segment/T wave is described by the concept of appropriate discordance, which suggests that the ST segment and T wave changes are located on opposite sides of the ECG baseline—a positively oriented QRS complex is associated with ST-segment depression and inverted T wave while, conversely, a negative QRS complex is associated with ST-segment elevation and upright T wave (**Figure 54.1A**).

Recognition of this QRS-ST/T discordance as the anticipated ECG presentation of uncomplicated RBBB is important—the clinician will not confuse the uncomplicated RBBB presentation with that of AMI. **Figure 54.1A** illustrates this issue quite well. **Figure 54.1B** demonstrates a very early STEMI, with subtle elevation of the J point and corresponding ST-segment elevation. **Figure 54.1C** shows an obvious STEMI with

Right Bundle Branch Block — ST Segment in Lead V₁

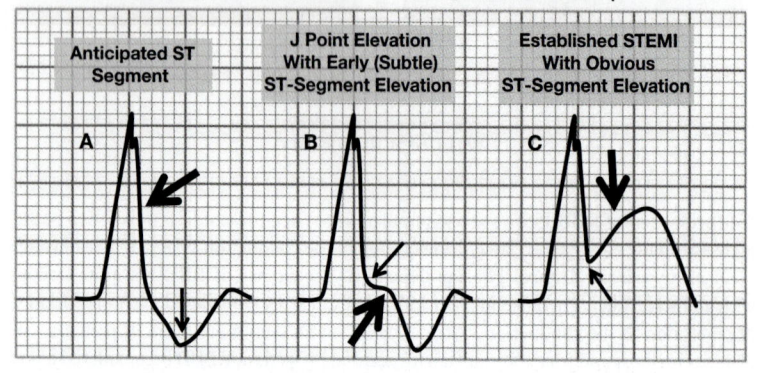

FIGURE 54.1 (**A**) Anticipated ST-segment configuration in lead V1 with RBBB. The ST segment is depressed (small arrow), on the opposite side of the electrocardiographic baseline from the major terminal portion of the QRS complex (large arrow). (**B**) J point elevation with early (Subtle) STEMI. The J point is elevated (small arrow) with corresponding ST-segment elevation (large arrow) rather than depressed and located on the same side of the electrocardiographic baseline as the major terminal portion of the QRS complex. (**C**) Established STEMI with obvious ST-segment elevation. The J point (small arrow) and ST segment (large arrow) are elevated, consistent with STEMI.

considerable concordant ST-segment elevation (ie, the QRS complex is positively oriented while the ST segment is elevated on the same side of the ECG baseline).

Patients with STEMI who have RBBB are at increased risk of adverse outcomes. RBBB complicates approximately 6% of all AMIs with a broad range of reported occurrences (from 3% to 30%); patients with RBBB-AMI tend to be older and frequently present with either proximal left anterior descending artery obstructive disease or multivessel coronary artery disease. Patients with RBBB are more likely to experience acute congestive heart failure, hypotension requiring treatment, cardiogenic shock, and cardiac arrest during their infarct-related hospitalization. Mortality is also markedly high in these patients at presentation and at 1-year follow-up.

The management of these patients with AMI is similar to that of those not presenting with RBBB. STEMI should be managed with either urgent percutaneous coronary intervention or fibrinolysis. NSTEMI presents across a spectrum of severity; management should be tailored to the patient's overall presentation. Consideration of the time course of the RBBB should impact management decisions with the new-onset right bundle branch block indicating a very high risk presentation and the corresponding need for an aggressive, early treatment approach.

PEARLS

- RBBB does not confound the ECG diagnosis of STEMI.

- An understanding of the anticipated ST segment and T-wave findings of uncomplicated RBBB is vital, allowing for the recognition of early STEMI.
- Close scrutiny of the J point and related ST segment is required in patients with RBBB suspected of AMI.
- New-onset RBBB, in the setting of evolving STEMI, is a marker of extreme risk, similar to LBBB.

Suggested Readings

Horton CL, Brady WJ. Right bundle branch block in acute coronary syndrome: diagnostic and therapeutic implications for the emergency physician. *Am J Emerg Med*. 2009;27:1130-1141.

Kleemann T, Juenger C, Gitt AK, et al. Incidence and clinical impact of right bundle branch block in patients with acute myocardial infarction: ST elevation myocardial infarction versus non-ST elevation myocardial infarction. *Am Heart J*. 2008;156:256-261.

55

High-Sensitivity Troponins—High Yield or High Risk

Wesley Zeger and Andrew Barnett

Ischemic heart disease continues to be the leading cause of death worldwide, and chest pain is one of the most common presenting complaints in EDs in the United States. Newer, hsTrop assays began incorporation into clinical practice around 2007. These high-sensitivity assays can detect serum troponin at 10 to 100× lower concentrations than traditional assays. As of 2021, most healthcare systems were still using traditional assays.

The definition of a type 1 acute myocardial infarction from the ESC Fourth Universal Definition of Myocardial Infarction (2018) is "acute myocardial injury with clinical evidence of acute myocardial ischemia." Acute myocardial injury requires detection of a rise and/or fall of cardiac troponin values with at least one value above the 99th percentile URL. Clinical evidence of myocardial ischemia requires at least one of the following:

- Symptoms of myocardial ischemia
- New ischemic ECG changes
- Development of pathologic Q waves
- Imaging evidence of a new loss of viable myocardium or a new regional wall motion abnormality in a pattern consistent with an ischemic etiology
- Identification of a coronary thrombus by angiography or autopsy

There are several important aspects (risks) to consider when integrating hsTrop into clinical decision-making for the assessment of ACS:

1) Is there an increase or decrease in resource utilization for non-ACS/low-risk patients (increased use of invasive or noninvasive testing, increase in hospitalizations, or increased length of stay)?
2) Is there a difference in mortality when hsTrop is implemented?
3) Do hsTrop values differ between populations?
4) Can hsTrop assays be safely integrated into risk stratification?

Medical screening tests with poor sensitivity result in missed disease diagnoses, and poor specificity could result in overuse of more invasive and higher risk procedures. This conundrum raises the important question of how we maximize hsTrop assay testing strengths and minimize the associated risks of adoption into the evaluation of chest pain concerning ischemia.

HsTrop is measured in nanograms per liter, and there are three important values to be aware of: the value at the 99th percentile, the LOD, and the difference between the initial and repeat tests (the delta value). Each of these values differs among assays, and the 99th percentile varies across genders with females having lower values. The LOD is the lowest amount of circulating troponin the hsTrop assay can detect. The real advantage of hsTrop assays is the sensitivity of the delta values to identify and exclude early ischemia (type 1 and type 2 MI). Delta values only require an initial and repeat measurement (typically at 2 or 3 hours). Delta values for various assays are found in the 2020 ESC guidelines with associated sampling timeframes.

The ability to detect small elevations has implications when the test is ordered for nonischemic (nonocclusive type 2 or type 3 MI). In these scenarios, elevated hsTrop could be reflective of right heart strain, myocarditis, endocarditis, etc, and should be interpreted within the constructs for why the test was ordered. For patients who are presenting with chest pain or a chest pain equivalent, where acute coronary occlusive disease is a concern, a structured evaluation process should be followed.

A structured assessment is recommended in patients with concerns of ischemic chest pain. The AHA and ESC have recommended this approach. Switching to hsTrop assays has been associated with:

- More echocardiography among persons with non–ST-segment elevation ACS but not among individuals with low-risk chest pain
- Less invasive coronary angiography among low-risk patients but similar use for patients with NSTE-ACS
- Among individuals with NSTE-ACS, hsTrop use was not associated with increased revascularization or in-hospital mortality.
- Shorter length of stay within a healthcare system

Further studies are needed to determine if these favorable outcomes persist across gender, race, and ethnicity.

Over the last decade, hsTrop assays have been extensively studied and are now being widely adopted in-hospital systems for the evaluation and risk stratification of acute ischemic chest pain. Early data have found these assays to be highly sensitive while better matching system resources compared to conventional troponin assays. Conversion from conventional assays to high-sensitivity assays has been high yield and low risk.

PEARLS

- Units of newer hsTroponin assays are now measured in nanograms per liter rather than micrograms per liter.
- hsTrop 99th percentile values differ in men and women.
- A single 2- or 3-hour delta value replaces serial troponins.
- High-sensitivity troponin implementation did not increase resource use for low-risk patients.

SUGGESTED READINGS

Collet JP, Thiele H, Barbato E, et al. 2020 ESC guidelines for the management of acute coronary syndromes in patients presenting without persistent ST-segment elevation. *Eur Heart J*. 2021;42(14):1289-1367.

Gulati M, Levy PD, Mukherjee D, et al. 2021 AHA/ACC/ASE/CHEST/SAEM/SCCT/SCMR guideline for the evaluation and diagnosis of chest pain: a report of the American College of Cardiology/American Heart Association Joint Committee on Clinical Practice Guidelines. *Circulation*. 2021;144(22):e368-e454.

Ioannides KLH, Sun BC, Baecker AS, et al. Not all HEART scores are created equal: identifying "low-risk" patients at higher risk. *J Am Coll Emerg Physicians Open*. 2020;1(6):1161-1167.

McCarthy C, Li S, Wang TY, et al. Implementation of high-sensitivity cardiac troponin assays in the United States. *J Am Coll Cardiol*. 2023;81(3):207-219.

Roffi M, Patrono C, Collet JP, et al. 2015 ESC Guidelines for the management of acute coronary syndromes in patients presenting without persistent ST-segment elevation: Task Force for the Management of Acute Coronary Syndromes in Patients Presenting Without Persistent ST-Segment Elevation of the European Society of Cardiology (ESC). *Eur Heart J*. 2016;37(3):267-315.

56

DO NOT FORGET THE NON-ACS CAUSES OF CHEST PAIN

JENNIFER MCGOWAN AND J. JEREMY THOMAS

There are numerous etiologies of chest pain that range from benign to life threatening. Delayed diagnosis of these time-sensitive conditions leads to increased morbidity and mortality.

TAD

The incidence of TAD is estimated to be three to four cases per 100,000 persons per year. Mortality rates of untreated TAD approach 1% per hour. The incidence of TAD peaks at age 70 and is more common in males and those with a history of hypertension. Patients younger than 40 years often have a history of connective tissue disease (ie, Marfan syndrome, Ehlers-Danlos syndrome), cocaine use, or a bicuspid aortic valve. Pregnancy, especially in the third trimester, is an established risk factor for TAD.

Abrupt onset of chest pain, especially severe pain that quickly reaches maximal intensity, isolated thoracic back pain, or symptoms that cross the diaphragm (ie, chest and abdominal pain) should raise concern for TAD. The characteristic physical examination findings in patients with TAD include a blood pressure differential between the extremities, an extremity pulse deficit, an aortic insufficiency murmur, or a focal neurologic deficit. These findings are variable and are often absent in patients with TAD.

CTA is the diagnostic imaging of choice in suspected TAD. A chest x-ray may show widening of the mediastinum or an abnormal aortic contour, but these classic x-ray findings are not present in most cases. D-dimer testing has sensitivity of 82% to 95% and poor specificity for TAD.

PE

Risk factors for PE include hypercoagulability, recent surgery, prolonged immobilization, connective tissue disease, and exogenous estrogen use. Patients with PE commonly present with chest pain, which is often pleuritic. Dyspnea is commonly reported. Other classic symptoms include lower extremity or calf pain, unilateral lower extremity swelling, cough, or hemoptysis. Patients with PE may have tachycardia, tachypnea, hypoxia, or none of these findings. With a massive PE, the patient may present with hypotension and signs of shock. A low-grade fever may be present in patients with PE, which can mislead clinicians toward a diagnosis of pneumonia.

The diagnostic evaluation for PE requires an understanding of current clinical decision rules. The emergency clinician should be able to risk stratify patients to low risk of PE with a combination of clinical gestalt and the pulmonary embolism rule-out criteria. Beyond these low-risk patients, one must understand and correctly apply risk stratification scores such as the Well criteria or revised Geneva score to calculate pretest probability and guide further evaluation with either a D-dimer test or CTA of the chest.

Tension Pneumothorax

The emergency provider should have a high index of suspicion for tension pneumothorax in patients with a history of trauma or recent instrumentation of the thorax, neck, or upper extremity regions. Tension pneumothorax almost always presents with a combination of acute chest pain and respiratory distress. Clinical features on the examination include unilateral absent breath sounds, tracheal deviation, and jugular venous distension. Vital sign abnormalities may include hypotension, tachycardia, and hypoxia.

Tension pneumothorax is a clinical diagnosis that requires rapid intervention to prevent decompensation and cardiac arrest. Bedside ultrasound demonstrating absent lung slide can be used to quickly confirm the diagnosis in patients with an equivocal exam. Although diagnosis is evident on both chest x-ray and CT, decompression should not be delayed to obtain imaging.

Cardiac Tamponade

In cardiac tamponade, a pericardial effusion increases pericardial pressure, decreases right ventricular filling, and decreases cardiac output. Etiologies of pericardial effusion include malignancy, trauma, infectious diseases, pericarditis, uremia, and acute myocardial infarction.

Patients with a pericardial effusion with development of tamponade often report chest pain, dyspnea, and fatigue. Diminished breath sounds or a pericardial friction rub are heard in only one-third of patients. The classic triad of hypotension, muffled heart sounds, and jugular venous distension is a late finding. The electrocardiogram in patients with a pericardial effusion can demonstrate low voltage, tachycardia, and electrical alternans.

Similar to tension pneumothorax, bedside ultrasound can be used to quickly confirm the diagnosis. The presence of an effusion with diastolic right ventricular collapse should lead to emergent pericardiocentesis.

Esophageal Rupture

Esophageal rupture is a rare diagnosis with high mortality. Common precipitants of esophageal rupture include iatrogenic (ie, esophagogastroduodenoscopy, esophageal dilation), severe emesis, trauma, caustic ingestion, and esophageal foreign body. Chest pain is most often retrosternal, severe, and frequently radiates to the back, neck, shoulders, or abdomen. Additional historical features may include dysphagia, dyspnea, and emesis. Patients with esophageal rupture often present in shock with tachycardia, hypotension, and signs of poor perfusion. Physical exam findings can include subcutaneous emphysema in the cervical and clavicular region. Patients with an intra-abdominal rupture may present with signs of a surgical abdomen.

Although a chest x-ray can demonstrate a pneumothorax, pneumomediastinum, or pleural effusion, the diagnosis of esophageal rupture is confirmed with CT of the chest. CT findings of esophageal rupture can include periaortic or periesophageal air, pleural effusions, or soft tissue stranding.

PEARLS

- Patients with TAD more commonly report the abrupt onset of sharp pain that quickly reaches maximal intensity.
- Patients with PE may not present with tachycardia, tachypnea, or hypoxia.
- Imaging should not delay definitive management for tension pneumothorax.
- The classic triad of hypotension, muffled heart sounds, and jugular venous distension is a late finding in patients with cardiac tamponade.
- The most common etiology of esophageal rupture is iatrogenic.

Suggested Readings

Asha SE, Miers JW. A systematic review and meta-analysis of D-dimer as a rule-out test for suspected acute aortic dissection. *Ann Emerg Med*. 2015;66(4):368-378.

Khandaker MH, Espinosa RE, Nishimura RA, et al. Pericardial disease: diagnosis and management. *Mayo Clinic Proc*. 2010;85(6):572-593.

Kline JA, Kabrhel C. Emergency evaluation for pulmonary embolism, Part 1: clinical factors that increase risk. *J Emerg Med*. 2015;48:771-780.

Thomson D, Kourounis G, Trenear R, et al. ECG in suspected pulmonary embolism. *Postgrad Med J*. 2019;95(1119):12-17.

57

PITFALLS IN ADULTS WITH CONGENITAL HEART DISEASE

SARAH K. WENDEL AND WILLIAM WOODS

Ninety percent of patients with severe CHD survive into adulthood due to new interventions and improvements in surgical outcomes. These patients are presenting to EDs more often. Understanding the general approach to presentations and common complications in these patients is imperative. Emergency clinicians should employ standard cardiac diagnostic testing and therapies while addressing aspects of care unique to this population. Clinicians should contact the patient's cardiologist after initial evaluation and management.

Most ED patients with CHD have a previously known diagnosis. However, some conditions may not be identified in adulthood until a sentinel event, such as aortic dissection (eg, bicuspid aortic valve), HF (eg, Ebstein anomaly or congenitally corrected transposition of the great arteries), or sudden cardiac arrest (eg, anomalous coronary arteries).

Patients with prior surgical repair(s) may have myocardial scarring leading to abnormal electrical conduction and abnormal baseline ECGs. Typical ECG forces do not always apply to patients with CHD, and it is critical to compare the ECG to previous ones. For example, patients with atrioventricular canal defects usually have a superior axis on their ECGs that will persist even after surgical repair. Arrhythmias and conduction delays are common in adults with corrected CHD. Both bradyarrhythmias and tachyarrhythmias can occur, and clinicians must thoroughly investigate reports of palpitations in these patients.

Patients with CHD have variable levels of pulmonary blood flow. These phenotypes can be classified as "wet" or "dry" and "warm" or "cold." "Wet" versus "dry" corresponds to the clinical assessment of pulmonary blood flow. "Wet" patients have excess pulmonary blood flow and present similarly to patients in decompensated HF, with rales, cough, and pulmonary edema. Both systemic and pulmonary venous congestion must be considered. Younger patients are more likely to have hepatomegaly rather than peripheral edema in right-sided HF. New elevations of hepatic transaminases may suggest new-onset HF. Room air oxygen saturation measurements are inadequate to make a distinction between "wet" and "dry." Some patients with CHD may have lower baseline oxygen saturations. Chest radiographs may be helpful to assess pulmonary vascularity status compared to the patient's baseline. "Dry" patients can have decreased or normal pulmonary blood flow. They present with desaturations and dark lungs on chest x-ray (decreased pulmonary blood flow).

"Warm" versus "cold" refers to the evaluation of adequacy of peripheral perfusion. Pre- and post-ductus arteriosus blood pressures and oxygen saturations (RUE + either LE) are useful to measure, even in adults. Patients with recurrence of aortic coarctation after repair can be identified with a measured BP higher in the RUE compared to the LE. Without pre-ductal blood pressure comparison in the patient with re-coarctation, the etiology of the apparent poor LE perfusion could be misassigned.

The overall goal is to achieve a "warm and dry" state. Patients who are "warm and wet" often need diuretics. Patients who are "cold and wet" need fluid resuscitation to address intravascular depletion and may benefit from vasopressors or inotropic support if there is depressed contractility on bedside echocardiography. These patients may need simultaneous diuresis and fluid resuscitation for intravascular depletion with pulmonary congestion. Patients who are "cold and dry" often need fluid resuscitation alone.

Patients born with hypoplastic left or right heart syndrome or versions of these require multiple surgeries throughout their lifetime and are considered "complex CHD." The three-step surgical process (Norwood, Glenn, and Fontan) separates the pulmonary and systemic systems. Patients with single-ventricle physiology have a lower risk of pulmonary edema because pulmonary blood flow is passively driven by central venous pressure. These patients may have difficulty tolerating positive pressure ventilation or hypovolemia when filling pressures are low, as in cases of dehydration or sepsis. In contrast, in patients with normal filling pressures, positive pressure ventilation may expand alveoli and decrease pulmonary vascular resistance, increasing pulmonary blood flow and cardiac output, and should be well tolerated.

Complications specific to repaired CHD include stenosis at the surgical anastomosis, arrhythmias, and endocarditis. Patients with complex CHD/single-ventricle physiology have additional risks, including preload dependency, since pulmonary blood flow passively flows from systemic central veins to the pulmonary artery anastomosis. These patients will nearly always be "dry" rather than "wet." Those with complex CHD/single-ventricle physiology carry an increased lifetime risk of venous and arterial thrombotic events (eg, pulmonary embolism, stroke). Patients with CHD with valvular surgery, patches, stents, or other post-procedural foreign material are also at an increased risk of endocarditis over time.

Patients with hypoplastic left heart progressively lose ventricular function over their lifetime. In this condition, the RV acts as the "systemic" ventricle. Over time, the RV does not tolerate the higher systemic pressures, resulting in ventricular dilation and decreased function with possible need for eventual transplant.

Patients with surgically corrected CHD have an increased risk of cardiovascular disease, with a higher operative risk for noncardiac surgical procedures. Risks and benefits must thus be explored before considering ED procedural sedation. Pregnancy may be a higher risk in patients with CHD, especially those with underlying pulmonary hypertension. These patients can have ischemic coronary artery disease at younger ages than nonaffected age-matched patients. Prompt specialist consultation may be warranted to identify risks of afterload reduction in patients who may have nonvalvular aortic stenosis (eg, Williams syndrome).

PEARLS

- Patients with CHD represent a heterogeneous group of pathologies with varied repairs and anatomy. Consider prompt cardiology consult.
- Physical examination can distinguish between cold, warm, wet, or dry presentations.
- Patients with complex CHD/single-ventricle physiology are exquisitely preload dependent and may need aggressive intravenous hydration to correct hypotension.
- Patients with corrected CHD have an increased risk of cardiovascular disease at younger ages and may be at higher risk for complications such as dissection, stenosis, and thrombosis.

Suggested Readings

Baumgartner H, De Backer J, Babu-Narayan SV, et al. 2020 ESC guidelines for the management of adult congenital heart disease. *Eur Heart J*. 2021;42(6):563-645.

Brickner ME, Hillis LD, Lange RA. Congenital heart disease in adults. *New Engl J Med*. 2000;342(5):334-342.

Opotowsky AR, Siddiqi OK, Webb GD. Trends in hospitalizations for adults with congenital heart disease in the U.S. *J Am Coll Cardiol*. 2009;54(5):460-467.

Shekhar S, Agrawal A, Pampori A, Lak H, Windsor J, Ramakrishna H. Mortality in adult congenital heart disease: analysis of outcomes and risk stratification. *J Cardiothorac Vasc Anesth*. 2022;36(8 Pt B):3379-3388.

58

Occlusion Myocardial Infarction: Time to Move Past the STEMI Paradigm

Christopher Thom

AMI is a critical diagnosis requiring prompt evaluation in the ED. For several decades, AMI has been subdivided into NSTEMI and STEMI, which is based on findings on the ECG. The treatment strategies of these two entities can be highly disparate, and yet there is overlap in the underlying disease. The finding of STEMI on ECG is meant to identify cases of AMI resulting from an acute coronary occlusion, wherein prompt reperfusion therapy, generally in the form of primary PCI or systemic thrombolytic therapy, is beneficial. However, acute coronary occlusion does not always produce STEMI morphology; it is crucial to identify these patients, as they may also benefit from reperfusion therapy.

STEMI-NSTEMI Paradigm

Historically, patients with STEMI on ECG had improved survival from emergent reperfusion therapy with a resultant paradigm that a STEMI indicated an acute coronary occlusion. In contrast, an NSTEMI on ECG is thought to represent an MI not arising from an acute coronary occlusion and therefore not needing immediate reperfusion. However, this paradigm leaves a large subgroup of patients with AMI improperly treated. Up to 30% of patients with NSTEMI have an acute coronary occlusion on delayed cardiac catheterization. These are patients with potentially salvageable myocardium who were not given timely reperfusion therapy because of the mistaken assumption that no STEMI equates to no acute coronary occlusion. In addition, 15% to 35% of STEMI cases are found to be false positives and not the result of an acute coronary occlusion.

OMI Versus NOMI Paradigm

The OMI/NOMI categorization has been suggested as a paradigm shift to replace the above STEMI/NSTEMI designation. Assigning "OMI" to denote an acute coronary occlusion instead of using a surrogate (ie, STEMI) is perhaps a step toward improved clarity. Recent work has shown that STEMI-negative patients who are found to have an OMI have similar characteristics to patients who are STEMI-positive. This includes similar clinical features, peak troponin levels, and echocardiographic findings. However,

TABLE 58.1	COHORT OF 282 PATIENTS WITH NSTEMI IN THE DIFOCCULT TRIAL WHOSE ECGs WERE CONSISTENT WITH ACUTE CORONARY OCCLUSION

ECG FINDING	% OF PATIENTS
Minor ST elevation with reciprocal depression	76
Hyperacute T waves or DeWinter pattern	12
Subtle anterior ST elevation	6
Nonconsecutive ST elevation	5

the time delay to the catheterization laboratory can be significant in patients with OMI without STEMI.

Investigations have begun into additional ECG criteria that move beyond the defined criteria of STEMI to provide a means to identify patients with an OMI without signs of STEMI on ECG. Findings that have been shown to be predictive of an OMI in cases who were "STEMI-negative" are shown in **Table 58.1**. These patients were found to have similar in-hospital and long-term mortality rates as compared to the STEMI cohort. Additional ECG findings that might be of use in OMI identification include subtle ST elevation inferiorly with coexistent ST depression in aVL, ST depression in leads V1 to V4, the Aslanger pattern, and the modified Sgarbossa criteria in the presence of left bundle branch block and ventricular paced rhythms.

In addition, the amount of ST elevation should take into account the relative QRS amplitude to help identify OMI; a lower QRS amplitude may imply that a lower degree of ST elevation could still be a relevant and acute finding. Overall, the diagnostic accuracy of the OMI/NOMI classification has the potential to surpass our current STEMI/NSTEMI categorization for the identification of acute coronary occlusions.

ECHOCARDIOGRAPHY

Echocardiography has been supported by the American College of Cardiology as a tool to clarify the diagnosis of STEMI and support risk stratification of patients with chest pain and uncertainty about the presence of a STEMI. The finding of RWMA, particularly in the setting of suspicious ECG findings in that anatomic area, can help clarify an acute coronary occlusion diagnosis. This can be, particularly, helpful in cases where the ECG does not meet STEMI criteria but might represent an OMI that would benefit from early reperfusion (**Table 58.1**). One should be wary of preexisting wall motion abnormalities and left bundle branch blocks when assessing for RWMA. Importantly, emergency physicians have been shown to accurately (78%-88%) detect RWMAs. Echocardiography can also rapidly evaluate the aortic root for dilatation or dissection in the rare case of a STEMI or OMI caused by an aortic dissection involving the aortic root. Echocardiography also has a much higher sensitivity (78%-100%) for aortic root dissection than chest x-ray. However, literature pertaining to emergency physician-performed echocardiography is still limited.

PEARLS

- The current STEMI/NSTEMI paradigm is an imperfect classification system for the identification of an acute coronary occlusion.
- A significant number of patients with an acute coronary occlusion will not have STEMI on ECG and thus will not receive timely reperfusion therapy.

- The OMI/NOMI paradigm seeks to clarify our understanding of acute myocardial infarction by seeking to identify those patients with an acute coronary occlusion.
- Findings suggestive of OMI that do not meet STEMI criteria include minor ST elevation with reciprocal depression, hyperacute T waves, and nonconsecutive ST elevation.
- Early echocardiography can help identify patients with an acute coronary occlusion without a definitive STEMI on ECG by identifying RWMA.

SUGGESTED READINGS

Aslanger EK, Meyers PH, Smith SW. STEMI: a transitional fossil in MI classification? *J Electrocardiol*. 2021;65:163-169.

Aslanger EK, Yıldırımtürk Ö, Şimşek B, et al. DIagnostic accuracy oF electrocardiogram for acute coronary OCClUsion resuLTing in myocardial infarction (DIFOCCULT Study). *Int J Cardiol Heart Vasc*. 2020;30:100603.

Meyers HP, Bracey A, Lee D, et al. Comparison of the ST-elevation myocardial infarction (STEMI) vs. NSTEMI and occlusion MI (OMI) vs. NOMI paradigms of acute MI. *J Emerg Med*. 2021;60(3):273-284.

Terlecki M, Wojciechowska W, Dudek D, et al. Impact of acute total occlusion of the culprit artery on outcome in NSTEMI based on the results of a large national registry. *BMC Cardiovasc Disord*. 2021;21(1):297.

Xu C, Melendez A, Nguyen T, et al. Point-of-care ultrasound may expedite diagnosis and revascularization of occult occlusive myocardial infarction. *Am J Emerg Med*. 2022;58:186-191.

59

IS A RECENT STRESS TEST HELPFUL IN THE ED PATIENT WITH CHEST PAIN?

JORDAN WARCHOL AND AARON BARKSDALE

Patients presenting to the ED with CP often present more of a disposition conundrum than a diagnostic one. In the high-risk patient, there is a baseline risk of MACE regardless of the quality or character of their presenting pain. For those with symptoms concerning for ACS, the results of recent cardiac stress testing are often cited as a reassuring factor for the absence of an emergency condition. However, the utility of this result and the time frame considered acceptable for a negative test to be considered helpful are topics of much debate in emergency medicine.

One caveat when determining whether a negative recent stress test is helpful to the EP is to recognize that the patient must have presented to a clinician previously with symptoms concerning for angina. Patients presenting with atypical symptoms of ischemic heart disease, such as women, older adults, and non-White patients, may exhibit a bias, where the presence of a prior stress test indicates a higher risk for ACS.

In addition, not all ischemic heart disease is detected by every type of stress testing. Several forms of testing do not account for functional changes and may miss nonobstructive or microvascular disease, thereby giving a false sense of reassurance when said to be a "negative" test.

The utility of a patient's recent stress test in determining the ED workup and disposition depends on the type of stress testing completed. Both functional and nonfunctional exams are commonly used, often with consideration of the patient's pretest probability, patient-specific characteristics such as ability to exercise, ordering provider's comfort, and availability of specific modalities, as deciding factors when determining the best test for each patient.

The most common forms of stress testing include:

- Exercise ECG—continuously records ECG while walking on a treadmill.
- Stress echocardiography—echocardiogram performed after exercise or after medication given to simulate exercise's effect on the heart.
- MPI using either SPECT or PET.
- cCTA and CT perfusion.
- Cardiac magnetic resonance imaging.
- Various combinations of the aforementioned tests.

Each of these methods varies in their specificity, sensitivity, and interrater variability as well as cost and availability. Generally, those tests that include imaging are more sensitive, though the specificity of the above-listed tests is approximately the same; very few studies have directly compared any two methods.

Relatively few studies exist that follow patients to a certain end point after cardiac stress testing, and fewer specifically utilize a population from the ED. A meta-analysis by Mehta et al examined the risk of MACE in ED patients with a negative troponin and reassuring ECG who subsequently had cardiac stress testing of various modalities (stress ECG/echocardiography, cCTA, or MPI). They concluded that low- and intermediate-risk patients (defined as TIMI ≤5 or HEART ≤6), a normal stress test or cCTA with lesser than 50% stenosis within 1 year of presentation to the ED with a chief complaint of CP, have a very low incidence of MACE and can be discharged without further risk stratification.

In May 2021, AEM published its "Guidelines for reasonable and appropriate care in the emergency department (GRACE)" for low-risk patients with recurrent CP visits. They recommend against repeat stress testing in those with a negative study in the past 12 months as a means to decrease MACE at 30 days. The consensus guidelines also report that a low-risk patient with cCTA absent of coronary stenosis in the last 2 years can be discharged following a single normal high-sensitivity troponin.

Regarding patients with suspected or known CAD, Smulders et al published a meta-analysis assessing the AER of MI and cardiac death following a negative noninvasive cardiac investigation. Their analysis reported a very low incidence of AERs across all modalities, ranging from 0.32% in cCTA to 1.66% for stress echocardiography.

The published findings previously described are also consistent with the 2021 clinical practice guidelines released by the American College of Cardiology/American Heart Association Joint Committee. They support a 2-year warranty period following normal cCTA without stenosis or plaque, and 1 year for an adequate normal stress test.

Finally, when determining the utility of a stress test for an ED patient with CP, one should consider whether able to view the full report or only patient's verbal recollection. Advancements in EMRs and the advent of HIEs can be helpful in increasing the availability of data for review, though not all systems are integrated in this way. Physicians

PEARLS

- In low-risk patients with recurrent ED visits for CP and who had a normal stress test within 12 months, AEM does not recommend repeat stress testing.
- In low-risk patients with recurrent ED visits for CP and cCTA with no coronary CAD within the prior 2 years, AEM suggests no additional testing except a single high-sensitivity troponin.
- ED patients with CP with low to intermediate risk with a normal stress test or cCTA with less than 50% stenosis can be discharged without further risk stratification.
- Patients with known or suspected CAD who have undergone a cCTA demonstrated less than 50% stenosis, normal stress test or MPI, have a low incidence of MI or cardiac death at 1 year.
- The stress test should be considered inadequate if a patient is unable to reach 85% of their MPHR.

SUGGESTED READINGS

Gulati M, Levy PD, Mukherjee D, et al. 2021 AHA/ACC/ASE/CHEST/SAEM/SCCT/SCMR guideline for the evaluation and diagnosis of chest pain: a report of the American College of Cardiology/American Heart Association Joint Committee on Clinical Practice Guidelines. *J Am Coll Cardiol*. 2021;78(22):e187-e285.

Mann A, Williams J. Consideration for stress testing performed in conjunction with myocardial perfusion imaging. *J Nucl Med Technol*. 2020;48(2):114-121.

Mehta P, McDonald, Hirani R, Good D, Diercks D. Major adverse cardiac events after emergency department evaluation of chest pain patient with advanced testing: systematic review and meta-analysis. *Acad Emerg Med*. 2021;29:748-768.

Pusey PI, Bellolio F, Upadhye S, et al. Guidelines for reasonable and appropriate care in the emergency department (GRACE): recurrent, low-risk chest pain in the emergency department. *Acad Emerg Med*. 2021:28:718-744.

Smulders MW, Jaarsman C, Nelemans PJ, et al. Comparison of the prognostic value of negative non-invasive cardiac investigations in patients with suspected or known coronary artery disease-a meta-analysis. *Eur Heart J Cardiovasc Imaging*. 2017;18:980-987.

60

KNOW THE MIMICS OF VENTRICULAR TACHYCARDIA

MITCHELL WEEMAN AND J. JEREMY THOMAS

VT is a WCT that is typically associated with coronary artery disease or other significant heart diseases. Diagnosis is entertained with three consecutive wide complexes and then further characterized as sustained VT (>30 seconds) or non-sustained VT

(<30 seconds). The rapid rate, often in conjunction with poor baseline cardiac function, can produce cardiovascular instability. Without prompt treatment, cardiovascular collapse will almost certainly ensue. This has led to the position of treating all WCTs as VT until proven otherwise. For management purposes, it is important to attempt to differentiate between VT and SVT with aberrant conduction. In some cases, the distinction between these two rhythms is not possible. As a result, management decisions must be made based on the patient's clinical situation and the ECG rhythm. The differential diagnosis of WCT is depicted in **Figure 60.1**.

Several conditions can mimic the appearance of VT on the ECG. These include, but are not limited to, SVT with aberrant conduction, AIVR, "reperfusion rhythm," WPW syndrome, artifact, metabolic disorders (eg, hyperkalemia), and toxic ingestions (ie, medications that block the sodium channel). In some of these conditions, the electrical impulse is delayed or slowed as it passes through the conduction system and ventricular myocardium. This results in a wide-QRS complex. The dysfunction in the intraventricular conduction system can be permanent or transient. In some cases, abnormal conduction may only be seen at higher heart rates. WCTs propose a broad differential and can be classified as either regular or irregular.

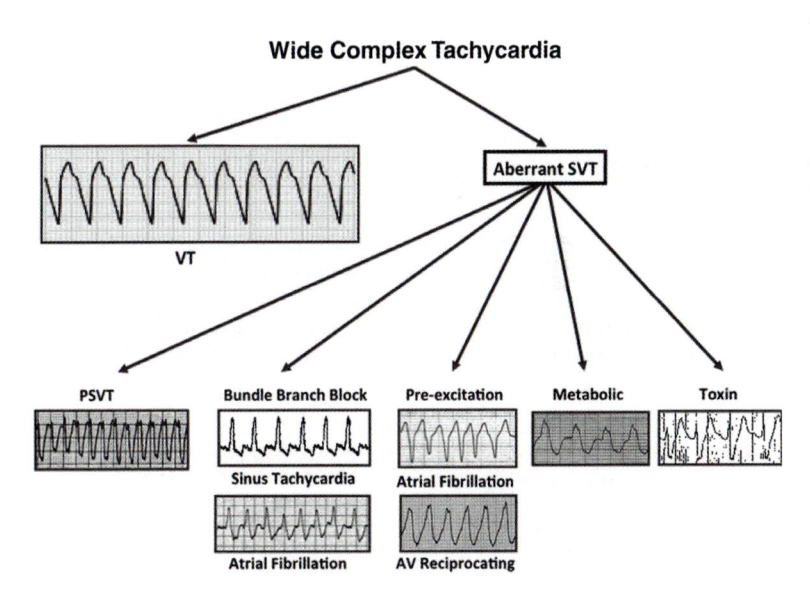

FIGURE 60.1 The differential diagnosis of wide complex tachycardia (WCT) with ventricular tachycardia and supraventricular tachycardia (SVT) with aberrant conduction. The dysrhythmias associated with SVT with aberrant conduction include paroxysmal SVT, sinus tachycardia, atrial fibrillation with rapid ventricular response, Wolf-Parkinson-White syndrome WCTs, and metabolic or toxicologic dysrhythmias.

Regular WCT can further be differentiated based on heart rate. Heart rates less than 120 beats/min classically occur with severe hyperkalemia and AIVR. AIVR usually occurs postarrest and should not be treated because it is self-limiting and treatment could induce dangerous dysrhythmias. The differential for regular WCT with heart rates greater than 120 beats/min includes VT and most types of SVTs with aberrancy. Aberrancy usually relates to underlying BBB. Common examples of SVT with aberrancy are atrial flutter, sinus tachycardia, and PSVT. Also, sinus tachycardia with an anterior ST-segment elevation myocardial infarction can mimic VT. Toxic and metabolite causes (eg, tricyclic antidepressants, acidosis, digoxin) can vary in heart rate. In cases of hyperkalemia or sodium channel blocker toxicity, administration of sodium bicarbonate can be both diagnostic and therapeutic.

Irregular WCTs are particularly interesting and can be due to ventricular fibrillation, SVTs with aberrancy (atrial fibrillation, atrial flutter with variable heart block, and multifocal atrial tachycardia), and polymorphic VT (torsades de pointes, non-sustained VT, and atrial fibrillation with WPW syndrome). WPW is a form of ventricular preexcitation that involves an accessory conduction pathway between the atria and ventricles. Patients with WPW are prone to develop a variety of supraventricular tachyarrhythmias, especially WPW-related atrial fibrillation and WCT. This is one of the reasons why first-line treatments of WCT are with procainamide and not AV node blockers. If AV blockers (eg, adenosine, beta-blockers, calcium channel blockers, digoxin, amiodarone) are used in atrial fibrillation with WPW, they can precipitate life-threatening dysrhythmias.

Lastly, ECG artifacts can be mistaken for VT. Patient movement, poor electrode application, equipment malfunction, or electromagnetic interference can all cause ECG artifacts and mimic the appearance of VT.

PEARLS

- SVT with aberrant conduction is a common mimic of VT.
- Consider hyperkalemia in any WCT where the heart rate is less than 120 beats/min.
- Tricyclic antidepressant toxicity is well known to cause a WCT and should be considered in the differential diagnosis of VT.
- Patient movement, equipment malfunction, and poor electrode placement or contact result in artifacts and mimic the appearance of VT.
- Consider WPW in the differential diagnosis of a WCT.

Suggested Readings

deSouza IS, Peterson AC, Marill KA, et al. Differentiating types of wide-complex tachycardia to determine appropriate treatment in the emergency department. *Emerg Med Pract.* 2015;17:1-22.

Jastrzebski M, Kukla P, Czarnecka D, et al. Comparison of five electrocardiographic methods for differentiation of wide-QRS tachycardias. *Europace.* 2012;14:1165-1171.

Mattu A. ECG Pearls: beware the slow mimics of ventricular tachycardia. *Emergency Physicians Monthly.* 2010. Accessed July 1, 2016. http://epmonthly.com/article/ecg-pearls-beware-the-slow-mimics-of-ventricular-tachycardia

61

Management of Ventricular Storm

Jakob Ottenhoff and Winston Wu

Ventricular, or electrical, storm is a pathologic state in which a patient suffers repeated bouts of malignant ventricular arrhythmias over a short period of time that leads to hemodynamic collapse. As such, it must be recognized quickly and intervened on rapidly. VS constitutes ≥ 3 episodes (or sustained) of ventricular tachycardia, ventricular fibrillation, or appropriate shocks from an AICD within 24 hours. Each episode must last > 30 seconds, involve hemodynamic compromise, or necessitate intervention to terminate the episode.

Typically, the nidus of VS is structural heart disease resulting in abnormal conduction patterns that are predisposed to generating malignant ventricular arrhythmias when triggered by a secondary insult. The most common type of structural heart disease in VS is ischemic cardiomyopathy, accounting for two-thirds of cases, followed by idiopathic dilated cardiomyopathy, arrhythmogenic right ventricular dysplasia, and other causes of infiltrative or structural disease. After the development of these arrhythmogenic regions, VS can then be triggered by a variety of inciting factors such as metabolic derangements, infection, and myocardial ischemia.

Patient presentations can vary significantly from palpitations to cardiac arrest, requiring a high index of suspicion for the condition, especially since a history of structural heart disease may not be known. In general, the workup consists of an ECG and telemetry monitoring as well as cardiac biomarkers including troponin and BNP, a metabolic panel, thyroid studies, and investigations directed at identifying the secondary insult. The workup is further complicated by the fact that the initial ECG will frequently be normal in the stabilized patient and should not exclude the diagnosis of VS. This highlights the need for continuous telemetry to capture the patient's rhythm should symptoms return.

Initial management of the patient in VS should focus on the patient's airway and circulatory state, similar to any critically ill patient. Standard ACLS interventions should be undertaken with priority given to electrical cardioversion for ventricular tachycardia or defibrillation for ventricular fibrillation. However, given that the physiology of the disease is defined by recurrent arrhythmias, initial attempts at correcting the rhythm may only be temporizing and may require further therapy in the form of antiarrhythmics, beta-blockade, and sympatholysis. In addition, inciting factors such as infection, ischemia, and metabolic disarray should be promptly treated (**Figure 61.1**).

Amiodarone is the antiarrhythmic of choice in most cases of VS. It decreases further ventricular arrhythmias, including cases refractory to other antiarrhythmics such as lidocaine. In addition, it decreases further ICD shocks and improves survival to hospital admission. Long-term side effects of amiodarone include hepatotoxicity and pulmonary fibrosis, but it has relatively few contraindications in the acutely decompensated patient and is considered safe in patient with systolic dysfunction. Amiodarone may cause minor inotropic reduction and potential AV nodal blockade, but these negative effects are generally outweighed by the benefit of decreasing malignant ventricular arrhythmias.

```
                    ≥3 Episodes of VF/VT/ICD shocks within
                                    24 h
                                     │
                                     ▼
                    Evaluate need for ACLS
                    interventions or immediate      ───►   Stabilize patient
                    cardioversion/defibrillation
                                     │
                                     ▼
                                   ECG
          ┌──────────────────────────┼──────────────────────────┐
          ▼                          ▼                          ▼
   Monomorphic VT/VF  ◄──── Polymorphic VT/torsades       Brugada syndrome
                                     │                          │
                                     ▼                          ▼
                             Normal QT                    Isoproterenol
                          (typically ischemia)
```

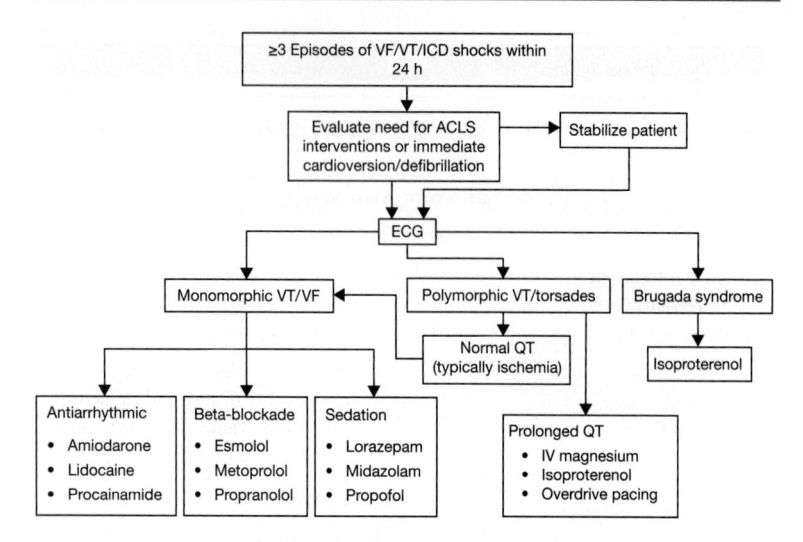

Antiarrhythmic	Beta-blockade	Sedation
• Amiodarone	• Esmolol	• Lorazepam
• Lidocaine	• Metoprolol	• Midazolam
• Procainamide	• Propranolol	• Propofol

Prolonged QT
- IV magnesium
- Isoproterenol
- Overdrive pacing

FIGURE 61.1 Management of ventricular storm. ACLS; ECG, electrocardiogram; ICD, implantable cardioverter defibrillator; IV, intravenous; VF, ventricular fibrillation; VT, ventricular tachycardia.

Lidocaine has shown benefit in the subset of patients where the underlying cause of VS is myocardial ischemia. However, in VS without myocardial ischemia as the inciting event, amiodarone has higher conversion rates and increased survival to hospital admission and is therefore the antiarrhythmic of choice.

Procainamide is another sodium channel–blocking agent that may be considered because of its efficacy in treating stable monomorphic ventricular tachycardia. However, because it has the potential to cause hypotension and QRS widening in patients with systolic dysfunction and kidney disease, its use in VS is limited to hemodynamically stable patients with normal systolic function.

Beta-blockade is a cornerstone of VS therapy and has been shown to increase survival. It decreases sympathetic tone to the heart and has been demonstrated to raise the threshold for ventricular fibrillation in animal models. Traditionally, propranolol and metoprolol are the most common agents used; however, there is a growing body of evidence to show esmolol may be beneficial as well. Due to its extremely short-acting effects, esmolol can be aggressively titrated and discontinued if adverse effects are noted. The choice of beta-blockade is ultimately tailored to the specific clinical situation and provider preference, but it is an essential component of therapy in addition to antiarrhythmics.

Patients in VS have incredibly high sympathetic activity because of the endogenous and exogenous catecholamines that come with the physical stress of multiple arrhythmias and their treatment. Beta-blockade attempts to decrease stress on the heart, but sedation can often provide significant sympatholysis as well and is an often-overlooked therapy. Adequate sedation can be accomplished with propofol or IV benzodiazepines. In patients who are intubated because of VS, propofol may be the preferred agent because it is rapidly titratable and deeply sedating. However, the use of propofol typically requires definitive airway management and therefore is not conducive for the relatively stable VS patient. In this case, IV benzodiazepines, either lorazepam or midazolam, may be more useful. There are no definitive guidelines regarding the ideal agent or depth of sedation.

Special consideration must also be given to two instances of VS: Brugada syndrome and prolonged QT syndromes. Prolonged QT syndromes that degenerate into VS typically manifest as polymorphic ventricular tachycardia (torsades de pointes) and should be treated with IV magnesium in addition to standard resuscitation to shorten the QT interval. Brugada syndrome that leads to VS should be treated with isoproterenol, as traditional antiarrhythmics may worsen VS in these patients.

PEARLS

- VS is a deadly clinical syndrome that may present with symptoms such as palpitations or lightheadedness, yet requires prompt recognition and management.
- Typically, patients will have underlying structural cardiac disease and an inciting event; however, the structural heart disease may not be known, therefore clinicians should not rely on this historical feature to make the diagnosis.
- Management consists of ACLS interventions (prioritizing cardioversion/defibrillation), antiarrhythmic therapy, and beta-blockade.
- Sedation is an underutilized way to decrease endogenous catecholamines and is a cornerstone of VS management.

Suggested Readings

Dyer S, Mogni B, Gottlieb M. Electrical storm: a focused review for the emergency physician. *Am J Emerg Med*. 2020;38(7):1481-1487. PMID: 32345562.

Martins RP, Urien J-M, Barbarot N. Effectiveness of deep sedation for patients with intractable electrical storm refractory to antiarrhythmic drugs. *Circulation*. 2020;142(16): 1599-1601. PMID: 33074763.

Nademanee K, Taylor R, Bailey WE, Rieders DE, Kosar EM. Treating electrical storm: sympathetic blockade versus advanced cardiac life support-guided therapy. *Circulation*. 2000;102(7):742-747. PMID: 10942741.

Nayyar S, Ganesan AN, Brooks AG, Sullivan T, Roberts-Thomson KC, Sanders P. Venturing into ventricular arrhythmia storm: a systematic review and meta-analysis. *Eur Heart J*. 2013; 34(8):560-571. PMID: 23264584.

62

In Pace of Emergency

Moira Smith and M. Kathryn Mutter

Transcutaneous Pacing

The goal of TcP is to maintain or restore myocardial depolarization as a temporary measure before the initiation of TvP or insertion of a permanent pacemaker.

Indications for TcP or TvP:

1) **Unstable bradycardia**. Unstable bradycardia can present with hypotension, altered mental status, recurring syncope, chest pain, or pulmonary edema. It is caused by physiologic or structural damage to the conduction system resulting in high-grade AV block (2° type II or 3° heart block) or ventricular escape rhythms. Bradycardias caused by underlying metabolic abnormalities (acidosis, hyperkalemia, toxins, and hypoxia) or hypothermia are less likely to respond to pacing, and the underlying derangement should be treated primarily.
2) **Overdrive pacing**. Examples of indications for overdrive pacing include recurrent monomorphic ventricular tachycardia and unstable supraventricular tachycardia after pharmacologic intervention and cardioversion have failed. Ventricular tachycardia or ventricular fibrillation can result from overdrive pacing, so DC cardioversion should be available.
3) There is no evidence to support pacing in bradyasystolic arrest.

PROCEDURE

Patients require continuous monitoring with pulse oximeter, cardiac monitor, and ECG leads in addition to adequate analgesia (IV fentanyl) and sedation (IV midazolam, ketamine, or etomidate) before initiation and for the duration of the procedure. Consider a dissociative dose of ketamine in cases of unstable bradycardia where hypotension limits the use of sedation. Be cautious as the combination of an unstable bradycardia and sedation may cause airway compromise.

It is recommended to apply external pacing pads in the anterior-posterior position as it minimizes transthoracic impedance and may lead to improved capture. Patients with existing pacemakers can be transcutaneously paced so long as the pacing pads are not placed directly over the pacemaker box.

If the pacemaker has both a demand/synchronous mode and a fixed/asynchronous mode, the demand/synchronous mode should be used (the pacemaker senses the intrinsic electrical impulses of the heart and paces only when the patient's HR falls below a specified rate). If capture fails while in demand/synchronous mode, then the pacemaker should be switched to the fixed/asynchronous mode. The risk of fixed/asynchronous mode pacing is the possibility of causing an R-on-T phenomenon resulting in ventricular tachycardia or ventricular fibrillation.

Initial settings should be a rate at 70 to 80 beats/min, or 30 beats/min above the intrinsic rate. Start the output at 70 mA and increase until pacing capture is achieved, then set the current at 5 to 10 mA above the threshold for capture. If pacing is not captured at a current of 120 to 130 mA, adjust the pad placement and repeat these steps with the starting current again at 70 mA. The pacing threshold may be higher in certain conditions such as obesity, myocardial ischemia, COPD, pleural or pericardial effusions, metabolic derangements, pneumothorax, and poor skin-to-electrode contact.

The pulse width (pulse duration) is adjustable in some devices. A wider pulse width can reduce the pacing threshold (mA) required to achieve successful capture and can minimize the discomfort of skeletal muscle stimulation.

The presence of a QRS complex after each pacing stimulus suggests electrical capture, though it is important not to mistake this as final confirmation of successful pacing. Confirm mechanical capture by palpating pulses or looking at the pulse oximetry wave as they should match the set pacing HR. Obtain an ECG to confirm the presence of a QRS complex after each pacer spike. Bedside echocardiogram can also be helpful for assessing capture by correlating the HR on M-mode.

Patients should be admitted to an intensive care unit at an institution where TvP can be initiated or a permanent pacemaker placed. Consider inserting a TvP before transfer. TvP will be required unless there is a reversible etiology, such as digoxin toxicity, for the patient's symptomatic bradycardia.

COMPLICATIONS

Complications of TcP include failure to pace (oversensing), failure to capture, and patient discomfort. Failure to pace occurs when the pacemaker incorrectly recognizes interferences (eg, muscle tremors, or nerve stimulators) as a normal cardiac electrical signal, thereby inhibiting external pacing.

Failure to capture occurs when the impulse generated by the pacemaker does not result in myocardial depolarization. Causes of failure to capture include poor pad placement, large body habitus, faulty electrical contact, pneumothorax, pericardial effusion, myocardial ischemia, and metabolic derangements. When failure to capture occurs, recheck lead connections to the pacing device, skin-electrode contact, and electrode placement. Troubleshooting measures include moving the electrodes, wiping the skin, and trimming excess body hair. Shaving body hair is not advised as this can create skin abrasions and result in increased pain during pacing. With prolonged pacing, failure to capture can occur as the pacing threshold may increase over time. If the pacing device allows for adjusting the pulse width, increase the pulse width to reduce the pacing threshold.

Pediatrics

Indications and contraindications for TcP in pediatric patients are similar to those of adult patients. Pacing is not indicated if bradycardia is due to respiratory failure and in that case the underlying cause should be addressed. Adult pacing pads can be used for pediatric patients weighing more than 15 kg in the anterior-posterior positioning to avoid pad overlap. Pediatric patients are at increased risk for pacing-induced burns due to their limited body surface area and thin skin.

PEARLS

- Anterior and posterior pad placement may lead to improved capture for most patients and is recommended as the initial pad placement.
- Metabolic causes of bradycardia are less likely to respond to TcP and the underlying cause should be addressed first.
- Moving the pacing pads, wiping the skin with alcohol, and trimming excess body hair can aid in achieving capture.
- Confirm capture by palpating pulses in addition to assessing for electrical capture (as noted by the presence of a QRS complex after every pacer spike).

SUGGESTED READINGS

Chan T, Brady W, Harrigan R. Diagnosis: pacemaker failure to capture. *Emerg Med News*. 2007;29(1):11.

Doukky R, Bargout R, Kelly RF, Calvin JE. Using transcutaneous cardiac pacing to best advantage: how to ensure successful capture and avoid complications. *J Crit Illn*. 2003;18(5):219-225.

Moayedi S, Patel P, Brady N, Witting M, Dickfeld TL. Anteroposterior pacer pad position is more likely to capture than anterolateral for transcutaneous cardiac pacing. *Circulation*. 2022;146(14):1103-1104.

Safavi-Naeini P, Saeed M. Pacemaker troubleshooting: common clinical scenarios. *Tex Heart Inst J*. 2016;43(5):415-418.
Singh HR, Batra AS, Balaji S. Pacing in children. *Ann Pediatr Cardiol*. 2013;6(1):46-51.

63

Management of Atrial Fibrillation: Rate Control Versus Rhythm Conversion

Aaron R. Kuzel and J. Jeremy Thomas

AF is the most commonly encountered dysrhythmia in emergency medicine, presenting variably from asymptomatic to hemodynamic collapse. Patients with AF may develop RVR (pulse >100). Untreated AF with RVR may increase the risk of myocardial infarction, stroke, thrombus formation, or HF. ED management of patients with AF with RVR often focuses on rate or rhythm control. Both strategies have demonstrated symptom improvement and reduction of thromboembolic events, though neither strategy has proven mortality benefits. For the majority of patients presenting with AF of unknown duration, rate control is preferred. However, rhythm control alone has resulted in lower rates of mortality from cardiovascular disease, stroke, and hospitalizations for ACS or HF.

Rate Control

BB and CCB are commonly used to achieve rate control by decreasing conduction at the atrioventricular node. Medication choice for rate control depends on individual patient specifics. Patients with AF and hypertension or compensated HF may be safely treated with a BB, whereas a CCB may be more appropriate for a patient with AF and COPD or asthma.

Both BB and CCB are equally efficacious at rate control. Some literature suggests that diltiazem (0.25 mg/kg IV) may be superior to metoprolol in achieving rate control. However, it may be more likely that diltiazem simply results in shortened time to rate control as compared to metoprolol.

Digoxin and amiodarone are also options for rate control. A positive inotrope, digoxin can be considered in patients with decompensated HF, patients intolerant to or refractory to CCB or BB, or patients with hypotension not amenable to cardioversion. Amiodarone is potentially useful in managing AF with RVR that is causing hemodynamic compromise and is either refractory to or not a candidate for electrical cardioversion. Importantly, amiodarone may also cardiovert AF to sinus rhythm, increasing the risk of thromboembolic event in patients not receiving anticoagulation.

Rhythm Control

Rhythm control may be more challenging in the acute setting and involves either chemical or electrical cardioversion. For patients without significant comorbid conditions presenting with AF less than 48 hours, rhythm control is reasonable, using either strategy. Before attempting rhythm control, it is critical to ascertain the duration of AF, which can be particularly challenging for patients with asymptomatic AF. Patients with AF for more than 48 hours or unclear duration should be adequately anticoagulated prior to rhythm control, due to risk of thromboembolism. Regardless of the method used to treat AF, it is important to assess the patient's need for long-term anticoagulation to prevent thromboembolic events. Younger patients (<60-65 years) with AF onset lesser than 48 hours who have been successfully cardioverted generally do not require long-term anticoagulation.

Prior to electrical or chemical cardioversion, a risk stratification score, such as CHADS2 or CHA_2DS_2-VASc, can help determine thromboembolism risk and need for anticoagulation. For high-risk patients, clinicians should consider anticoagulation with heparin before or immediately after electrical cardioversion with eventual bridge to oral anticoagulation.

Cardioversion to normal sinus rhythm is usually successful but is dependent on several factors: age, underlying health conditions, duration of AF, previous heart disease, and whether the AF was triggered by an underlying cause. Characteristics of patients with better cardioversion outcomes include younger (age <60 years), first AF episode, no underlying heart disease, shorter duration of symptoms, and precipitated by reversible cause. The American, Canadian, and European Cardiology AF Guidelines all support early cardioversion for AF with duration lesser than 48 hours. The Rate Control Versus Electrical Cardioversion Trial 7-Acute Cardioversion Versus Wait and See Trial found that in hemodynamically stable patients with onset of AF within 36 hours, delayed (48 hours) cardioversion was noninferior to earlier cardioversion. The 2020 ESC Guidelines acknowledged both delayed and early cardioversion as acceptable treatments to AF within 48 hours of AF onset.

Hemodynamic instability due to AF with RVR necessitates emergent electrical cardioversion. For ED patients requiring emergent electrical cardioversion, it is recommended to begin intravenous unfractionated or low-molecular-weight heparin prior to cardioversion, though this intervention may be impossible in emergent circumstances and of unproven benefit. Procedural sedation should be employed when possible. The combination of antiarrhythmic medications and electrical cardioversion has been demonstrated to be beneficial in patients with AF with RVR. The most effective antiarrhythmic medication in combination with electrical cardioversion is ibutilide, but class Ia, Ic, and III antiarrhythmics agents can also be effective.

PEARLS

- Electrical cardioversion is the treatment of choice for patients who are hemodynamically unstable due to AF with RVR.
- Rate control is the preferred treatment for with AF with RVR more than 48 hours from symptom onset; diltiazem and metoprolol are equally efficacious, yet diltiazem likely achieves more rapid rate control.
- Consider rhythm control for healthy patients who present within 48 hours from AF onset.
- Use the CHADS2 or CHA_2DS_2-VASc score to determine the stroke risk for patients with AF and decide upon anticoagulation.

Suggested Readings

Compagner CT, Wysocki CR, Reich EK, Zimmerman LH, Holzhausen JM. Intravenous metoprolol versus diltiazem for atrial fibrillation with concomitant heart failure. *Am J Emerg Med*. 2022;62:49-54.

January CT, Wann LS, Calkins H, et al. 2019 AHA/ACC/HRS Focused Update of the 2014 AHA/ACC/HRS Guideline for the management of patients with atrial fibrillation: a report of the American College of Cardiology/American Heart Association Task Force on Clinical Practice Guidelines and the Heart Rhythm Society. *J Am Coll Cardiol*. 2019;74(1):104-132.

Kirchhof P, Camm AJ, Goette A, et al. Early rhythm-control therapy in patients with atrial fibrillation. *N Engl J Med*. 2020;383(14):1305-1316.

Lan Q, Wu F, Han B, Ma L, Han J, Yao Y. Intravenous diltiazem versus metoprolol for atrial fibrillation with rapid ventricular rate: a meta-analysis. *Am J Emerg Med*. 2022;51:248-256.

64

Mismanagement of Atrial Fibrillation in Wolff-Parkinson-White Syndrome

Kellie A. Mitchell and William J. Brady

In the early 1930s, Wolff, Parkinson, and White characterized the combination of bundle branch block, shortened PR interval, and recurrent episodes of tachycardia occurring in young, healthy patients with structurally normal hearts. This combination of clinical and electrocardiographic findings distinguishes the ventricular preexcitation syndrome known as WPW syndrome. In WPW, an accessory pathway connects the atrial tissues to the ventricular myocardium and bypasses the AV node to create a direct electrical connection between the atria and ventricles and provide the substrate for dysrhythmia. Patients with WPW can experience a range of supraventricular tachydysrhythmias with resultant symptoms from unpleasant to disabling to, in extreme cases, cardiovascular collapse and death.

The electrocardiographic features of WPW in sinus rhythm include the classic triad:

1) Shortened PR interval (<0.12 seconds)
2) Delta wave, an initial slurring of the QRS complex
3) Minimally widened QRS complex (>0.10 seconds)

For the diagnosis of the WPW syndrome, patients must demonstrate the classic ECG triad and the presence of one of the three classic dysrhythmias: orthodromic (narrow QRS complex) AVRT (65%), antidromic (wide QRS complex) AVRT (10%), or WPW-related atrial fibrillation (25%).

Atrial fibrillation is the second most frequent dysrhythmia in the patient with WPW. The multiple foci in the atrial tissues generate impulses which are conducted to the ventricular myocardium via both the AV node and accessory pathway. The AV node controls the rate of impulse transmission to the ventricle but the accessory pathway transmits all impulses without delay. The resultant ventricular depolarization results from a combination, or fusion, of the two separate electrical impulses which arrive via the AV node and accessory pathway (**Figure 64.1C**). This form of atrial fibrillation is particularly dangerous as patients can experience extremely rapid ventricular rates and subsequent systemic hypoperfusion.

Unique features of the WPW-related atrial fibrillation can be identified in **Figure 64.1A and B**.

In addition, a delta wave can be seen in this form of atrial fibrillation resulting from the premature depolarization of a portion of the ventricular myocardium.

The management of WPW-related atrial fibrillation must be approached with a consideration of the hemodynamic status of the patient. This form of atrial fibrillation has a tendency to deteriorate and in the patient who is hemodynamically unstable, electrical cardioversion with sedation is the treatment of choice. In the stable patient, initial medication administration is reasonable, though electrical therapy and other resuscitation interventions should be immediately available. Procainamide is the primary agent for this rhythm dosed at 20 to 30 mg/min until one of the following end points are reached: development of hypotension, further QRS complex widening (prolonged by 50% from

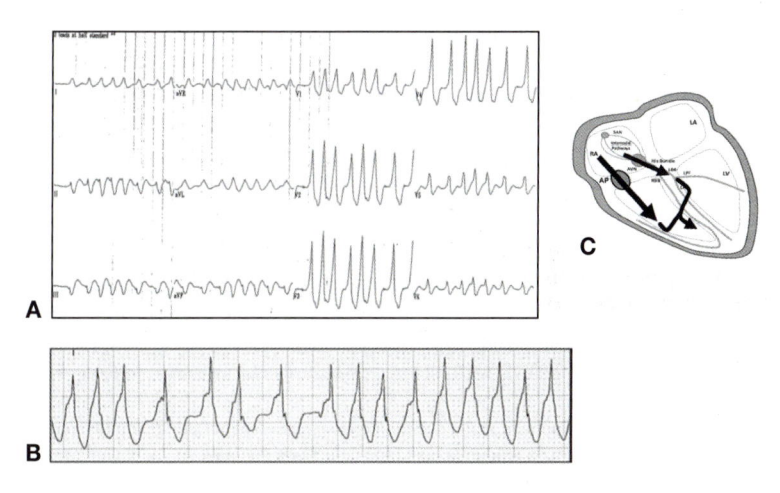

FIGURE 64.1 Atrial fibrillation in the Wolff-Parkinson-White syndrome. A. 12-lead ECG with a very rapid, irregularly irregular rhythm with widened QRS complex and beat-to-beat variation in the QRS complex morphology. B. ECG rhythm strip demonstrating the dysrhythmia; note the beat-to-beat variation in the QRS complex morphology and width, a key feature of WPW-related atrial fibrillation. C. Depolarization of the ventricle in a patient with WPW syndrome complicated by atrial fibrillation. AP, accessory pathway; AVN, atrioventricular node; LA, left atrium; LBB, left bundle branch; LPF, left posterior fascicle; LV, left ventricle; RA, right atrium; RBB, right bundle branch; SAN, sinoatrial node.

its original width), significant acceleration of the tachycardia, arrhythmia termination, or administration of a full loading dose (1 g). An alternative regimen is a loading dose of 17 mg/kg IV (intravenous) over approximately 45 minutes. Adverse effects include worsened tachycardia or hypotension. Both strategies of procainamide administration have a slow onset of action, not reaching therapeutic blood levels for 40 to 60 minutes. Sedated electrical cardioversion can be initially employed, even in the hemodynamically stable patient, with an initial synchronized shock of 100 J.

Caution should be exercised with the use of amiodarone in this type of rhythm presentation. Its diverse electrophysiologic effects, including beta-adrenergic, calcium channel, and fast sodium channel mechanisms with their acute impact on the accessory pathway, make rapid IV administration potentially problematic. Amiodarone can cause acceleration of the ventricular rate accompanied by cardiovascular collapse and/or ventricular fibrillation.

AV nodal blocking agents are also contraindicated in the patient with WPW with atrial fibrillation. Calcium channel antagonists, beta-adrenergic blocking agents, adenosine, and digoxin are contraindicated in this setting because they enhance conduction via the accessory pathway, subjecting the ventricle to excess rates, malignant ventricular dysrhythmia, and potential for cardiovascular collapse.

While general agreement exists on the management of tachyarrhythmia due to WPW, much debate exists about the management of asymptomatic patients incidentally found to have the classic ECG triad of WPW. While these patients do not technically have all the criteria for the WPW syndrome without any presenting tachyarrhythmia, many go on to undergo evaluation by a cardiologist, and some receive ablations as a result. In general, these patients do not require urgent cardiology evaluation—the risk of sudden cardiac death has been estimated in the range of 0.05% to 2% per year. Though the risk is higher at a younger age, whether ablation is necessary is still questioned. However, cardiology referral is recommended, and strict return precautions for symptoms should be given. Patients should be advised that strenuous physical activity predisposes to the occurrence of tachyarrhythmia and sudden cardiac death in this setting.

PEARLS

- WPW with atrial fibrillation can cause significant hemodynamic compromise and should be treated with sedated electrical cardioversion and/or IV procainamide.
- Medications with significant AV node-blocking effects including amiodarone, calcium channel antagonists, beta-adrenergic blocking agents, adenosine, and digoxin are contraindicated in WPW with atrial fibrillation.

SUGGESTED READINGS

Brady WJ. Wolff-Parkinson-White Syndrome. In: Brady WJ, et al, eds. *The ECG in Prehospital Emergency Care*. Wiley; 2012.

Obeyesekere MN, et al. Risk of arrhythmia and sudden death in patients with asymptomatic preexcitation. *Circulation*. 2012;125:2308-2315.

Wolff L, Parkinson J, White PD. Bundle-branch block with short PR interval in healthy young people prone to paroxysmal tachycardia. *Am Heart J*. 1930;5:685–704.

65

Pitfalls in Hypertensive Emergencies

Lauren M. Hunter and Aaron M. Blackshaw

Nearly half of American adults have hypertension, leading to an estimated 1 million annual ED visits. While elevated BP readings are common during ED patient encounters, true hypertensive emergencies are rare.

The diagnosis of hypertensive emergency requires two criteria: a significantly elevated BP *and* evidence of new or worsening end-organ damage. Most sources suggest BP measurements of more than 180/120 or that a MAP of more than 135 is required to define this disease process. However, the numeric values and oft-cited definitions are less important than the individual patient's baseline BP, the rate of BP rise, and patient symptomatology. No specific BP threshold constitutes a true hypertensive emergency.

The most typical presentation of hypertensive emergency is acute heart failure with pulmonary edema. Ischemic stroke, acute coronary syndrome, ICH, acute aortic syndrome, and hypertensive encephalopathy follow in order of decreasing incidence.

Nonadherence to prescribed antihypertensive medications is the most common precipitating factor for these hypertensive emergencies. Other potential triggers include increased dietary sodium intake, anxiety/panic, severe pain, urinary retention, and withdrawal from alcohol, benzodiazepines, clonidine, baclofen, or tizanidine. Medications that can elicit acute BP elevations include the over-the-counter variety (eg, nonsteroidal anti-inflammatory drugs, decongestants, certain supplements), prescription medications (eg, stimulants, glucocorticoids, and calcineurin inhibitors—like tacrolimus and cyclosporine), and illicit drugs (eg, cocaine, methamphetamines, and other sympathomimetic agents). Acute heart failure or stroke can be both a cause and a consequence of severe hypertension.

The primary goal in managing patients with hypertensive emergencies is careful BP control. There are no robust trials comparing different pharmaceutical agents and pressure goals in patients with a hypertensive emergency. However, the general aim is to induce a controlled and timely reduction in BP. The initial reduction of MAP by 20% to 25% within the first 1 to 2 hours of symptoms is reasonable. Conditions that require close attention to ICP and CPP may warrant more liberal BP goals, such as ischemic stroke with or without thrombolytics. However, conditions such as aortic dissection, ICH, and (pre)eclampsia require much more aggressive BP reductions. Regardless of the target reduction, evidence is clear that excessive BP reduction is associated with increased mortality rates related to organ hypoperfusion. **Table 65.1** lists common hypertensive emergencies with recommended BP goals and first-line therapeutic options.

The ideal medications to treat hypertensive emergencies have predictable hemodynamic effects, IV administration options, are readily titratable, and have short half-lives. For this reason, calcium channel blockers (eg, nicardipine, clevidipine) and beta-blockers (eg, labetalol) tend to be first-line therapeutic options in the emergency setting. Other therapeutic options should be customized based on specific patient circumstances. For instance, IV nitroglycerin works quickly as a potent vasodilator (decreases preload), is

TABLE 65.1 CONSENSUS BASED GUIDELINES OF HYPERTENSIVE EMERGENCIES

CLINICAL PRESENTATION	TREATMENT GOALS (MMHG)	FIRST LINE THERAPEUTICS
Ischemic stroke	<220/120[a]	Labetalol, nicardipine, clevidipine
Ischemic stroke receiving thrombolytic therapy	≤185/110 (before thrombolytics) ≤180/105 (after thrombolytics)	Labetalol, nicardipine, clevidipine
Intracerebral hemorrhage (initial SBP 150-220)	SBP <140[b] or <180[c]	Labetalol, nicardipine, clevidipine
Intracerebral hemorrhage (initial SBP >220)	SBP <220[b]	Labetalol, nicardipine, clevidipine
Hypertensive encephalopathy	Decrease MAP by 20-25%	Labetalol, nicardipine
Eclampsia and preeclampsia with severe features	130-150/80-100	Labetalol, hydralazine, nifedipine, magnesium sulfate[d]
Aortic dissection	SBP 100-120[e]	Esmolol and nicardipine/clevidipine, nitroglycerin
Acute coronary syndrome	SBP <140, keep DBP >60	Labetalol, metoprolol, nicardipine, clevidipine, nitroglycerin
Acute cardiogenic pulmonary edema	SBP <140 or decrease MAP by 20-25%	Nitroglycerin, loop diuretics, hydralazine

[a]Permissive hypertension is recommended in the 24 hours after an ischemic stroke not undergoing thrombolysis
[b]Reducing SBP <130 may increase the risk of cerebral hypoperfusion and other adverse outcomes, titrate carefully to avoid peaks and variability
[c]Target <140 if no pre-existing HTN or <180 if history of chronic HTN
[d]Magnesium sulfate is first line therapy in eclampsia but has very little acute effect on the BP
[e]Standard of care involves both aggressive SBP management and target HR <60 bpm

readily titratable, and is frequently used in cases of severe decompensated heart failure and pulmonary edema. Clevidipine is extraordinarily titratable and does not require hepatic or renal clearance, but availability may be limited. Benzodiazepines (along with calcium channel blockers and nitrates) are the first-line treatment for hypertensive emergencies resulting from cocaine abuse; beta-blockers should be avoided given the theoretical risk of unopposed alpha-adrenergic agonism. Hydralazine (a direct vasodilator) should be avoided for hypertensive emergencies as it causes reflex tachycardia, has unpredictable antihypertensive properties, and can have prolonged physiological effects up to 12 hours after dosing.

Adjunctive therapies are often necessary, especially if pressures are refractory to usual doses of antihypertensives. Addressing underlying potentiators of elevated BP with analgesics, antiemetics, and antianxiety medications may be warranted. In a hypertensive emergency patient with an uncommon diagnosis (eg, pheochromocytoma, severe autonomic dysfunction, thyroid storm, scleroderma renal crisis), early consultation from specialists and acute care pharmacists might be required.

In contrast, hypertensive urgency is an acutely elevated BP *without* end-organ damage. This term has fallen out of favor among many in the medical community, with a suggestion that it be replaced in the medical lexicon with "asymptomatic markedly elevated BP." The ACEP clinical policy states that routine screening for target organ damage in asymptomatic patients with markedly elevated BP is not indicated. Screening for kidney disease with serum creatinine only in patients with poor follow-up can be considered. The policy also states that initiating antihypertensive treatment based on BP reading alone can be detrimental to the patient. In particular, physicians should not aim to normalize asymptomatic BP elevations in the ED. While these patients do not need a diagnostic ED workup or treatment, they do warrant timely outpatient follow-up, given the detrimental effects of long-standing hypertension.

PEARLS

- Hypertensive emergency is end-organ damage caused by significantly elevated BPs. Although differing values are often cited, absolute numbers are less important than changes in the patient's baseline BP, the rate of rise of the BP, and the patient's symptomatology.
- Customize treatment based on the damaged end-organ system and the patient's relevant history, medications, allergies, and other comorbidities. Referencing ever-changing guidelines for specific disease states is also highly recommended.
- Aiming for an approximately 20% reduction in BP over the first 1 to 2 hours of most presentations is a reasonable and measured approach. Avoid excessive lowering of MAP, given the risk of inducing ischemia.
- Nicardipine and clevidipine or labetalol are the mainstay treatment for most patients presenting in a hypertensive emergency. Hydralazine has significant limitations in hypertensive emergencies and should be avoided.
- Adjunctive therapies, particularly treatment of anxiety and pain, can also help lower BP.
- Hypertensive urgency is a misnomer, as asymptomatic patients with elevated BPs do not typically require any diagnostic evaluation or treatment in the ED.

SUGGESTED READINGS

Astarita A, Covella M, Vallelonga F, et al. Hypertensive emergencies and urgencies in emergency departments: a systematic review and meta-analysis. *J Hypertension*. 2020;38(7):1203-1210.

Peixoto AJ. Acute severe hypertension. *N Engl J Med*. 2019;381:1843-1852.

Rossi GP, Rossitto G, Maifredini C, et al. Management of hypertensive emergencies: a practical approach. *Blood Press*. 2021;30(4):208-219.

Unger T, Borghi C, Charchar F, et al. 2020 International Society of Hypertension global hypertension practice guidelines. *Hypertension*. 2020;75(6):1334-1357.

Van den Born B, Lip GYH, Brguljan-Hitij J, et al. ESC Council on hypertension position document on the management of hypertensive emergencies. *Eur Heart J Cardiovasc Pharmacother*. 2019;5(1):37-46.

Wolf SJ, Lo B, Shih RD, Smith MD, Fesmire FM; American College of Emergency Physicians Clinical Policies Committee. Clinical policy: critical issues in the evaluation and management of adult patients in the emergency department with asymptomatic elevated blood pressure. *Ann Emerg Med*. 2013;62(1):59-68.

66

CHEST PAIN PLUS ... DON'T MISS AORTIC DISSECTION

J. David Gatz

Aortic dissection (AD) is a rare (estimated incidence of 4.4 per 100,000 person-years) but deadly condition that is often at risk of delayed diagnosis and misdiagnosis. While older patients often have traditional risk factors (eg, chronic hypertension, preexisting aortic/aortic valve abnormalities, atherosclerosis), younger patients may also suffer ADs in the setting of other risk factors like sympathomimetic use or connective tissue disorders.

Chest pain with additional features should raise suspicion for AD. Predictive historical and physical exam features are listed in **Table 66.1**. Recent studies found that generalized chest pain, the presence of abdominal pain, a "tearing" quality, and migrating pain were not significant predictors of AD. Although history of hypertension is associated with the development of dissection, the presence of hypertension on presentation is not a significant predictor. Findings of a new aortic regurgitation murmur and pulmonary edema are similarly unhelpful. Case reports describe chest pain in combination with a variety of additional symptoms: bowel ischemia, dysphagia, hemoptysis, hoarseness, Horner syndrome, limb ischemia, or even transient neurologic symptoms. While most patients with dissection have chest pain, a painless dissection is possible.

The absence of any one feature, such as asymmetric pulses or new neurologic deficit, does not exclude the possibility of AD. While specific, none of these findings are particularly sensitive and placing too much emphasis on their absence may contribute to misdiagnosis. In contrast, the presence of multiple features should greatly increase suspicion for AD.

TABLE 66.1 PREDICTIVE VALUE OF HISTORICAL AND PHYSICAL EXAMINATION FEATURES FOR AD

FEATURE	POSITIVE LIKELIHOOD RATIO	NEGATIVE LIKELIHOOD RATIO
Historical Features		
Syncope	1-2.4	NR
Severe pain	1.5-2.3	0.31-0.68
Acute onset	1.0-2.6	0.30-0.98
Back pain	1.0-23	0.64-0.99
Examination Features		
Focal neurologic deficit	4.3	NR
Pulse deficit	2.5	NR
Hypotension or shock	1.2-4.3	NR

NR, not reported.

Diagnosis

The preferred diagnostic imaging for AD is an emergent CTA. It is sensitive, specific, and accessible, and should be pursued without delay for renal function testing. Transesophageal echocardiogram and MR-based imaging are alternative modalities with limited use in the ED setting. Point-of-care US may expedite diagnosis but is technically challenging and cannot rule out disease. Observing a flap in the aorta on US is sufficient to empirically start treatment while awaiting definitive imaging. Chest radiographs lack sufficient sensitivity and specificity for acute aortic syndromes, although there may be suggestive findings (eg, mediastinal widening or abnormal aortic contour).

Laboratory studies, such as D-dimer and troponin, do not have a significant role in the diagnosis of AD but may be considered in the workup of alternative diagnoses. Acute coronary syndrome is a common misdiagnosis of patients with AD. While most ECGs will be nonspecific in AD, some may demonstrate a STEMI.

ED Management

The management of AD should be immediate and aggressive once diagnosed or highly suspected. While multiple classification systems exist, perhaps the most useful in the ED setting is the Stanford Type A versus Type B distinction based on the most proximal portion of the aorta involved. Type A involves the ascending aorta, while Type B only involves the descending aorta. Both types require immediate medical "anti-impulse" therapy to decrease aortic wall stress beginning with heart rate control and aggressive analgesia. Target a rate of 60 to 80 bpm, usually via an easily titratable beta-blocker such as esmolol. Clinicians should only add a vasodilator, such as nicardipine or clevidipine, if the blood pressure is not sufficiently controlled after beta-blocker use and analgesia. Clinicians should target a systolic blood pressure of less than 120 mm Hg, provided it still allows adequate end-organ perfusion and thus avoids iatrogenic obtundation, oliguria, and mottling. Initiation of a vasodilator first could result in a reflex tachycardia that is ultimately detrimental to the patient. Adequate analgesia with IV opioids is essential, given its possible impact on tachycardia and hypertension. Most patients will require an arterial line in whichever extremity is registering higher blood pressure and subsequent admission to either an operating room or ICU setting.

Surgical management varies by type of dissection and local practice. In general, Type A dissections require prompt surgical intervention and should be managed by cardiothoracic surgeons. Medical management should not delay surgical treatment. Type B dissections may require endovascular treatment with stenting or medical management alone and often should be discussed with a vascular surgeon.

Complications

ED clinicians must be prepared to manage a wide array of potential complications. Shock is possible through a variety of mechanisms, including cardiac tamponade, right ventricular myocardial infarction, aortic rupture, and acute severe aortic regurgitation. In the setting of cardiac tamponade, patients may require preload and vasopressor support. The role of percutaneous pericardiocentesis is controversial as aggressive drainage may ultimately worsen or kill the patient. Newer guidelines suggest withdrawing small amounts of fluid (just enough to restore perfusion in 5-10 mL aliquots) as a temporizing procedure.

Myocardial infarction is another possible complication if the dissection compromises a coronary artery ostium (classically the right, cutting off the RCA and resulting in an inferior STEMI). Patients presenting with a STEMI may result in premature diagnostic closure. While this scenario is fortunately rare, it can result in critical delays in the diagnosis of a Type A AD, which carries an untreated mortality rate of 1% to 2% per hour. Point-of-care US or even CTA may be considered before primary percutaneous coronary intervention if there is a specific clinical concern for AD.

PEARLS

- While traditionally thought of as an abrupt tearing pain that radiates to the back in older adults, AD may present in patients of any age and with a variety of symptoms or abnormal findings.
- CTA is the best imaging modality for rapid confirmation of AD and its complications.
- Most patients with a STEMI on ECG and/or positive troponin are experiencing a traditional myocardial infarction and benefit from emergent PCI. Consider US and/or CTA before cardiac catheterization if there is high suspicion for AD.
- Medical management of AD focuses first on heart rate control and aggressive analgesia. Blood pressure control can subsequently be initiated, if still needed.
- Immediate consultation with a cardiothoracic surgeon is appropriate for any confirmed or highly suspected ascending AD.

Suggested Readings

Carrel T, Sundt TM 3rd, von Kodolitsch Y, Czerny M. Acute aortic dissection. *Lancet*. 2023;401(22):773-788.

Hackett A, Stuart J, Robinson DL. Thoracic aortic syndromes in the emergency department: recognition and management. *Emerg Med Pract*. 2021;23(12):1-28.

Isselbacher EM, Preventza O, Hamilton Black J 3rd, et al. 2022 ACC/AHA guideline for the diagnosis and management of aortic disease: a report of the American Heart Association/American College of Cardiology Joint Committee on Clinical Practice Guidelines. *Circulation*. 2022;146(24):e334-e482.

Mehta CK, Son AY, Chia MC, et al. Management of acute aortic syndromes from initial presentation to definitive treatment. *Am J Emerg Med*. 2022;51:108-113.

Ohle R, Kareemi HK, Wells G, Perry JJ. Clinical examination for acute aortic dissection: a systematic review and meta-analysis. *Acad Emerg Med*. 2018;25(4):397-412.

67

Don't Overlook Atypical Risk Factors for ACS

Michael J. Yoo and Brit Long

Recognition of typical risk factors for ACS including hypertension, hyperlipidemia, and DM remains important in improving outcomes in heart disease. However, several nontraditional conditions also significantly increase the risk of ACS: CKD, rheumatologic disorders, malignancy, alcohol consumption, pregnancy, systemic infection, and HIV.

CKD

Patients with diminished GFRs have an increased risk for all-cause and CV mortality, with lower GFRs conferring the highest risks. Specifically, a GFR less than 60 mL/min/1.73 m^2 is an independent risk factor for CV mortality. Patients with a GFR of 45 to 59, 30 to 44, 15 to 29, and less than 15 mL/min/1.73 m^2 are 1.4, 2.0, 2.8, and 3.4 times as likely to experience a major adverse cardiac event. Furthermore, patients with decreased GFRs are more likely to present with NSTEMI and less than half report typical symptoms, such as chest pain or radiation of pain. Younger patients with CKD are more likely to present with single or two-vessel ACS, whereas older patients with CKD present with multivessel disease. Patients with CKD have a higher baseline of CAD and traditional risk factors; however, the additional chronic inflammation, coagulopathy, endothelial dysfunction, and accelerated arterial calcifications further elevate the risk for ACS. Patients undergoing hemodialysis also experience volume and electrolyte fluctuations that can cause direct myocardial injury. Finally, many disease-modifying drugs, such as statins, may be less efficacious at lower GFRs, also increasing the long-term risk of ACS.

Rheumatologic Disorders

Patients with rheumatologic disorders, primarily RA, SLE, and psoriasis, have up to a 3.7 times risk of MI. Furthermore, in contrast to patients without rheumatologic conditions, patients with rheumatologic disorders who present with ACS tend to be younger, predominantly women (67%), and have NSTEMI (77%). In addition, patients with underlying rheumatologic conditions and MI have a higher risk of all-cause mortality, heart failure, recurrent MIs, and need for reintervention compared to patients with ACS but without rheumatologic disease. This is likely due to a combination of a higher prevalence of typical risk factors such as hypertension, as well as a chronic inflammatory state, coagulopathy, and lipid dysregulation. Furthermore, these patients are more likely to be on systemic steroids, for which active use, especially in the first 30 days, and dosages exceeding 10 mg/day of prednisolone or equivalent increase the risk of ACS.

Cancer

CVD and ACS remain important causes of morbidity and mortality in the population with cancer, with a prevalence reported between 3% and 17%. Patients with a history of cancer represent up to 8.1% of patients admitted with ACS. Patients with cancer admitted with ACS have worse outcomes, with a 2.4 and 1.9 relative risk of in-hospital and 1-year cardiac death, respectively, likely due to increased comorbid conditions such as CKD. Furthermore, patients with cancer and non-cancer patients with CVD share several traditional risk factors for ACS, including hypertension, tobacco use, and decreased physical activity. The increased risk of ACS in cancer may also be attributable to a chronic inflammatory state, oxidative stress, and hypercoagulopathy. Patients with cancer with ACS are typically older males, more commonly present with STEMI, and have single or double vessel disease.

Several therapies are associated with cardiotoxicity, including ACS, with the most common inciting agents belonging to the anthracycline, alkylating, and fluoropyrimidine classes. Chemotherapy-associated cardiotoxicity occurs in 8.3% of patients, with coronary thrombosis and vasospasm being the most common culprits of ACS. Radiation therapy directly injures the endothelium but is a less frequent cause. Cardiotoxicity is also associated with the use of immunotherapy, though further data are needed given its relative novelty.

Alcohol Consumption

The effects of alcohol consumption on ACS have been controversial, including a possible risk reduction at lower doses of intake (<12 g of alcohol per day). Conversely, higher alcohol consumption including 12 to 24 g and greater than 24 g of alcohol/day is associated with a 2.7 and 5.4 times increased risk of developing ACS, respectively. Recent studies have also demonstrated that heavy alcohol consumption (>2 drinks per day) is an independent risk factor of in-hospital mortality in patients admitted with ACS, though heavier alcohol users have more comorbid conditions at baseline. The mechanism behind heavy alcohol use and increased risk of ACS is unclear, though it may be secondary to coronary microvascular damage. The deleterious effect of higher alcohol use is magnified in patients with underlying CAD, who are at high risk for worsening cardiac ischemia with alcohol consumption.

Pregnancy

ACS affects up to 10 in 100,000 pregnancies, translating to a 3 to 4 times increased risk compared to nonpregnant women of similar age. Mortality rates for ACS in pregnancy have been cited as high as 17%. Current data regarding the etiology of ACS in pregnancy are mixed, though atherosclerotic disease (27%-43%) and spontaneous coronary artery dissection (14%-43%) comprise most cases. Other etiologies include thrombosis (21%), vasospasm (5%), and embolism (4%). Of the patients with embolic disease, patients typically have underlying arrhythmias, including atrial fibrillation and valvular disease. The most common presentation of ACS in pregnant patients is NSTEMI (57.6%).

Age (>30 years old) and previous CVD are the strongest risk factors, with a 16.2 and 15.3 OR for ACS in pregnancy, respectively. Traditional risk factors also increase the risk of ACS in pregnancy; however, the development of preeclampsia and eclampsia, gestational hypertension, and gestational DM appear to be independent risk factors. Concomitant gestational hypertension and gestational DM are associated with a 2.4 times risk of developing CVD in the late postpartum period (>5 years after delivery).

Systemic Infection

Patients with systemic infections are 2 to 3 times more likely to experience any type of ACS. Bacteremia and respiratory infections demonstrate the strongest associations, though urinary tract and gastroenterologic infections also increase the risk of ACS. While the systemic inflammatory response in more severe infections plays a direct role in myocardial stress, inflammation may also cause acute worsening of preexisting atherosclerotic plaques. Specifically, endothelial damage, thrombosis, and free radicals promote acute coronary obstruction. Of note, patients with ACS and COVID-19 have a 4.95 OR of in-hospital mortality, likely due to the supraphysiologic inflammatory response and hypercoagulability.

HIV

CVD accounts for up to 22% of deaths in patients with HIV, and MI occurs 2 to 3 times more frequently compared to similarly aged HIV-negative individuals. The pathophysiology is likely multifactorial, including early onset CAD from chronic immune dysfunction and viremia along with unstable and noncalcified atherosclerotic plaques that are prone to premature rupturing. Antiretroviral drugs may increase the risk of ACS, with several common combination therapies increasing serum triglycerides, low-density lipoproteins, and total cholesterol levels. Taking ritonavir, lopinavir, efavirenz, and abacavir has been specifically associated with an increased risk of ACS, though the true causality is controversial. Notably, the population with HIV also has a significantly higher incidence of typical ACS risk factors such as hypertension and DM.

PEARLS

- Clinicians should maintain a low threshold for initiating a workup for ACS in patients with atypical risk factors.
- Patients with CKD have an increased risk of ACS, especially when the GFR is less than 60 mL/min/1.73 m^2, and typical anginal symptoms may not be present.
- Patients with rheumatologic conditions and ACS are likely to be younger women with NSTEMI.
- Cancer and its treatments are associated with coronary artery thrombosis, vasospasm, pericarditis, myocarditis, and heart failure.
- Pregnant women have a 3 to 4 times elevated risk of ACS compared to nonpregnant women.
- Systemic infections and HIV are associated with inflammatory states that increase the risk of premature plaque rupture.

Suggested Readings

Chronic Kidney Disease Prognosis Consortium, Matsushita K, van der Velde M, et al. Association of estimated glomerular filtration rate and albuminuria with all-cause and cardiovascular mortality in general population cohorts: a collaborative meta-analysis. *Lancet.* 2010;375(9731):2073-2081.

Corrales-Medina VF, Madjid M, Musher DM. Role of acute infection in triggering acute coronary syndromes. *Lancet Infect Dis.* 2010;10(2):83-92.

Durand M, Sheehy O, Baril JG, Lelorier J, Tremblay CL. Association between HIV infection, antiretroviral therapy, and risk of acute myocardial infarction: a cohort and nested case-control study using Québec's public health insurance database. *J Acquir Immune Defic Syndr.* 2011;57(3):245-253.

Echouffo Tcheugui JB, Guan J, Fu L, Retnakaran R, Shah BR. Association of concomitant gestational hypertensive disorders and gestational diabetes with cardiovascular disease. *JAMA Netw Open.* 2022;5(11):e2243618.

El-Qushayri AE, Dahy A, Benmelouka AY, Kamel AMA. The effect of COVID-19 on the in-hospital outcomes of percutaneous coronary intervention in patients with acute coronary syndrome: a large scale meta-analysis. *Am J Med Open.* 2023;100032.

Gevaert SA, Halvorsen S, Sinnaeve PR, et al. Evaluation and management of cancer patients presenting with acute cardiovascular disease: a Consensus Document of the Acute CardioVascular Care (ACVC) association and the ESC council of Cardio-Oncology-Part 1: acute coronary syndromes and acute pericardial diseases. *Eur Heart J Acute Cardiovasc Care.* 2021;10(8):947-959.

Go AS, Chertow GM, Fan D, McCulloch CE, Hsu C-Y. Chronic kidney disease and the risks of death, cardiovascular events, and hospitalization [published correction appears in N Engl J Med. 2008;18(4):4]. *N Engl J Med.* 2004;351(13):1296-1305.

Hansson GK, Robertson A-KL, Söderberg-Nauclér C. Inflammation and atherosclerosis. *Annu Rev Pathol.* 2006;1:297-329.

Jalnapurkar S, Xu KH, Zhang Z, Bairey Merz CN, Elkayam U, Pai RG. Changing incidence and mechanism of pregnancy-associated myocardial infarction in the State of California. *J Am Heart Assoc.* 2021;10(21):e021056.

James AH, Jamison MG, Biswas MS, Brancazio LR, Swamy GK, Myers ER. Acute myocardial infarction in pregnancy: a United States population-based study. *Circulation.* 2006;113(12):1564-1571.

Kang S, Han K, Jung J-H, et al. Associations between cardiovascular outcomes and rheumatoid arthritis: a nationwide population-based cohort study. *J Clin Med.* 2022;11(22):6812.

Koene RJ, Prizment AE, Blaes A, Konety SH. Shared risk factors in cardiovascular disease and cancer. *Circulation.* 2016;133(11):1104-1114.

Lai AC, Bienstock SW, Sharma R, et al. A personalized approach to chronic kidney disease and cardiovascular disease: JACC review topic of the week. *J Am Coll Cardiol.* 2021; 77(11):1470-1479.

Lima MAC, Brito HRA, Mitidieri GG, et al. Cardiotoxicity in cancer patients treated with chemotherapy: a systematic review. *Int J Health Sci (Qassim).* 2022;16(6):39-46.

Long B, Yoo MJ, Brady WJ, Holian A, Sudhir A, Gottlieb M. Chimeric antigen receptor T-cell therapy: an emergency medicine focused review. *Am J Emerg Med.* 2021;50:369-375.

Lucà F, Parrini I, Abrignani MG, et al. Management of acute coronary syndrome in cancer patients: it's high time we dealt with it. *J Clin Med.* 2022;11(7):1792.

Niccoli G, Altamura L, Fabretti A, et al. Ethanol abolishes ischemic preconditioning in humans. *J Am Coll Cardiol.* 2008;51(3):271-275.

O'Kelly AC, Ludmir J, Wood MJ. Acute coronary syndrome in pregnancy and the post-partum period. *J Cardiovasc Dev Dis.* 2022;9(7):198.

Pennefather C, Esterhuizen T, Doubell A, Decloedt EH. The 12-month period prevalence and cardiac manifestations of HIV in patients with acute coronary syndrome at a tertiary hospital in Cape Town, South Africa: a retrospective cross-sectional study. *BMC Infect Dis.* 2021;21(1):657.

Pitsavos C, Makrilakis K, Panagiotakos DB, et al. The J-shape effect of alcohol intake on the risk of developing acute coronary syndromes in diabetic subjects: the CARDIO2000 II Study. *Diabet Med.* 2005;22(3):243-248.

Roule V, Verdier L, Blanchart K, et al. Systematic review and meta-analysis of the prognostic impact of cancer among patients with acute coronary syndrome and/or percutaneous coronary intervention. *BMC Cardiovasc Disord.* 2020;20(1):38.

Sarnak MJ, Amann K, Bangalore S, et al. Chronic kidney disease and coronary artery disease: JACC state-of-the-art review. *J Am Coll Cardiol.* 2019;74(14):1823-1838.

Seecheran VK, Giddings SL, Seecheran NA. Acute coronary syndromes in patients with HIV. *Coron Artery Dis.* 2017;28(2):166-172.

Shibata T, Kawakami S, Noguchi T, et al. Prevalence, clinical features, and prognosis of acute myocardial infarction attributable to coronary artery embolism. *Circulation.* 2015;132(4): 241-250.

Smilowitz NR, Gupta N, Guo Y, et al. Acute myocardial infarction during pregnancy and the puerperium in the United States. *Mayo Clin Proc.* 2018;93(10):1404-1414.

Tersalvi G, Biasco L, Radovanovic D, et al. Heavy drinking habits are associated with worse in-hospital outcomes in patients with acute coronary syndrome: an insight from the AMIS plus registry. *Cardiology.* 2020;145(12):757-765.

Varas-Lorenzo C, Rodriguez LA, Maguire A, Castellsague J, Perez-Gutthann S. Use of oral corticosteroids and the risk of acute myocardial infarction. *Atherosclerosis.* 2007;192(2): 376-383.

Wassif H, Saad M, Desai R, et al. Outcomes following acute coronary syndrome in patients with and without rheumatic immune-mediated inflammatory diseases. *J Am Heart Assoc.* 2022;11(18):e026411.

Yoo MJ, Long B, Brady WJ, Holian A, Sudhir A, Gottlieb M. Immune checkpoint inhibitors: an emergency medicine focused review. *Am J Emerg Med.* 2021;50:335-344.

68

BE AGGRESSIVE WITH NITROGLYCERIN IN ACUTE CARDIOGENIC PULMONARY EDEMA

JAKOB OTTENHOFF AND GUSTAVO CARMEN LOPEZ

Acute heart failure is a common cause of presentation to the ED and accounts for a massive burden on the US healthcare system, with greater than one million hospital admissions in the United States every year. Traditional teaching suggests that progressive fluid retention from dietary factors and medication noncompliance leads to retention in the extravascular spaces resulting in signs and symptoms of clinical heart failure. The subsequent peripheral and pulmonary edema results in progressive dyspnea. Therefore, treatment strategies for acute decompensated heart failure have emphasized fluid restriction and diuresis to target the suggested underlying pathophysiology while using NIPPV and preload reduction as temporizing measures.

However, a second phenotype of acute cardiogenic pulmonary edema has been suggested in addition to the classic fluid overload syndrome. In this second scenario, an acute rise in the systemic vascular resistance leads to an increase in the LV filling pressure. While a healthy LV adjusts to a wide range of afterload presentations, an LV hampered by systolic and/or diastolic dysfunction has a narrower range of afterload that it can accommodate. The resulting LV function and afterload mismatch causes a rapid backflow of fluid into the pulmonary circulation and subsequent pulmonary edema. This mismatch is further exacerbated as decreased LV cardiac output leads to organ hypoperfusion, triggering a sympathetic response resulting in more vasoconstriction. A rapid cycle of deterioration ensues as the LV is unable to compensate for this increase in afterload and fluid is rapidly redistributed. In addition, the increase in sympathetic tone results in redistribution of fluid from vascular beds such as the splanchnic circulation to the pulmonary circulation. This manifests as acute pulmonary edema without evidence of significant peripheral edema. Patients present clinically with severe sudden dyspnea, marked hypertension, and scant peripheral edema; the constellation of symptoms is known as SCAPE.

Although both entities are caused by underlying heart failure, the distinction is important as they necessitate different treatment strategies. Targeting euvolemia through fluid restriction and diuresis in patients with SCAPE is unlikely to be successful as these patients may not be significantly fluid overloaded and the effects of diuretics have a delayed onset. A successful strategy focuses on rapid reduction of both preload and afterload, which are the underlying pathologic triggers. NIPPV can help reduce preload, but HDN more directly targets the malignant pathophysiology.

Nitroglycerin affects the vascular system by causing the release of nitric oxide, which results in relaxation of smooth muscle cells in the vessels. Low-dose nitroglycerin reduces preload by relaxing the smooth muscles of the venous vasculature in acute heart failure exacerbations and relieves anginal pain in acute coronary syndrome. In this setting, nitroglycerin is typically administered intravenously between 5 and 100 mcg/min, titrated to alleviate symptoms such as anginal chest pain. However, at rates greater than

250 mcg/min, nitroglycerin affects the arterial circulation, relaxing smooth muscle and reducing systemic vascular resistance. Thus HDN is an ideal therapeutic agent for patients with SCAPE as it targets both preload and afterload.

While there are no large prospective randomized trials comparing the use of HDN to standard therapy for acute treatment of SCAPE, there is a sizable body of literature demonstrating its efficacy and safety in this patient population. Studies have shown a decreased use of NIPPV, endotracheal intubation, ICU admission, and hospital length of stay with use of HDN versus standard care in cardiogenic pulmonary edema. There were no differences in complication rates, including hypotension, myocardial infarction, and worsening renal function. Continuous infusion at rates of HDN at 100 to 400 mcg/min, in contrast to bolus doses, has been shown to be safe and effective.

Cardiogenic pulmonary edema is a life-threatening presentation of acutely decompensated heart failure that requires prompt diagnosis and treatment and is distinct from the hypervolemic phenotype of heart failure. HDN terminates the cycle of LV function and afterload mismatch that shifts fluid into the pulmonary circulation and results in rapid pulmonary edema. Literature to date has clearly demonstrated the safety of HDN, and recent cardiovascular society guidelines have begun to endorse this approach. This strategy targets the underlying pathophysiology and should be used aggressively in patients with SCAPE given the high risk of cardiovascular collapse.

PEARLS

- Cardiogenic pulmonary edema is a life-threatening clinical entity that requires prompt recognition and management to prevent cardiovascular collapse.
- SCAPE is not typically a result of severe volume overload but caused by increased sympathetic tone and markedly increased afterload. These patients may actually be euvolemic.
- HDN is an ideal agent for the treatment of SCAPE as it exerts vasodilatory effects on both the arterial and venous circulation and more accurately targets the underlying pathophysiology.
- HDN is effective at decreasing ICU admissions, intubations, and length of stay. More importantly, it has been shown to be safe when compared to standard of care.

Suggested Readings

Bhatt DL, Lopes RD, Harrington RA. Diagnosis and treatment of acute coronary syndromes: a review [published correction appears in *JAMA*. 2022;327(17):1710]. *JAMA*. 2022;327(7):662-675. PMID: 35166796.

Heidenreich PA, Bozkurt B, Aguilar D, et al. 2022 AHA/ACC/HFSA guideline for the management of heart failure: a report of the American College of Cardiology/American Heart Association Joint Committee on Clinical Practice Guidelines. *Circulation*. 2022;145:e895-e1032.

Houseman BS, Martinelli AN, Oliver WD. High-dose nitroglycerin infusion description of safety and efficacy in sympathetic crashing acute pulmonary edema: the HI-DOSE SCAPE study. *Am J Emerg Med*. 2023;63:74-78. PMID: 36327753.

Lang RM, Goldstein SA, Kronzon I, Khandheria BK, Saric M, Mor-Avi V. *ASE's Comprehensive Echocardiography*. Elsevier, Inc; 2022.

McDonagh TA, Metra M, Adamo M; ESC Scientific Document Group. 2021 ESC guidelines for the diagnosis and treatment of acute and chronic heart failure [published correction appears in *Eur Heart J*. 2021;42(48):4901]. *Eur Heart J*. 2021;42(36):3599-3726. PMID: 34447992.

Wang K, Samai K. Role of high-dose intravenous nitrates in hypertensive acute heart failure. *Am J Emerg Med*. 2020;38(1):132-137. PMID: 31327485.

Wilson SS, Kwiatkowski GM, Millis SR. Use of nitroglycerin by bolus prevents intensive care unit admission in patients with acute hypertensive heart failure. *Am J Emerg Med*. 2017;35(1):126-131. PMID: 27825693.

69

WHEN GOOD VADs GO BAD

WILLIAM J. BRADY

With the development of the VAD, patients with end-stage cardiac failure have an increased survival rate and improved quality of life. The LVAD is the most common VAD in clinical practice, though a RVAD and a BiVAD are also available. Within the first year after implantation, one-third of patients have experienced complications or device malfunctions; approximately 80% will have such an adverse event by the end of the third year. With this high rate of complication, it is imperative for the EP to have a general awareness and understanding of VADs. Early consultation with VAD specialists is strongly encouraged.

Two basic pump types are encountered. The pulsatile pump, the earlier of the two models, produces a stroke volume that mimics systole; these pumps usually have a fixed stroke volume with a variable heart rate. The continuous flow pump, the most common type, is easier to implant, smaller in size, and quieter. It uses a central rotor without valves, producing continuous flow in non-physiologic manner yet providing better organ perfusion.

The LVAD system (**Figure 69.1**), regardless of the type, is composed of several common components, including the inflow cannula, pumping chamber, outflow cannula, percutaneous driveline, system controller, and power source. The percutaneous driveline, a frequent source of device-related infection, connects the pumping circuit to the system controller and power source. The system controller is the "brain" of the system, providing direction for function as well as an interface with the patient and healthcare team.

The ED evaluation of a patient on LVAD should begin with assessment of the patient's ABCs. Check for an audible hum, indicating that the device is functioning; the absence of an audible hum suggests dysfunction and the need for rapid assessment and resuscitation. The cardiac rhythm should be considered and viewed via standard electrocardiographic monitoring. Altered techniques are required to assess pulse and blood pressure. Current devices deliver a continuous flow and thus an absent pulse. The MAP should be used for BP assessment; the MAP can be obtained with a blood pressure cuff and Doppler ultrasound over the brachial or radial artery. The target range for MAP in patients on VAD is 70 to 90 mm Hg. End-tidal CO_2 should be measured; interpretation is the same in the patient on VAD. It is also important to evaluate additional signs of peripheral perfusion, such as mental status and skin color and warmth. Inspect the percutaneous driveline for evidence of infection. Additional information from the VAD that should be included in the initial assessment are the speed, flow, power, battery life of the device, and any alerts; these values are found in the system controller of the LVAD.

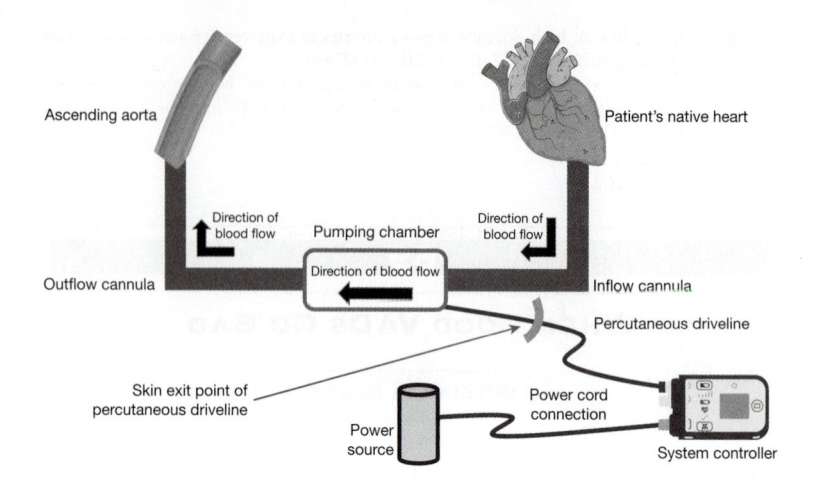

FIGURE 69.1 LVAD system.

Atrial or ventricular dysrhythmias occur in up to 50% of patients; it is important to obtain an ECG in most patients on VAD. Patients on VAD who are unstable due to a dysrhythmia should be managed appropriately, including cardioversion or defibrillation, if indicated. It is recommended to place the defibrillation pads in an anterior and posterior position. Stable patients on VAD with concerning dysrhythmias can receive antiarrhythmic medications and electrical therapy. Malignant dysrhythmias, such as ventricular fibrillation or ventricular tachycardia, should be managed expeditiously, even if the patient appears to be tolerating them. Patients can also receive intravenous fluids, if necessary.

Echo can be used to evaluate for pump thrombosis, RV failure, and "suction" events. Pump thrombus occurs in up to 2% of patients within 2 years after implantation; it reduces cardiac output, resulting in increased pump power readings. Patients on VAD with suspected thrombosis should receive anticoagulation with heparin. Acute RV failure can occur in up to 25% of patients and is usually seen soon after implantation. VADs are preload-sensitive and in low-flow states; the negative pressure produced by the VAD can cause leftward displacement of the intraventricular septum, producing a "suction" event. Suction events usually result from hypovolemia, but they can also occur with cardiac tamponade, dysrhythmias, and malposition of the inflow cannula. Initial management of a suction event includes intravenous fluids and echo with urgent consultation.

Bleeding occurs in up to 40% of patients on VAD. All patients on VAD are placed on anticoagulant and antiplatelet medications to decrease the rate of thromboembolic events. In addition, these patients develop an acquired von Willebrand syndrome in response to shear forces from the VAD. Finally, the decreased pulse pressure of the continuous flow contributes to arteriovenous malformations. Patients on VAD who are unstable due to hemorrhage should receive blood products and agents to reverse anticoagulation. Anticoagulation reversal in a stable patient on VAD, however, should be done in consultation with the device specialist.

Patients on VAD are at high risk for infection that can occur anywhere along the VAD including the surgical site, driveline, pump, or device pocket. VAD infections can be caused by a variety of organisms, including gram-positive organisms, gram-negative organisms, and fungi. Critically ill patients on VAD should receive broad-spectrum antibiotics.

Patients on VAD may present in cardiac arrest. In these patients, the controller should be quickly evaluated for battery life and proper connections. If available, echo can be evaluated for pericardial effusion, LV function, or RV dilatation. Chest compressions can be initiated if necessary; caution is advised in that dislodgement of the inflow cannula can occur.

PEARLS

- Contact the patient's VAD coordinator as soon as possible.
- Obtain an ECG early to evaluate for dysrhythmias.
- Consider bleeding and sepsis in any critically ill patient on VAD.
- Use echo to assess for pump thrombosis, RV failure, and suction events in the Patient on VAD.
- CPR is reasonable in cardiac arrest in the patient on VAD.

SUGGESTED READINGS

Long B, Robertson J, Koyfman A, Brady W. Left ventricular assist devices and their complications: a review for emergency clinicians. *Am J Emerg Med.* 2019;37:1562-1570.

Pratt AK, Shah NS, Boyce SW. Left ventricular assist device management in the ICU. *Crit Care Med.* 2014;42:158-168.

70

THE MYOCARDITIS MASQUERADE

TENNESSEE PARK AND JOSHUA EASTER

Myocarditis arises from inflammation of the myocardium. It is a challenging diagnosis, as it mimics multiple other conditions commonly encountered in the ED. Its underlying pathophysiology can be infectious, immune mediated, or toxic. The true prevalence of myocarditis is likely significantly higher than published estimates. The gold standard for diagnosis is endomyocardial biopsy, which is highly invasive and not routinely performed, thereby leading to underestimation of the incidence. Moreover, the incidence of myocarditis appears to have risen in the setting of COVID infection and vaccination. Myocarditis most frequently afflicts young adult males.

CLINICAL PRESENTATION

The presentation of myocarditis is highly variable, ranging from asymptomatic to cardiogenic shock. It often mimics other conditions and commonly entails a preceding nonspecific prodrome with malaise, fever, cough, nausea, and diarrhea (**Table 70.1**). The most common symptom is shortness of breath. Less commonly, patients report chest pain, which may be exertional or pleuritic. Other possible presentations of myocarditis include syncope or sudden cardiac death. In the subacute phase (>2 weeks after symptom onset), patients may have only nonspecific symptoms, such as fatigue, myalgias, or palpitations.

Table 70.1	Myocarditis often resembles more common conditions
Clinical Mimic	**Symptoms of Myocarditis**
Respiratory tract infection	Fever
	Malaise
	Cough
	Shortness of breath
Gastroenteritis	Vomiting
	Diarrhea
Acute coronary syndrome	Chest pain
	Shortness of breath
Arrhythmia	Fatigue
	Palpitations
Heart failure	Shortness of breath
	Peripheral edema
	Hepatomegaly
Vasovagal syncope	Lightheadedness
	Loss of consciousness

Diagnosis

Myocarditis is a diagnostic challenge, and the diagnosis is often missed or delayed. Clinicians should consider myocarditis in the differential for patients with:

- Infectious symptoms (eg, fever) and chest pain
- New and unexpected heart failure (eg, young adults)
- Persistent and unexplained tachycardia

Criteria have been proposed for diagnosing myocarditis, which include a clinical presentation consistent with myocarditis and relevant findings on ECG/telemetry, troponin testing, echocardiogram, angiography, or cardiac magnetic resonance imaging. While no single test or laboratory finding can rule out myocarditis, the combination of a normal troponin, CRP, and BNP substantially reduces the likelihood of myocarditis. Potential diagnostic clues include (**Table 70.2**):

Table 70.2	Diagnostic accuracy of various tests for myocarditis
Test	**Sensitivity (%)**
Abnormal ECG	47
Troponin I	34
Troponin T	53
BNP	50
CRP	78
Chest radiograph	20
Echocardiogram	69
Cardiac MRI	88

BNP, brain natriuretic peptide; CRP, C-reactive protein; ECG, electrocardiogram; MRI, magnetic resonance imaging.

- ECG—Nonspecific ST-segment or T-wave changes; patients may also have ischemic changes and tachy—or brady—arrhythmias.
- Troponin—Moderately sensitive and high-sensitivity troponin might be better.
- BNP—Elevations should increase suspicion for myocarditis.
- CRP or ESR—Might be elevated but not sensitive.
- Chest radiograph—Can be normal or have cardiomegaly, pulmonary edema, and effusions.
- Bedside echocardiogram—Can have depressed ventricular function, wall motion abnormalities, or pericardial effusions.
- CT—Might show delayed contrast enhancement.
- MRI—Most sensitive and specific noninvasive evaluation for myocarditis.

Importantly, regardless of which tests suggest myocarditis, *there must also be an absence of both angiographically detectable coronary artery disease, preexisting cardiovascular disease, or extra-cardiac causes that could explain the syndrome* (eg, valvular disease or congenital heart disease). Consequently, the definitive diagnosis of myocarditis is unlikely to occur in the ED.

TREATMENT

The treatment of myocarditis is primarily supportive and, therefore, depends on the presentation. This is helpful for clinicians in the ED, as therapy can be initiated before the definitive diagnosis is made. Potential therapies based on the clinical presentation include:

- Heart failure—Patients presenting with heart failure may require standard heart failure therapy, including diuretics and vasodilators.
- Arrhythmias—Amiodarone or cardioversion is appropriate for tachyarrhythmias. Beta-blockers should typically be avoided in patients with concomitant acute heart failure.
- Rescue measures—For critically ill patients that fail to improve with the aforementioned therapies, consider ECMO.
- Activity restrictions—Patients who are discharged should typically avoid exertion initially.

Other therapies should be administered in consultation with a cardiologist. In the ED, the etiology for the myocarditis is often unknown, and it is challenging to initiate these therapies. These potential therapies include:

- Immunosuppression—Only certain subtypes might benefit from such therapies.
- Antiviral drugs—These remain experimental.
- Immunoglobulin—In the pediatric population, immunoglobulin therapy may have a beneficial effect, although evidence is limited.
- Cardiac transplant—This tends to be reserved for patients with chronic myocarditis and cardiac dysfunction.

Importantly, murine models of NSAID therapy for myocarditis have demonstrated worsened mortality. Therefore, NSAIDs should be avoided.

PROGNOSIS

The prognosis for acute myocarditis varies. In patients presenting with mild symptoms and no left ventricular dysfunction, most (75%) will resolve completely in 2 to 4 weeks. However, others will experience persistent cardiac dysfunction or progression after the initial presentation. Overall, there are no definite clinical criteria to predict prognosis, and patients should follow up with a cardiologist.

For the emergency medicine physician suspecting myocarditis, a reasonable diagnostic and treatment algorithm is demonstrated in **Figure 70.1**.

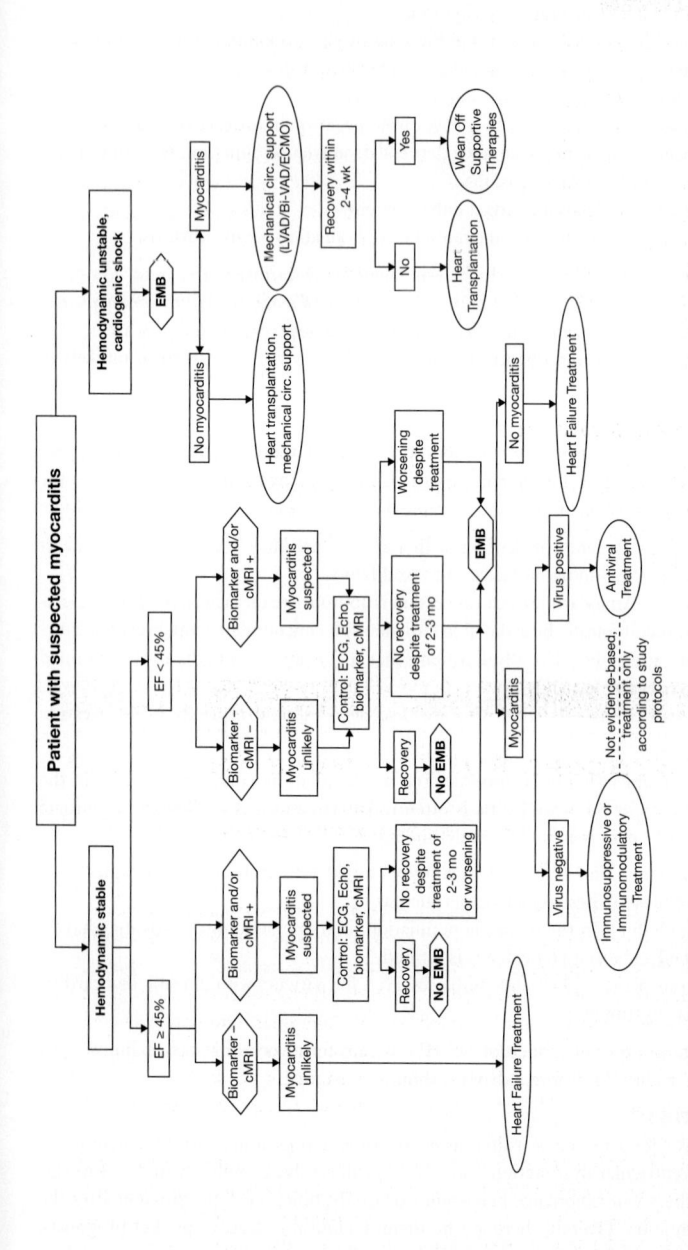

FIGURE 70.1 Consensus based diagnostic and therapeutic algorithm for myocarditis. Bi-VAD, biventricular assist device; cMRI, cardiac magnetic resonance imaging; ECG, electrocardiogram; Echo, echocardiography; ECMO, extracorporeal membrane oxygenation; EF, ejection fraction; EMB, endomyocardial biopsy; LVAD, left ventricular assist device. (Reprinted from Kindermann I, Barth C, Mahfoud F, et al. Update on myocarditis. *J Am Coll Cardiol.* 2012;59(9):779-792, Figure 5, with permission from Elsevier. Copyright © 2012 American College of Cardiology Foundation. Published by Elsevier Inc. All rights reserved.)

PEARLS

- Myocarditis commonly presents with nonspecific symptoms, such as shortness of breath, fatigue, or chest pain. It often mimics other clinical entities such as heart failure, ACS, and cardiac arrhythmias.
- Myocarditis should be included in the differential of unexplained and persistent tachycardia, unanticipated heart failure, or fever and chest pain.
- No single bedside finding or laboratory test can rule out myocarditis, but the combination of a normal troponin, CRP, BNP, and ECG reduces the likelihood.
- Management in the ED depends on the severity of symptoms and includes standard therapy for the presenting issues (eg, arrhythmia, shock, etc).
- Suspected myocarditis typically warrants consultation or follow-up with a cardiologist.

Suggested Readings

Basso C. Myocarditis. *New Engl J Med*. 2022;387(16):1488-1500.
Dancea AB. Myocarditis in infants and children: a review for the paediatrician. *Paediatr Child Health*. 2001;6(8):543-545.
Kindermann I, Barth C, Mahfoud F, et al. Update on myocarditis. *J Am Coll Cardiol*. 2012;59(9):779-792.

71

ONE SYNCOPE RULE TO RULE THEM ALL?

VANESSA KHOURY AND HEATHER LOUNSBURY

Syncope is a self-limited transient episode of loss of consciousness and postural tone that is a result of global cerebral hypoperfusion. It accounts for 3% of ED visits with up to half of these patients requiring hospitalization. The initial ED evaluation fails to uncover an apparent cause in at least half of patients presenting with syncope and makes accurate risk assessment a common challenge. Up to one-quarter of patients with unexplained syncope experience an adverse event within the next 30 days including cardiac arrhythmia, myocardial infarction, and death. At least nine syncope decision rules have been developed to assist in risk-stratifying patients with unexplained syncope and help guide disposition.

The SFSR assesses the risk of serious outcomes at 7 days post syncope and emphasizes the importance of an abnormal ECG and congestive heart failure in risk stratification. It is the most thoroughly investigated prediction rule for syncope. Although sensitivity in the initial derivation study was found to be 98%, this high level of sensitivity has not been replicated in external validation studies.

The CSRS assesses the 30-day risk of serious adverse events following syncope. High-risk factors include an abnormal ECG, a history of heart disease, and an elevated troponin. The CSRS has been externally validated on several patient cohorts both in Canada and internationally and, on systemic review, accurately stratifies low- and high-risk patients.

The ROSE Risk Score for syncope predicts 1-month serious outcomes and all-cause death. It was one of the first scores to incorporate BNP as a major risk stratification tool. Although it has high negative predictive value for low-risk patients, it has not accurately identified high-risk patients.

The FAINT Score predicts the 30-day risk of serious cardiac outcome post syncope. Unlike other scores, it was designed for patients above the age of 60 and focuses on predicting the risk of death and serious cardiac outcomes as opposed to all serious clinical outcomes. This score relies on cardiac biomarkers for risk stratification and suggests that an elevated NT-proBNP should be considered a strong clinical predictor of serious cardiac outcomes. It has not been externally validated.

The OESIL Score for syncope estimates the 12-month all-cause mortality. This score suggests considering outpatient evaluation for low-risk patients and admission for intermediate- to high-risk patients. Two validation cohorts have shown similar patterns of increasing mortality with increasing scores. However, on systemic review, this score lacked accuracy and subsequent validations were not able to reproduce similar results.

Although each decision rule has its limitations, several common themes for a greater risk of adverse outcomes post-syncope emerge. These include an abnormal ECG on presentation and a history of heart disease, particularly structural heart disease. Evidence-based guidelines published by the ACEP recommend admitting patients with acute decompensated heart failure or structural heart disease, as well as those with high-risk features such as age, certain ECG patterns, a cardiac history, hemoglobin less than 9 g/dL, sinus bradycardia, and lowest systolic blood pressure in the ED less than 90 mm Hg.

Some proposed reasons that these rules have yielded inconsistent results in validation studies include the vague definition of the patient population and lack of a clear definition of "abnormal ECG." When applying these scores, several caveats should be maintained: patients should reflect the population in which these scores were studied; ECG stratification may be subjective; and clinician judgment plays a vital role in the final decision. Emergency clinicians have excellent judgment regarding patient risk but still admit close to 30% of those who they consider low risk for adverse outcomes. Risk stratification scores play a valuable role in guiding disposition, especially in resource-limited settings.

The following approach to a patient with syncope is proposed. If the initial ED evaluation, including history, physical exam, ECG, and indicated diagnostic tests, reveals a clear cause of syncope, then disposition is determined based on the severity of the diagnosis. However, if the cause of syncope is unexplained, clinicians may use syncope scores, the ACEP syncope policy, or the presence of high-risk factors (**Table 71.1**) to risk-stratify patients for hospital admission. Low-risk patients who remain asymptomatic could be discharged with appropriate follow-up. Intermediate-risk patient disposition may depend on the availability of hospital resources (eg, consultants and observation unit beds) and whether timely outpatient follow-up can be arranged. High-risk patients should be admitted for further evaluation and close monitoring.

TABLE 71.1	HIGH-RISK FACTORS
Characteristics of syncope	During exertion, supine, with chest discomfort or dyspnea, preceded by palpitations
Patient history	Family history of sudden death, history of cardiac disease
Variables, symptoms, signs	Age >40, Hgb <9, lowest ED SBP <90 mm Hg, sinus bradycardia (<40 beats/min)
ECG findings	New or previously unknown left bundle branch block, new non-sinus rhythm, prolonged QTC, acute ischemia, Brugada pattern, bifascicular block with or without prolonged PR interval

ECG, electrocardiogram; ED, emergency department; Hgb, hemoglobin; SBP, systolic blood pressure.

PEARLS

- Each syncope rule has its limitations, and guidelines do not recommend any single decision rule.
- Use syncope scores in patients with unexplained syncope to risk-stratify patients.
- Syncope rules should be used as an adjunct to clinician judgment and not in isolation.
- Admit patients with syncope who have an abnormal ECG, heart failure, or structural heart disease.
- Syncope rules may play a more important role in the disposition of low-risk patients rather than determining high-risk patients and may be even more valuable in settings with limited hospital resources.

Suggested Readings

Safari S, Khasraghi ZS, Chegeni MA, Ghabousian A, Amini A. The ability of Canadian Syncope risk score in differentiating cardiogenic and non-cardiogenic syncope: a cross-sectional study. *Am J Emerg Med*. 2021;50:675-678.

Serrano LA, Hess EP, Bellolio MF, et al. Accuracy and quality of clinical decision rules for syncope in the emergency department: a systematic review and meta-analysis. *Ann Emerg Med*. 2010;56(4):362-373.e1.

Sweanor RA, Redelmeier RJ, Simel DL, Albassam OT, Shadowitz S, Etchells EE. Multivariable risk scores for predicting short-term outcomes for emergency department patients with unexplained syncope: a systematic review. *Acad Emerg Med*. 2021;28:502-510.

Werline L, Young A. Multicenter emergency department validation of the Canadian Syncope Risk Score. *J Emerg Med*. 2020;58(6):981.

SECTION V
GASTROENTEROLOGY

72

CAN APPENDICITIS BE TREATED WITH ANTIBIOTICS ALONE?

CLARE ROEPKE

Appendicitis is estimated to occur in 75 per 100,000 of the population per year. It occurs most commonly in patients 10 to 19 years of age and remains the most frequent cause of abdominal pain in children over the age of one, as well as the most common non-obstetric surgical emergency in pregnancy.

Traditionally, patients with a diagnosis of acute uncomplicated appendicitis require an immediate surgical consult for appendectomy. A nonoperative approach to acute appendicitis has typically been reserved for patients too sick or too high risk for emergent surgery. However, a nonoperative approach to appendicitis using antibiotics alone may be preferred and appropriate for a subset of patients.

WHICH PATIENTS ARE NOT APPROPRIATE FOR AN ANTIBIOTIC ALONE MANAGEMENT STRATEGY?

Antibiotic treatment alone for acute appendicitis is not recommended for patients with signs of sepsis, shock, peritonitis, those who are immunocompromised or pregnant, children less than 18 years of age, and adults older than 60 years. It is also not recommended for patients with the following radiologic features: fecalith, abscess, phlegmon, ascites, free air, or neoplasm.

WHICH PATIENTS MAY BE APPROPRIATE FOR ANTIBIOTICS ALONE?

Antibiotic treatment alone without surgical intervention is common in inflammatory conditions such as diverticulitis, neonatal enterocolitis, and salpingitis. The findings of recent randomized controlled trials suggest that up to 70% of patients with a first presentation of acute uncomplicated appendicitis could be treated with antibiotics alone. Other studies have suggested that up to 40% of those patients treated with antibiotics alone may have disease recurrence and require surgery within 5 years. It is, therefore, suggested that those patients deemed low risk (between the ages of 18 and 60 who do not have the complicating clinical or radiologic features in appendicitis as noted earlier) be counseled by their surgeon on surgical intervention compared with antibiotics alone in a shared decision-making process.

Pediatric Considerations

The current recommendation for children younger than 18 years with a diagnosis of appendicitis remains the same: appendectomy. Although antibiotics alone for acute uncomplicated appendicitis may be effective in adults, their use in pediatric patients remains controversial.

Antibiotic Treatment of Choice

Patients who are good candidates for antibiotics alone should be admitted and receive intravenous antibiotics for the first 24 to 72 hours. During this period, they should be monitored clinically for deterioration or worsening pain. Antibiotics should cover aerobic and anaerobic gram-negative organisms. Possible regimens include ampicillin/sulbactam, piperacillin/tazobactam, cefoxitin, or a combination of metronidazole plus ciprofloxacin.

PEARLS

- Managing appendicitis with antibiotics alone has been shown to be non-inferior to appendectomy in a subset of patients who are at low risk.
- Up to 40% of patients treated with antibiotics alone may have disease recurrence and require surgery within 5 years.
- Antibiotic treatment alone is not recommended for patients with signs of sepsis or shock, peritonitis, those who are immunocompromised or pregnant, children younger than 18 years, and adults older than 60.
- Antibiotic treatment alone is not recommended for patients with a fecalith, abscess, phlegmon, ascites, free air, or neoplasm on imaging.
- Antibiotics alone for acute, uncomplicated appendicitis in children remain controversial.

Suggested Readings

CODA Collaborative; Flum DR, Davidson GH, Monsell SE, et al. A randomized trial comparing antibiotics with appendectomy for appendicitis. *N Engl J Med.* 2020;383(20): 1907-1919. PMID: 33017106.

DeKoning E. Acute appendicitis. In: Tintinalli JE, Ma O, Yealy DM, Meckler GD, Stapczynski J, Cline DM, Thomas SH, eds. *Tintinalli's Emergency Medicine: A Comprehensive Study Guide.* 9th ed. McGraw Hill; 2020. Accessed February 15, 2023. https://accessmedicine-mhmedical-com.libproxy.temple.edu/content.aspx?bookid=2353&sectionid=206322423

Farooq A, Rouleau-Fournier F, Brown C. Antibiotics alone in the treatment of appendicitis. *CMAJ.* 2021;193(21):E769. PMID: 34035057.

Huang L, Yin Y, Yang L, Wang C, Li Y, Zhou Z. Comparison of antibiotic therapy and appendectomy for acute uncomplicated appendicitis in children: a meta-analysis. *JAMA Pediatr.* 2017;171(5):426-434. PMID: 28346589.

73

Don't Underestimate an Acute Variceal Hemorrhage!

Lee Plantmason

UGIB results from a variety of conditions that can vary from annoying to life threatening. The determination of nonvariceal versus variceal bleeding is critical as the tests and treatments vary depending on the etiology. AVH is the most common etiology of UGIB in patients with cirrhosis. It accounts for roughly 50% of cases and is associated with a mortality rate as high as 20%. Cirrhosis causes fibrotic changes in the hepatic parenchyma that decrease hepatic vascular compliance and increase portal vascular resistance. This, in turn, leads to dilatation of collateral vessels located at the gastroesophageal junction, that is, varices.

Presentation

Patients with a history of alcohol abuse, known cirrhosis, or a history of varices presenting with a UGIB should be presumed to have variceal bleeding and treated as such. Initial history taking should focus on the amount and route of hemorrhage. For hematemesis, is it coffee-ground or bright red? For blood by rectum, is it melena or hematochezia? Ask about other risk factors for UGIB such as a history of gastric/esophageal varices, use of anticoagulants and NSAIDs, and other comorbidities that may affect the patient's ability to cope with acute blood loss. Symptoms of chest pain, shortness of breath, pallor, decreased urine output, or confusion may portend worsening end-organ perfusion and shock.

Stabilization

Given their potential to decompensate quickly, patients require large-bore intravenous access and close monitoring. Large-volume hematemesis, altered mental status, and hemodynamic instability are indications for early airway management due to risks of aspiration and to facilitate endoscopy. Circulatory collapse in the case of a brisk hemorrhage should be addressed with crystalloids and blood products with a target hemoglobin greater than 7 g/dL (potentially higher transfusion targets for those at risk of end-organ dysfunction). Plasma or PCC and platelets should be given to correct coagulopathy with a goal INR less than 1.8 and platelets greater than 50,000. However, in rapid blood loss, there will be significant delay in the fall of the measured hemoglobin concentration, so treat the patient's hemodynamic and perfusion status, not the numbers from the laboratory!

Laboratory studies may include complete blood count (blood loss, platelets), coagulation factors (hepatic synthetic function), liver function tests (indication of hepatic dysfunction), basic metabolic panel (elevated BUN from blood in the alimentary canal and renal function), creatinine (renal function), and type and cross (transfusion). Bedside tests such as NGL and stool guaiac testing have classically been utilized in assessing an upper GI bleed. The utility of NGL, however, is questionable in all but the most severe cases of UGIB, and it causes great discomfort to patients.

TREATMENT

Pharmacologic interventions for variceal bleeding include the use of PPIs, somatostatin analogues (octreotide), and antibiotics (ceftriaxone). PPIs are commonly used empirically in the cirrhotic with UGIB because brisk bleeding from peptic ulcer disease is also quite common. Current guidelines recommend a bolus of 80 mg of pantoprazole with an infusion of 8 mg/h, but a recent meta-analysis in 2014 showed that intermittent bolus dosing was noninferior to bolus plus infusion for bleeding ulcers. Somatostatin analogues (namely, octreotide in the United States) are recommended to treat variceal bleeds to reduce portal hypertension. Octreotide is given as a bolus dose of 25 to 50 mcg IV with an infusion of 25 to 50 mcg/h. To date, studies show an increased rate of early hemostasis and 5-day hemostasis but no change in adverse events nor a decrease in mortality. Prophylactic antibiotics (commonly ceftriaxone 2 g IV) should be given to all acute variceal bleeds because they confer a mortality benefit in addition to decreasing rebleeding and hospital length of stay.

CONSULTATION AND DISPOSITION

Early consultation with the gastroenterology service is recommended for immediate endoscopy, given that only 50% of variceal bleeding will stop on its own. Most patients with AVH will require ICU admission: Indications include the need for emergent endoscopy, hemodynamic instability or altered mental status, evidence of active bleeding (hematemesis or large bloody lavage), or significant comorbidities (coronary artery disease, cancer, alcohol withdrawal, etc). Patients who fail endoscopic therapy may benefit from emergent TIPS to reduce portal pressure and achieve hemostasis.

Finally, in the case of the unstable patient without access to immediate endoscopy, balloon tamponade can be employed as a temporizing measure after the patient has been orotracheally intubated. Each commercially available balloon device has its own particular requirements for placement. The Sengstaken-Blakemore and Minnesota tubes have both a gastric balloon and an esophageal balloon. The Linton-Nachlas tube has only a single gastric balloon, which is usually sufficient to provide local tamponade of bleeding from gastroesophageal variceal bleeding. Complications can be severe and include esophageal rupture, airway obstruction, or aspiration pneumonia; however, balloon tamponade is potentially lifesaving when other options are unavailable.

PEARLS

- All patients with cirrhosis presenting with UGIB should be presumed to have AVH.
- These patients are sick and often require early airway management and resuscitation with multiple blood products.
- Endoscopic therapy (consult GI early) + medical therapy (PPI, octreotide, and ceftriaxone) are first-line treatments.
- Consider TIPS or balloon tamponade for uncontrolled bleeding.

Suggested Readings

Bhutta A, Garcia-Tao G. The role of medical therapy for variceal bleeding. *Gastrointest Endosc Clin N Am*. 2015;25:479-490.

Bosch J, Thabut D, Bendtsen F, et al. Recombinant factor VIIa for upper gastrointestinal bleeding in patients with cirrhosis: a randomized, double-blind trial. *Gastroenterology*. 2004;127:1123-1130.

Habib A, Sanyal AJ. Acute variceal hemorrhage. *Gastrointest Endosc Clin N Am*. 2007;17(2):223-252.

Imperiale TF, Birgisson S. Somatostatin or octreotide compared with H_2 antagonists and placebo in the management of acute nonvariceal upper gastrointestinal hemorrhage: a meta-analysis. *Ann Intern Med*. 1997;127:1062-1071.

Sreedharan A, Martin J, Leontiadis GI, et al. Proton pump inhibitor treatment initiated prior to endoscopic diagnosis in upper gastrointestinal bleeding. *Cochrane Database Syst Rev*. 2010;(7):CD005415.

74

High Risk: Acute Mesenteric Ischemia

Kalle J. Fjeld and Alison Marshall

AMI occurs when blood flow to the small intestine is not sufficient for normal bowel function. AMI is a high-risk diagnosis that carries an extremely high mortality rate (beyond 70%) if not recognized in a timely manner before bowel infarction occurs.

Etiologies

AMI can be divided into three different syndromes based on pathophysiology. It is important to distinguish these, as each one has different risk factors and different management strategies:

1) **Acute mesenteric arterial occlusion** (65%-70%) is the most common cause of AMI and carries the highest mortality. It is most often encountered in older patients. Acute mesenteric arterial occlusion is secondary to either an embolic or thrombotic event:
    a) **Embolic occlusion** results from embolization of clots from the heart to the SMA and its branches. Risk factors for this syndrome include atrial fibrillation, myocardial infarction and akinesis, vascular disease, and valvular heart disease including bacterial endocarditis.
    b) **Thrombotic occlusion** occurs due to an in situ thrombotic event in patients with severe atherosclerosis, most often at the proximal SMA. The pathophysiology resembles myocardial infarction. Consequently, associated risk factors (age, hypertension, and severe vascular disease) and patient history (exertional angina, in this case postprandial) resemble acute coronary syndrome.
2) **Nonocclusive mesenteric ischemia** (20%) is a multifactorial condition often seen in hospitalized patients without evidence of a vascular occlusion. Etiologies include

shock, decreased cardiac output, or adverse sequelae of medications such as AV nodal blockers and vasoconstrictors. Notably, nonocclusive mesenteric ischemia can occur with or without narrowing of the mesenteric vasculature. It is associated with high mortality, often due to the precipitating condition.

3) **Mesenteric venous thrombosis** (5%-15%) is the only category of AMI that tends to affect younger patients. The underlying pathophysiology is similar to other venous thromboembolic events and, subsequently, the majority of patients with this syndrome have a history of DVT and/or hypercoagulable states. While the mortality rate is lower than in the other categories of AMI, it is still approximately 20% to 50%.

CLINICAL PRESENTATION

The presentation of AMI varies by syndrome, but most patients complain of sudden onset of severe colicky, poorly localized abdominal pain that is often out of proportion to the examination findings. Associated diarrhea is common. Initially, patients may only complain of mild diffuse abdominal discomfort and have a benign abdominal exam. Abdominal distention and peritoneal signs are typically late findings that suggest that the bowel has already become necrotic. Septic shock and multiorgan dysfunction can develop well before bowel necrosis, which often occurs 10 to 12 hours after symptom onset. At this stage, mortality is about 70%.

DIAGNOSIS

First-line imaging in AMI is CT angiography (CTA) of the abdomen and pelvis, which includes both venous and arterial phases. Early identification of AMI requires a high index of suspicion that should be communicated directly to radiology for improved diagnostic accuracy. One study found that AMI was correctly identified by radiology 97% of the time when suspicion for AMI was noted as the indication for CTA versus only 81% of the time when AMI was not mentioned. Oral contrast should be avoided as it can obscure the view of the blood vessels.

There are no definitive diagnostic or screening laboratory studies on AMI. Lactate is commonly used as a screening lab but is a late finding suggestive of extensive bowel ischemia. Lactate therefore provides limited utility in the ED, where the goal is early detection and intervention. D-Dimer has been suggested as a possible screening test in thromboembolic AMI. However, while a negative D-dimer makes thromboembolic AMI of the SMA less likely, there is no clear threshold for its use in AMI and it is not recommended as a stand-alone screening test. Of note, lactate is less sensitive than D-dimer in ruling out AMI, further emphasizing why lactate should not be used as a screening test when pretest probability is high.

MANAGEMENT

Management of AMI centers on IV fluid resuscitation, IV antibiotics, nasogastric tube placement, avoidance of AV nodal blockers and vasoconstrictive medications, and early surgical consultation. If vasopressors are needed for resuscitation, alpha-agonists (such as phenylephrine) should be avoided. If there are peritoneal signs or bowel necrosis on CT, immediate laparotomy is indicated.

If no bowel necrosis is evident, specific management is dependent on the syndrome. If the cause is arterial occlusion, revascularization should be attempted by interventional radiology or, in some cases, angioplasty, surgical thrombectomy, and thrombolysis. If the cause is venous thrombosis, the patient should be anticoagulated (eg, IV heparin), unless contraindicated. For AMI without evidence of vascular occlusion, the underlying condition should be treated, and an intra-arterial vasodilator infusion can be considered.

PEARLS

- AMI is a deadly condition that should be considered early and intervened upon rapidly.
- A negative lactate or relatively benign abdominal exam does not exclude AMI.
- CTA is first-line imaging for diagnosis of AMI. To increase diagnostic accuracy, suspicion for AMI should be included in the indication for CTA.
- Specific treatment varies based on the etiology of AMI, but always includes prompt surgical consultation.

Suggested Readings

Jones J, Cudnik MT, Stockton S, Macedo J, Darbha S, Hiestand B. 59 The diagnosis of acute mesenteric ischemia: a systematic review and meta-analysis. *Ann Emerg Med.* 2012;60(4).
Kärkkäinen JM, Acosta S. Acute mesenteric ischemia (part I)—incidence, etiologies, and how to improve early diagnosis. *Best Pract Res Clin Gastroenterol.* 2017;31(1):15-25.
Kühn F, Schiergens TS, Klar, E. Acute mesenteric ischemia. *Visc Med.* 2020;36(4):256-263.
Oldenburg WA, Lau LL, Rodenberg TJ, Edmonds HJ, Burger CD. Acute mesenteric ischemia. *Arch Intern Med.* 2004;164(10):1054.

75

When Should You Image Patients With Acute Pancreatitis?

Kalle J. Fjeld and Alison Marshall

AP is a common ED presentation that often results in hospital admission. Use of CT has become increasingly common during the initial ED evaluation of AP, even in patients with clearly diagnostic biomarkers and mild severity scores. Is there utility in this emerging practice pattern, or are we routinely exposing patients to unnecessary and potentially harmful testing that may be avoided?

Utility of Imaging in the Diagnosis of AP

In patients with typical symptoms and diagnostic laboratory tests that confirm AP, CT and/or MRI are not required. Current guidelines state that abdominal pain typical of AP and elevated serum amylase and/or lipase is diagnostic for AP, and CT/MRI imaging is not indicated. Conversely, when the diagnosis is unclear due to equivocal laboratory findings or an atypical presentation, CT imaging of the abdomen and pelvis may be indicated to assess for alternative etiologies or complications, such as infection. US has limited utility in the diagnosis of AP, but is a critical tool in the assessment of an etiology and in management, as discussed as follows.

UTILITY OF IMAGING FOR MANAGEMENT AND PROGNOSIS

CT and MRI have limited utility in the management of acute, uncomplicated pancreatitis in the ED. Importantly, clinical scoring systems are as accurate as CT when evaluating for disease severity. Therefore, CT and MRI are primarily indicated when there is concern for complications of AP, such as pancreatic necrosis or pseudocysts that may warrant interventional drainage. These complications are typically present more than 48 hours after symptom onset and may require repeat CT or MRI even if initial imaging is obtained in the ED. Additionally, when complications are detected on CT or MRI, initial management recommendations are often supportive, with intervention typically reserved for fluid collections that fail to resolve spontaneously or pancreatic necrosis that is associated with infection.

One of the most common causes of AP is cholelithiasis, which can be rapidly ruled out by transabdominal US. Biliary US is a low-risk, low-cost imaging modality with concordant sensitivity and specificity between radiology and trained ED providers. If US illustrates dilation of the common bile duct or lab work suggests biliary obstruction, further imaging of the biliary tree with MRCP or EUS should be pursued to evaluate for choledocholithiasis. CT has limited sensitivity for biliary stones and is unlikely to provide additional insight if the CBD has already been visualized on US.

HAZARDS OF IMAGING

CT imaging of the abdomen and pelvis is associated with an increased risk of cancer, particularly in patients who undergo repeated scans. There is additionally the potential for significant expense incurred by patients who undergo CT or MRI. These imaging modalities should therefore be approached judiciously.

PEARLS

- Routine CT or MRI is not indicated for assessment of uncomplicated AP in the ED.
- Biliary US should be completed during the initial ED evaluation of AP to rule out cholelithiasis.
- Consider CT imaging if the diagnosis is unclear, the timeline is protracted, or there is concern for a complication.
- Abdominal CT is not a benign exam. It is associated with an increased risk of cancer, particularly in patients who undergo repeated scans.

SUGGESTED READINGS

Banks PA, Bollen TL, Dervenis C, et al. Classification of acute pancreatitis—2012: revision of the Atlanta classification and definitions by international consensus. *Gut*. 2013;62:102-111.

Bollen TL, Singh VK, Maurer R, et al. A comparative evaluation of radiologic and clinical scoring systems in the early prediction of severity in acute pancreatitis. *Am J Gastroenterol*. 2012;107:612-619.

Crockett SD, Wani S, Gardner TB, Falck-Ytter Y, Barkun AN; American Gastroenterological Association Institute Clinical Guidelines Committee. American Gastroenterological

Association Institute guideline on initial management of acute pancreatitis. *Gastroenterology*. 2018;154:1096-1101.
Dachs RJ, Sullivan L. Does early ED CT scanning of afebrile patients with first episodes of acute pancreatitis ever change management? *Emerg Radiol*. 2015;22:239-243.
Ross M, Brown M, McLaughlin K, et al. Emergency physician–performed ultrasound to diagnose cholelithiasis: a systematic review. *Acad Emerg Med*. 2011;18:227-235.
Shinagare AB, Ip IK, Raja AS, et al. Use of CT and MRI in emergency department patients with acute pancreatitis. *Abdom Imaging*. 2015;40:272-277.
van Dijk AH, de Reuver PR, Besselink MG, et al. Assessment of available evidence in the management of gallbladder and bile duct stones: a systematic review of international guidelines. *HPB*. 2017;19(4):297-309.

76

WHEN SHOULD YOU IMAGE PATIENTS WITH INFLAMMATORY BOWEL DISEASE?

JACK ALLAN

IBD is an increasingly diagnosed disease entity consisting primarily of UC and CD. As of 2015, the Centers for Disease Control estimates that approximately 1.3% of the US population carries an IBD diagnosis. UC is characterized by inflammation that is limited to the mucosal and submucosal colonic surfaces, generally found in the rectum, and extends proximally to a variable extent. In contrast, CD is characterized by transmural inflammation that can occur anywhere along the GI tract, which increases the risk for a variety of complications. It is also important to note that patients with IBD are at increased risk for extraintestinal processes, such as nephrolithiasis or sacroiliitis, that may be difficult to differentiate from GI complications.

The number of patients with IBD who present to the ED with concerns for acute complications continues to increase. CT is the most accessible imaging modality available in EDs nationwide, but it also exposes patients to high levels of ionizing radiation. Given the overall younger age of diagnosis of IBD, with many patients diagnosed in childhood, paired with the baseline increased risk for malignancy associated with IBD, increased CT utilization in the ED places patients at increased risk of future complications from radiation exposure. As such, it is important to carefully consider CT imaging of these patients in the ED.

TO IMAGE OR NOT?

There are no prospectively validated clinical decision-making tools to guide imaging in patients with IBD. However, there are several considerations that can aid in the decision to use emergent imaging, delayed imaging, or no imaging strategies.

The pathophysiology of UC has a lower risk of disease-specific complications. Therefore, the decision on emergent imaging can be guided by similar principles as patients without IBD, such as surgical history, clinical presentation, and physical exam. However, it is important to acknowledge that patients with UC with prior disease-related complications will continue to have a higher risk for future complications and will likely require emergent CT imaging. Patients with UC with suspected flare-related pain without concerning features, such as peritoneal signs or signs suggestive of a non-UC related surgical emergency, may benefit more from direct visualization with endoscopic evaluation rather than CT imaging. As such, management of patients with UC with concern for disease flares not adequately managed as an outpatient should be coordinated with gastroenterology consultation for consideration of inpatient endoscopic evaluation. In pediatric patients with UC, a similar imaging strategy is indicated, but care decisions may rely on AXR if there is concern for obstruction or other complications such as toxic megacolon.

In contrast to UC, patients with CD are at higher risk for disease-related complications that include fistula, abscess, obstruction, and stricture. Furthermore, CD is characterized by variable phenotypes of disease manifestation with variable locations along the GI tract as well as variable behavior patterns including penetrating (increased risk of abscess and fistula), fibrostenotic (increased risk of obstruction or stricture), or primarily inflammatory (limited to mucosal surfaces of the intestinal tract). Though this information is not always easily available to the ED provider, it should be considered if known.

One approach in the high-risk patient group with CD is to consider a variety of factors in choosing an appropriate imaging strategy. First, all acute abdomens should rapidly undergo CT imaging and/or surgical consultation. It is also reasonable to have a low threshold to obtain CT imaging in older patients in which further ionizing radiation exposure is of lower concern or in patients where a non-CD-related pathology is suspected. In contrast to the patient with concern for an acute abdomen, the decision to obtain CT imaging in stable patients with acute-on-chronic symptoms should take into account their specific disease features. A stable patient presenting with concern for obstruction may benefit from a delayed imaging strategy with inpatient MR imaging, as these patients will benefit more from disease-directed medical management over surgical management. Stable patients with CD known to be isolated to the colonic mucosa will benefit from nonimaging or delayed MR imaging strategies as the need for acute intervention is less likely. Stable patients with known isolated perianal disease with concern for fistula formation or abscess, delayed MR imaging, ultrasonography, or exam under anesthesia may help reduce radiation exposure. Patients presenting with primary changes in bowel movements likely do not require emergent imaging. In pediatric patients with CD, small bowel ultrasonography or MR imaging can be employed in stable patients, while AXR or pediatric surgical consultation may be warranted for more acute concerns.

Though various studies have explored specific indicators for imaging, there is currently no strong consensus in the literature. Some of these indicators include the history of obstruction or intra-abdominal abscess, history of IBD surgery, C-reactive protein greater than 5 mg/dL (though some sources suggest 2.5 mg/dL), white blood cell count greater than 12,000 (though some sources suggest 10,000), pulse rate greater than 100 beats/min, and low body mass index. History of biologic agent medication use is considered a negative predictor. These factors, as well as GI consultation, can augment decision making in murkier clinical presentations.

PEARLS

- Obtain emergent imaging for any patient with an acute abdomen, regardless of IBD history.

- Patients with UC are more likely to benefit from GI endoscopic evaluation if symptoms are thought to be disease-related.
- Patients with CD are at higher risk for disease-specific complications, but patient-specific disease features can inform imaging decisions to reduce ionizing radiation exposure.
- Select historical and lab findings may further inform imaging decisions in patients with CD.
- Ultrasonography or MR imaging, when available, should be preferential in pediatric or pregnant patients with IBD.

SUGGESTED READINGS

Griffey RT, Fowler KJ, Theilen A, Gutierrez A. Considerations in imaging among emergency department patients with inflammatory bowel disease. *Ann Emerg Med*. 2017;69(5):587-599.

Kilcoyne A, Kaplan JL, Gee MS. Inflammatory bowel disease imaging: current practice and future directions. *World J Gastroenterol*. 2016;22(3):917-932. PMID: 26811637.

77

CAN YOU DISCHARGE THAT PATIENT WITH ACUTE DIVERTICULITIS?

RYAN C. GIBBONS

Diverticula are focal outpouchings of the intestinal wall involving the mucosa, muscularis, and serosa. False diverticula do not contain the thick muscularis layer. The majority of colonic diverticula are false.

Diverticular disease includes a clinical spectrum from asymptomatic diverticulosis to acute diverticulitis and its associated complications. It is among the most frequently encountered gastroenterologic ailments, affecting 50% of individuals over the age of 60 nationwide. Surprisingly, the incidence in adults aged 40 to 49 years has increased more than 130% since 1980.

Of those patients with diverticular disease, 5% to 25% will experience an acute episode of diverticulitis, with a recurrence rate of 20% within a decade of the initial presentation. The likelihood of recurrence increases with each subsequent flare. Over 10% of patients will experience complications, most commonly abscess development. Other potential complications include perforation, obstruction, sepsis, and chronic stricture and fistula formation. Contrary to conventional wisdom, the risk of complications diminishes with repeated occurrences.

The pathophysiology of acute diverticulitis is poorly understood, but recent evidence implicates chronic inflammation and altered intestinal microbes as etiologies for

TABLE 77.1	RISK FACTORS FOR DIVERTICULAR DISEASE
Western diet (low in fiber; high in red meat and fat)	Obesity
Tobacco use	Sedentary lifestyle
NSAIDs	Corticosteroids
Sibling with diverticular disease	Opiate use

Nuts and seeds are not risk factors.

acute diverticulitis rather than the traditional teaching of diverticular obstruction that triggers localized ischemia, micro-perforation, and infection (**Table 77.1**).

ASSESSMENT

Left lower quadrant pain is the most common presenting symptom in acute diverticulitis. Other symptoms include fever, nausea with or without vomiting, and change in bowel movements. Urinary complaints and right-sided pain are less common but can be present. Given these nonspecific symptoms, the clinical acumen is less than 65% sensitive for the diagnosis of acute diverticulitis.

Inflammatory markers, such as CRP and WBC, may be normal or elevated. When elevated, patients are at higher risk of complications. Importantly, normal inflammatory markers do not exclude complicated presentations.

CT with IV contrast remains the gold standard for diagnosis of acute diverticulitis with a sensitivity that exceeds 95%. Oral and rectal contrast are rarely indicated. Magnetic resonance imaging should largely be reserved for pregnant patients. Plain films do not have a role in the diagnosis of acute diverticulitis. The diagnostic accuracy of ultrasound is variable and user dependent. **Table 77.2** lists the indications for CT imaging.

TABLE 77.2	INDICATIONS FOR CT[a] AND ANTIBIOTICS
Suspected complications	Decompensated liver disease
Immunocompromised	>70 years old
■ Malignancy	
■ HIV/AIDS	Unable to tolerate oral intake
■ Organ transplant	
■ Chronic steroid use	Failed outpatient treatment
Poorly controlled diabetes and those with evidence of end organ damage	Peritonitis
End stage renal disease	Sepsis
Recent cardiac event	>1 Systemic inflammatory response syndrome criteria
■ Acute myocardial infarction	Elevated inflammatory markers
■ Congestive heart failure	■ CRP
	■ WBC

[a]Scan all patients without previously diagnosed diverticular disease.

Management

Antibiotics, analgesia, and dietary modifications have been the traditional treatments for uncomplicated diverticulitis, with surgery reserved for complicated cases. However, these traditional treatments have been based solely on expert opinion. Recently, several large, multicenter, randomized trials have demonstrated a lack of benefit from antibiotics for uncomplicated diverticulitis in low risk, immunocompetent patients. Patients with complicated presentations, such as those detailed in **Table 77.2**, may warrant admission for IV antibiotics and surgical consultation.

Lifestyle modifications are important to limit recurrence. These include a high-fiber diet, exercise, weight loss, tobacco cessation, and NSAIDs avoidance. There is no role for mesalamine, probiotics, or rifaximin. All patients should have a colonoscopy 6 to 8 weeks following the first episode of acute diverticulitis and after each complicated occurrence.

PEARLS

- Consider discharge in low risk, immunocompetent patients with uncomplicated acute diverticulitis with a clear liquid diet and advance as tolerated. Encourage lifestyle modifications to limit recurrence and complications.
- In low risk, immunocompetent patients with known diverticular disease, limit unnecessary utilization of CT for suspected cases of uncomplicated acute diverticulitis.
- Do not routinely prescribe antibiotics for low risk, immunocompetent patients diagnosed with uncomplicated acute diverticulitis. If they have no clinical improvement at 48 to 72 hours, instruct the patient to return for imaging and antibiotics.
- Prescribe antibiotics for patients with the following:
  - Elevated inflammatory markers
  - Complicated cases
  - Immunocompromised
  - Comorbidities (see **Table 77.2**)
  - Above 70 years
- When prescribing antibiotics, the recommended regimen includes amoxicillin-clavulanate or a fluoroquinolone and metronidazole for a duration of 4 to 7 days.
- Facilitate follow-up colonoscopy 6 to 8 weeks after the first episode of diverticulitis and after each episode of complicated diverticulitis.

Suggested Readings

Au S, Aly EH. Treatment of uncomplicated acute diverticulitis without antibiotics: a systematic review and meta-analysis. *Dis Colon Rectum*. 2019;62(12):1533-1547.

Bolkenstein HE, Van De Wall BJ, Consten EC, Broeders IAMJ, Draaisma WA. Risk factors for complicated diverticulitis: systematic review and meta-analysis. *Int J Colorectal Dis*. 2017;32(10):1375-1383.

Epifani AG, Cassini D, Cirocchi R, et al. Right sided diverticulitis in western countries: a review. *World J Gastrointest Surg*. 2021;13(12):1721-1735.

Fugazzola P, Ceresoli M, Coccolini F, et al. The WSES/SICG/ACOI/SICUT/AcEMC/SIFIPAC guidelines for diagnosis and treatment of acute left colonic diverticulitis in the elderly. *World J Emerg Surg*. 2022;17(1):5.

Hall J, Hardiman K, Lee S, et al. The American Society of Colon and Rectal Surgeons Clinical Practice Guidelines for the treatment of left-sided colonic diverticulitis. *Dis Colon Rectum.* 2020;63(6):728-747.

Peery AF, Shaukat A, Strate L. AGA clinical practice update on medical management of colonic diverticulitis: expert review. *Gastroenterology.* 2021;160:906-911.e1.

Qaseem A, Etxeandia-Ikobaltzeta I, Lin JS, et al. Diagnosis and management of acute left-sided colonic diverticulitis: a clinical guideline from the American College of Physicians. *Ann Intern Med.* 2022;175(3):399-415.

Strate LL, Morris AM. Epidemiology, pathophysiology, and treatment of diverticulitis. *Gastroenterology.* 2019;156(5):1282-1298.e1.Nuts and seeds are not risk factors.ªScan all patients without previously diagnosed diverticular disease.

78

PITFALLS IN ESOPHAGEAL PERFORATION

JAMES VANDENBERG

Esophageal perforation is a rare condition that is difficult to diagnose and has significant mortality. Spontaneous esophageal perforation due to forceful emesis (ie, Boerhaave syndrome) was first described in the 1700s. Though this is often taught as the classic etiology, there are numerous causes of spontaneous perforation that include childbirth, straining, weight lifting, laughing, and seizures. Spontaneous etiologies of perforation account for up to 38% of cases. Overall, the most common etiology of esophageal perforation is iatrogenic and includes procedures such as intubation, transesophageal echocardiogram, esophagogastroduodenoscopy, thoracic surgery, and balloon tamponade device placement. Additional etiologies of perforation include trauma, caustic ingestions, and foreign body ingestion. The mortality rates of esophageal perforations are estimated to be 11.9% to 13.3%.

CLINICAL PRESENTATION

Esophageal perforation results in mediastinal contamination by gastroesophageal contents, which causes an inflammatory reaction and leads to mediastinitis and sepsis. Mortality doubles if the diagnosis is delayed more than 24 hours from onset. Unfortunately, over half of esophageal perforations are initially misdiagnosed as a result of nonspecific signs and symptoms. Common presenting symptoms of perforation include fever, dyspnea, nausea, hoarseness, dysphagia, and pain that can be in the chest, neck, back, abdomen, or shoulder regions. The classic presenting symptoms of Mackler's Triad (vomiting, chest pain, and subcutaneous neck emphysema) are uncommon and present in as few as 14% of patients.

Abnormal vital signs in esophageal perforation can take time to develop. Tachycardia and tachypnea may occur early, but signs such as fever or cardiopulmonary collapse are often delayed. The location of perforation can determine the abruptness of signs and symptoms, as distal perforations rapidly contaminate the mediastinum, whereas cervical perforations are more contained due to esophageal attachments to pre-vertebral fascia. Overall, sepsis is present at the time of admission in just 23% of patients. Classic findings such as subcutaneous emphysema are initially present in only 25% of cases. Other findings include Hamman's crunch, as well as decreased breath sounds due to a concomitant pleural effusion or pneumothorax.

DIAGNOSIS

There are no gold-standard tests for esophageal perforation. If obtained, pleural fluid may demonstrate a low pH and high amylase, suggesting contamination of gastric contents. CXR is neither sensitive nor specific, but can demonstrate findings such as pneumomediastinum, mediastinal widening, and subcutaneous emphysema. Other findings include pleural effusion, pneumothorax, and free air under the diaphragm (seen with intra-abdominal perforations). Quite simply, a CXR cannot be used to rule out esophageal perforation. Though it is also nondiagnostic, ultrasound may demonstrate pleural effusions, free intraperitoneal fluid, or pneumopericardium.

The recommended diagnostic test for esophageal perforation is CT of the chest with IV contrast. CT can detect the involvement of surrounding structures, identify alternative pathology, and does not require the patient to drink oral contrast. If CT of the chest cannot be obtained, a fluoroscopic esophagography using a water-soluble contrast (eg, Gastrograffin) can be performed. Barium contrast is not recommended, as it causes an inflammatory reaction if leaked into the mediastinum. If the initial studies are negative but high clinical suspicion remains, an endoscopy can be considered. This can be diagnostic and therapeutic but is limited, given the potential to worsen the perforation.

TREATMENT

All patients with suspected esophageal perforation should be made NPO and receive IV fluids and vasopressors, as necessary. Broad-spectrum antibiotics should be started and include coverage of gastrointestinal microbes. Consider antifungal medications for immunocompromised patients, prolonged proton pump inhibitor use, or previous fungal infections. For patients who present with respiratory distress, noninvasive positive pressure ventilation should be avoided, as positive pressure can worsen the perforation and expulse contaminants/air into the mediastinum. Early intubation should be considered for those in respiratory distress. Nasogastric tube placement is controversial and should be discussed with the surgical team, as there is a risk of worsening the perforation and it may induce gastroesophageal reflux.

Definitive treatment of esophageal perforation often requires surgical repair. Surgical consultation should be obtained when considering this diagnosis. Patients can sometimes be treated nonoperatively with antibiotics and observation, although this is typically limited to contained perforations without evidence of sepsis. Additional approaches to treatment include a variety of minimally and noninvasive techniques such as esophageal stenting. Definitive treatment decisions are best made in consultation with a surgical team.

PEARLS

- Delays in diagnosis of esophageal perforation are common and result in increased mortality.
- Maintain high suspicion in patients with chest pain and a history of forceful emesis or recent endoscopic procedure.
- Mackler's Triad is seen in less than 50% of cases.
- CT chest with IV contrast is the recommended test of choice.
- Definitive management necessitates a multidisciplinary approach; it is essential to obtain appropriate consultation early.

SUGGESTED READINGS

Allaway MGR, Morris PD, B Sinclair JL, Richardson AJ, Johnston ES, Hollands MJ. Management of Boerhaave syndrome in Australasia: a retrospective case series and systematic review of the Australasian literature. *ANZ J Surg.* 2021;91:1376-1384.

Biancari F, D'Andrea V, Paone R, et al. Current treatment and outcome of esophageal perforations in adults: systematic review and meta-analysis of 75 studies. *World J Surg.* 2013;37: 1051-1059.

Brinster CJ, Singhal S, Lee L, Marshall MB, Kaiser LR, Kucharczuk JC. Evolving options in the management of esophageal perforation. *Ann Thorac Surg.* 2004;77:1475-1483.

Derr C, Drake JM. Esophageal rupture diagnosed with bedside ultrasound. *Am J Emerg Med.* 2012;30:2093.e1-2093.e20933.

DeVivo A, Sheng AY, Koyfman A, Long B. High risk and low prevalence diseases: esophageal perforation. *AmJ Emerg Med.* 2022;53:29-36.

Eckstein M, Henderson SO. Thoracic trauma: esophageal perforation. In: Biros MH, Ling LJ, Danzl DF, et al, eds. *Rosen's Emergency Medicine Concept and Clinical Practice.* 8th ed. Elsevier Health Sciences; 2014:455-458.

Halani SH, Baum GR, Riley JP, et al. Esophageal perforation after anterior cervical spine surgery: a systematic review of the literature. *J Neurosurg Spine.* 2016;25:285-291.

Hess JM, Lowell MJ. Esophagus, stomach, and duodenum: esophageal perforation. In: Biros MH, Ling LJ, Danzl DF, et al, eds. *Rosen's Emergency Medicine Concept and Clinical Practice.* 8th ed. Elsevier Health Sciences; 2014:1172-1173.

Juhl-Olsen P. Air gap sign in ultrasound: rhythm is the answer. *A A Pract.* 2019;12:256-257.

Pickering O, Pucher PH, De'Ath H, et al. Minimally invasive approach in Boerhaave's syndrome: case series and systematic review. *J Laparoendosc Adv Surg Tech A.* 2021;31: 1254-1261.

Sainathan S, Andaz S. A systematic review of transesophageal echocardiography-induced esophageal perforation. *Echocardiography.* 2013;30:977-983.

Sdralis EIK, Petousis S, Rashid F, Lorenzi B, Charalabopoulos A. Epidemiology, diagnosis, and management of esophageal perforations: systematic review. *Dis Esophagus.* 2017;30:1-6.

Vidarsdottir H, Blondal S, Alfredsson H, Geirsson A, Gudbjartsson T. Oesophageal perforations in Iceland: a whole population study on incidence, aetiology and surgical outcome. *Thorac Cardiovasc Surg.* 2010;58:476-480.

79

WHAT ARE THE PRIORITIES IN PATIENTS WITH ACUTE LIVER FAILURE?

MATTHEW L. WONG

ALF is the combination of acutely abnormal liver function tests, coagulopathy, and altered mental status. This is a relatively rare entity, with roughly 2,000 cases per year in the United States. Without liver transplantation, the morbidity and mortality for patients with ALF are extremely high. Because it is so uncommon, ALF is an understudied condition with gaps in the literature. Management is generally supportive with few opportunities for targeted therapy or specific antidotes, and the relevant guidelines are predominantly based on expert opinion. Because of the dearth of evidence-based guidelines, these patients merit very close scrutiny, thoughtful consideration, and hospitalization in an intensive care unit.

Consider ALF When the More Common Illness Scripts Don't Fit

Given how infrequent ALF is, the diagnosis may not be at the forefront of the emergency physician's mind. Altered mental status and delirium are common in sick patients. Liver function test abnormalities are also very common and often nonspecific in other illnesses, or perhaps a hepatic function panel was never ordered as part of the initial workup. The most likely circumstance you'll encounter ALF, therefore, is when you initially start with a plan and a few diagnoses in mind, but the data don't fit neatly with what you had in mind. For example, a patient was initially suspected to have a bacterial infection (ie, urinary tract infection) causing their altered mental status, but the workup does not reveal a source.

On physical examination, the patient with ALF will often have jaundice, right upper quadrant tenderness, and stigmata of chronic liver disease. The altered mental status portion of the diagnostic triad of ALF may simply be changes in behavior with minimal change in level of consciousness. That is to say, patients with ALF need not be comatose and may only be subtly altered or confused. Many forms of critical illness can cause elevation in aspartate transaminase, alanine transaminase, and bilirubin. While there is no specific threshold that identifies ALF from other forms of acute illness, the AST and ALT will almost always be greater than 1,000 U/L. When the physical exam and laboratory tests are consistent with ALF, the physician should go back to the bedside and talk to the patient and get as much additional information as possible, specifically asking about any potential toxins and the risk for viral hepatitis.

Obtain a Detailed History for Hepatic Toxins, Particularly Acetaminophen

Acetaminophen toxicity is the leading cause of ALF. While there are many causes of ALF, the emergency physician should always have a high suspicion for acetaminophen toxicity. Acute ingestions that put the patient at risk of ALF are usually easier to diagnose based on the context, but histories of subacute and chronic toxicity may not be as forthcoming. Sending an acetaminophen level should be considered routinely in patients with liver dysfunction, and it should be remembered that the Rumack-Matthews nomogram applies only for acute ingestions.

Many medications, even taken weeks prior to presentation, can result in drug-induced liver injury. Confirm with the patient, and their pharmacy if possible, all medications taken within the past few months. The National Institute of Health's LiverTox website can be a useful resource to determine if a medication may have hepatotoxicity. It is also important to ask the patient about any over-the-counter supplements, herbal remedies, or other "traditional medicines." The patient may consider them benign or harmless and forget to disclose them unless specifically asked. Wild mushrooms are of particular concern, and those toxidromes have a high morbidity and mortality.

NAC, Right Upper Quadrant Ultrasound, and Supportive Care

When in doubt, start NAC. There is some data to support its use even in non-acetaminophen-related forms of ALF. The typical intravenous form is readily available and has a favorable risk-benefit profile. The administration of NAC is done in phases: a loading dose over the first hour and then a prolonged infusion at lower doses. This typically involves administering several separate physical bags of NAC. Practically speaking, the emergency physician should discuss the administration of NAC with the pharmacy to ensure adequate supply and proper administration.

Obtain a right upper quadrant ultrasound with Doppler to evaluate for preexisting liver disease (eg, signs of cirrhosis, abnormal liver tissue density and surface morphology, splenomegaly, ascites), as well as patent vascular flow, to rule out portal vein thrombosis or Budd-Chiari syndrome.

Supportive care for patients with ALF is critical. Because the patient's mental status should be closely monitored, avoid medications that may sedate the patient (eg, benzodiazepines, opioids) as much as possible. Increased intracranial pressure is one complication of ALF, so do not confound the patient's neurologic exam without good reason. Maintaining a mean arterial pressure of at least 65 mm Hg is important to maintain liver and cerebral perfusion.

Call a Consult

The advice of a specialist early in the patient's management may assist with treatment priorities and appropriate disposition. Many blood tests will be requested for the dual tasks of clarifying the etiology for ALF, as well as in preparation for possible liver transplant. If ALF is not due to acetaminophen toxicity, the differential diagnosis for ALF is extensive and includes other medications and toxins, viral syndromes (eg, HAV, HBV, HIV, CMV, HSV), autoimmune diseases, deposition diseases (ie, Wilson), or malignancy. In consultation with the hepatologist, the patient may be best served in an intensive care unit at an institution capable of liver transplant.

PEARLS

- Consider ALF when the more common illnesses don't fit.
- Take a detailed history for hepatic toxins, particularly acetaminophen.
- In the ED, give NAC, get a right upper quadrant ultrasound, and provide supportive care.
- Call a consult.
- Admission to the ICU at a hospital capable of transplant is often the best disposition.

Suggested Readings

AASLD Guidelines on the management of acute liver failure, 2011. https://www.aasld.org/practice-guidelines/management-acute-liver-failure

LiverTox: Clinical and research information on drug-induced liver injury [Internet]. National Institute of Diabetes and Digestive and Kidney Diseases; 2012. https://www.ncbi.nlm.nih.gov/books/NBK547852/

Nanchal R, Subramanian R, Karvellas CJ, et al. Guidelines for the management of adult acute and acute-on-chronic liver failure in the ICU: cardiovascular, endocrine, hematologic, pulmonary and renal considerations: executive summary. *Crit Care Med*. 2020;48(3):415-419.

80

Know When to Administer Antibiotics for Severe Acute Pancreatitis

Alyssa Karl

Acute pancreatitis is a common gastrointestinal complaint in the ED with increasing incidence. Patients often present with clinical symptoms of constant epigastric or left upper quadrant abdominal pain with radiation toward the back, chest, or flanks, and is typically associated with nausea and vomiting. The patient's clinical presentation is not related to the severity of the disease. Several different classification systems are used to help predict the severity of disease, including APACHE II, Ranson, Glasgow, Balthazar, and Atlanta. The most used grading system is the Atlanta Classification, or revised Atlanta Classification, where mild acute pancreatitis is defined as the absence of organ failure or local complications, moderately severe acute pancreatitis involves local complications and/or transient organ failure for less than 48 hours, and severe acute pancreatitis as persistent organ failure for more than 48 hours. While the overall mortality of acute pancreatitis is only 5%, the presence of multisystem organ failure increases the mortality rate to 47%.

Regardless of the severity of the disease or type of acute pancreatitis (interstitial edematous pancreatitis vs necrotizing pancreatitis), the initial treatment remains the same with early IV hydration and supportive care. Despite numerous different trials, no specific medication has proven effective in the treatment of acute pancreatitis. Antibiotic use in pancreatitis has remained controversial, and clinical practice varies greatly. Current guidelines recommend against the routine use of antibiotics in the treatment of acute pancreatitis. Additionally, antibiotic use in patients with sterile necrosis to prevent the development of infected necrosis is not recommended. The use of prophylactic antibiotics in acute pancreatitis without evidence of infection has not been shown to improve mortality, reduce systemic complications, or reduce the occurrence of infected necrosis.

Instead, the *American Journal of Gastroenterology* guidelines recommend that antibiotics should be used once the diagnosis of infected necrosis has been established. Fever, tachycardia, and elevated white blood cell counts may be present early in acute pancreatitis due to the SIRS response, which may make it difficult to distinguish from an infectious complication. About one-third of patients with pancreatic necrosis develop infected necrosis and up to as many as 20% of patients with acute pancreatitis will develop extrapancreatic infections. If antibiotics are started early in the course of acute pancreatitis due to concern for infection, whether intrapancreatic or extrapancreatic (ie, pneumonia, cholangitis, urinary tract infections, bacteremia), they should be stopped once cultures result as negative and an infectious source is not identified.

Infected necrosis typically occurs after the first 1 to 2 weeks in the course of acute pancreatitis and should be suspected in patients with necrosis whose condition worsens based on clinical instability, such as new or persistent fever, end-organ dysfunction, or increasing white blood cell counts or failure to improve after 7 to 10 days of hospital admission. CT imaging with findings of gas within the necrosis in the setting of clinical signs of infection is suggestive of infected necrosis and can be considered an indication to start antibiotics. CT-guided FNA may be utilized to obtain a culture in suspected infected necrosis; however, antibiotics should likely be started while awaiting results and can be discontinued if there is no growth.

Although surgical debridement of infected necrosis may ultimately be necessary, reports and case series have shown that antibiotics alone may successfully treat infection without the need for surgical intervention in a select group of patients. Infections in acute pancreatitis are typically monomicrobial and usually from typical gut flora, such as *Escherichia coli, Pseudomonas, Klebsiella,* and *Enterococcus.* The antibiotics given must also have the ability to penetrate pancreatic necrosis, which include carbapenems, quinolones, metronidazole, and high-dose cephalosporins. Surgery for debridement of the infected necrosis may then be performed promptly after antibiotics are started or be delayed, as some studies suggest that a prolonged course of antibiotics for patients with infected necrosis who are clinically stable was associated with decreased mortality. Guidelines from the International Association of Pancreatology and the American Pancreatic Association recommend that invasive interventions for infected necrotizing pancreatitis be delayed until at least 4 weeks after initial presentation. Delayed intervention allows for the infection to become more organized or "walled off" and the inflammatory response to decrease.

PEARLS

- Current guidelines do not recommend the routine use of antibiotics in the treatment of acute pancreatitis.
- Prophylactic antibiotics have not been proven to prevent the development of infected necrosis in necrotizing pancreatitis.
- Infected necrosis should be suspected when patients have persistent or worsening fever, leukocytosis, and end-organ dysfunction or fail to improve after 7 to 10 days.
- When antibiotics are given for infected necrosis, they should be capable of penetrating the pancreatic necrosis and cover for gut-derived organisms.

SUGGESTED READINGS

Banks PA, Freeman ML; Practice Parameters Committee of the American College of Gastroenterology. Practice guidelines in acute pancreatitis. *Am J Gastroenterol.* 2006; 101:2379-2400.

Dellinger EP, Tellado JM, Soto NE, et al. Early antibiotic treatment for severe acute necrotizing pancreatitis: a randomized, double-blind, placebo-controlled study. *Ann Surg.* 2007;245: 674-683.

Tenner S, Baillie J, DeWitt J, Vege SS; American College of Gastroenterology. American College of Gastroenterology guideline: management of acute pancreatitis. *Am J Gastroenterol.* 2013;108:1400-1415.

Working Group IAP/APA Acute Pancreatitis Guidelines. IAP/APA evidence-based guidelines for the management of acute pancreatitis. *Pancreatology.* 2013;13:e1-e15.

81

ACALCULOUS CHOLECYSTITIS: NO STONES, NO PROBLEMS?

CLARE ROEPKE

Emergency clinicians are familiar with acute calculous cholecystitis, which is classically defined as inflammation of the gallbladder caused by a mechanical obstruction, most commonly by a gallstone. In contrast, emergency clinicians tend to be less familiar with acute *acalculous* cholecystitis. Acute acalculous cholecystitis does not involve an obstructing gallstone and is caused by dysfunction or hypokinesis of gallbladder emptying. Another key difference between calculous and acalculous cholecystitis is the clinical presentation. Acalculous cholecystitis typically presents more gradually and is more common in critically ill patients.

Acalculous cholecystitis is a surgical emergency, and a good outcome hinges on early recognition and appropriate surgical treatment. It is estimated that acalculous cholecystitis comprises about 10% of all cholecystitis cases. In one study, within a 7-year period, 77% of all patients identified with acalculous cholecystitis presented in the outpatient setting. Importantly, 45% of those patients were ultimately admitted without the diagnosis of cholecystitis. If treatment is delayed, acute acalculous cholecystitis has a mortality rate as high as 65%, whereas, with early intervention, mortality is approximately 7%. In contrast, the mortality for calculous cholecystitis commonly ranges from 1.5% to 3%. Though acalculous cholecystitis is a rare entity, it is important to keep in mind in patients with sepsis due to an unclear source, especially in the setting of abdominal pain.

The pathophysiology of acute acalculous cholecystitis begins with dysfunction or hypokinesis of gallbladder emptying. This stasis of the gallbladder leads to increased distention, increased intraluminal pressure, and a localized inflammatory response, ultimately leading to inflammation and ischemia of the gallbladder wall. It is hypothesized that bile salts and their by-products are also toxic to the gallbladder during stasis. Stasis can also lead to a secondary bacterial colonization of the gallbladder, usually with coliforms and anaerobes (commonly *Escherichia coli* and *Klebsiella pneumoniae*). The exact nature and mechanism of the bacterial infection are not fully understood. Nevertheless, antibiotics are still considered a mainstay of treatment.

The clinical presentation of acalculous cholecystitis can be varied but most commonly consists of right upper quadrant abdominal pain, fever, jaundice, nausea, vomiting, and, occasionally, septic shock. Physical examination may reveal a palpable right upper quadrant mass, and laboratory tests may show leukocytosis and elevated liver enzymes. Inpatients are more apt to have well-known risk factors for acalculous cholecystitis, including burns, trauma, nonbiliary surgeries, the use of inotropes, mechanical ventilation, or childbirth. It is more difficult to identify these patients in the outpatient and ED settings. Acalculous cholecystitis is more common in males (1:1 to 2.8:1 male-to-female predominance), advanced age (average age is in the 60s), cardiovascular disease, diabetes, hypertension, peripheral vascular disease, alcoholic liver disease, and COPD. These cases can be complicated by the patient being demented or developmentally delayed, which may prevent an adequate history and physical examination. In children, acalculous cholecystitis may present as a complication of EBV infection. Patients with AIDS may also present with a nonspecific infectious prodrome and upper abdominal pain with acalculous cholecystitis secondary to an opportunistic infection, though it is more common for these patients to have cholangitis.

Diagnostic imaging is critical in making an early diagnosis of this condition. One study that evaluated imaging modalities for acalculous cholecystitis found that ultrasound (sensitivity 92%, specificity 96%) and CT (sensitivity 100%, specificity 100%) were both excellent diagnostic modalities but that scintigraphy suffered from poor specificity (38%). Often, at the time of diagnosis, the differential remains broad, and a CT scan may offer further diagnostic assessment for other possibilities on the differential.

Once the diagnosis is confirmed, the treatment remains similar to that of calculous cholecystitis. Antibiotics should be initiated to cover coliforms and anaerobes and typically includes a beta-lactam with a beta-lactamase inhibitor. Surgical consultation is necessary to decide whether the patient should be taken to the operating room for cholecystectomy versus an interventional radiology–guided cholecystostomy. This decision is usually dependent upon the patient's comorbidities and perioperative risk. Complications such as emphysematous cholecystitis and perforated gallbladder can drastically alter the patient's course and treatment plan, further reinforcing the importance of early diagnosis in the ED.

PEARLS

- Not all cholecystitis is caused by gallstones.
- Acalculous cholecystitis typically presents more insidiously and is typically more common in critically ill patients.
- Once the diagnosis is made, initiate broad-spectrum antibiotics and obtain early surgical consultation.

SUGGESTED READINGS

Jones MW, Ferguson T. Acalculous cholecystitis. In: *StatPearls [Internet]*. StatPearls Publishing; 2023 January. https://www.ncbi.nlm.nih.gov/books/NBK459182/

Mirvis SE, Vainright JR, Nelson AW, et al. The diagnosis of acute acalculous cholecystitis: a comparison of sonography, scintigraphy, and CT. *AJR Am J Roentgenol*. 1986;147:1171.

Savoca PE, Longo WE, Zucker KA, et al. The increasing prevalence of acalculous cholecystitis in outpatients. Results of a 7-year study. *Ann Surg*. 1990;211:433.

Wang AJ, Wang TE, Lin CC, et al. Clinical predictors of severe gallbladder complications in acute acalculous cholecystitis. *World J Gastroenterol*. 2003;9:2821.

Yi DY, Kim JY, Yang HR. Ultrasonographic gallbladder abnormality of primary Epstein-Barr virus infection in children and its influence on clinical outcome. *Medicine (Baltimore)*. 2015;94(27):e1120.

82

Who Needs an Emergent EGD in the ED?

Jessica Moore

EGD, also termed *upper endoscopy*, is a commonly performed procedure with various diagnostic, prognostic, and therapeutic functions. This chapter discusses emergent EGD indications relevant to the emergency physician.

Esophageal Obstruction

Esophageal obstruction mainly occurs in patients with underlying esophageal pathology. In adults, obstruction is typically caused by impacted foods, particularly meats. Objects causing complete esophageal obstruction should be removed emergently, due to the risk of aspiration as well as esophageal pressure necrosis. Preprocedural radiographic evaluation is not generally required if the food bolus is nonbony and the patient shows no evidence of associated complications (ie, perforation). Uncomplicated esophageal food impactions, which do not cause complete obstruction, may be treated by EGD on an urgent, rather than emergent, basis.

Foreign Body Ingestion

Foreign body ingestion is seen more commonly in children than adults. While many foreign bodies will pass without intervention or complication, a subset requires emergent endoscopic removal. Disk or "button" batteries in the esophagus should be removed immediately, due to the risk of rapid-onset liquefactive necrosis. Similarly, sharp objects in the esophagus should be removed emergently due to the risk of esophageal perforation. Any esophageal foreign body causing complete obstruction or respiratory compromise requires emergent removal.

Objects that should be considered for removal on an urgent, rather than emergent, basis include sharp objects in the stomach or duodenum, esophageal food impactions without complete obstruction, and objects greater than 6 cm in length. Ingested magnets require special consideration, as the force between multiple magnets (or a magnet and ingested piece of metal) can cause intestinal wall necrosis and subsequent complications, including perforation, fistula formation, and volvulus. Magnets within endoscopic reach should be removed. Most other ingested foreign bodies can be observed for spontaneous passage or removed nonemergently, assuming the patient has no evidence of associated gastrointestinal obstruction or perforation. Packets containing illicit substances should not be removed endoscopically due to the risk of rupture and related drug toxicity.

Caustic Ingestion

Ingestion of caustic materials can lead to esophageal necrosis and several related complications, including perforation, mediastinitis, and shock. Esophageal strictures are a common long-term complication of such injury. While the ED management of caustic esophageal injury is mainly supportive, EGD provides important diagnostic and prognostic information for such patients. Current guidelines recommend EGD for caustic esophageal injury within 12 to 24 hours. Endoscopy performed at 48 hours or more may be associated with an increased risk of esophageal perforation due to the development of tissue necrosis. EGD is contraindicated in patients with evidence of associated perforation.

BILIARY OBSTRUCTION

Biliary obstruction is now commonly treated endoscopically, via ERCP. Cholangitis may be a complication of conditions such as choledocholithiasis, biliary stricture, and malignancy. It can be a life-threatening condition that presents with jaundice and evidence of sepsis and shock.

While biliary decompression via ERCP is generally indicated in the management of cholangitis, optimal timing of the procedure remains controversial. Current guidelines suggest early (within 48 hours) as compared to delayed (>48 hours) ERCP; however, more studies are needed to determine the optimal time frame for ERCP in cholangitis. While awaiting ERCP, patients with cholangitis should be treated with antibiotics and aggressive supportive measures.

UPPER GIB

Upper GIB is a common reason for ED presentation, with peptic ulcer disease being the most common etiology. EGD has become mainstay in the evaluation and management of upper GIB. Endoscopy allows not only for the identification of the source of bleeding but also for targeted interventions, such as thermal coagulation, injection therapy, and variceal ligation.

While experts agree that EGD for patients with high-risk upper GIB should be performed within 24 hours, whether a shorter time window is superior continues to be an area of research and debate. ED management of patients with significant upper GIB includes supportive measures, such as blood transfusion, proton–pump inhibitors, and, in cases of suspected or confirmed varices, antibiotics and octreotide.

PEARLS

- Most ingested foreign bodies will pass spontaneously and do not require emergent intervention.
- Esophageal foreign bodies including button batteries, sharp objects, and those causing complete obstruction or respiratory compromise require emergent endoscopic removal; such cases should prompt immediate gastroenterology consultation.
- Caustic esophageal injury should be evaluated via endoscopy within 12 to 24 hours.
- Consider early consultation with gastroenterology in cases of significant upper GIB and cholangitis, acknowledging that many gastroenterologists will recommend medical resuscitation of the patient before performing endoscopy.

SUGGESTED READINGS

ASGE Standards of Practice Committee, Ikenberry SO, Jue TL, et al. Management of ingested foreign bodies and food impactions. *Gastrointest Endosc*. 2011;73(6):1085-1091.

Buxbaum JL, Buitrago C, Lee A, et al. ASGE guideline on the management of cholangitis. *Gastrointest Endosc*. 2021;94(2):207-221.e14.

Laine L, Barkun AN, Saltzman JR, Martel M, Leontiadis GI. ACG Clinical guideline: upper gastrointestinal and ulcer bleeding [published correction appears in *Am J Gastroenterol.* 2021;116(11):2309]. *Am J Gastroenterol.* 2021;116(5):899-917.

Lau JYW, Yu Y, Tang RSY, et al. Timing of endoscopy for acute upper gastrointestinal bleeding. *N Engl J Med.* 2020;382(14):1299-1308.

83

KNOW HOW TO DEAL WITH THE DISPLACED PEG TUBE

JULIE Y. VALENZUELA AND ROLANDO G. VALENZUELA

As the number of physicians capable of placing PEG tubes has increased, so has the number and type of PEG tubes being placed. A PEG tube is placed for feeding access as well as for gut decompression. Nearly 10% of patients with a PEG tube suffer some sort of malfunction, with dislodgement occurring in up to 4.4% of patients. The emergency clinician should be familiar with PEG tubes and comfortable with the evaluation and management when these patients come to the ED with PEG tube dislodgement.

The PEG tube consists of a single-lumen tube protruding into the stomach, with a fixed internal bolster and a sliding external bolster. Normally, there should be 1 to 2 cm of movement of the tube before reaching the external bolster. Gauze is usually placed between the skin and the external bolster to collect any moisture that may gather. Normally, the skin surrounding the wound should be without erythema, exudate, or drainage. Irritation dermatitis can occur at the insertion site but should typically only be mild redness. A common error in the evaluation of PEG tubes is misdiagnosis of an infection (redness, pain, warmth, drainage, fever) at the insertion site and ascribing symptoms and signs to irritation dermatitis. The two must be carefully differentiated. Abscess, wound infection, and necrotizing skin infection should be considered in patients who show systemic signs of infection. Importantly, patients who are immunocompromised may not manifest typical signs and symptoms of infection.

Dislodgement of a PEG tube occurs more frequently in agitated, demented, or delirious patients. The decision to replace the PEG tube in the ED depends on the amount of time elapsed since the PEG tube was placed, as well as the amount of time the PEG tube has been dislodged.

The PEG tube's initial placement involves controlled perforation of a hollow organ with the formation of a gastrocutaneous fistula. The PEG tube holds the anterior stomach to the peritoneal wall. Eventually, the stomach becomes attached to the abdominal wall as adhesions form. The tract is considered mature in approximately 10 to 14 days, although the literature describes a range of 1 week to 6 months. Maturation will take longer in older or malnourished patients as well as those with AIDS, cancer, or diabetes; those who have undergone radiation therapy; or those who have an otherwise compromised immune system.

When a tube becomes dislodged, a focused history from the patient or caregiver and examination are important. It is especially important to find out when the PEG tube was placed and how long it has been dislodged. Lack of maturation of the tract means that there is a high probability that the stomach has fallen away from the abdominal wall. The primary concern is intraperitoneal spillage of gastric contents with associated sepsis or peritonitis, necessitating urgent surgical exploration. However, in many cases, peritoneal contamination is minimal, and a more conservative approach can be adopted. With an immature tract, avoid blind placement of a PEG tube, which may result in the tube being placed in the peritoneum. Patients with an immature tract and a dislodged PEG tube should be considered to have a perforation. Broad-spectrum antibiotics should be initiated, a nasogastric tube placed, and surgical consultation obtained. In these cases, PEG tube replacement should be performed by a specialist using endoscopic techniques in a controlled setting.

A PEG tube that has been present for more than 1 month is considered mature, and a replacement PEG tube can be placed blindly into the fistula with minimal risk to the patient. Replacement should not be delayed, as the gastrocutaneous fistula will begin to close 4 to 48 hours after dislodgement. Be sure to inflate the interior balloon. If a replacement PEG is unavailable, a Foley catheter can be used to maintain the patency of the tract and can be used for feeding purposes until a replacement PEG tube can be inserted. It should be noted that the mechanism for dislodgement, that is, trauma, or external traction, can result in disruption of a mature tract and can result in peritoneal placement if a PEG is inserted blindly. For this reason, confirmation of placement should always be performed. This can be achieved using an abdominal x-ray with radiopaque contrast injected into the tube.

The most common errors in the ED management of these patients include (1) failure to consult a specialist when an immature fistula track exists and proceeding with blind replacement and (2) failure to promptly maintain the fistula track and prevent its closure with a Foley catheter or replacement PEG tube.

PEARLS

- Consider infection of the tract in a patient with redness and tenderness, especially when systemic signs of infection are present.
- Obtain a confirmatory study after PEG tube replacement in a patient with a mature fistula track.
- In patients with immature tracts (<4 weeks), specialist consultation should be obtained.

Suggested Readings

Jacobson G, Brokish PA, Wrenn K. Percutaneous feeding tube replacement in the ED—are confirmatory x-rays necessary? *Am J Emerg Med.* 2009;27(5):519-524.

Marshall JB, Bodnarcuk G, Barthel JS. Early accidental dislodgement of PEG tubes. *J Clin Gastroenterol.* 1994;18(3):210-212.

McClave S, Neff RL. Care and long-term maintenance of percutaneous endoscopic gastrostomy tubes. *JPEN J Parenter Enteral Nutr.* 2006;30:S27-S38.

Schrag S, Sharma R, Jalk NP, et al. Complications related to percutaneous endoscopic gastrostomy (PEG) tubes. A comprehensive clinical review. *J Gastrointestin Liver Dis.* 2007;16(4): 407-418.

84

Biliary POCUS Pitfalls

Ryan C. Gibbons

Ultrasonography is the diagnostic imaging modality of choice to evaluate biliary pathology. **Table 84.1** reviews the most common biliary abnormalities and their sonographic appearance (see also **Figures 84.1-84.5**).

Current literature validates the diagnostic accuracy of biliary POCUS. **Table 84.2** reviews the test characteristics of POCUS, evaluating the most common biliary pathology.

In brief, begin by orienting the low-frequency (*2-5 MHz*) curvilinear (*abdominal*) transducer in the longitudinal plane just below the xiphoid process. Slide or move laterally looking for a cystic structure along the liver edge. Do not mistake the first part of the duodenum for the gallbladder. The duodenum has an anechoic wall and displays peristalsis. In addition, intraluminal air creates "dirty" gray shadowing. In comparison, the gallbladder is a cystic structure with a hyperechoic wall encompassing anechoic fluid.

Perform a longitudinal sweep from the patient's right to left. Then rotate the transducer 90° counterclockwise to the transverse orientation and repeat a sweep in a cranial-to-caudal direction. At times, the gallbladder presents a challenge to locate. **Table 84.3** reviews common reasons to overlook the gallbladder, while **Table 84.4** provides tips to facilitate visualizing the gallbladder.

Take note of the subtle differences between a WES sign and porcelain gallbladder depicted in **Figures 84.7** and **84.8**. With a WES sign, one visualizes the hyperechoic anterior gallbladder wall above anechoic bile adjacent to hyperechoic stone(s) creating posterior acoustic shadowing, which obscures additional views of the gallbladder. In contrast, a porcelain gallbladder has a calcified, hyperechoic anterior wall, which conceals

TABLE 84.1   Biliary pathology

	Echogenicity	Shadowing	Mobile
Cholelithiasis	Hyper	x	x
Choledocholithiasis	Hyper	x	Impacted in gallbladder neck
Sludge	Hypo		Collects dependently
Polyps[a]	Hypo		
Adenomyomatosis[b]	Hyper		
Folds[c]	Hyper		
Septations	Hyper		

[a] Follow-up based on clinical characteristics and size.
[b] Displays ring-down artifact.
[c] Phrygian cap at fundus.

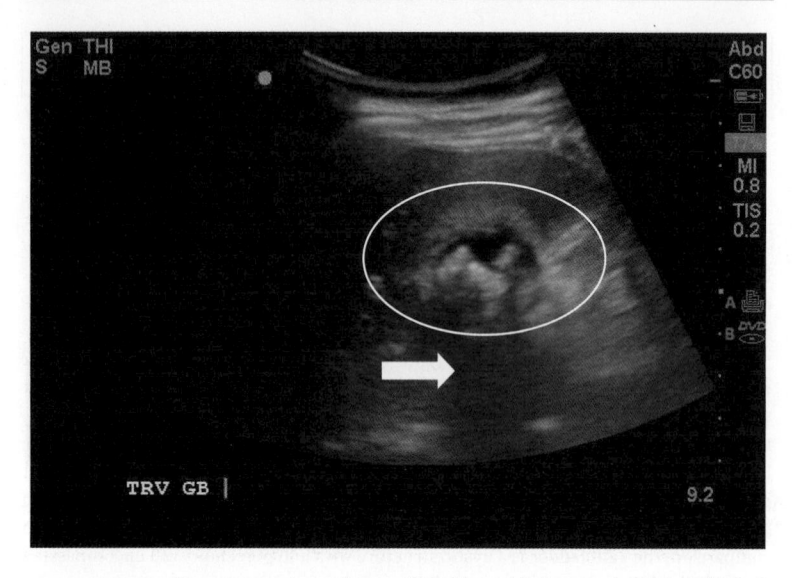

FIGURE 84.1 Transverse view of the gallbladder with hyperechoic cholelithiasis (circled) demonstrating posterior acoustic shadowing (arrow).

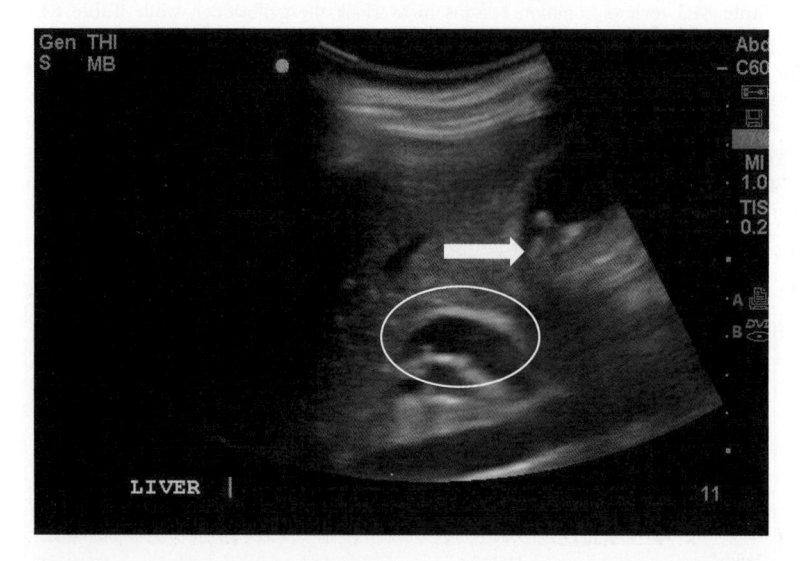

FIGURE 84.2 Hyperechoic cholelithiasis (arrow) with dilated CBD (circle). CBD, common bile duct.

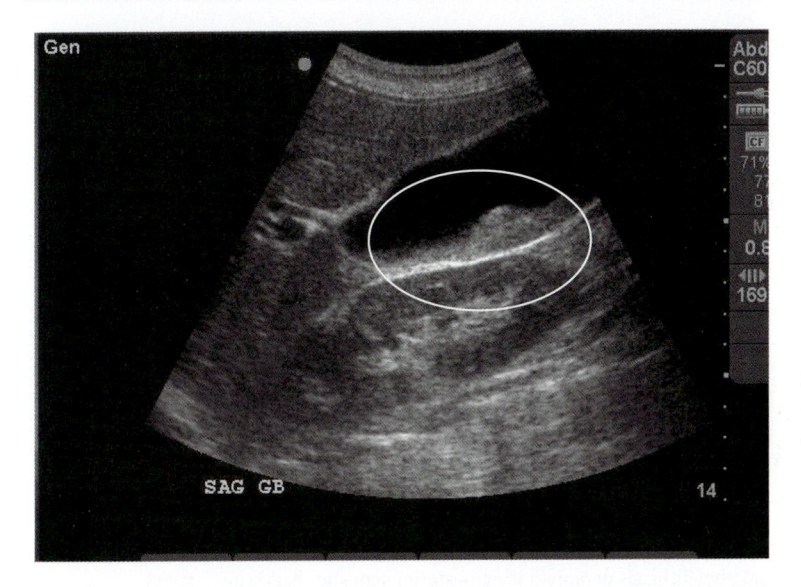

FIGURE 84.3 Longitudinal view of the gallbladder with hypoechoic sludge that layers dependently (circled). Sludge does not cause posterior acoustic shadowing.

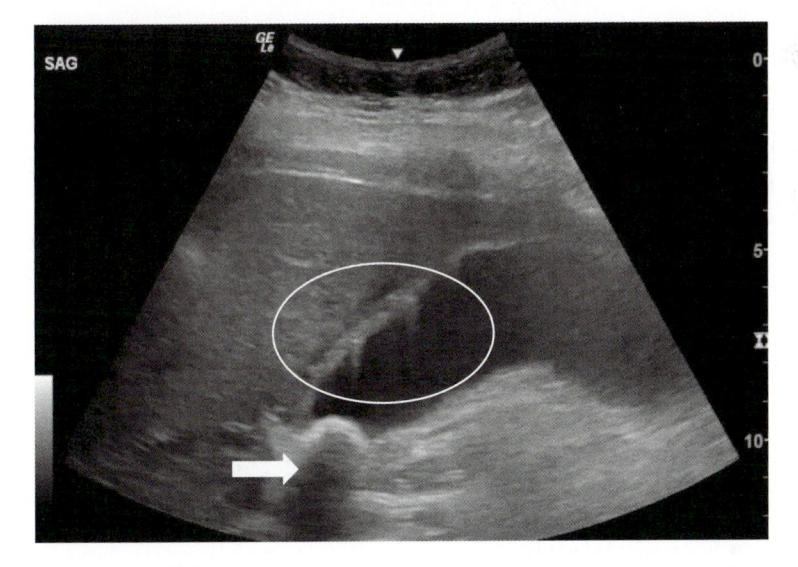

FIGURE 84.4 Longitudinal view of the gallbladder with adenomyomatosis along anterior wall demonstrating ring-down artifact (circled) and gallstone with posterior acoustic shadowing (arrow).

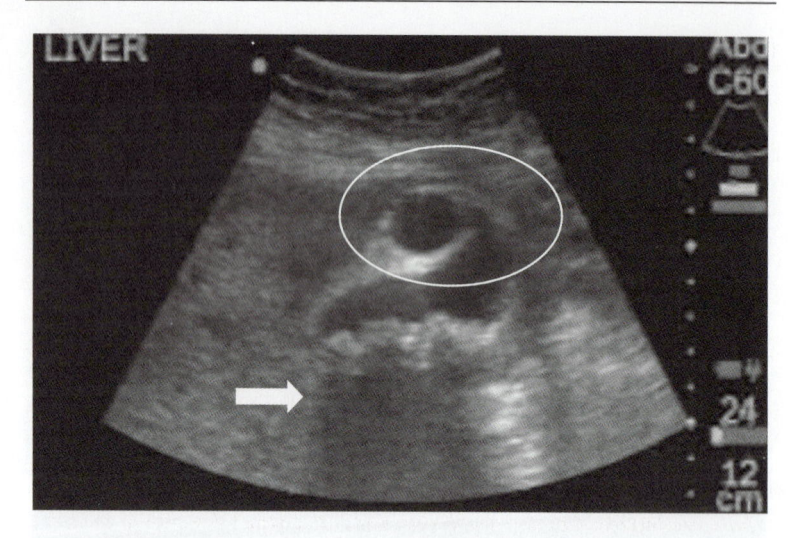

FIGURE 84.5 Longitudinal view of the gallbladder with Phrygian cap (circled) and cholelithiasis demonstrating posterior acoustic shadowing (arrow).

TABLE 84.2	BILIARY POINT-OF-CARE ULTRASOUND TEST CHARACTERISTICS					
	SENSITIVITY	SPECIFICITY	PPV	NPV	PLR	NLR
Cholelithiasis	89 (86-96)	88 (83-97)			7.5	0.12
Cholecystitis	86 (78-94)	71 (66-88)	92	99	3.32	0.18

NLR, negative likelihood ratio; NPV, negative predictive value; PLR, positive likelihood ratio; PPV, positive predictive value.

TABLE 84.3	CHALLENGES TO VISUALIZING THE GALLBLADDER

- Biliary agenesis
- Ectopic gallbladder
  - Retro- or intrahepatic
  - Left liver lobe
- Postprandial (*contracted gallbladder*)[a]
- Cholecystectomy
- WES sign[a]
- Porcelain gallbladder[a]
  - 50% associated with malignancy
- Obscured by bowel gas
- Body habitus

WES, wall echo shadow.

[a]See Figures 84.6 to 84.8.

Table 84.4 Tips for Visualizing the Gallbladder

- Deep inspiration
- Left lateral decubitus position
- Slide the transducer cranially
  - Utilize phased-array (cardiac) transducer[a]
    - Abdominal setting

[a]Smaller footprint for imaging within an intercostal space.

the remainder of the gallbladder. Remember, nearly 50% of porcelain gallbladders are malignant.

Once located, measure the most anterior gallbladder wall. The posterior wall appears thicker secondary to a common sonographic artifact known as posterior acoustic shadowing (**Figure 84.9**). A measurement exceeding 3 mm thickness is considered abnormal. Next, assess for the presence of gallstones, which appear as hyperechoic, mobile structures that display posterior acoustic shadowing. Beware that gallstones

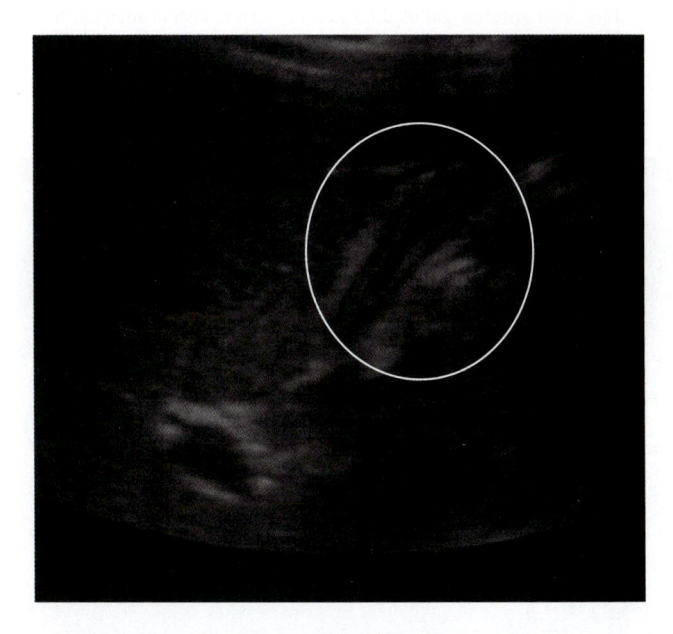

Figure 84.6 Postprandial (contracted) gallbladder.

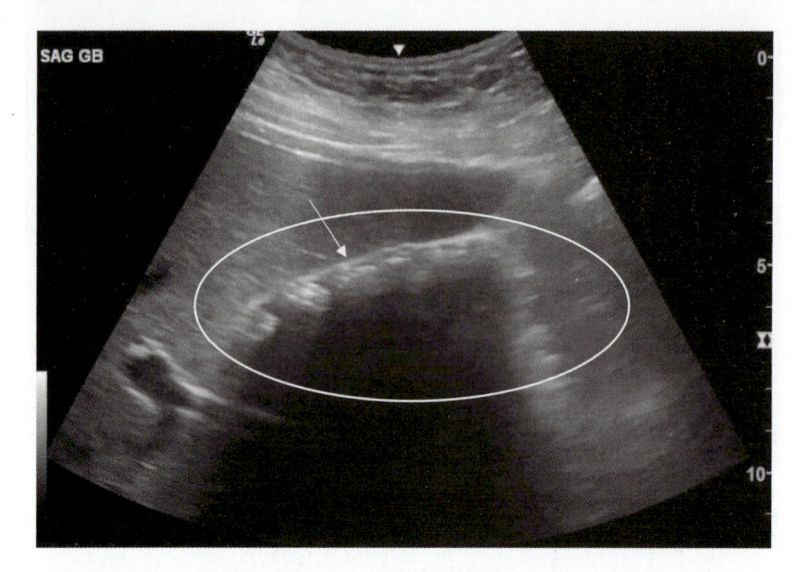

FIGURE 84.7 Longitudinal view of the gallbladder demonstrating the WES sign (circled). The most anterior gallbladder (arrow) wall is visible adjacent to anechoic biliary fluid layering above hyperechoic gallstones. WES, wall echo shadow.

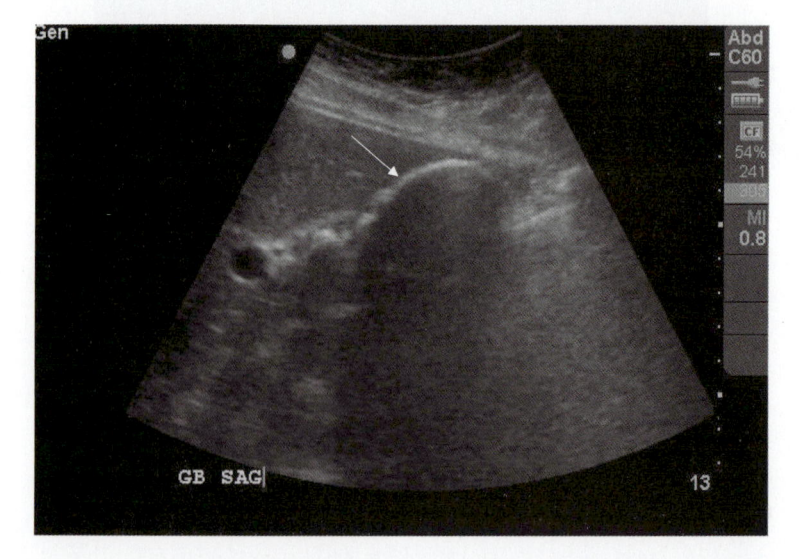

FIGURE 84.8 Porcelain gallbladder with hyperechoic anterior wall (arrow) obscuring visualization for gallbladder.

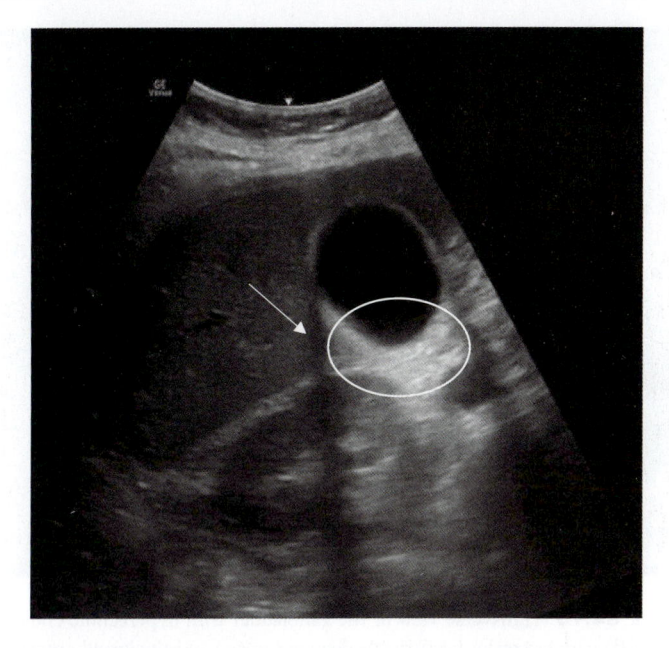

FIGURE 84.9 Edge artifact (arrow) with posterior acoustic enhancement (circle). Pericholecystic fluid (*anechoic*) lies adjacent to the gallbladder wall. The presence of cholelithiasis plus one of the following has a 92% positive predictive value for cholecystitis.

smaller than 4 mm may not shadow, and stones impacted within the neck render visualization challenging. The longitudinal orientation is best for evaluating the gallbladder neck. Moreover, edge artifact (**Figure 84.9**) can mimic gallstones. This sonographic aberration occurs along the edges of a cystic structure, such as gallbladder, cyst, and bladder. Simply, edge artifact is secondary to refraction and results in anechoic shadowing along the edges of cystic structures.

The presence of cholelithiasis plus one of the following has a 92% positive predictive value for cholecystitis.

- Anterior wall greater than 3 mm
- Pericholecystic (anechoic) fluid
- Sonographic Murphy sign (*maximal tenderness overlying the gallbladder*)

However, additional pathologies, including ascites, pancreatitis, hepatitis, congestive heart failure, cirrhosis, and adenomyomatosis, cause gallbladder wall thickening as well (**Figure 84.10**).

The CBD is assessed most easily in the longitudinal orientation. Locate the gallbladder. Then follow the hyperechoic main lobar fissure connecting the gallbladder with

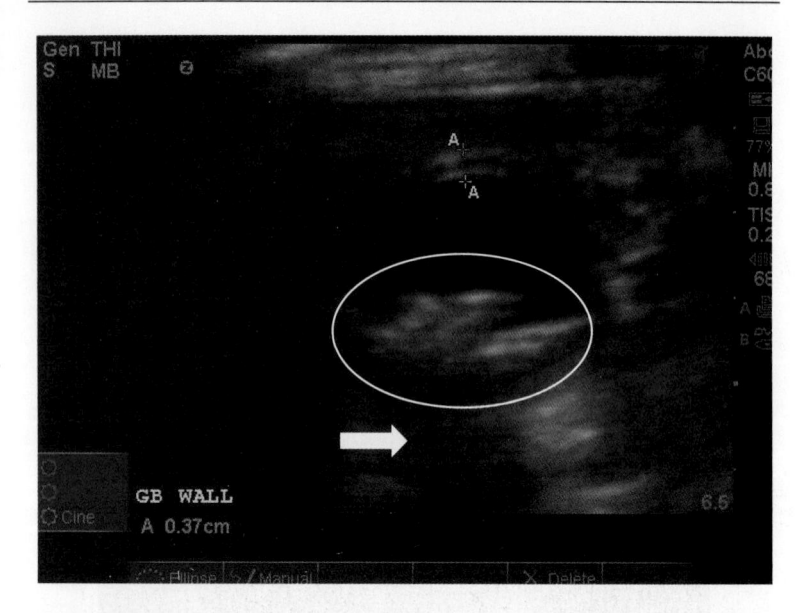

FIGURE 84.10 Transverse view of the gallbladder with hyperechoic cholelithiasis (circled) with posterior acoustic shadowing (arrow) and thickened anterior wall (*3.7 mm*).

the portal triad. The image often mimics an "exclamation point." The portal vein, common hepatic artery, and CBD create the appearance of a "Mickey Mouse" sign. Typically, the CBD is the most anterolateral structure. However, the CBD is anteromedial in up to 30% of patients.

Utilize color-flow Doppler to distinguish between vasculature and the biliary ducts. Tracking the structures aids in differentiating them as well. Once located, measure the largest diameter from inside wall to inside wall. A measurement greater than 5 mm is considered abnormal. However, with each decade over 50-years-old, an additional 1 mm is normal. Moreover, a CBD measuring 10 mm is within normal limits following a cholecystectomy. Nonetheless, remember to clinically correlate sonographic findings and assess laboratory values as an adjunct. There is some evidence suggesting limited utility in assessing the CBD without jaundice and/or abnormal liver function tests.

Acalculous (<5%) and emphysematous cholecystitis are less common clinical entities associated with severe illness. Emphysematous cholecystitis appears similar to adenomyomatosis. Be sure to clinically correlate the sonographic findings with the patient presentation. **Figures 84.11 to 84.13** portray each of these uncommon pathologies.

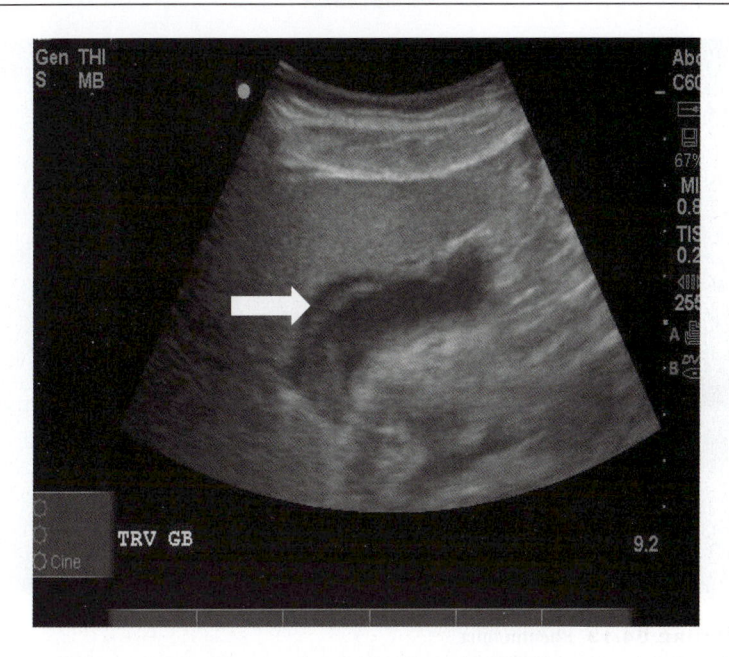

FIGURE 84.11 Acalculous cholecystitis with thickened wall and pericholecystic fluid. The arrow points to thickened gallbladder wall and pericholecystic fluid.

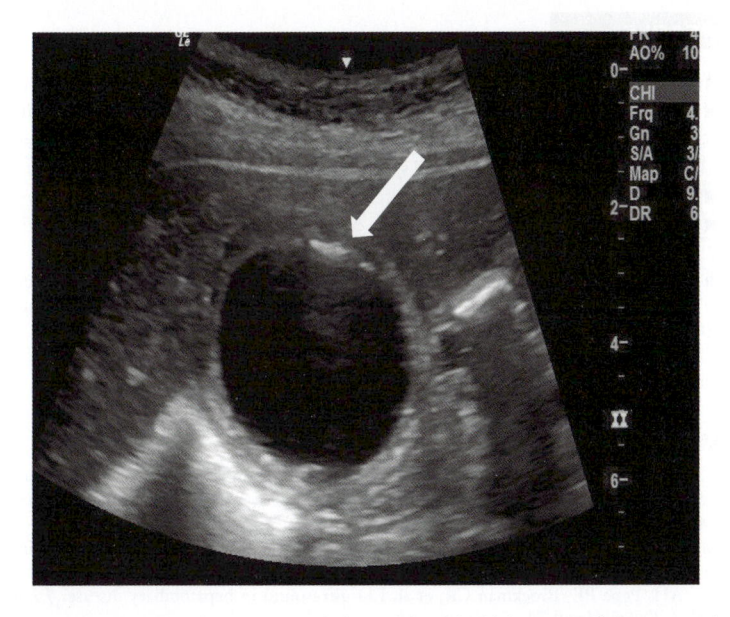

FIGURE 84.12 Emphysematous cholecystitis with thickened wall demonstrating air artifact. The arrow points to the air artifact.

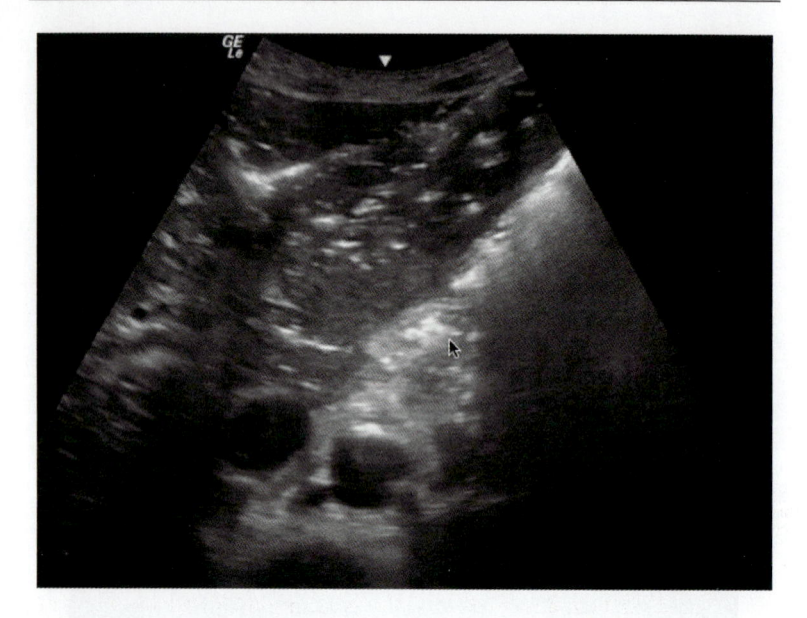

FIGURE 84.13 Pneumobilia.

PEARLS

- Measure the most anterior gallbladder wall to avoid posterior acoustic shadowing.
- Tips to visualize the gallbladder include asking the patient to inhale deeply, rolling the patient onto the left lateral decubitus position, and using the phased-array transducer within the intercostal space.
- Do not miss the WES sign or a porcelain gallbladder (*malignancy*).
- Wall thickness (>3 mm) is not always cholecystitis. Consider ascites, pancreatitis, congestive heart failure, and hepatitis.
- CBD less than 5 mm is within normal limits. Add 1 mm for every decade over 50-year-old. A CBD 10 mm or less is normal for patients status post cholecystectomy.

SUGGESTED READINGS

Jain A, Mehta N, Secko M, et al. History, physical examination, laboratory testing, and emergency department ultrasonography for the diagnosis of acute cholecystitis. *Acad Emerg Med*. 2017;24(3):281-297.

Lahham S, Becker BA, Gari A, et al. Utility of common bile duct measurement in ED point of care ultrasound: a prospective study. *Am J Emerge Med*. 2018;36(6):962-966.

Miller AH, Pepe PE, Brockman CR, et al. ED ultrasound in hepatobiliary disease. *J Emerg Med*. 2006;30(1):69-74.

Ross M, Brown M, McLaughlin K. Emergency physician–performed ultrasound to diagnose cholelithiasis: a systematic review. *Acad Emerg Med.* 2011;18(3):227-235.

Summers SM, Scruggs W, Menchine MD, et al. A prospective evaluation of emergency department bedside ultrasonography for the detection of acute cholecystitis. *Ann Emerg Med.* 2010;56(2):114-122.

85

TICKING TIME BOMB: THE GASTRIC BYPASS PATIENT WITH ABDOMINAL PAIN

DILLON WARR AND ZACHARY REPANSHEK

Obesity is a complex, multifactorial disease that has nearly tripled worldwide since 1975. In fact, more than a third of the world's population is now considered overweight or obese. It is well established that obesity increases the risk for multiple disease conditions, including diabetes, heart disease, and cancer, as well as negatively affects quality of life, work productivity, and healthcare costs. With this rise in obesity, so too has risen the popularity of weight-loss interventions, including bariatric surgery. There were 256,000 bariatric procedures performed in the United States in 2019 alone, a 61.7% increase from 2011, with the gastric sleeve, laparoscopic gastric banding, and the RYGB being the most popular. These options allow for either malabsorptive, restrictive, or combined approaches for weight loss. Unfortunately, despite their demonstrated benefit, these procedures are not without complications, often landing these patients in the ED. To ensure proper management, emergency clinicians must swiftly recognize and treat these complications.

SURGICAL PROCEDURE

The RYGB accounted for up to 20% of bariatric procedures in the United States in 2020 and is the most popular restrictive-malabsorptive procedure. This laparoscopic procedure involves creating a small gastric pouch from the stomach and then connecting this pouch to the jejunum, bypassing a portion of the stomach, the duodenum, and the upper jejunum (**Figure 85.1**). This results in reduced food intake and decreased calorie and nutrient absorption. However, this revised gut anatomy creates a unique set of potential complications. In fact, 5% of patients undergoing treatment for weight management visit the ED within 3 months of their initial surgery.

OVERALL APPROACH

The most common reason that bariatric surgery patients return to the ED within 3 months of surgery is abdominal pain, followed by vomiting and dehydration. These presentations can be challenging, as "bariatric surgery" is a catch-all for a suite of different procedures, each different in technique, that result in distinct structural anatomic changes that predispose patients to unique complications. The clinical examination can be unreliable in the postoperative RYGB patient due to truncal obesity, and in some cases, tachycardia is

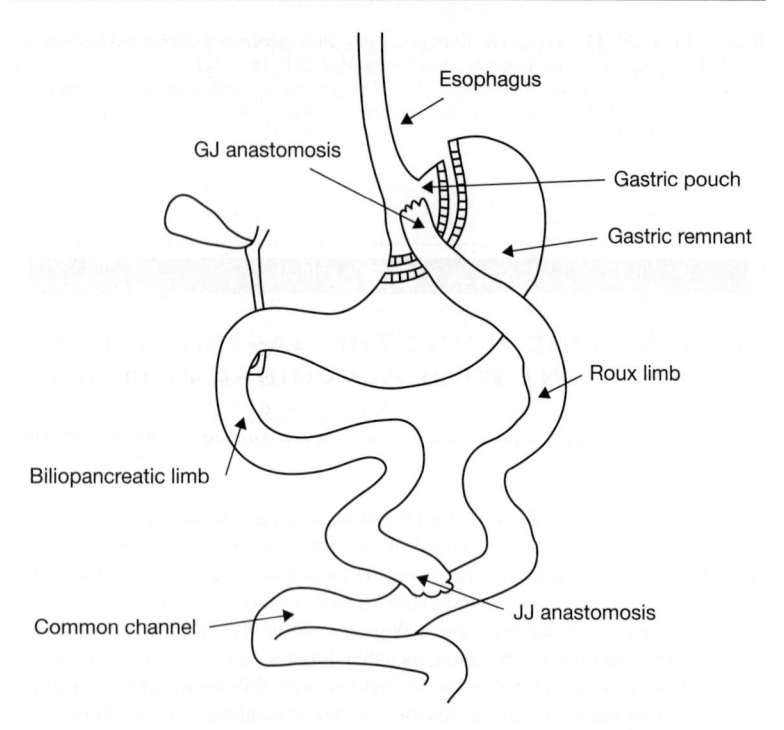

FIGURE 85.1 The Roux-en-Y gastric bypass. GJ, gastro-jejunal; JJ, jejuno-jejunal.

the only clinical sign of a possible surgical complication. The standard differential for abdominal pain, including metabolic and surgical pathologies, also still applies.

When evaluating the RYGB patient, the possible complications are based on the time from the surgery. Within the first month after their operation, patients are more likely to have bleeding, leakage, abscess formation, surgical wound infection, and anastomotic strictures. Presentations beyond postoperative day 30 have a higher likelihood of intra-abdominal infection, obstruction, herniation, ulceration, and nutritional deficiency.

If your suspicion is high for a surgical complication, particularly within the immediate postoperative period, it is important to contact the appropriate surgical consultant early in the clinical evaluation. This evaluation should include a broad laboratory workup and a very low threshold for CT imaging.

EVALUATION AND MANAGEMENT OF RYGB-SPECIFIC COMPLICATIONS

Anastomotic leak is the most concerning complication of RYGB, with a prevalence of approximately 2%. There are multiple suture lines at risk of leak, including the gastric pouch, the excluded stomach, the GJ, the JJ, and the staple closures of the small intestine division sites. The most common site of leakage is the GJ, accounting for over 50% of cases. In addition to abdominal pain, patients will often present with fever, tachycardia, nausea, vomiting, and hypotension. CT with PO and IV contrast is the recommended first-line imaging modality for this complication—one of the few indications for CT with

PO contrast in the ED. Second-line imaging typically involves a UGIS. If the diagnosis is confirmed, broad-spectrum antibiotics, fluid resuscitation, and surgical consultations should be performed. Although patients who are hemodynamically unstable will require emergent surgical exploration, stable patients may be able to be managed with percutaneous drainage or endoscopic procedures.

The most important aspect of the treatment of an anastomotic leak is early recognition, especially as the presentation can be subtle. One must have a low threshold for further investigation. In fact, tachycardia is often the only sign of an anastomotic leak, and persistent tachycardia greater than 120 beats/min requires hospital admission for fluid resuscitation, close monitoring, and possible surgical intervention, even with negative CT imaging, given the risk for sepsis and rapid deterioration.

Early anastomotic stricture can occur at either the GJ or the JJ anastomosis. JJ stenosis occurs early, most often in the first week postoperatively, while GJ stenosis occurs weeks to months later. Symptoms and management differ depending on location. In JJ stenosis, although the stricture causes obstruction, patients do not present with emesis. The biliary limb instead dilates, leading to gastric distension and eventual gastric perforation and peritonitis. This requires urgent surgical intervention with JJ reconstruction and gastric decompression. On the other hand, GJ stenosis presents with the typical symptoms of obstruction: nausea, vomiting, and abdominal pain. Treatment involves endoscopic balloon dilation in most cases. UGIS is the typical diagnostic test for both GJ and JJ stenosis.

Marginal ulceration occurs at the GJ anastomosis, with 50% occurring within the first 3 months. The pathophysiology may include some combination of jejunal exposure to unbuffered stomach acid, tension at the anastomosis, NSAID use, *Helicobacter pylori* infection, and smoking. Symptoms include epigastric pain, nausea, vomiting, dietary intolerance, hematemesis, and melena. Severe cases can lead to upper GI bleeding and perforation. Stable patients can be discharged from the ED with PPI therapy and outpatient GI follow-up for endoscopic diagnosis and management.

Small bowel obstruction after RYGB occurs due to internal hernia in 60% of cases, followed by postoperative adhesions. Although internal hernias can develop at any point postoperatively, they more commonly occur as a delayed complication, as the patient's resulting weight loss facilitates the creation of potential spaces in the mesentery within which the intestine can incarcerate. Diagnosis of an internal hernia can be challenging as the obstruction is often intermittent, with patients experiencing distinct periods of abdominal pain. This is further complicated by the frequent lack of emesis in patients post-RYGB. First-line imaging is an abdominal CT with PO and IV contrast performed during a painful episode. A similar approach to diagnosis can be used for obstruction caused by postoperative adhesions, which can also develop at any time postoperatively.

Dumping syndrome, while not a surgical emergency, occurs in nearly 75% of postgastric bypass patients and, thus, is an important cause of abdominal pain to consider in the RYGB patient. It occurs when high-carbohydrate meals pass rapidly into the small bowel without the anatomic barrier of the pylorus to control transit. It leads to bowel distension, fluid shifts, and GI hormone secretion. Patients can develop early (<30 minutes after eating) dumping symptoms defined by dehydration, tachycardia, hypotension, abdominal pain, and syncope from fluid shifting. Alternatively, they can develop late-dumping symptoms (2-4 hours after eating) defined by hypoglycemia from a postprandial insulin surge. ED treatment involves fluid and electrolyte repletion as well as dietary modification.

> **PEARLS**
>
> - Bariatric surgery refers to multiple different surgical procedures, each with distinct structural anatomic changes and unique complications.
> - The clinical examination can be unreliable in the postoperative RYGB patient, and tachycardia may be the only sign of a surgical emergency.
> - It is important to contact the appropriate surgical consultant early in the clinical evaluation, and there should be a very low threshold for CT imaging.
> - Postoperative abdominal pain in the RYGB patient is one of the few indications for CT with PO contrast in the ED.
> - Anastomotic strictures and internal hernias are both obstructive processes that can present without emesis in the RYGB patient.

SUGGESTED READINGS

Altieri MS, Wright B, Peredo A, Pryor AD. Common weight loss procedures and their complications. *Am J Emerg Med*. 2018;36(3):475-479.

Contival N, Menahem B, Gautier T, Le Roux Y, Alves A. Guiding the non-bariatric surgeon through complications of bariatric surgery. *J Visc Surg*. 2018;155(1):27-40.

Kassir R, Debs T, Blanc P, et al. Complications of bariatric surgery: presentation and emergency management. *Int J Surg*. 2016;27:77-81.

Lim R, Beekley A, Johnson DC, Davis KA. Early and late complications of bariatric operation. *Trauma Surg Acute Care Open*. 2018;3(1):e000219.

Luber SD, Fischer DR, Venkat A. Care of the bariatric surgery patient in the emergency department. *J Emerg Med*. 2008;34(1):13-20.

86

DON'T MISS AORTOENTERIC FISTULA: A RARE BUT LIFE-THREATENING CAUSE OF GASTROINTESTINAL BLEEDING!

NEENA KASHYAP AND ZACHARY REPANSHEK

AEF is a rare cause of GIB that should be considered in the differential diagnosis for patients with GIB. Classically taught as the triad of GIB, abdominal pain, and a pulsatile abdominal mass, this triad of symptoms is only present approximately 10% of the time. If AEF is missed or diagnosis delayed, mortality approaches 100%.

Primary AEF refers to a spontaneous fistulous connection between the aorta and any part of the bowel. The most common cause of primary AEF is an aortic aneurysm, but infection, tumor, foreign body ingestion, and radiation therapy have all been reported as causative etiologies. Primary AEF is exceedingly rare, with an incidence at autopsy of less than 0.1%.

Secondary AEF refers to the formation of a fistulous connection after aortic surgery and is more common than primary AEF. It most frequently occurs after emergent surgery for a ruptured aortic aneurysm but can happen after any aortic surgery, including elective AAA resection, aortic replacement or bypass for aortoiliac occlusive disease, and open or endovascular stent graft placement for aortic aneurysm. It is associated with aortitis from the initial surgery, intestinal flora translocation, or postoperative bacteremia from another source. Median time from initial surgery to secondary AEF formation is generally 2 to 4 years, though there have been reports of AEF occurring from 1 week to 26 years.

Both primary and secondary AEF have a distinct male predominance. Fifty to 70% of cases are associated with the third and fourth portions of the duodenum due to its retroperitoneal placement and proximity to the aorta.

GIB is the most common presentation of AEF, occurring in more than 90% of patients. Hematemesis is most common, though melena and hematochezia may also occur. Patients may present with a small bleed that is self-limited due to thrombus formation and vasospasm. This initial bleed has been termed a "herald bleed" and occurs in about 50% of cases of AEF. A herald bleed may precede further bleeding anywhere from hours to weeks later. Patients may also present with nonspecific symptoms, such as abdominal pain, back pain, fever, sepsis, or hypotension.

AEF should be considered and ruled out in any patient with a history of AAA or aortic repair who presents with GIB. If the patient is hemodynamically stable, CTA of the abdomen and pelvis is the recommended initial test of choice, with a sensitivity of 94% and specificity of 85%. Diagnostic signs of AEF on CTA include extravasation of contrast from the aorta into adjacent bowel, gas collections around aortic grafts, bowel wall thickening near an aortic graft, loss of the fat plane between the aorta and the intestine, and an intramural duodenal hematoma. If AEF is strongly considered and the patient cannot be stabilized for CT scan, prompt consultation with a vascular surgeon for exploratory laparotomy and repair is paramount.

Typical initial diagnostic procedures used in the admitted patient with GIB (endoscopy, colonoscopy) have limited utility in the diagnosis of AEF, with only 30% and 10% of patients diagnosed with AEF by endoscopy and colonoscopy, respectively. Twenty-three percent of patients with primary AEF in one series had concurrent gastric ulcers, which could be attributed as the source of GIB, confounding the diagnosis. Concern for AEF should be communicated to the gastroenterologist so they can attempt to evaluate down to the third or fourth portion of the duodenum.

Management of AEF follows the same principles as for any critically ill ED patient: at least two large-bore IVs, cardiac monitoring, and appropriate diagnostic lab testing, including type and cross. Blood products and IV fluids are important for stabilizing a patient with hypotensive bleeding; however, in AEF, one should consider permissive hypotension similar to the resuscitation of trauma patients or those with ruptured AAA. Temporary clots can form to temporize the bleeding, so permissive hypotension may be beneficial before operation.

In addition to emergency stabilization, broad-spectrum antibiotics directed to gram-positive and gram-negative bacteria should be initiated. These will typically be continued for at least 1 week even after negative operative cultures and 4 to 6 weeks if cultures are positive.

Definitive management of AEF is surgical, so early surgical consultation is essential. Hospitals without a vascular surgeon need to stabilize and then transfer these patients. Repair of AEF consists of obtaining vascular control and subsequent revascularization via in situ repair or bypass grafting. Thirty-day mortality has been historically reported at 30% to 40% after surgery, though one series from 1991 to 2003 reported a

21% 30-day mortality. Early mortality is significantly associated with patients presenting in hypovolemic or septic shock. In recent years, endovascular AEF repair (a minimally invasive interventional radiology procedure) has been employed as a temporizing measure with lower postoperative mortality. Nevertheless, endovascular repair is currently limited by the complications of recurrent infection and bleeding—perhaps a reflection of the fact that the fistula is not primarily repaired.

PEARLS

- Emergency clinicians should consider AEF in any patient with a history of aortic surgery or AAA who presents with a GIB.
- CTA of the abdomen and pelvis is key to the diagnosis in stable patients.
- Early vascular surgical consultation is critical.
- Additional ED management includes establishing vascular access, transfusion of blood products with consideration of permissive hypotension, and broad-spectrum antibiotics.

Acknowledgments

We gratefully acknowledge the contributions of previous edition author, Kristin Berona, as portions of their chapter have been retained in this revision.

Suggested Readings

Armstrong PA, Back MR, Wilson JS, et al. Improved outcomes in the recent management of secondary aortoenteric fistula. *J Vasc Surg*. 2005;42(4):660-666.
Bergqvist D, Björck M, Nyman R. Secondary aortoenteric fistula after endovascular aortic interventions: a systematic literature review. *J Vasc Interv Radiol*. 2008;19(2 Pt 1):163-165.
Ranasinghe W, Loa J, Allaf N, et al. Primary aortoenteric fistulae: the challenges in diagnosis and review of treatment. *Ann Vasc Surg*. 2011;25(3):386.e1-386.5.
Saers SJ, Scheltinga MR. Primary aortoenteric fistula. *Br J Surg*. 2005;92(2):143-152.
Tagowski M, Vieweg H, Wissgott C, et al. Aortoenteric fistula as a complication of open reconstruction and endovascular repair of abdominal aorta. *Radiol Res Pract*. 2014;2014:383159.

87

Don't Miss the Patient With Perforated Peptic Ulcer

Katey S. Cohen and Zachary Repanshek

The prevalence of PUD in the general population is 5% to 10%, while the risk of complications in patients with chronic PUD is 2% to 3%. There has been a consistent decrease in the incidence of complications of PUD in the United States, presumably due to the decline in *Helicobacter pylori* prevalence and increasing use of PPIs. Despite this downtrend, complications from PUD remain a significant source of morbidity and mortality due to the possibilities of bleeding, perforation, or obstruction. One study showed that of patients undergoing surgery for a perforated peptic ulcer, one in three patients died in the follow-up period. As such, early detection of PUD complications is critical in the ED setting.

Risk Factors for PUD and Its Complications

The development of PUD can be multifactorial, with *H. pylori* infection and NSAIDs as the most predominant causes. Studies have shown a dose-dependent relationship between bleeding ulcers and NSAID use, also noting that the risk was significantly higher in the first 30 days of NSAID use. Approximately half of perforated peptic ulcers involve NSAID use. Patients on corticosteroid therapy can also be at increased risk for the development of both PUD and its complications. Stress, malignancy, and critical illness are other potential risk factors. Patients with PUD taking antiplatelet or anticoagulant medications are at increased risk for bleeding.

When to Consider a Perforated Peptic Ulcer

The presentation of PUD can vary and is nonspecific but typically involves epigastric abdominal pain. Clinicians should maintain a high degree of suspicion for PUD in patients with risk factors presenting with abdominal pain. Pain occurring several hours after eating or awakening at night with pain relieved by food intake suggests PUD.

Perforated peptic ulcer should be considered in patients with symptoms suggestive of PUD, or a known history of PUD, who experience sudden, diffuse abdominal pain. Vital sign abnormalities may range from mild tachycardia to overt hemodynamic instability. Examination may reveal hypoactive bowel sounds, a distended abdomen, and signs of peritonitis, such as guarding and rigidity. Abdominal pain, rigidity, and tachycardia are a classic triad for perforation. However, perforations may be walled off, fibrotic, or retroperitoneal, leading to a seemingly less acute presentation. These patients may not be peritoneal.

Duodenal ulcer perforation typically presents with acute abdominal pain while gastric ulcer perforation may not and, therefore, are associated with increased mortality due to delays in diagnosis. Maintaining a high degree of clinical suspicion for a perforated gastric ulcer is crucial.

Diagnosis

When a perforated ulcer is suspected, prompt diagnosis and management is pivotal. CT scan is the best test for the detection of perforation, as it is both sensitive and specific with the added benefit of the ability to localize the ulcer site. CT findings may include pneumoperitoneum, intraperitoneal fluid, bowel wall thickening, and mesenteric fat streaking. If CT is not immediately available, bedside ultrasound or upright abdominal x-ray (KUB) can be utilized. Bedside ultrasound requires a trained clinician who could visualize free air under the diaphragm. KUB has a sensitivity of 50% to 70% for detecting free air, and the ability of a peritoneal patient to maintain an upright position for the study can be challenging. Lab testing is nonspecific, although it may show metabolic acidosis, elevated serum lactate, and leukocytosis.

Management

The first step in management is resuscitation. This will include IV fluids, broad-spectrum antibiotics, and NPO status. Restoration of hemodynamics is of the utmost importance, and resuscitative goals should include a mean arterial blood pressure greater than 65 mm Hg, urine output greater than 0.5 mL/kg/h, and lactate normalization. Hemodynamic monitoring such as invasive arterial lines may be indicated, and the use of vasopressors may be necessary. Electrolyte derangement is common, and the clinician should check a metabolic panel and replete as necessary. If there is concern for associated bleeding ulcers, a PPI should be started.

Early surgical consultation is necessary for PUD with perforation, and both operative and nonoperative management are options. Patients presenting with perforated peptic ulcers are often older with comorbidities, which can increase morbidity and mortality of surgical intervention. For operative patients, hemodynamic status as well as comorbidities are considered when deciding on the timing of intervention and surgical technique. Nonoperative management is also possible for small perforations, as the omentum can form adhesions and heal without surgical intervention.

PEARLS

- The classic triad of abdominal pain, tachycardia, and abdominal rigidity should prompt consideration of a perforation, especially with known history or risk factors for PUD.
- CT is the best imaging modality to detect perforation.
- Resuscitation and early management should include IV fluids, broad-spectrum antibiotics, NPO status, and hemodynamic monitoring.
- Early surgical consultation is essential.
- Both operative and nonoperative management are options depending on age, surgical risk factors, hemodynamic condition, and size of perforation.

Suggested Readings

Agarwal A, Jain S, Meena LN, Jain SA, Agarwal L. Validation of Boey's score in predicting morbidity and mortality in peptic perforation peritonitis in Northwestern India. *Trop Gastroenterol*. 2015;36(4):256-260.

Cho KC, Baker SR. Extraluminal air. Diagnosis and significance. *Radiol Clin North Am*. 1994;32(5):829-844.

Horowitz J, Kukora JS, Ritchie WP Jr. All perforated ulcers are not alike. *Ann Surg*. 1989;209(6):693-696.

Lanas A, Chan FKL. Peptic ulcer disease. *Lancet*. 2017;390:613-624.

Lanas A, García-Rodríguez LA, Arroyo MT, et al. Risk of upper gastrointestinal ulcer bleeding associated with selective cyclo-oxygenase-2 inhibitors, traditional non-aspirin non-steroidal anti-inflammatory drugs, aspirin and combinations. *Gut*. 2006;55(12):1731-1738.

Tarasconi A, Coccolini F, Biffl WL, et al. Perforated and bleeding peptic ulcer: WSES guidelines. *World J Emerg Surg*. 2020;15:3.

Thorsen K, Søreide JA, Søreide K. Long-term mortality in patients operated for perforated peptic ulcer: factors limiting longevity are dominated by older age, comorbidity burden and severe postoperative complications. *World J Surg*. 2017;41:410.

Wang YR, Richter JE, Dempsey DT. Trends and outcomes of hospitalizations for peptic ulcer disease in the United States, 1993 to 2006. *Ann Surg*. 2010;251:51.

Wong CS, Chia CF, Lee HC, et al. Eradication of *Helicobacter pylori* for prevention of ulcer recurrence after simple closure of perforated peptic ulcer: a meta-analysis of randomized controlled trials. *J Surg Res*. 2013;182(2):219-226.

88

Don't Be Fooled by a Subtle Presentation—SBP Can Be Deadly!

Alessandra Conforto

SBP is typically a complication of ascites in patients with advanced cirrhosis and is defined as the presence of infection in the ascitic fluid without any identifiable intra-abdominal source. Annually, approximately 25% of patients with ascites develop SBP, with the risk correlating to the severity of the underlying liver disease. Importantly, SBP is distinct from peritonitis secondary to another intra-abdominal process (eg, appendicitis, viscus perforation) and from peritonitis that develops in patients receiving peritoneal dialysis. Current mortality for SBP is reported as 20% to 30%. With early diagnosis and treatment, the prognosis improves dramatically.

Pathogenesis

SBP occurs when bacteria translocate from the intestinal lumen to the ascitic fluid, which causes infection typically with gram-negative enteric flora. The most common organisms in SBP are *Escherichia coli* (70%), *Klebsiella* species (10%), *Proteus* species (10%), *Enterococcus faecalis* (4%), and *Pseudomonas* species (2%). Approximately 35% of infections are due to an MDRO.

Examination

The clinical exam in patients with SBP is variable, with up to 13% of patients having no signs or symptoms of infection at the time of diagnosis. Presenting signs and symptoms of SBP may include fever (>37.8 °C or 100.0 °F), mild confusion or worsening hepatic encephalopathy, mild diffuse abdominal pain, nausea, vomiting, diarrhea, decreased urine output, gastrointestinal bleeding, sepsis, and shock. Patients with SBP will rarely have a rigid abdomen, so mild tenderness or pain should be taken seriously and investigated. Laboratory abnormalities such as leukocytosis, worsening renal function, and acidosis are ominous findings and should raise the concern for SBP.

Diagnosis

The presumptive diagnosis of SBP in the ED is based on the analysis of peritoneal fluid obtained by paracentesis. Paracentesis is a safe procedure, with a risk of bleeding reported between 1% and 3%, a risk of hollow viscus perforation of 1%, and overall risk of death less than 0.5%. The use of ultrasound to identify an appropriate pocket of ascites is recommended to reduce the rate of complications. Contraindications to performing a diagnostic paracentesis are relative and include untreated clinically apparent coagulation abnormalities and skin infection at the site. Ileus with abdominal distention and abdominal wall surgical scars pose an increased risk of bowel perforation. Recent guidelines indicate that neither an elevated INR nor thrombocytopenia require correction before the procedure. A potential exception to correction of thrombocytopenia is in patients with concomitant platelet dysfunction from renal impairment who may benefit from treatment with DDAVP.

The most commonly accepted criterion for the diagnosis of SBP is the presence of more than 250 PMN/mm^3 of ascitic fluid. If there is significant blood contamination

(>10,000 RBC/mm^3), a correction factor subtracting 1 PMN for every 250 RBCs can be used. Gram stains are rarely positive because the concentration of bacteria is usually low but can be helpful in identifying secondary peritonitis. In addition to the cell count, the pH of ascitic fluid (<7.35), a blood–ascitic fluid pH gradient 0.10 or more, as well as a serum-ascites albumin ratio 1.1 g/dL or more can help confirm the diagnosis of SBP in equivocal cases.

In contrast to SBP, secondary peritonitis should be suspected if ascitic PMNs are significantly more than 250/mm^3 or if two of the following criteria are present in ascitic fluid: glucose less than 50 mg/dL, protein more than 10 g/L, or ascitic LDH is greater than serum LDH. The suspicion of secondary peritonitis mandates broadening antibiotic coverage to include anaerobic organisms and the search for a surgically correctable source of peritonitis with immediate surgical consultation and advanced imaging.

Treatment

Early administration of appropriate antibiotic coverage and infusion of albumin are the foundations of treatment for SBP. Once septic shock develops, each hour of delay in antibiotic administration causes a 10% increase in mortality.

Third-generation cephalosporins (cefotaxime, ceftriaxone, or ceftazidime) are the antibiotics of choice. Oral fluoroquinolones may be prescribed for patients who are awake and not vomiting. Due to the emergence of MDROs, current guidelines recommend broader coverage in patients who are at risk for MDRO infections (critically ill patients in the ICU, patients with nosocomial infection or recent hospitalization). In these patients, piperacillin/tazobactam should be the first antibiotic with vancomycin added if a positive swab or a previous infection was due to methicillin-resistant Staph aureus. Daptomycin is added in the setting of suspected vancomycin-resistant enterococcus and meropenem is indicated if the patient has previously been treated with piperacillin/tazobactam.

Intravenous albumin plays a vital role in decreasing mortality in the setting of SBP, particularly in those patients with signs of decompensated liver disease (bilirubin >5 mg/dL) or renal insufficiency (BUN >30 mg/dL or creatinine >1 mg/dL). The recommended dosing is 1.5 g/kg on day 1, followed by 1 g/kg on day 3.

Due to the emergence of MDROs, current recommendation advocates for a repeat paracentesis within 48 hours to document an appropriate response to treatment, as evidenced by a decrease in the number of PMN/mL of 25% from baseline.

Positive Cultures in a Discharged Patient?

Bacterascites is a term used to describe ascitic fluid that is colonized with bacteria (culture positive) but with a PMN count less than 250/mm^3. The diagnosis is delayed, usually 3 days after the original paracentesis when the culture results become available. The current recommendation is to perform a repeat paracentesis on day 3. *Bacterascites* is treated as SBP if, on the second paracentesis, the PMN count is more than 250/mm^3, or if the second culture is also positive. If PMN count is less than 250/mm^3 and cultures remain negative, no further action is necessary.

PEARLS

- Maintain a high index of suspicion for SBP in all patients with cirrhosis. Clinical diagnosis of SBP is difficult, as patients present with nonspecific complaints.
- Patients with ascites who are admitted to hospital should receive a diagnostic paracentesis regardless of their presenting complaint.

- Do not delay the administration of antibiotics and make every effort to perform paracentesis and blood cultures before administering antibiotics.
- Don't forget to administer albumin in SBP.

Suggested Readings

Biggins SW, Anglei P, Garcia-Tsao G, et al. Diagnosis, evaluation and management of ascites, spontaneous bacterial peritonitis and hepatorenal syndrome: 2021 Practice Guidance by the American Association of the Study of Liver Diseases. *Hepatology*. 2021;74(2):1014-1048.

Koulaouzidis A, Bhat S, Saeed AA. Spontaneous bacterial peritonitis. *World J Gastroenterol*. 2009;15(9):1042-1049.

Lutz P, Nischalke HD, Strassburg CP, et al. Spontaneous bacterial peritonitis: the clinical challenge of a leaky gut and a cirrhotic liver. *World J Hepatol*. 2015;7(3):304-314.

Wong CL, Holroyd-Leduc J, Torpe KE, et al. Does this patient have bacterial peritonitis or portal hypertension? The rational clinical examination. *JAMA*. 2008;299:1166-1178.

89

Acute Cholangitis aka Biliary Sepsis

Prathap Sooriyakumaran

Acute cholangitis is a critical, time-sensitive illness that refers to a bacterial infection of the biliary system (biliary sepsis) and requires both obstruction and bacterial colonization of the biliary tract. Also known as *ascending cholangitis* (bacteria can enter an obstructed biliary system by "ascending" from the duodenum), it can be fatal if not appropriately and timely diagnosed and treated.

Normally, bile is sterile. Bile salts have bacteriostatic properties, and the sphincter of Oddi controls the direction of bile flow, acting as a barrier between the sterile bile duct and the bacteria-filled duodenum. Obstruction and the resulting increase in bile duct pressure lead to a breakdown of these defenses and subsequent bacterial colonization and infection. The most common bacteria identified in acute cholangitis include *Escherichia coli*, *Klebsiella*, *Enterobacter*, *Enterococcus*, *Pseudomonas*, *Bacteroides*, and *Citrobacter*. Without obstruction of the biliary system, acute cholangitis does not occur.

Biliary obstruction most commonly occurs from choledocholithiasis, followed by malignancy. Another important, though less frequent, etiology stems from the interference of the physiologic barrier between the bile duct and the intestine via surgery, ERCP, or PTC. Common causes of biliary obstruction in adults are outlined in **Table 89.1**. Importantly, children can also get ascending cholangitis. Pediatric patients who have undergone surgical Roux-en-Y procedures (such as the Kasai procedure for biliary atresia) and those with indwelling catheters or failure to thrive are at increased risk.

It is important to consider acute cholangitis in any patient with sepsis who has signs and symptoms of biliary tract disease (often subtle), especially if that patient is diabetic,

TABLE 89.1 CAUSES OF BILIARY OBSTRUCTION

Gallstones (choledocolithiasis, Mirizzi syndrome)

Malignant biliary strictures (pancreatic cancer, cholangiocarcinoma, gallbladder cancer, ampullary tumor, duodenal malignancy)

Post-ERCP, PTC, or surgical intervention

Benign biliary strictures (postsurgical, acute and chronic pancreatitis, primary sclerosing cholangitis, autoimmune cholangitis, congenital anomalies)

Parasitic infections

Duodenal diverticulum/Lemmel syndrome (more common in older patients)

AIDS cholangiopathy

Biliary stent obstruction

---

older, or debilitated. Charcot was one of the first physicians to describe cholangitis, or "hepatic fever," and noted a constellation of symptoms that make up Charcot triad of intermittent fever with chills, right upper quadrant pain, and jaundice. Reynolds pentad also includes mental status changes and shock and confers a much graver prognosis without prompt decompression. The most frequent symptoms with acute cholangitis are fever and abdominal pain (approximate incidence of 80% in most reports). Clinical jaundice is less frequently seen. Severe presentations (eg, with shock and altered mental status) are fortunately much less common. Cholangitis rarely presents classically, so it is an important consideration in any patient with sepsis without an obvious source. Importantly, the most severe cases are often the most difficult to detect as the patient may be too sick to provide the clinician with a good history or clear physical examination.

Ultrasound examination may be particularly helpful in this scenario as a screen for biliary pathology in the patient with sepsis with altered mental status, but CT has become the initial imaging study of choice to both confirm biliary obstruction and identify its source. The Tokyo guidelines, originally published in 2007 and revised in 2013 and 2018, provide a diagnostic framework for cholangitis and involves confirming systemic inflammation (fever and lab evidence of inflammation), cholestasis (jaundice and abnormal liver function tests), and imaging evidence of biliary dilation and evidence of an etiology of obstruction. Regarding labs in acute cholangitis, alkaline phosphatase is the most consistently elevated marker, and liver function tests are commonly elevated, but the elevations can range from mild to severe.

Once recognized, the keys to treatment include hemodynamic stabilization, broad-spectrum antibiotics, admission to a monitored setting (ICU often), and prompt biliary tract decompression (getting your GI consultants on board quickly is crucial). These patients are sick, and if you don't make the diagnosis, they will not do well!

PEARLS

- Consider ascending cholangitis in any patient with sepsis without an obvious source.
- Choledocolithiasis is the most common cause of obstruction in cholangitis.

- Think of risk factors that lead to obstruction of the biliary system, and include cholangitis in your differential for pediatric patients with sepsis.
- CT is the initial imaging study of choice to confirm biliary obstruction and identify the source of obstruction.
- Get your GI consultant involved early as prompt biliary decompression is key.

Suggested Readings

An Z, Braseth A, Sahar, N. Acute cholangitis: causes, diagnosis, and management. *Gastroenterol Clin North Am.* 2021;50(2):403-414.

Ely R, Long B, Koyfman A. The emergency medicine-focused review of cholangitis. *J Emerg Med.* 2018;54(1):64-72.

Mosler P. Diagnosis and management of acute cholangitis. *Curr Gastroenterol Rep.* 2001;13(2):66-72.

Sulzer J, Ocuin L. Cholangitis: causes, diagnosis and management. *Surg Clin North Am.* 2019;99(2):175-184.

Yokoe M, Hata J, Takada T, et al. Tokyo guidelines 2018: diagnostic criteria and severity grading of acute cholecystitis (with videos). *J Hepatobiliary Pancreat Sci.* 2018;25(1):41-54.

90

Beware of the Patient With Painless Jaundice

Rolando G. Valenzuela and Andrés Guzmán

Jaundice is defined as a yellowish discoloration of the skin and mucosa. It is the clinical manifestation of elevated serum bilirubin (>2.5 mg/dL), which is largely the product of degraded red blood cells. It is usually first appreciated in the sclera or in the oral mucosa at the hard palate or under the tongue. Elevated bilirubin can be due to unconjugated bilirubin in the plasma before it undergoes glucuronidation in the liver (prehepatic), through dysfunction of the liver itself (intrahepatic), or conjugated bilirubin after it has undergone glucuronidation (posthepatic) and is excreted from the liver in urine (as urobilinogen) or stool (stercobilin).

Important historical features in a patient with painless jaundice include an occupational history, history of toxin exposures, overseas travel, family history, a history of alcohol or IV drug misuse, or high-risk sexual activity. A history of significant weight loss, fevers, night sweats, and increasing abdominal girth can also lead the physician to specific diagnoses such as parasitic infections, autoimmune diseases, or neoplasms. Signs and symptoms of anemia, a history of melena, and any other suggestion of GI bleeding are very important.

On physical examination, there are certain findings that, in conjunction with jaundice, are concerning for an underlying *emergent* condition. These include any vital sign abnormalities and anemia. While mnemonics including triads and pentads are useful didactic tools, often ill patients rarely have all symptoms necessary to complete them and a healthy index of suspicion is warranted in working up the patient with jaundice. Avoid the temptation to attribute abnormal vital signs to an underlying chronic disease. Any degree of hypotension or fever, for example, should prompt an active search for a source of bleeding or infection. The practitioner must also carefully examine the patient's mental status, as hepatic encephalopathy can initially present as only mild confusion. Any signs of new or worsening altered mental status should be very concerning and warrant admission for further investigation. Initial testing should include serum glucose, a CBC, electrolytes, LFTs, type and screen, and fecal occult blood. If the bilirubin level is abnormal, one must distinguish between conjugated (direct) and unconjugated (indirect) bilirubin. Acute GI bleeding is a critical consideration and should be recognized as quickly as possible; portal hypertension due to liver dysfunction increases the risk of gastroesophageal varices and ulcers that may manifest initially with hemorrhage (acute or chronic).

Jaundice with unconjugated (prehepatic) hyperbilirubinemia in the presence of normal transaminases and alkaline phosphatase should raise concern for hemolysis. This may be due to a variety of reasons including infectious, drug-induced, autoimmune, or due to an inherited disorder. If hemolytic anemia is suspected, a peripheral smear should be ordered as well as reticulocyte count, haptoglobin, and LDH. A hematologist should be consulted, and admission is warranted. When direct hyperbilirubinemia is present a CBC with differential, LFTs, and a PT will help identify the presence of primary hepatic failure (intrahepatic causes), primary intraductal or biliary tree disease, or the presence of obstructive pathology (posthepatic causes). Painless jaundice with a posthepatic obstructive source should prompt a search for primary or metastatic malignancies of the liver, gallbladder, or pancreas. The presence of eosinophilia should raise suspicion for a parasitic process, especially in a recently returned traveler.

Viral hepatitis will typically cause direct (conjugated) hyperbilirubinemia along with transaminitis (with or without elevation of alkaline phosphatase), indicating a primarily hepatocellular process. Viral hepatitis may develop gradually, so that patients may only present when significant jaundice ensues. If a viral etiology is suspected, serologic studies should be performed. If an autoimmune disease is suspected, relevant tests should be ordered, though this may be done as an outpatient if close follow-up is arranged.

Toxin exposure can result in acute, chronic, or acute-on-chronic liver failure. A careful occupational history may reveal exposures to chemicals in the workplace (arsenic, carbon tetrachloride, vinyl chloride). Acutely ingested or chronically used over-the-counter medications (eg, acetaminophen, NSAIDs), commonly prescribed medications (isoniazid, amoxicillin-clavulanic acid, TMP-SMX, valproic acid, nitrofurantoin), and complementary, alternative, or herbal medications (ackee fruit, camphor, kava leaves) can all cause hepatic failure. As foraging for edible fungi and other plants increases, the clinician should know that subacute ingestion of plants or fungi (amanita mushrooms) can also result in hepatic failure.

There are several imaging modalities used to evaluate the liver, gallbladder, and biliary tree. Ultrasonography is an excellent tool to evaluate the presence of gallbladder stones and dilation of intrahepatic ducts, but it is operator dependent and lacks the sensitivity and specificity of ERCP in evaluating extrahepatic and common biliary ductal etiologies. Nevertheless, ultrasound is the initial imaging study of choice. CT does not identify gallstones as well as ultrasound or ERCP; however, it has better sensitivity and specificity for hepatic abscesses, hepatic neoplasms (primary or secondary), and periampullary neoplasms and masses. CT should be considered the modality of choice when suspicion is high for malignancy in obstructive disease.

The disposition of the patient will depend on the suspected underlying pathology as well as the patient's clinical condition. The asymptomatic patient who is tolerating oral food and fluids with jaundice can be discharged safely home if acute and acute exacerbations of chronic underlying processes are excluded; prompt ambulatory follow-up for further evaluation should be arranged. Patients with abnormal vital signs or encephalopathy should be admitted, and patients with signs of fulminant hepatic failure (transaminases >10 times normal, elevated) should be admitted to the ICU.

PEARLS

- Painless jaundice with anemia may be a manifestation of acute GI bleeding. The initial assessment should identify patients at risk for variceal bleeding and ulcers.
- Hemolytic anemia is potentially life threatening and presents with unconjugated hyperbilirubinemia.
- When studies suggest a posthepatic disease process, consider primary or secondary malignancies as well as parasitic infectious diseases.
- Toxins can produce liver failure with jaundice. Ask about acetaminophen intake, use of complementary and alternative remedies, teas, and plant-based medicines, and workplace chemical exposures.
- Explore all abnormal vital signs and carefully examine the patient with jaundice for subtle signs of early confusion or worsening mental status.

Suggested Readings

Lalani T, Couto CA, Rosen MP, et al. ACR appropriateness criteria jaundice. *J Am Coll Radiol*. 2013;10(6):402-409.

Pappas G, Christou L, Akritidis NK, et al. Jaundice of unknown origin: remember zoonoses! *Scand J Gastroenterol*. 2006;41(4):505-508.

Taylor T, Wheatley M. Jaundice in the emergency department: meeting the challenges of diagnosis and treatment. *Emerg Med Pract*. 2018;20(4):1-24.

Wheatley MA, Heilpern KL. Jaundice. In: Marx JA, Hockberger RS, Walls RM, eds. *Rosen's Emergency Medicine*. 8th ed. Elsevier/Saunders; 2014:232-237.

91

Twist and Shout! The Patient with Volvulus

Kraftin E. Schreyer

Volvulus, derived from the Latin *volvere*, meaning to turn or roll, refers to the rotation of a segment of the alimentary tract greater than 180°. In adults, this most commonly occurs in the sigmoid colon, followed by the cecum, although it can occur in any gastrointestinal location. In children, volvulus most commonly affects the small intestine. Although uncommon, volvuli are important etiologies of bowel obstructions. The intestinal torsion of volvulus can compromise the blood supply and potentially lead to bowel ischemia and necrosis. Mortality rates for volvulus have been reported to be as high as 40% to 60% if treated nonsurgically and 12% to 25% even with surgical interventions.

Volvulus can present in a variety of ways depending on the anatomic location, which also impacts the demographics of the population most affected and the extent and duration of the bowel rotation. Evaluation for volvulus should include imaging, most commonly abdominal CT, abdominal x-ray, contrast enema (if colonic volvulus), and ultrasound. Definitive treatment is endoscopic and surgical, but adequate resuscitation should be done before either intervention.

Sigmoid Volvulus

Sigmoid volvulus typically presents gradually, with abdominal pain and distention followed by nausea and vomiting. Most patients are older males and suffer from conditions that could contribute to an acquired lengthening of the mesentery and dilation of the colon, such as chronic constipation, neuroleptic medication use, and colonic dysmotility from underlying neurologic or myopathic disorders. Abdominal radiographs may demonstrate the "bent inner tube" or "coffee bean" appearance of the U-shaped distended colon extending from the pelvis into the right lower or upper quadrants. Abdominal CT may show a "whirl pattern" or "bird's beak" at the rotational axis of two colonic segments. Sigmoidoscopy is most often the initial treatment, unless contraindications such as bowel necrosis or perforation exist. Colonic resection is performed if sigmoidoscopy fails, but is also standard after successful sigmoidoscopy, given the high rate of recurrence and associated morbidity and mortality of sigmoid volvulus.

Cecal Volvulus

Cecal volvulus tends to occur in younger patients and is more common in females. The presentation is variable and can be gradual or acute. There are three types of cecal volvulus, all of which are predisposed by a mobile cecum and ascending colon, which can be congenital or acquired. Pregnancy, distance running, colonoscopy, adhesions, and colonic atony have all been described as the risk factors for cecal volvulus. Endoscopy can be attempted for treatment but is often unsuccessful. Surgical treatment often includes a right hemicolectomy with or without ostomy creation. Mortality rates for cecal volvulus have been reported to be higher than those for sigmoid volvulus.

Gastric Volvulus

Gastric volvulus is the most affected site external to the colon in adults and often results from diaphragmatic defects, including hernias. The clinical presentation is often variable. Acute gastric volvulus classically manifests with the triad of nonproductive retching, epigastric pain, and inability to pass a nasogastric tube. When diagnosed, gastric volvulus also requires endoscopic and surgical management, and mortality rates have been reported to be as high as 15% to 20%.

Pediatric Volvulus

Volvulus in children is most often the result of malrotation associated with congenital anatomic malformations, such as omphalocele, congenital diaphragmatic hernia, intestinal atresia, Meckel diverticulum, and Prune-belly syndrome. Pediatric volvulus most commonly impacts those less than 1 year of age but can occur later. Most commonly, malrotation of the small intestine around the superior mesenteric artery leads to extensive bowel ischemia. Vomiting is the most common presentation and is often bilious. Diagnosis is often made on imaging, of which ultrasonography is the preferred initial modality. All pediatric patients with volvulus require expedited surgical management.

PEARLS

- Volvulus can present in numerous ways and is associated with a high mortality rate.
- Although volvulus most commonly affects the sigmoid colon in older adults and the cecum in younger adults, any portion of the gastrointestinal tract is vulnerable.
- Treatment, barring complications, is endoscopy, which is then followed by definitive surgical management.
- Pediatric volvulus is associated with congenital intestinal malrotation and requires surgical intervention.

Suggested Readings

Elam A, Downs A, Burgess M, et al. A case of gastric volvulus in the emergency department. *Am J Biomed Sci Res.* 2021;14(2):158-162.

Le CK, Nahirniak P, Anand S, et al. Volvulus. In: *StatPearls[Internet]*. StatPearls Publishing; 2022. https://www.ncbi.nlm.nih.gov/books/NBK441836/

Tezel O, Salman N, Acar Y, Kaplan M, Şenocak R. Asymptomatic sigmoid volvulus: a rare case in emergency department. *Balk Mil Med Rev.* 2015;18(3):97-100.

92

Don't Be Afraid to Order a CT on a Pregnant Patient If They Really Need It

Jennifer Repanshek

Radiation exposure in pregnancy is a complex topic. Physicians remain cautious when weighing the need to image a pregnant patient versus the potential harm to an embryo or fetus. According to the ACR, the low amount of radiation in a plain film does not cause harm to a developing fetus. However, CT studies can vary in levels of exposure and should be used only after appropriate risk/benefit analysis.

The ACR has released a practice parameter to guide clinicians in determining which diagnostic studies to order when imaging pregnant or potentially pregnant patients with ionizing radiation. The ACOG has also released guidelines for imaging in pregnancy. According to ACOG, the possibility of radiation exposure to a fetus should never prevent medically indicated imaging for a pregnant patient. These guidelines were most recently updated in 2023 and 2017, respectively.

TABLE 92.1	ESTIMATED FETAL EXPOSURE FROM SOME COMMON RADIOLOGIC STUDIES
IMAGING STUDY	**FETAL EXPOSURE (mGy)**
Chest x-ray (two views)	0.0002-0.0007
Abdominal film (single view)	1
Hip film (single view)	0.07-0.20
Barium enema or small bowel series	20-40
CT scan of head or chest	<10
CT scan of abdomen and lumbar spine	35

CT, computed tomography.

1 mGy = 0.1 rad; amount of energy deposited per kilogram of tissue.

Adapted from American College of Obstetrics and Gynecology. Guidelines for diagnostic imaging during pregnancy and lactation. www.acog.org. Published October 2017. https://www.acog.org/clinical/clinical-guidance/committee-opinion/articles/2017/10/guidelines-for-diagnostic-imaging-during-pregnancy-and-lactation

The ACR has summarized radiation effects based on gestational age. The risk of radiation-induced CNS effects is greatest at 8 to 15 weeks of gestation. At any gestational age, radiation exposure of lesser than 50 mGy has not been shown to cause harm. Imaging that delivers 50 to 100 mGy in patients more than 18 weeks pregnant has also not been shown to cause harm to the developing fetus. Imaging with greater than 100 mGy may cause detrimental effects at all gestational ages. The ACR reports that a 20-mGy dose of radiation to the fetus represents an additional lifetime cancer risk of approximately 0.8%. **Table 92.1** shows radiation doses for common imaging studies. **Table 92.2** shows suspected radiation effects by dose at multiple gestational ages.

Ultrasound and MR are the preferred diagnostic modalities in pregnancy; however, MR is not always available. CT should not be withheld if needed to make a critical diagnosis. In addition, IV contrast should be ordered only if really necessary. There is some concern that it may interfere with fetal thyroid function as IV contrast does cross the placenta. Animal studies, however, have not shown teratogenic effects. According to ACOG, contrast agents are unlikely to cause harm.

CT imaging of the abdomen and pelvis in pregnant patients is most commonly ordered in the setting of suspected appendicitis and trauma. When evaluating a pregnant patient with possible appendicitis, the most common nonobstetric surgical emergency in pregnancy, ultrasound is the preferred first-line imaging modality. If the ultrasound is nondiagnostic, MR is recommended as the next best imaging study. If MR is unavailable, CT should be performed. In a stable patient with blunt abdominal trauma, x-ray and ultrasound are performed first. However, ultrasound has diagnostic limitations in the pregnant patient with trauma; CT remains the most accurate and cost-efficient tool when evaluating blunt abdominal trauma. Single-phase CT of the abdomen and pelvis usually delivers less than 35 mGy, and with dose-sparing protocols, the radiation dose is typically 10 to 25 mGy. There is no significant evidence that a single CT of the abdomen and pelvis will be detrimental to a growing embryo or fetus. However, dose-saving or adapted protocols should be used whenever possible.

Informed consent should always be obtained, and every effort should be made to decrease the amount of radiation required for the study. According to the ACR, when obtaining patient consent, a realistic overview of the limited risk and the beneficial role

TABLE 92.2 SUMMARY OF SUSPECTED IN UTERO INDUCED DETERMINISTIC RADIATION EFFECTS

Gestational Age	<50 mGy	50-100 mGy	>100 mGy
0-2 wk (0-14 d)	None	None	None
3rd and 4th wk (15-28 d)	None	Probably none	Possible spontaneous abortion
5th-10th wk (29-70 d)	None	Potential effects are scientifically uncertain and probably too subtle to be clinically detectable.	Possible malformations increasing in likelihood as dose increases
11th-17th wk (71-119 d)	None	Potential effects are scientifically uncertain and probably too subtle to be clinically detectable.	Risk of diminished IQ or of mental retardation, increasing in frequency and severity with increasing dose
18th-27th wk (120-189 d)	None	None	IQ deficits not detectable at diagnostic doses
>27 wk (>189 d)	None	None	None applicable to diagnostic medicine

IQ, intelligence quotient.
Adapted from ACR-SPR practice parameter for imaging pregnant or potentially pregnant patients with ionizing radiation. Revised 2023. https://www.acr.org/-/media/acr/files/practice-parameters/pregnant-pts.pdf

of the imaging should be explained to the patient in understandable language. They state, "Conveying information in a positive, rather than negative, format is useful in helping a patient understand an accurate perspective of risk."

PEARLS

- Any diagnostic imaging required to make a critical diagnosis should be ordered if the benefit to the patient outweighs the risk to the embryo or fetus.
- A single CT scan of the abdomen and pelvis is unlikely to cause fetal harm.

Suggested Readings

ACR-SPR practice parameter for imaging pregnant or potentially pregnant patients with ionizing radiation. Revised 2023. https://www.acr.org/-/media/acr/files/practice-parameters/pregnant-pts.pdf

ACOG. Guidelines for diagnostic imaging during pregnancy and lactation. www.acog.org. Published October 2017. https://www.acog.org/clinical/clinical-guidance/committee-opinion/articles/2017/10/guidelines-for-diagnostic-imaging-during-pregnancy-and-lactation

Mainprize JG, Yaffe MJ, Chawla T, Glanc P. Effects of ionizing radiation exposure during pregnancy. *Abdom Radiol (NY)*. 2023;48(5):1564-1578. PMID: 36933026.

Wieseler KM, Bhargava P, Kanal KM, et al. Imaging in pregnant patients: examination appropriateness. *Radiographics*. 2010;30(5):1215-1229.

SECTION VI

CUTANEOUS

93

IS THIS NECROTIZING FASCIITIS?

TRACY LEIGH LEGROS

NF is the most well-known NSTI. NF is also referred to as *gangrene foudroyante de la verge*, the flesh-eating disease, Meleney ulcer, suppurative fasciitis, and synergistic necrotizing cellulitis. It is a bacterial or fungal infection that enters the body, usually through a skin break, resulting in the rapid destruction of the soft tissues. Points of entry occur due to trauma, surgery, or cancer. The most common sites of infection are the lower legs and perineum. Metastatic abscesses may develop in the liver, lung, spleen, brain, pericardium, and skin.

CLASSIFICATION

There are four types of NSTIs, classified according to the causative etiologic pathogen (**Table 93.1**). In addition, each NSTI type has its own bodily geographic predilection. **Cervicofacial** NSTI occurs secondary to mandibular fractures or dental infection. **Fournier gangrene** is NF of the perineal, genital, and perianal regions. There are several **pediatric** NSTIs, including post-chickenpox (type II NSTI), omphalitis, necrotizing enterocolitis, and urachal anomalies.

TABLE 93.1 NSTI Types

NSTI TYPES	PATHOGENS	PATIENTS AT RISK
Type I Polymicrobial	*Staphylococcus aureus, Escherichia coli, Vibrio, Haemophilus, Bacteroides fragilis*	Older, diabetic
Type II "Flesh-eating disease"	Hemolytic group A strep and staph (including MRSA)	All age groups and health states
Type III Gas gangrene, myonecrosis	*Clostridium perfringens, Clostridium septicum, Vibrio,* and *Aeromonas*	Feces, malignancy, seafood, liver disease, marine exposure
Type IV Fungal	*Candida* spp., *Zygomycetes*	Trauma, immunocompetent, immunocompromised

DIFFERENTIAL DIAGNOSIS

The differential diagnoses of NF are especially broad. Early presentations mimic superficial infections or injuries, progress to localizing symptoms, and finally overwhelming toxicity and sepsis (Table 93.2).

CLINICAL PRESENTATION

NF presents with acute onset of severe pain, fever, vomiting, and a purple-colored bullous skin infection that rapidly spreads. The pathologic and clinical progression of NF, as well as NF risk factors, are shown in Table 93.3.

RISK FACTORS

Risk factors include immunocompromised state (HIV, cancer, diabetes, hepatitis, chemotherapy, chronic steroid use, IV drug use), obesity, malnutrition, alcoholism, peripheral artery disease, aspirin/NSAID use, advanced age, severe chronic illness, and malignancy.

EVALUATION

Efficient, swift evaluation of patients with NF is paramount. Rapid order sets for NF can be helpful (Table 93.4). Blood cultures are usually negative for *clostridial species*. However, fungal cultures should be taken liberally, as immunocompetent and immunocompromised patients are at risk. There is no need to start antifungal therapy but send the cultures.

ANTIBIOTIC THERAPY

Initiate broad-spectrum empiric antibiotics as soon as possible. The World Health Organization's latest recommendation for empiric therapy is piperacillin-tazobactam plus clindamycin. Once *Streptococcus pyogenes* is ruled out, consider ceftriaxone

TABLE 93.2 DIFFERENTIAL DIAGNOSES OF NF

DISEASE	TOXICITY
Cellulitis, abscess, chilblains, erysipelas, pyomyositis	Without systemic symptoms
Compartment syndrome, arterial insufficiency	Limb-threat
Phlegmasia alba/dolens, warfarin necrosis, pyoderma gangrenosum	Potential life-threat
Sepsis, toxic shock syndrome, toxic epidermal necrolysis, purpura fulminans, disseminated intravascular coagulopathy	Life-threat
Necrotizing cellulitis, necrotizing myositis	Life-threat, debridement
Clostridial myonecrosis (gas gangrene)	Life-threat, requires amputation

TABLE 93.3 CLINICAL PROGRESSION OF NF

INITIAL INJURY	PROGRESSION OF INJURY	OVERWHELMING SEPSIS
Day 1	Days 2-3	Days 4-5
Severe pain out of proportion, fever, vomiting, and malaise	Purplish skin, edema, fluid blisters, necrosis, crepitus; nerves die and pain lessens	Overwhelming sepsis, altered mental status, and shock

TABLE 93.4 RAPID ORDER SETS FOR NF	
LABS, STUDIES, AND MEDS	CULTURES AND SPECIAL TESTING
CBC, CMP, CK, PT/INR, ESR, CRP, UA, UPT, lactate	Blood, urine, and fungal cultures Gram stain, fungal stain
ABG, ECG, CXR	Deep tissue cultures and biopsies
CT scan with contrast/MRI	MRSA sensitivities and *Clostridium perfringens* testing
IV fluids (LR), IV antibiotics, pressor agents (sepsis protocol)	

and metronidazole. For suspicion of MRSA, add vancomycin to either of the abovementioned options. Recently FDA-approved alternatives include oritavancin, dalbavancin, and tedizolid.

DIAGNOSTIC IMAGING

CT scan with contrast has high sensitivity and spatial resolution, but lacks specificity, as some findings are seen in non-NF. CT scans identify bone involvement, infectious sources, and vascular complications and may guide surgical debridement and drainage. MRI is the gold standard for the diagnosis of NF, with a sensitivity of 93%. The T1-weighted images assess anatomy; T2 fat-saturated sequences reveal fascial thickening and edema. Post-gadolinium sequences delineate the extent of infection.

LRINEC SCORE

LRINEC is used to differentiate NSTIs from abscess or cellulitis utilizing laboratory data (CRP, WBC, Hg, Na, Cr, and glucose). However, LRINEC is not reliable in all cases. A 2022 meta-analysis of patients with extremity NF, LRINEC had a 49.39% sensitivity and an 83.17% specificity. The greatest utility of LRINEC may be to rule out (not in) NF.

HBO THERAPY

Adjunctive HBO therapy benefits for NF include reversing tissue ischemia, augmenting bactericidal leukocyte functions, enhancing fibroblast replication, increasing collagen formation, promoting neovascularization, inhibiting alpha-toxin formation, increasing flexibility of RBCs, preserving intracellular ATP, and terminating lipid peroxidation. HBO therapy for NF imparts a 9-fold increase in survival and an 11-fold controlled increase in survival. Moreover, HBO therapy for NF imparts an 8.9 odd ratio advantage and an exceptional number needed to treat of 3.

PEARLS

- NF is a surgical emergency. Immediate IV access, labs, cultures, and diagnostic imaging orders should be placed and a call to surgery initiated as soon as possible.
- Remember to order fungal cultures. Immunocompetent patients with fungal NF are not uncommon.
- Think about NF when a patient presents with a painful red or mottled wound and reports that antibiotics did not improve their infection.
- CT scan is the most utilized standard for diagnosis. However, MRI is the gold standard.

Suggested Readings

Escobar SJ, Slade JB Jr, Hunt TK, Cianci P. Adjuvant hyperbaric oxygen therapy (HBO2) for treatment of necrotizing fasciitis reduces mortality and amputation rate. *Undersea Hyperb Med.* 2005;32(6):437-443.

Hofmaenner DA, Wendel Garcia PD, Blum MR, et al. The importance of intravenous immunoglobulin treatment in critically ill patients with necrotizing soft tissue infection: a retrospective cohort study. *BMC Infect Dis.* 2022;22(1):168.

Hollabaugh RS, Dmochowski RR, Hickerson WL, Cox CE. Fournier's gangrene: therapeutic impact of hyperbaric oxygen. *Plast Reconstr Surg.* 1998;101(1):94-100.

Kadri SS, Swihart BJ, Bonne SL, et al. Impact of intravenous immunoglobulin on survival in necrotizing fasciitis with vasopressor-dependent shock: a propensity score-matched analysis from 130 US hospitals. *Clin Infect Dis.* 2017;64(7):877-885.

Ngan V. Necrotising fasciitis. DermNet Case Studies. 2003. Updated by Dr Jannet Gomez, Dr Amanda Oakley (Ed Chief). Accessed February 2016. https://dermnetnz.org/topics/necrotising-fasciitis.

Tarricone A, De La Mata K, Gee A, et al. A systematic review and meta-analysis of the effectiveness of LRINEC score for predicting upper and lower extremity necrotizing fasciitis. *J Foot Ankle Surg.* 2022;61(2):384-389.

Wilkinson D, Doolette D. Hyperbaric oxygen treatment and survival from necrotizing soft tissue infection. *Arch Surg.* 2004;139(12):1339-1345.

94

Cutaneous Bullous Pemphigoid vs Pemphigus Vulgaris

Tracy Leigh LeGros

Bullous pemphigoid (pemphigoid) and pemphigus vulgaris (pemphigus) are autoimmune disorders in which blistering of the skin is a primary symptom. Autoantibodies against hemidesmosomes cause the subepidermal blistering of pemphigoid, while autoantibodies against desmoglein cause intraepidermal blistering in pemphigus. Neither pemphigoid nor pemphigus is contagious. Pemphigus vulgaris is most common in the United States and Europe, though it is still a rare disease. It is also chronic and potentially fatal. Pemphigus is unique from pemphigoid in that the blistering can involve the mucous membranes as well as the skin and is rarely associated with myasthenia gravis. Both diseases are associated with high morbidity and mortality, with the most common cause of death being opportunistic infections from prolonged immunosuppression.

Definitions

Bullous pemphigoid involves pruritic bullae and/or urticarial plaques most commonly on the groin, axillae, and flexural areas. Oral involvement only occurs in one-third of cases. It usually presents as a sudden widespread eruption. Taking a medication history is paramount, as over 50 medications, such as antibiotics, NSAIDs, and diuretics have been reported to cause drug-induced bullous pemphigoid. Pemphigoid occurs more commonly with increasing age, with a median age of 80, with a 2:1 predominance for women. The risk of death is significantly less than pemphigus.

TABLE 94.1	BULLOUS PEMPHIGOID VERSUS PEMPHIGUS VULGARIS	
CHARACTERISTICS	**BULLOUS PEMPHIGOID**	**PEMPHIGUS VULGARIS**
Age of onset	≥60 yr	40-60 yr
Lesions	Tense bullae, urticarial plaques, some milia	Flaccid bullae, erosions, and flexural growths
Nikolsky sign	Negative	Positive
Lutz sign	"B" or "P" spread	Angled or "V" spread
Site of separation	Subepidermal	Intradermal
Involved areas	Extremities	Oral mucosa
Area of spread	Moves inward to the flexural surfaces and trunk	Moves widely to the face, scalp, flexural surfaces, and trunk
Diagnosis—Skin biopsy	**First biopsy:** edge of intact bullae (hematoxylin and eosin staining) **Second biopsy:** adjacent normal skin (immunofluorescence)	**Two biopsies:** Deep shave or punch biopsy from the edge of a new erosion shows acantholysis.
Differential diagnoses	**Non-bullous phase:** urticaria, atopic dermatitis, irritant contact dermatitis, eczema, and dermatitis herpetiformis **Bullous phase:** pemphigus foliaceus, epidermolysis bullosa, bullous lupus, prurigo, impetigo, erythema multiforme, Sweet syndrome, toxic epidermal necrolysis, and autotoxic pruritus	**Oral ulcers:** HSV, aphthae, lichen planus, cicatricial pemphigoid, or erythema multiforme **Skin findings:** pyoderma, impetigo, bullous pemphigoid, bullous lupus, linear IgA bullous dermatosis, bullous erythema multiforme, bullous drug reactions, dermatitis herpetiformis

HSV, herpes simplex virus; IgA, immunoglobulin A.

Pemphigus has flaccid, thin-walled bullae originating on the oropharyngeal mucosa. The bullae then spread to involve the face, scalp, chest, axilla, and groin, which then rupture. The erosions are intensely painful. Patients present with erosions with a positive Nikolsky sign. Both diseases have their own type of Lutz sign. Pemphigus is rare with a median age of 71 years. It also occurs twice as often in women but with a much higher mortality risk (**Table 94.1**).

Nikolsky sign: Superficial layers of skin can be separated from the deeper layers by mechanical pressure.

Lutz sign: also known as the bullae spread sign; identifies the type of lateral spread with pressed curved blister movement.

TREATMENT

Treatment goals for both conditions include decreasing or stopping blister formation, the healing of existing blisters and erosions, and controlling the associated pruritus and pain. Topical and systemic corticosteroids, other immunosuppressive, and anti-inflammatory agents are used. Although steroids act to reduce autoantibody production, alternative therapies vary between pemphigoid and pemphigus.

Bullous pemphigoid therapy includes topical steroid cream as a first-line measure. It is as effective or superior to systemic steroid therapy in those with moderate to extensive disease. Either oral or intramuscular steroids are reserved for patients with mucous membrane involvement. Oral prednisone dosage is 0.5 to 1 mg/kg/d and can be tapered within 1 to 2 years. Recalcitrant cases may respond to glucocorticoid-sparing agents such as azathioprine, cyclophosphamide, and mycophenylate mofetil.

Initial therapy for pemphigus vulgaris includes oral prednisone (1 mg/kg/d) and tapering once the patient begins to respond. For those with very limited disease, sublesional steroid injections with triamcinolone acetonide may be helpful. Patients unresponsive to steroids within 6 months (or with intolerable steroid side effects) should be advanced to the glucocorticoid-sparing agents listed for bullous pemphigoid. Truly refractory cases may require intravenous immunoglobulin, rituximab, or both. Highly aggressive cases may be responsive to plasmapheresis, which removes circulating antibodies.

Fluid management is essential for both diseases and patients should be treated similarly to burn patients. For those with significant comorbidities, no significant changes need to be made unless there is a contraindication to using the recommended medications.

Follow-up

Patients with pemphigoid and pemphigus require dermatologic follow-up to keep patients in remission. Instructions include an explanation that bullous pemphigoid is usually less severe and can resolve in 1 to 2 years and that pemphigus is a chronic and potentially fatal disease and patients should be counseled accordingly.

PEARLS

- Pemphigoid and pemphigus are both associated with high morbidity and mortality, with the most common cause of death being opportunistic infections from prolonged immunosuppression.
- Taking a medication history is paramount, as over 50 medications, such as antibiotics, NSAIDs, and diuretics have been reported to cause drug-induced bullous pemphigoid.
- Pemphigus vulgaris has a positive Nikolsky sign, and bullous pemphigoid has a negative Nikolsky sign. Both diseases have their own type of Lutz sign.
- Fluid management is essential and patients should be treated similarly to burn patients.

Suggested Readings

Chu KY, Yu HS, Yu S. Current and innovated managements for autoimmune bullous skin disorders: an overview. *J Clin Med.* 2022;11(12):3528.

Di Lernia V, Casanova DM, Goldust M, Ricci C. Pemphigus vulgaris and bullous pemphigoid: update on diagnosis and treatment. *Dermatol Pract Concept.* 2020;10(3):e2020050.

Kayani M, Aslam AM. Bullous pemphigoid and pemphigus vulgaris. *BMJ.* 2017;357:j2169.

Naldi L, Cazzaniga S, Borradori L. Bullous pemphigoid: simple measures for a complex disease. *J Invest Dermatol.* 2012;132(8):1948-1950.

Stavropoulos PG, Soura E, Antoniou C. Drug-induced pemphigoid: a review of the literature. *J Eur Acad Dermatol Venereol.* 2014;28(9):1133-1140.

95

COMMON CELLULITIS MIMICS

SHABANA WALIA

There are many dermatologic conditions that can be strikingly similar to cellulitis, especially on first presentation to the ED. While some diagnoses are more chronic and indolent, others are life-threatening and crucial for the emergency clinician to diagnose. Distinguishing between cellulitis and other skin conditions can lead to a decrease in antibiotic use and decrease in the development of antibiotic resistance, as well as expedited treatment of alternate and deadly diagnoses.

Cellulitis is an acute bacterial infection causing inflammation of the epidermis, dermis, and the underlying subcutaneous tissue. Group A beta-hemolytic *Streptococcus* and *Staphylococcus aureus* are the most common bacteria causing cellulitis. However, in children, and less commonly in adults who are not responding to initial treatment, one must think of other causes of cutaneous cellulitis. *Haemophilus influenzae* type B is a severe form of cellulitis that is accompanied by a respiratory infection. *H. influenzae* cellulitis can be differentiated from more common forms of cellulitis by physical examination, as the rash can have a characteristic blue-red-purple appearance. Other uncommon pathogens of cellulitis are *Vibrio vulnificus* and *Aeromonas hydrophila*, both of which are water-related organisms. *A. hydrophila* should be suspected if there is a history of exposure to freshwater, if treatment for streptococcal cellulitis fails, or if there are bullae and abscesses with foul-smelling exudates on physical examination. *V. vulnificus* should be suspected if there was an exposure to salt water, along with physical examination findings of large bullae and vesicles. In more aggressive and serious stages, *V. vulnificus* can progress to a necrotizing soft tissue infection.

Erysipelas is a type of superficial cellulitis that involves the epidermis, upper dermal layer, and the superficial lymphatic channels. On history, the patient may describe a more rapidly progressing infection than cellulitis. Similar to cellulitis, the infected area of skin can be erythematous, warm, and tender. In contrast, erysipelas can be differentiated by the raised margins and sharply demarcated edges due to the superficial nature of the infection versus the indistinct margins of cellulitis. Since group A *Streptococcus* is the most common cause of erysipelas, the treatment and clinical management is often the same as deeper forms of cellulitis.

Stasis dermatitis, an inflammatory condition commonly known as *varicose eczema*, is often misdiagnosed as cellulitis in the emergency setting. It is a complication of long-standing chronic venous insufficiency, leading to edema and extravasation of blood cells, which can result in decreased blood flow to the tissues. Patients with this condition will often have nontender, swollen, erythematous legs, with areas of hyperpigmentation and scaling ongoing for several months to years. Stasis dermatitis can be secondarily infected with a superimposed cellulitis or ulcers.

Lipodermatosclerosis or "sclerosing panniculitis" can be a complication of long-standing chronic venous insufficiency and stasis dermatitis. The proposed pathophysiology is similar to stasis dermatitis, resulting in decreased tissue perfusion, with the addition of further endothelial damage. This damage causes microvascular thrombi formation, which results in tissue infarction and the formation of fibroblasts and granulation tissue. As this disease typically affects the bottom third of the lower legs, on physical examination, you should notice tapering of the legs, resembling the upside-down "champagne bottle appearance." This finding may be the only differentiating factor from cellulitis in the acute phase as patients can also develop severe pain, warmth, and redness with indistinct margins of the skin similar to cellulitis. The chronic phase is characterized by erythematous-indurated skin with browning discoloration and sclerotic plaques, thus more easily differentiated from cellulitis.

Contact dermatitis is a skin reaction from an allergen or irritant that results in skin inflammation. Differentiating cellulitis from dermatitis can be simplified with a clear history from the patient. The presence of erythema or a rash at the site of an allergen exposure is a clue to diagnosing this condition. Patients may also complain of intense pruritus with the rash or have a history of allergies. Clinicians should inquire about the use of new soaps, detergents, or topical creams. Contact dermatitis is a type IV hypersensitivity reaction, thus usually occurring 1 to 2 days after the exposure. It improves with avoidance of the allergen, antihistamines, and mild steroid cream and should not require antibiotics. Papular urticaria is a common hypersensitivity reaction that can occur after an insect bite. It consists of pruritic papules surrounded by wheels or erythematous bases that can progress to blisters and ulcers and tends to be localized near the insect bite. Treatment consists of systemic antihistamines and a topical steroid.

The deadliest "can't miss" mimic of cellulitis is necrotizing fasciitis. Early on in the course of deep soft tissue infections, it can be extremely difficult to detect differences on physical examination as they can share many characteristics with cellulitis, such as erythema, warmth, localized swelling, and tenderness. Necrotizing fasciitis involves the deep subcutaneous tissues and spreads rapidly through the fascia and later can involve the muscle. Though the infection is most commonly caused by group A beta-hemolytic *Streptococcus*, a wide range of bacteria including Gram-negative, Gram-positive, and anaerobic bacteria, have been implicated. Pain out of proportion to the examination should always alert the physician that a deeper soft tissue infection may be occurring. The progression of the disease is much faster than other dermatologic conditions. Within hours, the skin layers can become erythematous, swollen, and crepitant and form abscesses. Gas can be seen on radiographs, but imaging should never delay diagnosis. Early administration of broad-spectrum antibiotics, including anaerobic coverage, and immediate surgical consultation and debridement are required to prevent amputation and mortality. The definitive diagnosis is often confirmed in the operating room by direct visualization of necrotic tissue.

Other conditions that can mimic the clinical presentation of cellulitis include deep venous thrombosis, thromboembolism, compartment syndrome, vasculitis, viral and drug-related exanthems, fungal infections, and malignancy. Most importantly, the patient should be instructed to follow up with a primary physician within 24 to 72 hours of initial presentation of an acute rash to ensure improvement or further evaluation. Dermatologic conditions in immunosuppressed individuals, those not responsive to initial treatment, or recurrent/chronic rashes should prompt admission or urgent dermatology follow-up.

PEARLS

- A thorough history and physical examination will most often direct the clinician in differentiating cellulitis from its mimics.
- Cellulitis most often presents unilaterally.

- Stasis dermatitis, the most common mimic of cellulitis, results from a long-standing history of chronic venous stasis and decreased tissue perfusion and is usually bilateral.
- Pain out of proportion to examination and a rapidly progressing cellulitis should prompt the emergency clinician to consider a necrotizing soft tissue infection.
- Observation and serial examinations will aid in treatment and, if no improvement, may necessitate evaluation for alternate diagnoses.

Suggested Readings

Blum CL, Menzinger S, Genné D. Cellulitis: clinical manifestations and management. *Rev Med Suisse*. 2013;9(401):1812-1815.

Hirschmann JV, Raugi GJ. Lower limb cellulitis and its mimics: part I. Lowerlimb cellulitis. *J Am Acad Dermatol*. 2012;67(2):163.e1-12.

Keller EC, Tomecki KJ, Alraies MC. Distinguishing cellulitis from its mimics. *Cleve Clin J Med*. 2012;79(8):547-552.

Westerman EL. Other disorders that mimic infectious cellulitis. *Ann Intern Med*. 2005;142:949.

Wolfson AB, Cloutier RL, Hendey GW, Ling LJ, Rosen CL, Schaider JJ. *Harwood-Nuss' Clinical Practice of Emergency Medicine*. 6th ed. Wolters Kluwer; 2015. Print.

96

Know When Should You Prescribe Antibiotics After I&D of an Abscess

Chance Anderson and Emily Rose

SSTIs are common, with an estimated six million cases seen annually in in the United States. The increase in SSTIs has resulted in increased antibiotic utilization, which is felt to contribute to the increase in antibiotic resistance. Antibiotic stewardship programs emphasize decreasing unnecessary prescriptions, targeting narrow-spectrum coverage, and limiting treatment duration.

Definitions

A skin abscess is a collection of pus within the dermis or subcutaneous space, while cellulitis is a breach in skin barrier that manifests as an area of skin erythema, edema, and warmth. Traditional teaching is that an abscess without cellulitis does not require antibiotics if adequately drained, whereas cellulitis requires antibiotics. However, many lesions are not clearly defined.

In 2014, the IDSA established guidelines for the prescription of antibiotics based on underlying comorbid conditions and clinical status. However, recent studies have shown that antibiotic therapy may reduce the rate of abscess recurrence, even in healthy patients. Clinical uncertainty remains because of these recent studies. Current recommendations state that it is reasonable to withhold antibiotics for patients with low illness severity as evidenced by the following:

- Single abscess that is less than 2 cm in diameter
- No cellulitis or minimal cellulitis
- No systemic signs of toxicity (ie, fever, hypotension, tachycardia)
- No immunosuppression or other uncontrolled comorbidities
- No prior clinical failure with I&D alone
- No indwelling medical device (ie, pacemaker, vascular graft)
- No risk for endocarditis

Patients who have more moderate illness severity, defined as those with abscesses greater than 2 cm, uncontrolled comorbid conditions, or immunosuppression who do not show systemic signs of infection, can be discharged after I&D and treated with oral antibiotics. Studies have found that patients with purulent soft tissue infections, the majority of whom had abscesses, had positive skin cultures for *Staphylococcus aureus* in approximately 80% of cases. Of those with positive skin cultures, approximately 80% grew MRSA. Given the prevalence of MRSA, recommended antibiotics include doxycycline, TMP-SMX, or clindamycin for a treatment duration of 5 to 10 days. Local resistance patterns should be considered when deciding which antibiotic to prescribe.

Patients with more severe illness severity, defined as those who are immunocompromised (ie, acquired immunodeficiency syndrome, active malignancy receiving chemotherapy), failed oral antibiotic therapy with signs of systemic infection, evidence of deeper space infection, or who meet criteria for sepsis require parenteral antibiotics, such as vancomycin or linezolid, intravenous fluids, and hospital admission.

While antibiotic therapy can reduce the rate of recurrence and lead to faster healing time, it is important to be judicious with antibiotic prescription to minimize community antibiotic resistance and its associated risks.

The decision of antibiotic initiation should be thoughtfully applied to each unique patient and based on the likelihood of recurrence, associated risk factors, patient preference, and underlying comorbid conditions. Each patient is different, and knowledge of the established guidelines and new literature can assist in making the right clinical decision for your patient. Antibiotic duration ranges from 7 to 10 days depending on the severity of illness and comorbidities. Wound monitoring within 48 hours assists in titrating the need for continued or escalating therapy. As with any discharge from the ED, patients should be provided anticipatory guidance and information about signs and symptoms that should prompt them to return for further evaluation, including recurrence or spread of lesions.

PEARLS

- Antibiotic therapy in patients with an abscess should be initiated when there is significant associated cellulitis; incomplete drainage of a lesion, with complex lesions; and associated patient comorbidities.
- Use established guidelines as a framework to guide your clinical management but utilize clinical judgment.
- Discharged patients should be seen for wound check within 48 hours to ensure appropriate healing.
- Always give good return precautions as infections do not always respond to initial treatment.

Suggested Readings

Daum RS, Miller LG, Immergluck L, et al. A placebo-controlled trial of antibiotics for smaller skin abscesses. *N Engl J Med.* 2017;376(26):2545-2555. PMID: 28657870.

Stevens DL, Bisno AL, Chambers HF, et al. Practice guidelines for the diagnosis and management of skin and soft tissue infections: 2014 update by the Infectious Diseases Society of America [published correction appears in *Clin Infect Dis.* 2015;60(9):1448. Dosage error in article text]. *Clin Infect Dis.* 2014;59(2):e10-52. PMID: 24973422.

Taira BR, Singer AJ, Thode HC Jr, Lee CC. National epidemiology of cutaneous abscesses: 1996 to 2005. *Am J Emerg Med.* 2009;27(3):289-292. PMID: 19328372.

Talan DA, Mower WR, Krishnadasan A, et al. Trimethoprim-sulfamethoxazole versus placebo for uncomplicated skin abscess. *N Engl J Med.* 2016;374(9):823-832. PMID: 26962903.

97

Chickenpox or Mpox? How Do I Tell the Difference?

Emily Rose and Kristina van de Goor

Mpox virus is an orthopoxvirus that has been endemic to Africa for many years. Cases diagnosed in other locations are usually traced to travel from endemic areas. However, since May 2022, the CDC has reported over 80,000 confirmed cases of mpox spanning over 100 countries, marking this new spread of mpox a global health emergency. Despite its low mortality, the sudden increase in cases, high transmissibility, long duration of painful lesions, and potential complications make diagnosis of mpox important and pertinent to the emergency physician. Differentiating mpox from other more commonly encountered infections with vesicular lesions, such as varicella-zoster virus (chickenpox), can be difficult. This chapter focuses on key differences between these two viruses, including transmission, incubation periods, and lesion appearance to aid in clinical decision making.

Assessing Risk Factors

During this most recent global outbreak, direct intimate contact has been the primary means of person-to-person transmission of mpox in the community, thereby making individuals who engage in sex with multiple partners at higher risk. Data suggest that men between the ages of 21 and 55 years who engage in sexual activities with other men currently make up most cases. Nevertheless, transmission of mpox can occur to any individual from direct contact with bodily fluids or lesions of an infected person, indirect contact through fomites, vertical transmission from mother to fetus, or respiratory droplets from close face-to-face contact with an infected person. Whereas children and adolescents make up less than 1% of diagnosed mpox infections and transmission is usually from a direct household contact, over 95% of chickenpox infections occur in individuals under the age of 20 years. Varicella is similarly transmitted via contact with aerosolized droplets, most commonly nasopharyngeal secretions, or direct contact with the skin lesion fluid, though intimate contact has not been reported as a primary means of transmission. Uniquely, primary varicella infections are mainly spread to individuals who have never had chickenpox or its vaccine before. This highlights the importance of screening patients for risk factors and potential exposures, as well as a history of prior primary varicella infection or vaccination status to help determine the likelihood of a certain infection.

Similarly, incubation periods and symptom onset can help differentiate between these two viruses. The mean incubation period for varicella is approximately 15 days from exposure, while during this current outbreak of mpox, data suggest an incubation periods of 7 to 10 days. Although the clinical prodrome of fever, chills, and malaise is well described in both infections, the eruption of skin lesions in varicella is usually seen within 1 to 2 days after fever onset, whereas in mpox infections, the lesions can arise up to 4 to 5 days after the initial systemic prodrome. Lymphadenopathy remains the main differentiator, being reported in more than 70% of confirmed mpox cases, while not a common presentation of uncomplicated chickenpox infections.

LESION APPEARANCE AND CHARACTERISTICS

It is important to consider the appearance and characteristics of each vesicular rash. Although there have been reports of atypical presentations of each infection, the classic appearance of the skin lesions in each infection has been well described and subtly differs. Mpox lesions are generally broader, deeper, and firmer than those of chickenpox. In addition, mpox lesions tend to be umbilicated, similar to molluscum contagiosum. Mpox lesions are considered pseudo-pustules, meaning they may appear like the pustular or vesicular lesions of chickenpox but do not actually contain any fluid. Meanwhile, the fluid-filled vesicles of chickenpox are more fragile and easily broken to reveal the vesicular fluid. Typically, chickenpox sores are primarily pruritic, whereas the lesions in mpox are extremely painful and may progress to being pruritic only in the healing stages when the lesions have scabbed over.

EVOLUTION OF LESIONS

Mpox lesions most commonly arise in the location of inoculation, such as perioral, perianal, or genital regions, and are usually all in the same stage of development. When involving the entirety of the body, lesions are more commonly found on the extremities and face. Meanwhile, chickenpox lesions primarily start on the face, back, and trunk, appearing in "crops," and, therefore, evolve in different stages of healing. Generally, new chickenpox lesions stop developing after 4 days and are crusted over and beginning to fall off within 1 week. The duration of symptoms also differs, with chickenpox usually self-resolving within 2 weeks and the sores of mpox may extend up to 4 weeks.

DIAGNOSTIC TESTING

Assessment of risk factors and consideration of lesion appearance may help distinguish mpox from chickenpox; however, due to the variety of presentations and overlapping symptomatology of the two viruses, confirmatory laboratory tests should be used in conjunction with clinical recognition. Due to its high sensitivity and specificity, PCR viral testing from unroofed lesions can be used to accurately diagnose both chickenpox and mpox. Serologic testing of antibodies is also available, though it has not been shown to be accurate. It should be noted that there have been accounts of coinfections with both mpox and chickenpox viruses, so careful consideration should be made when there is a high suspicion of a certain infection, even in the presence of other positive tests.

> **PEARLS**
>
> - The presence of cervical and inguinal lymphadenopathy is often a distinctive feature of mpox compared with varicella.
> - Mpox lesions are typically pseudo-pustules that do not contain fluid, while the easily breakable vesicles of chickenpox are fluid filled.
> - The lesions of mpox are typically broader, deeper, firmer, and more painful than those of chickenpox.
> - Mpox lesions are typically in the same stage of development, whereas varicella lesions arise in "crops" and are usually in different stages of development.
> - PCR viral testing is an important step in differentiating mpox infections from chickenpox when the clinical picture is unclear.

Suggested Readings

Brown K, Leggat PA. Human monkeypox: current state of knowledge and implications for the future. *Trop Med Infect Dis.* 2016;1(1):8. PMID: 30270859.

Ghazanfar A. Epidemiology, clinical features, diagnosis and management of monkeypox virus: a clinical review article. *Cureus.* 2022;14(8):e28598. PMID: 36185896.

Kim SB, Jung J, Peck KR. Monkeypox: the resurgence of forgotten things. *Epidemiol Health.* 2022;44:e2022082. PMID: 36228673.

98

Don't Miss Systemic Illnesses That Present With Cutaneous Signs and Symptoms

Annalise Sorrentino

Dermatologic complaints are common in the ED setting, comprising 4% to 12% of visits. While the vast majority of these patients will not have emergent medical conditions, it is important for the provider to be aware of underlying systemic illnesses that can initially present with cutaneous symptoms.

Neonatal HSV

During the first 3 months of life, the outermost layer of the epidermis (stratum corneum) undergoes restructuring, leaving newborns at risk for several cutaneous viral infections, with prematurity increasing that risk. One of the most devastating of these illnesses is neonatal HSV. While the majority of these infections are from perinatal transmission, a smaller percentage can occur postnatally. First episode primary maternal infection puts the infant at greatest risk as recurrent maternal infections are associated with some protective maternal antibodies.

Many of these patients will present with fever, but a percentage will present with only a vesicular rash. Lesions at areas of scalp electrode monitoring have been well described. Depending on the extent of HSV infection, these patients may also present with neurologic signs and symptoms, including seizures.

If neonatal HSV is suspected, cultures of the conjunctiva, nares, mouth, and anus should be collected in addition to any skin lesions. HSV PCR can also be obtained if available. Blood and cerebrospinal fluid should also be obtained and tested. Another risk factor is a serum alanine aminotransferase, and this should also be collected. Intravenous acyclovir should be administered pending culture and PCR results.

EN

EN, also referred to as an acute nodular septal panniculitis, can be a result of a hypersensitivity reaction but can also be indicative of underlying systemic illness, both infectious and inflammatory. More common in females, it can be caused by several different bacterial, viral, and fungal causes but also has an association with malignancies and IBD. In cases of IBD-associated EN, the severity of cutaneous findings is directly related to intestinal involvement and improves with treatment of the systemic condition.

Acute onset of reddish purple nodules, 1 to 5 cm in size on bilateral shins with tenderness, should alert you to EN. The prognosis of the rash is favorable with supportive treatment, but considerations should be made to evaluate for underlying causes depending on a constellation of presenting signs and symptoms. CBC and inflammatory markers should be strongly considered in these patients. A chest x-ray (to evaluate for possible pulmonary tuberculosis) and group A streptococcal testing can also be considered. Every attempt to ensure appropriate outpatient follow-up should be made.

LE

LE is an autoimmune disease that affects hundreds of thousands of people worldwide. Although most commonly encountered in women of childbearing age, it can also be seen in male and pediatric patients. Up to 80% of patients with SLE will have cutaneous symptoms, with about 25% having a dermatologic finding as their presenting sign. A percentage of these patients will go on to develop SLE, but some will also have isolated CLE. CLE can further be classified into acute, subacute, and chronic.

Most commonly, ACLE presents with the stereotypical butterfly facial erythema but can also manifest in a generalized manner. Typically seen on sun-exposed areas, it can appear urticarial or maculopapular. On the extensor surfaces of the hands, it spares the knuckles (an important difference from Gottron papules seen in dermatomyositis). There can also be mucosal involvement that is usually painless.

The diagnosis of CLE or SLE can be challenging, but if suspected, ANAs should be obtained. While a positive result doesn't confirm the diagnosis, a negative result has a high negative predictive value. Other labs that could be considered are anti-dsDNAs and anti-Smith antibodies. Complement levels may also be helpful. In the acute setting, labs to assess multiorgan involvement should be considered, including CBC, metabolic panels, and inflammatory markers. Urinalysis, including a urine protein-to-creatinine ratio, can also help with disposition.

DRESS

DRESS (also known as DIHS) is defined by a constellation of clinical and laboratory findings. It is characterized by maculopapular or morbilliform rash, fever, lymphadenopathy (≥ 2 cm in diameter at two or more sites), and hematologic abnormalities (typically eosinophilia or atypical lymphocytosis). Elevated transaminases and leukocytosis can also be seen.

The pathophysiology isn't completely understood, but viral reactivations (particularly Epstein-Barr virus, cytomegalovirus, and human herpesvirus 6) have been heavily implicated. Several drugs have been known to cause DRESS but most commonly encountered are anticonvulsants, antimicrobials, sulfonamides, and allopurinol.

If DRESS is suspected, CBC, inflammatory markers, and metabolic panels to include renal and hepatic function should be obtained. Additional systemic evaluation may include cardiac or viral testing and should be done if clinically indicated.

Initial and most important treatment in a patient with suspected DRESS is to stop the offending agent. The mainstay of therapy is primarily supportive with identification of possible comorbidities. Admission is typically recommended for close monitoring and serial labs and examinations. Systemic corticosteroids are the treatment of choice, and there is supportive evidence for both intravenous and oral preparations. IVIG has also been used with good results.

PEARLS

- Cutaneous complaints are very common in the ED, and while the majority will be benign and self-limited, a small percentage will be indicative of underlying systemic illness.
- Neonatal HSV should be considered in newborns with a suspicious rash, even in the absence of fever.
- Strongly consider obtaining a CBC and inflammatory markers in a patient you suspect to have EN.
- CLE is most commonly seen in women of childbearing age but can been seen in males and children as well.
- DRESS can be distinguished from other drug eruptions by the stereotypic lymphadenopathy.

Suggested Readings

Cardones AR. Drug reaction with eosinophilia and systemic symptoms (DRESS) syndrome. *Clin Dermatol.* 2020;38(6):702-711. PMID: 33341203.

Castillo SA, Pham AK, Dinulos JG. Cutaneous manifestations of systemic viral diseases in neonates: an update. *Curr Opin Pediatr.* 2017;29(2):240-248. PMID: 28134705.

Hafsi W, Badri T. Erythema nodosum. In: *StatPearls [Internet].* StatPearls Publishing; 2022. https://www.ncbi.nlm.nih.gov/books/NBK470369/

Herzum A, Gasparini G, Cozzani E, Burlando M, Parodi A. Atypical and rare forms of cutaneous lupus erythematosus: the importance of the diagnosis for the best management of patients. *Dermatology.* 2022;238(2):195-204. PMID: 34082424.

Kilic D, Yigit O, Kilic T, Buyurgan CS, Dicle O. Epidemiologic characteristics of patients admitted to emergency department with dermatological complaints; a retrospective cross sectional study. *Arch Acad Emerg Med.* 2019;7(1):e47. PMID: 31602430.

Malik TF, Aurelio DM. Extraintestinal manifestations of inflammatory bowel disease. In: *StatPearls [Internet].* StatPearls Publishing; 2022. PMID: 33760556.

Pérez-Garza DM, Chavez-Alvarez S, Ocampo-Candiani J, Gomez-Flores M. Erythema nodosum: a practical approach and diagnostic algorithm. *Am J Clin Dermatol.* 2021;22(3):367-378. PMID: 33683567.

Villalon-Gomez JM. *Pityriasis rosea*: diagnosis and treatment. *Am Fam Physician.* 2018;97(1):38-44. PMID: 29365241.

99

Staphylococcal Toxic Shock Syndrome

Hurnan Vongsachang and Emily Rose

STSS is a clinical illness that describes the rapid onset of fever, rash, hypotension, and, ultimately, multiorgan system dysfunction. STSS was initially described in a series of pediatric cases in 1978 and gained notoriety in the 1980s, with an explosion of cases in women. These cases were associated with the use of certain highly absorbent tampons. The subsequent removal of some brands of tampons from the market paralleled a decrease in incidence of STSS in the following years. However, any source of staphylococcal infection (eg, wound packing, indwelling catheter) can be associated with STSS.

Pathogenesis

Most cases of STSS are derived from methicillin-sensitive *Staphylococcus aureus*, but the incidence of methicillin-resistant *S. aureus* is rising as well. The driving factor behind the pathogenesis of STSS is the production of TSST-1, an exotoxin that has been implicated in 85% to 100% of menstrual-related STSS and 40% to 60% of nonmenstrual STSS. Exotoxins are superantigens that activate T cells, resulting in a cytokine storm. Endogenous pyrogens lead to high fevers and may induce muscle proteolysis, resulting in myalgias and elevated levels of serum creatine phosphokinase.

Individuals between 6 months and 2 years of age are more susceptible to STSS, as passive immunity is waning and active immunity is developing. Antibodies to TSST-1 were found in approximately 70% of cases in children aged 0 to 6 months, whereas only 30% were found in those aged 7 months to 2 years. By early adulthood, 70% to 80% of individuals have developed antibodies to TSST-1, and 90% by mid-adulthood.

Clinical Presentation

One of the defining features of STSS is its rapid clinical development, usually over the course of 48 hours. Clinical manifestation includes the following:

- Systemic findings: This includes fevers 38.9 °C or higher and chills. Serum blood tests often reveal neutrophilic predominance with or without the presence of leukocytosis.
- Hypotension: In adults, hypotension is defined as a systolic blood pressure of 90 mm Hg or less, and less than the fifth percentile by age in children aged 16 years and below. Hypotension in STSS may be unresponsive to large amounts of intravenous fluids, leading to shock and hypoperfusion of organs. This leads to tissue ischemia and, ultimately, multiorgan failure. Decreased systemic vascular resistance and increased vascular permeability secondary to the cytokine storm lead to the leakage of intravascular fluid into the interstitial space, manifesting as nonpitting edema.
- Rash: Various dermatologic findings have been described in STSS. The initial erythroderma has been described as erythema, macular, diffuse, and blanching that may resemble a sunburn and commonly affects the palms and soles. One to 3 weeks later, the rash may appear more pruritic and desquamate. Mucous involvement may include hyperemia of the vaginal and oropharyngeal mucosal as well as conjunctival scleral hemorrhage. When compared to toxic epidermal necrolysis (which also involves skin sloughing and erythroderma), the mucous membrane involvement with STSS is much less prominent.

- Multiorgan failure: One of the characterizing features of STSS is multiorgan dysfunction, typically resulting from the profound hypoperfusion and subsequent tissue ischemia. This is reflected in a variety of laboratory abnormalities.
  - Neurologic: A variety of neurologic findings have been described in patients with STSS, including headaches, confusion, irritability, disorientation, lethargy, agitation, hallucinations, and seizures.
  - Renal: An increase in BUN and creatinine is often found, reflecting both prerenal and intrinsic renal insult. Subsequent metabolic derangements may be found, including hyponatremia, hypoalbuminemia, hypophosphatemia, and hypocalcemia.
  - Hepatic: An increase in liver enzymes, such as transaminases and bilirubin, is often found in the setting of liver insult.
  - Gastrointestinal: Patients with STSS are often found to have gastrointestinal symptoms, including nausea, vomiting, diarrhea, and abdominal pain.
  - Hematologic: The first few days of illness are often characterized by thrombocytopenia and anemia. This may progress to frank DIC.
  - Muscular: Patients with STSS often report myalgias. Elevated levels of creatinine phosphokinase are commonly described, reflecting diffuse muscle proteolysis.
  - Other: Pulmonary edema, pulmonary effusions, and cardiac dysfunction have also been reported in cases of STSS.

Diagnostic Criteria

The US Centers for Disease Control and Prevention has established diagnostic criteria for STSS (https://ndc.services.cdc.gov/case-definitions/toxic-shock-syndrome-2011/). However, this is intended for epidemiologic data collection and surveillance and should not be used in substitution of clinical judgment.

Treatment

Management of STSS includes treatment of shock; surgical debridement, if necessary; removal of infected foreign bodies; and intravenous antibiotics.

- Treatment of shock: A hallmark of STSS is profound hypotension unresponsive to fluid resuscitation. Multiple liters of fluid and initiation of vasopressors are frequently required to maintain adequate tissue perfusion.
- Surgical debridement: Particularly in patients with recent surgeries, wounds should be explored and debrided for source control.
- Removal of infected foreign bodies: Foreign bodies are potential niduses for infection that must be removed for source control. These items may include tampons, other intravaginal items such as contraceptive devices, intrauterine devices, and wound packing/dressings.
- Antibiotic therapy: Prompt initiation of intravenous antibiotics is critical in the treatment of STSS. Empiric coverage awaiting culture results include vancomycin, clindamycin, and one of the following: a penicillin plus beta-lactamase inhibitor (eg, piperacillin-tazobactam), cefepime, or a carbapenem. Refer to local antibiogram once cultures have isolated methicillin-resistant versus methicillin-sensitive strains of *S. aureus*.

PEARLS

- STSS is defined as a rapid progression of fever, rash, hypotension, and multiorgan dysfunction.

- Dermatologic manifestations are highly variable and may involve the palms, soles, and mucosa. Consider STSS in the evaluation of a critically ill patient presenting with an erythematous rash.
- Laboratory markers are often abnormal and reflect the profound hypotension, resultant tissue ischemia, and organ dysfunction.
- Management of STSS includes treatment of shock, source control with wound exploration versus debridement or foreign body removal, and intravenous antibiotics.

SUGGESTED READINGS

Parsonnet J, Hansmann MA, Delaney ML, et al. Prevalence of toxic shock syndrome toxin 1-producing *Staphylococcus aureus* and the presence of antibodies to this superantigen in menstruating women. *J Clin Microbiol.* 2005;43(9):4628-4634.

Quan L, Morita R, Kawakami S. Toxic shock syndrome toxin-1 (TSST-1) antibody levels in Japanese children. *Burns.* 2010;36(5):716-721.

100

SHOULD YOU I&D THAT ABSCESS IN THE PATIENT WITH HIDRADENITIS?

MATTHEW ALAN DEMAREST AND EMILY ROSE

Hidradenitis suppurativa (HS) is a chronic inflammatory skin condition with both genetic predisposition and lifestyle-associated risk factors (ie, obesity, smoking). It most commonly occurs after puberty, with onset usually in the second to third decades of life. The pathophysiology of HS is incompletely understood but likely involves excessive ductal keratinocyte proliferation and keratin plugging of hair follicles. Mechanical stress exacerbates local inflammation. This ultimately leads to follicular rupture and triggers a localized inflammatory immune response. Cultures of ruptured lesions grow typical skin flora as well as Gram-negative rods and anaerobic bacteria. The role of bacteria in HS is controversial, as unruptured lesions are often sterile.

The axillary, inguinal, and other intertriginous areas (eg, genital and inframammary areas) are more prone to HS lesions. Recurrent lesions, malodorous drainage, and scarring often have significant psychological impact on patients.

CLINICAL PRESENTATION

This disease manifests clinically as chronic, recurrent, and painful nodules or abscesses. As HS progresses in time, recurrent abscesses result in severe scarring with characteristic skin tunnel (previously termed *sinus tract*) formation. Patients with HS typically present with new onset, or acute worsening, of inflammatory nodules, which represent acute flares that occur periodically throughout the course of this chronic disease.

HS is a clinical diagnosis. Acute HS flares are difficult to distinguish from other common skin and soft tissue infections. Clinical overlap with skin infections contributes to diagnostic delay. Features suggestive of HS include the location and shape of abscess. HS tends to affect the intertriginous areas. In contrast to boils or furuncles, HS lesions are deep and rounded without the classic purulent pointed head of other infections. In addition, HS abscesses are typically chronic, recurrent, and associated with other typical HS lesions, including scarring and skin tunnels.

HS in the pediatric population may lack the characteristic features seen in adults. Scarring and skin tunnel formation are both features of chronic disease. Children with endocrine disorders, such as precocious puberty or congenital adrenal hyperplasia, are predisposed to HS.

If there is suspicion of HS based on any of the abovementioned characteristics, it is important to ask about previous abscesses in the same area, as this can be an important clue in making the diagnosis.

I&D

Routine I&D of HS lesions is *not* recommended. I&D of HS abscess will provide short-term relief of acutely inflamed lesions. However, I&D will nearly always result in abscess recurrence. In addition, the procedure itself causes additional mechanical trauma to the epidermis and dermis, which can hasten disease progression.

I&D of HS abscesses may be considered in select clinical scenarios:

- To provide immediate symptomatic relief for intractable pain that is not responsive to oral or intravenous analgesic medications
- Superimposed bacterial infections especially those at risk for sepsis and clinical deterioration (eg, those with surrounding cellulitis, systemic symptoms, or significant comorbid conditions)

The preferred method of I&D is to use a punch biopsy tool, if available, to de-roof the abscess. This creates a larger defect than a traditional scalpel and allows the wound to heal by secondary intention. This may result in lower rates of recurrence.

ED Management and Definitive Therapy

The primary ED treatment for acute HS flares is topical and oral antibiotics. Antibiotics decrease skin bacterial load and also provide some anti-inflammatory properties. Topical clindamycin is the initial agent of choice, followed by an oral tetracycline, such as doxycycline. For patients younger than 8 years of age, a macrolide antibiotic such as azithromycin is a reasonable alternative to a tetracycline. Metformin and antiandrogenic medications (ie, oral contraceptives, spironolactone) are often used as adjunctive therapy. Warm compresses and intralesional corticosteroids may provide symptomatic relief.

Finally, all patients who have a suspected or confirmed diagnosis of HS should be instructed to follow up with a dermatologist upon discharge from the ED. Dermatologists have greater capabilities to offer long-term maintenance therapy for HS and can help prevent future ED visits.

PEARLS

- HS is a chronic, inflammatory skin condition that manifests as painful nodules and abscesses and will progress over time to severe skin scarring and skin tunnel formation.

- Abscess location, chronicity, and recurrence in the same location all suggest a diagnosis of HS rather than furuncle, carbuncle, or other skin and soft tissue infections.
- HS abscess should not be routinely incised and drained because of high rates of recurrence and because this procedure can hasten disease progression.
- I&D may be considered in rare cases where HS abscesses cause intractable pain or are associated with bacterial superinfection.
- A reasonable discharge regimen for HS flare includes oral doxycycline for adults or oral azithromycin for children less than 8 years in addition to topical clindamycin.

Suggested Readings

Alikhan A, Sayed C, Alavi A, et al. North American clinical management guidelines for hidradenitis suppurativa: a publication from the United States and Canadian Hidradenitis Suppurativa Foundations: part I: diagnosis, evaluation, and the use of complementary and procedural management. *J Am Acad Dermatol.* 2019;81(1):76-90. PMID: 30872156.

Okun MM, Flamm A, Werley EB, Kirby JS. Hidradenitis suppurativa: diagnosis and management in the emergency department. *J Emerg Med.* 2022;63(5):636-644. PMID: 36243614.

Patel K, Leszczynska M, Peña-Robichaux V, Diaz LZ. Caring for pediatric hidradenitis suppurativa patients in the emergency department. *Pediatr Emerg Care.* 2021;37(6):312-317. PMID: 34038925.

SECTION VII
ENDOCRINE/METABOLIC

101

A Normal Bicarbonate Value Does Not Exclude an Acid-Base Disturbance

Emily Miller and George C. Willis

Acid-base disturbances are commonly found in lab results in the ED. Being able to quickly discern if there is an acid-base problem is essential in practice. Failure to act or the act of misrecognition can lead to serious complications for patients. With acid-base disturbances, it is not quite as easy as evaluating the pH and bicarbonate (HCO_3^-) singly to discern if there is a disturbance. While pH and HCO_3^- are key components in determining an acid-base disturbance, neither can be looked at in isolation. pH, HCO_3^-, CO_2, and chronicity all play a role in acid-base physiology.

Acid-base problems are separated into two broad categories: metabolic and respiratory disturbances. By definition, metabolic disturbances cause a change in HCO_3^- while respiratory disturbances cause a change in CO_2, either leading to a change in pH. Although "pure" disturbances with one variable driving the changes do occur, frequently, changes in pH, HCO_3^-, and CO_2 occur together leading to a so-called mixed acid-base disturbance, in other words, a combination of both a metabolic and respiratory problem.

Plasma has electrical neutrality, or no net charge, meaning there is a balance in positive and negative charges from cations and anions, respectively. Sodium, chloride, and bicarbonate are the primary contributors to charge; however, there are several "unmeasured" cations (calcium, magnesium, and proteins) and anions (albumin, phosphate, sulfate, and organic acids) that play into electrical neutrality.

The AG equation is used to determine the etiology of a metabolic acidosis. An elevated AG indicates an accumulation of acids or "unmeasured" anions causing a compensatory decrease in HCO_3^-, while a normal AG indicates a primary loss of HCO_3^-.

$$AG = Na^+ - (Cl^- + HCO_3^-)$$

In most cases of normal AG metabolic acidosis or alkalosis, the serum bicarbonate will be altered. If the AG and the serum bicarbonate are both normal, there is unlikely to be an acid-base disturbance. If the AG is elevated, there is some form of AG metabolic acidosis present, either with a concomitant metabolic alkalosis or a non–AG metabolic acidosis.

In order to figure out the etiology, the change in bicarbonate and the change in AG must be calculated and compared. This is otherwise known as the delta-delta. The delta AG is the AG − 10. The delta bicarbonate is the serum bicarbonate − 24. If the delta AG is similar to the delta bicarbonate, then there is purely an AG metabolic acidosis present. If the delta AG is much lower than the delta bicarbonate, then there is a concomitant non–AG metabolic acidosis present. If the delta AG is much higher than the delta bicarbonate, then there is a concomitant metabolic alkalosis present.

Changes in HCO_3^- levels can be caused by direct gains/losses (metabolic acid-base disturbances) or by indirect compensatory responses to respiratory acid-base disturbances. Any change to the balance between acids and bases will drive the bicarbonate dissociation equation ($H^+ + HCO_3^- \leftrightarrow CO_2 + H_2O$) in the opposite direction. For example, an increase in CO_2 will drive the equation to the left, causing an increase in HCO_3^- and H^+, whereas an increase in acid (H^+) will drive the equation to the right resulting in increased CO_2.

While pH and CO_2 can fluctuate quickly with disturbances in respiratory status or other factors (ie, metabolic disturbances), HCO_3^- is regulated by the kidneys, which can take significantly more time to adjust in primary respiratory problems. The kidneys help manage the excretion and formation of HCO_3^- based on the acid-base status of the body. Changes in respiratory drive can adjust CO_2 concentration quickly based on HCO_3^- and pH; however, renal response to pulmonary disturbances requires hours to days to reach full equilibrium. Therefore, HCO_3^- can lag in compensation in respiratory problems and appear "normal," when in reality the body is in a state of disequilibrium.

Expected HCO_3^- compensation in respiratory disturbances is usually determined depending on the following equations:

Acute respiratory acidosis

Expected $[HCO_3^-] = 24 + (\text{actual } p_{CO_2} - 40)/10$

Usually increased by 1 for every increase of 10 of pCO_2

Chronic respiratory acidosis

Expected $[HCO_3^-] = 24 + 4(p_{CO_2} - 40)/10$

Usually increased by 4 for every increase of 10 of pCO_2

Eq 101.1

Acute respiratory alkalosis

Expected $[HCO_3^-] = 24 - 2(40 - p_{CO_2})/10$

Usually decreased by 2 for every decrease of 10 of pCO_2

Chronic respiratory alkalosis

Expected $[HCO_3^-] = 24 - 5(40 - p_{CO_2})/10$

Usually decreased by 5 for every decrease of 10 of pCO_2

If the predicted HCO_3^- does not match the actual HCO_3^-, then there is a concomitant metabolic acidosis or alkalosis present. This can lead to a normal HCO_3^-, although there is an obvious acid-base disturbance in terms of pCO_2 and pH. It is therefore important to evaluate for appropriate compensations in all acid-base derangements.

Bicarbonate levels reflect a complex balance in acid-base physiology designed to maintain a narrow physiologic range in pH. Evaluating for acid-base disturbances requires a thorough understanding of the multiple organ systems and compensatory mechanisms involved. Bicarbonate typically fluctuates with acute changes in metabolic and respiratory issues. However, as demonstrated, bicarbonate can be seemingly normal despite underlying acid-base disturbance. It is therefore important to realize that while bicarbonate can be normal, it does not rule out an underlying problem. These situations are clearly important to recognize for the practicing physician. Failure of recognition can lead to serious complications to patients and can further complicate care.

PEARLS

- HCO_3^- is a dynamic electrolyte that changes due to direct and indirect mechanisms in metabolic and respiratory derangements.
- Renal response to respiratory problems can take hours to days to have a compensatory change in HCO_3^-.
- Acid-base disturbances are not uncommonly "mixed," which can lead to normal bicarbonate and abnormal pH.

Suggested Readings

Hyneck M. Simple acid-base disorders. *Am J Hosp Pharm*. 1985;42(9):1992-2004.
Koh ES. Hidden acid retention with normal serum bicarbonate level in chronic kidney disease. *Electrolyte Blood Press*. 2023;21(1):34-43.
Kraut JA, Madias NE. Serum anion gap: its uses and limitations in clinical medicine. *Clin J Am Soc Nephrol*. 2007;2(1):162-174.
Narins R, Emmett M. Simple and mixed acid-base disorders: a practical approach. *Medicine*. 1980;59(3):161-187.
Rice M, Ismail B, Pillow MT. Approach to metabolic acidosis in the emergency department. *Emerg Med Clin North Am*. 2014;32(2):403-420.

102

Pitfalls in the Management of Adults With DKA

Anthony Roggio

DKA is one of the most serious acute complications associated with diabetes in both adults and children. The disease is a metabolic derangement defined by hyperglycemia and ketonemia, typically initiated by physiologic stressors (ie, acute illness, MI, sepsis), lack of insulin, iatrogenic disease from medications such as corticosteroids and SGLT2 inhibitors and sympathomimetic drugs such as cocaine. Current guidelines are complicated and practitioners often fall into cracks in managing this disease. Knowing these management pitfalls and how to avoid them is paramount in the care of these critically ill patients.

Fluid Choice

Current American Diabetes Association and International Society for Pediatric and Adolescent Diabetes guidelines discuss the importance of early fluid resuscitation, highlighting isotonic saline as a keystone of resuscitation strategy. While 0.9% saline is widely available, balanced electrolyte crystalloid solutions (such as lactated Ringers, PlasmaLyte A) have been studied as an alternative, demonstrating a more rapid closure of the anion gap and increases in MAP and urine output within the first 4 to 6 hours. A recent study has additionally shown that balanced solutions also contribute to a faster resolution of the acidosis and shorter duration of insulin infusion. These findings make sense: 0.9% saline has an average pH of 5.5 compared to 7.4 in balanced electrolyte solution. Moreover, chlorine concentration (154 mEq/L) in 0.9% saline is supraphysiologic and can result in a hyperchloremic metabolic acidosis with large infusion volumes. Because the serum chloride level will increase, the anion gap can close even when acidosis is still present. Balanced electrolyte solutions, on the other hand, have a more physiologic chloride concentration, limiting the chloride load given to patients, curbing this effect.

In addition, balanced solutions typically contain potassium, an electrolyte that is commonly depleted in patients with DKA. Literature has shown decreased incidence of hypokalemia in patients with DKA receiving balanced crystalloid. While no studies have yet demonstrated improved mortality with balanced fluids, we still recommend a balanced electrolyte solution as the initial fluid of choice based on the proven early benefits to the patient. If balanced solutions are not available, 0.9% normal saline is a reasonable alternative choice for initial resuscitation, especially since supplemental potassium and magnesium can be coinfused with the fluid when needed.

Insulin Management

Insulin administration is essential to correcting the acidosis by reversing the ketogenesis and glucose-generating metabolic processes that result in DKA. To optimize care, the provider must understand how to risk stratify patients correctly and navigate potential pitfalls in insulin administration management. Patients are stratified into one of three categories of severity (**Table 102.1**) as defined by pH, serum bicarbonate, and sensorium.

Old guidelines suggest giving a bolus of regular insulin before starting an insulin infusion. This was due to the belief that insulin wouldn't reach concentrated levels in the blood for at least 1 to 2 hours if a drip was started alone. New studies have shown that bolus insulin is not necessary to maintain insulin plasma concentrations and is not required if the patient's infusion rate is started at 0.1 U/kg/h. While likely unnecessary, insulin boluses are still safe in *adult* patients. Moreover, patients classified as being in mild or moderate DKA can be managed safely with intermittent subcutaneous short- or medium-acting insulin regimens (such as insulin lispro) in lieu of a continuous insulin infusion. However, subcutaneous insulin treatment regimens have not been safely

TABLE 102.1	INSULIN MANAGEMENT		
	MILD	MODERATE	SEVERE
pH	7.25-7.3	7-7.24	<7
Bicarbonate	15-18	10-14	<10
Sensorium	Alert	Alert/drowsy	Stupor/coma

demonstrated in severe DKA, so continuous IV insulin infusions should still be the treatment of choice in this cohort.

In patients with DKA, insulin administration needs to continue until the anion gap is closed and the acidosis is resolved, even if blood sugar levels have fallen to a more "normal" range. For this reason, once the serum glucose level is 250 mg/dL or less, fluids should be changed to dextrose-containing ones to maintain normoglycemia while the acidosis is being treated with the insulin infusion. After acidosis is resolved and the anion gap closed, long-acting subcutaneous insulin should be started. To prevent rebound hyperglycemia or ketoacidosis before long-acting insulin takes effect, the IV insulin infusion should be continued for 1 to 2 hours (at a minimum of 0.02-0.05 U/kg/h) post long-acting insulin administration.

Potassium Supplementation

Most patients with DKA will appear to have elevated potassium levels due to shifts of electrolytes from intracellular to intravascular spaces. However, the majority of patients are actually hypokalemic with loss of potassium in urine due to osmotic diuresis. When insulin is administered, extracellular potassium shifts into the cells across a large gradient and rapid decreases in serum potassium level can occur. Hypokalemia can be fatal, and to prevent this complication, potassium repletion should be initiated when potassium levels are less than 5 mEq/L at a rate of 20 to 30 mEq in each liter of fluid infused. If initial levels are less than 3.5 mEq/L, or drop to below that level during management with an insulin infusion, insulin should be held and potassium should be given to get serum concentrations above 3.5 mEq/L before initiating or restarting insulin therapy.

Utilization of Sodium Bicarbonate

Past guidelines restrict the use of sodium bicarbonate to severe DKA in adults and recognize *no* role for bicarbonate in DKA treatment in children. This is because literature demonstrates that bicarbonate therapy paradoxically worsens intracellular acidosis and is linked to development of cerebral edema in children. Furthermore, even in patients with severe DKA with a pH less than 7, bicarbonate therapy has not consistently shown improvements in morbidity, mortality, time to acidosis resolution, or other benefits. Given the lack of evidence for benefit and the demonstrated potential for harm, it is not recommended to use sodium bicarbonate as an adjunctive treatment in DKA except in cases of severe hyperkalemia, cardiac arrest due to profound acidemia, or refractory hypotension from decreased cardiac output due to acidemia.

PEARLS

- Balanced solutions are preferred to 0.9% normal saline and leads to faster resolution of acidosis in DKA.
- Subcutaneous insulin treatment regimens have not been safely demonstrated in severe DKA.
- After acidosis is resolved and the anion gap closed, long-acting subcutaneous insulin should be started 1 to 2 hours before stopping the IV infusion of insulin in order to prevent rebound hyperglycemia and ketoacidosis.
- Reserve sodium bicarbonate administration for critically ill patients rather than a pH value alone.

Suggested Readings

Catahay JA, Polintan ET, Casimiro M, et al. Balanced electrolyte solutions versus isotonic saline in adult patients with diabetic ketoacidosis: a systematic review and meta-analysis. *Heart Lung.* 2022;54:74-79.

Mahler SA, Conrad SA, Wang H, Arnold TC. Resuscitation with balanced electrolyte solution prevents hyperchloremic metabolic acidosis in patients with diabetic ketoacidosis. *Am J Emerg Med.* 2011;29(6):670-674.

Patel MP, Ahmed A, Gunapalan T, Hesselbacher SE. Use of sodium bicarbonate and blood gas monitoring in diabetic ketoacidosis: a review. *World J Diabetes.* 2018;9(11):199-205.

Self WH, Evans CS, Jenkins CA, et al. Clinical effects of balanced crystalloids vs saline in adults with diabetic ketoacidosis: a subgroup analysis of cluster randomized clinical trials. *JAMA Netw Open.* 2020;3(11):e2024596.

103

Do Not Rely on Orthostatic Vital Signs to Diagnose Volume Depletion

Mukund Mohan and Anand K. Swaminathan

OH is defined as when position change results in the following:

- Reduction of SBP of at least 20 mm Hg
- Reduction in diastolic BP of at least 10 mm Hg
- Increase in HR by greater than 30 beats per minute

Traditional teaching holds that orthostatic BP measurements are useful in determining volume status. Measurements should be obtained after standing from a supine position. Depending on the patient, optimal time of BP measurement will vary. Patients 60 years and older may display BP changes at 1 minute; however, those younger than 40 may take up to 5 minutes, or longer. In addition, a patient may instead feel symptomatic, light-headedness, dizziness, blurred vision, nausea, palpitations, headache, or weakness with erect position and these may resolve with recumbency. The presence of symptoms with position change regardless of vital sign changes represents symptomatic OH.

It is important to remember that OH is simply a physical exam finding and not a disease. A 1995 study demonstrated that neither SBP nor mean BP changes with standing predicted mortality at 10 years' follow-up; however, a diastolic drop of 10 mm Hg with standing was associated with increased vascular mortality (odds ratio 2.7, 95% CI, 1.3 to 5.6). When further analyzed, this association disappeared in multivariate analysis after adjusting for background factors such as underlying cardiovascular disease. It suggested that patients with a more labile diastolic pressure likely had underlying risk factors that predisposed them to increased vascular mortality such as stroke and MI. More recent studies have also confirmed no difference in composite 30-day serious outcomes in patients older than 60 years discharged from the ED who presented with syncope or near-syncope and had abnormal orthostatic vital signs.

To further investigate the screening efficacy of OH as a marker of volume depletion, a study performed tilt table testing in healthy volunteers after blood donation (moderate blood loss <600 mL). In adult patients younger than 65 years, a change in pulse greater than 20 beats per minute or a change in SBP greater than 20 mm Hg had a sensitivity/specificity of 47%/84% for volume depletion. Sensitivity and specificity were similar in those older than 65 years (41%/86%) and both groups showed similarly weak likelihood ratios (+) LR = 2.93 and (−) LR = 0.69. The results of this study suggest that a finding of OH is not sensitive or specific enough to state with confidence that moderate volume depletion has occurred and the absence of OH does not rule out significant volume depletion.

As clinicians, we have a bias toward overemphasizing OH in the older population. However, the data reveal that OH vital signs are common in both older and younger adults. Data from large studies on older nursing home patients demonstrate rates of OH ranging from 28% to 50%. Studies in adolescents show similar numbers, with approximately 44% of patients exhibiting orthostatic changes. Regardless of age group, OH vital signs aren't a useful clinical predictor of volume status.

Symptoms of OH have weak predictive value in regard to mild to moderate volume according to a systematic review. However, in patients with severe blood loss (defined as 600-1,100 mL), there was noted a dramatic increase of sensitivity 97% and specificity 98% in those patients who were unable to even stand for vital signs due to severe dizziness. In this subset of severely symptomatic patients, the inability to stand serves as an excellent clinical predictor of severe volume loss. Otherwise, simply the complaint of nausea or dizziness with standing is not clinically useful and, as such, should not be used as a surrogate marker of volume status.

PEARLS

- Based on the available literature, OH by measurement does not appear to be sensitive or specific for screening patients for moderate volume loss.
- Prevalence of baseline OH is common; between 28% and 50% of patients can be expected to have orthostatic vital signs.
- A finding of OH in the older population is not any more useful for clinical prediction of volume status than in the normal adult population.
- If the patient is symptomatic to the point of preventing measurement of upright vital signs, they have likely suffered severe volume loss.

Suggested Readings

American Autonomic Society, American Academy of Neurology Consensus Conference. Consensus statement on the definition of orthostatic hypotension, pure autonomic failure and multiple system atrophy. *Clin Auton Res.* 1996;6:125-126.

Aronow WS, Lee NH, Sales FF, Etienne F. Prevalence of postural hypotension in elderly patients in a long-term health care facility. *Am J Cardiol.* 1988;62:(4):336.

McGee S, Abernethy WB, Simel DL. Is this patient hypovolemic. *JAMA.* 1999; 281(11):1022-1029.

Ooi WL, Barrett S, Hossain M, Kelley-Gagnon M, Lipsitz LA. Patterns of orthostatic blood pressure change and the clinical correlates in a frail, elderly population. *JAMA.* 1997; 277:1299-1304.

Raiha I, Luutonen S, Piha J, Seppanen A, Toikka T, Sourander L. Prevalence, predisposing factors and prognostic importance of postural hypotension. *Arch Intern Med.* 1995;155: 930-935.

Stewart JM. Transient orthostatic hypotension is common in adolescents. *J Pediatr.* 2002;140: 418-424.

White JL, Hollander JE, Chang AM, et al. Orthostatic vital signs do not predict 30 day serious outcomes in older emergency department patients with syncope: a multicenter observational study. *Am J Emerg Med.* 2019;37(12):2215-2223.

Witting MD, Wears RL, Li S. Defining the positive tilt test: a study of healthy adults with moderate acute blood loss. *Ann Emerg Med.* 1994;23(6):1320-1323.

104

Hyperglycemic Hyperosmolar State: When High Sugar Gets You Down

Jaime Hope

A patient presents to your ED with elevated blood glucose readings and altered mental status. DKA should be on the differential but the glucose comes back extremely elevated. With good diagnostic acumen, you can avoid the common pearls and pitfalls in your patients with hyperglycemia.

Diabetes is a very common medical condition, affecting more than 37 million Americans, which is 1 in 10 people, according to the CDC. Approximately 95% of these people afflicted with diabetes have type 2 diabetes, which puts them at risk for diabetic HHS. From 1990 to 2018, the number of patients with diabetes has more than quadrupled and the rate of diabetes-specific ED visits increased by over 50% in the same time frame.

HHS is a life-threatening complication that primarily affects individuals with T2DM. It is characterized by severe hyperglycemia, marked dehydration, and an elevated plasma osmolality. HHS is distinct from DKA, which typically occurs more often in individuals with type 1 diabetes; both conditions can present with hyperglycemia. The mortality rate in HHS is 10 times higher than the mortality seen in DKA, so recognition is crucial.

HHS often develops due to a combination of precipitating factors, including insulin resistance, relative insulin deficiency, and increased glucose production by the liver. Precipitating factors may include infections, inadequate insulin therapy, noncompliance with medications, ischemia or infarctions of end organs such as myocardial infarctions or stroke, and certain medications such as glucocorticoids or diuretics. Infections, primarily urinary tract infections and pneumonia, were the most common precipitating factors for HHS in patients with T2DM.

The clinical presentation of HHS is characterized by the gradual onset of symptoms over several days or weeks, which is different from the more typical fast onset seen in DKA. Patients may experience polyuria, polydipsia, weakness, weight loss, and visual disturbances. As the condition progresses, neurologic symptoms such as altered mental status, seizures, and focal deficits may occur, which differentiates HHS from simple hyperglycemia.

Altered mental status is the most common presenting symptom in patients with HHS, followed by dehydration and focal neurologic deficits. As HHS is more common in the older population with type 2 diabetes, it can be challenging, at times, to recognize if this alteration in mental status is acute. The altered mental status can be mistaken for baseline dementia, especially in the debilitated nursing home patient with minimal history.

Patients with dementia or physical debility are at high risk for developing HHS as they are often on many medications that can lead to profound dehydration and they may not be able to easily communicate symptoms such as thirst or discomfort. Also, they are often bedbound and lack mobility or insight to stay adequately hydrated. Therefore, clinicians should maintain a high index of suspicion for HHS in older patients with elevated glucose levels, with chief complaints of altered mental status, confusion, or lethargy.

A finger-stick glucose should be a sixth vital sign in any patient with altered mental status and can be helpful in establishing the early diagnosis of HHS. HHS may be missed because the symptoms can mimic other pathology, such as sepsis, CNS pathology, thyroid emergencies, toxicologic pathology, and other medical emergencies and be difficult to distinguish from baseline dementia in patients who are chronically impaired.

The next conundrum is to determine whether the HHS is the "chicken or the egg" question, or, in other words, the cause or the result of a patient's neurologic condition. Patients with HHS can mimic the symptoms of patients with stroke having focal neurologic deficits, including hemiparesis. It is important to remember that stressors, such as stroke, can also exacerbate hyperglycemia, which can develop into HHS. Therefore, providers should be aggressive in working up these patients for their neurologic presentations with appropriate imaging and lab studies. As these patients are often poor historians, it is important to consider a wide differential as to the etiology of their HHS. ECG, CBC, troponin, lactic acid, CT of the head, chest imaging, drug levels, cultures, and abdominal imaging may be useful in determining an underlying serious cause of HHS.

The diagnosis of HHS is based on a combination of clinical and laboratory findings. According to the ADA, the diagnostic criteria for HHS include plasma glucose levels greater than 600 mg/dL (33.3 mmol/L), serum osmolality greater than 320 mOsm/kg, absence of significant ketosis, and pH greater than 7.3. The most common missed laboratory abnormality is the sodium as it is commonly in the normal range, which, in a patient with severe hyperglycemia, is very bad. Recall that sodium contributes the most to serum osmolarity, so the corrected sodium in these patients is often severely elevated. In addition, arterial or venous blood gas analysis may reveal a high serum bicarbonate concentration. An elevated BUN and creatinine are commonly observed due to dehydration and prerenal azotemia.

The management of HHS involves prompt fluid resuscitation, correction of electrolyte imbalances, and initiation of insulin therapy. Intravenous fluid therapy is crucial to correct dehydration and improve hemodynamic stability. A standardized HHS protocol with an initial bolus of 1 to 2 L of 0.9% sodium chloride followed by continuous intravenous fluid infusion was associated with reduced mortality rates and shorter hospital stays. Use caution in patients with poor heart function or at risk for pulmonary edema and respiratory compromise.

Insulin therapy should be initiated once adequate fluid replacement is achieved. Regular insulin is the preferred agent, administered as an intravenous infusion. A gradual, not rapid, reduction in blood glucose levels is crucial to prevent cerebral edema, and blood glucose should be monitored frequently to ensure optimal control. The ADA recommends a target glucose reduction rate of 50 to 75 mg/dL/h to give time for hydration. Potassium levels should be closely monitored and replaced as necessary to prevent or correct hypokalemia.

In summary, HHS is a severe and potentially fatal complication of T2DM. Prompt recognition, appropriate management, and prevention strategies are essential to minimize morbidity and mortality associated with HHS. Early fluid resuscitation, correction of electrolyte imbalances, and gradual glucose reduction through insulin therapy are key components of management.

PEARLS

- ED visits for hyperglycemia are common, having increased by more than 50% over the past few years.
- The mortality rate in HHS is 10 times higher than the mortality seen in DKA.
- The symptoms of HHS may be gradual and mimic other pathology.
- Altered mental status distinguishes HHS from simple hyperglycemia.
- Management includes prompt but judicious fluid resuscitation.
- Rapid correction of glucose levels can be dangerous.
- Closely monitor glucose, corrected sodium, and potassium during treatment.

Suggested Readings

Adeyinka A, Kondamudi NP. Hyperosmolar hyperglycemic syndrome [Updated 2023 Aug 12]. In: *StatPearls [Internet]*. StatPearls Publishing; 2023. https://www.ncbi.nlm.nih.gov/books/NBK482142/

Kitabchi AE, Umpierrez GE, Miles JM, Fisher JN. Hyperglycemic crises in adult patients with diabetes. *Diabetes Care*. 2009;32(7):1335-1343.

Munro JF, Campbell IW, McCuish AC, Duncan LJ. Euglycaemic diabetic ketoacidosis. *Br Med J*. 1973;2(5866):578-580.

Pasquel FJ, Umpierrez GE. Hyperosmolar hyperglycemic state: a historic review of the clinical presentation, diagnosis, and treatment. *Diabetes Care*. 2014;37(11):3124-3131.

Umpierrez GE, Kitabchi AE. Diabetic ketoacidosis: risk factors and management strategies. *Treat Endocrinol*. 2003;2(2):95-108.

Uppal TS, Chehal PK, Fernandes G, et al. Trends and variations in emergency department use associated with diabetes in the US by sociodemographic factors, 2008-2017. *JAMA Netw Open*. 2022;5(5):e2213867.

105

VBG Wizardry: The Down and Dirty on Interpreting the VBG

Joshua (Josh) Nichols and William F. Taber

The "ABG versus VBG" decision historically polarized the field of emergency medicine. Maybe clinicians trained with an attending who beat them for mention of a VBG, or.... Maybe they ride motorcycles and quote EM podcasts, thumbing their proverbial nose at the ABG. Regardless of where providers fall on the spectrum, a VBG in place of an ABG can save time and spare the patient pain, potential thrombosis, and arterial injury. However, clinicians need to know how to interpret either and distinguish when one test or the other is appropriate.

INTERPRETING THE pH OF A VBG

Overall, the pH of the VBG correlates well with the ABG. In two large meta-analyses, authors showed that the mean difference between venous and arterial pH is between 0.033 and 0.035. This difference has shown good correlation in patients with acidosis, such as diabetic ketoacidosis, and with alkalosis, such as COPD exacerbations, with studied pH ranges from 7.05 to 7.61.

There are three clinical instances where the provider must be wary of the pH of a VBG: patients with mixed acid-base disorders, the patient with hypotension, and in the case of cardiac arrest. These concerns are based on there being a lack of evidence supporting correlation between the two studies. Several studies in the past 5 years demonstrated a large discrepancy in pCO_2 in patients in shock and during cardiac arrest. In addition, a few studies that correlate venous and arterial pH in the patient with hypotension (<90 mm Hg systolic) have been conducted. In one small study, authors showed that arterial-venous pH difference increased slightly in patients with hypotension compared to those who are normotensive; however, this increase was not statistically significant.

INTERPRETING THE pCO_2 OF A VBG

The pCO_2 of the VBG is an important measurement; however, it does not correlate well enough with pCO_2 of the ABG at all levels to be used as a surrogate marker. At normal pCO_2 levels, the VBG and ABG pCO_2 do correlate well; however, they disassociate in hypercapnia. How then can we use the pCO_2 of a VBG clinically? The answer is that the pCO_2 from a VBG is a useful screening tool for hypercapnia. A venous pCO_2 of less than 45 mm Hg has a 100% NPV for arterial pCO_2 of greater than 50 mm Hg. Therefore, if the VBG pCO_2 is normal, hypercapnia has been effectively ruled out. If venous pCO_2 is greater than 45 mm Hg, obtain an ABG to determine the arterial pCO_2 to check whether there is a clinically relevant hypercapnia.

INTERPRETING THE HCO_3^- OF A VBG

As with pH, the VBG HCO_3^- correlates well with arterial HCO_3^-. In two large meta-analyses, the mean difference between venous and arterial HCO_3^- was 1.03 to 1.41. The small mean difference and a narrow confidence interval make venous estimation of arterial HCO_3^- clinically useful in most cases. However, the clinician must be cognizant of the patient's underlying medical conditions. In one study comparing venous and arterial pH in patients with COPD presenting with hypercapnic respiratory failure, individual arterial and venous HCO_3^- measurements could differ by as much as -6.24 to $+10.0$ mmol/L, making the VBG less useful in these patients. Although not entirely clear, this poor level of agreement may be due to patients' underlying COPD, causing a baseline chronic metabolic alkalosis combined with an acute respiratory acidosis. This finding again highlights the poor understanding of VBG and ABG correlation in mixed acid-base disorders. Therefore, in these cases, the clinician should consider ordering an ABG.

INTERPRETING THE LACTATE OF A VBG

Venous lactate correlates well with arterial lactate at normal levels (<2 mmol/L). In support of this, a systematic review showed that at normal levels, mean difference between venous and arterial lactate is 0.25 mmol/L. However, the authors noted that in studies that included hemodynamically unstable trauma patients and patients with higher lactate levels, there was poorer correlation between arterial and venous lactate.

PEARLS

- The VBG is appropriate for estimating arterial pH and HCO_3^- unless the patient is hypotensive or there is suspicion of a mixed acid-base disorder.
- The VBG pco_2 can only be used to rule out hypercapnia. There is poor correlation with arterial pco_2 at greater than 45 mm Hg.
- The VBG lactate correlates best with ABG lactate at values less than 2 mmol/L. VBG lactate can be used as an estimate of arterial lactate except in patients with hypotension or severe trauma.
- ABG is preferable to VBG in patients with shock, severe trauma, and mixed acid-base disorders.

SUGGESTED READINGS

Baskin S, Brewer T. Cyanide poisoning. In: Sidell F, Takefuji E, Franz D, eds. *Medical Aspects of Chemical and Biological Warfare*. Office of the General Surgeon; 1997:271-286.

Bloom BM. The role of venous blood gas in the emergency department: a systematic review and meta-analysis. *Eur J Emerg Med*. 2014;21:81-88.

Byrne AL. Peripheral venous and arterial blood gas analysis in adults: are they comparable? A systematic review and meta-analysis. *Respirology*. 2014; 19(2):168-175.

Chong WH, Saha BK, Medarov BI. Comparing central venous blood gas to arterial blood gas and determining its utility in critically ill patients: narrative review. *Anesth Analg*. 2021;133(2):374-378.

Kelly A-M. Validation of venous pco_2 to screen for arterial hypercarbia in patients with chronic obstructive airway disease. *J Emerg Med*. 2005;28(4):377-379.

Kelly A-M. Review article: can venous blood gas analysis replace arterial in emergency medical care. *Emerg Med Australas* 2010;22(6):493-498.

Zeserson E, Goodgame B, Hess JD, et al. Correlation of venous blood gas and pulse oximetry with arterial blood gas in the undifferentiated critically ill patient. *J Intensive Care Med*. 2018;33(3):176-181.

106

BICARBONATE USELESS? CURRENT INDICATIONS FOR THE USE OF BICARBONATE THERAPY

KIMBERLY BOSWELL

The use of sodium bicarbonate therapy in the ED has varied over the past several decades. From treating DKA to being prophylaxis for "renal protection" prior to the administration of intravenous contrast, bicarbonate has had many roles. Studies have challenged the utility and safety of bicarbonate administration for several disease processes, but there is a place for bicarbonate in several others. Currently, there are only a few indications for administering bicarbonate in the ED and many of the prior indications continue to be controversial. Given here are the current standards and discussion surrounding the utilization of bicarbonate therapy in the ED.

Mainstays of treatment of DKA include aggressive fluid resuscitation, electrolyte management (specifically potassium repletion), and insulin. Bicarbonate is no longer recommended to treat the acidosis associated with DKA unless the patient's pH is below 6.9. If bicarbonate is given for a pH less than 6.9, it should be given in small aliquots (100 mEq) and infused over a 1- to 2-hour period. The venous pH should be checked every 2 hours and bicarbonate should be stopped when the pH is 7.0 or higher. The controversy surrounding bicarbonate therapy in DKA is primarily 2-fold. First, there is little evidence to support the benefit of its administration and there are several possible side effects including a paradoxical decrease in the cerebral pH and a further decrease of the serum potassium. Second, there is evidence to suggest that it slows the clearance of ketones. Also, important to note, its use in pediatrics is discouraged due to its association with cerebral edema. The routine use of bicarbonate therapy in DKA should no longer be considered a pillar of treatment and should only be reserved for the most critically ill patients.

Lactic acidosis can be the result of many underlying disease processes or injuries. The use of exogenous bicarbonate to treat acidosis is controversial and generally should be considered only when a patient has a severe acidosis, defined by a pH less than 7.1 and a serum bicarbonate less than 6. Data supporting the use of bicarbonate in severe acidosis are lacking but its administration is recommended to mitigate the negative physiologic effects of acidosis. Acidosis results in a reduction in left ventricular contractility, decreases the response to catecholamines, and can lead to arrhythmias. Treating the underlying cause of lactic acidosis in patients with a pH greater than 7.1 is recommended as lactate can be cleared and serum bicarbonate levels can increase relatively quickly. Several studies have suggested there is little difference in the administration of bicarbonate compared to saline with respect to the increase in cardiac output, mean arterial pressure in patients with a pH greater than 7.1. In fact, it is important to remember that the administration of exogenous bicarbonate can have several effects on electrolyte balance including causing hypocalcemia and hypernatremia. It also has a direct effect on the serum potassium levels. In addition, exogenous bicarbonate stimulates arterial and tissue production of P_{CO_2}. The goal of bicarbonate treatment in severe acidosis is simply to achieve a pH greater than 7.1, but not fully normalize the pH, while simultaneously treating the etiology of the acidosis.

Hyperkalemia, when hemodynamically significant and life-threatening, continues to be an indication for the use of bicarbonate. Bicarbonate results in a shift of extracellular potassium intracellularly in order to maintain an electrically neutral environment. Interestingly, there have been no studies that actually demonstrate an immediate or significant benefit (acute change in the serum potassium level), but the recommendation to administer bicarbonate still exists. It is important to note that administration of bicarbonate should not be the only intervention employed in the acute treatment of hyperkalemia, but therapy should include calcium, insulin and glucose, and beta-2 agonists.

The use of sodium bicarbonate in the setting of cardiac arrest has been a mainstay of treatment for years. However, recent literature has suggested that routine use of bicarbonate may not convey a clinical benefit and, in some cases, may actually worsen outcomes. Literature review of both the adult and pediatric cardiac arrest populations over the past several years has demonstrated that there is a trend against the use of routine use of bicarbonate during resuscitation and is associated with a significantly decreased rate of survival to hospital discharge, respectively. The use of sodium bicarbonate in cardiac arrest related to hyperkalemia or tricyclic antidepressant overdose is still recommended. In addition, the AHA 2022 Guidelines for Cardiopulmonary Resuscitation and Emergency Cardiovascular Care recommend against the routine use of sodium bicarbonate in resuscitation.

Aggressive correction of pH regardless of the etiology (DKA, shock leading to lactic acidosis, or treatment of hyperkalemia) with bicarbonate therapy has a limited role in the ED and we continue to learn more about its risks, benefits, limitations, and the proper use.

PEARLS

- Bicarbonate is no longer used in treatment of DKA unless pH is less than 6.9.
- Lactic acidosis with pH less than 7.1 should be treated with bicarbonate while treating the underlying cause of the acidosis.
- There are no data to support the use of bicarbonate in the treatment of hemodynamically significant hyperkalemia, but it is still done.
- Routine use of sodium bicarbonate during cardiac arrest is no longer recommended unless the arrest is suspected to be related to hyperkalemia or tricyclic antidepressant overdose.

SUGGESTED READINGS

Blumberg A, Weidmann P, Ferrari P. Effect of prolonged bicarbonate administration on plasma potassium in terminal renal failure. *Kidney Int*. 1992;41(2):369-374.

Chang CY, Wu PH, Hsiao CT, et al. Sodium bicarbonate administration during in-hospital pediatric cardiac arrest: a systematic review and meta-analysis. *Resuscitation*. 2021;162: 188-197.

Kraut JA, Kurtz I. Use of base in the treatment of severe acidemic states. *Am J Kidney Dis*. 2001;38(4):703-727.

Kraut JA, Madias NE. Treatment of acute metabolic acidosis: a pathophysiologic approach. *Nat Rev Nephrol*. 2012;8(10):589-601.

Latif KA, Freire AX, Kitabchi AE, et al. The use of alkali therapy in severe diabetic ketoacidosis. *Diabetes Care*. 2002;25(11):2113-2114.

Panchal AR, Bartos JA, Cabañas JG, et al. Adult Basic and Advanced Life Support: 2020 American Heart Association Guidelines for Cardiopulmonary Resuscitation and Emergency Cardiovascular Care. *Circulation*. 2020;142(16):S366-S468.

Velissaris D, Karamouzos V, Pierrakos C, et al. Use of sodium bicarbonate in cardiac arrest: current guidelines and literature review. *J Clin Med Res*. 2016;8(4):277-283.

107

Pass the Steroids: Don't Miss Adrenal Insufficiency

William Caputo and Sarah Lee

The adrenal glands normally produce three classes of hormones: glucocorticoids, mineralocorticoids, and androgens. Adrenal steroid secretion is tightly regulated at multiple levels in the human body. The hypothalamic-pituitary-adrenal axis regulates cortisol production in response to stress and numerous other inputs. Aldosterone is the main mineralocorticoid produced by the adrenal glands and helps regulate sodium and potassium levels, blood volume, and blood pressure. Aldosterone production is mainly regulated by the renin-angiotensin system.

Adrenal insufficiency occurs when the adrenal glands produce an insufficient amount of one or more of these classes of hormones. Adrenal insufficiency can result in significant patient morbidity and mortality. However, due to the range of signs and symptoms, variable clinical course, and many possible etiologies, it can be challenging to diagnose and manage.

Acute adrenal crisis is the severe result of decompensated adrenal insufficiency. It is a potentially fatal condition resulting from the absence of the adrenal gland hormones, cortisol and aldosterone, as well as insufficient catecholamines for the shock state present. Patients in adrenal crisis may be in severe distributive shock, presenting with hypotension and on the edge of cardiovascular collapse. The mortality rate of adrenal crisis ranges from 6% to 15%.

Patients at Risk

Adrenal insufficiency can manifest at any age, but often presents between the ages of 20 and 50 years. Infections that can cause adrenal insufficiency are tuberculosis, meningococcemia, HIV/AIDS-related infections, and fungal infections. Patients with amyloidosis or those on chronic steroid courses are also at increased risk. Certain cancers can metastasize to the adrenal gland and can cause adrenal insufficiency, including renal cell carcinoma, melanoma, lung cancer, colon cancer, and lymphoma.

Signs and Symptoms

Patients with a history of adrenal insufficiency classically experience weakness, changes in pigmentation of skin, and weight loss. The gastrointestinal symptoms that can be seen include abdominal pain, vomiting, constipation, and diarrhea. The neurologic symptoms that can be seen include syncope and impaired consciousness, which can range from delirium all the way to obtundation and coma.

When to Suspect

Clinical symptoms, history, medication use, lab abnormalities, and vital signs serve as important clues to the diagnosis of adrenal insufficiency. Possible triggers of adrenal crisis, such as infections, should also be considered. Gastroenteritis is frequently cited as a precipitant and can be particularly dangerous since vomiting and diarrhea impair the absorption of oral medication and may also exacerbate dehydration. Other common triggers include recent surgery or trauma, pregnancy, myocardial infarction, hypoglycemia, withdrawal or reduction of glucocorticoid therapy, and strenuous physical activity or emotional stress.

The following patient presentations should clue the clinician to a possible diagnosis of adrenal crisis:

- Steroid withdrawal syndrome: patient on chronic or recent prolonged steroid course for more than 2 weeks
- Hypotension refractory to high-dose single vasopressor or multiple vasopressors
- Refractory hypoglycemia despite glucose repletion
- Dehydration or hypotension out of proportion to the severity of current illness
- Hyponatremia, hyperkalemia, non–anion gap metabolic acidosis
- New changes in skin color, especially on the face, neck, and back of hands

Workup in Adrenal Crisis

Assessment of renal and liver function, electrolytes, serum glucose, venous blood gas, and complete blood count are recommended in any patient with suspected adrenal insufficiency or adrenal crisis. Serum cortisol and thyroid function studies can be sent from the ED but results may not be available promptly or influence immediate management. Cosyntropin stimulation testing is classically taught as the confirmatory test for adrenal insufficiency. However, this is only recommended in the clinically stable patient. Otherwise, the patient should be treated presumptively with stress dose steroids.

The classic findings of adrenal insufficiency include hyponatremia, hyperkalemia, and a non–anion gap metabolic acidosis. Hypercalcemia may also be present. Hypoglycemia, which can be refractory to glucose repletion, can also be seen and is more common in children than adults. The complete blood count can show normocytic anemia, neutropenia, eosinophilia, and lymphocytosis.

Management

Assess and address the airway, breathing, and circulation in your patient. Obtain an immediate finger-stick glucose level. Treatment for adult patients includes prompt administration of IV hydrocortisone, given as a 100-mg bolus, followed by 200 mg every 24 hours, with subsequent doses tailored to the clinical response. Waiting for the confirmatory labs is not recommended. If the clinician is concerned about affecting the results of confirmatory testing, dexamethasone 4 to 8 mg IV is an effective alternative to hydrocortisone that does not interfere with confirmatory testing. It is also important to give electrolyte replacement and dextrose, as needed. Rehydrate with rapid IV infusion of 1,000 mL of isotonic saline infusion within the first hour, followed by further IV rehydration as required (usually 4-6 L in 24 hours in adults; monitor for fluid overload in case of renal impairment and in older patients). It is important to always treat the underlying problem that precipitated the crisis.

PEARLS

- Signs and symptoms of adrenal insufficiency are often nonspecific, but diagnosis is important to make for the Emergency Medicine provider. Beware of

generalized weakness, weight loss, and skin changes, as these are extremely common in adrenal insufficiency.
- Clues to the diagnosis of adrenal crisis include hypotension out of proportion to illness, hypotension refractory to vasopressors, hyponatremia, hypoglycemia, hyperkalemia, volume depletion, and recent or chronic steroid use.
- Adrenal crisis is often precipitated by triggers, with gastroenteritis and infections being common triggering events.
- Adrenal crisis requires resuscitation with hydrocortisone or dexamethasone and IV fluids, correction of glucose and electrolyte abnormalities, treatment of the underlying acute trigger, and inpatient hospitalization.

Suggested Readings

Husebye ES, Pearce SH, Krone NP, Kämpe O. Adrenal insufficiency. *Lancet*. 2021; 397(10274):613-629.

Lentz S, Collier KC, Willis G, Long B. Diagnosis and management of adrenal insufficiency and adrenal crisis in the emergency department. *J Emerg Med*. 2022;63(2):212-220.

Rushworth RL, Torpy DJ, Falhammar H. Adrenal crisis. *N Engl J Med*. 2019;381(9):852-861.

The Crashing Infant: Don't Miss Inborn Errors of Metabolism

Kyra Paticoff and Danielle Langan

When it comes to managing the crashing infant in the ED, it is crucial to have a high level of suspicion for IEMs as a potential diagnosis. IEMs encompass a broad range of metabolic disorders that may be inherited or spontaneous, which typically involve failure of the metabolic pathways. Although these disorders individually are rare, the likelihood of an infant having a metabolic disorder is 1 in 2,500 births, making this diagnosis more common than most perceive. Presentation of IEMs can occur at any age. Neonatal screening tests exist to try to identify IEMs early. However, different states and hospitals use various types of screening panels. There are thousands of different types of inborn errors, yet screening tests can only identify between 8 and 50 specific disorders depending on the diagnostic test. In addition, screening can yield false-negative results if tested too early. It is important to remember that although IEMs are typically diagnosed within the neonatal period, about 50% do not present until adulthood.

Classification

IEMs can be broken down into three broad categories: (1) disorders leading to intoxication (eg, urea cycle defects); (2) disorders involving energy metabolism (eg, hypoglycemia), and (3) errors involving synthesis or catabolism of complex molecules (eg, lysosomal storage disorders).

Making the Diagnosis/Clinical Presentation

IEMs present with features commonly seen in other causes of the crashing infant. Therefore, obtaining a detailed history is a vital step in narrowing your differential. Family history of IEMs or multiple unexplained early deaths in the family should raise suspicions for this diagnosis. Patients may arrive at the ED due to deterioration; neurologic abnormalities such as loss of milestones, poor tone, seizure, and decreased activity; and GI symptoms such as vomiting, dehydration, hepatomegaly, and exercise intolerance.

An infant with hypoglycemia, bradydysrhythmias and tachydysrhythmias, hyperpyrexia, seizures, or poor tone, may appear to have sepsis. However, severe errors in carbohydrate metabolism, typically seen in the neonatal period, also have these features. In intoxicated, lethargic infants with altered mental status, vomiting, seizures, and elevated ammonia, severe errors in excretion pathways should be considered. Some IEMs are associated with difficulty accessing stored energy. Infants with this error, who maintain carbohydrate intake, are usually asymptomatic. Triggers such as GI illness or diet changes such as stopping night feeds can lead to hypoglycemia and seizures in these previously well-appearing children.

A thorough physical exam is another important step for diagnosing these patients. Your examination should incorporate a cardiac, abdominal, neurologic, and genital investigation, as well as an ophthalmologic and a hearing exam. Facial features should also be observed. Physical exams may reveal cataracts, cardiac murmurs, myopathy, hepatomegaly, and ascites. Many IEMs are associated with dysmorphic features including macrocephaly, hypospadias, and rocker bottom feet.

Workup

Although a definitive diagnosis is unlikely in the ED, there are several laboratory tests helpful for narrowing your differential diagnoses. The first set of labs for the crashing infant should include glucose, blood gas with lactate, serum chemistry with BUN and creatine, and a CBC with differential. The results of those initial tests will guide your next step. If suspicious for IEM, additionally obtain an ammonia level, CK, and serum or urine ketones.

There are laboratory patterns visible for different IEMs. If blood gas results reveal respiratory alkalosis or are normal, consider urea cycle disorders. In this group of disorders, glucose, lactate, and ketones will be normal and ammonia will be elevated. When the blood gas shows high anion gap metabolic acidosis, the next step is to look at lactate levels. Elevated lactate levels suggest mitochondrial disorders of pyruvate metabolism. Hypoglycemia, ketosis, and normal CK levels may or may not be observed. Patients with a normal lactate level in the setting of high anion gap metabolic acidosis should have urine ketones measured. Absent urine ketones point you toward fatty acid oxidation disorders (eg, carnitine palmitoyl transferase deficiency). This diagnosis will also present with hypoketotic hypoglycemia, abnormal liver function tests, and elevated CK. If urine ketones are present, the likely diagnosis is organic acidemias or MSUD. Ketotic hypoglycemia and neutropenia are associated with organic acidemias, while patients with MSUD have ketotic hypoglycemia with or without elevated plasma leucine, isoleucine, and valine. In these latter cases, essential analysis would be required for serum and urine amino acids and organic acids.

Tip: If your clinical suspicion for IEMs is high, draw extra labs for any further serum amino acid and organic acid testing. If a lumbar puncture is to be performed, gather extra CSF for any further testing.

TREATMENT/MANAGEMENT

When treating these crashing infants, it is important to remember the basics. Your first step will be to stabilize the infant using PALS/ACLS resuscitation. After the patient is stabilized, these patients often require a D10 bolus to treat hypoglycemia. Lastly, when IEM is suspected, patients should be made NPO. Intravenous D10 at 1.5 maintenance can be given to patients, especially those with poor caloric intake. Insulin may need to be given to manage hyperglycemia caused by the fluids. Exogenous glucose also serves to halt catabolic processes that contribute to the accumulation of amino acids, organic acids, and even ammonia. If the infant is presenting with elevated ammonia levels, nitrogen scavengers such as sodium benzoate or sodium phenylacetate should be given. Ammonia levels over 600 require dialysis. These patients will require further management in the pediatric intensive care unit and may require transfer to a specialized children's hospital.

PEARLS

- Individually, IEMs are rare, but as a group they are common, making IEM an important differential diagnosis in the crashing infant.
- A good history, including family history and thorough physical exam, is key to diagnosing these patients.
- When drawing labs, draw extra for any further testing that may need to be done.
- Remember the basics of treating crashing infants. The first step in treatment is stabilizing your patient.

SUGGESTED READINGS

El-Hattab AW. Inborn errors of metabolism. *Clin Perinatol.* 2015;42(2):413-439.
Jeanmonod R, Asuka E, Jeanmonod D. Inborn errors of metabolism. In: *StatPearls [Internet].* StatPearls Publishing; 2023. https://www.ncbi.nlm.nih.gov/books/NBK459183/
MacNeill EC, Walker CP. Inborn errors of metabolism in the emergency department (undiagnosed and management of the known). *Emerg Med Clin.* 2018;36(2):369-385.

109

FEVER AND ALTERED MENTAL STATUS: DON'T FORGET THYROID STORM

SHOROK HASSAN AND HALLIE TIBURZI

Patients presenting to the ED with fever and altered mental status are not a rare occurrence. In this current environment of recognizing sepsis early, most emergency clinicians are in tune with the rapid evaluation and management of patients with these symptoms. However, not all patients with these symptoms have an infectious source *and* sometimes infection is a trigger for a much rarer and sneaky diagnosis: thyroid storm. Thyroid storm is a very rare, acute, and severe condition in patients with a history of hyperthyroidism, diagnosed or undiagnosed. It most commonly occurs in patients with Graves disease but can also occur in patients with toxic multinodular goiter and toxic thyroid adenoma. Thyroid storm is primarily triggered by a stressor, which can be infection, surgery, trauma, pregnancy, infarction (ie, cardiac, pulmonary, cerebral, mesenteric), or another endocrinopathy. The most common thyroid-related triggers include thyroid surgery, noncompliance with antithyroid medications, or overdose of thyroid hormone. However, about 30% of patients with thyroid storm do not have an identifiable cause. If left untreated, it may result in multiorgan failure and death. Thyroid storm mortality rates are estimated to be as much as 25%. Due to its rarity and diverse presentation, it may not be readily considered by the clinical team; therefore, educating clinicians in an emergent setting of the various signs and symptoms may reduce thyroid storm case severity and mortality.

DIAGNOSIS

The diagnosis of thyroid storm can be challenging as it typically presents as a mimic of more common disease processes including infectious (cholangitis, sepsis), neurologic (psychosis, meningitis, and hyperthermia), or cardiac (sepsis, heart failure, atrial fibrillation with tachycardia) abnormalities. Signs and symptoms of thyroid storm are listed in **Table 109-1**.

To delineate these symptoms, there are five situations in which thyroid storm should be considered:

1) When a patient with a known history of hyperthyroidism presents with any acute illness
2) In patients with new-onset atrial fibrillation and dilated cardiomyopathy
3) In patients with new-onset altered mental status or psychosis in combination with abnormal vital signs including fever and tachycardia
4) In patients with hyperthermia (temperature >40 °C) of unknown etiology
5) In patients appearing to have sepsis without a known source of infection

The B-W criteria is a scoring system for thyroid storm and can be referenced in patients presenting with one or more of these situations in order to identify the likelihood of thyroid storm and whether storm management should be initiated. It should be noted, however, that the B-W scoring system is sensitive but not specific to the diagnosis of thyroid storm. The Japanese Thyroid Association came up with a different scoring system

TABLE 109.1 SIGNS AND SYMPTOMS OF THYROID STORM

CARDIAC	NEUROLOGIC	HYPERTHERMIA	GASTROINTESTINAL	OTHER
■ Tachycardia (including atrial fibrillation) ■ High output, distributive heart failure ■ Systolic heart failure ■ Systolic hypertension	■ Delirium ■ Agitation ■ Psychosis ■ Stupor ■ Coma	■ Temperature up to 40-41 °C	■ Diarrhea ■ Nausea ■ Vomiting ■ Abdominal pain ■ Jaundice	■ Weight loss ■ Tremor, restlessness ■ Goiter ■ Exophthalmos

that involves the use of thyroid laboratory testing and clinical signs to make the diagnosis. This scoring system is more specific but was shown to miss more thyroid storm than the B-W scoring system. If the clinical suspicion is high and the patient is presenting with symptoms of hyperthyroidism, thyroid storm management should be initiated as it is still an effective treatment for the continuum of thyroid symptoms that occur before the storm.

On initial evaluation, thyroid testing should be done including a TSH and a free T4. In addition, basic laboratory studies including glucose, electrolytes including calcium/magnesium/phosphorus, liver function tests, CBC, coagulation studies, and creatinine kinase should be ordered. Have a low threshold to obtain blood cultures and initiate an infectious workup. A chest x-ray may help assess heart failure, a head CT can be useful in ruling out neurologic etiology in applicable patients, and an ECG is performed to monitor for arrhythmias.

Laboratory values are consistent with uncomplicated hyperthyroidism and are not indicative of thyroid storm. Key lab findings include low TSH, elevated free T4 and free T3, and may include hyperglycemia, hypercalcemia, high or low white blood cell count, and abnormal liver function test results.

MANAGEMENT

Management includes administration of systemic blockade, stress dose steroids, thionamide (methimazole or propylthiouracil), iodine, or lithium. Cardiovascular stabilization is essential in the initial management of a thyroid storm and includes volume repletion based on echocardiography, lung sonography, and patient history. Beta-blockers are classically used for systemic blockade. However, their use should be held until a point-of-care ultrasound is performed to assess for left ventricular function as beta-blockade may exacerbate cardiogenic or distributive shock in patients with reduced EF. Tachycardia around 130 bpm may be allowed to persist in patients with systolic heart failure and thyroid storm to achieve adequate perfusion. Heart rate control agents including propranolol or esmolol may be administered if hemodynamic evaluation deems it safe. Glucocorticoids decrease the conversion of T4 to T3 and should be used in patients with severe symptoms. Thionamides should be administered early as well and there is no significant clinical difference between propylthiouracil and methimazole. Iodine should be administered *at least 60 minutes after thionamide administration* as iodine can increase thyroid hormone levels. Hyperthermia management includes acetaminophen and the use of cooling blankets. Salicylates and NSAIDs should be avoided as they may increase free thyroid hormone levels. Agitation can be managed by the administration of benzodiazepines.

Following the appropriate management, clinical improvement should be seen within 24 to 46 hours. Once a thyroid storm has been survived, patients should receive definite therapy for their preexisting hyperthyroidism to avoid recurrences. However, some patients do not respond to management or improve. Refractory thyroid storm treatment thus includes therapeutic plasma exchange or thyroidectomy.

PEARLS

- Thyroid storm is primarily triggered by a stressor.
- Have a low threshold to check a TSH in patients with a high risk for thyroid storm.
- Use a point-of-care ultrasound to assess for left ventricular function before administration of beta-blockade.

- Management should proceed in a stepwise manner.
- Iodine should be administered at least 60 minutes after thionamide administration.

SUGGESTED READINGS

Chiha M, Samarasinghe S, Kabaker AS. Thyroid storm. *J Intensive Care Med*. 2013;30(3): 131-140.
Farkas J. Thyroid storm. EMCrit Project. Retrieved January 13, 2023. https://emcrit.org/ibcc/tstorm/
Pokhrel B, Aiman W, Bhusal K. Thyroid storm. In: *StatPearls [Internet]*. StatPearls Publishing; 2022. https://www.ncbi.nlm.nih.gov/books/NBK448095/

110

KNOW HOW TO RECOGNIZE AND TREAT MYXEDEMA COMA

KEVIN MOLYNEUX AND CHEN HE

Myxedema coma (MC) is a rare, but life-threatening form of decompensated hypothyroidism. The incidence is between 0.22 and 1.08 cases per million per year and is more common in the older population and in women. MC has an in-hospital mortality between 30% and 60%, with higher mortality among older patients (>65 years), and those presenting with coma, cardiac complications, sepsis, hemodynamic instability, and requiring pressors and mechanical ventilation. Given its rarity, insidious onset, and wide range of presentations, it often goes undiagnosed in the ED, with about 50% of patients being missed during their ED visit.

In terms of clinical findings, MC is a bit of a misnomer. Myxedema commonly is thought to refer to the nonpitting edema often found on the pretibial surface of the lower extremity. However, myxedema can occur anywhere, including the face and airway and is not always present at initial presentation. In addition, the term *coma* in "*myxedema coma*" refers to patients who may present not yet in a coma but who have impaired mental status, lethargy, psychosis, confusion, and disorientation. Many patients will not present with coma, and this can lead to missed or delayed diagnosis. The most common findings in MC are rather decreased mental status and hypothermia.

Patients may enter a myxedema crisis for various reasons. Infection is the leading precipitant. Normothermia may be seen in patients with MC with a concomitant infection. A patient with an afebrile infection should prompt consideration of MC, and similarly a patients with normothermic MC should prompt an infectious workup and broad-spectrum antibiotic administration. Other precipitating events include GI hemorrhage, hypoglycemia, hypothermia, CO_2 retention, trauma, burns, stroke, and medications, including beta-blockers, opioids, benzodiazepines, and steroids.

Once suspected, MC should be treated on the basis of clinical suspicion alone and not delayed while awaiting blood test results. With high clinical suspicion, the level of TSH elevation should not exclude MC. There can be wide ranges of TSH values in MC, and the TSH may not be as elevated in older patients or those with hypothyroidism due to TSH deficiency. A low free T4 level is confirmatory for hypothyroidism. It is imperative that the clinician additionally search for and manage any precipitating event based on the presentation. Complete blood count, comprehensive metabolic studies, urine studies including culture, blood cultures, chest x-ray, and electrocardiogram should be obtained, with further workup tailored to the individual patient. Consider a CT of the head for those with altered mental status, given the MC-induced coagulopathy.

Regarding management, resuscitation takes precedence. Fluid expansion for hypotension should be done carefully, as patients can easily become fluid overloaded, and should be done with isotonic fluids with dextrose given the high rates of hypoglycemia. Intubation can be required but should be approached cautiously due to the increased potential for peri-intubation hemodynamic collapse due to hypotension, metabolic derangements, hypercapnia, and hypoxemia. In addition, the intubation can be technically difficult due to laryngeal edema, macroglossia, and angioedema. External rewarming can manage hypothermia, but vitals must be closely monitored as the resultant vasodilation can cause hypotension. Patients should receive antibiotics in case of infection and comprehensive care of multiorgan dysfunction.

There is an increased incidence of concomitant adrenal insufficiency with MC, so stress-dose steroids should be administered. IV glucocorticoid therapy should be administered prior to levothyroxine. The standard approach is to give hydrocortisone at 50 to 100 mg every 6 to 8 hours until a concomitant adrenal insufficiency can be ruled out. Initial thyroid hormone replacement for MC is IV levothyroxine (T4), with a loading dose of 200 to 400 mcg, followed by a daily replacement dose of 1.6 mcg/kg PO, reduced to 75% if being given IV. Lower doses may be given for smaller or older patients and those with a history of coronary disease or arrhythmia.

IV liothyronine (T3) may be given in addition to levothyroxine at a loading dose of 5 to 20 mcg and maintenance dose of 2.5 to 10 mcg every 8 hours. The theory behind this is that MC can decrease thyroxine conversion to triiodothyronine, but strong evidence is lacking. Further, there is an increased rate of arrhythmia and cardiac ischemia in patients with underlying coronary artery disease after administration.

Because of the high rates of morbidity and mortality with these patients, they often require close monitoring and management in an intensive care unit.

PEARLS

- The cardinal signs are decreased mental status and hypothermia, but the presentation can be highly variable, so the clinician must maintain a high index of clinical suspicion for MC.
- Provide hemodynamic support with warming, IV fluids, and vasopressors.
- Initiate treatment immediately when suspected. TSH levels may not be available to the clinician, and may be normal depending on the patient.
- Initiate treatment with IV hydrocortisone and IV levothyroxine (T4). Consider IV liothyronine (T3).
- When diagnosed, search for and manage the precipitating event that triggered the MC.

Suggested Readings

Beynon J, Akhtar S, Kearney T. Predictors of outcome in myxoedema coma. *J Crit Care*. 2008;12:111.

Bridwell RE, Willis GC, Gottlieb M, et al. Decompensated hypothyroidism: a review for the emergency clinician. *Am J Emerg Med*. 2021;39:207-212.

Chen YJ, Hou SK, How CK, et al. Diagnosis of unrecognized primary overt hypothyroidism in the ED. *Am J Emerg Med*. 2010;28:866-870.

Dubbs SB, Spangler R. Hypothyroidism: causes, killers, and life-saving treatments. *Emerg Med Clin N Am*. 2014;32:303-317.

Jonklaas J, Bianco AC, Bauer AJ, et al. Guidelines for the treatment of hypothyroidism. *Thyroid*. 2014;24(12):1670-1751.

Mathew V, Misgar RA, Ghosh S, et al. Myxedema coma: a new look into an old crisis. *J Thyroid Res*. 2011;2011:493462.

Ono Y, Ono S, Yasunaga H, et al. Clinical characteristics and outcomes of myxedema coma: analysis of a national inpatient database in Japan. *J Epidemiol*. 2017;27:117-122.

Rodríguez I, Fluiters E, Pérez-Méndez LF, et al. Factors associated with mortality of patients with myxedema coma: prospective study in 11 cases treated in a single institution. *J Endocrinol*. 2004;180:347-350.

Wartofsky L. Myxedema coma. *Endocrinol Metab Clin N Am*. 2006;35:687-698.

111

Know Causes of Ketoacidosis in the Patient Without Diabetes

Tyler Yates and Irina Aleshinskaya

Ketone bodies (acetoacetate, beta-hydroxybutyrate, and acetone) are formed in the liver by the breakdown of fatty acids. Their production commonly occurs during periods of fasting and is triggered through a decreased insulin-to-glucagon ratio. Normally, ketone production equals the rate of ketone utilization, maintaining serum ketone levels at low levels (<0.6 mmol/L). Because ketone bodies are acidic, they contribute to an elevated anion gap metabolic acidosis (ie, an anion gap >12 mEq/L). In high quantities, they can create a serious condition called *ketoacidosis* (loosely defined as a blood ketone level >3.0 mmol/L and a bicarbonate concentration <18 mEq/L). Diabetic ketoacidosis is the most common cause of ketoacidosis seen in the ED, but there are several other critical causes of ketoacidosis that should not be missed.

Alcoholic Ketoacidosis

The development of ketoacidosis is seen in the context of chronic alcohol abuse and its development is multifactorial. Nutritional deficiency and starvation cause depleted protein and glycogen stores and a subsequent reliance upon ketone bodies for energy. The metabolism of alcohol is reductive in nature where NAD+ is used to oxidize ethanol first to acetaldehyde and then to acetic acid. The resultant elevated NADH-to-NAD+ ratio further worsens hypoglycemia by decreasing liver gluconeogenesis and shunts acetyl-CoA toward ketogenesis. In addition, acute physiologic stressors, such as vomiting and hypovolemia, can cause an increase in sympathetic activity and an increase in glucagon and cortisol. These hormonal changes increase the release of free fatty acids, further precipitating ketone body formation.

Ingestion of toxic alcohols by patients with chronic alcohol abuse can further complicate the presentation of alcoholic ketoacidosis, as these molecules are not detected by routine blood ethanol levels. Methanol and ethylene glycol poisoning results in a high anion gap metabolic acidosis. Their metabolism in the liver follows the same pathway as alcohol and exhausts NAD+ stores, which can worsen existing hypoglycemia and ketosis. In methanol toxicity, metabolism to formic acid further contributes to the gap acidosis. Toxic alcohols can be differentiated depending on their tendency to cause considerably elevated osmolar gaps (ie, the measured osmolar concentration minus the calculated osmolar concentration). Treatment of toxic alcohols requires blockade of alcohol metabolism with fomepizole, as it is their metabolites that cause the characteristic toxicities (eg, retinopathy or oxalic acid calculi). In severe concentrations, hemodialysis may be warranted.

Starvation Ketoacidosis

In a healthy person who is on a restricted carbohydrate diet (eg, a ketogenic diet), ketosis can be a benign finding. Ketosis can also be seen in patients with an acute episode of starvation, such as during gastroenteritis or fasting for religious observations. Although uncommon, these events can become severe enough to cause serious ketoacidosis. Starvation ketoacidosis is more likely in individuals with elevated glucose requirements at baseline, such as young children or pregnant or lactating females. Pregnant women have increased ketone levels and insulin resistance due to human placental lactogen increasing sugar availability for the metabolically active fetus. Lactation is also a metabolically demanding activity, and lactose production is reliant upon glucose as a substrate. Additional physiologic stressors (eg, GI illness, hypovolemia, or intense exercise) can make starvation ketoacidosis much more likely in these susceptible populations. These risk factors can certainly exacerbate each other; case reports have found dangerously high metabolic acidosis in pregnant or lactating women on restricted carbohydrate diets. Treatment of starvation ketoacidosis is with dextrose-containing IV fluids.

Salicylate Ingestion

In addition to abdominal complaints, tinnitus, and tachypnea, salicylate poisoning can result in ketoacidosis. Following an acute ingestion, there is an initial primary respiratory alkalosis. After approximately 12 to 24 hours, there is a shift toward a high anion gap metabolic acidosis. This is due to many mechanisms, including the uncoupling of oxidative phosphorylation (and therefore an increase in anaerobic metabolism and lactate) and increased lipolysis. An increase in free fatty acid concentration increases ketogenesis by the liver. Treatment is with bicarbonate infusion to enhance the elimination of salicylates in the urine. Hemodialysis may be indicated in severe overdose scenarios.

IEMs

Ketoacidosis in pediatric patients may be due to IEMs and involve the enzymes critical for the breakdown of ketone bodies. Mitochondrial acetoacetyl-CoA thiolase deficiency (formerly known as beta-ketothiolase deficiency) is an IEM that causes loss of an enzyme that metabolizes both isoleucine and ketone bodies. It is the second step in ketolysis. Loss of this enzyme can cause ketoacidosis, in addition to elevated blood and urinary levels of isoleucine metabolites (eg, 2-methyl-3-hydroxybutyric acid). Onset is typically within the first 2 years of life with a presentation of vomiting, dehydration, and potential neurologic symptoms including coma. Genetic testing is required to confirm the diagnosis, and treatment involves lifelong avoidance of fasting or high-fat diets that could promote ketone formation. SCOT deficiency is the first and rate-limiting step of ketolysis but its deficiency is a far rarer IEM. Presentation is generally within the first few years of life, and diagnosis is with an enzyme activity test.

PEARLS

- Alcoholic ketoacidosis typically corrects rapidly with dextrose. Do not forget the thiamine!
- The presence of an osmolar gap greater than 25 (and especially >50) in an anion metabolic acidosis is fairly specific for toxic alcohol ingestion.
- Isopropanol may be metabolized directly to acetone, a ketone body, but is not a source of acidosis.
- In starvation ketoacidosis, the metabolic acidosis should improve with IV fluids containing dextrose alone. Do not expect a considerable improvement when treating with NS or LR with bicarbonate additive.
- A quick bedside test: Adding a few drops of ferric chloride to the patient's urine will make it turn purple if there are salicylates.

SUGGESTED READINGS

Alfadhel M, Babiker A. Inborn errors of metabolism associated with hyperglycaemic ketoacidosis and diabetes mellitus: narrative review. *Sudan J Paediatr.* 2018;18(1):10-23.
Al Alawi AM, Falhammar H. Lactation ketoacidosis: case presentation and literature review. *BMJ Case Reports* 2018;2018:bcr2017223494.
Bartels PD, Lund-Jacobsen H. Blood lactate and ketone body concentrations in salicylate intoxication. *Hum Toxicol.* 1986;5(6):363-366.
Grünert SC, Foster W, Schumann A, et al. Succinyl-CoA:3-oxoacid coenzyme A transferase (SCOT) deficiency: a rare and potentially fatal metabolic disease. *Biochimie.* 2021;183:55-62.
Höjer J. Severe metabolic acidosis in the alcoholic: differential diagnosis and management. *Hum Exp Toxicol.* 1996;15(6):482-488.
Sass JO. Inborn errors of ketogenesis and ketone body utilization. *J Inherit Metab Dis.* 2012;35(1):23-28.
Wiener SW. Toxic alcohols. In: Hoffman RS, Howland M, Lewin NA, Nelson LS, Goldfrank LR, eds. *Goldfrank's Toxicologic Emergencies*, 10th ed. McGraw Hill; 2015.

112

PITFALLS IN HYPERKALEMIA

STEVEN POLEVOI

The recognition of hyperkalemia is treacherous and errors in management are common. However, successful recognition and management of this condition is among the most dramatic and rewarding experiences for the well-prepared emergency physician. This is truly one of the few conditions where patients can be near death yet successfully resuscitated in mere minutes with the correct treatment. The key clinical questions when evaluating patients with hyperkalemia are as follows:

1) Does the ECG show signs of hyperkalemia?
2) Once recognized, how is the hyperkalemia best treated?

Understanding the pathophysiology of hyperkalemia is helpful to both identification and management. Most potassium in the body is found in the intracellular compartment. As the extracellular potassium concentration rises, the resting membrane potential of the myocyte is decreased (less negative) as this potential is critically dependent on the concentration gradient between the intracellular and extracellular compartments. Initially, this reduction in resting membrane potential increases myocyte excitability as the threshold potential for activation is more quickly reached. At greater extracellular concentrations of potassium, the rate of rise of the phase 0 portion of the cardiac action potential is attenuated and depression of cardiac conduction occurs.

The earliest ECG sign of hyperkalemia is reported to be a tall, narrow-based, symmetric T wave, bearing a sharp point: the so-called *peaked* T wave. For reference, T-wave amplitude is normally less than 0.5 mV in the limb leads or 1.5 mV in the precordial leads. Importantly, peaked T waves are the least sensitive finding for hyperkalemia as well as the least likely to result in short-term adverse events, with a relative risk of 0.7 compared to other ECG findings. As the serum potassium rises, lengthening of the P-R interval and a reduction of P-wave amplitude occurs. With further increases in potassium concentration, widening of the QRS complex occurs with subsequent development of various intraventricular conduction abnormalities including atypical bundle branch blocks. Ultimately, an "M-"shaped QRS-ST-T complex develops and, without intervention, VF or asystole develops. Importantly, these changes don't always appear in a sequential manner as the potassium rises.

Unfortunately, the ECG is neither sensitive nor specific as a tool for determining the serum potassium concentration. In a study of experienced acute care physicians, sensitivity of the ECG for hyperkalemia was at best 0.43 and specificity was 0.86. In the same study, sensitivity of the ECG was only 0.62 when limited to those patients with a K^+ greater than 6.5 mmol/L. Furthermore, it has been demonstrated that the ECG is particularly insensitive to elevations in potassium concentration in patients with ESRD. This places such patients at risk as physicians may depend on the classic findings of hyperkalemia and may be reassured in the absence of these findings even in the presence of marked elevations of potassium concentration.

As cardiac conduction is depressed with increasing concentrations of serum potassium, patients become symptomatic and hemodynamically compromised. At moderate to severe elevations in potassium, bradycardia and various AV blocks are a common presentation in the acute care setting (**Figure 112.1**). It is critical that practitioners both recognize and treat bradycardia with or without hemodynamic compromise aggressively with close cardiac monitoring to prevent VF and cardiac standstill.

The management of life-threatening hyperkalemia can be organized into three distinct phases that should be performed sequentially (**Table 112.1**). First, *antagonize* K^+ with calcium salts, then *shift* K^+ intracellularly with insulin, glucose, and beta-2 agonists, and finally *remove* K^+ from the body with cation exchange resins, IV fluids, or loop diuretics depending on volume status and ability to urinate, and hemodialysis if the patient has ESRD or is anuric.

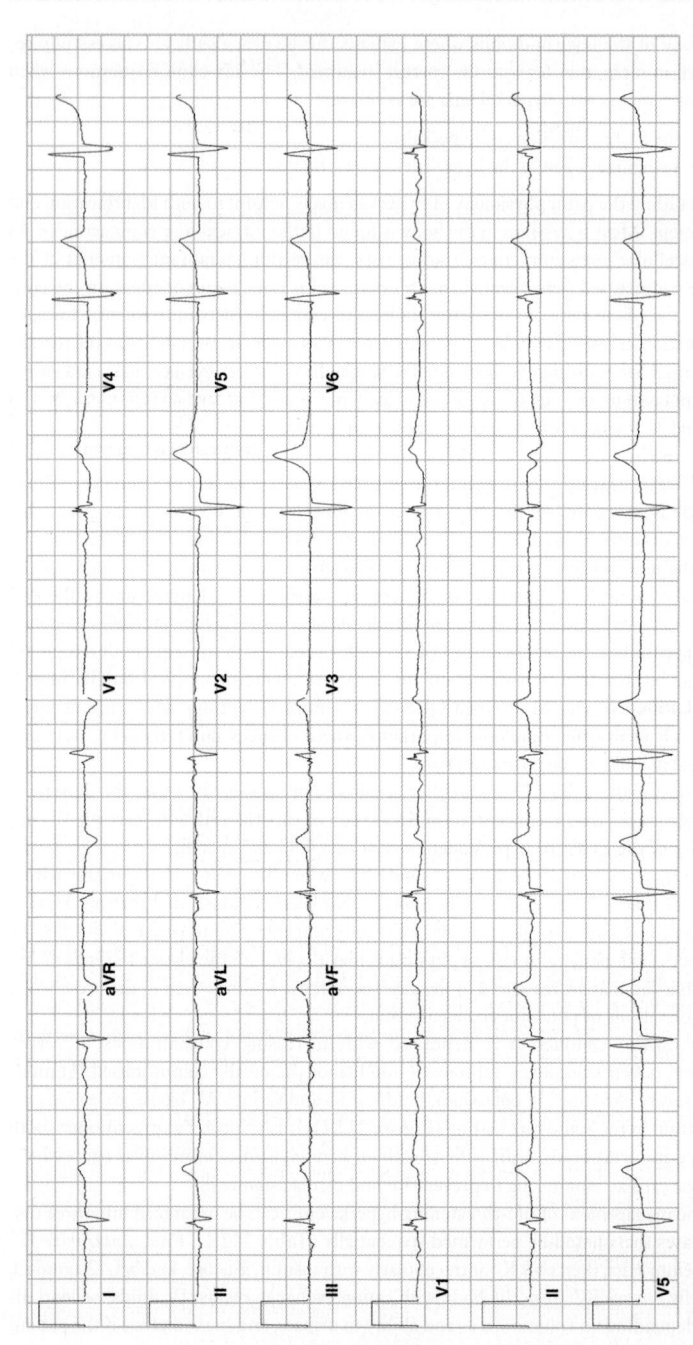

FIGURE 112.1 Sinus bradycardia with sinus arrhythmia with first-degree AVB, slightly widened QRS, and minimal T-wave peaking ($K^+ = 8.8$).

TABLE 112.1	MANAGEMENT OF LIFE-THREATENING HYPERKALEMIA			
AGENT	DOSE	ONSET	DURATION	COMMENTS
Antagonize the effect of K^+ on excitable cell membranes				
Calcium gluconate (10%)	2-3 g IV	Seconds to 3 min	30-60 min	Controversial in digoxin toxicity
Calcium chloride (10%)	1 g IV	Seconds to 3 min	30-60 min	Extravasation risk; use in cardiac arrest or via central line.
Shift K^+ from extracellular to intracellular spaces				
Insulin (short acting)	10 units IV	20 min	30-60 min	Hypoglycemia risk; give with at least 2 amps of D50 IV in CKD.
Beta-2 agonists (albuterol)	10-20 mg nebulized	30 min	2 h	Tachycardia is common.
Sodium bicarbonate (8.4%)	1 mL/kg IV	Hours	Hours	Uncertain efficacy; not first-line therapy
Remove K^+ from the body				
Cation exchange resin (sodium zirconium cyclosilicate)	10 g PO	1 h	Days	Sodium polystyrene sulfonate no longer advised
Loop diuretics (furosemide or bumetanide)	40-80 mg IV, 1-2 mg IV	15 min	2-3 h	Ineffective if anuric
Hemodialysis		Immediate	3 h	Requires catheter or preexisting fistula

The timing and indication for each step is important. With confirmed severe hyperkalemia greater than 6.5 mEq/L and hemodynamic compromise plus ECG findings (not just T-wave changes), *all* of these therapies should be given immediately. Repeat doses of calcium salts may be needed if ECG changes and hemodynamic compromise persist. In patients who are hypovolemic with hyperkalemia, diuresis with loop diuretics would be harmful and, therefore, IV fluids should be administered, although with caution, in patients with ESRD or who are anuric. In addition, insulin is renally cleared and has the potential for longer action in patients with renal insufficiency, putting these patients at high risk for hypoglycemia. Therefore, two doses of dextrose should be administered, once immediately prior to insulin administration and once 30 minutes after administration. For other patients with less severe hyperkalemia, treatment that shifts and removes K^+ is the logical response.

PEARLS

- The ECG is neither sensitive nor specific in the diagnosis of hyperkalemia.
- Peaked T waves are not reliably seen in severe hyperkalemia.

- Patients with weakness or hemodynamic compromise undergoing dialysis have hyperkalemia until proven otherwise.
- Bradycardia in the setting of hyperkalemia is ominous and should be treated aggressively.

SUGGESTED READINGS

Ahmed J, Weisberg L. Hyperkalemia in dialysis patients. *Semin Dial.* 2001;14:348-356.

Aslam S, Friedman EA, Ifudu O. Electrocardiography is unreliable in detecting potentially lethal hyperkalaemia in haemodialysis patients. *Nephrol Dial Transplant.* 2002;17:1639-1642.

Durfey N, Lehnhof B, Bergeson A, et al. Severe hyperkalemia: can the electrocardiogram risk stratify for short-term adverse events? *West J Emerg Med.* 2017;18(5):963-971.

Montague BT, Ouellett JR, Buller GK. Retrospective review of the frequency of ECG changes in hyperkalemia. *Clin J Am Soc Nephrol.* 2008;3:324-330.

Parham WA, Mehdirad AA, Biermann KM, Fredman CS. Hyperkalemia revisited. *Tex Heart Inst J.* 2006;33:40-47.

Weisberg L. Management of severe hyperkalemia. *Crit Care Med.* 2008;36:3246-3251.

113

PITFALLS IN THE MANAGEMENT OF HYPONATREMIA

KELLY-ANN MUNGROO AND ABBAS HUSAIN

Hyponatremia is defined as a serum sodium concentration less than 135 mEq/L. The management of hyponatremia can be challenging because the timing of treatment is as crucial, if not more so, than the treatment itself. Inappropriately rapid correction of hyponatremia can result in ODS, which doesn't always present acutely and can present 2 to 6 days after the correction has occurred. It is important to note that the goal of treatment is not simply to correct hyponatremia but rather to address the underlying conditions. Causes of hyponatremia include SIADH, adrenal insufficiency, diuretics, hypovolemia, and others. Consideration of the underlying disease will guide treatment and prevent complications such as ODS.

In managing hyponatremia, it is important to consider the classification of hyponatremia. Timing is a key factor in this classification. If the hyponatremia has developed in less than 48 hours, it is considered acute and requires close monitoring to avoid overcorrection. In addition, the treatment of chronic hyponatremia (with an onset beyond 48 hours) less than 105 mEq/L also carries an increased risk of developing ODS.

In addition to determining acuity, the severity of symptoms should guide management. The severity of hyponatremia symptoms can range from mild to severe (**Table 113.1**) depending on the extent and speed of sodium loss and the patient's overall health status.

TABLE 113.1	CLASSIFICATIONS AND SYMPTOMS OF HYPONATREMIA	
MILD HYPONATREMIA (NA 130-135 MEQ/L)	MODERATE HYPONATREMIA (NA 120-129 MEQ/L)	SEVERE HYPONATREMIA (NA <120 MEQ/L)
Nausea	Severe headache	Seizures
Headache	Nausea and vomiting	Coma
Fatigue	Confusion and disorientation	Elevated ICP
Muscle cramps	Seizures	Cardiac arrest
Confusion		

Patients that have acute and severely symptomatic hyponatremia should receive 3% hypertonic saline with the goal of increasing the sodium concentration by 2 to 3 mEq/L in the first hour and no more than 8 mEq/L in the first 24 hours. Initial dosing for 3% hypertonic saline in the patient who is acute and severely symptomatic is a 100-mL IV bolus for more than 10 minutes. A study showed that rapid intermittent boluses worked as well as slow continuous infusion, but there was less need for sodium relowering in the rapid intermittent bolus group. If hypertonic saline is not readily available, an ampule of sodium bicarbonate is a reasonable alternative. Each ampule of 8.4% sodium bicarbonate that is stocked in code carts contains 50 mEq of sodium, comparable to 51.3 mEq of sodium found in 100 mL of 3% sodium chloride. Repeat sodium levels should be performed after the bolus to evaluate if repeat dosing is necessary. If the sodium level has increased less than 3 mEq, a repeat dose should be given. If the sodium level has increased 3 mEq or more and the patient remains symptomatic, hyponatremia is unlikely to be the etiology and an alternative source of symptoms should be investigated.

For patients with mild to moderate symptoms, a careful calculation of fluid rate should be done:

$$\text{Fluid rate, mL/h} = \frac{(1{,}000 \times \text{Desired rate of sodium correction, mEq/L/h})}{(\text{Change in serum sodium, mEq})} \quad \text{EQ 113.1}$$

where "change in serum sodium" is the expected change of serum sodium after administration of 1 L of the chosen fluid:

$$\text{Change in serum sodium, mEq} = \frac{(\text{Fluid sodium, mEq/L} - \text{Serum sodium, mEq/L})}{\text{Total body water} + 1} \quad \text{EQ 113.2}$$

Total body water is a fraction of body weight that varies by age and gender. For children, total body water is 60% of total body weight; for younger men, 60%; younger women, 50%; older men, 50%; older women, 45%.

However, whether this is necessary depends on the cause of hyponatremia. For example, hypovolemic hyponatremia requires volume repletion by isotonic fluids in small amounts at a time. Careful consideration of the sodium concentration in the fluids to be administered is important in the management of these patients. The use of hypertonic saline in these patients is likely to overcorrect sodium and increase the risk of developing ODS. It is important that with any course of treatment sodium levels be monitored every 1 to 2 hours to ensure sodium is being repleted at an appropriate rate. Some other etiologies requiring treatments other than hypertonic saline that should be considered are listed in **Table 113.2**.

Table 113.2 Treatment Approaches by Etiology

Causes of Hyponatremia	Treatment Approach and Considerations
Adrenal insufficiency	Hydrocortisone administration to correct sodium concentration Use cortisol level to guide diagnosis.
SIADH	Restrict fluid intake. Identify and stop medications that may be causing SIADH, such as thiazide diuretics, analgesics, and antipsychotics.
Hypervolemia	Restrict fluid intake. Loop diuretics to correct sodium concentration Consider in patients with heart failure, cirrhosis, and renal failure.
Psychogenic polydipsia	Restrict fluid intake.
Beer potomania	Improve nutrition. Increase salt and protein intake.

Beyond the abovementioned scenarios, special attention should be paid to certain groups of patients that are at increased risk of developing ODS. Patients that are chronically hyponatremic, especially those with a sodium concentration less than 105 mEq/L or have concurrent hypokalemia, hypoxia, malnutrition, or a history of cirrhosis, should be managed carefully because of their predisposition to ODS. These patients are best managed with very slow correction over a period of days, oftentimes simply with fluid restriction.

PEARLS

- Hyponatremia (Na <135 mEq/L) can be classified into mild, moderate, or severe depending on the timing of hyponatremia development.
- Inappropriately rapid correction of hyponatremia can result in ODS, which can take up to 6 days to develop.
- Treatment of hyponatremia should be guided by severity of symptoms and timing of development of hyponatremia.
- Finding the underlying cause is paramount in developing the approach to treatment.

Suggested Readings

Adrogué H, Madias NE. Aiding fluid prescription for the dysnatremias. *Intensive Care Med.* 1997;23(3):309-316.

Adrogué HJ, Madias NE. Hyponatremia. *N Engl J Med.* 2000;342(21):1581-1589.

Ball S, Barth J, Levy M. Society for Endocrinology Endocrine Emergency Guidance: emergency management of severe symptomatic hyponatremia in adult patients. *Endocr Connect.* 2016;5(5):G4-G6.

Hoorn EJ, Zietse R. Diagnosis and treatment of hyponatremia: compilation of the guidelines. *J Am Soc Nephrol.* 2017;28(5):1340-1349.

Wakil A, Atkin SL. Serum sodium disorders: safe management. *Clin Med (Lond).* 2010;10(1):79-82.

SECTION VIII

ENVIRONMENTAL

114

ACCLIMATIZE, DESCEND, OR DIE!

KEVIN HANLEY

Most emergency clinicians will not encounter altitude emergencies within their department. However, we chose a fast-paced and high-stakes profession, and unsurprisingly, many of us are often allured to high-altitude endeavors. Therefore, whether you are taking a test or are on a mountain, it is crucial that ED clinicians understand how to diagnose, prevent, and treat altitude emergencies. In all cases, you either acclimatize, descend, or die!

AMS AND HACE

Diagnosis of AMS requires a setting (rapid ascent of an unacclimatized person to ≥2000 m) plus symptoms. The hallmark symptom of AMS is a headache that is throbbing, bitemporal or occipital, and worse with Valsalva, bending over and at night. The Lake Louise consensus definitions are useful when diagnosing AMS and other altitude illnesses. AMS typically occurs 1 hour to 2 days after ascent and can be associated with GI disturbance, fatigue, lassitude, and/or dizziness. Oliguria is a concerning sign, and a person who infrequently urinates should be watched closely for AMS.

AMS is often thought to be on a continuum with HACE, which is diagnosed in a patient with progressive neurologic deterioration, most importantly ataxia or ALOC. HACE occurs 1 to 3 days after ascent and has been reported at as low as 2500-m elevation. HACE can rarely present with focal neurologic deficits, such as a third or sixth cranial nerve palsy; generally, focal neuro deficits suggest a diagnosis other than HACE. Many other diagnoses can present similarly to HACE, including stroke, cerebral hemorrhage, electrolyte disturbance, dehydration, and CO poisoning, among others.

HIGH-ALTITUDE PULMONARY EDEMA

HAPE carries the highest mortality of altitude illnesses. Symptoms typically begin during or after the second night at a new altitude. Early diagnosis is critical in preventing bad outcomes: a dry cough with decreased exercise tolerance is enough to suspect HAPE. Patients can also have localized rales, most commonly in the right middle lobe of the lung, that generalize as the disease worsens and can be induced with exercise. The amount of tachycardia and tachypnea correlates to the severity of disease.

Resting oxygen saturation in HAPE also tends to be 10% to 20% lower than expected for a given altitude. As "normal" oxygen saturation decreases as altitude increases, one trick to establish "normal" for a given altitude is to average the oxygen saturation among those feeling well. Medications for HAPE prevention are recommended in those who have had a prior episode or are at high risk, including those with baseline cardiac or respiratory disease. These patients are also at higher risk of other diagnoses that can cause dyspnea, so keep a broad differential and workup of patients for pneumonia, pulmonary embolism, acute coronary syndrome, or acute exacerbations of chronic diseases where appropriate.

PREVENTION AND TREATMENT

Acclimatization

A graded ascent is a safe and effective way to prevent altitude-related emergencies. Many sources recommend sleeping between 2500 and 3000 m for two to three nights before ascending further and increasing sleeping altitude by no more than 500 m/d thereafter. One should avoid overexertion, alcohol, and other respiratory depressants as these will make acclimatization more difficult. People who are at high risk for or have a history of AMS, HACE, or HAPE are recommended to have a more conservative approach and use prophylactic medications.

Descent

The most important therapy for AMS, HACE, or HAPE is immediate descent. Descending at least 1000 m should reliably reduce symptoms, but there is no limit to the rate or amount of descent. The patient should not descend alone, and they should maintain normothermia and minimize exertion as cold and exertion worsen HAPE. If descent is unfeasible, hyperbaric bags can be used to simulate a 1500-m drop in altitude, though they require constant tending by providers and symptoms can recur once use is discontinued.

Medications

All treatments in **Table 114.1** should be accompanied by descent whenever possible.

Pediatrics

Pediatric patients at higher risk for altitude illnesses include those with congenital cardiopulmonary diseases, those with Down syndrome, and those with systemic diseases that compromise respiratory function. The treatments for pediatric patients experiencing an altitude illness use the same strategy as in the table with changes in dosing of dexamethasone (0.15 mg/kg/dose q6h, max 4 mg) and acetazolamide (2.5 mg/kg/dose BID).

Table 114.1 Prevention and Treatment

	AMS	HACE	HAPE
Prevention	■ Acetazolamide 125 mg BID started 1 d before ascent and continued for 2 d at maximum altitude	■ Same as for AMS	■ Nifedipine is first line, 20 mg q8h or 30 mg BID in extended-release formulation ■ Dexamethasone can be used (8 mg q12h started 2 d before ascent). Acetazolamide may be useful, though only anecdotal evidence exists.
Treatment	■ Dexamethasone is first line for the treatment of moderate-to-severe AMS (8 mg loading, then 4 mg q6h) ■ Acetazolamide 62.5-250 mg BID can be used, though inferior to other treatments ■ Oxygen should improve a headache from AMS within 10-15 min of administration. Nocturnal O_2 of 0.5-1 L/min is effective for mild AMS. ■ Can also consider symptomatic treatment for headache and nausea	■ Oxygen (goal saturation >90%) and dexamethasone (8 mg loading dose, then 4 mg q6h) ■ Acetazolamide can be used as an adjunct (250 mg BID) but is insufficient alone ■ Hypertonic saline, loop diuretics, and mannitol may be helpful if admitted	■ Oxygen is mainstay of therapy with goal saturation >90%. Bed rest plus oxygen may be sufficient for mild-moderate cases in a monitored setting. ■ If the abovementioned are not available, can consider nifedipine, PDE-5 inhibitors, dexamethasone, CPAP/EPAP. Can also combine these with abovementioned therapies (do not use nifedipine and PDE-5 inhibitors together for risk of hypotension).

PEARLS

- The key to diagnosing altitude illness is recent rapid ascent plus symptoms. (Refer to the Lake Louise consensus definitions.)
- Initial symptoms tend to be vague—having a high suspicion for illness can save lives.
- The key therapy ALWAYS includes descent; other treatments are stopgaps if descent is unfeasible.
- Consider alternate diagnoses—if the patient is not improving as expected, remember many other diagnoses can present similarly.

Suggested Readings

Luks AM, Beidleman BA, Freer L, et al. Wilderness Medical Society clinical practice guidelines for the prevention, diagnosis, and treatment of acute altitude illness: 2024 update. *Wilderness Environ Med*. 2023:S1080-6032(23)00167-9.

115

SMOKE INHALATION: COMMONLY OVERTREATED AND UNDERTREATED ASPECTS

DENNIS ALLIN

Smoke inhalation is the most common cause of death from fires, increasing the mortality of a 30% TBSA burn by 70%. Smoke inhalation injury generally occurs through the inspiration of superheated gases in enclosed spaces, and treatment involves the management of multiple mechanisms of injury including thermal burns, effect of inhaled chemical irritants, and inhaled systemic toxins.

THERMAL BURNS

In most cases, thermal burns will occur in the oropharynx with dissipation of heat protecting the lower airways. However, smaller size particles can still pass into the lower airway structures. The findings suggesting upper airway thermal injury include:

1) Stridor
2) Hoarseness
3) Carbonaceous sputum
4) Visible burns to the mucosa and/or face

In patients involved in an enclosed space fire with signs of potential upper airway involvement, elective endotracheal intubation should be considered early and before signs of overt airway obstruction as deterioration of the airway can occur very rapidly and, once present, make intubation nearly impossible due to swelling of the glottic and supraglottic structures. Methods to evaluate the glottis include rapid sequence induction, awake laryngoscopy or bronchoscopy with local anesthesia, and video laryngoscopy depending upon the skill of the practitioner and availability of resources. Another advantage of early endotracheal intubation is the opportunity to place an 8.0 endotracheal tube for subsequent bronchoscopies necessary for pulmonary toilet.

SYSTEMIC TOXINS

CO is the product of incomplete combustion of carbon compounds and thus a common component of smoke inhalation. Toxicity results from hypoxic stress secondary to the binding of hemoglobin by CO with leftward shift of the oxygen dissociation curve. There are, however, additional immunologic and inflammatory pathologic processes that evolve over time and result in delayed neurologic sequelae including dizziness, motor weakness, imbalance, and cognitive deficits.

The diagnosis of acute CO toxicity is suspected in patients with potential exposure to CO who display any of the symptoms of headache, nausea, dizziness, altered mental status, loss of consciousness, or metabolic acidosis. Diagnosis is confirmed by carboxyhemoglobin levels of greater than 10% in a smoker, or greater than 4% in a nonsmoker, measured in either venous or arterial samples. Importantly, the level of CO measured in the ED has a poor correlation to the patient's level of toxicity, thus patients displaying symptoms of toxicity with any elevated level of carboxyhemoglobin should be started on 100% oxygen therapy with a nonrebreather face mask.

The role of hyperbaric oxygen therapy in CO toxicity remains somewhat controversial, but the generally accepted indications to refer a patient for hyperbaric oxygen treatment include loss of consciousness, neurologic dysfunction, or cardiovascular dysfunction. The principal purpose of hyperbaric oxygen therapy is to prevent the development of delayed neurologic sequelae by mitigating the inflammatory and immunologic effects of CO; thus, the patient should be stable from an airway, cardiopulmonary, and hemodynamic status before being considered for transfer to a hyperbaric center. Only 30% of hyperbaric centers can provide 24/7 coverage for emergency indications, so the treating physician needs to carefully weigh the risk versus benefit of overemphasizing the transfer of a patient for hyperbaric oxygen therapy before managing the life-threatening complications of thermal burns to the airway and skin as well as the pulmonary injuries, especially if this entails a long-distance transfer. Consultation with the hyperbaric medicine physician can aid in this risk assessment.

Cyanide exposure is common in patients with smoke inhalation from building fires, released during the combustion of many common fabrics. Cyanide exerts its toxic effects through binding of cytochrome c oxidase resulting in cellular hypoxia and subsequently causing lactic acidosis, headache, nausea, altered mental status, hemodynamic instability, and coma. Although these symptoms are very similar to CO poisoning, cyanide toxicity is frequently overlooked, However, if left untreated, cyanide toxicity is often fatal. With no rapid confirmatory test available, it is reasonable to consider treating smoke inhalation patients empirically for cyanide toxicity if they have coma, altered mental status, acidosis, or hemodynamic instability. Several cyanide antidotes are available, but hydroxocobalamin is commonly used by ED and prehospital providers due to its relative lack of adverse effects. Hydroxocobalamin rapidly acts through the binding of cyanide to form cyanocobalamin which is excreted in the urine.

PEARLS

- Do not wait for obvious signs of airway obstruction in patients exposed to enclosed space fires if they display smoke inhalation. The airway can obstruct very rapidly leaving cricothyroidotomy as the only airway alternative.
- Smoke inhalation patients with altered mental status and acidosis should be considered for hydroxocobalamin treatment for cyanide toxicity empirically. This could prove lifesaving.
- Standard pulse oximetry is a poor marker for CO levels, and ED venous measures of carboxyhemoglobin will have a poor correlation with the degree of toxicity. Carboxyhemoglobin levels in the ED indicate exposure to CO, but they may not provide a precise measure of the degree of exposure.
- Emergency hyperbaric therapy is relatively limited in availability and may require long transport times. The priorities in smoke inhalation patients are airway management, prevention of hypoxia, and treatment of thermal burns. Patients with concomitant CO toxicity, meeting criteria for hyperbaric therapy, should be treated when otherwise stable and if available within a reasonable distance.

Suggested Readings

Bagley BA, Senthil-Kumar P, Pavlik LE, et al. Care of the critically injured burn patient. *Ann Am Thorac Soc*. 2022;19(6):880-889.

Hamad E, Babu K, Bebarta VS. Case files of the University of Massachusetts Toxicology fellowship: does this smoke inhalation victim require treatment with cyanide antidote? *J Med Toxicol*. 2016;12(2):192-198.

116

Exercise-Associated Hyponatremia: Drinking Yourself to Death (With Water)

Emily Pearce

Low serum sodium levels in the acute setting of exercise or exertion are uncommon but important to recognize; the identified prevalence of EAH has increased over recent decades in the setting of more extreme athletic endeavors such as ultramarathons and endurance events. Here, we will discuss the causes, diagnoses, and treatments for EAH.

Pathophysiology

EAH is an acutely low serum sodium that can lead to rapid osmotic shifts and cerebral edema. It is due to a combination of overhydration and ADH secretion, in which ADH levels are acutely stimulated by external stressors including heat, stress, anxiety, pain, nausea/vomiting, and extreme exertion or physical activity.

Identification and Diagnosis

EAH has been identified with a wide range of activities—including hiking, backpacking, running, in ultramarathon and endurance athletes, as well as football players and the military. The most important first step in identifying EAH is obtaining an accurate history of fluid and food intake. It is important to consider the volume of fluid consumed, over what period of time, and in the setting of the patient's body weight. Large volumes of isotonic or hypotonic fluid consumed over a short period of time in conjunction with limited food intake should be concerning for EAH. You should consider EAH when there is hydration that exceeds 1,000 mL/h. This has been seen in high school football players during preseason two-a-days in the summer and has also been seen in hikers, backpackers, endurance athletes, or military trainings during high ambient temperatures, like in the summer or desert environment. EAH has also been diagnosed in cold weather physical activities. If you are overseeing an athletic or endurance event, obtaining baseline participant weights before the event can be helpful as weight gain can indicate EAH when you don't have access to laboratory tests.

Patients may be asymptomatic or have a similar presentation to dehydration or mild heat illness, with fatigue, headache, nausea, and vomiting. ADH secretion leads to urinary retention, and this lack of urine output can be confused for dehydration. The key to identifying mild-to-moderate EAH before laboratory results is a clear history of overhydration over a short period of time, often over a period of hours, and generally less than 24 hours. You will find that mild-to-moderate EAH presents with a serum sodium level of 125 to 134 mEq/L.

More severe symptoms of EAH include ataxia, confusion, and a decreased level of consciousness and can progress to seizures in the setting of acute cerebral edema. Altered mentation is the key symptom in severe EAH and most commonly occurs at a serum sodium level below 124 mEq/L.

It is uncommon for EAH to be fatal; however, there are known cases of mortality in EAH; deaths have been confirmed in high school football players, military members, and endurance athletes. It can lead to prolonged intensive care hospitalizations if not identified and treated appropriately and death can occur from cerebral edema if not recognized.

TREATMENT OF EAH

Primarily, EAH can be prevented by discouraging overhydration. Fortunately, treatment of suspected mild-to-moderate EAH is very straightforward. Removal of the stressors contributing to ADH secretion is remarkably effective due to the short half-life of ADH (approximately 20 minutes). Simply having a patient rest, cooling them if they are showing signs of heat illness, and eating real, simple foods (chips, crackers, pretzels, etc) can lead to the patient auto-diuresing and self-correcting on their own. Small sips of water are acceptable, but patients should be fluid-restricted for at least the first hour or until the patient begins urinating consistently. As the effect of ADH clears, the patient is able to diurese and will likely correct the remainder of their hyponatremia on their own. A hypertonic oral sodium solution may also improve serum sodium. This can be simple as a ramen flavor packet or bouillon cube. Symptomatic treatment of nausea and vomiting with antiemetics can also be helpful. This author has reviewed multiple cases of EAH in which patients received large isotonic fluid boluses over short periods of time, which worsened mild EAH to altered mental status or seizures requiring more invasive interventions.

Severe EAH with altered mental status and confirmed serum sodium of less than 124 mEq/L should be treated with three boluses of 100 mL of 3% HTS over a total of approximately 30 minutes. Each 100 mL of 3% HTS has been shown to improve serum sodium by approximately 1 to 2 mEq/L. Seizures in the setting of suspected or confirmed severe EAH should be treated immediately with the same dose of HTS infused as quickly as possible. One ampoule of sodium bicarbonate is equivalent to approximately one 100 mL bolus of 3% HTS. Increasing serum sodium by 3 to 6 mEq/L should be sufficient, and the remainder of the hyponatremia correction should be allowed to occur spontaneously via urinary output. Benzodiazepines can be considered for the termination of seizure activity, but it is important to recognize that treating the cause of the seizures will most effectively treat them and prevent recurrent seizures or status epilepticus. Proper identification and treatment of EAH can prevent the need for intubation and advanced airway management, potentially saving the patient a prolonged and expensive ICU hospitalization. There are no documented cases of osmotic demyelination occurring in acute EAH. It is important to ensure this is not chronic hyponatremia before giving hypertonic saline. Consider a more chronic etiology in the older adults, patients on many sodium-influencing medications, and those with severely low serum sodium levels. In this author's experience of both treating and reviewing hundreds of confirmed cases of EAH while working as a search and rescue paramedic at Grand Canyon National Park, there were no documented cases of EAH occurring with serum sodium levels lower than 112 mEq/L. Severely low serum sodium levels, less than 110 mEq/L, should be concerning for alternative pathologies, and you should be extremely cautious in considering hypertonic saline in these circumstances.

PEARLS

- Safe hydration guidance during exertion ("drink to thirst") can help prevent overhydration.
- Mild-to-moderate EAH and dehydration can present similarly, and an accurate fluid intake history is critical in differentiating these pathologies when laboratory studies are unavailable.
- Simple interventions and time will treat most cases of mild-to-moderate EAH.
- Severe EAH should be considered in patients with an immediate history of intense physical activity and altered mental status or seizures.
- You should not delay in administering HTS to suspected severe EAH if there will be a delay in obtaining lab results; there are no documented cases of osmotic demyelination occurring with the administration of HTS for EAH.

Suggested Readings

Jonas CE, Arnold MJ. Exercise-associated hyponatremia: updated guidelines from the wilderness medical society. *Am Fam Physician*. 2021;103(4):252-253.

Klingert M, Nikolaidis PT, Weiss K, et al. Exercise-associated hyponatremia in marathon runners. *J Clin Med*. 2022;11(22):6775.

Rosner MH, Myers T, Bennett B, Lipman G, Hew-Butler T. Exercise-associated hyponatremia in the grand canyon: preventing fatalities through early recognition, timely therapy, and education. *Clin J Am Soc Nephrol*. 2023. Online ahead of print.

117

A Deep Dive on Decompression Illness

Michael Tom

In SCUBA diving, widely varied injuries occur from processes related to the physiologically foreign underwater environment. Herein, we will focus on diving injuries related to pathologic bubbles. DCS, or "the bends," and AGE are distinct diving injuries together making up the umbrella term DCI and are the diving diagnoses where HBOT is indicated.

Briefly, we will review three simplified laws of physics whose concepts are necessary to understand DCI. Keep in mind that descending in water corresponds to increasing ambient pressure, while ascending in water corresponds to decreasing ambient pressure.

First, Boyle's law states that pressure and volume are proportionally and inversely related. This primarily affects airspaces such as the middle ear. Middle ear barotrauma during descent is the most common albeit minor diving injury. On ascent from depth, decreasing ambient pressure corresponds to an increase in volume of airspaces such as the lungs. This is fundamental to AGE as we will discuss.

Second, Dalton's law describes partial pressures in gas mixtures. An example of a "gas mixture" is air, which is primarily oxygen and nitrogen. According to Dalton's law, increased total pressure at depth equates to increased partial pressures of both oxygen and nitrogen. Increased Po_2 is toxic in advanced forms of diving while increased P_{N_2} increases the risk for DCS and causes narcosis in deep diving. Finally, Henry's law states that more gas can dissolve in solution at higher ambient pressure. Conversely, as ambient pressure decreases, dissolved gas comes out of the solution as bubbles. This is why bubbles form in a soda bottle after opening and is the same process whereby nitrogen bubbles form in the blood of an ascending diver.

DCS is bubble overload. As a consequence of Dalton's (higher P_{N_2}) and Henry's (more gas dissolved in blood) laws, nitrogen accumulates in divers' tissues while breathing compressed air underwater. The deeper and longer the dive, the more nitrogen accumulation. On ascent, the decreasing ambient pressure leads to nitrogen bubble formation. Bubbles have been sonographically demonstrated in asymptomatic divers and are usually without clinical consequence, as small quantities are filtered by pulmonary capillaries. In DCS, the diver's depth and time profile is such that too much accumulated nitrogen results in too many bubbles. The pulmonary capillary filter is overwhelmed, and tissue injury ensues. Symptoms of DCS commonly manifest as rash, musculoskeletal aches (quintessential "bends"), dyspnea, or neurologic compromise with paresthesia, vertigo, or even paraplegia.

Unlike DCS, AGE is not dependent on diving too deep or too long. AGE occurs when SCUBA divers rapidly ascend while holding their breath, often due to panic. Boyle's law leads to pulmonary overexpansion. Pulmonary barotrauma allows gas to escape alveoli and embolize. Loss of consciousness is common and cerebral embolization can cause stroke-like symptoms such as hemiplegia. Severe AGE with intracardiac gas can cause "vapor lock" and cardiac arrest. AGE has been documented in as little as 3 feet of water, so shallow dives are not inherently safe as is frequently incorrectly assumed. AGE can be iatrogenic, so consider AGE in the setting of stroke-like symptoms that start immediately after an invasive procedure. *Transient* improvement following AGE is common. Thus, hyperbaric medicine consultation for AGE is still prudent even with apparent improvement in symptoms.

The history and physical examination for a diver are unique. A dive history must include the timing of symptoms, depth, duration, number of dives, water temperature, and breathing gas. Determining the presence or absence of rapid ascent, flying after diving, exertion during the dive, and thermal protection is also necessary. When used, dive computers can provide accurate dive profile data. Dive buddies and masters are useful historians in the obtunded or altered patient. On examination, a detailed neurologic exam with attention to balance, coordination, eye movements, and sensation is needed. Fully exposing the patient to evaluate for rash is important.

Timing of symptoms is most telling. AGE will manifest 0 to 5 minutes and no later than 10 minutes after a diver surfaces. DCS will manifest 0 to 24 hours after surfacing with most cases manifesting within 3 hours and more severe cases having earlier onset. Rarely, DCS can onset beyond 24 hours; however, the workup should broaden to consider non-diving etiologies in this time frame. Symptoms that occur while descending or at depth are unlikely to be DCI. Inner-ear barotrauma, gas toxicity, and cardiovascular events are diagnoses to consider in events occurring at depth.

Most diving is in austere, resource-limited locations. On scene, care should include oxygen supplementation and hydration. In the patient with obtundation, a recovery position is recommended with supportive airway measures, as resources allow. The head-down position previously thought to prevent further embolization of bubbles is not recommended. Modern teaching argues against any effect on bubble embolization and instead, there is a potentially injurious increase in intracranial pressure.

In the ED, DCI is a clinical diagnosis based on the timing of symptoms in relation to diving. Pneumomediastinum on chest x-ray and corresponding physical examination are common in AGE. Intracranial air can be noted on neuroimaging, though the absence of radiographic air does not exclude DCI. Definitive treatment for DCI is HBOT. The earlier HBOT is started, the better are patient outcomes. As such, discussion with a dive medicine specialist and transfer to an HBOT-capable facility should be mobilized as soon as DCI is suspected. HBOT benefits include bubble compression, nitrogen off-gassing, tissue oxygenation, and attenuation of perivascular inflammation. Outside 24 hours from symptom onset, treatment benefit diminishes, but HBOT should still be considered.

The only absolute contraindication to HBOT is an *untreated* pneumothorax, which can occur from pulmonary barotrauma intrinsic to AGE. Chest x-ray is therefore an essential prerequisite for HBOT. Patients with pneumothorax can still receive HBOT following chest tube placement.

DAN (Author has no financial relationship to DAN.) is a resource worth noting. DAN is available internationally, by phone, 24/7 to triage dive cases and help coordinate HBOT. Whether DCI is suspected or not, consultation with DAN or a dive medicine physician is recommended for any diving-related injury.

PEARLS

- Treatment for DCS and AGE (collectively DCI) is HBOT, which needs to start as soon as possible after onset of symptoms. Consult a dive medicine expert or DAN for any diving injury.
- DCS is from diving deeper and longer than allowable limits and excess nitrogen bubbles. AGE is from rapid ascent and pulmonary barotrauma.
- Shallower diving does not equate to safer diving. AGE can occur in as little as 3 feet of water.
- Relative to a standard ED examination, a robust neurologic exam is required for the injured diver where DCI may be suspected.
- Timing of onset symptoms is critical in determining a proper diagnosis in diving injuries.

Acknowledgments

We gratefully acknowledge the contributions of previous edition authors, Michael Iacono and Tracy Leigh LeGros, as portions of their chapter have been retained in this revision.

Suggested Readings

Bove AA, Davis JC. *Diving Medicine*. 2nd ed. WB Saunders; 1990.
Lampropoulou DI, Papageorgiou D, Pliakou E. Diving medicine: an exciting journey through time and future prospects. *Cureus*. 2024;16(3):e56947. PMID: 38665707.
Mitchell SJ. Decompression illness: a comprehensive overview. *Diving Hyperb Med*. 2024; 54(1Suppl):1-53. PMID: 38537300.
Vann RD, Butler FK, Mitchell SJ, Moon RE. Decompression illness. *Lancet*. 2011;377(9760): 153-164. PMID: 21215883.

118

Dry Drowning Is Not a Thing, So Stop Blowing Smoke!

Justin Sempsrott

"At Amsterdam on the 17th of September, 1767, an old Woman was taken out of the Rokin, a deep canal, in which she had sunk a considerable time, and being supposed dead, was to be carried away to a Hospital for burial: but Sybrand Yserman, a Skipper of Gouda, who had read the Society's Advertisement, believing that Tobacco-smoke might recover her, made the trial with a lighted pipe he had in his mouth: he put it up her anus, and taking the bowl in his mouth, blew up the smoke of it, and of another pipe after it, which by degrees so far recovered her, and she was able soon after to be carried home." (Alexander Johnson, 1773)

Some of the earliest documented treatments for drowning are tobacco enemas, bloodletting, brandy (oral and topical), emetics, cathartics, and hanging patients upside down or rolling them over a barrel. While these sound ridiculous now, they seemed to sometimes work, which led to a lot of misunderstanding of the treatment for drowning. In modern medicine, there still exists significant confusion about how to manage the person that has drowned, but doesn't need full resuscitation.

Drowning is the *process* of respiratory impairment from submersion or immersion in a liquid. Submersion is when the entire head is below water, immersion is when just the airway is covered, like someone in heavy surf or whitewater even while wearing a life jacket. There are only three outcomes of the drowning process—death or survival with morbidity or survival without morbidity, usually in the form of neurologic sequelae from cerebral anoxia. Terms such as *dry*, *wet*, *delayed*, *secondary*, and *near*-drowning have no accepted medical definition and should not be used. These terms only serve to distract from the final common pathway—cerebral anoxia. The treatment for all drowning is to get them oxygen as quickly as possible, it's that simple.

Drowning is a process, not an outcome. You wouldn't say that someone who survives a stroke, MI, or GSW had a near-MI, near-stroke, or near-GSW. Rather, you would say that they had a stroke and survived with or without residual deficit. Similarly, the proper terminology for someone who has drowned and survived is nonfatal drowning with or without morbidity.

Drowning is a spectrum from mild to moderate to severe, ultimately resulting in cardiac arrest. In the ED, we all know what to do with the patient in cardiac arrest, and with drowning there is no difference. We focus on airway, breathing, circulation, and follow the usual ACLS or PALS guidelines, doing what we can to provide the highest oxygen level possible to fight the patient's hypoxemia. Once intubated, follow standard ARDS ventilation strategies to reduce barotrauma.

Predicting outcomes can be difficult from the ED but, generally, those that arrive awake and alert do well and survive without morbidity. Patients that arrive obtunded can run the gamut and often need a few days in the ICU to identify those with severe anoxic brain injury. The factor most predictive of outcome is duration of submersion—independent of water temperature, age, salinity, or witnessed status.

What about those that arrive conscious with or without respiratory distress? Can symptoms develop after a completely asymptomatic period? It is these mild and moderate cases that create confusion and misunderstanding. Most cases of drowning are mild and need only minimal observation with or without oxygen. These are the cases that wind up with ill-defined modifiers such as "dry," "wet," "near," "delayed," "flush," and "parking lot" drowning.

In the case of mild drowning, patients often experienced a brief submersion/immersion and present with a cough with or without rales on auscultation. Routine labs are not beneficial unless you are looking for a precipitating etiology to the drowning (eg, hypoglycemia, syncope). Chest x-ray is usually normal and does not predict outcome; let symptoms be your guide. In limited published case series, patients either got better or worse in the first few hours after the incident. An observation period of 6 hours is sufficient to identify clinical deterioration. There are no case reports of *asymptomatic* patients later developing symptoms. The rare cases of seemingly delayed deterioration are in patients that displayed minimal symptoms that were initially overlooked.

In the case of moderate drowning, patients will have a cough, rales on auscultation, foam in the mouth or nose, and dyspnea without severe respiratory distress. Administer oxygen at the highest concentration available and monitor for worsening. NIPPV can be used if their mental status permits. NIPPV can be definitive or a bridge to endotracheal intubation (DSI). Sometimes, after moderate drowning, patients improve significantly and can be discharged home from the ED if they return to baseline after 6 hours off oxygen (**Table 118.1**).

The folklore of someone developing symptoms 12, 24, or 72 hours later just isn't supported by clinical experience or the literature. If someone presents with new respiratory

TABLE 118.1 DROWNING TREATMENT STRATEGIES

MILD	MODERATE	SEVERE
Conscious and alert; cough with normal lung auscultation, no dyspnea ■ Observe for 6 h post drowning. ■ Discharge if vital signs, symptoms, lung exam, and mentation remain normal.	Conscious and alert; cough/dyspnea with rales ■ Provide oxygen. ■ If improving, observe up to 6 h off oxygen. ■ Discharge if vital signs, symptoms, lung exam, and mentation return to baseline. ■ Admit if worsening.	Respiratory distress/obtunded ■ Provide high oxygen. ■ Manage according to usual respiratory distress pathway. ■ Follow ACLS/PALS. Use *ARDSNet* lung protective ventilation.

symptoms more than 6 hours after a submersion event and had been completely asymptomatic up to that point, seek alternative diagnoses. There are cases of viral myocarditis, cholecystitis, RSV, spontaneous pneumothorax, UTI, pneumonia, or MI that have been misdiagnosed as "dry" or "delayed" drowning, sometimes with fatal consequences.

Fortunately, we've come a long way from bloodletting, forcing brandy down a patient's throat, or smoke up the rectum. Let's leave terms such as *near*, *dry*, *wet*, *delayed*, and so on in the past with blowing smoke and focus on what's important: getting oxygen to the patient as soon as possible at the highest concentration available.

PEARLS

- The treatment for all drowning is to provide oxygen as quickly as possible; it is that simple.
- Discharge home if normal respiratory effort and no hypoxia 6 hours after exiting the water.
- Labs/imaging in mild and moderate cases only helpful if needed to identify inciting etiology.
- Respiratory symptoms due to drowning are present immediately after exiting the water and get better or worse over the next several hours. There is no asymptomatic period with a later decompensation.
- If the patient presents with respiratory symptoms that started more than 6 hours after being in the water, seek alternative diagnoses (URI, cholecystitis, spontaneous pneumothorax, myocarditis, UTI, pneumonia, MI, PE, etc).

SUGGESTED READINGS

Bierens J, Abelairas-Gomez C, Barcala Furelos R, et al. Resuscitation and emergency care in drowning: a scoping review. *Resuscitation*. 2021;162:205-217.

Bierens JJ, Lunetta P, Tipton M, Warner DS. Physiology of drowning: a review. *Physiology (Bethesda)*. 2016;31(2):147-166.

Johnson A. A short account of a society at Amsterdam instituted in the year 1767 for the recovery of drowned persons; with observations shewing the utility and advantage that would accrue to Great Britain from a similar Institution Extended To Cases Of Suffocation BY Damps In Mines, Choking, Strangling, Stifling, And Other Accidents. *Eighteenth century collections online*. 1773;[4]:56,55-140p.; 8°

119

PITFALLS IN HEAT STROKE MANAGEMENT

CHRISTOPHER G. WILLIAMS

In April 2009, a 26-year-old male firefighter commenced his 2-month certification program at a Texas firefighter training academy. A week later, the trainee participated in a 7 km jog as part of the physical fitness portion of the program. The temperature was approximately 73 °F with 87% relative humidity. According to reports, "About 50 feet from the finish line, the trainee became unsteady and told a crew member that he 'just wanted to finish'." Immediately thereafter, he stumbled, was assisted to the ground, and became unconscious. Vital signs revealed SBP of 60 mm Hg and HR of 170 beats/min. An ambulance arrived, established an IV, began crystalloids, and strategically placed ice packs. In the ED, a rectal temperature of 40.7 °C was documented; this was 45 minutes after the initial collapse, and more than 30 minutes after ice packs were placed on his skin.

Despite treatment in the ED and hospital for exertional heatstroke, the trainee died 5 days later. The autopsy report listed the cause of death as 'complications of hyperthermia and dehydration'.[1]

HS is the leading cause of morbidity and mortality among US high school athletes, as well as military recruits during training. Heat waves annually kill many thousands, predominantly among the extremes of age and those of lower socioeconomic means. Heat illness, in general, should be viewed as a spectrum involving minor symptoms such as heat edema, heat rash, heat cramps, heat syncope, or moderate-to-severe symptoms, namely heat exhaustion, heat injury (implying end-organ damage), and HS (CNS impairment).

HS is a misnomer in that there is no cerebrovascular impairment, but a patient suffering from HS will display many similar features: ataxia, confusion, speech impairment, and eventually a decreased level of consciousness, coma, and death. Typically, HS manifests with T_C (core temperature) above 40 °C; however, anyone suspected of heat injury who is also manifesting any CNS dysfunction should be treated as HS. The presence/absence of sweating should not factor into the diagnosis, nor should an inability to obtain a core temperature delay the diagnosis. Typically, HS is subdivided into two categories: classic and exertional. Classic HS includes those whose hyperthermic impairment is due to passive exposure to high environmental temperatures. Exertional HS results from hyperthermia occurring during strenuous exercise.

The main physiologic response to hyperthermia is vasodilation and sweating, which increase heat dissipation through radiation, convection, and evaporation. Even relatively minor elevations in T_C can increase blood flow to the skin by 7 or 8 L/min. Maintaining adequate blood pressure despite vasodilation and evaporative losses requires significantly increased cardiac output. To compensate, blood is shunted away from the gut; renal and splanchnic perfusions reduce by more than 30%.

Current research is lending more credence to the theory that this hypoperfused gut may have a significant contribution to the development of life-threatening HS. Many endurance athletes have completed races with T_C above 41 °C and no symptoms of heat injury. Yet, there are many cases of fatal HS occurring with core temperatures below that. So clearly, HS pathophysiology is more than a function of core temperature. As the gut becomes hypoperfused, its barrier role diminishes, allowing bacteria and their toxins (eg, LPS) to enter the bloodstream. This also explains the inflammatory storm and SIRS response that have been recognized in HS victims for decades. As T_C rises

---

[1] *NIOSH Fire Fighter Fatality Investigation and Prevention Program.* June 2010.

above 42 °C, proteins unfold and cellular structures disintegrate. This one-two punch of leaky-gut-induced systemic inflammatory response and thermal destruction results in multiorgan failure.

Due to its time-sensitivity and high-stakes potential for catastrophe or recovery, the recognition and treatment of acute HS can be a harrowing experience for emergency physicians. Treatment begins with cooling. Don't allow efforts to obtain IV access, run diagnostics, or get a core temperature to inhibit whole-body cooling. These important interventions can usually be done in parallel with active cooling.

Traditionally, hospitals have relied on evaporative/convective cooling as their primary method. This can be simple: wetted bedsheets and a large fan. (Remember to remove clothing and keep the sheets wet.) The best evaporative setup will drop the T_C by 0.08 °C/min at most. Many will try to augment this cooling with ice packs placed over the large vessels of the groin, axillae, and neck. Multiple studies have been unable to show significant heat reduction with ice packs alone. In fact, placing the ice packs on the palms, soles, and cheeks has elicited double the cooling rate over the traditional "major vessel" locations. The bottom line is the more surface area of the body exposed to the conductive effects of ice and cold water, the more rapid the cooling, which brings us to CWI. Whole-body CWI has long been used in the military and sports medicine for the treatment of exertional HS. It is proven to be equally effective for classic HS. The myth that rapid cooling of a patient with hyperthermia will induce vasoconstriction, shivering, and a consequential elevation in temperature has been discussed elsewhere. With CWI, one may achieve cooling rates of 0.25 °C/min—more than an order of magnitude faster than any other traditional method. This author has found that the most elegant solution for CWI in an ED is laying the patient in an open body bag and filling the bag with a slurry of water and ice. Take care to keep the patient's head above the water by propping it up with towels. A drawback of immersing your patient is difficulty accessing IV catheters, bladder catheters, and monitor leads; another concern is defibrillation or cardioversion. If the patient with HS is showing evidence of arrhythmia or impending cardiac arrest, consider covering the patient with as many ice packs as feasible; these could then be quickly removed if required.

Those with experience using the traditional evaporative/convective method will know that active cooling efforts last well over an hour. Since CWI is so effective, one must be aware of the expected cooling rate. Active cooling efforts should stop once the T_C drops below 39 °C. This may mean taking your patient out of the body bag of ice water slurry after only 10 to 15 minutes. This also presses the need for real-time core temperature measurement, preferably a temp-probe Foley catheter.

Medications that should be considered in HS are still a topic of debate. As the leaky-gut model gains traction, antibiotics and dexamethasone are becoming standard of care. Animal models have shown profound improvements in outcomes utilizing these drugs. Antipyretics are discouraged in treating HS; acetaminophen has shown no benefit, and NSAIDs may actually be harmful. Dantrolene, which has a role in treating malignant hyperthermia, has no place in HS.

Other active cooling methods, such as gastric or peritoneal lavage or bladder irrigation with ice water, have been shown efficacious in case reports, but data on cooling rates are lacking. Furthermore, none have purported to be superior to CWI. Chilled IV fluids may be a worthwhile adjuvant to active cooling efforts. One improvised method utilized by this author is to coil an extension of the IV tubing in a basin or bucket filled with an ice slurry.

> **PEARLS**
>
> - Anyone suspected of heat injury who is also manifesting any CNS dysfunction should be treated as HS.
> - CWI is the superior method to rapidly lower core temperature.
> - Active cooling efforts should cease when the core temperature is below 39 °C.
> - Due to splanchnic hypoperfusion and subsequent leaky gut with bacterial transmigration, patients with HS develop SIRS and "heat sepsis."
> - Along with active cooling, consider adjuvants such as chilled IV fluids, antibiotics, and steroids.

SUGGESTED READINGS

Lim CL. Heat sepsis precedes heat toxicity in the pathophysiology of heat stroke: a new paradigm on an ancient disease. *Antioxidants (Basel)*. 2018;7(11):149.

Lipman GS, Gaudio FG, Eifling KP, et al. Wilderness medical society clinical practice guidelines for the prevention and treatment of heat illness: 2019 update. *Wilderness Environ Med*. 2019;30(4S):S33-S46.

120

WHEN, HOW, AND WHY TO CALL YOUR FRIENDLY NEIGHBORHOOD HYPERBARIC DOC

MICHAEL TOM

To say that emergency-capable HBOT facilities are few and far between is an understatement. Of the estimated 1,500 clinical HBOT facilities in the United States, fewer than 8% treat emergent indications. This roughly translates to one emergency HBOT facility per 43 EDs! Many patients have never heard of HBOT until they need it, and many practitioners have not thought about it since they last took their board examinations. Depending on geography, CO poisoning may be a once-a-year diagnosis, while diving injuries can be a once-a-career diagnosis for the ED clinician. While generally rare in ED presentations, the cases that do benefit from HBOT are always time sensitive, and a delay in or omission of HBOT can be detrimental in terms of morbidity and mortality.

WHAT IS AN EMERGENCY-CAPABLE HBOT FACILITY?

The primary types of hyperbaric chambers are multiplace (Class A) and monoplace (Class B). A noteworthy difference is that care providers can be physically inside the much larger multiplace chambers and provide direct care. There is space for a single, recumbent patient in monoplace chambers which are typically acrylic cylinders. Multiplace chambers allow for hands-on reassessment and care during HBOT. With some exceptions, hyperbaric chambers accepting emergent and critical care referrals are facilities with multiplace chambers. Critical care in monoplace chambers requires specialized training and is facility dependent.

Emergent HBOT Indications

HBOT is primary therapy for three well-established indications and needs to be initiated emergently in these cases:

- AGE
- CO poisoning
- DCS

Evidence for each of these etiologies suggests the best patient outcomes when HBOT is started as soon as possible post-injury. Treatment effect wanes outside of 24 hours post-injury, and permanent neurologic injury can ensue with delay to HBOT. Transfer to an HBOT facility can be time consuming, so consulting a hyperbaric specialist is encouraged as soon as any of these diagnoses are suspected. The criteria for which cases of AGE, CO poisoning, and DCS require HBOT are covered in separate chapters. Keep in mind that AGE can be iatrogenic. Consider AGE when neurologic deficits or syncope occurs during or shortly after invasive procedures such as central venous catheters, lung biopsies, or cardiopulmonary bypass.

Urgent HBOT Indications

The remaining HBOT indications with relevance to emergency medicine are also time sensitive but are usually not referred directly from the ED to HBOT. These are:

- *Clostridial* myonecrosis
- Compartment syndrome
- Compromised tissue flaps and grafts
- Crush injury
- Necrotizing fasciitis

In these predominantly surgical diagnoses, HBOT is considered adjunctive, where standard medical and surgical interventions should be prioritized. While not required, the ED provider can facilitate hyperbaric medicine consultation if the admitting surgical service is amenable. Evidence for this category of HBOT indications suggests reduction in mortality, amputations, and number of reoperations with adjunctive HBOT.

Why Does HBOT Help in These Indications?

In brief, hyperoxygenation of ischemic tissues, controlled oxidative stress, altered neutrophil-mediated inflammatory response, attenuated ischemia-reperfusion injury, reduced lipid peroxidation, and varied antimicrobial effects are the primary HBOT mechanisms in emergency indications. Specific to AGE and DCS, compression of ectopic bubbles during HBOT is therapeutic.

An important note regarding hyperoxia is that oxidative stress does not imply oxidative injury. HBOT leads to a *brief* increase in ROS and RNS. ROS and RNS are generated as part of normal cellular metabolism. Upregulation of innate antioxidant pathways in response to HBOT is part of the therapeutic benefit. Brief, intermittent periods of hyperoxia characteristic of HBOT are distinctly different from unnecessary and prolonged normobaric oxygen administration which has been recognized as injurious in cardiac literature such as the AVOID study.

New Indications and the Frontiers of HBOT

CRAO is an indication recently approved by the UHMS but not ubiquitously integrated into HBOT practices. Treatment is logistically challenging in coordination with neurology, ophthalmology, and hyperbaric services. Some centers treating CRAO with HBOT have found success in the activation of "stroke alert" pathways for CRAO to mobilize resources and reduce the time to HBOT. HBOT for CRAO is an emergent indication, where immediate HBOT is indicated and benefit wanes if HBOT is initiated outside of 24 hours from symptom onset. Patients with CRAO typically have poor vision outcomes, and there is no other effective treatment. HBOT is generally considered safe and should be considered on an emergent basis if facility policy allows. Current researchers aptly refer to CRAO as the "eye stroke" and have ongoing investigations in thrombolysis and HBOT for CRAO.

Active multicenter trials are investigating adjunctive HBOT for acute TBI. Severe and mild TBI are being investigated separately. Evidence supporting HBOT for acute TBI is presently limited. High-quality evidence would need to emerge to recommend HBOT as adjunctive therapy for acute TBI. Other diagnoses with active HBOT research in progress include avascular necrosis of the hip, inflammatory bowel disease, and hypospadias.

How to Contact Hyperbaric Medicine

Emergency-capable HBOT facilities are available for consultation 24/7. If unsure how to contact hyperbaric medicine, Poison Control (800-222-1222) or Divers Alert Network (919-684-9111) are good resources. Both organizations can assist in cases of CO poisoning and diving injuries, respectively, by facilitating contact with the nearest emergency-capable HBOT facility.

Other HBOT Indications

Diabetic foot ulcers and delayed radiation injuries are the most common non-emergent indications treated with HBOT. Thermal burns are an indication supported by the UHMS but are difficult to treat since few burn centers also have critical care HBOT facilities. Other rare conditions where HBOT is indicated are idiopathic sudden sensorineural hearing loss, severe anemia (where the patient cannot receive transfusions), intracranial abscess, and rhinocerebral *mucormycosis*.

Conditions Where HBOT Is Not Indicated

Patients and families will frequently ask about HBOT for Lyme disease, fibromyalgia, musculoskeletal recovery, antiaging, chronic TBI, and sacral decubitus ulcers. Available literature does not support HBOT for these indications.

PEARLS

- All acute care HBOT is time sensitive. Emergent indications need HBOT within hours. Urgent indications need HBOT as soon as possible and this is often postoperative.
- Emergent indications are AGE, CO poisoning, and DCS. Where possible per hospital policy, CRAO is a part of this category.
- Urgent indications where HBOT is adjunctive are compartment syndrome, compromised tissue flap or graft, crush injury, gas gangrene, and necrotizing infections.

- HBOT mechanisms are hyperoxygenation, controlled oxidative stress, altered neutrophil inflammatory response, antimicrobial benefits, and reduced ischemia-reperfusion injury.
- Contact Poison Control (800-222-1222) or Divers Alert Network (919-684-9111) if unsure of how to contact the nearest HBOT facility.

121

ACCIDENTAL HYPOTHERMIC CARDIAC ARREST

GRAHAM BRANT-ZAWADZKI

"Accidental hypothermia" refers to a pathologic drop in core temperature below 35 °C (95 °F). Patients suffering from hypothermia may present at any time of year in any climate. Decreases in core temperature below 28 °C (82 °F) may lead to circulatory collapse and even cardiac arrest. AHCA most commonly occurs in the setting of some combination of injury, medication use, substance abuse, underlying critical illness, and environmental exposure; though any one of these insults alone may lead to severe hypothermia. In contrast to other causes of cardiac arrest, survival rates of patients who experience AHCA have been reported as high as 73%, with most of those survivors experiencing a favorable neurologic outcome. These superior outcomes are likely due to the protective physiologic effects of hypothermia and a readily reversible physiologic insult. The potential for neurologically intact survival underscores the importance of rapid recognition and treatment of accidental hypothermic arrest.

PHYSIOLOGY, SIGNS, AND SYMPTOMS

As core temperature decreases, central and peripheral neurologic function, tissue metabolism, and the spontaneous depolarization of cardiac pacemaker cells also diminish. These changes may manifest as clinical signs and symptoms such as progressive bradycardia, bradypnea, hyperglycemia, mydriasis, and declining mental status. Cardiovascular status typically remains stable in mild-to-moderate hypothermia, as the prolonged ventricular contraction and vasoconstriction experienced in mild and moderate hypothermia may paradoxically increase the contractile force of the heart up to 40%. As core temperature drops below 30 °C, however, cardiac output decreases markedly and bradycardia worsens. By the time core temperature drops as low as 28 °C, the metabolic demand of most tissues may drop to low as 50% of normal. In this setting, even a severely bradycardic sinus rhythm may still provide adequate perfusion to these quiescent tissues. Atrial and ventricular dysrhythmias are common at this point. As core temperatures drop below 24 °C, the risk for developing asystole increases markedly.

TREATMENT/MANAGEMENT

The approach to the victim of AHCA varies notably from that of other causes of cardiac arrest. *Once a patient is found to be hypothermic, rewarming efforts should begin immediately.* In the setting of severe hypothermia (temperatures <82 °F/28 °C), signs of life may be difficult to detect. The initial pulse and respiratory assessment should be carefully and patiently performed for at least 1 minute, with particular attention paid to identifying severe bradycardia and weak central pulses that may be difficult to palpate. This assessment should include assessment for electrical cardiac activity, end-tidal CO_2 monitoring, and evaluation with ultrasound if available. Incidents of mechanically stimulated ventricular dysthymias and cardiocirculatory collapse in patients initially stable with severe hypothermia have been reported. It is thus crucial to properly assess for the presence of organized cardiac activity before initiating other interventions, and particular care should be taken to avoid sudden, jarring movements. If a perfusing rhythm is identified, assess the blood pressure next. Most patients with hypothermia will benefit from IV fluid replacement with warmed fluid. Hypovolemia is common and systemic vascular resistance often decreases with rewarming, resulting in hypotension. If hypotension is refractory to fluid resuscitation, external cardiac pacing may be effective if available. If asystole or another non-perfusing state including VF, VT, or PEA is identified, immediate high-quality CPR should be initiated. There is no cutoff temperature for resuscitation, and patients have survived temperatures as low as 9 °C with good neurologic outcomes. Prolonged CPR may also be appropriate in the setting of AHCA. Multiple cases have been reported of successful resuscitations with full neurological recovery, including some individuals who underwent up to 6.5 hours of CPR following AHCA. Many cases of AHCA occur in locations where continuous CPR during patient extraction may be impractical or impossible. In these settings, strategies of "intermittent CPR" have been successfully applied. No clinical trial has been conducted to determine the most effective strategy for intermittent CPR, but expert opinion recommends alternating periods of compression (lasting a minimum of 5 minutes) interspaced by brief periods of interruption (not exceeding 5 minutes) until continuous CPR is possible. If a defibrillator device is available and identifies a shockable rhythm, one shock should be given at maximum power. No further shocks should be given until the patient's core temperature rises above 30 °C (86 °F), as defibrillation has been shown to have diminished efficacy below this temperature. Vasoactive and antidysrhythmic medications typically recommended in ACLS are similarly thought to be less effective in the patient with hypothermia, though evidence supporting or refuting this remains limited. Caution should be taken with administration of these or any other medications to the patient with hypothermia owing to decreased drug metabolism and increased protein binding. Medications administered during this state may have limited effect at the time, but increase activity as the patient warms.

Once assessment and treatment efforts have begun, rescuers must determine the most appropriate destination for their patients. Patients with severe hypothermia at risk for, or already demonstrating, ventricular dysrhythmias, hypotension, or cardiac arrest should be transferred immediately to a center capable of providing extracorporeal life support (ECLS). ECLS may be utilized for controlled warming and to provide any needed oxygenation and hemodynamic support during that process. In areas without access to ECLS, transport to the closest facility where other rewarming and resuscitation methods and screening for serum potassium are warranted. As a marker of cell lysis and death, serum potassium levels have been recommended as a screening test for the presence of hypoxia before arrest and prognostic indicator. Resuscitation efforts can be terminated for patients found to have a serum potassium level greater than 12 mmol/L.

PEARLS

- The initial examination of the patient with severe hypothermia must place special emphasis on assessment for subtle signs of life for at least 1 minute.
- Patients found to have suffered AHCA should receive immediate, high-quality CPR. If continuous CPR is not practical, intermittent CPR may be utilized. Prolonged CPR may be appropriate in this setting.
- If a defibrillator is available and a shockable rhythm present, a single shock should be delivered. Further ALS interventions may be withheld until core temperature rises above 30 °C. After this point, typical ACLS care should be initiated.
- Patients with hypothermia with risk factors for imminent cardiac arrest, ventricular dysrhythmias, hypotension, or who are already in cardiac arrest should be transferred directly to an ECLS center.

SUGGESTED READINGS

David EK. Accidental Hypothermia and Cardiac Arrest: Physiology, Protocol Deviations, and ECMO. ALiEM; December 12, 2018. https://www.aliem.com/accidental-hypothermia-cardiac-arrest-physiology-protocol-deviations-ecmo/

Dow J, Giesbrecht GG, Danzl DF, et al. Wilderness Medical Society Clinical Practice Guidelines for the out-of-hospital evaluation and treatment of accidental hypothermia: 2019 update. *Wilderness Environ Med*. 2019;30(4S):S47-S69.

Hymczak H, Gołąb A, Kosiński S, et al. The role of extracorporeal membrane oxygenation ECMO in accidental hypothermia and rewarming in out-of-hospital cardiac arrest patients—a literature review. *J Clin Med*. 2023;12(21):6730.

Lott C, Truhlář A, Alfonzo A, et al.; ERC Special Circumstances Writing Group Collaborators. European Resuscitation Council Guidelines 2021: cardiac arrest in special circumstances. *Resuscitation*. 2021;161:219-219.

Paal P, Pasquier M, Darocha T, et al. Accidental hypothermia: 2021 update. *Int J Environ Res Public Health*. 2022;19(1):501.

Takiguchi T, Tominaga N, Hamaguchi T, et al. Etiology-based prognosis of extracorporeal CPR recipients after out-of-hospital cardiac arrest: a retrospective multicenter cohort study. *Chest*. 2023. S0012-3692(23)05667-2.

122

DON'T BE BITTEN BY THE BITE

NICHOLAS B. HURST

Since antiquity, humankind has been fascinated by snakes. Whether feared or revered, the complex relationship between our species has led to many myths around the animals themselves as well as methods of treatment. This chapter will focus on the treatment of envenomation by North American pit vipers. The wide variation in presentation can make recognition and management of this disease challenging, but with the right "tools," one can avoid being "bitten by the bite!"

North American Pit Vipers

North American pit vipers is the collective name for multiple species of snakes from the genera *Agkistrodon*, *Crotalus*, and *Sistrurus* and include both rattlesnakes and non-rattlesnakes. Some common names include the western diamondback, copperhead, and massasauga, to name a few. Their venoms contain a mixture of enzymes and small molecules that have hemotoxic, cytotoxic, and neurotoxic effects. The relative proportions of venom components can differ between species, within the same species, and there are even ontogenic changes in an individual snake. These variations are part of what makes every patient with a pit viper envenomation unique.

Clinical Presentation

Pit viper envenomation presents with some combination of local injury (cytotoxicity), coagulopathy (hemotoxicity), and systemic toxicity (neurotoxicity). The predominate symptoms depend on the species involved as well as the geographic area, due to the variations mentioned in the "North American Pit Vipers" section. The most common presenting symptoms are pain and swelling. The cytotoxic components disrupt basement membranes causing capillary leakage and ecchymosis. Hemorrhagic bullae may form. Rhabdomyolysis can also be seen. Hemotoxic components can cause thrombocytopenia, elevated PT/INR, and hypofibrinogenemia. Frank bleeding is rare. Patients with neurotoxicity can present with autonomic instability, nausea, vomiting, diarrhea, respiratory muscle weakness, and myokymia.

Most patients will present with a history of hearing a rattle and seeing the snake along with associated symptoms. On examination, there may be one, two, or even four fang marks. As the front fangs begin to wear, replacement fangs will move up to take their place, sometimes resulting in multiple punctures from a single bite.

Treatment

First steps include removing any jewelry and restrictive clothing from the affected site. The leading edge of pain/edema should be marked. IV access should be established and blood drawn for labs to include a CBC, PT/INR, PTT, and fibrinogen. Pain management strategies should avoid NSAIDS for the theoretical risk of bleeding in the setting of a hemotoxic envenomation. The affected limb should also be elevated to help reduce edema and pain. Tetanus vaccination should be updated as necessary. Expert advice in management can be obtained by calling the local Poison Control Center at 1-800-222-1222. They can be a great resource in these cases, and they help provide a vital role in public health.

If the patient is exhibiting signs of envenomation, such as local injury, coagulopathies, or neurotoxicity, then the next step in treatment is antivenom. There are two FDA-approved antivenoms for the treatment of North American pit viper envenomation. The dosing is different between them, but the indications are the same. The treatment paradigm for how and when to use antivenom is also the same. Care is divided into three phases. The first phase is to gain initial control by giving a loading dose of antivenom over 1 hour. At the end of the infusion, you assess for signs of improvement or progression. If there has been progression of local injury, hemotoxicity, or continued signs of neurotoxicity, another loading dose should be infused. This is repeated until progression has stopped; there are no signs of neurotoxicity, and coagulopathies are reversed or trending toward normal. Once initial control is achieved, the observation phase starts. One of the antivenoms recommends maintenance doses of two vials every 6 hours for a total of three doses, and the other product does not. Both recommend a period of 18 hours of observation for new or returning signs of envenomation. During this period, if initial control is lost, a PRN dose of antivenom is indicated. It is infused over the same time period as the loading dose but consists of a different number of vials. During the initial treatment, re-dose until control is again achieved. The last phase is the discharge planning phase. The patient should be evaluated by physical therapy and occupational therapy, and follow-up should be arranged. There may be a need for outpatient labs to be obtained as late coagulopathies have been reported, putting the patient at risk for bleeding.

PEARLS

- Envenomation by North American pit vipers causes symptoms in three categories, cytologic, hemotoxic, and neurotoxic. These should be investigated in every patient.
- Because of venom variation, every envenomation is unique and may not follow the usual injury pattern.
- Antivenom is the only effective treatment for pit viper envenomation.
- Up to 25% of bites are thought to be "dry," where there are no apparent venom effects. If suspected, these patients should be observed for 8 to 12 hours, as delayed effects have been reported in the literature.
- Cytotoxicity from envenomation may mimic compartment syndrome. True compartment syndrome is exceedingly rare. Pressures should be measured first and antivenom administered before fasciotomy.
- Pediatric patients are treated the same as adults. Antivenom doses are the same but can be reconstituted in smaller volumes.

SECTION IX
HEAD, EARS, EYES, NOSE, AND THROAT (HEENT)

123

RECOGNIZING ZOSTER OPHTHALMICUS AND HOW TO TREAT IT

KELLI ROBINSON

Herpes zoster ophthalmicus (HZO) is varicella zoster virus (VZV) reactivation (shingles) in the V1 distribution of the trigeminal nerve with ocular involvement. Prompt recognition and treatment are imperative because of potential loss of vision. Over half of patients with VZV in the V1 dermatome will have ocular involvement. Dermatomes V2 and V3 are seldom affected.

HZO can affect any structure within the eye. The majority (two-thirds) will develop corneal involvement. Areas for potential visual morbidity include the cornea due to corneal thinning and perforation, the anterior chamber due to uveitis with subsequent glaucoma and cataract formation, and the retina due to retinal detachment and necrosis. Furthermore, patients diagnosed with HZO may have an increased risk of stroke within 1 year following their diagnosis compared to patients diagnosed with herpes zoster without ocular involvement.

PRESENTATION

HZO can affect any person; however, the typical patient will be older or immunocompromised (eg, HIV/AIDS, organ transplant). Chronologically, the typical patient narrative will begin with a weeklong history of prodromal flulike symptoms, followed by a unilateral vesicular rash with crusting lesions and pain in the unilateral V1 distribution. If the rash involves the tip of the nose (Hutchinson sign), it is highly specific for ocular involvement. This duplicate involvement is because the nasociliary branch of V1 innervating the tip of the nose is the same branch that innervates the globe. Ocular symptoms can range from tearing, redness, photophobia, and visual disturbances to lid droop. Ocular involvement may be delayed with respect to the onset of the rash; however, most ocular involvement presents within 2 weeks of the rash. Lack of a preceding vesicular rash does not preclude a diagnosis of HZO; a minority of patients will present with ocular involvement only. Patients with HIV/AIDS can have a generalized rash and appear more severely ill.

Varicella zoster is the primary cause of ARN and PORN. PORN is a severe version of ARN, usually found in patients with immunodeficiency. ARN will present as blurred vision and pain. Rapid loss of vision ensues due to retinal detachment, a common complication of ARN.

Visual acuity, eyelid evaluation, fluorescein staining, slit-lamp examination, and intraocular pressure measurement are key components in the evaluation of HZO. A slit-lamp examination is a necessity to evaluate for corneal involvement, as this finding is key in making the diagnosis.

HZO examination findings include punctate or pseudodendrite lesions and cell and flare in the anterior chamber. Pseudodendrites stain minimally, have a raised appearance, and lack terminal end bulbs. This is in contrast to HSV-induced true dendrites, which stain brightly and have terminal end bulbs. Decreased corneal sensation is suspicious for both HSV and VZV. A dilated fundoscopic examination is needed to evaluate for ARN and PORN.

The differential diagnosis for unilateral eye pain includes viral conjunctivitis (HSV, adenovirus), bacterial conjunctivitis (*Neisseria gonorrhoeae*, *Chlamydia*), allergic conjunctivitis, HSV keratitis, *Acanthamoeba* keratitis (in contact lens wearers), traumatic iritis, uveitis, and optic neuritis caused by systemic inflammatory/autoimmune disorders.

TREATMENT

1) HZO with skin lesions fewer than 7 days old, adult: acyclovir 800 mg PO 5×/day OR famciclovir 500 mg TID OR valacyclovir 1000 mg TID ×7 to 10 days. Treatment of VZV is most effective in decreasing both healing time and the formation of new lesions if initiated within the first 3, and up to 7, days of symptom onset.
2) HZO with skin lesions fewer than 7 days old, pediatric: use weight-based acyclovir dosing (20 mg/kg q8h) if younger than 12 years or under 40 kg. Older children or those greater than 40 kg can utilize adult dosage.
3) HZO with skin lesions greater than 7 days old or no active lesions: antibiotic ophthalmic ointment (erythromycin or bacitracin) BID and warm compresses to periocular skin TID
4) Conjunctivitis: erythromycin 0.5% ophthalmic ointment or bacitracin ophthalmic ointment BID
5) Iritis (suggested by photophobia): prednisolone acetate 1% one drop q1h to q6h; BEWARE: using topical steroids in HSV keratitis is contraindicated and consultation with ophthalmology is important.
6) Pain: cycloplegic agents (cyclopentolate 1% one drop TID) and cool compresses
7) Severe cases including those with ARN/PORN and all immunocompromised patients require strong consideration for admission and IV acyclovir. ARN/PORN requires over 3 months of both PO and IV acyclovir along with corticosteroids.

Immunocompetent patients without evidence of ARN/PORN or other severe features such as acute vision loss and corneal perforation can be discharged with ophthalmology follow-up within 2 days. VZV vaccine is noted to decrease the frequency and severity of HZO compared to placebo. Patients younger than 40 years need to pursue an outpatient workup for immunosuppression.

PEARLS

- Over half of patients with varicella zoster in the V1 dermatome will have ocular involvement.
- Vesicular lesions on the tip of the nose (Hutchinson sign) are highly suggestive of VZV ocular involvement.

- A slit-lamp examination must be performed for thorough evaluation of the cornea and anterior chamber to distinguishing HZO from other diagnoses.
- Initiating treatment within 72 hours of rash onset can provide symptomatic relief and may reduce the risk of visual morbidity.
- Ophthalmology should be consulted before steroid use. AVOID steroid ophthalmic drops in HSV keratitis.

Suggested Readings

Bagheri N, Wajda BN. *The Wills Eye Manual: Office and Emergency Room Diagnosis and Treatment of Eye Disease*. 7th edition. Lippincott Williams and Wilkins, a Wolters Kluwer business; 2017.

Lau CH, Missotten T, Salzmann J, et al. Acute retinal necrosis features, management, and outcomes. *Ophthalmology*. 2007;114:756-762.

Lin HC, Chien CW, Ho JD. Herpes zoster ophthalmicus and the risk of stroke: a population-based follow-up study. *Neurology*. 2010;74(10):792-797.

Pavan-Langston D. Herpes zoster ophthalmicus. *Neurology*. 1995;45(suppl 8):S50-S51.

Shaikh S, Ta C. Evaluation and management of herpes zoster ophthalmicus. *Am Fam Physician*. 2002;66(9):1723-1730.

Tintinalli J. Ocular emergencies. In: Cline DM, Kelen GD, Stapczynski JS, eds. *Tintinalli's Emergency Medicine Manual*. 8th ed. McGraw-Hill Medical; 2016:1561-1562.

124

Killer Sore Throats: Epiglottitis

Diane Rimple

The evolution of epiglottitis from an illness of children to one of adults since the introduction of the HiB vaccine is not news. The presentation of the disease in adults can be different from the classic picture of the toxic, drooling, distressed child. The "new" epiglottitis has a spectrum of presentations from mild illness with sore throat and odynophagia to the more classic, toxic appearance. This variability makes the disease more difficult to diagnose. In an adult with stridor, drooling, fever, and distress, the provider should immediately prepare for a difficult airway. But what about the patient presenting before they are in extremis? Maintaining a high index of suspicion in adults presenting with a sore throat without obvious signs of tonsillitis or pharyngitis will prevent one from missing this critically important diagnosis.

Invasive HiB disease still affects adults and children in the United States, though an estimated 75% of HiB infections now involve adults. Epiglottitis in adults can be due to other bacteria as well, including group A strep, *Streptococcus pneumoniae*, *Streptococcus pyogenes*, and *Staphylococcus aureus*. It is unusual for viruses to cause epiglottitis; however, a recent systematic review has identified many SARS-CoV-2 (COVID) associated cases.

Epiglottitis can also be triggered by caustic inhaled agents or thermal airway injuries. There are reports of epiglottitis being precipitated by inhaling crack cocaine, steam, or even by drinking hot beverages. There is a male predominance of the disease, the average age is in the 50s, and smoking seems to predispose to the disease, along with diabetes and other immunocompromised states.

While mortality has dropped from 7% to 1% in the pediatric population, the mortality rate has remained at 7% in adults for the past two decades. The morbidity and mortality of epiglottitis are closely related to late (emergent) airway management, which may be due to late presentation or a delay in diagnosis.

Patients with epiglottitis present with sore throat and odynophagia. Most will also have a fever. The onset in adults tends to be less dramatic than in children. Instead of hours, many adults with epiglottitis have several days of symptoms before presenting for care. Interestingly, those who present earlier (within hours) seem to have a more aggressive disease course and are more likely to need intubation.

The oropharyngeal examination will likely be unremarkable without edema or exudates. This should be a red flag for a deeper neck infection in a patient with a sore throat! Stridor is the sign most predictive of the need for acute airway management. Diabetes and obesity are other risk factors for severe disease requiring intubation.

The differential diagnosis for a patient with epiglottitis includes upper respiratory infection, viral pharyngitis, strep throat, peritonsillar abscess, retropharyngeal abscess, foreign body perforation, and head and neck cancer.

A CT of the soft tissue of the neck with IV contrast is an excellent way to identify epiglottitis while ruling out other diagnoses. The CT, however, requires the patient to lie flat. These patients are more comfortable sitting upright and may not tolerate lying flat long enough for imaging. Providers should perform a trial of supine positioning before sending the patient to CT and remain with them throughout the examination. A soft tissue lateral neck x-ray is performed upright and can be substituted if epiglottitis is suspected and a CT cannot be performed. While the specificity of x-rays is good (88%-100%), there is a false-negative rate of up to 20%. The best way to diagnose epiglottitis is through direct visualization with fiberoptic nasopharyngoscopy.

Management of severe epiglottitis presenting with stridor or other signs of airway compromise (drooling, tripoding, hypoxia) involves early definitive airway management. A difficult airway, including a surgical airway, must be prepared for and anticipated. Otolaryngology, anesthesia, or surgery should be called for backup, if available. Awake fiberoptic nasopharyngeal intubation is the preferred technique. Consider using a bougie to circumvent the engorged epiglottis if performing oral endotracheal intubation. A supraglottic device may actually make airway compromise worse by flattening the epiglottis over the trachea. Always be prepared to perform a cricothyrotomy should other intubation techniques fail.

Medical management includes steroids and broad-spectrum antibiotics, such as a third-generation cephalosporin (eg, ceftriaxone, cefuroxime, and cefotaxime) plus MRSA coverage, if the patient has an abscess or risk factors. The use of inhaled racemic epinephrine is controversial and has not been studied in any recent or adult patient literature. Admission to an ICU for close airway observation of the nonintubated patient is typically warranted.

PEARLS

- Maintain a high index of suspicion for epiglottitis in an adult presenting with a sore throat and a normal oropharynx examination.
- Stridor, drooling, and tripoding are signs of impending loss of airway, regardless of etiology.
- A negative lateral neck x-ray does not rule out epiglottitis.
- Direct visualization with a nasopharyngeal scope is the gold standard for diagnosing epiglottitis and is relatively quick, easy, and well tolerated by adults.
- When epiglottitis is suspected, request help early. Airway management, if necessary, should never be delayed for diagnostic studies.

SUGGESTED READINGS

File TM. Infections of the upper respiratory tract. In: Grippi MA, Elias JA, Fishman JA, eds. *Fishman's Pulmonary Diseases and Disorders.* 5th ed. McGraw-Hill; 2015.

Isakson M, Hugosson SJ. Acute epiglottitis: epidemiology and Streptococcus pneumoniae serotype distribution in adults. *J Laryngol Otol.* 2011;125(4):390-393.

Lindquist B, Zachariah S, Kulkarni A. Adult epiglottitis: a case series. *Perm J.* 2017; 21:16-089.

Sideris A, Holmes TR, Cumming B, et al. A systematic review and meta-analysis of predictors of airway intervention in adult epiglottitis. *Laryngoscope.* 2020;130(2):465-473.

125

CONSIDER A DEEP NECK SPACE INFECTION IN A CHILD WITH FEVER AND NECK PAIN OR TORTICOLLIS

NATALIE J. TEDFORD

Sore throat and neck pain are common complaints of children seeking care in the ED. Most children will have mild and self-limiting illnesses, although a life-threatening deep neck space infection can occasionally be present. Subtle clues and a high level of suspicion can help the ED provider identify which children have a potentially more serious pathology.

The two most common deep neck space infections are RPAs and PPAs. These occur either by direct penetrating trauma or through the spread of infection from a contiguous area. Both are typically complications of upper respiratory tract infections. The spread of infection and subsequent suppuration of the retropharyngeal or parapharyngeal lymph nodes leads to RPAs and PPAs, respectively.

Pediatric deep neck space infections have historically been associated with significant morbidity and mortality due to airway obstruction, mediastinitis, jugular vein thrombosis, aspiration pneumonia, or carotid artery aneurysm. Yet, advances in imaging and antibiotic treatment have significantly reduced these complications. As a result, deep neck space infections seldom lead to long-term consequences if detected early.

RPA is more common in boys, and the mean age at diagnosis is 4 years. The retropharyngeal lymph nodes are thought to involute around 5 years of age, making an abscess an uncommon finding in an older child unless it is related to trauma. At presentation, the most common symptoms of deep neck space infections are fever, neck pain, torticollis, dysphagia, neck mass, sore throat, and, less commonly, respiratory distress and stridor. The physical examination frequently reveals restricted neck mobility and cervical lymphadenopathy. RPA can present in preverbal children, so obtaining an accurate symptom history may be challenging. Nevertheless, restricted neck mobility in a child with a fever is the sentinel clinical clue to diagnosing RPA or PPA. Avoid attributing resistance to movement or painful neck movement in a child to benign pharyngitis or torticollis.

An adequate oral examination is critical when evaluating children for a deep neck space infection, although potentially challenging due to patient cooperation. The oropharyngeal examination may be normal; thus, a normal oropharynx in a symptomatic child should be worrisome for a deeper infection! A posterior pharyngeal bulge may be seen with an RPA, but its absence does not rule out the diagnosis. A peritonsillar abscess can present with similar symptoms; however, a unilateral bulge in the posterior aspect of the soft palate with contralateral uvular deviation should be readily apparent.

The relatively broad differential diagnosis for children with limited or painful neck mobility includes pharyngitis, stomatitis, cervical lymphadenitis, and meningitis. In cases with respiratory distress or stridor, the differential includes croup and epiglottitis.

A lateral neck radiograph may aid in the diagnosis of RPA. The child's neck should remain in slight extension during inspiration to avoid a false-positive thickening of the retropharyngeal space. Findings consistent with an RPA on plain films include a prevertebral space that is increased in depth compared with the anteroposterior measurement of the adjacent vertebral body or a retropharyngeal space that is greater than 7 mm at C2 or 14 mm at C6. Alternatively, the width of the prevertebral space should measure no more than half the thickness of the vertebral body from C1 to C4 or the total thickness from C5 to C7. The prevertebral space can change with crying (particularly in infants), swallowing, and ventilation, so plain x-rays are generally not the recommended radiologic study unless the patient is not stable enough for a CT. A neck CT with IV contrast is the imaging modality of choice for RPA and PPA with a sensitivity of 72% to 81% and specificity of 57% to 59% to detect a neck abscess.

When a high clinical suspicion is present or an abnormality is seen on imaging, it is essential to consult with an ENT specialist to help guide management. Surgical drainage was previously considered the standard treatment for RPA and PPA; however, current literature supports an initial trial of IV antibiotics unless the patient is unstable or has an abscess with rim enhancement with an axis greater than 20 mm on a CT scan. Medical management benefits include avoiding iatrogenic injury to cranial nerves or great vessels without potentially increasing the duration of hospitalization.

The cultures from abscess drainage are often polymicrobial. The organisms most commonly recovered from intraoperative cultures are *Staphylococcus aureus*, including MRSA, *Streptococcus pyogenes* (group A streptococcus), and respiratory anaerobes. Therefore, initial antibiotic therapy should target these organisms and may consist of ampicillin-sulbactam or clindamycin.

Whether treated medically or surgically, the length of hospital stay averages 3 to 5 days for pediatric deep neck space infections. Relapse rates are below 5%. Therefore, children with deep space infections typically have excellent outcomes when detected early and appropriately treated.

PEARLS

- Consider a deep neck space infection in a child with fever and limited neck mobility or torticollis.
- CT of the neck with IV contrast is the imaging modality of choice.
- Early consultation with an ENT specialist is essential to plan treatment.
- In a stable child with an abscess less than 20 mm on CT, an initial trial of IV antibiotics is the current treatment recommendation.

Suggested Readings

Carbone PN, Capra GG, Brigger MT. Antibiotic therapy for pediatric deep neck abscesses: a systematic review. *Int J Pediatr Otorhinolaryngol*. 2012;76:1647-1653.

Chang L, Chi H, Chiu NC, et al. Deep neck infections in different age groups of children. *J Microbiol Immunol Infect*. 2010;43(1):47-52.

Cheng J, Elden L. Children with deep space neck infections: our experience with 178 children. *Otolaryngol Head Neck Surg*. 2013;148(6):1037-1042.

Demongeot N, Akkari M, Blanchet C, et al. Pediatric deep neck infections: clinical description and analysis of therapeutic management. *Arch Pediatr*. 2022;29(2):128-132.

Elsherif AM, Park AH, Alder SC, et al. Indicators of a more complicated clinical course for pediatric patients with retropharyngeal abscess. *Int J Pediatr Otorhinolaryngol*. 2010;74(2):198-201.

Hoffmann C, Pierrot S, Contencin P, et al. Retropharyngeal infections in children. Treatment strategies and outcomes. *Int J Pediatr Otorhinolaryngol*. 2011;75(9):1099-1103.

126

Now Hear This: First Do No Harm When Treating Tympanic Membrane Perforation

John Herrick

There are many causes of TM perforation including infection, penetrating trauma, foreign bodies, blunt trauma, barotrauma, and iatrogenic injury. While the treatment is often straightforward, there are some common mistakes to avoid.

Most perforations are caused by infection. With otitis media (OM), fluid and pressure build behind the TM, causing pain. Eventually, the membrane ruptures, resulting in otorrhea. The presence of otorrhea in the setting of acute OM, and in the absence of otitis externa, confirms perforation. The presence of pain also suggests infection, as simple perforations do not cause pain. Due to the release of the middle ear pressure, patients with OM often feel relief when the TM perforates.

Cleaning the ear with cotton tip applicators or other instruments are a common cause of penetrating traumatic TM perforation. Physicians and providers can also cause perforation with overzealous irrigation or instrumentation for cerumen impaction or foreign body removal. The risk increases with poor visualization and with patient movement during the procedure. For this reason, strongly consider procedural sedation prior to attempting irrigation or instrumentation, especially in the pediatric population. Iatrogenic perforations are often large and are associated with delayed or incomplete healing.

Foreign bodies pose a risk of TM perforation, both through their presence and during attempts at removal. A button battery lodged in the ear can result in TM perforation within 2 hours. If not removed promptly, it can result in destruction of the ossicles and permanent hearing damage. Do not blindly irrigate clots or foreign bodies until TM perforation can be excluded.

A direct blow to the ear from an open hand, a head strike against water, lightning strikes, blast injuries, and burns through the TM from stray welding slag are other well-documented causes of TM perforation. TM ruptures that result from scuba diving or water sports injury are at increased risk of infection due to contaminated water entering the middle ear. For these injuries, antibiotic prophylaxis is indicated. Do not clean the ear with soap as it lowers the surface tension of the contaminating water and allows for easier penetration through the perforated TM.

Diagnosing TM perforation involves close inspection with an otoscope. A previous perforation may heal with a thin pseudomembrane. This may retract and be misdiagnosed as a persistent or new perforation. Air insufflation demonstrates decreased motion of the TM in the setting of perforation and may induce vertigo by pushing air into an injured otic capsule. Hearing can be tested with Rinne and Weber testing to help differentiate conductive and sensorineural hearing loss, although neither is sensitive nor specific. Patients with nystagmus, ataxia, and vertigo with head movement may have deeper injury. Hemotympanum, bloody drainage, or leaking cerebrospinal fluid may suggest a basilar skull fracture.

If there is concern for other trauma or infection associated with the TM perforation, a CT with fine cuts of the temporal bone is preferred to evaluate for bony abnormalities and fracture. CT with contrast can detect abscess or sinus thrombosis, but MRI is the test of choice for infectious complications such as intracranial abscess or sinus thrombosis.

Treatment with systemic antibiotics for OM with perforation should follow standard OM treatment guidelines. Traumatic perforations that do not show signs of infection and have not been exposed to contaminated water do not require antibiotics; however, keeping the TM moist using ofloxacin otic drops may promote healing. Topical therapy is a viable treatment for chronic suppurative OM but there are no studies to support its use in acute OM with perforation. Fluoroquinolone (ciprofloxacin or ofloxacin) drops are first line and the only FDA-approved topical agents. Aminoglycosides such as gentamicin and neomycin/polymyxin B/hydrocortisone (Cortisporin Otic) are considered ototoxic and are not recommended since aminoglycosides can cause sensorineural hearing loss due to cochlear damage. Patients should take precautions to keep water out of the ear such as placing a petroleum jelly–coated cotton ball in the outer portion of the ear when showering.

Patients with new, traumatic, or large TM perforation should be referred to an otolaryngologist for evaluation and audiometry testing. Most perforations will heal without treatment, but the size and location of the perforation helps predict who may need repair.

Indications for urgent consultation are ataxia, vertigo, significant hearing loss, facial nerve impairment, basilar skull fracture, CSF leak, ossicular disruption, and perilymph fistula.

In the office, an otolaryngologist may patch the eardrum with paper, use a fat plug, fibrin glue, or an absorbable sponge. A tympanoplasty requires anesthesia and involves placing a graft in place of the injured TM. Surgery has a risk of further impairing hearing, so the risks and benefits must be assessed, as many patients live with perforations without difficulty.

PEARLS

- Clean, noninfected perforations do not require antibiotics.
- Fluoroquinolone eardrops are considered safe and are FDA approved for TM perforation treatment.
- Consider using procedural sedation for otic foreign body removal in anxious or uncooperative patients to avoid iatrogenic perforation of the TM.
- Do not irrigate an ear with a known or suspected TM perforation.
- Early discussion and follow-up with an otolaryngologist can facilitate surgery when needed and lessen the chance of permanent hearing loss.

Suggested Readings

Carniol ET, Bresler A, Shaigany K, et al. Traumatic tympanic membrane perforations diagnosed in emergency departments. *JAMA Otolaryngol Head Neck Surg.* 2018;144(2):136-139.

Lou Z, Lou Z, Tang Y, Xaio J. The effect of ofloxacin otic drops on the regeneration of human traumatic tympanic membrane perforations. *Clin Otolaryngol.* 2016;41(5):564-570.

Marin JR, Trainor JL. Foreign body removal from the external auditory canal in a pediatric emergency department. *Pediatr Emerg Care.* 2006;22(9):630-634.

Orji FT, Agu CC. Determinants of spontaneous healing in traumatic perforations of the tympanic membrane. *Clin Otolaryngol.* 2008;33(5):420-426.

Suzuki K, Nishimura T, Baba S, et al. Topical ofloxacin for chronic suppurative otitis media and acute exacerbation of chronic otitis media: optimum duration of treatment. *Otol Neurotol.* 2003;24(3):447-452.

127

Know the Can't Miss Causes of a Red Eye

Gregory Jasani

Red eyes are often painful, and both the discomfort and appearance can be distressing to a patient. Causes range from the benign that require only reassurance to those that are vision-threatening and require immediate intervention. Critical pathology must be identified in order to initiate the appropriate treatments in a timely manner.

Key History

As always in emergency medicine, obtaining a thorough history is a crucial first step to determining whether a patient's presentation represents an ophthalmologic emergency.

- **Onset**: Acute onset often points to an emergent diagnosis. For example, acute angle–closure glaucoma often presents suddenly, typically after being in a dark environment.
- **Progression**: If the redness involves either the entire eye or both eyes, ask whether this has always been the case or if it evolved over time.
- **Pain**: A painful red eye can be a sign of an ocular emergency, such as acute angle–closure glaucoma, scleritis, or uveitis. Painless red eyes are often, although not always, more benign compared to painful ones.
- **Vision changes**: Inquire if the patient feels their vision has been affected by their symptoms, particularly vision out of the affected eye.
- **Past medical and past surgical history**: Obtain an accurate past medical and relevant ocular surgical history. Immunosuppressing and autoimmune conditions increase the risk of developing inflammatory conditions, such as uveitis or scleritis.

Key Physical Examination

A focused ocular examination is paramount not only for determining whether a presentation is emergent but also will provide critical information to convey to an ophthalmologist should it be necessary to consult them.

- **Visual acuity**: Visual acuity should be checked for both eyes as well as each eye individually so differences in the affected versus unaffected eye can be determined. Visual acuity should be performed with the patient wearing any glasses or contact lenses they wear at baseline.
- **Intraocular pressure**: For patients where there is concern for acute angle–closure glaucoma, an intraocular pressure should be calculated. An intraocular pressure of greater than 20 mm Hg is concerning for acute angle–closure glaucoma and warrants immediate ophthalmologic consultation.
- **Pupillary reactivity**: A fixed and nonreactive pupil is highly concerning for acute angle–closure glaucoma and warrants immediate ophthalmologic consultation.
- **Slit-lamp examination**: If there is concern for uveitis, a slit-lamp examination should be performed. On slit-lamp examination, white blood cells and flare are seen in the anterior chamber, and a hypopyon will develop as the purulent debris settles.

Consulting Ophthalmology

Ophthalmology should be consulted any time there is concern for an acute, sight-threatening disease process. In general, call ophthalmology immediately if there is vision loss, severe pain, precipitous onset of symptoms, or pupillary asymmetry.

Conditions that require immediate ophthalmology consult are listed as follows:

- **Acute angle–closure glaucoma**: Signs include firmness of the orbit palpated through the closed lid and a nonreactive, **dilated pupil**. Intraocular pressure–lowering medications (timolol, brimonidine, and acetazolamide) and emergent ophthalmology involvement are critical.
- **Acute anterior uveitis**: Physical examination reveals redness where the iris meets the sclera and **pupillary constriction** with sluggish pupillary reactivity. On slit-lamp examination, white blood cells and flare are seen in the anterior chamber, and a hypopyon

will develop. This can progress to glaucoma, pupil abnormalities, cataracts, macular dysfunction, and vision impairment. Consult ophthalmology early regarding the decision to initiate topical steroids. Antibiotics are only indicated in rare cases if there is concern for an infectious cause of uveitis.

- **Hyperacute (gonococcal) conjunctivitis**: This condition progresses rapidly and involves copious exudate, lid swelling, and preauricular lymphadenopathy. Symptoms can be unilateral or bilateral. Both topical (bacitracin, erythromycin, or ciprofloxacin) and systemic (ceftriaxone IM and either oral doxycycline or azithromycin for chlamydia coverage) treatments are needed. Patients should also be tested for STIs. Consult ophthalmology to evaluate for corneal ulceration, which could lead to perforation and vision loss.

    Neonatal gonococcal conjunctivitis presents 2 to 5 days after delivery. Treat with one dose of ceftriaxone (cefotaxime if the baby has jaundice), and admit for close monitoring of potential corneal compromise.

- **Inclusion (chlamydial) conjunctivitis**: This condition mimics typical bacterial conjunctivitis. Suspect it in sexually active adults, especially those with associated genitourinary symptoms or preauricular lymphadenopathy. Conjunctival follicles (round collections of lymphocytes) are often seen. Treat the underlying chlamydia with oral azithromycin or doxycycline. Strongly consider ceftriaxone for gonococcal coverage.

    Neonates will present 5 to 14 days after delivery with mucopurulent bloody discharge and/or pseudomembranes. Treat with azithromycin for 3 days.

- **Scleritis**: This disorder presents with redness of the sclera itself and deeper pain than episcleritis. Like episcleritis, it is likely autoimmune in etiology; however, scleritis poses a threat to vision and requires urgent ophthalmology consult for likely systemic steroids or other immunosuppressive agents. NSAIDs can be used for symptomatic management.

PEARLS

- Ask about the onset, progression, presence of pain, and vision changes to identify the vision-threatening causes of a red eye.
- Visual acuity, pupil reactivity, and intraocular pressures are key parts of the eye examination.
- Call ophthalmology immediately if there is vision loss, severe pain, precipitous onset of symptoms, pupillary asymmetry, or findings suggestive of hypopyon.

SUGGESTED READINGS

Abdel-Aty A, Gupta A, Del Priore L, et al. Management of noninfectious scleritis. *Ther Adv Ophthalmol*. 2022;14.

Azari AA, Arabi A. Conjunctivitis: a systematic review. *J Ophthalmic Vis Res*. 2020;15(3): 372-395.

Flores-Sánchez BC, Tatham AJ. Acute angle closure glaucoma. *Br J Hosp Med (Lond)*. 2019; 80(12):C174-C179.

Harthan JS, Opitz DL, Fromstein SR, et al. Diagnosis and treatment of anterior uveitis: optometric management. *Clin Optom (Auckl)*. 2016;8:23-35.

Kimberlin DW. Chlamydia trachomatis. In: Kimberlin DW, ed. *Red Book: 2015 Report of the Committee on Infectious Diseases*. 30th ed. American Academy of Pediatrics; 2015:288.

Zhang Y, Amin S, Lung KI, Seabury S, Rao N, Toy BC. Incidence, prevalence, and risk factors of infectious uveitis and scleritis in the United States: a claims-based analysis. *PLoS One*. 2020;15(8):e0237995.

128

EYEING THE CAUSES OF ACUTE ATRAUMATIC VISION LOSS

GREGORY GAFNI-PAPPAS

Acute vision loss requires prompt diagnosis to maximize the chance of vision recovery. Time-sensitive treatment may impact visual outcomes. Etiologies are based on the anatomic location of the pathology and include the media (anterior to the retina), retina, and neural visual pathways (posterior to the retina).

Key questions to ask include whether the acute vision loss is painful or painless, if the patient has a red eye, and whether the vision loss is monocular or binocular (**Table 128.1**). Important elements of the ocular examination include visual acuity, pupillary exam, visual fields, IOP, extraocular movements, slit-lamp examination, and fundoscopic examination.

CAUSES OF ACUTE VISION LOSS

Acute Angle-Closure Glaucoma
Acute monocular painful vision loss that often has an associated headache, nausea, and halos around light. The classic presentation is an older patient with eye pain that begins in a darkened room. Examination shows a mid-dilated nonreactive pupil with conjunctival injection. IOP is significantly elevated, usually greater than 40 mm Hg. Immediate treatment, including timolol, brimonidine, and acetazolamide, is indicated to lower IOPs. Emergent ophthalmology consultation is required.

TABLE 128.1 DIFFERENTIAL DIAGNOSIS FOR VISION LOSS

	PAINFUL	PAINLESS
Unilateral vision loss	■ Acute angle-closure glaucoma ■ Endophthalmitis ■ Hyphema ■ Keratitis ■ Optic neuritis ■ Uveitis ■ Trauma	■ Central retinal artery or vein occlusion ■ Ischemic optic neuropathy ■ Retinal detachment ■ Vitreous detachment or hemorrhage
Bilateral vision loss	■ UV keratitis	■ Chiasmal and retrochiasmal disorders ■ Giant cell arteritis ■ Medication side effects ■ Metabolic derangement ■ Psychogenic

UV, ultraviolet.

Central Retinal Artery Occlusion

Acute monocular painless vision loss with profoundly poor visual acuity, most often caused by carotid artery atherosclerotic embolism. Classic exam findings include an afferent pupillary defect, a pale white retina with a cherry red fovea, and "box-carring" of the retinal vessels. Immediate treatment should be initiated, including digital ocular massage, IOP lowering, ophthalmology consult, and potential hyperbaric treatment. Consider thrombolytics in consultation with neurology.

Giant Cell Arteritis

Acute monocular painless vision loss associated with headache, ipsilateral scalp tenderness in the area of the temporal artery, and ipsilateral jaw pain/claudication. ESR and CRP can be significantly elevated. GCA can cause retinal artery occlusion and retinal ischemia leading to vision loss in up to 30% of patients. Immediate treatment includes IV high-dose corticosteroids and immunosuppressive agents, as well as emergent ophthalmology consultation.

Keratitis

Acute monocular painful red eye with vision loss caused by inflammation of the cornea. Keratitis can be bacterial, viral, fungal, parasitic, or noninfectious. Examination shows corneal opacities or ulcers that may be visible to the naked eye. Slit-lamp examination can show fluorescein uptake as well as cell and flare in the anterior chamber. Immediately discontinue the use of contact lenses, if applicable. Same-day ophthalmologic consultation or referral is required for cultures and treatment.

Endophthalmitis

Acute monocular painful red eye and vision loss caused by an infection of the vitreous or aqueous humor, usually resulting from organisms introduced by trauma, surgery (including cataract removal), or an extension of keratitis. Classic exam findings include hypopyon (white blood cells layering in the anterior chamber) and a hazy view of the retina. Urgent ED ophthalmologic consultation is required for intravitreal aspiration and intravitreal antibiotics.

Uveitis

Acute monocular painful red eye and vision loss caused by inflammation of the iris, ciliary body, or choroid. Examination can show a ciliary flush or injection around the iris, photophobia, consensual photophobia, and cell and flare on slit-lamp examination. Topical corticosteroids and mydriatics are the mainstay of treatment. Consult ophthalmology for evaluation within 24 hours.

Vitreous Hemorrhage

Acute monocular painless vision loss that can occur in the setting of trauma or spontaneously, especially with sickle cell disease, anticoagulation use, or pathologic neovascularization in diabetes. Decreased red reflex may be present, and red blood cells may be evident on slit-lamp examination in the anterior chamber. Fundoscopic exam can show neovascularization of retinal vessels, and ultrasound may reveal hemorrhage in the posterior segment. Consult ophthalmology early.

Retinal Detachment

Acute monocular painless vision loss, described as a curtain over the eye. This is often preceded by "floaters" and flashes of light. Retinal detachment can be visualized on point-of-care ultrasound. Consult ophthalmology early.

Central Retinal Vein Occlusion

Acute monocular painless vision loss often occurring in older patients with a history of atherosclerotic disease. Fundoscopic examination shows multiple retinal hemorrhages termed "blood and thunder." Consult ophthalmology early.

Optic Neuritis

Acute monocular painful vision loss caused by inflammation of the optic nerve, most often caused by a demyelinating disease. Patients often present with progressive eye pain and central vision loss that is worse with eye movement. On examination, optic disc edema may be present, and there will always be an afferent pupillary defect. Consult neuro-ophthalmology urgently for high-dose IV corticosteroids.

Chiasmal and Retrochiasmal Disorders

Acute binocular painless vision loss that affects the neural visual pathways and can cause visual field deficits depending on the location of the lesion. Chiasmal lesions classically cause bitemporal hemianopsia while retrochiasmal lesions cause homonymous hemianopsia. Treatment is based on the etiology, which is most commonly pituitary adenoma in chiasmal disorders and ischemic stroke in retrochiasmal disorders. Consult neurology for management.

PEARLS

- Vision loss often requires time-sensitive treatment to prevent permanent loss of vision.
- Consult ophthalmology early for all cases of acute complete or partial vision loss.
- Conditions that require immediate treatment include acute angle-closure glaucoma, central retinal artery occlusion, and GCA.
- A complete ocular examination including visual acuity, visual field testing, slit-lamp examination, retinal examination, and IOP measurement can help to make a prompt diagnosis.
- Point-of-care ultrasound is a helpful adjunct when assessing vision loss from retinal detachment and vitreous hemorrhage.

Suggested Readings

Bennett JL. Optic neuritis. *Continuum (Minneap Minn)*. 2019;25(5):1236-1264.

Cabrera-Aguas M, Khoo P, Watson SL. Infectious keratitis: a review. *Clin Exp Ophthalmol*. 2022;50(5):543-562.

England E, Gafni-Pappas G. Chiasmal and retrochiasmal disorders. In: Mattu A, Swadron S, eds. *CorePendium*. CorePendium, LLC. Accessed May 2, 2023. https://www.emrap.org/corependium/chapter/recmyowsEwVBkMSZp/Chiasmal-and-Retrochiasmal-Disorders

Gervasio K, Peck T. *The Wills Eye Manual*. 8th ed. Lippincott Williams and Wilkins; 2021.

Hammond Victoria M. Endophthalmitis. In: Mattu A, Swadron S, eds. *CorePendium*. CorePendium, LLC. Accessed May 27, 2022. https://www.emrap.org/corependium/chapter/recNhH1BhePzp8Vpx/Endophthalmitis

Jasani G, Hammond Victoria M. Uveitis. In: Mattu A, Swadron S, eds. *CorePendium*. Accessed June 22, 2022. CorePendium, LLC. https://www.emrap.org/corependium/chapter/recdkyLdFQpheQmw7/Uveitis

Shaikh N, Srishti R, Khanum A, et al. Vitreous hemorrhage—causes, diagnosis, and management. *Indian J Ophthalmol*. 2023;71(1):28-38.

129

Digging for Gold: Some Nuggets About Epistaxis

Shahrzad Woodbridge and Eric R. Swanson

Patients with epistaxis can have an impressively wide range of presentations. Although there are no universally accepted guidelines, it is important to have an algorithmic approach. This includes a stepwise progression that combines anesthesia, pressure, vasoconstrictors, and cautery. It is imperative to know what tools are available in your ED and how to retrieve them quickly.

Most textbooks divide epistaxis into anterior and posterior etiologies. This division is not necessarily helpful to the ED clinician because anterior epistaxis may be copious and refractory to initial tamponade efforts, and similarly, posterior epistaxis may respond well to a large nasal tampon. It is more useful to think of epistaxis that can be controlled easily in the ED and refractory epistaxis requiring more advanced intervention.

There are many causes of epistaxis including URI, nose picking, minor trauma, dry air, supplemental oxygen, nasal steroids, cocaine, arteriovenous malformation, and coagulopathies. Because of the wide spectrum of presentations, the ED provider must know multiple options for its treatment. Below is a sample algorithm for use in the ED.

Step 1: Initial Measures

If the patient is hemodynamically unstable, prioritize IV access and resuscitation.

If the patient is stable, extend the head gently and spray copious oxymetazoline into the bilateral nares using an atomizer. Other vasoconstrictors may be used, such as atomized epinephrine or topical cocaine, though oxymetazoline is widely available and safe. Oxymetazoline-soaked gauze can also be inserted into the affected nare(s). Apply an anterior nasal clamp to the cartilaginous portion of the nose and leave it in place for approximately 20 minutes. One can fashion a clamp by taping two tongue depressors together, or have the patient pinch their nose (instruct them not to release until told). Most epistaxis will resolve after these measures.

Step 2: Reassessment

Using a nasal speculum with a light source or an otoscope, examine the nasal vestibules for any obvious source(s) of bleeding.

If hemostasis is maintained after 20 to 30 minutes and no further workup is needed based on the clinical context, you may safely discharge the patient home. Discharging the patient with petroleum jelly to apply to their anterior nares, additional oxymetazoline and a nasal clamp may be helpful for future episodes.

If an obvious source of bleeding is visualized, atomize approximately 2 mL of lidocaine with epinephrine into the affected nare or temporarily insert a cotton pledget soaked in a combination of oxymetazoline and 4% lidocaine. Once adequately anesthetized, if the bleeding source is visualized in an otherwise bloodless field, cauterize the site with silver nitrate sticks. This form of chemical cautery has the least amount of recurrence. Do not perform cautery to both sides of the septum or use electric cautery, as this increases the risk of septal perforation.

If the bleeding source is not visualized, a procoagulant can be tried. Insert a cotton pledget or nasal tampon soaked in 500 mg/5 mL TXA. This rivals traditional anterior packing. Additional procoagulant alternatives include "FloSeal," "Gelfoam," or "Surgicel," which are bioabsorbable and will not need to be removed.

Step 3: Packing

If bleeding continues, pack the affected naris with a nasal tampon or nasal balloon catheter. Each type has varying instructions including soaking or lubricating before insertion as well as balloon inflation after placement. Several brands are available and are equally effective. Use the largest size available that will fit into the patient's naris and aim posteriorly (not caudally) on insertion. Review specific instructions on packaging before insertion.

Monitor the patient for another half hour and check for bleeding around the tampon or in the back of the throat. For continued bleeding, attempt to use a larger tampon or a nasal balloon, or insert a second tampon into the contralateral naris to provide additional tamponade. Patients with comorbidities, symptomatic anemia, or requiring bilateral packing should be admitted. Otherwise, you may safely discharge the patient home with ENT follow-up in 2 to 3 days. Antibiotics are usually not necessary and have not been shown to reduce the incidence of toxic shock syndrome or sinusitis.

Step 4: Persistent Bleeding

Though 90% of epistaxis is anterior, consider a posterior source if the epistaxis is unrelenting. Most posterior epistaxis products use a double-balloon system—a large balloon for the anterior naris and a smaller balloon for the posterior naris. Insert the device to its hub and then inflate the posterior balloon; apply gently traction on the device and then inflate the anterior balloon.

If a double-balloon posterior device is not available, a Foley catheter can be used. Insert the Foley into the nose until the balloon is seen in the oropharynx. Inflate the balloon and then pull forward to lodge the balloon against the posterior vessels. An anterior tampon may then also be inserted around the tubing. This is extremely uncomfortable and requires analgesia and anxiolysis (though beware of hemodynamic instability and vagal events). Following insertion, maintain gently forward traction and secure the Foley using a hemostat or umbilical clamp so that the balloon cannot migrate posteriorly into the oropharynx.

Patients with posterior, or ongoing anterior, bleeds need urgent ENT consultation and should be admitted to the ICU or step-down unit to observe for airway obstruction, hemodynamic stability, and vagal events. In all cases, if your patient is anticoagulated, obtain coagulation labs and consider reversal for serious bleeding.

PEARLS

- Most epistaxis is controlled through a combination of vasoconstriction and tamponade.
- Topical procoagulants can be used to facilitate hemostasis.
- Posterior epistaxis (10% of epistaxis) will not be controlled with manual compression or anterior packing and requires a device with a posterior nasal balloon.
- Consider reversing anticoagulation agents.

Suggested Readings

Badran K, Malik TH, Belloso A, et al. Randomized controlled trial comparing Merocel and RapidRhino packing in the management of anterior epistaxis. *Clin Otolaryngol*. 2005;30(4):333-337.

Côté D, Barber B, Diamond C, et al. FloSeal hemostatic matrix in persistent epistaxis: prospective clinical trial. *J Otolaryngol Head Neck Surg*. 2010;39(3):304-308.

Janapala RN, Tran QK, Patel J, et al. Efficacy of topical tranexamic acid in epistaxis: a systematic review and meta-analysis. *Am J Emerg Med*. 2022;51:169-175.

Murano T, Brucato-Duncan D, Ramdin C, et al. Prophylactic systemic antibiotics for anterior epistaxis treated with nasal packing in the ED. *Am J Emerg Med*. 2019;37(4):726-729.

Newton E, Lasso A, Petrcich W, et al. An outcomes analysis of anterior epistaxis management in the emergency department. *J Otolaryngol Head Neck Surg*. 2016;45:24.

Singer AJ, Blanda M, Cronin K, et al. Comparison of nasal tampons for the treatment of epistaxis in the emergency department: a randomized controlled trial. *Ann Emerg Med*. 2005;45(2):134-139.

130

Properly Treating Dental Infections

Kinjal Sethuraman

Risk factors for dental infections include diabetes, other immunocompromised states, poor dental hygiene, and limited access to outpatient dental care.

History and Physical Exam

Patients often present to the ED for evaluation of facial or dental pain, swelling, or fever. They may describe a foul taste or odor. Decreased oral intake due to pain or trismus may be present. Pain is often described as a toothache exacerbated by temperature changes. As inflammation progresses to infection, pain may be described as continuous and severe. Fever, decreased oral intake, trismus, limited or painful neck motion, and tongue elevation are hallmarks of a severe infection.

The provider must evaluate the entire head and neck region for facial swelling and tenderness, trismus, drooling, and areas of fluctuance. Lymphadenopathy should be assessed. The intraoral exam, performed with gloves and tongue blade, includes examination of each tooth for tenderness to percussion, mobility, and obvious caries. Gums should also be examined for pain, erythema, and swelling. Palpate the gingival mucosal areas on both the buccal (cheek) and lingual (tongue) sides of each tooth for the presence of a fluctuant mass. Inspection and palpation for firmness under the tongue are important to identify soft tissue infection in the submental space. Trismus is often caused by spasms, pain, or swelling and can limit the intraoral examination. Painful neck range of motion may suggest a severe deep neck space infection in the submental or submandibular spaces that may compromise the airway.

Imaging

Uncomplicated dental pain and inflammation do not need imaging in the ED. Panoramic x-ray, if available, is useful for identifying caries, and CT of the face and neck with IV contrast will identify a fluid collection. In a study of 4,209 patients with emergent odontogenic visits, 49% had infections, and 20.8% had abscesses. Of those with abscesses, the inflamed tooth was clinically identified in most and treated with trepanation and antibiotics.

When clinically indicated, a CT scan with IV contrast can be utilized to identify the causative teeth and the presence of an abscess. The most commonly involved cervical space infections are in the masticator space, followed by the submandibular area.

MANAGEMENT

Odontogenic infections originate from plaque on the tooth surface. Plaque can enter through the gingival margin and lead to a periodontal abscess. Alternatively, plaque can enter through the tooth itself, cause caries through pulp invasion, disrupt the surrounding bone, and cause a periapical abscess with risk of extension into the deep spaces of the neck. A periodontal abscess differs from a periapical because its source is the gums, not the tooth, and can be seen even in the absence of tooth decay. Periapical and periodontal abscesses can both lead to severe soft tissue infections and both need antibiotics. Abscess drainage and irrigation can be performed in the ED before discharge.

The most benign dental infection is pulpitis. Patients will have *prolonged* pain after cold or heat exposure; a short burst of pain is normal. Pulpitis can be categorized as reversible (intermittent pain), irreversible (severe pain), periapical abscess (intractable pain), and necrotic pulp (no pain). Treatment for reversible and irreversible pulpitis, gingivitis (inflammation of the gums), and the more advanced periodontitis (chronic inflammation and loss of gum tissue) is anti-inflammatory medications for pain control and improved dental hygiene. These conditions do not need antibiotics.

Post-extraction alveolar osteitis (dry socket) results from tooth extraction and local inflammation of the alveolar bone. Treatment includes oral analgesics, dental block, and, sometimes, antibiotics. Pericoronitis involves gingival inflammation around an erupting tooth. It is treated by controlling pain and implementing proper dental hygiene. This condition can become severe and lead to infection requiring antibiotics.

Patients who are malnourished or severely immunocompromised are at risk for ANUG. This condition presents as painful oral ulcers and involves gingival spaces. Hallmark findings on exam are lymphadenopathy, fever, halitosis, bleeding gums, and fatigue. In severe cases, the infection may invade the surrounding bone. All cases require antibiotics and debridement of the gingiva or abscess. If the patient appears clinically unwell, admit for IV hydration and antibiotics.

Ludwig angina and parapharyngeal abscesses are the most severe odontogenic infections. These conditions require airway protection, emergency surgical consultation, timely broad-spectrum IV antibiotics, and admission.

Most patients with dental pain and infection do not require emergency care beyond pain control. However, they do need prompt dental follow-up and education on proper dental hygiene. Antibiotics should be reserved for only severe infections or intractable pain.

PEARLS

- One-third of Americans lack access to proper dental care; a disproportionate number of these people are older and of poor socioeconomic status.
- Odontogenic infections can lead to severe soft tissue infections requiring airway protection and prompt surgical consultation.

- Initial treatment includes pain and inflammation management, and abscess drainage, if present.
- Pulpitis does not require antibiotics.
- All patients with dental pain and infections need timely dental follow-up.

Suggested Readings

Costain N, Marrie TJ. Ludwig's Angina. *Am J Med*. 2011;124(2):115-117.
Daly B, Sharif MO, Newton T, et al. Local interventions for the management of alveolar osteitis (dry socket). *Cochrane Database Syst Rev*. 2012;12:CD006968.
Folayan MO. The epidemiology, etiology, and pathophysiology of acute necrotizing ulcerative gingivitis associated with malnutrition. *J Contemp Dent Pract*. 2004;5(3):28-41.
Jafarzadeh H, Abbott PV. Review of pulp sensibility tests. Part I: general information and thermal tests. *Int Endod J*. 2010;43(9):738-762.
Mahmoodi B, Weusmann J, Azaripour A, et al. Odontogenic infections: a 1-year retrospective study. *J Contemp Dent Pract*. 2015;16(4):253-258.
Oh JH, Kim Y, Kim CH. Parapharyngeal abscess: comprehensive management protocol. *ORL J Otorhinolaryngol Relat Spec*. 2007;69(1):37-42.
Wabik A, Hendrich BK, Nienartowicz J, et al. Odontogenic inflammatory processes of head and neck in computed tomography examinations. *Pol J Radiol*. 2014;79:431-438.

131

Fishing for Foreign Bodies

Eunhye (Grace) Kim and Molly K. Estes

FBs in the ears, nose, and throat can present in adult and pediatric populations with a variety of objects and complexity. Having optimal visualization and awareness of available equipment in your ED are key components of successful removal. Knowledge of potential complications and methods to minimize them can further ensure a successful removal.

Seeing Is Believing

In most cases of ear and nasal FBs, direct visualization with an otoscope can be sufficient. Given that most FBs are in patients less than 6 years old, procedural sedation may be advantageous in optimizing viewing and minimizing the risk of injury during removal. FBs in the ear are more often found on the right (dominant hand) side and at sites where the ear canal narrows. A nasal speculum is useful in locating nasal FBs that are commonly found on the floor of the nares or just anterior to the medial turbinate.

Neck and chest PA and lateral inspiratory-expiratory x-rays can be used to confirm, but not rule out, aspirated FBs. In 25% to 50% of cases, x-rays will appear negative, and CT should be considered if a high index of suspicion remains. Case reports have shown that POCUS can be used to evaluate for FBs in instances such as radiolucent objects or to minimize radiation exposure in children.

Choosing Your Lure

The most appropriate tool for object removal is highly dependent on the composition of the FB (**Table 131.1**). The most common aural FBs in children are paper and beads; and in adults, it is cotton wool.

For Aspirated FBs

Airway FB can pose potentially life-threatening situations. Aspirated FBs are in the upper airway in 20% of cases and in the bronchus in 80% of cases. In addition to children, populations at higher risk include those with impaired swallowing ability, developmental delay, alcohol use, and older patients. Aspirations causing complete airway obstructions and respiratory compromise require emergent intervention. Methods can be as simple as

TABLE 131.1　COMMON TOOLS FOR FB REMOVAL

FOREIGN BODY	INTERVENTION	DESCRIPTION
Solid objects	Alligator forceps	Commonly available tool with pincer mechanism to grasp rigid FB
Metal, magnetic objects, or batteries	Telescoping magnet	Elongating metal rod with magnetic head with a diameter typically <7.5 mm
Round objects	Swab stick and medical glue	Apply a few drops of adhesive to wood end of cotton swab, then wait 20-30 sec after attachment to the FB before gentle removal
Round objects	Frazier suction/Schuknecht suction catheter	Elongated suction device connected to low continuous suction. Can also be useful for objects at risk of fragmentation
Round objects	Right-angle hook	Insert past objects, hook, and gently retract
Soft objects	Water irrigation	Attach an angiocatheter (without needle) to 60-mL syringe filled with warm saline. Contraindicated in batteries, materials that may swell, or in suspected TM perforation
Ear wax, soft objects	Ear curette	If available, Bionix ear curette has built-in light source. Avoid metal curettes that may injure TM
Ear wax, soft objects	Cerumen loop	Mostly useful for ear wax removal
Styrofoam, superglue	Acetone	Dissolves Styrofoam and superglue
Live objects/insect	Mineral oil 2% lidocaine Hydrogen peroxide	Immobilize/euthanize live object before removal attempts. Combine with irrigation and suction for removal
Nasal FB	Parent's kiss BMV	Have parent form a tight seal over child's mouth while holding contralateral nare closed. Instruct parent to blow air forcefully into patient's mouth. Alternatively, use a BVM with a tight seal around mouth
Nasal FB	Balloon catheter/Katz extractor	Use a 5-6F Foley catheter and insert past object. Inflate a balloon and gently pull out. Useful for posterior FB

BMV, bag mask valve; FB, foreign body; TM, tympanic membrane.

back blows for infants and Heimlich maneuvers for others. For removal under direct or video laryngoscopy, tools such as Magill, alligator, or sponge stick forceps can be used. If the patient is stable, consider secretion reduction with glycopyrrolate 0.1 to 0.2 mg IV or atropine 0.5 mg IV given 20 to 30 minutes beforehand and anesthetizing the airway with 4% atomized lidocaine. Objects below the glottis can be retrieved with rigid bronchoscopy under procedural sedation. If intubation is required, consider using a larger endotracheal tube to facilitate bronchoscopy. Intubation can potentially be therapeutic by dislodging the object into a distal bronchus, changing a complete obstruction to a partial obstruction. Cricothyrotomy can be considered for objects lodged proximal to the cricothyroid.

Reel It In

FB removal by otolaryngology should be considered for limited visibility, sharp objects, incomplete removal, unsuccessful attempts, TM injury, button batteries (due to risk of liquefactive necrosis), and need for intervention under general anesthesia.

Complications

Multiple or traumatic attempts of ear FB removal can result in significant swelling, damage to the ear canal, and possible TM perforation. If a patient with an aural FB presents with associated drainage, TM rupture, or presence greater than 24 hours, ear drops (ciprofloxacin + dexamethasone) may be prescribed. The most common adverse event with nasal FB is epistaxis. Consider using oxymetazoline or 0.5% phenylephrine for vasoconstriction. Other complications include infection, septal perforation, pressure necrosis, and possible aspiration. Aspiration can have additional complications of pneumonia, bronchiectasis, tracheobronchial fistula, pneumomediastinum, and mediastinitis. Steroids can be administered to reduce postmanipulation subglottic edema. Admission for observation should be considered on a case-to-case basis.

PEARLS

- Always check the opposite ear and nares for additional FBs.
- Consider the composition of FB and choose the appropriate retrieval tool.
- Refer to otolaryngology for sharp objects, batteries, failed removal, or poor visualization.
- Airway FB can be visualized through multiple modalities, including x-ray, ultrasound, CT, and direct laryngoscopy.

Suggested Readings

Cetinkaya E, Arslan I, Cukurova I. Nasal foreign bodies in children: types, locations, complications and removal. *Int J Pediatr Otorhinolaryngol*. 2015;79(11):1881-1885.
Hsiang-Jer Tseng TN, Hanna WS, Majid Aized FK, Linnau KF. Imaging foreign bodies: ingested, aspirated, and inserted. *Ann Emerg Med*. 2015;66(6):570-582.
Kozaci N, Avci M, Pinarbasili T, et al. Ingested foreign body imaging using point-of-care ultrasonography: a case series. *Pediatr Emerg Care*. 2019;35(11):807-810.
Mazcuri M, Ahmad T, Shaikh KA, et al. Rigid bronchoscopy: a life-saving intervention in the removal of foreign body in adults at a busy tertiary care unit. *Cureus*. 2020;12(8):e9662.
Prasad N, Harley E. The aural foreign body space: a review of pediatric ear foreign bodies and a management paradigm. *Int J Pediatr Otorhinolaryngol*. 2020;132:109871.

132

Don't Miss the Tracheoinnominate Fistula

Sierra Tackett and Sara Manning

In the United States, approximately 85,000 adult tracheostomies and 5,000 pediatric tracheostomies are performed annually. Indications for tracheostomy include anatomic or functional airway obstruction or the need for prolonged ventilator support. They can be performed via an open surgical approach or a modified Seldinger-based percutaneous technique.

TIFs represent a direct connection between the innominate artery and the airway. They are a rare but deadly complication of tracheostomies occurring in 0.4% to 1% of patients, with mortality of 80% to 100%. Most TIFs occur within 1 to 4 weeks of tracheotomy placement.

Relevant Anatomy

Fistulas may be formed between the trachea and multiple vascular sources. The innominate artery (also known as the *brachiocephalic trunk*) is the most common culprit vessel. Other vascular structures, including the carotid artery, aortic arch, right subclavian artery, superior and inferior thyroid arteries, and innominate vein, have also been reported as sources of fistulas.

Appropriate tracheostomy placement is crucial. In most patients, the innominate artery overlies the anterior trachea at the level of the ninth tracheal ring, but anatomic variations with higher positioning are observed. If the tracheostomy is placed below the fourth tracheal ring, the inferior aspect of the cannula carries an increased risk of erosion into the innominate artery.

Risk Factors

Risk factors include excessive cuff pressures, low placement of tracheostomy, frequent head movements or prolonged neck extension, longer duration of tracheostomy presence, anatomically high-lying innominate artery, local infection, hypotension during placement, malnutrition, and corticosteroid use.

Three of four TIFs occur within the first month of placement with the remainder occurring at any point in the lifetime of the tracheostomy. Therefore, TIF must be considered in patients presenting with a bleeding tracheostomy regardless of the age of the tracheostomy. Patients below 40 years with chronic tracheotomies are at higher risk of a TIF presentation.

Presentation—Sentinel Bleed and Catastrophic Hemorrhage

Approximately 50% of patients with a TIF will experience a "sentinel bleed" days to weeks before massive hemorrhage. Sentinel bleeds vary in presentation from scant bleeding noted on suctioning to frank hemoptysis. Given this variation, it is incumbent upon clinicians to thoroughly evaluate any bleeding tracheostomy to exclude the presence of TIF, particularly in the high-risk early postoperative window.

Catastrophic hemorrhage from TIF is unmistakable. Patients will present in extremis with large-volume bleeding from the airway. Massive TIF hemorrhage is acutely life threatening in two distinct ways. Hemorrhage into the airway can produce rapid airway obstruction with resultant respiratory failure, and rapid blood loss can result in hemorrhagic shock. In those with controlled bleeding, physical exam findings include a low-lying tracheostomy and pulsatile movement of the device.

Diagnostics

Stable patients with resolved bleeding should undergo further diagnostics. CTA is a widely available and frequently utilized modality; however, TIF with a resolved sentinel bleed may be missed. Direct visualizations via flexible bronchoscopy or local exploration in the OR are definitive options but are limited by the availability of specialists and resources. High concern for TIF in a resource-limited setting should prompt consultation and rapid transfer to a referral center with ENT services.

Acute Management for Ongoing Hemorrhage

Evaluate any tracheostomy patient with concern of bleeding in a resuscitation room equipped with advanced airway supplies and suction. For large-volume bleeding, first overinflate the tracheostomy cuff by gradually instilling 35 to 50 mL of air to compress the anterior wall of the trachea with the balloon. Balloon overinflation can control bleeding in approximately 85% of cases. Uncuffed tracheostomies should be removed and replaced with either a cuffed tracheostomy or ET tube, via orotracheal intubation or through the stoma. The cuff then is overinflated.

If bleeding persists, the clinician may manually compress the innominate artery by inserting a finger through the stoma and applying pressure anteriorly toward the deep surface of the manubrium (Utley maneuver). Patients should be orally intubated with the cuff advanced beyond the stoma. A bronchoscope may be used to advance the ET balloon distal to the source of bleeding.

ED management should focus on securing the airway, volume resuscitation, and immediate transport to the OR for definitive management. Aggressive supportive care includes blood replacement utilizing massive transfusion protocols and reversal of any anticoagulation. Surgical teams (ENT, cardiovascular, general) should be emergently mobilized during resuscitation. Definitive treatment of the TIF involves median sternotomy, direct ligation, and sometimes vascular grafts. Patients may require ECMO to allow for sternotomy and bleeding control. In some cases, endovascular techniques can also be effective.

Conclusion

TIF is a rare but deadly complication of tracheostomies. The resulting massive hemorrhage is immediately life threatening due to acute airway obstruction as well as hemorrhagic shock. Rapid, well-coordinated care is essential to save the patient's life. This includes securing the airway, direct attempts to stop hemorrhage, and mobilization of operative services for definitive management. All resuscitative actions taken in the ED are limited and temporizing. Even small amounts of bleeding should raise concern for TIF. As many as half of all patients with TIF report a sentinel bleed before a major hemorrhage event, therefore all bleeding must be thoroughly evaluated to rule out TIF.

PEARLS

- While most common in the first month after tracheostomy placement, TIF can occur at any time.

- TIF should be considered after *any bleeding* from a tracheostomy and should be considered a sentinel bleed until proven otherwise.
- Direct pressure via an overinflated cuff can control bleeding in 85% of cases.
- Patients may require orotracheal intubation to secure the airway and allow manual compression of the fistula through the stoma.
- Aggressive supportive care including transfusion, correction of coagulopathy, and rapid mobilization of operative services is critical.

SUGGESTED READINGS

Bontempo LJ, Manning SL. Tracheostomy emergencies. *Emerg Med Clin North Am.* 2019;37(1):109-119.

Fernandez-Bussy S, Mahajan B, Folch E, et al. Tracheostomy tube placement: early and late complications. *J Bronchology Interv Pulmonol.* 2015;22(4):357-364.

Lewis CW, Carron JD, Perkins JA, Sie KCY, Feudtner C. Tracheotomy in pediatric patients: a national perspective. *Arch Otolaryngol Head Neck Surg.* 2003;129(5):523-529.

Long B, Koyfman A. Resuscitating the tracheostomy patient in the ED. *Am J Emerg Med.* 2016;34:1148-1155.

Scalise P, Prunk SR, Healy D, et al. The incidence of tracheoarterial fistula in patients with chronic tracheostomy tubes: a retrospective study of 544 patients in a long-term care facility. *Chest.* 2005;128(6):3906-3909.

133

HOW TO SUCCESSFULLY REPLACE A DISLODGED TRACH

MELISSA BACCI

EPs pride themselves on being the masters of airway management, ready to deal with even the most difficult of situations. While tracheostomy and laryngectomy airway emergencies are not common, they present a high-risk situation that may be uncomfortable for even the most experienced EP. Second only to tube obstruction, the dislodgement of a tracheostomy tube is a common complication that EPs need to be prepared to handle.

A tracheostomy is an airway placed surgically or percutaneously, usually between the second and third tracheal rings, below the location of where a cricothyrotomy would be performed. Tracheostomies are performed for several reasons, including the inability to manage secretions, inability to protect the airway, upper airway obstruction (such as from a tumor), or the need for long-term mechanical ventilation. Tracheostomy tube features include the outer cannula diameter, the brand or type of tube, and the presence or absence of an inflatable cuff. Most adult tubes have an inner cannula which can be removed to assist with secretion clearance and suctioning. Pediatric tubes do not have an inner cannula due to the smaller diameter tubes required for pediatric patients. Both adult and pediatric tubes come with an obturator (a solid, rigid device) used for initial placement and replacements of the tube.

When a tracheostomy tube is dislodged, there are key pieces of information that need to be obtained. The most important questions are how long ago was the tracheostomy initially placed and for how long has the tube been dislodged. It is also helpful to know the indication for the tracheostomy, the size, and the cuffed/uncuffed status of the tracheostomy tube that was in place. It is essential to understand that a patient who has had a total laryngectomy (as opposed to a tracheostomy) has a *complete disconnection* between their trachea and their nose and mouth. Patients who have undergone laryngectomy cannot be orally intubated and airway management must occur through their stoma.

Similar to the approach to all airways, it is key to follow an organized approach to managing the surgical airway. Necessary supplies include PPE, suction with a variety of catheter devices, a supplemental oxygen source and delivery devices (face mask, BVM, trach collar), difficult airway supplies (supraglottic airways and oral and nasal airway adjuncts), lubrication, several sizes of endotracheal tubes, and laryngoscopy equipment. In addition, one needs tracheostomy supplies, including a replacement tracheostomy tube the same size as what previously was in place and one 0.5 and 1 size smaller, as well as smaller endotracheal tubes (consider 5.0 or 6.0), a gum elastic bougie, a fiberoptic bronchoscope, and a cricothyrotomy kit.

The first step in airway management is to apply high-flow oxygen and support patient ventilation with a BVM, if necessary. In patients with a tracheostomy, it is important to apply oxygen to both the face and the stoma. If BVM ventilation is necessary, one must occlude the stoma if ventilating through the mouth/nose and occlude the mouth/nose if ventilating through the stoma.

If the tracheostomy is fewer than 7 days old, blind reinsertion puts the patient at high risk of false passage due to an immature tracheostomy tract. When a tracheostomy is this immature, one can either intubate orally or attempt to re-cannulate under direct visualization, ideally with a fiberoptic intubating bronchoscope. If fiberoptic visualization is not readily available or is outside of the practitioner's skill set, oral intubation should be attempted and a difficult intubation should be anticipated. Following successful oral intubation, the stoma site should be covered with an occlusive dressing.

If the tracheostomy is mature (over 7 days old), attempt tracheostomy tube reinsertion through the stoma. Placing the patient supine with a rolled towel under their scapulae can help extend the neck and allow easier access to the stoma. A new, well-lubricated tracheostomy tube with the obturator in place should be inserted into the stoma, followed by removal of the obturator and insertion of the inner cannula. Alternatively, a bougie can be placed through the stoma into the trachea. A tracheostomy tube can then be placed via the Seldinger technique, and once in place, the bougie removed and replaced with the inner cannula. If tube placement is unsuccessful, the bougie allows for alternate-size tube placement to be attempted. It is reasonable to start with the patient's prior-sized tracheostomy tube or with one 0.5 size smaller. If positive-pressure ventilation is anticipated, a cuffed tracheostomy must be used. A comparably sized endotracheal tube may also be utilized if tracheostomy tubes are not readily available. If utilizing an endotracheal tube, be cognizant to insert the tube just until the cuff disappears. The risk of right mainstem intubation is high given the close proximity of the stoma to the carina. If the initial tube, whether it be tracheostomy or endotracheal, encounters significant resistance and is unable to be placed, a smaller tube should be attempted. If this is unsuccessful, the patient may require oral intubation.

A chest radiograph and end-tidal capnography should be utilized for tube confirmation. If available, tube placement confirmation with fiberoptic visualization is ideal. If present, the cuff should be inflated, which allows for positive-pressure mechanical ventilation. The patient should be monitored with continuous capnography and should be frequently assessed for subcutaneous emphysema, which may indicate the presence of a false tract into the soft tissue.

As always, know what resources are available, and do not hesitate to involve ENT or anesthesia for backup, if needed. Tracheostomy tube replacement is well within the scope of practice of Emergency Medicine, and familiarity with the procedure in a critical situation can absolutely save a life.

PEARLS

- Key historical elements include when the tracheostomy was placed, the indication for placement, and the type/size of tube.
- Supplemental oxygen should be applied to both the face and the stoma.
- Do not blindly reinsert a tracheostomy tube if the stoma is fewer than 7 days old.
- Fiberoptic guidance is the gold standard for tracheostomy tube replacement.
- Patients with a laryngectomy have no connection between their oro/nasopharynx and their trachea.

SUGGESTED READINGS

Bontempo LJ, Manning SL. Tracheostomy emergencies. *Emerg Med Clin North Am*. 2019; 37(1):109-119.

Long B, Koyfman A. Resuscitating the tracheostomy patient in the ED. *Am J Emerg Med*. 2016; 34(6):1148-1155.

McGrath BA, Bates L, Atkinson D, et al. National Tracheostomy Safety Project. Multidisciplinary guidelines for the management of tracheostomy and laryngectomy airway emergencies. *Anaesthesia*. 2012;67(9):1025-1041.

Morris LL, Whitmer A, McIntosh E. Tracheostomy care and complications in the intensive care unit. *Crit Care Nurse*. 2013;33(5):18-30.

134

KNOW HOW TO PERFORM A LATERAL CANTHOTOMY WITH CANTHOLYSIS

MICHAEL D. SULLIVAN AND CHEYENNE FALAT

A lateral canthotomy with cantholysis is performed in emergent situations to relieve OCS. Most often occurring in cases of trauma with a retro–orbital hematoma, OCS is the result of increasing pressure in the orbit, leading to pressure ischemia of the optic nerve and retinal artery pressure ischemia. This can cause an acute loss of vision in the affected eye. A rapidly performed lateral canthotomy with cantholysis can be vision saving in cases of OCS.

INDICATIONS AND CONTRAINDICATIONS

Primary indications for a lateral canthotomy with cantholysis include a suspected or confirmed retrobulbar hematoma with the affected eye having a measured IOP greater than 40 mm Hg, proptosis, decreased visual acuity, or less compressibility of the globe (when palpated over a closed eyelid) when compared to the contralateral eye. Secondary indications include an afferent pupillary defect, ophthalmoplegia, or severe eye pain. OCS is a clinical diagnosis, and a lateral canthotomy with cantholysis should not be delayed for imaging or other diagnostics. The only contraindication to a lateral canthotomy is a globe rupture.

The recommended window for performing a lateral canthotomy is within 90 minutes from the time of injury.

SUPPLIES AND PROCEDURE

The recommended supplies are as follows:

- Lidocaine (preferably with epinephrine for hemostasis)
- Syringe with 23- to 25-gauge needle
- Hemostat or needle driver
- Iris or suture scissors
- Forceps
- Normal saline to irrigate the lateral canthal area

Position your patient with their head elevated approximately 10° to 15°. In an awake or agitated patient, assistance or sedation may be required to facilitate the procedure. Clear away debris and irrigate the orbital and periorbital areas with saline to prevent infection and improve visualization. Inject the lateral canthus region with 1 to 2 mL of lidocaine with epinephrine for analgesia and hemostasis. When injecting, insert the needle into the lateral canthus and point it toward the lateral orbital rim (away from the globe) to avoid globe puncture.

Next, apply a hemostat to the lateral canthus by inserting one jaw of the hemostat under the skin of the lateral canthus, then clamping the hemostat. Leave it clamped for approximately 30 to 90 seconds to devascularize the skin, and mark the area to incise. After removing the hemostat, insert scissors in the same manner and carefully cut the skin of the lateral canthus outward toward the lateral orbital rim (cut should be ~1 cm in length). This is known as the "lateral canthotomy," but by itself is insufficient to relieve OCS. It must be followed by cantholysis.

The lateral canthal ligament splits into an inferior crus and a superior crus. Use forceps to retract the lower eyelid downward to expose the inferior crus. The lateral canthal tendon is more easily palpated than visualized. Using the tip of the scissors, "strum" across the area of the inferior crus to identify the structure. Direct the scissors inferiorly and laterally while avoiding the globe, and cut the inferior crus of the lateral canthal ligament (**Figure 134.1**). If successful, the eye may become more proptotic, and this step may be sufficient to relieve the pressure of OCS. Reassess the IOP. If the IOP decreases to less than 40 mm Hg and/or the patient can verbalize improved visual acuity, the procedure can be terminated. If symptoms and/or elevated IOP persist, the superior crus of the lateral canthal ligament should be cut in a similar manner, but angling the scissors superiorly and laterally.

Lateral canthal tendon (superior crus)

Orbital rim

Incision line

Lateral canthal tendon (inferior crus)

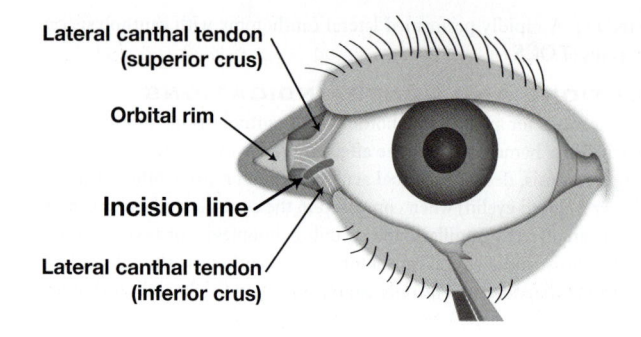

FIGURE 134.1 Eye anatomy showing the location of the lateral canthal tendons and location of first incision for a lateral cantholysis.

COMPLICATIONS AND FOLLOW-UP

Complications from this procedure include bleeding, infection, lacrimal gland injury, injury to the globe or lateral rectus muscle, cosmetic issues, or visual loss in the setting of a delayed procedure or incomplete cantholysis.

Patients should receive emergent ophthalmology consultation after a lateral canthotomy with cantholysis is performed for suspected or confirmed OCS.

PEARLS

- An emergent lateral canthotomy with cantholysis is most commonly performed to treat OCS due to orbital trauma with an associated retro-orbital hematoma.
- OCS is characterized by decreased visual acuity, afferent pupillary defect, ophthalmoplegia, and/or eye pain with an IOP greater than 40 mm Hg.
- A lateral canthotomy with cantholysis should be performed within 90 minutes of the development of OCS to maximize the chance of vision salvage.
- The canthal ligaments are often more easily palpated than visualized.
- A suture kit generally contains the required supplies to perform a lateral canthotomy with cantholysis.

SUGGESTED READINGS

Amer E, El-Rahman Abbas A. Ocular compartment syndrome and lateral canthotomy procedure. *J Emerg Med.* 2019;56:294-297.

McInnes G, Howes DW. Lateral canthotomy and cantholysis: a simple, vision-saving procedure. *CJEM.* 2002;4:49-52.

Rowh AD, Ufberg JW, Chan TC, Vilke GM, Harrigan RA. Lateral canthotomy and cantholysis: emergency management of orbital compartment syndrome. *J Emerg Med.* 2015;48:325-330.

Tyler MA, Citardi MJ, Yao WC. Management of retrobulbar hematoma. *Oper Tech Otolayngol Head Neck Surg.* 2017;28:208-212.

Vassallo S, Hartstein M, Howard D, Stetz J. Traumatic retrobulbar hemorrhage: emergent decompression by lateral canthotomy and cantholysis. *J Emerg Med.* 2002;22:251-256.

135

Beware of the Post-Tonsillectomy Bleed

Lia C. Cruz and Joseph Cruz

There are few presentations to the ED as deceptively insidious as the post-tonsillectomy bleed. Incidence of any hemorrhage is approximately 7.8%; however, the incidence of minor bleeding escalating to severe bleeding is about 41%. What may initially appear as a minor presentation can have a significant risk of catastrophe, occurring nearly instantaneously.

Risk Factors and Anatomic Changes

The reason for the tenuous postoperative stability is due to anatomy. There are five primary arteries that supply the tonsil. Since the surrounding tissues do not compress themselves, post-tonsillectomy hemorrhage must rely on the patient's inherent ability to produce hemostasis.

Integral questions are as follows:

- What is the postoperative day?
- Was adenoidectomy included with the tonsillectomy?
- How many prior episodes of tonsillitis did the patient have?
- Were there any intraoperative complications?
- Is there a personal, or family, history of abnormal bleeding?

The highest risk time for bleeding is on postoperative days 5 to 7 when the fibrin clot is expected to detach, leaving the vascular bed exposed. Other factors increasing risk include concurrent adenoidectomy, history of recurrent tonsillitis, intraoperative complications, operative technique, and personal or family history of abnormal bleeding or anticoagulation use. Significant post-tonsillectomy bleeding can even uncover the diagnosis of bleeding disorders (eg, von Willebrand disease). This is particularly true in pediatric patients where this may be the child's first episode of significant bleeding.

Preparation and Intervention

It is important to respect the potential for rapid deterioration in patients post a tonsillectomy. Patients may develop respiratory distress from airway obstruction due to bloody secretions and clots or from vomiting after swallowing blood. Patients may also quickly develop hemorrhagic shock. Adequate preparation must include contingencies for these potential life-threatening situations.

Necessary equipment includes the following:

- IV access
- Cardiopulmonary monitoring
- Suction
- Spit basin
- Oxygen

Table 135.1	Interventions for Ongoing Post-Tonsillectomy Hemorrhage
Primary measures	■ Cold water gargle and rinse ■ Benzocaine spray
Secondary measures[a]	■ Atomized TXA 500-1,000 mg ■ Nebulized racemic epinephrine ■ Systemic IV TXA ■ Consider DDAVP
Tertiary measures	■ Direct pressure to the tonsillar bed with gauze soaked in lidocaine with epinephrine ■ Direct application of thrombin powder or other topical coagulating agent

[a]ENT specialist should be on the way urgently at this point, and airway measures should be prepared.
TXA, tranexamic acid; DDAVP, desmopressin acetate.

- Airway cart with difficult airway equipment
- Access to massive transfusion protocol products

As with all potentially serious presentations in the ED, one should be prepared with several treatment options. Effective treatments may vary on a case-to-case basis and may be limited by the available resources. Nevertheless, there are several options for hemorrhage control (**Table 135.1**). Otolaryngology should be consulted early for any post-tonsillectomy bleeding regardless of whether the bleeding has been controlled.

THERAPEUTICS

Patients need reliable IV access for fluid or blood administration. Consider antiemetics to reduce the risk of vomiting, which can interfere with attempts at hemostasis.

Visualization of the pharyngeal space is mandatory in evaluating a post-tonsillectomy bleed, but the clinician must take particular care not to disrupt any clot seen in the surgical bed. Suctioning of the area is contraindicated unless there is high-volume bleeding. Clot manipulation will likely cause bleeding to worsen.

There are no large, randomized controlled trials for the use of inhaled TXA for the indication of post-tonsillectomy hemorrhage; however, a growing body of literature shows very good outcomes with successful hemostasis. There are also minimal to no incidences of adverse events reported. Some early systematic reviews showed no benefit to nebulized TXA; however, almost all early meta-analyses evaluated nebulized TXA in the immediate postoperative period, and not in the hemorrhage presenting following discharge. The best modality for delivering TXA to the tonsillar bed is via an atomizer. If an atomizer is not available, then an alternative form of delivery is via nebulizer. Use of a mouthpiece is preferred over the use of a face mask to decrease the amount of aerosol deposited onto the nose, eyes, and face.

Despite anecdotal success using nebulized racemic epinephrine, intravenous TXA, and direct application of thrombin or TXA to the bleeding site, there is scant literature studying the indications, efficacies, and standard dosing in this setting. However, knowledge about the use of these techniques for abating any serious, or potentially serious, hemorrhage should be kept in the clinician's armamentarium.

All patients with bleeding that cannot be controlled, have airway complications, or an overall declining status need to return to the OR. In addition, with rare exceptions, all patients with post-tonsillectomy high-volume hemorrhage should return to the OR to examine the operative bed and control exposed vessels. This applies even if the hemorrhage was transient.

A post-tonsillectomy hemorrhage can be a time bomb that can deteriorate rapidly in the ED. Armed with the knowledge that minor bleeds frequently progress to major hemorrhage and having, a prepared array of varying therapeutic treatment options, and otolaryngology and anesthesia support, these potential catastrophes can be avoided.

PEARLS

- Avoid the temptation to remove clots from the surgical bed during physical examination.
- The riskiest time for rebleeding is postoperative day 5 to 7 when fibrin clots detach and leave the vascular bed exposed.
- Normal appearance of the surgical bed is a thick gray coat by post-op day 5. A "blackberry" appearance is a visible clot with high risk for hemorrhage.
- About 41% of severe bleeding is preceded by a minor bleeding episode.
- Options for severe bleeding include nebulized TXA, nebulized racemic epinephrine, lidocaine with epinephrine-soaked gauze, and thrombin powder. Ultimately, patients should return to the OR.

Suggested Readings

Liu JH, Anderson KE, Willging JP, et al. Posttonsillectomy hemorrhage: what is it and what should be recorded? *Arch Otolaryngol Head Neck Surg.* 2001;127(10):1271-1275.

Osborne MS, Clark M. The surgical arrest of post-tonsillectomy haemorrhage: hospital episode statistics 12 years on. *Ann R Coll Surg Engl.* 2018;100(5):406-408.

Sarny S, Ossimitz G, Habermann W, et al. Hemorrhage following tonsil surgery: a multicenter prospective study. *Laryngoscope.* 2011;121(12):2553-2560.

Thejas SR, Vinayak R, Sindu M. Hydrogen peroxide as a hemostatic agent in tonsillectomy: is it beneficial? *Saudi J Otorhinolaryngol Head Neck Surg.* 2021:23(1):36-40.

Wall JJ, Tay KY. Postoperative tonsillectomy hemorrhage. *Emerg Med Clin North Am.* 2018; 36(2):415-426.

136

Expertly Manage Dental Trauma

Elizabeth Pontius

Dental trauma is a common complaint presenting to the ED. Dental pain, loose teeth, chipped teeth, missing teeth, and bleeding gums may all require urgent intervention that is readily within the scope of practice for the emergency clinician.

Pain Control

Acetaminophen or NSAIDs should be first-line medications for analgesia. At times, more pain control is needed, although opiates should rarely be necessary. Nonopioid options for pain control include topical anesthetics and dental blocks. Topical anesthetics such as benzocaine and lidocaine can be useful for painful oral lesions or used on the oral mucosa before administering a dental block. There are two types of dental blocks: supraperiosteal infiltration, used to numb a single tooth, and regional nerve blocks, which provide anesthesia to a larger area and are particularly useful in dental trauma when multiple teeth are involved.

Trauma

Facial trauma can lead to a fractured tooth, a luxated tooth, or an avulsed tooth. Tooth fractures were previously described by the Ellis classification; however, the current trend is to describe the fracture based on the layers of the tooth involved. Enamel fractures (Ellis Class I) are painless cosmetic injuries and do not require emergent intervention. Sharp edges can be filed, and patients can follow up with their dentist for cosmetic repair.

Next are fractures that involve the dentin (Ellis Class II). Dentin is ivory yellow in color and is created by the pulp of the tooth throughout life; thus, in children, the pulp layer is larger than the dentin layer, and the reverse is true in adults. Dentin is porous, so if the remaining dentin layer is thin (<0.5 mm), bacteria can pass through the dentin and invade the pulp. Fractures that involve the pulp (Ellis Class III) expose the neurovascular supply of the tooth to oral bacteria. To determine whether the pulp is exposed, wipe the surface of the tooth with a piece of gauze and then look for appearance of blood on the surface of the tooth, which indicates pulp involvement. Fractures that expose the pulp can be quite painful if the nerve is exposed, or completely painless if the trauma disrupted the neurovascular supply at the apex of the tooth. Since it can be challenging to differentiate dentin from pulp fractures, the safest option is to cover both types with calcium hydroxide paste and have the patient follow up with their dentist within 36 hours. If calcium hydroxide paste is unavailable, use cyanoacrylate glue to cover the fracture, followed by foil to cover the tooth. Though there are no data to support the use of prophylactic antibiotics to prevent pulp infection, it is recommended by many consultants.

A luxated tooth, or a tooth that is loose or partially displaced in the socket, can be stabilized by application of a periodontal pack. An avulsed tooth has been completely torn from the socket. Primary teeth are not replaced in children. Children can follow up with their dentist for a prosthetic until the secondary tooth erupts. Time is of the essence when faced with an avulsed permanent tooth; the periodontal ligament cells generally die after 60 minutes. Handle the tooth only by the crown and rinse it gently with saline or water. Do not scrub or wipe the tooth. Reimplant it in the socket as soon as possible. If the tooth must be transported, transport it in sterile water or milk. Once reimplanted, the tooth should then be stabilized by application of a periodontal pack.

To make a periodontal pack, mix equal parts of base and catalyst, place the mixture into a cup of sterile water, then mold it into two strips, each long enough to cover the involved tooth and two teeth on either side. Dry the patient's gingiva and teeth with gauze and use moistened gloves to mold the strip over the anterior and posterior surfaces of the five teeth. Have the patient close their mouth until the mixture hardens. If a periodontal pack is unavailable, take the metal nose piece off a nonrebreather face mask and use cyanoacrylate glue to secure it to the affected tooth and two teeth on either side. Patients can be discharged with a soft diet to follow up with a dentist within 24 hours.

Alveolar fractures can be associated with dental fractures and luxated or avulsed teeth. These fractures often occur in multitooth segments and may be apparent on examination by identifying malalignment of a segment of teeth or bone fragments at the base of the teeth. Alveolar fractures are stabilized by arch bars, which is beyond the scope of the emergency clinician. Urgent consultation with an oral surgeon or dentist is indicated.

BLEEDING

Controlling gingival bleeding can be difficult, especially in patients on anticoagulants. Bleeding after minor procedures or trauma can usually be controlled with 10 to 15 minutes of direct pressure. If bleeding persists, consider either topical application or local infiltration of a vasoconstrictor, such as lidocaine with epinephrine, or topical coagulating agents such as Gelfoam or Surgicel, followed by direct pressure. In severe cases, soaking a piece of gauze in tranexamic acid and applying direct pressure can help achieve hemostasis. A commonly recommended trick is to apply a moistened caffeinated teabag over the area of bleeding and hold pressure; tannins in tea do have hemostatic properties, so this can be considered if the abovementioned measures are not available.

PEARLS

- Dental blocks are a good option for opioid-sparing management of dental pain.
- Cover dental fractures that involve the dentin or pulp with calcium hydroxide paste, and discharge the patient to follow up with their dentist in 24 to 36 hours.
- An avulsed secondary (permanent) tooth should be replaced as soon as possible and secured with a periodontal pack, but primary teeth do not need to be replaced.
- Control gingival bleeding with direct pressure and/or with topical vasoconstrictors, local infiltration of vasoconstrictors, topical coagulating agents, or topical tranexamic acid.

SUGGESTED READINGS

Benko KR. Emergency dental procedures. In: Roberts JR, Custalow CB, Thomsen TW, eds. *Roberts and Hedges' Clinical Procedures in Emergency Medicine and Acute Care.* 7th ed. Elsevier; 2019:1384-1404.

Hammel JM, Fischel J. Dental emergencies. *Emerg Med Clin North Am.* 2019;37(1):81-93.

Pedigo RA. Oral medicine. In: Walls RM. *Rosen's Emergency Medicine: Concepts and Clinical Practice.* 10th ed. Elsevier; 2023:732-749.

Piccininni P, Clough A, Padilla R, Piccininni G. Dental and orofacial injuries. *Clin Sports Med.* 2017;36(2):369-405.

Sethuraman KN, Caplash JM. Dental trauma. In: Mattu A, Swadron S, ed. *CorePendium.* Emergency Medicine: Reviews and Perspectives; 2023. https://www.emrap.org/corependium/chapter/recmpEcW2rcijsYLl/Dental-Trauma

Spangler RM, Abraham MK. Regional anesthesia of the head and neck. In: Roberts JR, Custalow CB, Thomsen TW, eds. *Roberts and Hedges' Clinical Procedures in Emergency Medicine and Acute Care.* 7th ed. Elsevier; 2019:545-559.

137

POCUS Pearls for the Eye

Brianna Klucher and Samantha A. King

Ocular ultrasound is increasingly being integrated into ED practice, aiding in expeditious evaluation and diagnosis in patients presenting with eye pain, vision loss, headaches, and trauma. Numerous pathologies can be detected with high sensitivity and specificity. Ocular ultrasound scanning success can be improved with the methods described here.

Preparing to Scan

Ocular ultrasound is typically performed with a high-frequency linear probe. However, an endocavitary probe set to a short depth can also be utilized. One of the most important parts of setting up for an ocular ultrasound is ensuring the use of the proper setting. Most machines will have an "ocular" setting or a "small parts" setting that should be utilized. These settings reduce the mechanical and thermal index, minimizing potential damage or bioeffects on the eye.

For optimal scanning, place the patient in a recumbent or semi-recumbent position to allow a copious amount of gel to be used. Consider covering the patient's closed eye with a transparent film dressing, such as Tegaderm, which will prevent ultrasound gel from entering the eye. While ultrasound gel is not toxic to the eye and the cover may increase patient comfort, it can negatively impact image quality from air pockets trapped underneath the dressing. Place copious amounts of gel over the dressing. Float the probe within the gel and avoid placing pressure on the eye. Pressure on the eye may be uncomfortable for the patient and may trigger the oculocardiac reflex leading to bradycardia and, potentially, syncope. Importantly, if there is high suspicion or risk of globe rupture, ocular ultrasound should be avoided. Although minimal pressure is applied to the eye when performed as intended, any additional pressure may exacerbate a rupture.

Scanning Technique Tips

It is important to anchor the probe hand while scanning the eye. The fifth finger or ulnar aspect of the hand may be rested on the forehead, nasal bridge, or zygomatic arch. If the suspected injury is traumatic in nature, use careful hand placement so as not to worsen injury or discomfort. After gently placing the probe onto the prepared gel, visualize the orbit in transverse and sagittal planes, panning to visualize the entire orbit in both views. While in each view, the patient should be instructed to move their eyes in all directions to fully assess extraocular movements. This technique can serve as an adjunct to the physical exam in patients with extensive periorbital edema. In addition, increase the gain to visualize pathology that otherwise may be missed such as visualizing hemorrhage and retinal detachments. Next, visualize the tissues deep into the orbit to evaluate for fluid collections concerning for a retrobulbar hematoma. Lastly, measure the optic nerve by angling the probe about 10° to 15° toward the nasal bridge to best align with the optic nerve, which should be visualized as a linear hypoechoic structure extending from the posterior of the eye to the bottom of the screen. Center and freeze the image to measure the optic nerve width. The width should be measured at a depth of 3 mm from the posterior aspect of the orbit.

Diagnostic Findings

Optic Nerve
Ocular ultrasound is useful in assessing ICP. When measured as previously described, an optic nerve diameter greater than 6 mm is predictive of increased ICP. Measuring ICP can be useful for assessing elevated pressure in patients with suspected or confirmed intracranial hemorrhage or mass, or idiopathic intracranial hypertension.

Vitreous Hemorrhage
Vitreous hemorrhage can be detected on ocular ultrasound as echogenic material in the posterior chamber. A "washing machine sign" can be detected with eye movement as swirling of the echogenic debris. Remember that increasing the gain allows for improved visualization of debris that can otherwise be easily missed.

Retinal Detachment
Retinal detachment can be best visualized on ocular ultrasound during extraocular movements under high-gain settings. The mobile retina will appear as a hyperechoic membrane floating in the posterior chamber. The detached membrane will be anchored at the optic nerve, with large detachments giving a "V-shape" appearance.

Posterior Vitreous Detachment
Similar to retinal detachment, posterior vitreous detachments will appear as a hyperechoic membrane in the posterior chamber. However, as the retina is still intact, the membrane can cross the optic nerve and will not anchor, appearing as a "U-shape." In early detachments, it may be difficult to visualize, and ophthalmologic consultation should be obtained.

Pupillary Reflex
The pupillary reflex can be assessed under ultrasonography that can be particularly helpful in orbital trauma and periorbital edema when the pupil cannot otherwise be visualized. The presence or absence of this reflex can be detected by placing the probe on the inferior border of the lower eyelid and fanning up to view the pupil in transverse. One can then shine a light in the unaffected eye looking for constriction of the pupil on ultrasound.

Retrobulbar Hematoma
Appears as a hypoechoic collection posterior to the eye. May give the eye a "guitar-pick" appearance.

PEARLS

- Use copious amounts of gel to perform the ultrasound to avoid additional pressure to the orbit.
- Steady your hand by resting it on a portion of the patient's face such as the forehead, nasal bridge, or zygomatic arch.
- Use high-gain settings to detect subtle vitreous hemorrhages and signs of retinal detachment.
- Measure the optic nerve width at a depth of 3 mm from the optic disc; a width greater than 5 mm is abnormal and greater than 6 mm is indicative of increased ICP.

- Retinal and posterior vitreous detachments are distinguishable by where they anchor in the eye. In large detachments, retinal detachments will be anchored at the optic nerve, but posterior vitreous detachments will cross the optic nerve.

Suggested Readings

Amini A, Kariman H, Arhami Dolatabadi A, et al. Use of the sonographic diameter of optic nerve sheath to estimate intracranial pressure. *Am J Emerg Med*. 2013;31(1):236-239.

Blaivas M, Theodoro D, Sierzenski PR. A study of bedside ocular ultrasonography in the emergency department. *Acad Emerg Med*. 2002;9(8):791-799.

POCUS 101. *Ocular Ultrasound Made Easy: Step-By-Step Guide*. POCUS 101. https://www.pocus101.com/ocular-ultrasound-made-easy-step-by-step-guide/

Skidmore C, Saurey T, Ferre RM, Rodriguez-Brizuela R, Spaulding J, Lundgreen Mason N. A narrative review of common uses of ophthalmic ultrasound in emergency medicine. *J Emerg Med*. 2021;60(1):80-89.

Wiswell J, Bellamkonda-Athmaram V. Sonographic consensual pupillary reflex. *West J Emerg Med*. 2012;13(6):524.

SECTION X
HEMATOLOGY/ONCOLOGY

138

THROMBOTIC THROMBOCYTOPENIC PURPURA AND HEMOLYTIC UREMIC SYNDROME: BLOODY ZEBRAS WITH A BAD BITE

NAILLID FELIPE

TTP and HUS are rarely seen platelet aggregation disorders involving the deposition of fibrin and tiny clots in capillaries and arterioles. This leads to MAHA through the shearing of RBCs and to a systemic depletion of platelets, accompanied by end-organ damage due to reduced circulation.

Although TTP and HUS are similar disorders, TTP is more common in adults. HUS is often seen in children and renal effects predominate.

TTP

In TTP, ADAMTS13 (an enzyme that breaks down von Willebrand factor) is inhibited, which leads to the formation of microemboli. About 40% of cases appear to be secondary to other conditions, including cancer, pregnancy, autoimmune diseases, HIV, and certain medications (quinine, acyclovir, clopidogrel, and some immunosuppressants). There is a female, Black race, and obesity predominance. There also is a hereditary form of the disorder.

TTP is rare and is challenging to diagnose. The "classic" pentad of TTP, which is only present in less than 7% of cases, is as follows:

1) Fever
2) Thrombocytopenia (10,000-50,000 plts/mcL), with purpura
3) MAHA with evidence of fragmentation of RBCs
4) Fluctuating neurologic signs that may include subtle neurologic findings such as headache, transient confusion, or more severe signs such as stroke, seizures, altered mental status, and coma (of note, one-third of patients may not have neurologic signs)
5) Renal compromise, although often the creatinine remains normal or shows only an insignificant, transient rise

The anemia seen with TTP will usually manifest with a hematocrit below 20, and schistocytes (fragmented red cells) can often be detected on smears. Platelets will frequently be below 30,000. Markers of hemolysis include decreased haptoglobin, increased reticulocyte count, and increased LDH. The degree of renal involvement can vary from hematuria and proteinuria to frank acute renal failure. The PLASMIC score serves as a screening scoring tool to be used for evaluation of TTP.

The use of plasma exchange in the treatment of TTP has markedly improved the prognosis of this condition. In addition to plasma exchange, initial therapy may include steroids. Platelet transfusion must be avoided unless there is life-threatening hemorrhage, as it could cause more harm. The same platelet-destructive process will affect transfused platelets and cause additional thrombi to form in the microcirculation. If there is delay in plasma exchange (>6 hours), it is recommended to start plasma infusion.

Before plasma replacement infusion became widespread, mortality from TTP reached as high as 90%. With modern treatment, the mortality from this condition has fallen below 20%. Relapse is not uncommon and has been observed to occur in 20% to 50% of patients. Emergency physicians must keep a sharp eye out for the return of signs and symptoms in patients with a prior history of TTP.

HUS

HUS is one of the most common causes of acute renal failure in childhood. The clinical triad consists of a MAHA, renal failure, and thrombocytopenia. A typical presentation includes bloody diarrhea, crampy abdominal pain, and fever. Three to 8 days after onset of symptoms, patients often experience increased abdominal pain, bloody stools (colitis), hemolytic anemia, thrombocytopenia, and acute renal insufficiency with possible progression to renal failure.

The most common causative agent of HUS is *Escherichia coli* serotype 0157:H7, a STEC that can be contracted from undercooked meat, contaminated water and vegetables, contact with infected animals, or person-to-person spread. The Shiga toxin causes endothelial damage, leukocyte activation, platelet activation, and widespread inflammation. These processes promote the formation of thrombi in small vessels and lead to MAHA and thrombocytopenia. Other causes of HUS include primary disorders of complement regulation (referred to as *aHUS*), other infections including *Streptococcus pneumoniae* and HIV, as well as drug toxicity, particularly in patients with cancer or solid organ transplants. aHUS presentation is similar to that of HUS but without bloody diarrhea and is as common in adults as well as children. About 10% to 20% of aHUS is seen in pregnant patients. Overall, aHUS tends to have a worse prognosis.

The treatment of HUS is primarily supportive and includes early intravenous fluids for rehydration. Platelet or RBC transfusion is recommended only for severe active bleeding. Dialysis may be necessary in up to 50% of patients. Antimotility drugs should be avoided as these may lead to toxic megacolon. Antibiotics may increase the release of Shiga toxin from the bacteria and should be avoided as well. Although neurologic symptoms are less prominent than in TTP, they can be seen in up to 25% of patients with HUS.

The good news is that early dialysis and supportive therapy result in return to baseline renal function in about 90% of patients. In contrast to TTP, recurrence of HUS is very uncommon.

DIFFERENTIATING THE ZEBRAS

Diagnosis of these two conditions is based on the spectrum of clinical symptoms as well as diagnostic testing. Since TTP is associated with ADAMTS13 inhibition, a lab test showing less than 5% of normal ADAMTS13 levels is indicative of TTP. ADAMTS13 levels greater than 5% plus Shiga toxin–positive stool studies point toward typical HUS, while patients who are Shiga negative with levels greater than 5% may have atypical HUS.

TABLE 138.1	COMPARISON OF HUS VERSUS TTP	
	HUS	**TTP**
Age	Children	Adults
CBC	Anemia	Anemia
	Thrombocytopenia	Thrombocytopenia
Peripheral smear	MAHA	MAHA
	Schistocytes	Schistocytes
Clinical treatment	Predominantly renal	CNS and renal at end-stage disease
	Supportive	Plasmapheresis
	Dialysis	Steroids
Prognosis	Better	Worse

Here follows a table that compares and contrasts these two rare but crucial to recognize conditions (**Table 138.1**).

PEARLS

- Think TTP or HUS when confronted with anemia, thrombocytopenia, and schistocytes.
- TTP is more common in adults and significant risk factors include female sex, Black race, and obesity.
- TTP is treated with plasma exchange therapy, steroids, and monoclonal antibodies.
- HUS is a common cause of renal failure in children.
- The most common causative agent of HUS is a Shiga toxin–producing *E. coli* (0157:H7).
- HUS is treated supportively (with dialysis as needed) and has a better prognosis than TTP.

Acknowledgments

We gratefully acknowledge the contributions of previous edition author, Stephen A. Manganaro, as portions of their chapter have been retained in this revision.

Suggested Readings

Long B, Bridwell RE, Manchanda S, Gottlieb M. Evaluation and management of thrombotic thrombocytopenic purpura in the emergency department. *J Emerg Med*. 2021; 61(6):674-682.

Paydary K, Banwell E, Tong J, Chen Y, Cuker A. Diagnostic accuracy of the PLASMIC score in patients with suspected thrombotic thrombocytopenic purpura: a systematic review and meta-analysis. *Transfusion*. 2020;60(9):2047-2057.

Tsai HM. Atypical hemolytic uremic syndrome: beyond hemolysis and uremia. *Am J Med*. 2019;132(2):161-167.

Walsh PR, Johnson S. Treatment and management of children with haemolytic uraemic syndrome. *Arch Dis Child*. 2018;103(3):285-291.

139

HIGH TEMPS AND LOW COUNTS: TREAT PATIENTS WITH FEBRILE NEUTROPENIA WITH EARLY AND APPROPRIATE ANTIBIOTICS

Matthew W. Connelly, Steven Roumpf, and Molly K. Estes

When faced with neutropenic fever, many emergency medicine physicians wage chemical warfare on any and all possible infectious causes. As nearly half of these patients will have an identifiable source of infection, efficient evaluation and recognition are key to early initiation of treatment. The clinical challenge in treating patients with neutropenic fever lies in carefully managing the balance between early, sufficiently broad antibiotic coverage and the ever-increasing rates of antibiotic-resistant organisms. The 2018 update from the American Society of Clinical Oncology and Infectious Disease Society of America guidelines continues to promote early empiric antibiotic treatment in the patient with febrile neutropenia; however, more emphasis is now being placed on selecting proper antimicrobial therapy on a case-by-case basis rather than a "shotgun" approach. Stratifying patients with febrile neutropenia into high- and low-risk categories, based on various presenting factors, may help direct physicians to the appropriate empiric treatment agents and disposition.

Neutropenic fever is most commonly defined as an ANC less than 1,000 cells/mm^3 or an ANC that is expected to decrease below 1,000 cells/mm^3 during the next 48 hours as well as a single oral temperature measurement greater than 38.3 °C (101 °F) or a temperature greater than 38.0 °C (100.4 °F) sustained over a 60-minute period. Neutropenia is further classified as severe when the ANC falls below 500 cells/mm^3 and profound for cell counts below 100 cells/mm^3. Providers must also be able to recognize signs of infection in the patients with afebrile neutropenia and treat them similarly to those with documented fever. Once patients meeting these definitions have been identified, chest x-ray and pan-cultures, including blood from peripheral and central lines (all ports), urine, sputum, and CSF if there is concern for meningitis, should be obtained and individuals can be stratified into low- and high-risks groups based on multiple factors.

The Multinational Association of Supportive Care in Cancer risk-index score has been established and validated to quantify the likelihood of serious complications using objective criteria as well as subjective patient clinical status as determined by the provider. Low-risk characteristics in the otherwise healthy, well-appearing patient include age younger than 60, outpatient status, solid tumors, or hematologic malignancy with no history of fungal infection. Further criteria include ability to tolerate oral medications and expected improvement of ANC within the next 7 days. This can be predicted, in consultation with oncology, by considering ANC response to previous chemotherapy, timing of future treatment, and administration of bone marrow–stimulating medications. High-risk patients are characterized by age older than 60, history of COPD, acute gastrointestinal and neurologic symptoms, and signs of dehydration or hypotension. Profound neutropenia expected to last longer than 7 days and patient history of increased duration of neutropenia have also been found to have high rates of serious infection. Once stratified and stable, options regarding treatment and disposition can be discussed with the patient and their oncologist.

Low-risk patients with the proper home support structure and close follow-up (within 24 hours) may be discharged home on oral fluoroquinolone (ciprofloxacin or levofloxacin) plus amoxicillin/clavulanic acid (or clindamycin if the patient has a penicillin allergy) after discussion with their oncologist. The first dose of therapy should be administered in the ED and the patient observed for at least 4 hours prior to discharge. Early differentiation of the cliché "sick versus not sick" may help save these patients the cost and side effects associated with IV antibiotic therapy. For patients deemed to be at high risk for significant infection, no literature currently exists regarding a single superior empiric IV antibiotic regimen; however, numerous monotherapies have shown a high level of efficacy despite increasing incidence of antibiotic-resistant organisms. Empiric antibiotic dosing should ideally be administered within 1 hour of patient arrival to the ED. An expanding body of evidence has supported monotherapy with antipseudomonal beta-lactam agents such as piperacillin-tazobactam, carbapenems (meropenem or imipenem-cilastatin), or cefepime, keeping in mind institutional pathogen susceptibility. For patients with a history of severe penicillin allergy, empiric treatment with ciprofloxacin *plus* clindamycin or aztreonam *plus* vancomycin is recommended. As coagulase-negative staphylococci are the identifiable causative agent in the majority of bacteremia in patients with neutropenia, and will be covered by beta-lactams, vancomycin should not be part of standard empiric therapy and has not been shown to significantly alter mortality rates in this population. Addition of vancomycin (or linezolid/daptomycin in cases of known VRE) should be considered in cases of hemodynamic instability, radiographic pneumonia, suspected vascular catheter or soft tissue infection, or history of MRSA colonization. Aminoglycosides (gentamicin, tobramycin) may be considered as an addition to standard monotherapy in the critically ill patient with concern for resistant gram-negative bacteria. Antivirals and antifungals should be considered in patients with persistent fever or clear signs of active infection (eg, herpetic lesions or *Candida* esophagitis) but are often outside the scope of ED empiric treatment.

As the treatment of cancer trends more toward outpatient therapy, neutropenic fever will become a far more common occurrence in the ED. As the front line of evaluation and treatment for these patients, it is imperative that emergency medicine physicians readily diagnose and manage neutropenic fever aggressively but appropriately in consultation with infectious disease and hematology/oncology providers. Early treatment with targeted antibiotic regimens, determined by individual clinical presentation along with institutional antibiograms and protocols, will help more effectively treat neutropenic fever while minimizing the cost and risks of bacterial resistance that is often associated with broad-spectrum IV antibiotics.

PEARLS

- Recognize patients with neutropenia with fever and signs of infection, obtain pan-cultures, and treat early with antibiotics.
- Low-risk patients: Discuss with patient/oncologist the option of outpatient therapy with oral antibiotic regimen (ciprofloxacin *and* amoxicillin/clavulanic acid *or* clindamycin).
- High-risk patients: Start IV monotherapy with antipseudomonal beta-lactams.

- Vancomycin should *not* be standard empiric treatment unless there is hemodynamic instability, radiographic pneumonia, suspected vascular catheter or soft tissue infection, GPCs seen on preliminary blood culture or history of MRSA colonization.
- Viral and fungal coverage should not be routinely started in the ED without evidence of active disease but should be considered in high-risk patients after discussion with consultants.

SUGGESTED READINGS

Freifeld AG, Bow EJ, Sepkowitz KA, et al. Clinical practice guideline for the use of antimicrobial agents in neutropenic patients with cancer: 2010 update by the Infectious Diseases Society of America. *Clin Infect Dis.* 2011;52(4):e56-e93.

Klastersky J, Paesmans M, Rubenstein EB, et al. The multinational association for supportive care in cancer risk index: a multinational scoring system for identifying low-risk febrile neutropenic cancer patients. *J Clin Oncol.* 2000;18(16):3038-3051.

Paul M, Dickstein Y, Borok S, et al. Empirical antibiotics targeting gram-positive bacteria for the treatment of febrile neutropenic patients with cancer. *Cochrane Database Syst Rev.* 2014;(1):CD003914.

Taplitz RA, Kennedy EB, Flowers CR. Outpatient management of fever and neutropenia in adults treated for malignancy: American Society of Clinical Oncology and Infectious Diseases Society of America clinical practice guideline update summary. *J Oncol Pract.* 2018;14(4):250-255. PMID: 29517953.

140

MY CHEST! MY BACK! MY SICKLE CELL ATTACK!

KARLY LEBHERZ AND SALVADOR J. SUAU

Pain can be an indication of life-threatening pathology in a patient with SCD. VOE is the most common complication of SCD. However, it is a diagnosis of exclusion that requires ruling out other emergent sequelae of SCD. Complications of SCD are varied and risk changes throughout a patient's lifetime. Without any objective way to diagnose VOE, a thorough patient history and physical examination is of paramount importance. As SCD predominately affects people of African descent, clinicians must recognize the influence of structural racism and implicit bias when providing care for these patients who have been neglected by the health care system. This chapter is not a comprehensive review of SCD, but it highlights life-threatening complications that could be mistaken for VOE.

ACS

VOE often precedes or is concomitant with ACS. Roughly half of all patients with SCD will experience ACS, and it is also the leading cause of death. Mortality from a single episode of ACS is as high as 9% in adults with SCD. Given this significant mortality, ACS should be on the differential for any patient presenting with SCD.

ACS is defined by acute respiratory symptoms and fever with new density on chest imaging. The most common symptoms of ACS include fever, cough, chest pain, shortness of breath, extremity pain, and wheezing. Pediatric patients are less likely than adults to present with pain, but they more commonly have fever and wheezing. The emergency provider should assess the patient for common presenting signs and symptoms such as rales (the most common physical examination finding), oxygen saturation less than 92%, diminished basilar breath sounds (consistent with pleural effusion), or tachypnea greater than 30 breaths/min. One should be reluctant to attribute a patient's tachypnea to pain. Simply attributing these symptoms to a VOE could lead to serious morbidity and mortality.

Classically, ACS has been assessed using CXR, but sensitivity is poor early in the disease course. Patients presenting with symptoms of ACS often do not have radiographic evidence on CXR until days 5 to 6 of hospitalization. Lung POCUS has been shown to identify concerning findings for ACS, such as consolidation and effusion earlier than CXR. In pediatric patients, lung POCUS is superior to CT scan in identifying pneumonia.

When assessing chest pain in a patient with SCD, keep your differential wide and do not exclude other common causes of chest pain seen in the general population such as acute myocardial infarction, pulmonary embolus, pneumothorax, and, more recently, COVID-19. In fact, the most common presenting symptoms of patients with SCD and COVID are pain and fever. Rapid detection and proper treatment of COVID, and anticipation of further complications, enable a favorable prognosis.

STROKE

It is crucial to test for disability during the primary assessment of a patient with SCD presenting to the ED. VOE is not confined to the peripheral circulation; these patients are at high risk for stroke due to cell adhesion and inflammatory changes in cerebral vasculature. A thorough assessment of mental status and neurologic deficits should be promptly performed.

SCD is the leading cause of ischemic stroke in children. Children with SCD between 2 and 9 years old are at significant risk for stroke. Caregivers are the best source of information about changes in neurologic status for young children who are unable to participate in a neurologic examination. Routine screening of cerebral blood flow velocity via transcranial Doppler ultrasound and prophylactic RBC exchange transfusions to maintain HbS less than 30% has considerably reduced the risk of ischemic stroke. Information about the patient's history with these therapies can be helpful in assessing stroke risk.

SEQUESTRATION

Patients with SCD, particularly children, are at increased risk for acute life-threatening anemia. The most common cause of acute anemia in children with SCD is due to splenic sequestration of RBC and platelets.

Patients with acute splenic sequestration may present with left upper quadrant abdominal pain, hypotension, fatigue, weakness, abdominal distension, or back pain refractory to pain medication. You may palpate a tender, enlarged spleen on examination. A decrease in a patient's hemoglobin by 2 g/dL or more from baseline, thrombocytopenia (<150,000/mcL), and reticulocytosis is concerning for sequestration. If the spleen is not palpable, but suspicion is high, consider a bedside ultrasound, which may reveal an enlarged, hypoechoic spleen.

The spleen is a dangerously capable reservoir for blood, able to enlarge several times its normal size due to pooling. Splenic sequestration is therefore equivalent to major hemorrhage. Autosplenectomy from splenic infarction/vaso-occlusion is typically complete by 5 years old in patients with SCD, so splenic sequestration has primarily been a childhood diagnosis. However, disease-modifying therapies are lengthening the lifetime of spleens in patients with SCD. Therefore, it will be important to keep this on your differential for older children and young adults.

Hepatic sequestration may also occur, which presents similarly to splenic sequestration but also includes elevated transaminases, right upper quadrant pain, hepatomegaly, and fever.

Early detection of sequestration of blood cells enables early transfusion and prevention of severe shock. Another cause of acute anemia, particularly for pediatric patients with SCD, is aplastic crisis. Unlike splenic or hepatic sequestration, reticulocyte count will be inappropriately normal or decreased. Parvovirus B19 is well known to abruptly halt hematopoiesis and can be life-threatening to a patient with SCD.

Do not falsely attribute tachycardia to pain and delay identification of acute anemia. Continuous monitoring of vital signs and having an extremely low threshold for IV access in pediatric patients should be standard. Do not underestimate the information that a CBC, CMP, reticulocyte count, or POCUS could provide in making the correct diagnosis. Utilize POCUS as an extension of your physical examination to help elucidate these potentially fatal complications of SCD.

INFECTION

Infection is a common contributory factor to the RBC sickling that triggers a VOE. As mentioned earlier, most patients with SCD are functionally asplenic by adulthood, impairing defense against encapsulated bacteria, such as *Streptococcus pneumoniae*, *Neisseria meningitidis*, and *Salmonella* species. Penicillin prophylaxis and immunization have been instrumental in reducing mortality from infection. However, be mindful that adherence to penicillin prophylaxis is low, and many young children will not have completed vaccinations.

Maintaining a high level of vigilance for nidus of infection when a patient is presenting with VOE is crucial. Scrutinize for signs of meningitis, osteomyelitis, and septic arthritis. Obtain blood and urine cultures, followed by prompt administration of empiric antibiotics in patients who present with fever.

For all complications of SCD, early involvement of a hematologist in the treatment plan is important for patient outcome and transition of care from the ED.

PEARLS

- VOE is a diagnosis of exclusion; keep a wide differential for causes of pain in a patient with SCD. ACS should be the differential for any patient with SCD presenting to the ED.
- Initiate continuous pulse oximetry, obtain a CXR, and take advantage of POCUS early if you are concerned about ACS.
- Patients with SCD are at risk for stroke from RBC sickling. Always assess for neurologic disability. Although stroke is rare in children, pediatric patients with SCD have a much higher risk.
- Hypotension, abdominal distension, and back pain refractory to pain medication can be signs of acute splenic sequestration.

Suggested Readings

Buchanan GR, Yawn BP. Managing acute complications of sickle cell disease. In: *Evidence-Based Management of Sickle Cell Disease*. National Heart, Lung, and Blood Institute (NHLBI); 2014:31-54.

Ogu UO, Badamosi NU, Camacho PE, Freire AX, Adams-Graves P. Management of sickle cell disease complications beyond acute chest syndrome. *J Blood Med*. 2021;12:101-114.

Power-Hays A, McGann PT. When actions speak louder than words—racism and sickle cell disease. *N Engl J Med*. 2020;383(20):1902-1903.

141

Emergent Anticoagulant Reversal: A^2—Appropriately Aggressive

Keith Azevedo and Isaac Tawil

In the setting of life-threatening hemorrhage, the standard ABCs may be reconsidered as A^{2}BC, with the additional "A" representing concomitant anticoagulant reversal. The patient on anticoagulants with life-threatening hemorrhage does not allow time for nuanced discussions of maundering inhibitions, as reversal is a time-sensitive action. ICH provides a classic scenario of life-threatening hemorrhage requiring emergent anticoagulant reversal, where time is of the essence. We extrapolate recommendations for other hemorrhages from this often-studied patient group. The objectives of this chapter are to (1) explore the rationale for rapid anticoagulant reversal in life-threatening hemorrhage; (2) discuss the reversal of the historically common anticoagulant, warfarin; (3) discuss DOACs as well as antiplatelet agents and proposed reversal strategies; and (4) provide a practical reference guide that can be utilized on one's next shift.

Anticoagulants and Hemorrhage

Previously, the most common oral anticoagulant was the VKA, warfarin. DOACs, which include factor Xa inhibitors, and DTIs are now the most frequently prescribed oral anticoagulants due to lack of required monitoring and greater anticoagulation reliability. Other common antithrombotic agents include antiplatelet agents. **Table 141.1** summarizes the MOA and half-lives of common antithrombotic agents. While the relative safety of all these anticoagulation agents has been demonstrated, there remains a risk of life-threatening hemorrhage, including ICH. The incidence of ICH increases in the setting of anticoagulants as does hematoma expansion and resultant neurologic morbidity. A large systematic review and meta-analysis estimates ICH mortality at approximately 40%, and increasing to approximately 60% when complicated by anticoagulation. When such life-threatening hemorrhage is recognized, reversal of the anticoagulation is key in mitigating the situation.

Warfarin Reversal

Reversal of warfarin anticoagulation can be achieved through various agents, each differing in time of onset and duration of action: vitamin K, PCC, and FFP (**Table 141.1**). IV

TABLE 141.1 ANTITHROMBOTIC MOA/HALF-LIFE

ANTITHROMBOTIC AGENT	MOA	HALF-LIFE
Warfarin	VKA/epoxide reductase inhibitor, preventing synthesis of factors II, VII, IX, X	36 h
Rivaroxaban, apixaban, and edoxaban	Direct Xa inhibitors	7-21 h normal renal function
Dabigatran	Direct thrombin (IIa) inhibitor	14-17 h
Aspirin	Irreversible acetylation of COX-1 and fibrinogen	15-30 min, 5-7 d for full platelet recovery
Clopidogrel, prasugrel: thienopyridine derivatives	Irreversible inhibition of platelet ADP and platelet activity	7-8 h, 5-7 d for full platelet recovery

MOA, mechanism of action.

vitamin K has an onset of action of 2 to 6 hours and requires up to 24 hours to achieve reversal. PCC is a concentrate of vitamin K–dependent factors II, VII, IX, and X, plus protein C and S as well as a small amount of heparin and can be aPCC or inactivated PCC. Originally developed for hemophilia B treatment, PCC has been used in much of the developed world for emergent warfarin reversal due to rapidity of onset and reliable INR correction. Published in *Circulation* in 2013 by Sarode et al, a randomized trial of vitamin K + PCC versus vitamin K + FFP for VKA-associated hemorrhage compared hemostatic efficacy and INR correction. In this industry-sponsored noninferiority study, PCC reversal was more rapid and had fewer adverse effects, the most common of which was plasma-related volume overload. Thrombotic complications did not differ between groups. This study led to the FDA approval of PCC for urgent VKA reversal in the setting of major bleeding. A subsequent randomized trial by Goldstein et al (Lancet, 2015) of PCC versus plasma for rapid VKA reversal to facilitate urgent invasive procedures demonstrated four-factor PCC's noninferiority and superiority to plasma for rapid INR reversal and effective hemostasis. While mortality data are lacking, there are several reasons why PCC could be the preferable agent over plasma. The major downside of an FFP reversal strategy is the delay to INR correction owing to the required thawing of FFP and the unpredictable INR normalization. Additional complications include TACO from the colloid load and TRALI. Of note, in these emergency reversal settings, vitamin K is always given along with factor repletion to prevent rebound coagulopathy as the half-life of warfarin exceeds that of the repleted factors. Thus, the AHA recommendations for VKA-associated ICH include IV vitamin K plus PCC as preferable over FFP.

DOACs and Antiplatelet Agents

These agents can be placed into two categories based on their MOA: DTI and factor Xa. DTIs include the oral agent dabigatran and three parenteral agents bivalirudin, argatroban, and desirudin. Xa inhibitors in clinical use include rivaroxaban, apixaban, and edoxaban. Although there is a paucity of rigorous clinical evidence to guide reversal of the DOAC class, recommendations are based on some existing trials and expert opinion. For reversal of Xa inhibitors, andexanet alfa (a recombinant Xa protein that sequesters Xa inhibitors) or PCC should be considered. Evidence is lacking to recommend one option over the other. In the case of DTI-associated bleeding, although clearance by hemodialysis

TABLE 141.2	ANTICOAGULANTS
ANTITHROMBOTIC AGENTS	**REVERSAL AGENTS**
Warfarin	Vitamin K IV *plus either* PCC *or* FFP
Direct Xa inhibitors: rivaroxaban, apixaban, and edoxaban	PCC Andexanet alfa
Direct thrombin (IIa) inhibitor: dabigatran	Idarucizumab Activated PCC (FEIBA) PCC
Aspirin	Desmopressin (DDAVP)
Thienopyridine derivatives: clopidogrel, prasugrel	Consider platelets.

is possible, this is often time consuming and impractical in the emergency setting. Therefore, the antibody fragment idarucizumab, which reverses the anticoagulation effect of dabigatran, can be used. If idarucizumab is unavailable, aPCC, otherwise known as FEIBA, is recommended; and if aPCC is not available, then PCC should be used.

Consensus on how to address reversal or mitigation of antiplatelet agents is less clear. Despite the lack of robust evidence, many experts assert that since antiplatelet agents tend to increase bleeding, their action should similarly be reversed. The platelet transfusions for intracerebral hemorrhage (PATCH) trial showed platelet transfusion for spontaneous ICH in patients on antiplatelet agents, primarily aspirin therapy alone, did not reduce bleeding and was associated with an increased mortality and morbidity at 3 months. Platelet transfusion is also unlikely to reverse the effect of ticagrelor. The utility of platelet transfusion to reverse potent agents such as prasugrel or that of dual antiplatelet therapy remains in question but is a common practice given the known bleeding potentiation of these drugs. DDAVP (desmopressin) induces the release of von Willebrand factor and factor VIII, augmenting hemostasis in the setting of medication-induced platelet dysfunction. DDAVP administration is recommended by the Neurocritical Care Society and Society of Critical Care Medicine as a one-time dose in patients on antiplatelet therapy with ICH. Consider **Table 141.2** on your next shift when a patient on anticoagulants presents with life-threatening bleeding.

PEARLS

- Rapid anticoagulant reversal is critical in life-threatening hemorrhage.
- A warfarin reversal strategy should include 10 mg IV vitamin K plus PCC or FFP.
- DOAC reversal currently includes aPCC, PCC, and idarucizumab.
- While controversial, antiplatelet agent reversal includes DDAVP and consideration of platelet transfusion.

Suggested Readings

Greenberg SM, Ziai WC, Cordonnier C, et al. 2022 guideline for the management of patients with spontaneous intracerebral hemorrhage: a guideline from the American Heart Association/American Stroke Association. *Stroke*. 2022;53(7):e282-e361.

Sarode R, et al. Efficacy and safety of a 4-factor prothrombin complex concentrate in patients on vitamin K antagonists presenting with major bleeding: A randomized, plasmacontrolled, phase IIIb study. *Circulation*. 2013;128(11):1234–1243.

Tomaselli GF, Mahaffey KW, Cuker A, et al. 2020 ACC Expert Consensus Decision Pathway on management of bleeding in patients on oral anticoagulants: a report of the American College of Cardiology Solution Set Oversight Committee [published correction appears in *J Am Coll Cardiol*. 2021;77(21):2760]. *J Am Coll Cardiol*. 2020;76(5):594–622.

142

Know How to Evaluate and Manage the CAR-T Patient

Monica Kathleen Wattana and Brian Cameron

CAR-T therapy is a novel, rapidly expanding immunotherapy treatment modality. The process for CAR-T involves infusing a patient's own genetically altered T-cells to target specific cancer cell antigens.

There are multiple toxic side effects that can develop from CAR-T therapy, most being variations of various inflammatory syndromes, but the two that emergency medicine practitioners should be able to recognize, evaluate, and manage are CRS and ICANS.

CRS

CRS is the most common life-threatening CAR-T toxicity affecting up to 90% of patients who receive CAR-T infusions. It most often occurs 4 to 5 days after infusion and peaks in the subsequent 1- to 2-week period (although later occurrences have been known to occur).

At its essence, CRS is a systemic inflammatory response arising from infused CAR-T cells effecting a massive release of various pro-inflammatory cytokines and interleukins. This results in the patient presenting with a sepsis-like picture that can include fever, hypoxia, hemodynamic instability, and evidence of end-organ damage. It is a diagnosis of exclusion that if not promptly recognized and treated, it carries a 5% to 15% 30-day reported mortality.

ICANS

ICANS is the second most common acute CAR-T toxicity usually occurring within 4 to 5 days after infusion, but it has been shown to present more than 3 weeks after infusion in approximately 10% of patients. The mechanism leading to ICANS is less known but is likely related to cytokines resulting from CAR-T-cell treatment crossing the bloodbrain barrier. ICANS can present with or without CRS but more commonly occurs after CRS has subsided. The clinical presentation of ICANS encompasses a progressive spectrum of neurologic symptoms. Mild presentations may be subtle with word finding difficulty or mild confusion, while severe presentations can occur with decreased levels of consciousness, seizures, and cerebral edema. ICANS is a clinical diagnosis with an ED workup more often used to rule out alternative diagnoses. High-dose corticosteroids and IL-6 inhibitors are the management of choice for ICANS and are combined with supportive care measures that are based on symptom severity.

Diagnosis

Recognizing the possibility of CRS and ICANS is the initial step in treatment and should be considered in any patient with a history of CAR-T therapy. Since these are clinical diagnoses, additional lab work and imaging in the ED are useful for excluding alternative diagnoses. It should be stressed that since CAR-T is so new, most of these patients are followed very closely by their oncology team who should be included in any assessment and management decision whenever possible.

CRS Assessment and Management

These patients present with signs suggesting sepsis, which may or may not also be present. Therefore, initial steps include usual sepsis management such as supplement oxygen, fluids, and empiric antibiotics/fluid cultures as indicated. Additional treatment interventions, such as with glucocorticoids and IL-6 inhibitors, are based on symptom severity, so a complete history and physical examination are imperative in these patients (**Table 142.1**).

ICANS Assessment and Management

Inherent to ICANS assessment is the ICE grading system which is a 10-point score that is used to assess the degree of associated neurologic involvement.

By helping to assess neurologic toxicity, the ICE grading score then helps guide treatment (**Table 142.2**).

Table 142.1 CRS Assessment and Management

	Symptoms	Management
Grade 1	Fever >38 °C and constitutional symptoms	Supportive treatment with acetaminophen, IV fluids, antibiotics for possible sepsis *Consider* IL-6 inhibitors (tocilizumab), especially if fever >3 d.
Grade 2	Above grade PLUS mild hypotension and/or mild hypoxia	All the above, plus supplemental low-flow O_2 support *Consider* IL-6 inhibitors (tocilizumab) *and* a glucocorticoid (methylprednisone 1 mg/kg/d).
Grade 3	Above grades PLUS moderate hypotension requiring vasopressor and/or moderate hypoxia requiring high-flow oxygen	All the above, plus vasopressor and high-flow oxygen support IL-6 inhibitor (tocilizumab) *and* a glucocorticoid (methylprednisone 1 mg/kg/d). May need to repeat IL-6 inhibitor ICU admission
Grade 4	Above grades PLUS severe hypotension requiring multiple pressors and/or severe hypoxia with advanced respiratory support for respiratory failure	All the above, plus mechanical ventilation (positive pressure ventilation/intubation) IL-6 inhibitor (tocilizumab) *and* a glucocorticoid (methylprednisone 1 mg/kg/d) and *an additional* glucocorticoid (dexamethasone 10 mg every 6 h). May need to repeat IL-6 inhibitor ICU admission

ICU, intensive care unit; IL-6, interleukin-6; IV, intravenous.
Note: Of the IL-6 inhibitors, tocilizumab is the most common and is given 8 mg/kg IV.

IMMUNE EFFECTOR CELL-ASSOCIATED ENCEPHALOPATHY (ICE) GRADING SYSTEM

Points	Assessment
4	Orientation: to year, month, city, and hospital
3	Naming: ability to name three objects (eg, point to pen, table, glass)
1	Following commands: ability to follow simple commands (eg, "close your eyes" or "show me three fingers")
1	Writing: ability to write a standard sentence (eg, "A butterfly uses its wings to fly.")
1	Attention: ability to count backward by 10 from 100

TABLE 142.2 ICANS ASSESSMENT AND MANAGEMENT

Grade	Symptoms	Management
1	Encephalopathy and depressed consciousness (ICE score 7-9)	Supportive care *and* IL-6 inhibitor (tocilizumab) *and* glucocorticoids (methylprednisone 1 mg/kg/d) if associated with CRS Obtain an MRI of brain (or CT without contrast), neurology consult, EEG.
2	Encephalopathy and depressed consciousness (ICE score 3-6)	Supportive care *and* IL-6 inhibitor (tocilizumab) *and* glucocorticoids (methylprednisone 1 mg/kg/d) if associated with CRS Obtain MRI of brain (or CT without contrast), neurology consult, EEG.
3	Above PLUS brief rapidly resolving seizures Neuroimaging may show focal cerebral edema. (ICE score 0-2)	Supportive care *and* IL-6 inhibitor (tocilizumab) *and* glucocorticoid (methylprednisone 1 mg/kg/d) if associated with CRS Benzodiazepine as needed for seizure activity Obtain an MRI of brain (or CT without contrast), neurology consult, EEG. Consider ICU admission.
4	Above PLUS deep focal motor weakness (hemiparesis), prolonged seizures, and/or neuroimaging with diffuse cerebral edema (ICE score 0)	Supportive care *and* IL-6 inhibitor (tocilizumab) *and* a glucocorticoid (methylprednisone 1 mg/kg/d) *and* an additional *g*lucocorticoids dose (dexamethasone 10 mg every 6 h) if associated with CRS Possible intubation, reduce intracranial pressure ICU admission

CRS, cytokine release syndrome; CT, computed tomography; EEG, electroencephalogram; ICU, intensive care unit; IL-6, interleukin; MRI, magnetic resonance imaging.

Note: Seizures usually respond to benzodiazepines (lorazepam) and/or levetiracetam, and/or phenobarbital. Also important to replete any low magnesium and/or thiamine.

Summary

Patients with CAR-T-related CRS and/or ICANS toxicities have favorable prognoses and are expected to recover without persistent side effects if symptoms are recognized early and managed rapidly. These toxicities are relatively reversible and require prompt collaboration between the ED provider, oncologist, and other specialists.

PEARLS

- Of all the possible CAR-T toxicities, emergency medicine practitioners should be most familiar with diagnosing and managing CRS and ICANS.
- Since CRS and ICANS are diagnosed clinically, providers need a high index of suspicion in patients who have previously received CAR-T treatment.
- Management decisions should ideally include the patient's oncology team.
- Sepsis is difficult to distinguish from CRS initially, so providers should start empiric treatment for sepsis while concomitantly evaluating them for CRS.
- A 4-point gradation algorithm, which is based on symptoms and interventions, is used to guide treatment for both CRS and ICANS.

Suggested Readings

Brown AR. *How to Survive a Car Crash – Recognition and Management of Car T-Cell Therapy Toxicites*. MD Anderson Pharmacy Grand Rounds Online; 2017.
Garcia Borrega J, Gödel P, Rüger MA, et al. In the eye of the storm: immune-mediated toxicities associated with CAR-T cell therapy. *HemaSphere*. 2019;3(2):e191.
Neelapu SS. Managing the toxicities of CAR T-cell therapy. *Hematol Oncol*. 2019;37(S1):48-52.
Rees, J.H. Management of immune effector cell-associated neurotoxicity syndrome (ICANS). In: Kröger N, Gribben J, Chabannon C, et al. eds. *The EBMT/EHA CAR-T Cell Handbook*. Springer; 2022.
Riegler LL, Jones GP, Lee DW. Current approaches in the grading and management of cytokine release syndrome after chimeric antigen receptor T-cell therapy. *Ther Clin Risk Manag*. 2019;15:323–335.
Sheth VS, Gauthier J. Taming the beast: CRS and ICANS after CAR T-cell therapy for ALL. *Bone Marrow Transplant*. 2021;56:552-566.

143

All Aboard! Don't Miss TRALI and TACO

Darcy James Mainville and Jessica Muñoz

It was my first night on call as a senior resident at the Veterans Hospital. My first page at 2 AM was for an 80-year-old patient with hypoxic respiratory distress in the setting of recent surgery that had required a post-op blood transfusion. I walked into the patient's room and saw she was tachypneic, hypoxic and tachycardic. Her distress had started about 30 minutes after the blood products were hung, so I asked the nurse to stop the blood and start her on oxygen. My brain attempted to remember the pathophysiology of TACO or TRALI in order to figure out my next steps.

An acute transfusion reaction should always be considered in your differential when your patient develops adverse signs and symptoms during or after transfusion. The most severe reactions tend to occur within the first 15 minutes of the transfusion. TACO and TRALI are the top transfusion reactions leading to patient mortality. These transfusion reactions may present with nonspecific symptoms as well as overlapping with the patient's comorbid conditions, making the diagnosis challenging. Your first step when encountering a patient with severe signs and symptoms after or during a transfusion include assessment of oxygenation status and if the patient is hypoxemic, starting oxygen; stopping the transfusion; rapid chest x-ray; and if you suspect your patient looks volume overloaded, starting diuresis.

Interestingly, the main risk factor for onset of TRALI may not be the transfusion of packed red blood cells, but rather the transfusion of fresh frozen plasma. According to data from the France Hemovigilance Network, as well as other monitoring bodies, the highest risk of TRALI exists from transfusion of plasma (non solvent/detergent pooled), followed by platelets and then packed red blood cells. It is important to keep this in mind during any blood product transfusion with acute respiratory changes. In the US, there is no central database for TRALI reporting currently but all suspected incidents must be reported to the blood bank that provided the products used for tranfusion.

The basic definition of TACO is the new onset of dyspnea that occurs within 12 hours of a transfusion. You should suspect TACO in a patient that develops acute respiratory distress and hypoxemia with or without hypertension during or within 12 hours of completing a transfusion. TACO can occur with a transfusion of any blood product: platelets, fresh frozen plasma, red blood cells, cryoprecipitate, or other products.

TACO—new onset or exacerbation of three or more of the following symptoms (within 12 hours of transfusion and without alternative explanation):

- Respiratory distress (tachypnea, hypoxemia, tachycardia)
- Pulmonary edema diagnosed clinically or on imaging
- Elevated BNP
- Elevated central venous pressure
- High blood pressure

A chest x-ray will show evidence of pulmonary edema in patients with TACO. Individuals who are at higher risk for this circulatory overload include patients with end-stage renal disease, heart failure, and low body weight. TACO signs and symptoms tend to respond well to diuresis.

In some cases, it may be obvious if the patient appears overloaded but sometimes both TACO and TRALI may occur simultaneously. TRALI is basically indistinguishable from ARDS in that the transfusion creates an endothelial injury that leads to vascular leakage and ultimately pulmonary edema. The diagnosis can be made by looking for "acute, noncardiogenic pulmonary edema associated with hypoxia" that occurs during or after a transfusion. True TRALI will present in a patient that has absolutely no other reason to sustain an ALI, such as sepsis, pneumonia, aspiration, or other undifferentiated shock. TRALI will present with hypoxemia, hypotension, and a chest x-ray that demonstrates bilateral infiltrates without elevated atrial pressures. Remember that pulmonary congestion can also be seen in TACO. The clinical presentation of TRALI includes severe hypoxemia, with the patient likely desaturating to less than 90% on room air and also potentially developing hypotension, fever, and tachycardia, with rales on physical exam due to airway secretions. On chest x-ray, pulmonary infiltrates will be evident within 6 hours of the transfusion. The treatment for TRALI is airway support and fluid resuscitation with early intubation and mechanical ventilation using lung protective protocols being directly linked to improved patient outcomes.

Another transfusion-related reaction to keep on your differential includes a febrile nonhemolytic reaction. Symptoms may be a similar presentation to TACO and TRALI but you tend to see fevers as well as chills, headache, and myalgias. Febrile nonhemolytic transfusion reactions are clinically benign and tend to be self-limited when compared to TACO and TRALI. They can be treated with antipyretics, and we can reduce this reaction by using leukocyte-reduced red cells. Apart from these transfusion reactions, don't forget your more common respiratory distress diagnosis including a pulmonary embolism, myocardial infarct, sepsis, and anaphylaxis.

PEARLS

- If any new symptoms develop during transfusion, immediately stop the transfusion.
- Consider TACO and TRALI when your patient develops respiratory distress during or immediately following transfusion.
- Volume overload with or without hypertension, think TACO.
- Sudden pulmonary infiltrates with hypotension, think TRALI.
- Remember all the blood products can lead to TRALI. Transfusions of plasma and platelets are actually considered higher risk than red blood cells.

SUGGESTED READINGS

Renaudier P, Schlanger S, Vo Mai MP, et al. Epidemiology of transfusion related acute lung injury in France: preliminary results. *Transfus Med Hemother*. 2008;35:89-91.
Roubinian N. TACO and TRALI: biology, risk factors, and prevention strategies. *Hematology Am Soc Hematol Educ Program*. 2018;2018(1):585-594.
Wiersum-Osselton JC, Whitaker B, Grey S, et al. Revised international surveillance case definition of transfusion-associated circulatory overload: a classification agreement validation study. *Lancet Haematol*. 2019;6(7):e350-e358.

144

WHEN SHOULD YOU TRANSFUSE BLOOD PRODUCTS AND FACTORS?

NICHOLAS ANDREW AND MATTHEW P. BORLOZ

Transfusion in the ED is performed to address blood loss and replace dysfunctional or deficient coagulation factors. Donated blood products are combined with an anticoagulant and a preservative, tested for blood-borne pathogens, and often separated into various components before transfusion. Safe transfusion practices require informed consent and verification of patient identity with the correct blood product before transfusion in stable patients.

RISKS AND COMPLICATIONS OF BLOOD TRANSFUSION

Blood transfusion carries risks, such as transfusion-related infection and transfusion reactions (covered in Chapter[143]). Donor blood is screened for infectious agents, but a small risk remains. In the United States, blood is screened for syphilis, hepatitis B and C, HIV, human T-cell lymphotropic virus, West Nile virus, Chagas disease, Babesia and Zika virus.

TYPE, SCREEN, AND CROSSMATCH

Transfusion requires matching blood type (ABO, Rh) and screening for recipient antibodies to minor antigens. Typing takes approximately 15 minutes, and screening uses a prepared mix of important minor RBC antigens. If an antibody screen is positive, a crossmatch is performed between the recipient's plasma and the intended unit for transfusion.

WHOLE BLOOD

Whole-blood transfusion has garnered recent interest, especially in trauma, as it provides all components lost during hemorrhage. Stored whole blood has a shelf life of 21 to 35 days and is generally type O with a low titer of anti-A and anti-B antibodies. As emergent whole-blood transfusion is unmatched, females of child-bearing potential should receive Rh- products. All other patients may be given Rh+ products. Whole-blood transfusion has been used by the military since the Korean War, but its use in civilian practice is still being explored.

PRBCs

One unit of PRBCs for an adult patient measures 250 mL and is expected to raise the patient's hemoglobin by approximately 1 g/dL. The initial pediatric dose of PRBCs of 10 mL/kg is expected to raise the hemoglobin by 2 g/dL. Most adult patients are transfused below a hemoglobin of 7 g/dL, though patients with preexisting cardiovascular disease or undergoing surgery may be transfused at a threshold of 8 g/dL. One unit of PRBCs is generally transfused over 1 to 2 hours in stable patients. Treated PRBCs are used in specific applications (**Table 144.1**).

TABLE 144.1 TREATED PRBCs AND THEIR APPLICATIONS

Leukocyte reduced	■ 70%-85% of WBCs removed ■ Decrease febrile reactions and prevent HLA sensitization in bone-marrow-transplant candidates
Irradiated	■ Eliminate T-lymphocyte proliferation ■ Transplant patients (graft vs host), patients who are immunocompromised
Washed	■ Removes residual plasma ■ IgA deficiency, persistent febrile reactions
Frozen	■ RBCs are cryopreserved to extend shelf life to 10 yr. ■ Extremely rare blood groups, storage for high-demand situations such as mass-casualties and war

HLA, human leukocyte antigen; IgA, immunoglobulin A; PRBC, packed red blood cell; RBC, red blood cell; WBC, white blood cell.

Platelets

Platelets are transfused to prevent or treat bleeding due to inadequacy of platelet quantity or function. Most (>90%) platelets transfused in the United States are apheresis or single-donor-derived platelets. Some centers pool several units of random-donor or whole-blood-derived, platelets into a single bag, often called a "six-pack." These pooled units contain platelets from 4 to 6 donors. Each unit, apheresis or pooled, supplies 3×10^{11} platelets or more and should raise an adult's platelet count by approximately 30,000/mcL. Pediatric platelet transfusions are dosed at 5 to 10 mL/kg.

Platelet transfusion is recommended for levels less than 20,000/mcL before most invasive ED procedures (eg, paracentesis, central venous catheter insertion, tube thoracostomy) and less than 50,000/mcL for lumbar puncture (though some guidelines maintain <20,000/mcL). Transfusion thresholds for patients destined for surgical intervention are at the discretion of the operator.

Platelet transfusion is recommended to prevent spontaneous bleeding when platelets are less than 10,000/mcL. Those with bleeding at a noncompressible site should be transfused when the platelets are less than 50,000/mcL or when pharmacologic platelet dysfunction contributes to ongoing bleeding. Thromboelastography may assist with assessment of platelet function.

When possible, ABO- and Rh-matched units should be used, though recommendations and institutional policies vary. Except in cases of life-threatening hemorrhage, platelet transfusion should be avoided in conditions with concomitant thrombosis and hemorrhage (eg, disseminated intravascular coagulopathy, thrombotic thrombocytopenic purpura).

Plasma (Frozen and Liquid)

FFP is the component left after separating cell components from whole blood, which is then frozen for storage. FFP may be stored for up to 5 days and when needed for transfusion, takes 20 to 40 minutes to thaw. One unit of FFP measures approximately 250 mL and is expected to raise factor levels by 3% to 5%. Among other proteins, Factors I (fibrinogen), II, V, VII, VIII, IX, X, XI, XII, and XIII, as well as von Willebrand factor, antithrombin III, protein C, and protein S, are found in FFP, though concentrations of active protein vary by unit and decrease with time. FFP should be ABO-compatible, but Rh-compatibility is unnecessary; type AB is the universal donor for FFP. The INR of FFP is 1.5, and FFP administration to reverse coagulopathy may be indicated in patients with an INR 1.8 or more. Applications of FFP infusion include reversal of vitamin K antagonists and direct oral anticoagulants if PCC is unavailable, replacement of multiple coagulation deficiencies, hereditary angioedema by replacing deficient C1-esterase inhibitor, and plasma exchange. For conditions in which a single coagulation factor is missing, such as hemophilia A or B (Factor VIII and Factor IX, respectively), factor concentrates should be used for replacement whenever possible.

Cryoprecipitate

Cryoprecipitate is the principal source of fibrinogen available for clinical use, though it also contains factors VIII and XIII, as well as von Willebrand factor and fibronectin. Each unit of cryoprecipitate contains 150 mg of fibrinogen or more and should not be used for single-factor replacement unless concentrated factor is unavailable and bleeding is catastrophic.

Adult dosing is typically 5 to 10 units, which should raise the fibrinogen level by 50 to 100 mg/dL. Pediatric dosing is 1 unit/10 kg. Rh-compatibility is not necessary, though ABO compatibility may be required at some facilities.

Factors VIII, IX

Factors VIII and IX are deficient in patients with hemophilia A and B, respectively. For moderate-to-severe bleeding, 50 units/kg of factor VIII (hemophilia A) or 100 units/kg of factor IX (hemophilia B) should be given, assuming there are no known inhibitors. One-quarter to one-half of these doses may be used for minor bleeding that persists despite conservative measures. Patients with known factor inhibitors may be given recombinant factor VIIa or activated PCC.

PEARLS

- A numerical threshold should never be the sole determinant of blood product transfusion.
- Whole-blood transfusion is not widely available but is being studied for use in cases of large-volume hemorrhage such as major trauma.
- Hemorrhage source control, as well as pharmacologic mitigation of coagulopathy, is at least as important as blood product transfusion in the setting of life-threatening hemorrhage.
- Conditions with concomitant thrombosis and hemorrhage are challenging and may require subspecialty consultation to guide safe and effective therapy.
- Though some products do not require ABO- and Rh-compatibility testing, early type and screen prevent delays in product availability and ensure safe administration.

Suggested Readings

Bachowski G, Brunker P, Goldberg C, et al; American Red Cross Medical Office. *A Compendium of Transfusion Practice Guidelines*. 4th ed. 2021.

Carson JL, Stanworth SJ, Dennis JA, et al. Transfusion thresholds for guiding red blood cell transfusion. *Cochrane Database Syst Rev*. 2021;12(12):CD002042.

Long B, Koyfman A. Red blood cell transfusion in the emergency department. *J Emerg Med*. 2016;51(2):120-130.

145

Know This Clinical Presentation of Leukemia in the Pediatric Patient

B. Barrie Bostick

The diagnosis of leukemia is life-changing for a family and their child; however, this diagnosis can be difficult as the presenting symptoms are usually vague. It is better when the diagnosis can be made early, so it is important to identify red flags that should prompt further investigation.

Epidemiology

The diagnosis of childhood cancer is rare, with approximately 14,000 to 16,000 cases of all types of pediatric cancer diagnosed every year. Acute leukemia makes up approximately one-third of those diagnoses. The initial diagnosis of pediatric leukemia is usually made between the ages of 3 and 15 years, with poorer prognosis for those newly diagnosed out of that age range. There have been many advances in the treatment of pediatric leukemia, and the 5-year survival is reported to be more than 85%. Per the National Cancer Institute, the death rate for childhood leukemia for the year of 2020 was 0.5 per 100,000 children.

Symptoms

The presenting symptoms for leukemia are vague and caused by lymphoblast infiltration into the bone marrow, periosteum, lymph system, or CNS. They can include fever, weight loss, bone pain, fatigue, or pallor. Some of these symptoms can overlap with normal processes in children. Patients with isolated musculoskeletal symptoms, such as joint pain and bone pain, can have symptoms for months before diagnosis due to misdiagnosis of strain or growing pains. If the pain is persistent or frequent, worse at night, or associated with fever, it would be reasonable to obtain blood work. Similarly, fatigue and fever can be common in children with frequent viral infections. It would be helpful to pay attention to the chronicity of these symptoms, as well as their symptoms between illnesses, such as persistent fatigue or fevers without other associated symptoms. The infiltration of blasts into the bone marrow causes disruption of normal hematopoiesis, leading to anemia and thrombocytopenia. This usually results in pallor, petechiae, easy fatigability, and exercise intolerance in patients. Infiltration into the lymph system can cause hepatomegaly, lymphadenopathy, and splenomegaly. Patients can also experience a mediastinal mass, which can cause shortness of breath. It is also possible to experience neurologic symptoms, such as vomiting, headache, papilledema, or cranial nerve palsy, which can stem from infiltration into the CNS or, in late stages, leukostasis from hyperleukocytosis.

Physical Examination

The physical examination should examine for signs of easy bruising, petechiae, and pallor. These should always prompt further evaluation. There may also be signs of hepatomegaly and splenomegaly. It is important to assess for cervical, axillary, and inguinal lymphadenopathy. Patients can also have signs of testicular enlargement. Musculoskeletal findings might include tenderness over the extremities, joint effusions, or limp without a history of injury.

Laboratory Evaluation

CBC with manual differential is the best initial test to obtain when evaluating for anemia, thrombocytopenia, or leukemia. Lymphoblasts on manual differential are indicative of abnormal hematopoiesis, with increased specificity for leukemia if lymphoblasts are greater than 25%. When there is suspicion for leukemia, laboratory evaluation should include a CMP and a type and screen. With severe leukocytosis, it is possible for patients to present with TLS; if this is a clinical concern, uric acid, phosphate, lactic acid, and LDH should also be obtained.

Editor's note: It is more common to see hyperviscosity syndrome in acute leukemia than in TLS; TLS is usually induced by induction of chemotherapy, not with initial presenting syndrome.

If the CBC is abnormal, a peripheral smear for pathology review and flow cytometry should be ordered. The findings on CBC typically associated with leukemia are an elevated WBC with lymphoblasts on manual differential with a decrease in the hemoglobin and the platelet count; however, there can be a wide array of results depending on where the patient is in the disease process. Early consultation with hematology/oncology will be helpful for further management. Ultimately, the final diagnosis will be made with a bone marrow aspirate.

DIFFERENTIAL DIAGNOSIS

There is a large array of hematologic/oncologic entities that can mimic a similar presentation to leukemia, both in clinical presentation and laboratory findings. Differentials for pancytopenia can include aplastic anemia (both acquired and congenital), myelofibrosis, drug-induced cytopenia, and viral suppression of the bone marrow. Bone pain, arthralgia, and arthritis can all be symptoms of juvenile arthritis and other autoimmune disorders. Many of the symptoms of leukemia, such as fatigue, weight loss, and fever, can overlap with other oncologic diseases (eg, neuroblastoma, rhabdomyosarcoma, and Ewing sarcoma). Laboratory findings of anemia can be a sign of transient erythroblastopenia or hemolytic anemia. Petechiae with isolated thrombocytopenia can be commonly seen with idiopathic thrombocytopenic purpura.

ONCOLOGIC EMERGENCIES

It is important to be aware of different emergent presentations of leukemia. Leukostasis can be caused by hyperleukocytosis (WBC >100,000) that can cause decreased perfusion to the tissues, especially affecting the CNS and respiratory systems. Decreased perfusion to tissues can also be exacerbated by severe anemia. Rarely, patients with hyperleukocytosis can present with spontaneous TLS. If a patient shows signs of TLS or leukostasis, early consultation with the ICU and hematology/oncology would be recommended. Patients with thrombocytopenia can present with bleeding, although severe bleeding is rare in the initial presentation of leukemia, even with profound thrombocytopenia.

DISCUSSION WITH FAMILY

Emergency medicine providers are accustomed to delivering bad news in the ED. There are some special considerations when discussing this type of diagnosis with the family. Families will be already anxious based on their child's symptoms and worries for their child. Even with abnormal CBC, there is still a wide differential diagnosis for bone marrow dysfunction. Some parents will want to know all the possibilities, including leukemia, in order to prepare themselves, others will prefer to wait for a final diagnosis. Ask the parents their preference. It would also be beneficial to consider the developmental stage of the child. Is this a child who will be worried if the parents are upset? Perhaps consider having a discussion outside of the room. Is the child mature enough to understand what is going on? Will they have their own questions? Fortunately, this is a rare diagnosis in the ED; however, it should remain in our minds when caring for young patients.

PEARLS

- Chronicity of symptoms, atraumatic musculoskeletal symptoms, which are worse at night, fatigue, frequent fever without other symptoms, or petechiae, should prompt clinical concern for hematologic malignancy and prompt further laboratory workup.

- Consult hematology/oncology early in the process if malignancy is suspected.
- New diagnosis of leukemia can present with emergent complications, such as leukostasis or TLS.

Suggested Readings

Belay Y, Yirdaw K, Enawgaw B. Tumor Lysis syndrome in patients with hematological malignancies. *J Oncol.* 2017;2017:9684909. PMID: 29230244.

Bernard SC, Abdelsamad EH, Johnson PA, Chapman DL, Parvathaneni M. Pediatric leukemia: diagnosis to treatment—a review. *J Cancer Clin Trials.* 2007;2(2):1-3.

Esparza S, Sakamoto K. Topics in pediatric leukemia—acute lymphoblastic leukemia. *MedGenMed.* 2005;7(1):23.

Kaplan J. Leukemia in children. *Pediatr Rev.* 2019;40(7):319-331.

Mitchell C. Acute leukemia in children: diagnosis and management. *BMJ.* 2009;338:1491-1495.

Tubergen D, Bleyer A, Ritchey A. The leukemias. In: Kliegman R, ed. *Nelson Textbook of Pediatric.* Elsevier; 2011.

SECTION XI

IMMUNOLOGY

146

THERE ARE *NO* ABSOLUTE CONTRAINDICATIONS FOR EPINEPHRINE IN ANAPHYLAXIS

JOSEPH H. ASH AND ROBERT OLYMPIA

Anaphylaxis is a potentially fatal allergic reaction often requiring treatment in the ED. Prompt recognition of anaphylaxis is critical. Epinephrine is the cornerstone and first-line treatment in the management of anaphylaxis in both children in adults. Delayed time to administration of epinephrine has been associated with worse outcomes and more severe reactions. There has traditionally been some concern surrounding the use of epinephrine in certain patient populations such as those with preexisting cardiovascular disease or uncontrolled hypertension as well as concerns regarding medication interactions. However, these concerns are largely theoretic, whereas there has been a demonstrated increase in mortality when there are delays in administration of epinephrine or lack of administration altogether in anaphylaxis.

The NIAID/FAAN developed the following widely accepted criteria for the diagnosis of anaphylaxis. These criteria have a sensitivity of 97%, a specificity of 83%, a negative predictive value of 98%, and a positive predictive value of 69%. The diagnosis of anaphylaxis is *highly* likely when *one* of the following three criteria is demonstrated:

Criterion 1: Acute onset of symptoms involving the skin and mucosa *plus* either respiratory compromise or reduced blood pressure (or associated signs and symptoms of end-organ damage). This is considered the classic presentation of anaphylaxis with acute pruritus, flushing, lip/tongue swelling, hives, dyspnea, bronchospasm, stridor, hypoxemia, syncope, and mental status changes.

Criterion 2: The second criterion is more subtle. The patient will have two or more of the following symptoms after exposure to a *suspected allergen*: skin/mucosal tissue involvement, respiratory compromise, reduced blood pressure (or associated symptoms), and persistent GI symptoms. The patient may not have skin involvement. It is important to note that there will be no skin symptoms in 20% of cases of anaphylaxis.

Criterion 3: This requires exposure of a *known allergen* to the patient. The only symptom in this category is reduced BP; in adults, SBP less than 90 mm Hg (or 30% decrease from baseline if known). For children younger than 10 years, hypotension is defined as 70 mm Hg + 2 × age in years. Clinically, the patient may present with syncope as a sign of hypotension. It is important to remember this category, as it can often be missed.

Epinephrine is typically given via autoinjector outside the hospital and frequently in the hospital as well. Autoinjectors have been found to prevent dosing errors associated with prefilled syringes of epinephrine or manual calculation and drawing of epinephrine. Weight-based dosing in children is 0.01 mg/kg with a maximum of 0.3 mg in children and up to a maximum of 0.5 mg in adults. This dose is given IM, commonly in the anterolateral thigh. Doses of IM epinephrine can be given up to every 5 minutes with a maximum of three doses. In cases of refractory anaphylaxis and refractory anaphylactic shock, the patient may also require initiation of IV epinephrine, which is dosed as a continuous infusion at 0.05 to 2 mcg/kg/min. IV epinephrine has more predictable absorption and titration in shock states as the systemic absorption and distribution from IM administration can be affected by decreased peripheral perfusion.

There have been concerns related to possible adverse events related to epinephrine in those that have underlying cardiovascular disease. However, not only is this more typically associated with IV administration rather than IM administration, there is additional evidence that anaphylaxis itself poses greater risk of morbidity and mortality to those with underlying disease than exposure to epinephrine.

Factors associated with fatal anaphylactic reactions include missed or delayed diagnosis, either of which leads to delay in receipt of epinephrine. Outside of the hospital setting, there are additional barriers that may reduce the access. These include cost of autoinjectors, education on their use, and inconsistent availability during the initial onset of anaphylaxis if the patient has not been carefully counseled to carry it with them at all times. It is therefore critical that patients always be prescribed an autoinjector at ED discharge as well as thorough education on its use. In addition, biphasic anaphylactic reactions may occur, with the most recent literature describing an incidence of 0.4% to 4.5%. Biphasic reactions may occur up to 72 hours after the initial reaction.

When considering the potential risks and benefits associated with epinephrine use in the setting of anaphylaxis, there continue to be no absolute contraindications to the use of epinephrine in anaphylaxis in both the prehospital and ED settings.

PEARLS

- Prompt diagnosis and initiation of treatment is crucial for preventing morbidity and mortality in anaphylaxis.
- Understanding the NIAID/FAAN criteria will help identify atypical anaphylaxis presentations.
- There are no absolute contraindications to treatment with epinephrine in anaphylaxis.
- Prescribe self-injectable epinephrine for all patients with anaphylaxis or who may be at risk of future anaphylaxis and carefully instruct the patient on its use.

SUGGESTED READINGS

Campbell RL, Bellolio MF, Knutson BD, et al. Epinephrine in anaphylaxis: higher risk of cardiovascular complications and overdose after administration of intravenous bolus epinephrine compared with intramuscular epinephrine. *J Allergy Clin Immunol Pract*. 2015; 3(1):76-80.
Lieberman P, Nicklas RA, Randolph C, et al. Anaphylaxis—a practice parameter update 2015. *Ann Allergy Asthma Immunol*. 2015;115(5):341-384.
McHugh K, Repanshek Z. Anaphylaxis: emergency department treatment. *Emerg Med Clin North Am*. 2022;40(1):19-32.
Prince BT, Mikhail I, Stukus DR. Underuse of epinephrine for the treatment of anaphylaxis: missed opportunities. *J Asthma Allergy*. 2018;11:143-151.

147

SECOND-LINE MEDICATIONS IN ANAPHYLAXIS ARE JUST THAT—SECOND LINE!

LEKHA BAPU AND AALAP SHAH

Anaphylaxis is a serious, life-threatening, often misdiagnosed problem that requires immediate attention in the ED setting. Death from anaphylaxis will usually occur quickly secondary to airway obstruction and cardiovascular collapse. The key to better outcomes is early recognition and intervention. A thorough history and physical can be essential to diagnosis and recognition. It is critical to also use the guidelines mentioned in Chapter 146 as well as clinical judgment in determining whether to administer epinephrine to patients with suspected anaphylaxis.

Initial evaluation should focus on airway, breathing, and circulation. Immediate management should include IM epinephrine administration, removal of the inciting agent, placement of the patient in the supine position (unless in respiratory distress), supplemental O_2, large-bore IV access, and volume resuscitation. Patients with hypotension should receive a crystalloid bolus for cardiovascular support. The airway should be secured without delay if there are signs of airway compromise.

IM injection, given in the anterolateral thigh, is the preferred modality for delivery of epinephrine. There are no absolute contraindications to epinephrine administration in patients with suspected anaphylaxis. If a patient has refractory symptoms despite three appropriate epinephrine doses, a continuous IV infusion should be started.

Several second-line medications have been suggested for use in patients experiencing anaphylaxis, including inhaled bronchodilators, antihistamines, and glucocorticoids. In patients experiencing symptoms of persistent bronchoconstriction following IM epinephrine administration, adjunctive use of bronchodilators such as inhaled albuterol can be considered. Similarly, for patients experiencing refractory laryngeal or upper airway edema, nebulized epinephrine can be considered. These treatments should not delay or be used as a substitute to initial or repeat IM epinephrine administration.

Antihistamines are considered second line and are not used to treat conditions requiring emergent management, such as airway obstruction, respiratory compromise, and hypotension. They lack the bronchodilatory, vasoconstrictive, inotropic, and mast cell stabilization effects of epinephrine. These medications can be considered for symptom relief of primarily cutaneous manifestations. Time to onset of action for antihistamines is 30 to 80 minutes, limiting their benefit in the acute setting. There has been concern that inappropriate focus on treatment with antihistamines may delay initial or repeat epinephrine dosing.

While glucocorticoids theoretically decrease the production of inflammatory mediators in the body, they have a slow onset of action and have not been shown to have a useful effect in treatment of anaphylaxis or prevention of biphasic reactions. Given the lack of benefit and potential for delay of emergent therapy, experts have emphasized that glucocorticoids should have a limited role in treatment of acute anaphylaxis.

Review your patients' medications. Antihypertensive medications including beta-blockers may blunt the response to epinephrine and may prompt higher doses of epinephrine or glucagon administration.

In approximately 1% to 7% of individuals, biphasic reactions can occur. Generally, this can occur up to 72 hours following the initial episode. Risk factors for biphasic reactions include those with higher initial severity of anaphylaxis, such as hypotension or wide pulse pressure, and those who require more than 1 dose of epinephrine prior to resolution. These episodes should be treated similarly to the initial episode. While steroids and antihistamines have commonly been used in an attempt to prevent these biphasic reactions, data supporting their use for this purpose are lacking. Experts suggest against routine administration or prescription of these medications for this purpose.

Patients who have complete resolution of anaphylaxis following treatment can be discharged home following observation in the ED or inpatient setting. Experts have suggested a 1- to 8-hour period of observation as reasonable. The observation period should also be individualized depending on factors including the severity of the initial symptoms, age, cardiovascular or respiratory comorbidities, and history of biphasic reactions. In addition, factors such as barriers to appropriate patient education, as well as the patient's access to medications and medical care, should be considered.

Patient education prior to leaving your ED is of utmost importance due to the possibility of biphasic anaphylaxis or reexposure to the allergen. The patient should be instructed to immediately return to the ED if any of the symptoms recur. The patient should be discharged only after training in symptom recognition and epinephrine autoinjector use. Patients should be prescribed an epinephrine autoinjector at discharge.

PEARLS

- Immediate management of anaphylaxis should include ABCs, removal of the inciting agent, IM epinephrine, supplemental O_2, and volume resuscitation.
- There is no absolute contraindication to the administration of epinephrine in suspected anaphylaxis.
- Antihistamines and glucocorticoids have not been found useful for the treatment of anaphylaxis or prevention of biphasic reactions and should be considered as second-line treatment.

- There is no clear consensus on the length of the observation period prior to discharge, and this should be individualized depending on patient factors.
- It is critical that patients be prescribed epinephrine autoinjectors and be trained in their use prior to discharge.

SUGGESTED READINGS

Cardona V, Ansotegui IJ, Ebisawa M, et al. World allergy organization anaphylaxis guidance 2020. *World Allergy Organ J.* 2020;13(10):100472.
Long B, Gottlieb M. Emergency medicine updates: anaphylaxis. *Am J Emerg Med.* 2021; 49:35-39.
Loprinzi Brauer CE, Motosue MS, Li JT, et al. Prospective validation of the NIAID/FAAN criteria for emergency department diagnosis of anaphylaxis. *J Allergy Clin Immunol Pract.* 2016;4(6):1220-1226.
Muraro A, Worm M, Alviani C, et al. EAACI guidelines: anaphylaxis (2021 update). *Allergy.* 2022;77(2):357-377.
Shaker MS, Wallace DV, Golden DBK, et al. Anaphylaxis—a 2020 practice parameter update, systematic review, and Grading of Recommendations, Assessment, Development and Evaluation (GRADE) analysis. *J Allergy Clin Immunol.* 2020;145(4):1082-1123.

148

AVOID THESE PITFALLS IN THE MANAGEMENT OF ACE-INHIBITOR ANGIOEDEMA

AALAP SHAH AND JOSEPH J. MOELLMAN

PITFALL: CONFUSING DIFFERENT TYPES OF ANGIOEDEMA

Angioedema is a nonpitting, localized swelling of subcutaneous and submucosal tissues of the skin, upper respiratory tract, and gastrointestinal tract. Fluid accumulation is the result of increased vascular permeability by one of two mechanisms: histamine mediated or bradykinin mediated.

In histamine-mediated angioedema, histamine release from an IgE-mediated response results in increasing vascular permeability, leading to tissue edema. In bradykinin-mediated angioedema, excessive bradykinin is responsible for increased tissue edema by stimulation of bradykinin receptors (B2), which increases vascular permeability. Distinguishing between the two is paramount since the treatments are vastly different.

ACE-inh-induced angioedema has an incidence of only 0.1% to 0.7% in patients on pharmacotherapy, but accounts for more than 30% of angioedema cases seen in the ED. ACE-inhs act by blocking bradykinin degradation, leading to increased bradykinin levels. Typically, the patient with ACE-inh-induced angioedema will present with asymmetric, nonpitting edema of the lips, tongue, and airway structures. These side effects typically occur within the first week of drug initiation but can occur at any time. Compared to histamine-mediated angioedema, ACE-inh-induced (bradykinin-mediated) angioedema will generally have a slower onset, more prolonged duration (48-72 hours) and will not typically present with urticaria, pruritus, or wheezing. In addition, ACE-inh-induced angioedema is less likely to present with hypotension or shock and typically does not respond to epinephrine, steroid, or antihistamine therapy. These differences can be helpful in differentiating the two clinically.

Pitfall: Relying on Labs or Imaging to Diagnose ACE-inh-Induced Angioedema

Diagnosis and differentiation of angioedema types should be made clinically. History should focus on identifying associated symptoms, speed and pattern of disease progression, personal and family history, as well as medications and any possible allergic exposure or environmental triggers.

Imaging and blood work are largely unnecessary and delay proper treatment. Only in cases of diagnostic uncertainty will such diagnostic tests be useful. In those patients requiring cross-sectional imaging, care must be taken to ensure the airway is protected before the patient is sent for CT scan. In patients with multiple chronic presentations in whom providers suspect HAE, assessing complement levels (C4 and C1 inhibitor levels) may assist outpatient diagnosis.

Pitfall: Treating ACE-inh-Induced Angioedema the Same as Anaphylaxis

There are no specific guidelines for pharmacologic treatment of ACE-inh-induced angioedema. Patients with bradykinin-mediated angioedema do not respond to epinephrine, steroids, and antihistamines, and this approach may delay appropriate treatment. An American Academy of Emergency Medicine 2021 Clinical Practice Committee statement recommends against routine use of these medications (**Table 148.1**).

Although these medications have efficacy in treating histamine-mediated reactions, they have not shown benefit in bradykinin-mediated angioedema. It may be appropriate to administer these medications in cases of diagnostic uncertainty. Clinical response would strongly suggest histaminergic angioedema.

Table 148.1 Rescue Treatment

	Adult Dosing	Pediatric Dosing
IM epinephrine (1:1,000) to thigh every 15-20 min	0.3-0.5 mg	0.03 mg/kg (max 0.5 mg)
Oxygen		
Initial normal saline bolus	1-2 L	20 mL/kg
Diphenhydramine IV if skin involvement	25-50 mg	1-2 mg/kg (max 50 mg)
Ranitidine IV	50 mg	1 mg/kg (max 50 mg)
Methylprednisolone IV	125 mg	1-2 mg/kg (max 125 mg)

Pitfall: Relying on Adjunct Medications to Reverse the Disease Process

A number of medications that may act on bradykinin-mediated angioedema have been identified. These medications are primarily indicated in HAE. Studies on the efficacy of these medications in ACE-inh-induced angioedema have shown mixed results and there is an overall lack of data to support their routine use (**Figure 148.1**).

TXA

TXA functions as an inhibitor in the conversion of plasminogen to plasmin, which reduces bradykinin production. In theory, reducing bradykinin production may reduce symptoms in ACE-inh-induced angioedema. While generally deemed to have a low risk of adverse effects, studies showing efficacy are lacking.

Kallikrein Inhibitors

Kallikrein inhibitors, such as ecallantide, reduce the release of bradykinin. Originally FDA approved for HAE, large-scale studies have failed to show a benefit in management of ACE-inh-induced angioedema and they are not recommended in this population.

C1 Esterase Inhibitor Concentrate

These act on several areas of the kallikrein-bradykinin pathway, also aiming to reduce plasma bradykinin levels. Originally developed to replace deficiency in C1 esterase inhibitor for some types of HAE, they have also been suggested for use in ACE-inh-induced angioedema. However, large-scale studies evaluating their efficacy in this population are lacking, and studies to date have failed to show a benefit.

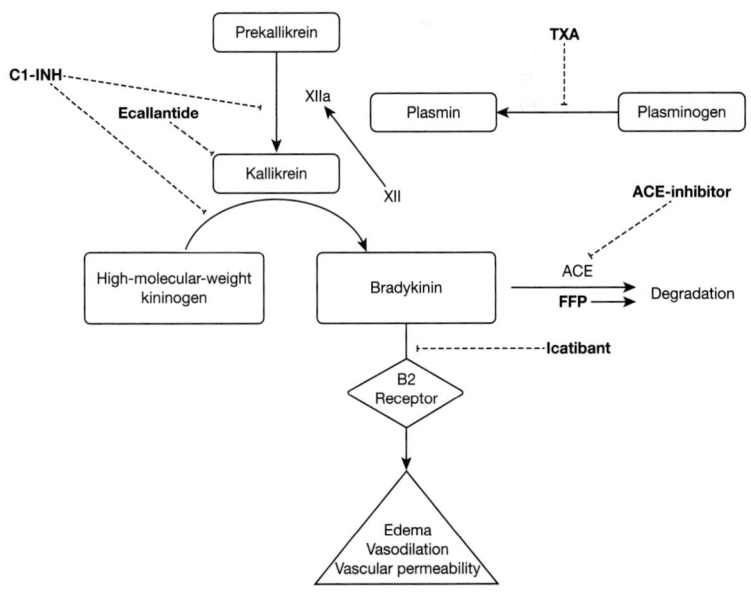

Figure 148.1 Bradykinin pathway with current pharmacologic inhibitors.

FFP

FFP has been used historically for treatment of angioedema, as it contains the C1 esterase inhibitor. However, it also contains prekallikrein and factor XII, which can increase bradykinin production. Prior studies have shown mixed results, with some reports of disease worsening.

B2 Receptor Antagonists

Icatibant acts as a competitive antagonist at the B2 receptor with the aim of reducing the effect of circulating bradykinin. It was FDA approved for treatment of HAE. Studies evaluating its use in ACE-inh-induced angioedema are mixed and have largely failed to show a benefit.

PITFALL: FAILURE TO PERFORM EARLY AIRWAY ASSESSMENT AND INTERVENTION

The greatest risk in patients with ACE-inh-induced angioedema is decompensation due to asphyxiation. It is essential to perform a thorough and timely evaluation of airway involvement. Intervening early is key as the rapidity of progression can be unpredictable.

All patients with ACE-inh-induced angioedema with suspected airway involvement should undergo evaluation of laryngeal structures via nasopharyngoscopy if possible, as it is difficult to predict the presence of posterior oropharyngeal involvement or laryngeal swelling based on external exam alone. Risk factors predicting need for airway intervention are tongue/palate/laryngeal swelling, as well as voice changes or hoarseness, drooling, globus sensation, stridor, or apparent respiratory distress.

When the need for intubation is predicted, early intervention in a controlled setting is recommended. All such patients should be considered a "difficult airway." Airway manipulation may worsen swelling. Awake, fiberoptic, or video-assisted approaches to the airway are preferred, and neuromuscular paralysis should be avoided. Preparation for a surgical airway is critical, as traditional rescue methods may not be effective due to anatomic obstruction. When available, the team should consider additional resources such as transfer to an operating room environment with assistance from anesthesia or ENT departments.

PITFALL: INAPPROPRIATE DISCHARGE FROM THE ED

ACE-inh-induced angioedema is self-limited. Localized swelling will resolve in 24 to 72 hours after cessation of the offending agent. Patients with isolated lip and facial swelling can likely be safely discharged home with return precautions after a 4- to 6-hour observation period in the ED. Those with oropharyngeal or laryngeal involvement may require longer periods of observation in an inpatient critical care setting.

Patients who are discharged must avoid all ACE-inhs in the future. Use of angiotensin receptor blockers in these patients is controversial and may carry a higher risk of angioedema. Patients should be provided clear return instructions regarding recurring symptoms.

PEARLS

- While most adverse drug reactions to ACE-inhs occur in the first week of treatment, angioedema can present many years later. Immediately discontinue ACE-inhs in all patients with signs of angioedema.
- ACE-inh-induced angioedema is diagnosed clinically. Labs are generally considered unnecessary.

- Medications such as epinephrine, steroids, and antihistamines, as well as TXA, FFP, and bradykinin pathway antagonists are unlikely to be of benefit in ACE-inh-induced angioedema.
- Asphyxiation is the primary etiology of morbidity and mortality in patients with angioedema, and initial evaluation should center around assessment of airway patency, with a low threshold to secure the patient's airway for any worrisome signs including voice change, hoarseness, dyspnea, and stridor.
- All patients with angioedema should be considered to have a difficult airway, and awake, fiberoptic, or video-assisted methods are preferred with preparation for surgical airway as a backup.

Suggested Readings

Mudd PA, Hooker EA, Stolz U, Hart KW, Bernstein JA, Moellman JJ. Emergency department evaluation of patients with angiotensin converting enzyme inhibitor associated angioedema. *Am J Emerg Med*. 2020;38(12):2596-2601.

Rosenbaum S, Wilkerson RG, Winters ME, Vilke GM, Wu MYC. Clinical practice statement: what is the emergency department management of patients with angioedema secondary to an ACE-inhibitor? *J Emerg Med*. 2021;61(1):105–112.

Wilkerson RG, Winters ME. Angiotensin-converting enzyme inhibitor-induced angioedema. *Emerg Med Clin North Am*. 2022;40(1):79-98.

149

Know How to Identify Immune-Based Therapy Toxicities

David Locke and Catherine A. Marco

mAbs are a therapeutic modality that utilizes the production of IgG antibodies from a B-cell clone to specifically target either one or two epitopes to be recognized by the mAb. Once the mAbs bind to their target, they can provide therapeutic benefit by inducing apoptosis, blocking specific channels, modulating signaling pathways, or assisting the immune system in identifying cells to be targeted. Based on their adaptability, they are being used as targeted cancer treatments, autoimmune condition therapies, drug reversal agents, transplant rejection modification, infectious disease treatment, and more. In this chapter, we discuss some of the most commonly used mAbs as well as those with ED-relevant side effect profiles.

Anti-CD20 mAbs

This category includes medications such as rituximab (Rituxan), ocrelizumab (Ocrevus), and others that target CD20 on B cells, leading to cytotoxicity among B cells. They have been approved for the treatment of autoimmune conditions including rheumatoid arthritis, myasthenia gravis, ITP, and some cancers. Use of rituximab is known to be associated with infusion reactions, causing shortness of breath, hypotension, and infections. In the ED, if one identifies a patient with recurrence of herpetic lesions, signs of hepatitis B, or neurologic examination and magnetic resonance imaging findings consistent with PML, you should order a panel of Ig levels and consider early Ig replacement with immunology consultation. In addition, severe reactions such as SJS/TEN, and tumor lysis syndrome may occur as a result of decreased B cells from anti-CD20 mAbs.

ANTI-TNF MABS

This group includes medications such as adalimumab (Humira), certolizumab pegol (Cimzia), and infliximab (Remicade). The mechanism of action is blocking the physiologic effects of TNF alpha, which plays a key role in granuloma formation and maintenance, as well as in recruiting other immune cells to areas of inflammation. Reactivation of latent TB is a well-known concern for those on anti-TNF mAbs. Roughly 25% of patients on anti-TNF mAbs develop a cutaneous complication including orange-red psoriasiform eczema, alopecia, skin cancer, and palmoplantar pustulosis. Eczema associated with anti-TNF mAb usage may become superinfected by *Staphylococcus aureus*. Current recommendations are to continue use of mAbs in most patients with dermatologic side effects but to be aware of their heightened risk for development of these conditions and their decreased ability to mount an immune response to superinfection. In addition, neurologic complications including optic neuritis, multiple sclerosis, and demyelinating processes of the CNS and PNS have been identified. The rate of their occurrences has primarily come from uncontrolled studies, and so a definitive association has yet to be drawn, but in those who begin to have unexplained neurologic symptoms and are taking one of these medications, this medication class as an etiology should be considered. Ceasing these medications has not been found to improve neurologic status. Management should include appropriate consultation with dermatology and neurology with intravenous Ig and corticosteroids to reverse and stabilize their condition.

VEGF MABS

Medications in this class include bevacizumab (Avastin), brolucizumab (Beovu), faricimab (Vabysmo), and more. Bevacizumab is a recombinant humanized IgG1 mAb that inhibits VEGF by binding to VEGF1 and VEGF2 receptors. These medications are used in the treatment of metastatic renal cell carcinoma, metastatic colorectal cancer, hepatocellular carcinoma, and some other cancers. While they have an excellent impact on tumor angiogenesis, they are associated with inducing hypertension and proteinuria, for which the mechanism is unknown. Proteinuria has been noted in 21% to 41% and hypertension in 3% to 43% of patients taking this medication, with a relative risk of hypertension in those taking it compared to those who are not, of 7.5. If a patient presents with hypertensive crisis, bevacizumab should be discontinued and antihypertensives should be initiated. Appropriate treatment options include nitrates, beta- or alpha-blockade, angiotensin-converting enzyme inhibitors, or angiotensin-receptor blockers. Some antihypertensive drugs induce VEGF secretion including nondihydropyridine CCBs and nifedipine, and these should be avoided in this population.

PEARLS

- Patients on anti-CD20 mAbs are at risk for hypogammaglobulinemia; if their symptoms cannot be explained otherwise or are indicative of

immunocompromise-associated infection, obtain an Ig panel and replace their Igs as indicated to decrease morbidity and mortality from hypogammaglobulinemia-associated infections.
- PML is classically found in patients with HIV, but use of anti-CD20 mAbs has also been found to be associated with the development of PML in patients without HIV and it is symptomatic of altered mental status, motor deficits, limb and gait ataxia, and seizures in late stages.
- Roughly 25% of patients taking anti-TNF alpha medications will develop a cutaneous complication such as psoriasiform eczema and may need Ig replacement and corticosteroids in order to reverse and stabilize their condition.
- Patients taking anti-VEGF mAbs are prone to developing hypertension and proteinuria. If they develop this, avoid nondihydropyridine CCBs and nifedipine for decreasing blood pressure acutely. Once they are stabilized, their antihypertensives should be adjusted by their primary care physician.

SUGGESTED READINGS

Barmettler S, Ong MS, Farmer JR, Choi H, Walter J. Association of immunoglobulin levels, infectious risk, and mortality with rituximab and hypogammaglobulinemia. *JAMA Netw Open*. 2018;1(7):e184169.

Bosch X, Saiz A, Ramos-Casals M. Monoclonal antibody therapy-associated neurological disorders. *Nat Rev Neurol*. 2011;7(3):165-172.

Breedveld FC. Therapeutic monoclonal antibodies. *Lancet*. 2000;355(9205):735-740.

Connor V. Anti-TNF therapies: a comprehensive analysis of adverse effects associated with immunosuppression. *Rheumatol Int*. 2011;31(3):327-337.

Izzedine H, Ederhy S, Goldwasser F, et al. Management of hypertension in angiogenesis inhibitor-treated patients. *Ann Oncol*. 2009;20(5):807-815.

Quintanilha JC, Wang J, Sibley AB, et al. Bevacizumab-induced hypertension and proteinuria: a genome-wide study of more than 1000 patients. *Br J Cancer*. 2022;126(2):265-274.

Segaert S, Hermans C. Clinical signs, pathophysiology and management of cutaneous side effects of anti-tumor necrosis factor agents. *Am J Clin Dermatol*. 2017;18(6):771-787.

Tan CS, Koralnik IJ. Progressive multifocal leukoencephalopathy and other disorders caused by JC virus: clinical features and pathogenesis. *Lancet Neurol*. 2010;9(4):425-437.

150

DAZED AND CONFUSED: IMMUNE-MEDIATED ENCEPHALITIDES

AESHA SHAH AND JESSICA DEITRICK

Immune-mediated encephalitis describes a group of heterogeneous autoimmune conditions in which the development of antibodies for different neuroreceptors leads to encephalitis. Symptoms can mimic a number of neurologic and psychiatric conditions.

Autoimmune encephalitis may be associated with viral triggers, paraneoplastic syndromes, or underlying autoimmune conditions. Often, these conditions begin with a prodrome of viral-like symptoms including fever, headache, and malaise before transitioning to a constellation that may include marked behavioral changes, memory loss, seizures, and dysautonomia. This disease process can present at any age and demographic but occurs most commonly in females younger than 45 years old.

PATHOPHYSIOLOGY

Pathophysiology varies depending on the underlying mechanism of the encephalopathy. In cases triggered by viral infection, immune response to common viruses is theorized to trigger development of autoantibodies to cell surface proteins, neuroreceptors such as dopamine-2 receptors, or myelin components such as NMDA and AMPA. The action of these autoantibodies leads to inflammatory changes in the CNS. Alternatively, in paraneoplastic encephalopathy, the underlying neoplasm develops antigens typically found in the CNS that act intracellularly, causing an immune response resulting in neuronal injury and destruction. Last, encephalopathy may be triggered by underlying autoimmune disease secondary to the creation of autoantibodies.

CLINICAL PRESENTATION

Patients may present to the ED with a wide variety of chief complaints including confusion, disorientation, memory deficit, and delusions or hallucinations or other symptoms mimicking psychiatric complaints. Late in the disease course, seizures, movement disorders including rigidity, tremor, and bradykinesia are possible. Later still, autonomic instability including temperature dysregulation, hypoventilation, blood pressure instability, or cardiac arrhythmia may develop. Classically, symptoms are progressive, from vague or generalized early in the disease process to more striking later in the course.

Prodromal viral or viral-like symptoms have often resolved by the time symptoms of encephalitis present and may therefore not be uncovered without a careful history. Classically, viral-like symptoms precede encephalopathy by at least 1 to 2 weeks. As symptoms can range from minor behavioral changes to catatonia and coma depending on the time of presentation, family or other contacts may be the only available source of history. In some cases, paraneoplastic encephalopathy may be the presenting symptom of malignancy. A thorough examination to rule out infection and toxic or metabolic encephalopathy is important and a careful neurologic exam is particularly critical. Overall, an emergency physician must have a high index of suspicion when evaluating patients demonstrating sudden changes from their baseline associated with subtle neurologic signs and symptoms.

DIAGNOSIS

Overall, proposed diagnostic criteria include subacute onset of personality change or change in level of consciousness including memory deficit, psychiatric symptoms, or seizures. Classically these symptoms progress within a time frame of a few weeks, but less than 3 months. At least one of the following—focal clinical CNS event, abnormal EEG, abnormal MRI, or CSF pleocytosis—is needed to firmly make the diagnosis and exclusion of alternate causes.

Patients with unexplained encephalopathy require a broad workup to identify reversible causes of altered mental status. It is reasonable to obtain electrolytes, thyroid studies, and screen for toxic substances. Likewise, a thorough infectious workup is recommended. It is reasonable to pursue a lumbar puncture for CSF analysis. CSF analysis may reveal lymphopleocytosis and elevated protein levels or can be completely normal. In the case of ADEM, oligoclonal bands or white blood cell pleocytosis may be seen. Assessing specifically for oligoclonal bands may increase the likelihood of diagnosis early in the course as the remainder of the CSF studies will typically be normal.

Neuroimaging should be pursued for patients with unexplained altered mental status. At minimum, a noncontrast CT of the head should be performed, although contrasted studies are indicated in immunocompromised patients or those with risk factors for focal CNS infection. Venography, either CT or MRI, should be considered in patients with risk factors for hypercoagulability. Ultimately, an MRI study with and without contrast with T2/FLAIR will be needed to make the diagnosis. Suggestive findings include intracellular edema manifesting as a T2 hyperintense signal. In patients with risk factors for HSV encephalitis, the MRI will often show abnormalities in the temporal lobes. In some cases, even an MRI can be negative.

Often, a broad workup in the ED will reveal no abnormalities. Formal diagnosis requires specific receptor testing and autoantibody testing in CSF or brain biopsy. From the perspective of the emergency physician, this is a diagnosis of exclusion.

MANAGEMENT

Management in the ED should be focused on stabilization and may chiefly consist of controlling symptoms to facilitate a safe and complete workup. This may include pharmacologic treatment of agitation, hallucinations, anxiety, or delirium. Pharmacologic treatment of seizures in these cases is identical to the management of other seizures with benzodiazepines and second- and third-line antiepileptics as needed. Medication options for agitation include first/second-generation antipsychotics, benzodiazepines, or ketamine. Airway management may be required if the patient requires sedating doses of medication to prevent harm to themselves or others. If a viral trigger or concurrent bacterial or fungal infection is identified, treat with the appropriate antimicrobials. Treatment with IVIG or plasmapheresis may be induced but are rarely started in the ED and should only be considered on the advice of neurology. Screening for occult neoplasm may be done after admission. Finally, persistent alteration in consciousness in the setting of a negative workup, particularly if the clinical suspicion is high for encephalitis, should prompt the emergency physician to seek the consultation of neurology and transfer if necessary.

DISPOSITION

Virtually all patients with unexplained encephalitis or multifocal unexplained neurologic findings will require admission. Advanced neuroimaging may require sedation, and CSF testing beyond basic evaluation for cell count, glucose, protein, and culture will take time to return. If these resources are not available, the patient should be transferred once it is safe to do so.

PEDIATRIC CONSIDERATIONS

Immune-mediated encephalitis, particularly ADEM, should also be considered in children with multifocal neurologic deficits and acute encephalopathy. The typical age of presentation is 3 to 7 years and there is a female predominance. ADEM in children classically presents after infection or vaccination. Common infections associated with ADEM include varicella, measles, smallpox, herpes simplex virus, enterovirus, coxsackievirus, EBV, CMV, *Campylobacter jejuni*, mycoplasma, Lyme disease, *Streptococcus pyogenes*, and malaria. Vaccines associated with ADEM include those for measles-mumps-rubella, smallpox, diphtheria-pertussis-tetanus, hepatitis B, rabies, and human papillomavirus.

Symptoms at presentation include fever, seizures, and ataxia as well as pyramidal symptoms including spasticity, weakness, hyperreflexia, and bradykinesia. In the very young, findings of inappropriate irritability or lethargy may be the only signs suggestive of encephalitis. As in adults, other causes of encephalopathy including infection or toxidrome must be ruled out prior to establishing the diagnosis. Likewise, CSF studies, EEG, and MRI are ultimately needed to verify the diagnosis.

The first-line treatment for ADEM in children is high-dose corticosteroids with the second line consisting of IVIG therapy or plasma exchange. Pediatric patients should be admitted or transferred to a center with child neurology availability.

PEARLS

- Consider the diagnosis of immune-mediated encephalopathy in patients who present with viral prodromal symptoms or headache and fever followed by marked behavioral changes/psychiatric illness and dysautonomia over a period of weeks to a few months.
- Multiple different, common viruses have been associated with acute encephalitis as have paraneoplastic syndromes and autoimmune diseases.
- ED workup should exclude other causes of acute altered mental status, particularly reversible causes; urgent consultation with neurology or transfer to a facility with neurology services available is indicated.
- ADEM is a diagnosis to consider in children, especially if they are presenting with multifocal neurologic deficits and encephalopathy after recent infection or vaccination.

Suggested Readings

Ball C, Fisicaro R, Morris L, et al. Brain on fire: an imaging-based review of autoimmune encephalitis. *Clin Imaging*. 2022;84:1-30.

Graus F, Titulaer MJ, Balu R, et al. A clinical approach to diagnosis of autoimmune encephalitis. *Lancet Neurol*. 2016;15(4):391-404. PMID: 26906964.

Hermetter C, Fazekas F, Hochmeister S. Systematic review: syndromes, early diagnosis, and treatment in autoimmune encephalitis. *Front Neurol*. 2018;9:706. PMID: 30233481.

Kassif O, Orbach R, Rimon A, Scolnik D, Glatstein M. Acute disseminated encephalomyelitis in children—clinical and MRI decision making in the emergency department. *Am J Emerg Med*. 2019;37(11);2004-2007.

Massa S, Fracchiolla A, Neglia C, Argentiero A, Esposito S. Update on acute disseminated encephalomyelitis in children and adolescents. *Children (Basel)*. 2021;8(4):280. PMID: 33917395.

Newman MP, Blum S, Wong RC, et al. Autoimmune encephalitis. *Intern Med J*. 2016;46(2): 148-157. PMID: 26899887.

Venkatesan A, Michael BD, Probasco JC, Geocadin RG, Solomon T. Acute encephalitis in immunocompetent adults. *Lancet*. 2019;393(10172):702-716. PMID: 30782344.

151

How Should You Evaluate Shortness of Breath in a Patient Post Lung Transplant?

Nathan J. Morrison and Jordan B. Schooler

Lung transplantation remains an approach to improve the overall health, quality of life, and life expectancy in patients suffering from COPD, ILD, CF, non-CF bronchiectasis, PAH, thoracic malignancy, and other end-stage lung diseases. The criteria and considerations of lung transplantation are an evolving field, with 2,597 adult and 36 pediatric recipients across 68 medical centers in the United States in 2020. These transplants are associated with a variety of complex complications that can be seen in EDs across the world.

Shortness of breath in patients that have received a lung transplant must be evaluated in the context of the initial impression, timing since transplantation, and suspected source, with consideration of their physiologic and immunologic changes after transplantation.

Initial Impression

As with any patient presenting to the ED, the primary survey and interpretation of vital signs are of the utmost priority. Immediate life threats such as pulmonary embolism, myocardial infarction, tension pneumothorax, and cardiac tamponade must not be overlooked. A key difference in the patient post a lung transplant is immunosuppression: This both increases the risk of infection as well as alters the normal response, increasing the likelihood of atypical presentations. Immunosuppression also causes unique complications of its own. After initial stabilization, it is essential that the clinician consider a broad differential diagnosis and has a low threshold for testing.

Infection and Malignancy

Infection is the most common complication in lung transplant recipients. The advancement of antirejection regimens has decreased the risk of organ rejection at the cost of worsening potential immunosuppression. In the acute phase, or the first 30 days after transplant, donor organ bacteria including MRSA, VRE, tuberculosis, *Candida*, and toxoplasmosis or Chagas disease can be considered as sources. Nosocomial infections including aspiration pneumonia or superinfection of lung graft tissue may also contribute. In the subacute phase, or 1 to 6 months following transplant, opportunistic infections begin to predominate. *Pneumocystis jirovecii*, *Histoplasmosis*, *Coccidioides*, CMV, tuberculosis, EBV, or host reactivation of infections becomes common. Six months after transplantation, community-acquired infections tend to predominate, including common respiratory viruses, such as influenza virus, coronaviruses, and RSV, and bacterial pneumonias including pneumococcus and *Legionella*. In addition, immunosuppressive agents increase the risk of new malignancy, occurring in 24% of recipients within 5 years of lung transplantation. Posttransplant lymphoproliferative disorder is the most common transplant-associated malignancy, often but not always associated with EBV infection.

Rejection

The most feared complication for organ recipients is rejection of the donor organ, which can present with shortness of breath, occurring in up to 30% of recipients within the first year. Common immunosuppressive agents include calcineurin inhibitors such as tacrolimus, as well as mycophenolate and prednisone. Rejection is classically divided into three stages: Hyperacute rejection occurs in minutes to hours and involves preexisting antibodies; acute rejection occurs within 6 months and is divided into acute cellular rejection involving lymphocytes or antibody-mediated rejection; and chronic rejection is after 6 months, again both cell and antibody mediated.

Rejection may present only with dyspnea or with other respiratory symptoms such as cough or wheezing. These patients will often display eosinophilia, and changes may be seen on CT chest but definitive diagnosis generally requires biopsy.

Mechanical Complications

The surgical technique to graft donor lungs involves the anastomosis of the donor to recipient trachea, donor right atrium to recipient right atrium, and pulmonary veins via atrial cuff to the left atrium. Tracheal or bronchial stenosis may occur secondary to inflammation and the formation of granulation tissue, typically weeks to months after transplant with prevalence up to 30%. Airway anastomotic dehiscence is rarer at 2% to 18%, presenting with pneumothorax. Both pulmonary arterial and venous anastomoses may also have dehiscence leading to bleeding, or stenosis can cause hypoxia, right heart strain, and graft loss. Of note, chronic right heart strain may have been present preoperatively and so interpretation of bedside or formal echocardiography may be difficult in this population. In an estimated 3% to 9% of cases, phrenic nerve injury may occur during operative placement of the lungs, presenting as dyspnea, hypoventilation, and hemidiaphragm elevation, although this would normally be seen in the immediate postoperative period.

Management

A primary survey of the patient may determine the hospital course if early intubation and mechanical ventilation is required for airway protection. Remember that occult pneumothorax may occur, leading to decompensation of lung transplant recipients requiring positive pressure ventilation. Broad-spectrum antibiotics should be started promptly following blood cultures in such recipients presenting to the ED with dyspnea. These should include coverage for MRSA and pseudomonas as well as atypical organisms; vancomycin, piperacillin-tazobactam, and azithromycin would be one reasonable set, although culture data for the patient should be utilized if available. Consultation with the patient's transplant team is strongly advised, as they may have insight into the patient's course and particular risk factors and be able to assist with disposition from the ED. Transfer to a transplant center and hospitalization is often necessary. These patients often require bronchoscopy with bronchoalveolar lavage and biopsies to identify infectious organisms, evaluate for rejection, and visualize tissue changes within the respiratory tract.

Considerations for laboratory testing include the following:

- *Imaging*: Chest x-ray should always be done. If the finding is negative or equivocal, then CT chest is advised as this may reveal occult pneumonia and may also better characterize findings as likely bacterial, fungal, atypical, or rejection.
- *Blood*: Order CBC with differential, complete metabolic panel, blood cultures, lactic acid level, CMV PCR, *Coccidioides*, *Aspergillus* antigen, and PPD or QuantiFERON

assay. Levels of immunosuppression medication are often ordered, but these are only clinically useful if timed as a trough or if adherence is in question.
- *Urine*: urine *Legionella*, histoplasmosis, and pneumococcal antigens
- *Respiratory*: respiratory viral panel, acid-fast bacillus and fungus smear and culture

PEARLS

- The number of lung transplant recipients continues to rise, making it important to be aware of their unique challenges.
- Immunosuppression increases the likelihood of infection or malignancy in transplant recipients, and these conditions may present atypically.
- Maintain a low threshold for lab testing, CT imaging, and broad-spectrum antibiotic coverage in these patients.
- Early consultation with the patient's transplant team will improve outcomes and assist in disposition.

Suggested Readings

Leard LE, Holm AM, Valapour M, et al. Consensus document for the selection of lung transplant candidates: an update from the International Society for Heart and Lung Transplantation. *J Heart Lung Transplant*. 2021;40(11):1349-1379.

Long B, Koyfman A. The emergency medicine approach to transplant complications. *Am J Emerg Med*. 2016;34(11):2200-2208.

Park MS. Medical complications of lung transplantation. *J Chest Surg*. 2022;55(4):338-356.

Suh JW. Surgical complications affecting the early and late survival rates after lung transplantation. *J Chest Surg*. 2022;55(4):332-337.

Valapour M, Lehr CJ, Skeans MA, et al. OPTN/SRTR 2020 annual data report: lung. *Am J Transplant*. 2022;22(Suppl 2):438-518.

Weill D. Lung transplantation: indications and contraindications. *J Thorac Dis*. 2018;10(7): 4574-4587.

152

What Do You Need to Know About the Sick Liver Transplant Patient?

David Basile and Annahieta Kalantari

The liver is the second most commonly transplanted organ after the kidney. The number of liver transplants has steadily increased since the first successful case in 1963, with more than 8,000 procedures done in 2020 and more than 90,000 living liver transplant recipients. The overall survival rate is 90% at 1 year and 70% at 5 years. Up to 40% of them will present to the ED within the first year of transplant, with a 75% admission rate. These patients can present with several issues including rejection, infection, drug

TABLE 152.1	SIGNIFICANCE OF TIMING IN A TRANSPLANT	
TIME	COMPLICATION	CONSIDERATIONS
Younger than 1 mo	■ Postsurgical bleeding ■ Postsurgical infections or health care–acquired infections ■ Common infections	■ Assess for tachycardia, hypotension, shortness of breath, dizziness, and fatigue. ■ Assess incision site redness or purulence and any drains in place. ■ Consider other infectious sources.
1-6 mo	■ Biliary complications: leakage, stricture, bile duct obstruction, biloma ■ Vascular complications: hepatic artery thrombosis, portal vein thrombosis, hepatic artery stenosis ■ Common infections ■ Opportunistic infections caused by *Candida*, *Aspergillus*, *Cryptococcus*, *Pneumocystis*, *Nocardia*, *Toxoplasma*, *Cryptosporidium*, *Giardia*, and *Clostridium difficile* ■ Viral infections: CMV, EBV, polyomavirus/BK (more common in the kidney) ■ Acute rejection (within first 12 mo)	■ Biliary: Assess for jaundice, obtain hepatic panel with direct bilirubin, and may need ERCP. ■ Vascular: ultrasound with Doppler; consider vascular surgery consultation. ■ Infectious workup including CBC, blood cultures, urine, and chest x-ray, can consider serologies but less helpful in the ED ■ Rejection: hepatic panel including GGT; may need biopsy
Older than 1 yr	■ Chronic rejection ■ Common infections ■ Opportunistic infections ■ Reactivation illnesses: hepatitis B and C, tuberculosis, varicella, PSC, PBC, autoimmune hepatitis, HCC	■ Consider metabolic changes from transplant surgery as causes. ■ Inquire why the patient underwent transplant. Recurrence illnesses will likely require biopsies for confirmation.

toxicities, and postoperative complications. The timing of the patient's transplant is critical in determining the possible etiology of complications (**Table 152.1**).

ASSESSING THE LIVER TRANSPLANT RECIPIENT

Caring for the sick post liver transplant patient requires consideration of a broad differential diagnosis, as they are prone to common illnesses in addition to illnesses and complications related to their transplant status. Overall, initial resuscitation is similar to that in nontransplant cases when addressing ABCs including medication choice in intubation, as well as, fluid and vasopressor choices in hypotension and shock. Notably, however, patients presenting in acute graft failure are more likely to be coagulopathic and hypoglycemic. Inquire about symptoms, such as fever, rash, diarrhea, jaundice, and abdominal pain, although many of these symptoms are nonspecific.

In the early postoperative period, bleeding, thrombosis, graft dysfunction, and infections can occur. Most bleeding in the early postoperative period is due to dehiscence of vascular anastomoses. Typically, this occurs while the patient is still admitted posttransplant, but later hepatic artery rupture can present with acute hypovolemic shock. Upper or lower GI bleeding should be managed as usual but these can be signs of graft dysfunction. Hepatic artery thrombosis that causes necrosis of bile ducts with subsequent graft failure, bile leak, abscess, and sepsis as well as portal vein thrombosis, which can present with abdominal pain, dyspepsia, ascites, and fever, can also be early complications. Acute graft failure can present similarly to acute liver failure with hypoglycemia, encephalopathy, coagulopathy, and hemodynamic instability. Graft failure typically occurs in the first weeks after transplant and is commonly caused by graft nonfunction with unclear cause. Early biliary complications can include bile leaks and obstruction. These often present with peritonitis and intra-abdominal abscess. Acute rejection within the first few weeks typically presents with jaundice, right upper quadrant pain, malaise, and fever; but these may be asymptomatic, with elevations in liver enzymes being the only clue.

Later complications, occurring more than a year after transplantation, include chronic rejection that may present indolently with low-grade fever, jaundice, right upper quadrant pain, and fatigue. Progressive development of dark urine and clay-colored stools may also occur.

Post the transplant, patients can still experience drug-induced, viral, or autoimmune acute liver failure. Inquire about sick contacts, travel, exposures to foods and animals, and prior infections. Ask about current medications, dosages, recent changes in medication, medication adherence, and history of rejection. Also, review other medical problems and medications as immunosuppressants can cause renal insufficiency, hypertension, diabetes mellitus, and bone density changes through a form of posttransplant metabolic syndrome.

Conduct a thorough physical exam. Review vital signs looking for fevers, tachycardia, or hypotension. In the early postoperative period, it is important to assess surgical sites for signs of infection. Jaundice within the first year of transplant can indicate postoperative complications such as biliary strictures, leaks, or bilomas. Signs of rejection can include tenderness at the graft site, jaundice, fever, ascites, and hepatosplenomegaly. Graft-versus-host disease can also present with painful or pruritic maculopapular rash along the palms, soles, shoulders, ears, or neck. Some immunosuppressive medications can cause neurologic changes, such as psychosis, tremors, seizures, and altered mental status.

Transplant recipients require broader workups compared to other patients, both due to anatomic changes from surgery and their immunosuppressed status. At a minimum, one should obtain a CBC, CMP, lipase, and PT/INR. Measurement of GGT and direct bilirubin may be helpful. All can serve as markers of rejection and graft dysfunction, especially when compared to previous baseline measurements.

If infection is a concern, brisk initiation of broad-spectrum antimicrobials is indicated. Obtain blood cultures, urinalysis with culture, lactic acid, chest x-ray, and CT imaging of the abdomen/pelvis. CT can also assess for anatomic changes. Sampling and culture of ascites is also indicated. Ultrasound duplexes are better at identifying vascular complications, such as thrombosis or artery stenosis. If there is a suspected neurologic infection, then a head CT before a lumbar puncture should be considered. Immunosuppression drug levels can be obtained, such as tacrolimus levels, but have limited use if not obtained at the therapeutic trough window (12 to 24 hours from last dose). Serologic titers for viruses can be obtained with herpes viruses being the most common, especially CMV. It is not uncommon for an ERCP to be needed to fully assess the liver transplant anatomy. Lastly, biopsy is the definitive diagnostic to assess for rejection.

PEDIATRICS

Liver transplants in children are commonly seen in those younger than 2 years of age and adolescents, and account for 7% to 8% of all transplants each year. Biliary atresia is the most common condition necessitating transplant in children followed by acute liver failure, which is commonly either drug induced or undetermined in etiology. Survival is at 95% at 1 year and 85% at 5 years. Children can experience the same complications from liver transplant as adults. Abnormal liver enzymes are common in long-term pediatric liver transplant survivors.

Adolescents are less likely to be adherent to their immunosuppressive regimens, placing them at increased risk for rejection.

PEARLS

- Resuscitate liver transplant recipients as you would any other patient, while also accounting for possible coagulopathy from graft failure.
- Establish a timeline since transplant to guide workup for possible etiologies of the patient's presentation and involve the patient's transplant team.
- Overall, consider infectious and other causes of liver injury as well as transplant rejection.
- Utilize CT imaging for anatomic changes and pathology and ultrasound for vascular complications.

Suggested Readings

Choudhary NS, Saigal S, Bansal RK, et al. Acute and chronic rejection after liver transplantation: what a clinician needs to know. *J Clin Exp Hepatol*. 2017;7(4):358-366.

Long B, Koyfman A. The emergency medicine approach to transplant complications. *Am J Emerg Med*. 2016;34(11):2200-2208. https://www.clinicalkey.es/playcontent/1-s2.0-S0735675716305411

McElroy LM, Schmidt KA, Richards CT, et al. Early postoperative emergency department care of abdominal transplant recipients. *Transplantation*. 2015;99(8):1652-1657.

Rawal N, Yazigi N. Pediatric liver transplantation. *Pediatr Clin North Am*. 2017;64(3):677-684.

SECTION XII
INFECTIOUS DISEASE

153

Don't Miss Acute Retroviral Syndrome

Sally Graglia

ARS is the clinical manifestation of an acute infection with HIV. The term ARS is often used interchangeably with a variety of other terms including acute HIV and primary HIV. Regardless of semantics, ARS is due to a surge in viremia and refers to the symptomatic illness during the initial virus-host interaction.

ARS is estimated to occur in more than 50% and up to 93% of patients with new HIV but is challenging to diagnose. Common symptoms of ARS are nonspecific including fever, fatigue, myalgias, lymphadenopathy, pharyngitis, rash, and headache. Present in more than 70% of cases, fever and malaise are the most common symptoms. Lymphadenopathy is nontender and can be present in the axillary, cervical, and occipital nodes. Pharyngitis usually presents without tonsillar enlargement or exudates. The rash is generally morbilliform or maculopapular and often involves the trunk. Headaches are commonly retrobulbar, exacerbated by eye movement. Gastrointestinal symptoms include nausea, diarrhea, and anorexia with associated weight loss. Whether related to HIV or a concurrent STI, painful mucocutaneous ulcerations of the oral mucosa, anus, penis, or esophagus are among the most distinctive manifestations. In rare cases, ARS can present as organ failure, stroke-like syndromes with cranial or peripheral nerve palsies, anemia, thrombocytopenia, the unmasking of malignancies, and even OIs.

Importantly, the clinical manifestation of ARS can be easily attributed to a variety of viral illnesses such as COVID-19, influenza, infectious mononucleosis, CMV, EBV, herpes, varicella, or hepatitis. Because of the nonspecific presentation, it is likely no surprise that the diagnosis of ARS is missed in up to 75% of patients.

Signs and symptoms typically occur 1 to 4 weeks following HIV exposure and can last from a few days to several weeks. Patients may not feel comfortable disclosing personal risk factors for the acquisition of HIV or may not know that certain activities such as receptive oral sex place them at risk for HIV. Thus, clinician suspicion for the disease, recognition of possible clinical manifestations, and a low threshold to screen patients can lead to early detection, notification, and treatment.

The laboratory diagnosis can seem as elusive as the presenting symptoms and signs of ARS. HIV RNA is the first laboratory finding in an acute HIV infection, detectable 10 to 11 days after acute infection. p24 antigen is the next marker, detectable 4 to 10 days later. IgM antibodies become detectable 3 to 5 days after that and are gradually replaced by IgG antibodies, which appear 2 to 6 weeks after initial HIV RNA. Since ARS is seen in patients immediately after acquisition of HIV, they will generally have a high HIV RNA level at the time of presentation but will not have detectable p24 antigens or HIV antibodies. Thus, a patient with ARS will likely not yet have a positive HIV-1/2 antigen-antibody immunoassay. Despite this, the CDC and the APHL recommend HIV-1/2 antigen-antibody immunoassays as the preferred initial HIV screening test. Given these timeframes and the potential for false negatives, providers should also test for serum HIV RNA-1/2 in any patient with a high concern for ARS.

ART is recommended for all individuals with HIV and should be initiated as soon as possible after an HIV diagnosis, ideally on the same day. First, initiation of ART can mitigate ARS symptoms. Second, the rapid initiation of treatment can minimize immunologic damage during the acute phase of the infection. Third, there is evidence to suggest that early treatment initiation can diminish the size of the latent HIV reservoir, which has implications on future care. Finally, and perhaps most importantly from a public health perspective, immediate initiation of treatment can decrease the viral load of patients with ARS and increase awareness of HIV-positive status. Both of these factors can save lives and greatly limit the spread of HIV. Due to the high viral load associated with ARS, the highest HIV transmission rates are a result of individuals with acute HIV who are unaware of their status. Accordingly, the CDC estimates that 37.6% of all new HIV infections in 2016 were the result of individuals who did not know their HIV status.

If a diagnosis of ARS is made, screening for other STIs should be performed if it was not already done. Genotypic drug resistance testing should be obtained in all patients with a new diagnosis of HIV; however, ART can be initiated prior to these results with the eventual referral and involvement of ID specialists for ongoing management. The following ART regimen options are recommended for individuals diagnosed with ARS in whom resistance is not known:

- Bictegravir-tenofovir alafenamide-emtricitabine
- Dolutegravir with tenofovir alafenamide or tenofovir DF plus emtricitabine or lamivudine
- Boosted darunavir with tenofovir alafenamide or tenofovir DF plus emtricitabine or lamivudine

Of note, patients with symptoms and signs of OIs or active tuberculosis should have thoughtful management of concurrent conditions prior to management with ARTs and in collaboration with an ID specialist. Patients who were on PrEP and those who are pregnant or have child-bearing potential should be given special consideration.

PEARLS

- ARS should be considered as a part of the differential diagnosis in all patients presenting with nonspecific symptoms or being diagnosed with a nonspecific viral illness.
- The diagnosis of ARS is missed in up to 75% of patients.
- HIV RNA will be positive in ARS but traditional antibody testing may not yet be positive early in the disease process.
- For individuals diagnosed with ARS, early ART may improve symptoms and is critical in reducing the transmission of HIV.
- Genotypic drug resistance testing should be ordered but should not delay initiation of ART.

Acknowledgments

I gratefully acknowledge the contributions of previous edition authors, Adeolu Ogunbodede and Joseph P. Martinez, as portions of their chapter have been retained in this revision.

Suggested Readings

Clinicalinfo.gov. Guidelines for the use of antiretroviral agents in adults and adolescents with HIV. Accessed March 2023. https://clinicalinfo.hiv.gov/en/guidelines/hiv-clinical-guidelines-adult-and-adolescent-arv/early-acute-and-recent-hiv-infection

Fauci A. Immunopathogenic mechanisms of HIV infection. *Ann Intern Med.* 1996;124:654-663.

Kahn JO, Walker BD. Acute human immunodeficiency virus type 1 infection. *N Engl J Med.* 1998;339:33-39.

National HIV Curriculum. https://www.hiv.uw.edu

National HIV Curriculum. Acute and recent HIV infection. https://www.hiv.uw.edu/go/screening-diagnosis/acute-recent-early-hiv/core-concept/all#clinical-manifestations-acute-retroviral-syndrome

National HIV Curriculum. HIV diagnostic testing. https://www.hiv.uw.edu/go/screening-diagnosis/diagnostic-testing/core-concept/all#timing-laboratory-markers-following-hiv-infection

Pilcher C. Detection of acute infections during HIV testing in North Carolina. *N Engl J Med.* 2005;352:1873-1883.

154

Understand When and How to Initiate HIV Post-Exposure Prophylaxis in the Emergency Department

Philana H. Liang and Stephen Y. Liang

ART has revolutionized the treatment and prevention of HIV infection. Individuals can become infected with HIV through condomless sex in consensual, nonconsensual, and transactional contexts, or through percutaneous and body substance exposures. PEP and PrEP are important tools in HIV prevention. Emergency physicians should be able to recognize high-risk exposures, know when to initiate HIV PEP, and refer patients for postexposure follow-up when appropriate.

Exposures Associated With HIV Transmission

Sexual transmission of HIV is greatest with receptive anal intercourse (138 infections per 10,000 exposures), followed by insertive anal intercourse (11 infections per 10,000 exposures), receptive penile-vaginal intercourse (8 infections per 10,000 exposures), and insertive penile-vaginal intercourse (4 infections per 10,000 exposures). The likelihood of HIV transmission with receptive oral or insertive oral intercourse is even lower, but not zero. Factors that impact HIV transmission include the presence of acute retroviral syndrome, advanced HIV, high viremia, concomitant genital ulcer disease, and involvement of traumatic injuries or wounds. Sexual assault involving anal or genital trauma or multiple assailants has also been associated with increased risk of HIV transmission.

Exposure to blood, tissue, and certain body fluids (eg, cerebrospinal, synovial, pleural, pericardial, peritoneal, or amniotic fluid; semen or vaginal secretions) may result in nonsexual HIV transmission. Saliva, nasal secretions, sputum, sweat, tears, urine, emesis, and feces are unlikely to harbor HIV unless visibly bloody. Exposures involving blood present the greatest risk. With needle sharing during injection drug use, the rate of infection is 63 per 10,000 exposures to an infected source. The risk of HIV transmission with percutaneous exposures (eg, needlestick) is 23 infections per 10,000 exposures. Transmission after percutaneous exposure is more likely with deep penetration, penetration with a device that is visibly contaminated with blood, penetration with a needle placed directly into a vein or an artery, penetration with a hollow-bore needle, or penetration involving a person with advanced HIV or viremia. The risk of HIV transmission from a body substance exposure (eg, splash) involving direct inoculation of mucous membranes or nonintact skin is less than 0.09%. Intact skin is effective protection against HIV infection; therefore, contamination of intact skin with blood or other body fluids is not considered a significant exposure.

INITIATION OF HIV PEP IN THE ED

PEP should be started if the exposure occurred within 72 hours of ED presentation and involves a body fluid known to transmit HIV at a body site capable of serving as a point of entry for HIV. However, initiation of PEP immediately or within the first hours of a significant exposure should be strongly considered whenever possible.

The CDC and the U.S. Public Health Service PEP guidelines recommend a combination of a dual nonnucleoside/tide reverse transcriptase inhibitor with either an integrase inhibitor or a protease inhibitor for 28 days, as highlighted in **Table 154.1**.

Emergency physicians should consult current PEP guidelines to confirm appropriate first-line and alternative regimens, particularly as single tablet regimens become increasingly accessible and accepted. Infectious disease specialists and the National Clinician's Post-Exposure Prophylaxis Hotline (1-888-448-4911) can also aid PEP decision making. Health care work–related exposures should be reported immediately to occupational health. Adherence to and completion of the full 28-day course should be strongly encouraged to maximize benefit. Patients should also be counseled regarding potential side effects. Gastrointestinal intolerance is not infrequent and antiemetic and antidiarrheal medications may improve adherence.

TABLE 154.1 RECOMMENDED HIV PEP REGIMENS FOR CREATININE CLEARANCE IN HEALTHY ADULTS AND ADOLESCENTS

PREFERRED REGIMENS	ALTERNATIVE REGIMEN
Tenofovir DF 300 mg/emtricitabine 200 mg once daily *and* raltegravir 400 mg twice daily	Tenofovir DF 300 mg/emtricitabine 200 mg once daily *and* darunavir 800 mg once daily *and* ritonavir 100 mg once daily
Tenofovir DF 300 mg/emtricitabine 200 mg once daily *and* dolutegravir 50 mg once daily	

The creatinine clearance values mentioned are greater than 60 mL/min.

Patients starting PEP should have a baseline rapid HIV test; however, testing should not delay the first dose. A pregnancy test should be done in patients of childbearing potential. Serum liver enzymes and BUN/creatinine should be performed in the ED as well as at 2 and 4 weeks following PEP initiation to evaluate for drug toxicity. STI screening for chlamydia, gonorrhea, and syphilis should be considered in exposures involving sex or injection drug use. Additional baseline testing for other blood-borne pathogens including hepatitis B and C may also be warranted in these instances as well as after an occupational exposure.

When the HIV status of the source is unknown but the source is available for testing, rapid HIV testing using a high-sensitivity assay should be performed along with testing for hepatitis B and C; syphilis testing may also be considered. If test results are not readily available, initiation of PEP should not be delayed. If a known HIV-infected source has been adherent to ART with an undetectable viral load, the likelihood of HIV transmission is likely low, but PEP should still be offered.

THE IMPORTANCE OF POST-ED VISIT FOLLOW-UP

Most seroconversions occur within 3 months of exposure. Referral to and coordination of postexposure care is critical to optimize patient outcomes and provide appropriate counseling and follow-up testing. Patients who receive PEP may also be offered PrEP on completion. PrEP involves taking antiretroviral medications *before* sexual contact or injection drug use to prevent HIV infection. While there is insufficient evidence demonstrating the effectiveness of PEP in preventing HIV infection from injection drug use, PrEP may be considered a better prevention strategy. When possible, emergency physicians should connect patients to PrEP resources anytime PEP is being considered after a potential HIV exposure.

PEARLS

- PEP is most likely to be effective when started within 72 hours of a high-risk exposure associated with HIV transmission.
- Testing should not delay initiation of PEP in the ED when clinically appropriate.
- Close follow-up for patients started on PEP is needed to monitor for medication adherence, drug toxicities, seroconversion and to provide postexposure counseling.
- PrEP should be considered anytime PEP is being considered following a potential HIV exposure.

SUGGESTED READINGS

Dominguez KL, Smith DK, Vasavi T, et al. Updated guidelines for antiretroviral postexposure prophylaxis after sexual, injection drug use, or other nonoccupational exposure to HIV—United States, 2016. Accessed January 1, 2023. https://stacks.cdc.gov/view/cdc/38856

Kuhar DT, Henderson DK, Struble KA, et al. Updated U.S. Public Health Service guidelines for the management of occupational exposures to human immunodeficiency virus and recommendations for post exposure prophylaxis. *Infect Control Hosp Epidemiol*. 2013; 34(9):875-892.

Patel P, Borkowf CB, Brooks JT, et al. Estimating per-act HIV transmission risk: a systematic review. *AIDS*. 2014;28(10):1509-1519.

155

Toxic Shock Syndrome: Do Not Hesitate—Resuscitate

Olena Kostyuk

TSS is an acute, toxin-mediated illness characterized by fevers, hypotension, multiorgan dysfunction, and a diffuse rash with subsequent desquamation. The annual incidence of TSS varies from 1.5 to 11 cases per 100,000 people, with older adults and young children being the most affected groups.

TSS is most commonly caused by *Staphylococcus aureus* and *Streptococcus pyogenes*. Other less common bacteria that can trigger TSS include *Streptococcus agalactiae*, *Streptococcus viridans*, *Clostridium sordellii*, and Group C and G streptococci. TSS results from an immune response to bacterial toxins that act as superantigens. These superantigens bypass the usual T-cell activation pathways, leading to a cytokine storm and uncontrolled activation of T and B cells. The risk of developing TSS is considerably reduced if one has antibodies against these superantigens. For instance, antibodies against TSST-1, a key superantigen in staphylococcal TSS, are present in more than 90% of adults but are much less common among children.

While TSS was previously associated with the use of high-absorbency tampons, the range of potential triggers has expanded since these products were withdrawn from the market in the early 1980s. Beyond menstrual cases, TSS can now manifest in a variety of scenarios, including, but not limited to, skin and soft tissue infections, localized infections such as pneumonia and pharyngitis, complications from surgical wounds, and postpartum and abortion-related complications, as well as burns. The condition is also associated with the use of foreign objects such as nasal packing or dialysis catheters. Compared to staphylococcal TSS, streptococcal TSS is more often linked to invasive infections, such as cellulitis or necrotizing fasciitis, and generally has a higher rate of severe illness and death.

Presentation

Patients with TSS often exhibit a variety of symptoms due to both toxin secretion and the site of infection. The condition is usually acute in onset and is characterized by a high fever, rash, and hypotension. A prodromal phase may precede this, presenting with chills, myalgias, and gastrointestinal symptoms (nausea, vomiting, diarrhea, and abdominal pain), as well as headaches and a sore throat. This stage is frequently misdiagnosed as a flulike or viral illness, leading to delayed treatment. Initial symptoms can quickly escalate, progressing to diffuse erythroderma accompanied by a rash, watery diarrhea, oliguria, and extremity edema. Neurologic manifestations may include confusion, somnolence, or agitation, with severe neurologic conditions often being attributed to cerebral edema. Cardiopulmonary symptoms may encompass pulmonary edema, decreased cardiac contractility, and pleural effusions. Reduced vascular resistance and increased intravascular leakage contribute to hypotension, which is a key diagnostic criterion.

The characteristic rash in TSS typically presents as a diffuse, red, macular pattern that resembles a sunburn and may be pruritic. The rash often worsens over a 2-week period and can extend to mucous membranes such as the conjunctiva, vaginal mucosa, and oral mucosa. In severe cases, superficial ulcerations may form on these mucosal surfaces, and the rash usually progresses to full-thickness skin peeling within 1 to 3 weeks.

Diagnosis

Early diagnosis is crucial, yet the disease's subtle initial symptoms often make timely identification difficult, contributing to high morbidity and mortality rates. The mortality rate for streptococcal TSS can exceed 50%, while the rate for non-streptococcal TSS is considerably lower, generally falling below 3%. The Centers for Disease Control and Prevention developed diagnostic criteria based on a compilation of physical and laboratory findings. These criteria have been shown to be useful for research but have two main limitations in clinical settings: They are not optimized for early diagnosis and not all cases meet these criteria as the disease evolves.

There is no specific lab test for TSS, but the findings usually reflect the severity of the illness. Laboratory tests may show elevated white blood cell counts with a left shift and neutrophil predominance. Anemia, thrombocytopenia, and abnormal coagulation profiles may mimic disseminated intravascular coagulation. Elevated BUN and creatinine levels indicate renal impairment, while muscle injury can lead to rhabdomyolysis. Common electrolyte imbalances include hyponatremia, hypocalcemia, and hypophosphatemia.

Management

Due to the rapid progression of TSS to multiorgan failure, immediate and aggressive IV hydration is crucial and is often supplemented by respiratory and inotropic support. Initial treatment should focus on source control of soft tissue infections such as necrotizing fasciitis, myositis, and cellulitis, which are frequent origins of the disease, particularly in streptococcal TSS. Rapid diagnostic efforts should concentrate on identifying these sources, which may necessitate emergent CT or MRI scans. Prompt removal of foreign objects is vital, as is surgical consultation for decisions regarding wound debridement.

Initial antibiotic therapy should be broad spectrum, especially in areas where MRSA is prevalent. Vancomycin or linezolid are common first-line options. In addition, several studies have demonstrated improved survival when clindamycin is added to existing antibiotic regimens, owing to its ability to inhibit toxin production. However, clindamycin should not be the sole antibiotic used due to its bacteriostatic nature and the increasing issue of bacterial resistance. Given the risk of polymicrobial infections, the initial antibiotic protocol should also cover gram-negative bacteria. Antibiotics should be adjusted depending on culture results, with the note that blood cultures yield positive results in about 60% of streptococcal TSS cases but in fewer than 5% of staphylococcal TSS cases.

IVIG, administered as a single dose at 1 to 2 g/kg, may be a useful supplementary treatment for neutralizing toxin activity and thereby inhibiting cytokine release, especially in treatment-resistant cases. While most supporting evidence comes from observational studies, IVIG has been linked to lower mortality rates. Corticosteroids may also offer potential benefits, although the supporting data are limited.

> **PEARLS**
>
> - TSS is an acute, toxin-mediated illness primarily due to *S. aureus* and *S. pyogenes*.
> - Beyond its known association with high-absorbency tampons, TSS can result from skin infections, surgical wounds, and foreign objects.
> - Immediate treatment includes aggressive IV hydration, broad-spectrum antibiotics, and respiratory and inotropic support. Supplementary treatments, such as IVIG and, possibly, corticosteroids, may be considered, especially in resistant cases.
> - TSS is a rapidly progressive, life-threatening condition that demands immediate medical action. Its varied triggers and subtle initial symptoms challenge timely diagnosis, emphasizing the need for ongoing research and public awareness.

Suggested Readings

Centers for Disease Control and Prevention. Streptococcal toxic shock syndrome. https://www.cdc.gov/groupastrep/diseases-hcp/Streptococcal-Toxic-Shock-Syndrome.html

Centers for Disease Control and Prevention. Toxic shock syndrome (other than Streptococcal) (TSS) 2011 case definition. https://ndc.services.cdc.gov/case-definitions/toxic-shock-syndrome-2011/

Cook A, Janse S, Watson JR, Erdem G. Manifestations of toxic shock syndrome in children, Columbus, Ohio, USA, 2010-2017. *Emerg Infect Dis*. 2020;26(6):1077-1083.

Gottlieb M, Long B, Koyfman A. The evaluation and management of toxic shock syndrome in the emergency department: a review of the literature. *J Emerg Med*. 2018;54(6):807-814.

Wilkins AL, Steer AC, Smeesters PR, Curtis N. Toxic shock syndrome—the seven Rs of management and treatment. *J Infect*. 2017; 74(Suppl 1):S147-S152.

156

Meningitis Doesn't Have to Be a Pain in the Neck!

Nicholas Macaluso

Infectious meningitis can be caused by a variety of organisms and should be on the differential for any patient with a headache, altered mental status, neck stiffness, or fever, as patients can present along a spectrum from overall well appearing to toxic and nonverbal. Bacterial and viral organisms account for the most common types of infectious meningitis, with fungal and parasitic pathogens representing more rare causes. In general, viral meningitis is a self-limited disease that resolves with supportive care. In contrast, bacterial meningitis is associated with significant morbidity and mortality. This chapter focuses on pearls and pitfalls in the diagnosis and treatment of patients with bacterial meningitis.

PHYSICAL EXAMINATION

It is commonly taught that patients with bacterial meningitis will have nuchal rigidity or present with either the Kernig or Brudzinski signs. Unfortunately, these classic physical examination findings are of limited value in the evaluation of patients with suspected meningitis. In fact, the sensitivity of Kernig, Brudzinski, and nuchal rigidity for meningitis is very low; these signs are present in less than 33% of patients with meningitis. Furthermore, large studies have reported that the classic triad of fever, neck stiffness, and altered mental status is present in just 36% to 58% of patients with meningitis. A comprehensive review by Attia et al evaluated the utility of the physical examination in the diagnosis of patients with confirmed meningitis and found that no individual clinical finding had significant sensitivity or specificity to exclude meningitis. In this study, the highest pooled sensitivities were for headache (0.50; CI, 0.32-0.68) with nausea and vomiting (0.30; CI, 0.22-0.38) following behind. In contrast to nuchal rigidity, Kernig sign, and Brudzinski sign, jolt accentuation (headache exacerbation with horizontal rotation of the head at two rotations per second) has been shown to increase the probability of meningitis in patients with a fever and headache. In fact, the sensitivity of jolt accentuation in the diagnosis of meningitis has been found to be 100%, with a specificity of 54%.

DIAGNOSTIC TESTING

Given the limitations of the physical examination, an LP should be performed to confirm the diagnosis of meningitis. The LP should be performed as soon as possible to maximize the diagnostic yield of a culture of the CSF. The CSF can be sterilized within hours of initiating antibiotic therapy. Importantly, antibiotic administration should not be delayed to perform the LP.

An elevated opening pressure, cloudy CSF, CSF pleocytosis (ie, elevated white blood cell count), elevated CSF protein, low CSF glucose, and a CSF glucose-to-blood glucose ratio of less than 0.4 support the diagnosis of bacterial meningitis. In general, these CSF studies should be considered as methods to confirm the diagnosis of meningitis (positive likelihood ratios >10) rather than methods to exclude the diagnosis (negative likelihood ratios <0.1). Normal or low CSF white blood cell counts may be seen in immunocompromised patients, those presenting with early bacterial meningitis, or those who have been partially treated (ie, with oral antibiotics).

For most patients with meningitis, a CT of the head is not required prior to the performance of an LP. Concerning patient characteristics and findings that should prompt a CT head prior to LP include immunosuppression, history of CNS disease (ie, mass lesion, stroke, or focal infection), focal abnormality on the neurologic examination, papilledema on funduscopy, or new-onset seizure that occurs within 1 week of presentation.

TREATMENT

In most cases, the clinical presentation and results of CSF analysis are sufficient to guide treatment and disposition. For patients in whom there is clinical ambiguity, it is best to administer antimicrobial therapy while awaiting the results of CSF culture, as any delay in antibiotics in cases of confirmed meningitis is associated with a significant increase in mortality. Importantly, antibiotic medications are given at higher doses when there is concern for meningitis. For example, 2 g of ceftriaxone or 2 g of cefotaxime should be administered to immunocompetent patients younger than 50 years to treat meningitis due to *Streptococcus pneumoniae* or *Neisseria meningitidis*. Vancomycin should be administered in suspected cases of methicillin-resistant *Staphylococcus aureus*, whereas ampicillin should be administered to patients with meningitis due to suspected *Listeria monocytogenes*. Prophylaxis for close contacts of those diagnosed with *N. meningitidis*—commonly defined as those with prolonged exposure (>8 hours) within 3 feet of the patient—can be achieved with a single dose of intramuscular ceftriaxone (250 mg for 15 years or older, and 125 mg for younger than 15 years).

In addition to antibiotic therapy, the administration of dexamethasone should be considered in cases of bacterial meningitis. Corticosteroids have been shown to reduce hearing loss and neurologic sequelae in patients with bacterial meningitis. Importantly, corticosteroids have not been shown to reduce patient mortality and have even been associated in some studies with increased mortality in meningitis caused by *Listeria*.

PEARLS

- Do not exclude bacterial meningitis based on the absence of classical findings such as nuchal rigidity, Kernig sign, or Brudzinski sign.
- The presence of jolt accentuation increases the likelihood of meningitis in patients with fever and headache.
- Perform an LP to confirm the diagnosis of meningitis.
- Obtain a CT head prior to LP in immunosuppressed patients or those with a history of CNS, focal neurologic abnormalities, findings of papilledema, or new-onset seizures that occur within 1 week of presentation.
- Have a low threshold to administer antibiotics in patients with suspected meningitis—don't wait on the LP.

Acknowledgments

I gratefully acknowledge the contributions of previous edition authors, Nick Tsipis and Liesl A. Curtis, as portions of their chapter have been retained in this revision.

Suggested Readings

Attia J, Hatala R, Cook DJ, et al. Does this adult patient have acute meningitis? *JAMA*. 1999;282:175-181.

Bhimraj A. Acute community-acquired bacterial meningitis in adults: an evidence-based review. *Cleve Clin J Med*. 2012;79(6):393-400.

Hasbun R. Progress and challenges in bacterial meningitis: a review. *JAMA*. 2022;328: 2147-2154.

Hasbun R, Abrahams J, Jekel J, et al. Computed tomography of the head before lumbar puncture in adults with suspected meningitis. *N Engl J Med*. 2001;345:1727-1733.

Proulx N, Fréchette D, Toye B, et al. Delays in the administration of antibiotics are associated with mortality from adult acute bacterial meningitis. *QJM*. 2005;98:291-298.

Thomas KE, Hasbun R, Jekel J, et al. The diagnostic accuracy of Kernig's sign, Brudzinski's sign, and nuchal rigidity in adults with suspected meningitis. *Clin Infect Dis*. 2002;35:46-52.

157

Avoid These Common Pitfalls in Influenza Treatment

Maryann Mazer-Amirshahi

Influenza is an infectious disease caused by the influenza A and B viruses and results in yearly outbreaks, most notably during the winter months. In general, influenza is a self-limited disease that manifests as respiratory symptoms, myalgias, fatigue, and fevers. Influenza can result in significant morbidity and mortality in high-risk populations, particularly older adults, young children, pregnant women, patients with chronic medical conditions (such as diabetes and underlying lung disease), and the immune compromised. Additional high-risk populations are listed in **Table 157.1**.

The CDC recommends seasonal vaccination against influenza for nearly all patient populations. When acute influenza treatment or prophylaxis is required, there are several therapeutic options, including the neuraminidase inhibitors and baloxavir marboxil, a cap-dependent endonuclease inhibitor. The CDC recommends that patients with suspected or confirmed influenza who require hospitalization, have evidence of a prolonged or complicated infection (ie, pneumonia), and are at high risk receive a neuraminidase inhibitor. The adamantanes (eg, amantadine, rimantadine) are no longer recommended for the treatment of influenza due to limited spectrum of activity and high rates of resistance. For patients without risk factors for complicated illness who present within 48 hours of symptom onset, the emergency provider must weigh the risks, benefits, and availability and cost of therapy.

The neuraminidase inhibitors available in the United States include oseltamivir, zanamivir, and peramivir. Indications, dosing, and adverse effects of all recommended medications are listed in **Table 157.2**. It is important to consider surveillance data, local resistance patterns, and individual patient factors when selecting a medication.

TABLE 157.1 HIGH-RISK POPULATIONS THAT REQUIRE ANTIVIRAL THERAPY

Age younger than 2 yr or older than 65	Metabolic disease (including diabetes mellitus)
Cardiovascular disease (except isolated hypertension)	Morbid obesity (BMI >40)
Chronic liver disease	Nursing home or chronic care facility residents
Chronic renal disease	
Hematologic disease (including sickle cell disease)	Neurologic and neurodevelopmental disease
	Pulmonary disease
Immune compromised states	Pregnant women (or <2 weeks postpartum)
Long-term salicylate therapy	Racial and ethnic minority groups

BMI, body mass index.

TABLE 157.2 COMPARISON OF MEDICATIONS USED FOR INFLUENZA TREATMENT AND PROPHYLAXIS (ADULTS)

DRUG	DOSING	COMMON ADVERSE EFFECTS	SPECIAL CONSIDERATIONS
Baloxavir (oral)	Treatment and prophylaxis: Weight <80 kg: one 40-mg dose Weight >80 kg: one 80 mg dose	Nausea, vomiting, diarrhea, headache; similar to placebo	Avoid administration with cations (calcium, magnesium) as this decreases absorption
Oseltamivir (oral)	Treatment: 75 mg twice daily × 5 d Prophylaxis: 75 mg daily × 5 d	Nausea, vomiting Rare neuropsychiatric effects and skin reactions	First line in pregnancy Dose adjustment for renal impairment
Peramivir (IV)	Treatment: 600 mg IV infusion × 1 dose Not approved for prophylaxis	Diarrhea, injection site reactions Rare neuropsychiatric effects and skin reactions	Alternative for patients that cannot take oral oseltamivir Infuse over 15 min Dose adjustment for renal insufficiency
Zanamivir (inhalation)	Treatment: 10 mg twice daily × 5 d Prophylaxis: 10 mg once daily × 5 d	Bronchospasm Rare neuropsychiatric effects and skin reactions	Avoid in asthma, COPD

COPD, chromic obstructive pulmonary disease.

Oseltamivir (Tamiflu) is administered orally, is well tolerated, and can decrease the time to symptom improvement by approximately 16 hours in outpatients. Additional studies in high-risk and hospitalized patients suggest a decrease in influenza complications, including days hospitalized, mechanical ventilation, and ICU admission. The greatest benefit is noted when therapy is initiated within 48 hours of symptom onset; however, delayed benefits have also been identified.

Zanamivir (Relenza) is administered by inhalation and can reduce time to symptom improvement by approximately 14 hours in outpatients. Zanamivir has not been shown to reduce hospitalizations or influenza complications. Zanamivir can cause bronchospasm and should be avoided in patients with lung disease.

Peramivir (Rapivab) is the most recently approved neuraminidase inhibitor. It is administered as a single intravenous dose of 600 mg. Peramivir was found to be noninferior to oseltamivir for use in outpatients. Peramivir should be considered in patients who cannot take oral medications and when there is concern for medication nonadherence.

Baloxavir (Xofluza) has a unique mechanism of action and is approved as a single dose for the treatment of influenza and for prophylaxis in high-risk individuals. Data demonstrating improved outcomes in hospitalized patients are lacking.

One important consideration that has emerged in recent years is the overlap between influenza and COVID-19 infection. Symptomatic patients should be tested for both viruses as it is difficult to distinguish between the two clinically. While coinfection with influenza and COVID-19 is uncommon, observational studies suggest outcomes are worse than in the setting of infection with a single virus and patients require treatment for both.

Given the variable effectiveness of the influenza vaccine, treatment should not be withheld in high-risk patients when there is a high clinical suspicion of influenza. Hospitalized patients should be treated, preferably with oseltamivir. High-risk patients who are discharged from the ED with antiviral treatment should have close outpatient follow-up.

PEARLS

- While coinfection with COVID-19 is rare, data suggest outcomes are worse, so test for both viruses and treat accordingly.
- Treat all high-risk and hospitalized patients with confirmed influenza regardless of the time of symptom onset.
- Oseltamivir is the treatment of choice in hospitalized patients, as data demonstrating improved outcomes in this population are lacking for the other agents.
- Consider the benefits and harms of treatment in low-risk patients presenting within 48 hours of symptoms onset. Do not treat patients if they present after 48 hours.
- Oseltamivir has been frequently impacted by drug shortages, so consider therapeutic alternatives when access is limited.

Suggested Readings

Chartrand C, Leeflang MM, Minion J, et al. Accuracy of rapid influenza diagnostic tests: a meta-analysis. *Ann Intern Med*. 2012;156(7):500-511.

Dobson J, Whitley RJ, Pocock S, et al. Oseltamivir treatment for influenza in adults: a meta-analysis of randomized controlled trials. *Lancet*. 2015;385(9979):1729-1737.

Muthuri SG, Venkatesan S, Myles PR, et al. Effectiveness of neuraminidase inhibitors in reducing mortality in patients admitted to hospital with influenza A H1N1pdm09 virus infection: a meta-analysis of individual participant data. *Lancet Respir Med*. 2014;2(5):395-404.

Pawlowski C, Silvert E, O'Horo JC, et al. SARS-CoV-2 and influenza coinfection throughout the COVID-19 pandemic: an assessment of coinfection rates, cohort characteristics, and clinical outcomes. *PNAS Nexus*. 2022;1(3):pgac071.

Uyeki TM, Bernstein HH, Bradley JS, et al. Clinical practice guidelines by the Infectious Diseases Society of America: 2018 update on diagnosis, treatment, chemoprophylaxis, and institutional outbreak management of seasonal influenza. *Clin Infect Dis*. 2019;68(6):895-902.

158

Treating Pneumonia in COPD

Diana Ladkany and Jeffrey Dubin

COPD is a general term used to describe several diseases characterized by loss of pulmonary elasticity, alveolar destruction, chronic airway inflammation, fibrosis, and mucous hypersecretion. Most commonly, COPD refers to emphysema and chronic bronchitis.

Chronic pulmonary infections and environmental exposures, most notably cigarette smoking, are the most frequent factors predisposing patients to COPD. This condition is fraught with complications and significant morbidity and mortality including frequent ED visits, hospitalizations, intensive care unit admissions, and noninvasive and invasive mechanical ventilation.

Patients with COPD are particularly susceptible to pulmonary infections and pneumonia, and this is, in part, related to their altered lung flora. These patients are frequently colonized with resistant organisms, and the condition is likely worsened by the chronic use of inhaled corticosteroids that alter the lung epithelium and immunity, providing bacteria a perfect location for proliferation. Viruses are also common culprits and can precipitate a viral pneumonia that is primed for secondary bacterial superinfection. Although *Streptococcus pneumoniae* is the most common pathogen that causes community-acquired pneumonia, many other pathogens play a role in patients with COPD with pneumonia. These include *Haemophilus influenzae*, *Moraxella catarrhalis*, and *Pseudomonas aeruginosa*. These patients are also at high risk for *S. aureus* and gram-negative bacterial infections.

Antibiotics should be chosen to target these common microbes; therefore, a combination regimen is usually selected until sputum culture results (if obtained) can help guide/tailor more specific therapy. Recommended combinations include a beta-lactam or a cephalosporin in conjunction with a macrolide or doxycycline. Monotherapy treatment utilizes a respiratory fluoroquinolone such as levofloxacin or moxifloxacin. Influenza is important to consider during peak seasons as targeted therapy with oseltamivir is available and recommended.

Acute exacerbations of COPD are defined by a rapid increase in COPD symptoms (notably dyspnea) outside of normal variations. Frequent triggers for exacerbations include environmental allergens and infections, especially viral illnesses and pneumonia. Prevention and early appropriate treatment of exacerbations is critical due to the accelerated risk of morbidity and mortality. Azithromycin has been found to have added benefit with reduced exacerbations and improved quality of life and can be considered as an adjunct to treatment during an acute exacerbation. Otherwise, antibiotic choices for pneumonia during an acute exacerbation are the same. Some studies have shown improved outcomes with early antibiotic administration for inpatients admitted for COPD exacerbations and are empirically recommended for those patients that are most likely to have an infectious etiology for their exacerbation, particularly in patients with a change in their sputum production or quality.

PEARLS

- Patients with COPD are particularly susceptible to pulmonary infections and are frequently colonized with resistant organisms.
- Inhaled corticosteroids alter the lung epithelium and immunity, providing bacteria a perfect location for proliferation.
- Sputum culture results can help guide more specific antibiotic therapy.
- Antibiotics are empirically recommended for those patients that are most likely to have an infectious etiology for their COPD exacerbation, particularly in patients with a change in their sputum production or quality.

Suggested Readings

Christenson SA, Smith BM, Bafadhel M, Putcha N. Chronic obstructive pulmonary disease. *Lancet*. 2022;399(10342):2227-2242.

GOLD REPORT 2023. Global initiative for chronic obstructive lung disease. Accessed February 15, 2023. https://goldcopd.org/2023-gold-report-2/

Mandell LA, Wunderink RG, Anzueto A, et al. Infectious Diseases Society of America/American Thoracic Society guidelines on the management of community acquired pneumonia in adults. *Clin Infect Dis*. 2007;44(Suppl 2):S27-S72.

Metlay JP, Waterer GW, Long AC, et al. Diagnosis and treatment of adults with community-acquired pneumonia. An official clinical practice guideline of the American Thoracic Society and Infectious Diseases Society of America. *Am J Respir Crit Care Med*. 2019;200(7):e45-e67.

Restrepo M, Mortensen EM, Pugh JA, et al. COPD is associated with increased mortality in patients with community acquired pneumonia. *Eur Respir J*. 2006;28(2):346-351.

Sethi S, Murphy TF. Acute exacerbations of chronic bronchitis: new developments concerning microbiology and pathophysiology—impact on approaches to risk stratification and therapy. *Infect Dis Clin North Am*. 2004;18(4):861-882.

Sethi S, Murphy TF. Infection in the pathogenesis and course of chronic obstructive pulmonary disease. *N Engl J Med*. 2008;359(22):2355-2365.

159

Know When to Immunize for Mpox

Dan Im

After a prolonged period under the COVID-19 pandemic, our society recently faced another infectious disease threat. Mpox is caused by an orthopoxvirus, similar to smallpox. Mpox has an incubation period of 5 to 21 days. After the incubation period, patients present with varying symptoms such as fevers, chills, and myalgias as well as rashes of different stages. These rashes can be found in several anatomic locations including anogenital and perioral areas. The rash typically begins as painful macules and evolves into papules, vesicles, and pustules that often have central umbilication. The lesions then crust over, dry, and the scab falls off over a course of 1 to 2 weeks. Residual scarring may persist.

Treatment of mpox is largely supportive in nature. Lesions on the oral mucosa, pharynx, and perianal areas can cause significant pain, and those at risk for dehydration may require hospitalization. Tecovirimat, an antiviral therapy that was approved for smallpox, is currently being used for treatment of mpox. Tecovirimat is indicated in those with severe disease such as hemorrhagic disease, large numbers of lesions that become confluent, sepsis, encephalitis, ocular or periorbital infections, or other conditions requiring hospitalization. It is also indicated when the lesions affect anatomic areas that, if scarred or strictured, might result in serious complications, such as the pharynx and anogenital areas. It should be also considered for those who are at high risk, including those who are immunocompromised, patients younger than 1 year, pregnant patients, and those with other skin comorbidities.

Fortunately, a vaccine against both smallpox and mpox had been already approved in the United States in 2019. The JYNNEOS vaccine is a live attenuated smallpox vaccine that has shown efficacy in preventing mpox disease in adults 18 years or older. It is given twice subcutaneously, with 4 weeks between injections. Immunocompromised individuals may have a diminished immune response to the vaccine, but it is not contraindicated in these patients. As of December 2022, a CDC study of males between the ages of 18 and 49 showed that the incidence of mpox was estimated to be 7 to 10 times higher in unvaccinated persons compared to those who received only the first dose and those who were fully vaccinated, respectively.

Current CDC guidelines recommend vaccination against mpox for people who meet the following:

- Have a known or suspected exposure to mpox; it is best to administer the vaccine within 4 days of exposure, but it can be given up to 14 days after exposure.
- Have had a sex partner in the past 2 weeks who was diagnosed with mpox.
- Are gay, bisexual, or other men who have sex with men; or a transgender, nonbinary, or gender-diverse person who in the past 6 months has had either one of the following:
  - A new diagnosis of a sexually transmitted disease
  - More than one sex partner
- Have had sex at a commercial sex venue in the past 6 months.
- Have had sex related to a large commercial event or in a geographic area where mpox virus transmission is occurring.
- Have had a sex partner with any of the abovementioned risks.
- Anticipate experiencing any of the abovementioned risks.
- Have HIV or other causes of immune suppression and have recently had or anticipate any of the abovementioned risks.
- Work in a setting where they may be exposed to mpox.

Health care professionals who are interested in providing mpox vaccinations to their patients can refer them to the local health department to see what options are available in their community. In some large cities, the vaccines may be available at the health department, public health clinics, hospitals, or even at large social gatherings or venues.

PEARLS

- Mpox is caused by orthopoxvirus, similar to smallpox.
- Vaccines previously developed for smallpox have shown efficacy against mpox.
- It is best to administer postexposure immunization within 4 days of exposure.
- Be familiar with the indications for mpox immunization and the treatment regimen.

Suggested Readings

Centers for Disease Control and Prevention. Mpox vaccination basics. Accessed August 31, 2023. https://www.cdc.gov/poxvirus/mpox/vaccines/index.html

Poland GA, Kennedy RB, Tosh PK. Prevention of mpox with vaccines: a rapid review. *Lancet Infect Dis.* 2022;22(12):e349-e358.

160

Diagnostic Delays in the Diagnosis of Osteomyelitis

Kenneth Lee

Osteomyelitis is defined simply as infection of the bone. It is primarily categorized by the way the infection reaches the bone, whether via hematogenous or nonhematogenous spread. It is also frequently classified by the duration of illness, ranging from acute (with a duration of a few days to a few weeks) to chronic (long-standing infection over months to years). Although osteomyelitis in the ED is often associated with the peripheral extremities and especially with diabetic foot ulcerations, nearly any bone can be involved in this disease process, including the vertebrae, pelvis, and sacrum.

Untreated osteomyelitis can result in a myriad of local and systemic complications. Clinical manifestations of osteomyelitis vary by degree of spread. Patients with local infection often initially present with pain, swelling, redness, warmth, and difficulty bearing weight but can quickly develop bony malformations that put them at increased risk of fractures. Infection that has spread to adjacent tissues can lead to abscess formation (often with sinus tracts in cases of chronic disease) and in more serious cases to necrotizing soft tissue infections. As with many types of infection, osteomyelitis also has the propensity to reach the bloodstream and result in bacteremia and sepsis.

Given the vast array of complications, prompt diagnosis and treatment of osteomyelitis is critical for wound healing and in reducing length of stay and overall morbidity in these patients. In the ED in particular, diagnostic delays remain, perhaps in part because of variable availability of the diagnostic imaging of choice—MRI. Luckily, the diagnosis of osteomyelitis is not solely dependent on MRI, and delays can easily be avoided even in facilities with limited MRI availability.

High clinical suspicion is the most important factor in preventing delays in the diagnosis of osteomyelitis. In patients with large (>2 cm) ulcerations and a positive probe-to-bone test result, nonhematogenous osteomyelitis needs to be considered. Hematogenous osteomyelitis should be considered in patients with known bacteremia or sepsis with new or worsening musculoskeletal pain.

As noted in **Table 160.1**, outside of a bone biopsy, the diagnosis of osteomyelitis can be made with classic clinical and radiographic findings (summarized in **Table 160.2**) in combination with either positive blood culture findings or elevated inflammatory markers. After the clinical evaluation, suggested workup includes both lab work, namely, inflammatory markers including ESR and CRP, as well as screening x-ray imaging. Classic

---

TABLE 160.1 DIAGNOSTIC CRITERIA FOR OSTEOMYELITIS

1. Clinical or radiographic findings consistent with osteomyelitis *and* positive blood culture findings *or* elevated inflammatory markers
2. Bone biopsy consistent with osteomyelitis

TABLE 160.2 FINDINGS CONSISTENT WITH OSTEOMYELITIS

Clinical exam findings
1. Skin ulceration >2 cm
2. Probes to bone

Inflammatory markers
1. Elevated ESR >70

Radiographic findings
1. Osteopenia
2. Bony destruction
3. Periosteal reaction

---

imaging findings for osteomyelitis include bony erosions in the region of concern, although secondary signs such as periosteal reaction may also be suggestive. It should be noted that x-ray sensitivity and specificity for osteomyelitis are relatively low, at approximately 54% and 68%, respectively. X-ray findings also frequently lag behind the onset of disease, particularly if less than 2 weeks of symptoms. If x-ray findings are negative and the clinical suspicion remains high, other radiographic options include MRI (sensitivity ~96%, specificity ~82%), or PET-CT (~84%, ~93%). CT can also be considered in cases of chronic osteomyelitis; however, sensitivity and specificity are reported to be low (~67%, ~50%).

Although the gold standards for diagnosis (MRI, bone biopsy) are sometimes inaccessible in the ED setting, osteomyelitis remains a pathology with serious complications when not treated in a timely manner. With high clinical suspicion and mastery of the appropriate screening tests, emergency physicians can play a meaningful role in limiting time to diagnosis and improving outcomes in patients with osteomyelitis.

PEARLS

- Left untreated, osteomyelitis can progress to significant complications including necrotizing soft tissue infection and fulminant sepsis.
- High clinical suspicion in patients with large ulcerations or lesions that probe to bone can reduce diagnostic delays and reduce morbidity.
- Although MRI and bone biopsy are the gold standards for diagnosis, osteomyelitis can be diagnosed through other more available modalities as well.

SUGGESTED READINGS

Dinh MT, Abad CL, Safdar N. Diagnostic accuracy of the physical examination and imaging tests for osteomyelitis underlying diabetic foot ulcers: meta-analysis. *Clin Infect Dis*. 2008;47(4):519-527. PMID: 18611152.

Llewellyn A, Kraft J, Holton C, Harden M, Simmonds M. Imaging for detection of osteomyelitis in people with diabetic foot ulcers: a systematic review and meta-analysis. *Eur J Radiol*. 2020;131:109215. PMID: 32862106.

Termaat MF, Raijmakers PG, Scholten HJ, Bakker FC, Patka P, Haarman HJ. The accuracy of diagnostic imaging for the assessment of chronic osteomyelitis: a systematic review and meta-analysis. *J Bone Joint Surg Am*. 2005;87(11):2464-2471. PMID: 16264122.

161

Don't Forget These Conditions in the Febrile Traveler

Richard Diego Gonzales y Tucker and Nathan Jasperse

Epidemiology

Annually, 50 million people travel to the developing world, with up to 19% seeking medical care for travel-associated illnesses. Among those seeking medical care, fever is a common chief complaint, with nearly 20% of travelers to the developing world reporting fevers on their return to the United States. Many will present to EDs, necessitating a fundamental knowledge of the etiologies of fevers in the returning traveler. The most common causes of fevers in patients with a travel-associated illness are *malaria*, *dengue*, *rickettsial diseases*, and *enteric fever (typhoid)*. **Table 161.1** lists some other etiologies of

TABLE 161.1	INCUBATION PERIODS FOR COMMON CAUSES OF FEVER IN THE RETURNING TRAVELER
INCUBATION PERIOD	**DISEASE**
<14 d	Acute HIV: 7-21 d
	Arboviruses (eg, chikungunya, Zika): 2-10 d
	COVID-19: 5-6 d
	Dengue: 4-8 d
	Enteric fever (typhoid): 7-18 d
	Leptospirosis: 7-12 d
	Influenza: 1-3 d
	Malaria
	Plasmodium falciparum: 6-30 d
	P. vivax/ovale: 12 d-12 mo
	Measles: 10-14 d
	Rickettsioses: 2-14 d
	Viral hemorrhagic fever: 2-21 d
	Viral gastroenteritis (eg, norovirus, rotavirus): 1-2 d
14 d-6 wk	Amebic liver abscess: weeks-months
	Bartonellosis: 2-14 mo
	Brucellosis: 3 wk-several mo
	Hepatitis A: 28-30 d
	Hepatitis B: 60-150 d
	Rabies: weeks-months
	Rubella: 14-21 d
	Schistosomiasis: 28-60 d
	Tuberculosis: weeks (primary infection)
	Visceral leishmaniasis: 2-10 mo

d, day; HIV, human immunodeficiency virus; mo, month; wk, week.

fevers in the returning traveler. As the differential is broad, and fever may be the only early sign of potentially deadly disease, an exhaustive history and thorough physical exam are crucial.

HISTORY

A thorough but targeted history is necessary for an accurate diagnosis in the febrile traveler, and it is important to consider both travel-associated illness as well as common diseases frequently found in the developed world (such as pneumonia and UTIs). More than 20% of patients presenting with a fever after travel will not receive a definitive diagnosis, highlighting that a consistent diagnostic approach and broad initial differential are requisite during an initial patient evaluation.

The clinician should ask whether the patient received appropriate predeparture vaccinations and whether they took any chemoprophylaxis. Depending on their itinerary, vaccinations against meningococcus, typhoid, yellow fever, and hepatitis A may be indicated. Malaria requires chemoprophylaxis, and many regimens require continuation upon return from travel abroad. Importantly, prescription of chemoprophylaxis does not imply compliance. Notably, up to 75% of patients do not adhere to their malaria prophylaxis regimens secondary to side effects. In addition, vaccination administration or adherence to chemoprophylaxis is not 100% protective against disease, as with typhoid.

An accurate itinerary of the patient's travel is crucial in developing an appropriate differential. In travelers to sub-Saharan Africa, malaria is the most common etiology of systemic febrile illness. Dengue is more common in South Asia and malaria and dengue are equally prevalent in South and Central America. It is important to establish an accurate timeline of travel and fever onset to determine the incubation time, which can be used to rule in or out disease (**Table 161.1**). The physician should inquire about reasons for travel (eg, tourism, business, visiting family). Travelers classified as VFR, visiting friends and relatives, often visit rural areas and are less likely to receive indicated vaccines or take chemoprophylaxis.

Additional pertinent history includes exposure to mosquitoes or other insects (eg, fleas, mites, ticks) and use of protective clothing, mosquito nets, and DEET-containing insect repellent. Physicians should inquire about animal bites, exposure to fresh water, diet history (eg, tap water, fresh vegetables, undercooked/raw meat), sexual history while abroad, body fluid exposure (eg, tattoos, piercings), and sick contacts. Emergency providers should inquire about any medications taken while traveling and if the patient interacted with the medical system while abroad, as hospital multidrug-resistant organisms are increasingly prevalent internationally.

Finally, the clinician should take a detailed history of the fever and any associated symptoms. If a rash is present, the clinician should ask about the time of onset. **Table 161.2** summarizes the presenting findings for the most common causes of fevers in travelers. The clinician should also consider other common or "cosmopolitan" infections such as UTIs, viral gastroenteritis, and influenza as well as noninfectious etiologies of fever in a traveler, such as venous thromboembolism. Early in the ED evaluation, the emergency physician should have a low threshold to place the patient in isolation to prevent propagation of disease.

PHYSICAL EXAM/WORKUP

A complete physical exam should begin with accurate vital signs, with consideration for a core temperature measurement. Both dengue and enteric fever may present with Faget sign or pulse-temperature dissociation (relative bradycardia in the setting of fever).

TABLE 161.2 **CHARACTERISTICS AND ASSOCIATED SYMPTOMS OF COMMON ETIOLOGIES OF FEVER IN RETURNING TRAVELERS**

DISEASE	FEVER	RASH	DIAGNOSIS
Dengue	"Breakbone fever" (arthralgias)	Petechial Early in disease course	Clinical May see eosinopenia
Enteric fever	Initially low grade High grade by 2nd week of illness	Rose spots	Clinical; may be diagnosed with blood, stool, or urine cultures May cause leukopenia and thrombocytopenia
Malaria	Can be paroxysmal *Plasmodium falciparum*: continuous	N/A	Thick and thin smear
Rickettsia	Presents first, followed by rash	Maculopapular Onset 3-5 days after other symptoms	Blood, stool, or urine culture

The abdominal and skin exams are particularly important. Splenomegaly may be found in malaria and enteric fever, while dengue can cause hepatosplenomegaly. The patient should be fully undressed for a complete skin exam, including examination for ticks or tick bites, which cause rickettsial illness. A maculopapular rash can be found in rickettsial disease, dengue, and enteric fever. Petechiae or purpura should raise a concern for viral hemorrhagic fever (eg, Ebola, Marburg), dengue hemorrhagic syndrome, or meningococcemia. Enteric fever classically causes cutaneous "rose spots," but these are transient and may be difficult to identify.

Diagnosis of most travel-associated febrile illnesses is clinical. Laboratory workup should focus on identifying patients with esoteric laboratory abnormalities (eg, eosinophilia) that suggest a specific diagnosis, or significant laboratory derangement, indicating severe illness and need for aggressive resuscitation. Initial workup should include a complete blood count with differential, complete metabolic panel, coagulation studies, and inflammatory markers; see **Table 161.2** for diagnostic tests for the common causes. Malaria is diagnosed by a thick and thin smear and should be ordered on every patient returning from travel with fever. Malaria can be challenging to identify, and interpretation of blood smear is dependent on lab technician expertise and the degree of parasitemia at the time of the blood draw. Diagnosis therefore requires a high index of suspicion, and frequently sending repeated thick and thin smears every 6 to 12 hours for up to 48 hours to ultimately identify the *Plasmodium* species. In many febrile travelers, no definitive diagnosis will be made despite comprehensive evaluation.

PEARLS

- An accurate chronologic travel history is crucial for evaluation of the returning febrile traveler.
- Geographic locations of travel and timing of fever onset are important for the development of appropriate differential diagnoses.

- Malaria, dengue, enteric fever, and rickettsial diseases are the most common travel-associated causes of fever from the developing world.
- Cosmopolitan diseases such as UTI, viral respiratory infections (such as COVID-19), and bacterial pneumonia are also common causes of fever in travelers and should not be overlooked.
- Twenty percent of returning travelers with a febrile illness will not be definitively diagnosed, necessitating a high index of suspicion for infectious disease.

SUGGESTED READINGS

Feder HM Jr, Mansilla-Rivera K. Fever in returning travelers: a case-based approach. *Am Fam Physician*. 2013;88(8):524-530.

Kotlyar S, Rice BT. Fever in the returning traveler. *Emerg Med Clin North Am*. 2013 Nov;31(4):927-44. Epub 2013 Sep 18. PMID: 24176472.

162

SYPHILIS IS BACK! OR WAS IT EVER GONE?

ELISE MOLNAR

Syphilis, the Great Imitator, has impacted medicine for more than five centuries without any signs of abating any time soon. According to the CDC, the rates of primary and secondary syphilis have increased steadily since the year 2000, with a 6.8% increase from 2019 to 2020. While most recent primary and secondary syphilis cases disproportionately affect MSM, the rates among women and heterosexual men continue to rapidly increase.

On its own, syphilis can progress to severe and morbid disease, but with coinfection with HIV, which represents 30% to 60% of syphilis cases, individuals tend to have more varied symptoms with faster progression to secondary and tertiary stages, particularly neurosyphilis. It is also important to note that stages may also overlap, so the delineation is not always clear cut. **Table 162.1** highlights the different stages of syphilis and their timeline of presentation after infection.

DIAGNOSTIC TESTING

Given the wide array of symptoms and physical exam findings, the threshold for diagnostic testing should be very low. Both the VDRL and RPR tests can be used for screening. Because these tests detect antibodies against cardiolipin, they can be falsely positive with increased age, pregnancy, SLE, malignancy, and other infections. Once the finding is positive for either the RPR or VDRL tests, an individual will test positive for life. In cases of reinfection, an RPR with titer can help guide treatment decisions. A titer increase of *two* dilutions (ie, 1:1-1:4) would indicate reinfection. The State Health Department can

TABLE 162.1 STAGES OF SYPHILIS AND ASSOCIATED SYMPTOMS

Presentation[a]		Timeline (After Infection)
Primary	■ Chancres (single, painless, demarcated ulcers with a clean base) that occur on penile, vulvar, cervical, anal, or oral mucosa ■ Localized, painless lymphadenopathy	3 wk
Secondary	■ Generalized lymphadenopathy ■ Nonpruritic, "copper-colored" maculopapular rash involving the palms and soles ■ Painless erosive ulcers in the mouth ■ Condylomata, papules, and ulcerations of the genital mucosa ■ Headache, fevers, malaise, nausea, decreased appetite	3-5 mo
Latent	■ Asymptomatic ■ Early latent syphilis: infection within 12 mo ■ Late latent syphilis: initial infection >12 mo ago ■ Latent syphilis of unknown duration: unclear if the infection occurs within the previous 12 mo	
Tertiary	*(30% of untreated cases)*	5-25 yr
Benign	■ Painless indurated nodules called *gummas* that occur over skin, liver, spleen, and bone	
Cardiovascular	■ Syphilitic aortitis that can lead to aortic regurgitation, ascending aortic aneurysms, or aortic rupture	

Neurosyphilis	■ Early
	  ■ Asymptomatic meningitis
	  ■ Syphilitic meningitis
	■ Late
	  ■ Meningovascular syphilis
	  ■ Mood changes, seizures, altered mental status, focal deficits
	■ Tabes dorsalis
	  ■ Argyll Robertson pupil, sensory ataxia, loss of temperature sensation, neuropathy, positive Romberg, distal neuropathies
	■ Paresis	

[a] Given the wide array of presentations, only common and particularly morbid presentations have been included.

also verify if there has been a previous positive RPR result and record of treatment. Although not usually available in the ED, confirmatory tests include serum FTA-ABS and dark-field microscopy. Refer to hospital and regional policies for reporting of positive test findings.

In patients with a positive RPR finding and a suspicion for cardiovascular syphilis, CT angiography of the aorta or a TEE should be performed; a cardiothoracic or vascular surgery consultation may be necessary if the imaging reveals aortic pathology. For those patients with a positive RPR finding and neurologic symptoms, a lumbar puncture should be performed as CSF VDRL with an associated elevated CSF lymphocyte count is diagnostic for neurosyphilis. If there is ocular involvement, a prompt consultation with ophthalmology is critical. Cases should also be managed in concert with infectious disease experts as they can help guide management decisions based on symptoms and available laboratory results.

Finally, due to the incidence of coinfection, all newly diagnosed individuals with syphilis should receive screening for other sexually transmitted infections including HIV, gonorrhea, chlamydia, and hepatitis B.

TREATMENT

The most recent CDC recommendations for treatment of the various stages of syphilis in adults are provided in **Table 162.2**.

TABLE 162.2 TREATMENT REGIMENS FOR THE VARIOUS STAGES OF SYPHILIS

Syphilis treatment for adults	
Primary and secondary syphilis	■ Benzathine penicillin G 2.4 million units IM once
Latent syphilis	■ Early: benzathine penicillin G 2.4 million units IM once ■ Late: benzathine penicillin G 2.4 million units, three doses at weekly intervals
Tertiary syphilis	■ With a normal CSF examination: benzathine penicillin G 2.4 million units, three doses at weekly intervals
Neurosyphilis, ocular syphilis, or otosyphilis	■ Aqueous crystalline penicillin G 18-24 million units per day, administered as 3-4 million units IV every 4 h or continuous infusion for 10-14 d ■ Procaine penicillin G 2.4 million units IM daily *plus* ■ Probenecid 500 mg orally 4 times daily for 10-14 d
Penicillin allergies	
Primary and secondary syphilis	■ Doxycycline (100 mg orally 2 times daily for 14 d) ■ Tetracycline (500 mg orally 4 times daily for 14 d) ■ Ceftriaxone (1 g daily either IM or IV for 10 d) ■ Consider desensitization.
Late latent or syphilis of unknown duration	■ Doxycycline (100 mg orally 2 times daily for 28 d) ■ Tetracycline (500 mg orally 4 times daily for 28 d)
Syphilis during pregnancy or tertiary syphilis with neurologic/ocular findings	■ Desensitization

CSF, cerebrospinal fluid; IM, intramuscular; IV, intravenous.

While primary and secondary stages can be treated and discharged from the ED, latent cases will need follow-up for continued treatment. In patients where the stage is unclear (eg, early vs late latency, syphilis of unknown duration), consult with infectious disease specialists or the health department to determine whether a longer course of therapy and follow-up is needed. Patients with suspected tertiary syphilis with neurologic or ocular involvement should be admitted for intravenous penicillin therapy.

Individuals receiving treatment for syphilis, especially in early stages, may experience the Jarisch-Herxheimer reaction, which is a constellation of fevers, secondary rash, headache, pharyngitis, and malaise that occurs in response to the release of *Treponema pallidum* lipoproteins from lysing organisms, and usually happens within 12 hours of initiation of antibiotic treatment. This is not an allergic reaction and can be managed with symptomatic treatment, namely, acetaminophen.

Finally, individuals exposed to *T. pallidum* through sexual contact should be evaluated clinically and serologically for treatment. Serologic test results may be negative in early exposure, so empiric treatment should be considered in high-risk individuals. Health departments may recommend notification and presumptive treatment of sex partners of persons with syphilis of unknown duration who have high serologic titers (ie, >1:32), as high titers can reflect early syphilis. Long-term sexual partners of persons with latent syphilis should be evaluated clinically and serologically and treated accordingly.

PEARLS

- Syphilis is common and has a wide array of presenting symptoms; providers should have a low threshold for screening.
- Once the result is positive, VDRL and RPR will remain positive. It is helpful to check previous RPR titers whenever possible (if available), or contact the health department.
- Any neurologic or ocular finding should be thoroughly evaluated for neurosyphilis.
- Penicillin is typically the recommended therapy, usually via the intramuscular route. However, ocular and neurologic disease requires intravenous antibiotic therapy.
- Coinfection with HIV can cause accelerated progression with an overlap in stages.

Suggested readings

Dourmishev LA, Dourmishev AL. Syphilis: uncommon presentations in adults. *Clin Dermatol*. 2005;23(6):555-564.
Hazra A, Collison MW, Davis AM. CDC sexually transmitted infections treatment guidelines, 2021. *JAMA*. 2022;327(9):870-871.
Read PJ, Donovan B. Clinical aspects of adult syphilis. *Intern Med J*. 2012;42(6):614-620.
Singh AE, Romanowski B. Syphilis: review with emphasis on clinical, epidemiological, and some biologic features. *Clin Microbiol Rev*. 1999;12(2):187-209.
Tintinalli JE. *Emergency Medicine: A Comprehensive Study Guide*. 9th ed. McGraw-Hill; 2019:1013-1019.

163

BY LAND, BY SEA, BY AIR: KNOW THESE BEST-PRACTICE STRATEGIES TO PREVENT INFECTIOUS SPREAD

LISA BELL

Hand hygiene is the single most effective measure to prevent infectious spread, regardless of whether the health care provider is wearing gloves. This should be performed with either alcohol-based hand disinfection or with soap and water before and after patient contact. Alcohol-based disinfection is likely the preferred method in the busy ED setting because it is less time intensive; however, soap and water are recommended when hands are visibly soiled or when providing care to patients with suspected *Clostridium difficile* infections. Frequency and consistency of hand hygiene is key. Standard/universal precautions for any patient involve frequent hand hygiene, as well as the use of gowns, gloves, and eye protection when there is anticipated exposure to blood or bodily secretions.

APPROPRIATE SELECTION OF ISOLATION PRECAUTIONS

Preventing Contact Transmission

Contact precautions are used in patients that may be colonized with multidrug-resistant bacteria, such as MRSA, ESBL organisms, and VRE. In addition, these precautions are used if direct contact with the patient would increase likelihood of transmission, such as in *C. difficile* infections, infectious conjunctivitis, and gastroenteritis (especially if working with patients who are incontinent, where there is an increased risk of exposure to stool). If possible, these patients should be in private rooms. A gown and gloves should be worn if direct contact with the patient is anticipated (including when entering the patient's room). Patients should ideally have dedicated medical equipment so that items such as thermometers, stethoscopes, or otoscopes do not become fomites of transmission from patient to patient.

Preventing Droplet Transmission

Droplet precautions are used when interacting with patients who are suspected or confirmed to have infections that generate large-particle respiratory droplets (such as those generated from coughing or sneezing). These respiratory secretions are greater than or equal to 5 microns and only remain suspended in the air for seconds to minutes, leaving a limited duration of time for susceptible individuals to be exposed to infection. Some infections/pathogens that fall under this category are *Neisseria meningitidis*, pertussis, *Streptococcus*, *Mycoplasma*, rhinovirus, influenza, and novel coronavirus SARS-CoV2 (COVID-19; apart from specific exceptions). The primary measure taken to avoid droplet transmission is wearing a surgical mask if the provider is within 6 feet of the patient.

Preventing Airborne Transmission

Airborne precautions are used for patients who are suspected or confirmed to have infections that may be transmitted via the airborne route, that is, pathogens with droplet nuclei of less than 5 microns that can remain in the air for hours, increasing the duration of time for possible exposure and for which droplet precautions will not provide adequate protection. For example, the measles virus can remain present in a room for up to 2 hours. Other infections with airborne transmission are tuberculosis, smallpox, disseminated zoster, and chickenpox. It is also recommended that airborne precautions be implemented when performing aerosolizing procedures on patients infected with SARS and COVID-19. Recommended infection control measures include placing a mask on the patient, placing the patient in a negative pressure isolation room, the use of a well-fitted N95 mask while in the room, and minimizing entry/exit into the room as well as the number of personnel required to enter the room.

Preventing Blood-Borne Transmission

Precautions against blood-borne pathogens are in place to prevent transmission of microorganisms in the blood that may cause disease in humans, including HIV, hepatitis B, and hepatitis C. Universal precautions are used to prevent blood-borne pathogen transmission. This includes use of gowns, gloves, and eye protection when handling bodily fluids of any kind; in addition, this includes avoidance of bodily fluid exposures such as needlesticks, splashes, and contact with mucosal surfaces or broken skin.

Approximately one-third of needlestick injuries occur during disposal of sharps. Monitoring sharps during and after procedures is essential to prevent blood-borne transmission through needlesticks. In addition, maintaining up-to-date hepatitis B vaccination is crucial in reducing transmission to providers.

What to do if exposed to body fluids:

1) Wash the needlestick or cut with soap and water. If a mucosal surface is exposed, irrigate copiously.
2) Report the incident immediately to your employer/supervisor; this expedites medical evaluation as well as identification of any potential source of infection.
3) Seek prompt medical evaluation, including laboratory evaluation following your institution's guidelines.
4) Initiate postexposure prophylaxis medications, if indicated.

PEARLS

- Hand hygiene is an essential part of infection prevention.
- Contact precautions include the use of a gown and gloves when performing tasks with direct patient contact.
- Droplet precautions include the use of a surgical mask when within 6 feet of patients with diseases transmitted via large-particle respiratory droplets.
- Airborne precautions include the use of an N95 mask and a negative pressure isolation room when exposure to droplets less than 5 microns is anticipated.
- Always be aware of any sharp implements during use and disposal.

SUGGESTED READINGS

Centers for Disease Control and Prevention. Accessed February 13, 2023. www.cdc.gov
Occupational Safety and Health Administration. Accessed February 13, 2023. www.osha.gov

Antibiotic Timing in Sepsis: What Really Matters?

Sean Denny

Prompt administration of antibiotics is widely accepted as a key component in the treatment of sepsis. However, the timeframe within which these antibiotics must be given has been a matter of debate and research.

Surviving Sepsis Campaign and SEP-1

The recommendation from the 2021 update to the Surviving Sepsis Campaign Guidelines is that antibiotics be given within 1 hour of recognition of sepsis in patients with or without shock. For patients with possible sepsis in shock, the recommendation is that antibiotics be administered within 1 hour. For patients with possible sepsis but not in shock, the recommendation is that a rapid evaluation be performed to delineate infectious versus noninfectious causes, followed by the administration of antibiotics within 3 hours for those who are still suspected to have sepsis after this evaluation.

The Centers for Medicare and Medicaid Services developed the SEP-1, which requires the administration of antibiotics within 1 hour for patients with either sepsis or septic shock.

Alternative Viewpoints

The IDSA has expressed concerns about the potential for SEP-1 to drive the overuse of antibiotics, based on the issue that it does not account for sepsis overdiagnosis and recommends antibiotics for any patient with possible sepsis, regardless of illness severity or certainty of diagnosis. In a 2018 article discussing the IDSA's concerns, they recommended limiting SEP-1 to patients with septic shock, as this subgroup of patients has the strongest data supporting the benefit of administration of antibiotics within 1 hour of sepsis recognition.

In 2021, the ACEP released a policy statement regarding the early care of adults with suspected sepsis in the ED. Within this statement, they note that data are mixed regarding the impact of the exact timing of antibiotic administration on mortality. Overall, they agreed that antibiotics should be rapidly given once the diagnosis of sepsis is made, and that collective data support a shorter time window for the administration of antibiotics in patients with septic shock, but note that the available data did not support a singular time target that clearly improves outcomes for all patients.

What Do Some of the Latest Studies Show?

In 2017, Liu et al published a retrospective study of 35,000 randomly selected patients in Northern California who were treated for sepsis between 2010 and 2013. They found an increased risk of in-hospital mortality for each elapsed hour between registration and antibiotic administration, but the mortality benefit was variable depending on severity of illness, with the least benefit noted in patients with sepsis without shock (a 0.3%-0.4% increase in absolute mortality for each hour's delay in antibiotic administration) and the most benefit in patients in septic shock (a 1.8% increase in absolute mortality for each hour's delay in antibiotic administration).

In 2020, Seok et al published a prospective cohort study of 482 patients treated for sepsis at one ED in Korea between 2016 and 2019. The time to and appropriateness of initial antibiotics were not associated with 7-, 14-, and 28-day mortality.

In 2022, Im et al published a prospective cohort study that included 3,035 patients who presented in 2019 to 2020 to any of the 19 participating hospitals in Korea and were diagnosed with sepsis or septic shock in the ED. They found that administration of antibiotics within 1 hour of sepsis recognition improved in-hospital mortality for patients with septic shock but did not find a statistically significant benefit for administration of antibiotics within 1 hour for patients with sepsis without shock. Among patients in septic shock who received antibiotics within 3 hours, there was an increased risk of mortality for every hour of delay in antibiotic administration.

PEARLS

- Patients in septic shock are most likely to have a mortality benefit from administration of antibiotics within 1 hour of recognition.
- Data are mixed and controversy remains regarding the exact timing of antibiotic administration in patients with suspected sepsis to achieve a mortality benefit.
- Be aware of your hospital's policy and if they require adherence to SEP-1 or the Surviving Sepsis Campaign 2021 Guidelines.

SUGGESTED READINGS

Evans, L, Rhodes A, Alhazzani W, et al. Surviving sepsis campaign: international guidelines for management of sepsis and septic shock 2021. *Crit Care Med*. 2021;49(11):e1063-e1143.

Im Y, Kang D, Ko RE, et al. Time-to-antibiotics and clinical outcomes in patients with sepsis and septic shock: a prospective nationwide multicenter cohort study. *Crit Care*. 2022;26(1):19.

Liu VX, Fielding-Singh V, Greene JD, et al. The timing of early antibiotics and hospital mortality in sepsis. *Am J Respir Crit Care Med*. 2017;196(7):856-863.

Rhee C, Chiotos K, Cosgrove SE, et al. Infectious Diseases Society of America Position Paper: recommended revisions to the National Severe Sepsis and Septic Shock Early Management Bundle (SEP-1) Sepsis Quality Measure. Clin Infect Dis. 2021;72(4):541-552.

Seok H, Song J, Jeon JH, et al. Timing of antibiotics in septic patients: a prospective cohort study. *Clin Microbiol Infect*. 2020;26(11):1495-1500.

Yealy DM, Mohr NM, Shapiro NI, Venkatesh A, Jones AE, Self WH. Early care of adults with suspected sepsis in the emergency department and out-of-hospital environment: a consensus-based task force report. *Ann Emerg Medicine*. 2021;78(1):1-19.

TIMELY SOURCE CONTROL IN SEPSIS

JOHN STOCKTON

Sepsis is among the most common critical illnesses seen in the ED. While the initial approach focuses on early identification, antibiotic administration, and fluid resuscitation, timely source control is a fundamental pillar in the management of patients with sepsis.

What Is Source Control?

Source control is defined as any intervention that controls or removes an infection and restores optimal function to the affected area. This may be broken down into three general categories: drainage, debridement, and removal, all of which aim to definitively control the source of infection. Drainage may range from an uncomplicated incision and drainage of a soft tissue abscess, to an interventional radiology-guided drainage of an intra-abdominal fluid collection, placement of a surgical drain, removal of an obstruction, or open surgical exploration. The classic example of debridement is the removal of gangrenous tissue in necrotizing fasciitis but may also include the elimination of surrounding tissue in conditions such as necrotizing pancreatitis or bowel infarction. Finally, device removal includes removing a urinary Foley catheter or central line (where a dangerous bacterial biofilm may have grown) or objects such as spinal hardware or a prosthetic heart valve.

The most recent Surviving Sepsis Guidelines recommend rapid identification of infections requiring source control and implementation of source control interventions as soon as it is medically and logistically possible. Just as successful treatment of sepsis is often contingent on timely antibiotics and fluid resuscitation, it is also important to recognize if a patient may benefit from an intervention such as those described earlier (drainage, debridement, or removal of an infected device).

Who Needs Source Control?

While the presence of a source is sometimes obvious (in, say, a soft tissue infection that is apparent on physical exam), this is not always the case. Sometimes, imaging is needed and this decision is typically guided by the overall clinical picture. For example, if a patient presents with right upper quadrant pain and a fever, an ultrasound is a good first choice to evaluate for an infected gallbladder. Alternatively, if the patient recently underwent a colostomy and now presents in septic shock, a CT scan may help show the culprit fluid collection or leak. In general, the patients that benefit from source control are those with soft tissue infections, intra-abdominal infections, and infected devices. **Table 165.1** lists common infections that require source control by anatomic location.

While no procedure is without risk, the intervention that source control requires should be weighed against the potential dangers for the patient. After the initial steps of resuscitation and stabilization, the decision to pursue such an intervention should be discussed with the appropriate specialist as soon as possible.

What Makes Source Control Timely?

The optimal timing of source control depends on the nature of the infection. In necrotizing fasciitis, for example, source control via surgical debridement is the definitive treatment and should be performed as soon as possible. Alternatively, for a suspected intra-abdominal abscess, imaging may help with operative planning, and thus serve as a reasonable cause for delay.

In general, timing in source control has been considered a difficult thing to study, likely contributing to the overall lack of data on the topic. There are some studies that show source control within 6 hours is associated with reduced mortality, while others suggest the optimal timing to be within 6 to 12 hours. Although the best time frame may remain somewhat unclear, putting together a cohesive plan with the appropriate specialist for timely source control is essential in the management of sepsis.

TABLE 165.1	ANATOMY OF COMMON INFECTIONS REQUIRING SOURCE CONTROL
ANATOMY	**SOURCE OF INFECTION**
Head/neck	■ Brain abscess ■ Infected ventriculoperitoneal shunt ■ Dental, peritonsillar, or retropharyngeal abscess ■ Epidural abscess
Chest	■ Endocarditis ■ Pericarditis ■ Prosthetic heart valve ■ Mediastinitis ■ Lung empyema ■ Infected pacemaker ■ Infected indwelling catheter/PICC
Abdomen	■ Cholecystitis ■ Cholangitis ■ Liver abscess ■ Appendicitis ■ Bowel perforation or post-op anastomotic leak ■ NEC or necrotic bowel ■ Necrotizing pancreatitis ■ Intra-abdominal abscess
Pelvis	■ Tubo-ovarian abscess ■ Infected kidney stone ■ Retained products of conception ■ Infected urinary catheter ■ Perirectal/anal abscess
Soft tissue	■ Necrotizing fasciitis/myositis/cellulitis ■ Infected wound ■ Soft tissue abscess
Joints	■ Septic arthritis ■ Infected joint prosthesis

NEC, necrotizing enterocolitis; PICC, peripherally inserted central catheter.
Adapted from De Waele JJ, Girardis M, Martin-Loeches I. Source control in the management of sepsis and septic shock. *Intensive Care Med*. 2022;48(12):1799-1802.

PEARLS

- Source control generally consists in drainage, debridement, or removal of an infected device.
- Consider the need for source control in all patients presenting with sepsis.
- Patients that benefit from source control are typically those with soft tissue infections, intra-abdominal infections, and infected implanted devices.
- The need for source control should be weighed against the risks of invasive intervention, a decision best made in consultation with specialists.
- For those that would benefit from source control, it is important to initiate the process as soon as possible, ideally within 6 to 12 hours.

Suggested Readings

De Waele JJ, Girardis M, Martin-Loeches I. Source control in the management of sepsis and septic shock. *Intensive Care Med*. 2022;48(12):1799-1802.

Evans L, Rhodes A, Alhazzani W, et al. Surviving sepsis campaign: international guidelines for management of sepsis and septic shock 2021. *Crit Care Med*. 2021;49(11):e1063-e1143.

Kim H, Chung SP, Choi SH, et al. Impact of timing to source control in patients with septic shock: a prospective multi-center observational study. *J Crit Care*. 2019;53:176-182.

Lagunes L, Encina B, Ramirez-Estrada S. Current understanding in source control management in septic shock patients: a review. *Ann Transl Med*. 2016;4(17):330.

Marshall JC. Principles of source control in the early management of sepsis. *Curr Infect Dis Rep*. 2010;12(5):345-353.

Reitz KM, Kennedy J, Li SR, et al. Association between time to source control in sepsis and 90-day mortality. *JAMA Surg*. 2022;157(9):817-826.

SECTION XIII

MUSCULOSKELETAL (NONTRAUMA)

166

UGH! ANOTHER REPEAT VISIT FOR BACK PAIN?! KEEP EPIDURAL ABSCESS ON THE DIFFERENTIAL!

AUBREY BETHEL AND HAEDAN DOTY

Despite being one of the most common presenting complaints, the evaluation of back pain is rarely straightforward. The discerning physician must determine whether the patient simply needs anti-inflammatory medications versus blood work, MRI of the total spine, and antibiotics. The key to appropriate management is diagnosis. In this chapter, the authors focus on the physical exam, laboratory workup, and imaging modalities used to make the diagnosis of SEA.

SEA is a rare diagnosis but can have devastating consequences for the patient and provider if missed. Approximately half of patients with an SEA present with vague, nonspecific complaints and are discharged to eventually return for a second ED visit.

A careful history and knowledge of specific red flags can help make the diagnosis during the initial visit. Common risk factors for SEAs include IV drug use, recent hospitalization, diabetes mellitus, end-stage renal disease, cancer, alcoholism, and anything that may cause immunosuppression. Spinal procedures such as injections, lumbar punctures, and epidurals also predispose patients to SEAs. Beware red herrings in the history such as recent minor trauma or chronic back pain as they may obscure a more insidious cause for the back pain. Don't let them trip you up.

Signs and symptoms are crucial. A textbook presentation for an SEA is a patient who is febrile, uses IV drugs, and presents with back pain and neurologic deficits. Unfortunately, this classic triad is rare and seen in less than 20% of patients. In fact, only about one-third of patients have fever! A patient's symptoms and their progression are useful: worsening back pain, weakness, incontinence, decreased sensation, and paralysis. Any patient who reports back pain, neurologic deficits, and infectious symptoms should be considered to have an SEA until proven otherwise, as early identification may prevent progressive deterioration.

A thoughtful and well-documented physical exam protects both the patient and physician, especially in the setting of a return visit to the ED. Unfortunately, many clinicians neglect to document a thorough physical exam in the medical record. Documentation of a thorough physical exam, including a full neurologic exam as well as a DRE to evaluate sphincter tone, is especially helpful if the patient returns for the same chief complaint. The patient's sensation, motor strength, cerebellar function, and reflexes should be documented. Sensory exam should also include evaluation for saddle anesthesia. In addition, a thorough examination of the back should be done, looking for areas of redness, increased warmth, or swelling especially in the setting of a recent procedure. The patient may have midline back pain, which may worsen with percussion of their spinous processes. Take the time to make sure the patient is changed into a hospital gown so that an examination of the patient's skin can be done.

The finding of urinary retention in a patient is more sensitive than other findings on the physical examination. If there is concern for overflow urinary incontinence, a bladder scan should be done before and after the patient urinates to check for PVR. The general consensus for a normal PVR is less than 100 mL, and, certainly, retention greater than 150 mL is concerning for spinal compression.

A complete blood count, a comprehensive metabolic panel, an ESR, and C-reactive protein, along with two sets of blood cultures should be obtained, especially if the patient is febrile and has urinary incontinence. Importantly, just 60% of patients with an SEA have an elevated WBC count. Do not be falsely reassured if the patient has a normal WBC count. ESR will likely be elevated in the setting of SEA, which is often followed up to assess disease progression or resolution.

The gold standard imaging study is an MRI. MRI of total spine with IV contrast will identify the SEA, reveal the extent of the abscess, and may help rule in other diagnoses such as malignancy, transverse myelitis, hematomas, or a bulging disk. If you do not have MRI capabilities or the patient cannot have an MRI done, then the next best option is CT myelography.

If your suspicion for SEA is high, start antibiotics early, especially in the setting of sepsis. The most common organism in SEA is *Staphylococcus aureus*, but broad-spectrum antibiotics should be administered to also cover *Escherichia coli* and *Pseudomonas aeruginosa*. One recommended regimen is vancomycin plus cefepime or meropenem. It is important to advocate for the patient and obtain an MRI as soon as possible. The sooner the SEA is diagnosed, the sooner the patient can get to the operating room. Small abscesses may be drained by interventional radiology, but your spinal surgeon should be contacted first. If your hospital does not have a spine surgery service, the patient should be transferred as quickly as possible to a center that has one. Delays in transferring may mean development or worsening of neurologic deficits, which can cause irreparable damage to a patient and their functional status.

PEARLS

- Think of a spinal epidural abscess any time a patient returns to the ED for back pain.
- The classic triad of fever, back pain, and neurologic deficits is uncommon, so a good history and knowledge of risk factors will aid in making the diagnosis.
- The physical examination should include a DRE if the patient reports incontinence or saddle anesthesia. Remember to document this!
- Normal temperature and WBC count are commonly seen in patients with confirmed SEA, so their absence cannot be used to rule out the condition.
- An MRI of the entire spine with IV contrast should be ordered as soon as possible.
- If suspicion is high and the patient has sepsis, start IV antibiotics and consult with a spinal surgeon.

Suggested Readings

Ameer MA, Knorr TL, Munakomi S, et al. Spinal epidural abscess. In: *StatPearls* [Internet]. StatPearls Publishing. Updated February 12, 2023. https://www.ncbi.nlm.nih.gov/books/NBK441890/

Chao D, Nanda A. Spinal epidural abscess: a diagnostic challenge. *American Family Physician*. Published April 1, 2002. Accessed August 13, 2023. https://www.aafp.org/pubs/afp/issues/2002/0401/p1341.html

Mackenzie AR, Laing RBS, Smith CC, et al. Spinal epidural abscess: the importance of early diagnosis and treatment. *J Neurol Neurosurg Psychiatry*. 1998;65:209-212.

Rosc-Bereza K, Arkuszewski M, Ciach-Wysocka E, Boczarska-Jedynak M. Spinal epidural abscess: common symptoms of an emergency condition: a case report. *Neuroradiol J*. 2013;26(4):464-468.

Tetsuka S, Suzuki T, Ogawa T, Hashimoto R, Kato H. Spinal epidural abscess: a review highlighting early diagnosis and management. *JMA J*. 2020;3(1):29-40.

167

Under Pressure: Rapidly Diagnosing and Treating Acute Compartment Syndrome of the Extremities

Darren Stapleton and Anna L. Waterbrook

ACS is a true life- and limb-threatening surgical emergency that requires a high degree of clinical suspicion to make the diagnosis. If it is recognized and treated early, it may prevent permanent damage to limb tissues that may result in paralysis, contractures or loss of limb, rhabdomyolysis, kidney damage, and possibly death.

ACS occurs anytime there is increased pressure in a musculoskeletal compartment that compresses muscles, nerves, and vessels and results in decreased tissue perfusion, ischemia, and eventually cell death. While it may affect any enclosed tissue space, it most commonly occurs in the muscle compartments of the arms and legs. In fact, approximately 40% of ACS cases occur in the lower extremities. The lower leg contains four compartments surrounding the tibia and fibula, which are the anterior, lateral, superficial posterior, and deep posterior compartments. The forearm contains both a volar or flexor compartment and a dorsal or an extensor compartment and are the next most affected. Other areas, such as the hands, feet, and thigh, may also be affected, but much less commonly.

While there are many potential causes of ACS, it most often occurs following a fracture. The most common fractures associated with ACS include tibia, humeral shaft, forearm, and supracondylar fractures. Other causes include prolonged limb compression or immobilization (ie, comatose, intubated, prolonged surgeries, casts, tourniquets), excessive exertion, crush injuries, reperfusion injury, burns, intravenous drug use, coagulopathy, and envenomation.

ACS is largely a clinical diagnosis, and one needs a high degree of suspicion to recognize it. Symptoms usually rapidly progress over a few hours but can be delayed up to 48 hours after the initial event. The textbook signs and symptoms of ACS are the "5 P's": pain, paresthesias, paresis, pallor, and pulselessness. However, these are not sensitive or specific for ACS and only rarely will all be present. Pain out of proportion to the exam is the most sensitive finding in ACS. The patient will often experience pain even with passive stretch. Most commonly, the affected compartment will be swollen, firm, and tender with squeezing by the examiner and is often described as "woody." Paresthesias may begin within 2 to 4 hours of elevated compartment pressures. Paresis (weakness) may often be subtle and missed because it is attributed to pain. Pallor and pulselessness are late findings. Usually, the arterial circulation is present, and the affected extremity will still be warm and have a pulse. When pulselessness does occur, it is usually long after tissue necrosis and ischemia have occurred.

Whenever the diagnosis is considered, it is essential to measure compartment pressures. Normal compartment pressure is less than 10 mm Hg. Classic teaching is that compartment pressures that exceed 30 mm Hg need fasciotomy. However, current literature suggests the use of a "delta pressure," rather than an absolute pressure, when evaluating for ACS. Delta pressure, or Δp, is defined as the diastolic pressure minus compartment pressure. Several studies have suggested that a Δp of less than 30 mm Hg is an indication of fasciotomy. It has been demonstrated that the use of Δp decreases the chances of unnecessary fasciotomies while not leading to increased morbidity or mortality. This is because compartment pressures necessary for injury vary depending on systemic blood pressure. Patients who are hypertensive may require much higher elevations for tissue ischemia to occur, while they may have tissue damage at much lower pressures.

Compartment pressures may be tested with a commercially available device, which includes a manometer, a needle, and a syringe with normal saline. It is important to not only measure the compartment in question but also the surrounding compartments. To measure compartment pressures, place the needle in the appropriate compartment, inject a couple of drops of normal saline, and record the pressure. It is recommended to check each compartment twice. If there is an associated fracture, it is important to measure the compartment pressure within 5 cm of the fracture site. If a commercially available device is unavailable, it is also possible to measure compartment pressures using an 18-gauge needle attached to an arterial line setup. It is important to remember that a normal pressure does not rule out ACS. If clinical suspicion is high, perform serial measurements and obtain early surgical consultation. While there is limited evidence on the utility of serum biomarkers aiding in the diagnosis of ACS, there may be times when serum lactate, troponin, and urine myoglobin may be of benefit.

Treatment of ACS is aimed at preventing irreversible tissue damage and its subsequent complications. Early surgical consultation for fasciotomy is essential and the only definitive treatment. Permanent damage is unlikely to occur if ACS is treated within 6 hours of injury; however, irreversible damage results when there has been more than 8 hours of tissue ischemia. Initial treatment includes reduction of displaced fractures as this can help decrease associated edema, removal of any compressive dressings or casts, analgesics, supplemental oxygen, and a normal saline bolus if the patient is hypotensive to improve tissue perfusion. It is also important to keep the affected limb at the level of the torso (ie, the heart), in order to maximize perfusion.

PEARLS

- ACS is a true life- and limb-threatening surgical emergency and can be a difficult diagnosis to make.

- ACS is primarily a clinical diagnosis. Do not rely on normal compartment pressures if clinical suspicion is high.
- The most sensitive signs and symptoms in ACS are pain out of proportion to the exam and a tense compartment.
- Use a Δp (diastolic blood pressure − intercompartmental pressure) less than 30 mm Hg to help determine whether fasciotomy is necessary.
- Any delay in diagnosis or treatment can lead to significant morbidity; thus, early surgical consultation for fasciotomy in any suspected case is essential.

Suggested Readings

Long B, Koyfman A, Gottlieb M. Evaluation and management of acute compartment syndrome in the emergency department. *J Emerg Med*. 2019;56(4):386-397.

McQueen MM, Christie J, Court-Brown CM. Compartment pressure after intramedullary nailing of the tibia. *J Bone Joint Surg Br*. 1990;72:395-397.

McQueen MM, Christie J, Court-Brown CM. Compartment pressure monitoring in tibial fractures. *J Bone Joint Surg Br*. 1996;78:99-104.

Mubarak SJ, Owen CA, Hargens AR, et al. Acute compartment syndromes: diagnosis and treatment with the aid of the wick catheter. *J Bone Joint Surg Am*. 1978;60:1091-1095.

Osborn CPM, Schmidt AH. Management of acute compartment syndrome. *J Am Acad Orthop Surg*. 2020;28(3):e108-e114.

Osborn PM, Schmidt AH. Diagnosis and management of acute compartment syndrome. *J Am Acad Orthop Surg*. 2021;29(5):183-188.

White TO, Howell GED, Will EM, et al. Elevated intramuscular compartment pressures do not influence outcome after tibial fracture. *J Trauma*. 2003;55:1133-1138.

168

Don't Get Broken Up About Muscle Breakdown—Rhabdomyolysis

Amir Rombod Rahimian and Isaac J. Farrell

Rhabdomyolysis is a systemic injury state secondary to muscle tissue necrosis with release of intracellular contents into the circulation. In the United States, approximately 25,000 people are diagnosed with rhabdomyolysis annually. The majority of cases involve Na+/K+ ATPase disruption and, ultimately, calcium exchange resulting in myocyte necrosis and cell content release.

Risk factors for rhabdomyolysis include immobilization, electrocution, burns, polytrauma, rigors, excessive muscle movement, drowning, heat stroke/exhaustion, hypothermia, neuroleptic malignant syndrome, intoxication, agitation, infection, adverse medication reactions, and venoms and toxins. These conditions induce myolysis secondary to a combination of tissue ischemia, hypoperfusion, intracellular electrolyte disequilibrium, and ATP depletion. Given this extensive list of causes, it is important to consider rhabdomyolysis on the differential diagnosis of myriad clinical complaints and scenarios.

Symptoms can be variable, with the classic presentation of rhabdomyolysis categorized as muscle weakness, back and leg muscle aches, and reddish brown urine. These symptoms can be accompanied by low-grade fever, peripheral edema, and myoedema. In more moderate to severe cases, decreased urinary output, abdominal pain, nausea, vomiting, altered mental status, and encephalopathy occur. When assessing patients with these complaints and findings, be sure to obtain a detailed history including medications, recent trauma or increased physical activity, and social history including alcohol and drug use.

On examination, be sure to evaluate the temperature, heart rate, and rhythm. Assess musculoskeletal strength and palpate the muscle compartments for weakness, pain, or tense compartments. Skin examination can demonstrate dry mucous membranes, burns, bruising, soft tissue swelling/edema, or crush injury.

For the critical patient with rhabdomyolysis, establish intravenous access, provide supplemental oxygen, and place them on continuous cardiac monitoring. Assess the patient's airway, breathing, circulation, disability, and expose them. If the patient requires intubation, consider the risk of hyperkalemia and avoid succinylcholine. Treat agitation and initiate supportive care.

An electrocardiogram and a point-of-care potassium are beneficial in rapidly ruling out hyperkalemia and dysrhythmias. Labs for rhabdomyolysis should include CK, urinalysis, coagulation tests, phosphorus, magnesium, complete metabolic panel, and complete blood count, as well as uric acid. Evaluate the patient for any other exacerbating factors of their rhabdomyolysis, including sepsis or trauma.

CK is crucial in establishing this diagnosis and the degree of injury. Rhabdomyolysis is defined as an elevation 5 times (>1,000 IU/L) the upper limit of normal (20-200 IU/L). Increases appear within 12 hours of injury with a half-life of 1.5 days and can correlate with the muscle injury severity. Urinalysis is used to detect myoglobinuria secondary to myoglobinemia. Microscopic urine exam can differentiate between hemoglobinuria and myoglobinuria, with an absence of RBCs in rhabdomyolysis. Coagulation studies can detect a critical complication of rhabdomyolysis, disseminated intravascular coagulation. The release of intracellular contents including potassium, phosphorus, calcium, uric acid, creatinine, and transaminases necessitates the importance of investigating with a complete metabolic panel and uric acid and electrolyte levels. A complication of rhabdomyolysis is acute renal failure. Monitoring renal labs (BUN, creatinine), urine output, and the aforementioned labs will guide management of the patient. Patients with CK levels greater than 5,000 IU/L are at higher risk of acute renal injury.

ED management necessitates identification and treatment of any inciting factors, including discontinuation of medications that may be causing this condition, treating infection, warming or cooling the patients with environmental exposure, and damage control surgeries. Prevent further nephrotoxicity by stopping nephrotoxic medications and avoiding beta-blockers that may decrease renal blood flow. Fluid resuscitation is dependent on the fluid status of the patient. Resuscitation in patients with hypovolemia guided by urine output is recommended. Aggressive fluid resuscitation in patients with hypervolemia may cause fluid overload, increasing acute kidney injury risk and can increase the risk of compartment syndrome. Stabilization and management of acute electrolyte derangements is vital, particularly the treatment of hyperkalemia. Alkalinization of urine with sodium bicarbonate in rhabdomyolysis is controversial and can be initiated in a patient with metabolic acidosis. When monitoring kidney status, the McMahon score may be utilized by examining inciting factors, age, sex, creatinine, calcium, CK, phosphate, and bicarbonate levels to predict the need for renal replacement therapy.

Patient disposition is dependent on the disease severity. Healthy individuals experiencing exertional rhabdomyolysis with decreasing CK levels following fluid resuscitation and no other exacerbating factors may be discharged from the ED with outpatient follow-up and strict return precautions that include worsening weakness, swelling, decreased urinary output, or muscle pain. In patients with trauma, sepsis, dehydration, environmental exposure, intoxication, and increasing CK levels after fluid resuscitation will likely require hospital admission for further resuscitation and close monitoring.

PEARLS

- Clinical manifestations of rhabdomyolysis include muscle tenderness, weakness, and dark urine.
- Rhabdomyolysis should be considered in a variety of clinical histories including traumatic or crush injuries, drug abuse, seizures, and heat exposure.
- Diagnosis is confirmed by elevation in serum CK levels. Monitoring of serum levels will show a peak in 1 to 2 days with decline after 3 days, if inciting etiology has been corrected.
- Initial ED management includes the identification and correction of offending etiology, electrolyte management, and fluid resuscitation to prevent more severe sequelae of renal injuries.

SUGGESTED READINGS

Brown JV, Falat C. Rhabdomyolysis. In: Mattu A, Swadron S, eds. *CorePendium*. CorePendium, LLC. Updated June 30, 2022. Accessed April 23, 2023. https://www.emrap.org/corependium/chapter/reca40wRJ2SAEcJhB/Rhabdomyolysis#h.xwwapx7s6qp

Farkas J. Rhabdomyolysis. *Internet Book of Critical Care (IBCC)*. Accessed November 4, 2022. https://emcrit.org/ibcc/rhabdo/#Preamble

Hager HH, Burns B. Succinylcholine chloride. In: StatPearls [Internet]. StatPearls Publishing. Updated February 20, 2023. https://www.ncbi.nlm.nih.gov/books/NBK499984/

Long B, Koyfman A, Gottlieb M. An evidence-based narrative review of the emergency department evaluation and management of rhabdomyolysis. *Am J Emerg Med*. 2019; 37(3):518-523.

McMahon GM, Zeng X, Waikar SS. A risk prediction score for kidney failure or mortality in rhabdomyolysis. *JAMA Intern Med*. 2013;173(19):1821-1828.

Stanley M, Chippa V, Aeddula NR, et al. Rhabdomyolysis. In: *StatPearls* [Internet]. StatPearls Publishing. Updated January 16, 2023. https://www.ncbi.nlm.nih.gov/books/NBK448168/

Zimmerman JL, Shen MC. Rhabdomyolysis. *Chest*. 2013;144(3):1058-1065.

When Back Pain Is an Emergency

James Bohan and Manzy Byrd

Back pain is an extremely common complaint in every ED. In most cases, the diagnosis is nonspecific back pain that is treated with conservative management. Notwithstanding, it is important to consider emergent causes of back pain that may result in permanent neurologic dysfunction or even death. Several of these time-sensitive, emergent causes of back pain include cauda equina syndrome, epidural abscess, malignancy, and ruptured AAA.

Cauda equina syndrome is a rare but serious cause of back pain. It is most commonly the result of a massive central disk herniation that compresses multiple nerve roots. Other causes include malignancy, spinal hemorrhage, trauma, epidural abscess, and postoperative complications. The most common presenting symptom is urinary retention, with or without overflow incontinence, along with perineal anesthesia. Bilateral sciatica pain, sensory changes in the lower extremities, bowel dysfunction, and sexual dysfunction should also raise suspicion for cauda equina syndrome. As with any patient with acute back pain, it is important to conduct a thorough physical exam when considering cauda equina. On the physical examination, assess for altered bladder or bowel function, loss of rectal tone, saddle sensory deficits, lower extremity reflexes and motor function. A critical finding in cauda equina is urinary incontinence, which is overflow incontinence from a neurogenic bladder. If patients report or demonstrate urinary incontinence, check a postvoid residual with ultrasound, a bladder scan, or straight catheterization. A postvoid residual greater than 200 mL increases the likelihood of cauda equina syndrome. Importantly, not all symptoms are present at the time of clinical presentation, so it is important to maintain a high degree of suspicion for this condition. An emergent MRI should be obtained when concerned about cauda equina. Definitive treatment is surgical decompression. As such, it is important to consult your pertinent surgical service as soon as the diagnosis is considered or confirmed. Outcome is improved if decompression occurs within 2 days of symptom onset.

Epidural abscess is a back pain emergency that has significant morbidity and mortality if the diagnosis is delayed or missed. Patients at risk for epidural abscess include those who use IV drugs, are immunosuppressed, have diabetes, have had a recent spinal surgical intervention, and are alcoholics. Epidural abscess can result from hematogenous spread of bacteria from a remote site, from direct inoculation following a spinal procedure, or local extension from infections such as a disk space infection. *Staphylococcus aureus* is the most common bacterial cause, accounting for more than 60% of cases. In approximately one-third of cases, no portal of entry is found. The classic triad of epidural abscess is fever, back pain, and neurologic deficit. Unfortunately, this triad is rarely present upon initial presentation. Often, patients will present without fever and have no neurologic deficits. On physical examination, there may be tenderness to percussion in the area affected. Laboratory studies that may be helpful include an ESR, CRP, and CBC. Importantly, patients with an epidural abscess may not demonstrate a leukocytosis. If the ESR, CBC, and CRP findings are all normal, then the risk of an epidural abscess is low. The gold standard for diagnosis of epidural abscess is an MRI of the entire spine with contrast. A CT myelogram can also be ordered in place of an MRI in patients with contraindications to MRI. Once diagnosed, epidural abscesses are treated with surgical decompression and antibiotics. Given that many cases of epidural abscess are due to hematogenous spread, blood cultures should be obtained prior to antibiotic administration. Broad-spectrum antibiotics should include coverage for MRSA/MSSA and gram-negative organisms, especially in patients who use IV drugs.

Spinal epidural metastasis due to malignancy is another emergent etiology of back pain that is often missed during the initial evaluation. Metastatic lesions in the spine can result in cord compression and permanent neurologic deficits. Back pain is the most common presenting complaint. Classically, the pain is insidious in onset, worse at night, and partially relieved by activity. Sudden onset of pain may be the result of a pathologic fracture. CT of the spine will demonstrate bony detail best; however, MRI of the entire spine is indicated if there are signs and symptoms of cord compression. MRI with contrast will show the extent of epidural disease, edema around any fracture, and small lesions that may be missed on CT. Treatment includes high-dose steroids and neurosurgical consultation.

Finally, it is important to keep ruptured AAA in your differential of acute back pain. An AAA does not typically cause symptoms unless it is rapidly expanding or ruptures. Risk factors for AAA include male sex, age older than 50 years, and tobacco use. Ruptured AAA may present as only back or flank pain with no abdominal complaints. This can often be misdiagnosed as renal colic. Bedside ultrasound or CT with IV contrast can be used to confirm the diagnosis. Treatment requires emergent surgical consultation with operative or endovascular repair.

PEARLS

- Consider cauda equina in patients with acute back pain, saddle anesthesia, and a PVR greater than 200 mL.
- The classic triad of epidural abscess is rarely present at the time of initial presentation.
- Patients at high risk for epidural abscess include IV drug users, recent spinal procedure, patients with diabetes, and the immunocompromised.
- Spinal epidural metastasis often presents with insidious back pain that is worse at night.
- Ruptured AAA may present only with flank pain and can be misdiagnosed as renal colic.

Suggested Readings

Angus M, Curtis-Lopez CM, Carrasco R, *et al.* Determination of potential risk characteristics for cauda equina compression in emergency department patients presenting with atraumatic back pain: a 4-year retrospective cohort analysis within a tertiary referral neurosciences centre *Emergency Medicine Journal* 2022;39:740-746

Della-Giustina D. Evaluation and treatment of acute back pain in the emergency department. *Emerg Med Clin North Am.* 2015;33(2):311-326.

Gitelman A, Hishmeh S, Morelli BN, et al. Cauda equina syndrome: a comprehensive review. *Am J Orthop.* 2008;37(11):556-562.

Himmel W, Steinhart B, Helman A. Low back pain emergencies. *Emergency Medicine Cases*. Published September 2012. https://emergencymedicinecases.com/episode-26-low-back-pain-emergencies/

Reihsaus E, Waldbaur H, Seeling W. Spinal epidural abscess: a meta-analysis of 915 patients. *Neurosurg Rev*. 2000;23(4):175-204; discussion 205.

170

WHAT WORKS FOR MSK LOW BACK PAIN? STEROIDS, MUSCLE RELAXERS, OPIOIDS?

JONATHAN P. COSS AND PRITI RAWANI-PATEL

Approximately 80% of adults have low back pain at some time in their lives and this accounts for nearly 5% of total ED visits. This chapter discusses treatment recommendations for nontraumatic MSK low back pain.

MSK low back pain is defined as any pain, stiffness, and soreness between the 12th rib and the gluteal folds. Pain arises from one or more of the following anatomic structures: vertebrae, vertebral disks, facet joints, ligaments, and muscles. Symptoms commonly are described as dull, gnawing, tearing, burning, or electrical pain/spasms. Some patients present well appearing and ambulatory and may only need reassurance and resources for outpatient care. EM clinicians also see patients with debilitating pain unable to maintain their own ADLs and need admission. As the clinician tasked to initiate treatment, proper evaluation is critical.

The diagnosis of MSK low back pain should be made after excluding time-sensitive causes of back pain, such as infection, fracture, and neoplasm with cord compression. Chronicity of symptoms is also important. Most guidelines divide back pain into acute (<4 weeks), subacute (4-12 weeks), and chronic (>12 weeks). History consistent with MSK back pain often includes overuse, pain secondary to a lifting event, prolonged position changes, or poorly fitting backpacks in the pediatric population.

A thorough physical exam should be performed. Motor, sensory, reflexes, sphincter function, and postvoid residual measurements are crucial elements to evaluate in the patient with acute back pain. When confident the etiology of the pain is from an MSK source, diagnostic and laboratory tests are not indicated. The process of obtaining a thorough history, physical exam, and rapport building leads to a situation where true team decision-making with the patient can be done to avoid overworking/treating these conditions.

Current consensus practice guidelines recommend nonpharmacologic management as first-line treatment in patients with MSK low back pain. This includes rapport building, education, early return to normal activity/mobilization, temperature-based treatments, and gentle stretching. Rapid return to normal activity has been shown to lead to improved outcomes compared to bed rest. Massage, acupuncture, physical therapy, spinal manipulation, multidisciplinary rehabilitation, mindfulness-based stress reduction, tai chi, yoga, motor control exercise, progressive relaxation, biofeedback, low-level laser therapy, and cognitive behavioral therapy may be recommended as adjuncts and may be as effective as medications.

Reassuringly, 30% to 60% of patients recover in 1 week, 60% to 90% in 6 weeks, and 95% in 12 weeks. Approximately 40% of patients have a relapse at 6 months. In the ED, pharmacologic options are frequently utilized. Current guidelines allow for individualized medication management. Most start with medications that relieve pain/inflammation. NSAIDs, acetaminophen, muscle relaxants, and topical agents are first-line regimens. NSAIDs, acetaminophen, and skeletal muscle relaxants have shown good evidence for short-term effectiveness for acute pain, as well as tricyclic antidepressants for chronic pain. In cases of severe or uncontrolled pain, second-line therapy options include opioids, muscle relaxants, benzodiazepines, and gabapentin. Each class involves weighing benefits and harms with side effects. Notably, there is good evidence that systemic corticosteroids are ineffective for acute back pain. For disposition, all discharged patients should be recommended follow-up with a primary care physician within 1 to 2 weeks and given strict return precautions and education.

The treatment of MSK low back pain is truly an art and individualized. It is important to ask questions such as, "Where does the patient live? What type of work do they do? What type of transportation do they have?" Ultimately, the goal is to evaluate and treat any emergent pathologies and subsequently set the patient up for success to manage their concerns appropriately. We do this by combining team decision-making with clinical evidence. Clinically we look at outcomes including pain resolution, back function, quality of life, reduction of disability/return to work, global improvement, number of episodes and time between episodes, patient satisfaction, and adverse events.

PEARLS

- Individualized, case-by-case team decision-making is vital for treatment of nontraumatic MSK low back pain in the ED.
- Nonpharmacologic treatment should be used initially for most patients with acute or subacute low back pain.
- Stepwise pharmacologic treatment starting with NSAIDs and skeletal muscle relaxants should be used in conjunction with nonpharmacologic measures.
- Patient satisfaction seems to be more related to their perception that a careful history and physical examination have been conducted and that the provider has clearly explained the diagnosis and care plan rather than to receiving imaging/testing.

Suggested Readings

Balagué F, Mannion AF, Pellisé F, Cedraschi C. Non-specific low back pain. *Lancet*. 2012;379(9814):482-491.

Carey TS, Garrett J, Jackman A, et al. The outcomes and costs of care for acute low back pain among patients seen by primary care practitioners, chiropractors, and orthopedic surgeons. The North Carolina Back Pain Project. *N Engl J Med*. 1995;333:913-917.

Chou R, Huffman LH; American Pain Society; American College of Physicians. Medications for acute and chronic low back pain: a review of the evidence for an American Pain Society/American College of Physicians clinical practice guideline [published correction appears in *Ann Intern Med*. 2008;148(3):247-248]. *Ann Intern Med*. 2007;147(7):505-514.

Deyo RA, Weinstein JN. Low back pain. *N Engl J Med*. 2001;344:363-370.
Edlow JA. Managing nontraumatic acute back pain. Ann Emerg Med. 2015;66(2):148-153.
Edwards J, Hayden J, Asbridge M, Gregoire B, Magee K. Prevalence of low back pain in emergency settings: a systematic review and meta-analysis. *BMC Musculoskelet Disord.* 2017;18(1):143.
Friedman BW, Chilstrom M, Bijur PE, Gallagher EJ. Diagnostic testing and treatment of low back pain in United States emergency departments: a national perspective. *Spine (Phila Pa 1976)*. 2010;35(24):E1406-E1411.
Gianola S, Bargeri S, Del Castillo G, Corbetta D, Turolla A, Andreano A, et al. Effectiveness of treatments for acute and subacute mechanical non-specific low back pain: a systematic review with network meta-analysis. *Br J Sports Med.* 2022;56(1):41-50.
Malmivaara A, Hakkinen U, Aro T, et al. The treatment of acute low back pain—bed rest, exercises, or ordinary activity? *N Engl J Med.* 1995;332:351-355.
National Institute of Neurological Disorders and Stroke. Low back pain fact sheet. U.S. Department of Health and Human Services. https://www.ninds.nih.gov/low-back-pain-fact-sheet.

171

KNEE PAIN? DON'T FORGET TO CHECK THE HIP!

ALEXANDRA BARBOSA

Knee pain is a frequent reason for pediatric patients to present to the ED. The differential diagnosis can be extensive and include fractures, inflammatory and infectious etiologies, and malignancy. Delayed diagnosis can be detrimental and can lead to lifelong disability or delayed development. Referred pain from other locations and the inability of younger children to voice their complaints may further confound the diagnosis. A careful history and physical exam is needed to ascertain the primary cause of pain, especially in knee pain.

HISTORY

Age should guide the clinical history. For infants, the history should be obtained from a parent or the primary caregiver. Mechanism of injury should be considered in the context of development. For example, a fall from "walking" in a 6-month-old child should raise concern for nonaccidental trauma since developmentally this is very unlikely. In the older child, the onset, character, location of pain (eg, hip, pelvic, knee, or thigh), and occurrence of trauma are critical elements of the history, as is fever. Hip pathology may also present with altered gait or refusal to bear weight. Collateral information should be obtained from caregivers.

History questions should target the involved joint, as well as the joint above and below the area. It is well-recognized that children may present with knee pain that is referred from hip pathology. For example, 15% to 50% of patients with SCFE or Perthes disease will have knee pain at initial presentation, with up to 20% having a missed or delayed diagnosis. Given the risk of misdiagnosis, hip pathology should be considered in all patients with knee pain or with gait abnormalities.

EXAMINATION

The exam should begin with a gait analysis of truncal movement, pelvic tilt, hip and knee flexion and extension, and length of step. Children with advanced hip pathology may demonstrate truncal sway or Trendelenburg gait (pelvic tilt toward the ambulatory side with walking from weakness in the stationary side). Inability to bear weight in the affected limb after analgesia should raise concern for serious pathology that necessitates laboratory studies, imaging, and may include arthrocentesis to assess for septic arthritis.

It is important to assess bilateral joints, muscle groups, and nerve distributions. The initial examination should occur at rest. Patients with hip effusion, hemarthrosis, or hip fracture will often present with the hip resting in flexion, abduction, and external rotation. Examination also involves assessing skin changes, perfusion, and pulses distal to the site, followed by sensory and motor evaluation with passive and active range of motion of the joint. Internal rotation limitations may indicate hip joint disease. Serious pathology is not eliminated by an initial negative examination.

All ligaments of the knee should be tested for laxity. Active and passive range of motion of the knee should be used to further isolate involved ligaments and muscle groups. If no abnormality is found, referred pain should be considered in the differential diagnosis and other joints evaluated. In the setting of hip pathology, the back, groin, and abdomen should be evaluated as genitourinary pathology, acute abdomen, or lumbar disease may masquerade as hip pain.

WORKUP AND IMAGING

Laboratory and imaging studies should be guided by physical exam. The Kocher criteria can be used to assess the risk of transient synovitis versus septic arthritis. The Kocher criteria is defined as an erythrocyte sedimentation rate greater than 40 mm/h, white blood cell count more than 12,000 cells/mm^3, refusal to bear weight, and fever. The addition of CRP to the Kocher criteria may improve sensitivity for septic arthritis. Although low yield, blood cultures should be obtained and can confirm the diagnosis and guide management in some cases. Concern for rheumatologic etiologies may necessitate immunologic lab markers.

Plain radiographs are considered first-line imaging and may demonstrate widening of joint spaces, fracture, and bone density irregularities. SCFE, typically seen in the early adolescent and obese boys, is assessed with radiographs. The Klein line, a line normally extending from the superior edge of the femoral neck and crossing the superior femoral head epiphysis lateral aspect, on AP radiographs is measured. Without that intersection, SCFE is likely. AP and frog leg views with bilateral hip imaging should be used as SCFE may be bilateral in 20% of cases.

POCUS can assess the periarticular tissue and joint space if there is concern for effusion but cannot distinguish between pyogenic or sterile effusions. Ultrasound allows for dynamic evaluation of the joint space and tissues but is still considered inferior to MRI. MRI with intra-articular contrast can assess joint space abnormalities and the synovium. MRI allows for the best visualization of the joint space, synovium, labrum, and surrounding musculature and is considered superior to CT for evaluation of soft tissues. However, MRI can be cost and resource intensive, as children may require procedural sedation to obtain images.

> **PEARLS**
>
> - Primary hip pathology should be considered in the differential for knee pain.
> - The joint above and below the area of interest should be evaluated with musculoskeletal complaints.
> - Examination and the differential should guide workup, including labs and imaging.

SUGGESTED READINGS

Chiamil SM, Abarca CA Imaging of the hip: a systematic approach to the young adult hip. *Muscles Ligaments Tendons J*. 2016;6(3):265-280.

Houghton KM. Review for the generalist: evaluation of pediatric hip pain. *Pediatr Rheumatol*. 2009;7:10.

Karkenny AJ, Tauberg BM, Otsuka NY. Pediatric hip disorders: slipped capital femoral epiphysis and Legg-Calvé-Perthes disease. *Pediatr Rev*. 2018;39(9):454-463.

Kocher MS, Mandiga R, Zurakowski D, Barnewolt C, Kasser JR. Validation of a clinical prediction rule for the differentiation between septic arthritis and transient synovitis of the hip in children. *J Bone Joint Surg Am*. 2004;86(8):1629-1635.

Matava MJ, Patton CM. Knee pain as the initial symptom of slipped capital femoral epiphysis: an analysis of initial presentation and treatment. *J Pediatr Orthop*. 1999;19(4):455-460.

Mick NW, Valasek AE. Pediatric orthopedic emergencies. in Orthopedic Emergencies: Expert Management for the Emergency Physician. Cambridge University Press 2013: 165-177.

Neville DN, Zuckerbraum N. Pediatric nontraumatic hip pathology. *Clin Pediatr Emerg Med*. 2016;17(1):13-28.

Song KM, Halliday S, Reilly C, Keezel W. Gait abnormalities following slipped capital femoral epiphysis. *J Pediatr Orthop*. 2004;24(2):148-155.

172

AVOID THESE PITFALLS IN THE DIAGNOSIS OF SEPTIC JOINT

DELANEY FISHER AND PRITI RAWANI-PATEL

Any patient with an acute monoarticular arthritis should be considered to have septic arthritis until proven otherwise. Prompt diagnosis in the ED is essential, since cartilage can be destroyed within days, leading to permanent disability. As if permanent joint destruction was not bad enough, the mortality rate for in-hospital septic arthritis is high; 7% to 15% despite antibiotic use. Predisposing factors include advanced age, preexisting joint disease (crystalline arthropathies, rheumatoid arthritis, prosthetic joints), recent joint surgery or injection, overlying skin or soft tissue infection, injection drug use, and immunosuppression.

Septic arthritis most commonly arises from hematogenous spread. The synovial tissue lacks a basement membrane, meaning that bacteria can easily pass from blood into the synovial fluid. Keep in mind that bacteremia is more likely to localize in a joint with preexisting disease. Other modes of infection include direct inoculation into the joint or spread from an adjacent soft tissue or bone infection.

In decreasing order, septic arthritis most commonly affects the knee (50% of cases), hip, shoulder, and elbow; however, any joint can become infected. Septic arthritis is usually monomicrobial, with *Staphylococcus aureus* (including methicillin-resistant *S. aureus*) being the most common cause in healthy adults. Streptococci species are also important causes of infection. Infection with a gram-negative bacillus typically occurs in older patients, immunocompromised, and injection drug users.

Unfortunately, the ED clinician cannot rely solely on physical examination findings and blood work to differentiate a septic joint from an inflamed joint. The classic teaching is that patients will present with an erythematous, swollen, painful joint with decreased range of motion; however, the absence of these symptoms does not rule out a septic joint. Most will obtain bloodwork, including blood cultures, CBC with differential, and inflammatory markers, and although a leukocytosis and elevated ESR/CRP may raise our suspicion for a septic joint, the lack of these findings does not reliably rule out the diagnosis. The definitive test is an arthrocentesis.

When septic arthritis is suspected, arthrocentesis is mandatory. Synovial fluid should be sent for cell count and differential, glucose and protein, culture, and light microscopy for crystals. Generally, a synovial fluid WBC count of greater than 50,000 with a neutrophil predominance is suggestive of an infectious process. The presence of crystals does not exclude septic arthritis, as patients with gout and pseudogout are at higher risk for concomitant septic arthritis. After arthrocentesis, prompt antibiotic administration is crucial. Treatment is divided into gonococcal and nongonococcal coverage. A third-generation cephalosporin, such as ceftriaxone, is treatment of choice for gonococcal disease. For nongonococcal disease, initial antibiotic treatment should also include vancomycin to target gram-positive cocci. Orthopedic surgery should be consulted, and all patients should be admitted for continued antibiotic therapy and possible surgical management.

PEARLS

- Septic arthritis is a form of acute, destructive arthritis. Prompt diagnosis is essential to avoid permanent joint destruction and mortality. Maintain a high index of suspicion.
- Do not rely solely on history and physical examination findings to rule in or rule out the diagnosis.
- If abnormal, blood work may help corroborate a suspicion of septic arthritis but should not be used alone to rule in or rule out the diagnosis.
- Arthrocentesis is the only definitive diagnostic test and required to confirm a septic joint.

Suggested Readings

Carpenter CR, Schuur JD, Everett WW, Pines JM. Evidence-based diagnostics: adult septic arthritis [published correction appears in *Acad Emerg Med.* 2011;18(9):1011]. *Acad Emerg Med.* 2011;18(8):781-796. PMID: 21843213.

Hanlon D, Meyer J. Septic arthritides. In: Mattu A, Swadron S, eds. *CorePendium*. CorePendium, LLC. 2023. Accessed July 11, 2023. https://www.emrap.org/corependium/chapter/rechjM70gyPsnPomE/Septic-Arthritides#h.wak5jz4oldqm

Long B, Koyfman A, Gottlieb M. Evaluation and management of septic arthritis and its mimics in the emergency department. *West J Emerg Med*. 2019;20(2):331-341. PMID: 30881554.

Margaretten ME, Kohlwes J, Moore D, Bent S. Does this adult patient have septic arthritis? *JAMA*. 2007;297(13):1478-1488. PMID: 17405973.

Mathews CJ, Coakley G. Septic arthritis: current diagnostic and therapeutic algorithm. *Curr Opin Rheumatol*. 2008;20(4):457-462. PMID: 18525361.

173

DON'T MISS (INFECTIOUS) FLEXOR TENOSYNOVITIS

SAM KAPLAN AND NICOLA BAKER

Infectious flexor tenosynovitis is a surgical emergency that cannot be missed in the ED. Flexor tenosynovitis can be difficult to distinguish from other hand infections or pathologies, and a delay in diagnosis can lead to substantial morbidity to the patient. Since flexor tenosynovitis is mainly a clinical diagnosis, it is the job of the emergency physician to quickly diagnose the condition in order to initiate appropriate antibiotics and disposition of the patient to a hand specialist. In this chapter, we focus on the etiologies, signs/symptoms, workup, and treatment of infectious flexor tenosynovitis.

Flexor tenosynovitis is inflammation of a flexor tendon sheath in the hand. This inflammation is not always infectious and can be due to systemic disease. Infectious, or pyogenic, flexor tenosynovitis is due to bacterial infection within the enclosed tendinous sheath. This is most commonly a result of direct inoculation following penetrating trauma. It can less commonly be caused by hematogenous spread from another infection (such as a felon, septic joint, or deep space infection).

History questions should focus on risk factors, such as recent trauma, animal/human bites, IV drug use, or, in rare cases, water exposure that can cause tenosynovitis due to *Mycobacterium marinum*. It is also important that you ask about factors that may predispose them to infection or poor wound healing, such as immunosuppression or diabetes, as well as any sexual risk factors for disseminated gonococcal disease. Be sure to inquire when they received their last tetanus booster.

Patients will typically present to the ED with complaints of redness, swelling, and pain of the digit and/or hand. The pain is often worse with movement. The symptoms are usually localized to the affected digit on the palmar aspect. Patients can present in a delayed manner approximately 24 to 48 hours after the inciting event, so quick recognition is imperative. First and foremost, ensure that the infected digit is neurovascularly intact. The emergency physician should then examine the digit/hand for the following four Kanavel cardinal signs of flexor tenosynovitis:

1) Pain with passive extension of the digit
2) Tenderness to palpation along the flexor tendon sheath

3) Uniform symmetric swelling of the digit ("sausage" digit)
4) Digit held in flexion at rest

The Kanavel signs have a high sensitivity (91%-97%) but a low specificity (51%-69%) for flexor tenosynovitis. The presence of all four Kanavel signs should certainly cue the emergency physician to suspect flexor tenosynovitis. However, given the consequence of a missed diagnosis, even the presence of some of the Kanavel signs should raise suspicion for the disease.

The tendon sheaths in the second through fourth digits are closed spaces, so infections in these digits should be contained. However, the tendon sheaths of the first and fifth digits can connect via bursae at the wrist, leading to a "horseshoe abscess." To assess for this condition, palpate the volar aspect of the wrist for any signs of tenderness, fluctuance, or induration.

Although flexor tenosynovitis is predominately a clinical diagnosis, general infectious laboratory work is recommended and can be useful to support the diagnosis. Workup can include a CBC, CRP, ESR, and x-ray of the affected digit. Radiographs can be helpful to evaluate for a foreign object and to screen for osteomyelitis. An MRI is sometimes done to determine the extent of the ongoing infection and/or to guide surgical planning and evaluate for osteomyelitis. However, MRI cannot accurately delineate infectious versus inflammatory tenosynovitis. POCUS can be a helpful adjunct in the diagnosis of flexor tenosynovitis by demonstrating peritendinous fluid and thickened synovial sheath. The use a water bath can aid in ultrasound imaging of the hand. Identification of peritendinous fluid on POCUS can be useful to distinguish between cellulitis, abscess, and flexor tenosynovitis in instances where all four Kanavel signs are not present.

Once you suspect infectious flexor tenosynovitis, immobilize the affected area and give empiric IV antibiotics. Empiric antibiotic therapy should cover gram-positive (including MRSA) and gram-negative organisms. Gram-negative coverage can be guided by the mechanism of injury and the history obtained from the patient. Vancomycin plus ampicillin/sulbactam or vancomycin plus ceftriaxone are common empiric regimens. If the patient is diabetic or there is a concern for pseudomonas, IV piperacillin/tazobactam can be substituted as the second agent. If exposure to seawater occurred, consider covering for marine exposure to *M. marinum* with either doxycycline or sulfamethoxazole/trimethoprim.

The definitive treatment for infectious flexor tenosynovitis is surgical exploration and incision and drainage of the tendon sheath by general orthopedics or a hand specialist. Suspected infectious flexor tenosynovitis should be transferred for consultation if one is not available. Failure to recognize and treat infectious tenosynovitis can lead to ischemia, skin/tendon necrosis, contracture, and amputation.

This high-risk condition cannot be missed in the ED. This is a surgical emergency, so recognition of the cardinal Kanavel signs with immediate initiation of antibiotics, appropriate surgical consultation, and admission to the hospital is extremely important.

PEARLS

- The four cardinal Kanavel signs are critical to the diagnosis.
- Immediately start broad-spectrum antibiotics that cover common skin and soft tissue organisms.
- An emergent orthopedics/hand consult is necessary in the ED.

- Laboratory studies can increase suspicion for the condition but cannot exclude it.
- Imaging is not required. MRI may help determine the extent of infection, guide surgical management, or determine associated osteomyelitis.

Suggested Readings

Chapman T, Ilyas AM. Pyogenic flexor tenosynovitis: evaluation and treatment strategies. *J Hand Surg Am.* 2019;44(11):981-985.

Goyal K, Speeckaert AL. Pyogenic flexor tenosynovitis: evaluation and management. *Hand Clin.* 2020;36(3):323-329.

Hermena S, Tiwari V. Pyogenic flexor tenosynovitis. In: *StatPearls* [Internet]. StatPearls Publishing; 2023. https://www.ncbi.nlm.nih.gov/books/NBK576414/

Jardin E, Delord M, Aubry S, Loisel F, Obert L. Usefulness of ultrasound for the diagnosis of pyogenic flexor tenosynovitis: a prospective single-center study of 57 cases. *Hand Surg Rehabil.* 2018;37(2):95-98.

SECTION XIV
NEUROLOGY

174

DIAGNOSING CERVICAL ARTERY DISSECTION IN THE ED: A REAL PAIN IN THE NECK!

AMIR A. ROUHANI, KELLIE KITAMURA, AND STEVEN LAI

CAD is a condition characterized by a tear or rupture of the intimal wall of a cervical artery, resulting in a partial or complete interruption of blood flow. The two subtypes of CAD include carotid artery dissection and vertebral artery dissection. Carotid artery dissection is the underlying cause of 2.5% of all strokes and up to 20% of strokes in children and young adults. In contrast, the annual incidence of vertebral artery dissection is far less common, occurring in as few as 1 in 100,000 patients. While the overall incidence of CAD is low, a high index of suspicion and prompt diagnosis in the ED are crucial, given the risk of rapid progression of thromboembolic complications leading to devastating adverse outcomes.

CAD is often classified by its mechanism, either traumatic or spontaneous. Traumatic CAD occurs as a direct result of significant trauma. Spontaneous CAD generally occurs "spontaneously" in patients with an underlying predisposition. The term *spontaneous CAD*, however, is somewhat of a misnomer as many instances are also associated with minor trauma. Therefore, a more appropriate term *provoked spontaneous* CAD has been suggested.

The traumatic factors implicated in CAD include blunt neck trauma as well as "minor" neck stressors, such as vomiting, painting a ceiling, practicing yoga, chiropractic neck manipulations, and/or sneezing. Approximately 15% to 20% of patients with CAD will also have an underlying condition that predisposes to vascular abnormalities, such as fibromuscular dysplasia, Marfan syndrome, autosomal polycystic kidney disease, or osteogenesis imperfecta.

The clinical presentation of CAD is variable, making it challenging to diagnose in the ED. Patients with carotid artery dissection may present with anterior circulation stroke symptoms, including hemiparesis, dysarthria, or Horner syndrome. Vertebral artery dissection can manifest as a posterior circulation stroke syndrome, with ataxia, diplopia, or dysarthria. Many patients, however, present only with isolated headache, neck pain, or facial pain, emphasizing the need for a high index of suspicion. Because current therapy for CAD involves early initiation of anticoagulation to prevent thromboembolic complications, prompt diagnosis with advanced angiographic imaging with CT or MRI at this early stage is essential to prevent poor outcomes.

Carotid Artery Dissection

The most characteristic presentations of carotid artery dissection are those where patients present with findings of both pain and neurologic symptoms. The combination of carotid artery–specific focal neurologic deficits along with neck pain (25%-50%), facial pain (50%), or headache (44%-69%) should alert the clinician toward the diagnosis of carotid artery dissection. The neck pain in carotid artery dissection tends to be ipsilateral and is located in the upper anterolateral cervical region, while the facial pain most typically involves the orbital region. The headache can be frontal, frontal-temporal, frontal-parietal, or posterior. The headache is most often gradual and throbbing but can also present as sudden and severe in onset.

The classic triad described for carotid artery dissection of headache, anterior cerebral stroke, and Horner syndrome is present in only 8% of patients. The most common neurologic deficits in these patients are anterior cerebral and retinal ischemic deficits. Amaurosis fugax, or transient monocular vision loss, occurs in approximately 3% of patients with carotid artery dissection and generally precedes the cerebral infarct. Dissection of the arterial wall can also lead to compromise of ascending sympathetic fibers, causing a complete or incomplete Horner syndrome. Cranial nerve palsies occur in approximately 12% of patients, with the hypoglossal (XII) nerve most frequently affected. Isolated dysgeusia, although rare, can be highly suggestive of carotid artery dissection. Multiple cranial nerve findings that occur simultaneously have also been reported. Finally, pulsatile tinnitus has been reported, and a cervical bruit can sometimes be auscultated on examination.

The following combination of pain and neurologic symptoms should immediately raise suspicion for carotid artery dissection:

- Pain and anterior cerebral ischemia
- Pain and complete or partial Horner syndrome
- Pain and cranial nerve palsies
- Pain and pulsatile tinnitus

Vertebral Artery Dissection

Vertebral artery dissection is associated with a different constellation of symptoms compared to carotid artery dissection. The head and neck pain is generally posterior in location, and the accompanying neurologic signs and symptoms involve deficits characteristic of compromise to the posterior circulation. Posterior circulation deficits include ataxia, diplopia, dysarthria, locked-in syndrome, and lateral medullary syndrome. Neurologic deficits in vertebral artery dissection can also result from compressive aneurysmal dilation leading to unilateral radicular weakness in the C5-C6 distribution.

Patients With No Neurologic Findings

In the most challenging of clinical circumstances, a patient with a CAD may present with only headache, facial pain, or neck pain in the absence of specific neurologic findings. Several studies have shown that isolated headache is a common presentation in patients with CAD, with up to 44% presenting with this lone complaint. In these cases, the only "clue" of CAD may be the new onset of headache or neck pain in a typical distribution, preceded by a concerning mechanism (often minor!) and/or occurring in a patient with an underlying predisposition, such as a connective tissue disease.

Table 174.1 summarizes the clinical features of both types of CAD.

TABLE 174.1	CLINICAL FEATURES OF CERVICAL ARTERY DISSECTION	
	CAROTID ARTERY DISSECTION	**VERTEBRAL ARTERY DISSECTION**
Pain symptoms	Frontal headache Facial or orbital pain Anterior or lateral neck pain	Occipital headache Posterior neck pain
Neurologic symptoms	Anterior circulation stroke Partial or complete Horner syndrome Amaurosis fugax Cranial nerve palsies (including tongue deviation and isolated dysgeusia) Pulsatile tinnitus	Posterior circulation stroke ■ Hemianopsia ■ Ataxia ■ Diplopia ■ Dysarthria ■ Locked-in syndrome Lateral medullary syndrome Upper extremity radiculopathy

PEARLS

- CAD can result from injury to the intimal wall of the carotid or vertebral artery and can be traumatic or spontaneous.
- Consider CAD in patients with a new onset of headache or neck pain after blunt neck trauma or any activity that results in minor trauma, stress, or manipulation of the neck.
- CAD can present with or without neurologic deficits.
- Carotid artery dissection can present with any combination of head/facial/neck pain with or without anterior circulation stroke symptoms, Horner syndrome, amaurosis fugax, cranial nerve palsies, or pulsatile tinnitus.
- Vertebral artery dissection can present with any combination of head/neck pain and posterior circulation stroke symptoms.

SUGGESTED READINGS

Arnold M, Cumurciuc R, Stapf C, Favrole P, Berthet K, Bousser MG. Pain as the only symptom of cervical artery dissection. *J Neurol Neurosurg Psychiatry*. 2006;77(9):1021-1024.

Debette S, Leys D. Cervical-artery dissections: predisposing factors, diagnosis, and outcome. *Lancet Neurol*. 2009;8(7):668–678.

Patel RR, Adam R, Maldjian C, et al. Cervical carotid artery dissection: current review of diagnosis and treatment. *Cardiol Rev*. 2012;20(3):145-152.

Robertson JJ, Koyfman A. Cervical artery dissections: a review. *J Emerg Med*. 2016; 51(5):508-518.

Robertson JJ, Koyfman A. Extracranial cervical artery dissections. *Emerg Med Clin North Am*. 2017;35(4):727-741.

Shea K, Stahmer S. Carotid and vertebral arterial dissections in the emergency department. *Emerg Med Pract*. 2012;14(4):1-23; quiz 23-24.

175

UNDERSTAND THE UTILITY AND LIMITATIONS OF DIAGNOSTIC IMAGING IN NONTRAUMATIC SUBARACHNOID HEMORRHAGE

MIGUEL LEMUS

Headache is the chief complaint for 2% of ED patients each year. Only 1% of those will ultimately be diagnosed with a nontraumatic SAH. The diagnosis of SAH is challenging but essential in the ED as the disease is potentially catastrophic if not identified in a timely manner. On the first day of illness, patients with nontraumatic SAH have a 12% mortality. This increases to an alarming 40% by 1 month after the event. If a diagnosis of aneurysmal rupture is missed, the risk of rebleed and significantly higher morbidity and mortality is imminent. To ensure appropriate diagnosis of this life-threatening disease, we should understand the utility and limitations of the various diagnostic imaging modalities currently employed in patients with suspected SAH.

Fortunately, the combination of negative noncontrast CT of the head followed by negative LP adequately rules out SAH. Subarachnoid blood seen on CT or a CSF specimen sample with either nonclearing red blood cells or xanthochromia is highly suggestive of SAH.

Noncontrast CT has a high sensitivity for ruling out SAH when obtained very early after the onset of headache but drops rapidly with time. There is a nearly 100% sensitivity in ruling out SAH with a negative noncontrast CT head with the following caveats: (1) the headache must have clearly started less than 6 hours before imaging, (2) the CT used is at least a 3rd-generation multidetector scanner, and (3) the read is finalized by an attending radiologist (either a neuroradiologist or a general radiologist with routine exposure to CT head). The sensitivity of a negative head CT drops to 93% at 12 to 24 hours and to less than 60% at 24 hours to 5 days. A negative head CT after 6 hours requires additional diagnostic evaluation.

Some physicians have advocated for the use of CTA in lieu of the traditional noncontrast CT/LP approach as LPs are time consuming, have a low diagnostic yield, a high rate of traumatic taps, a high rate of uninterpretable test results, and are associated with a relatively high rate of procedural pain and of post-LP headaches. CTA has some desirable characteristics to support its use: It is fast, easy to obtain, and minimally invasive. Moreover, CTA has a sensitivity of 98% in ruling out aneurysms greater than 3 mm, but it must be recognized that the CTA will not show bleeding, as it only images the vascular lumen. The strategy of utilizing CTA in place of CT/LP does pose some additional considerations. These include an increased exposure to ionizing radiation, contrast exposure with possible reactions, and most importantly, the diagnosis of incidental (asymptomatic) aneurysms. The prevalence of aneurysms in the general population is 2%, while the incidence of SAH is exceedingly low (0.01%). Therefore, most aneurysms detected on CTA are *incidental*—they pose little or no risk of rupture. Simply identifying these "nonculprit" aneurysms can pose potential downstream harm to the patient in the form of unnecessary neurosurgical evaluation, further imaging, and the potential for unnecessary surgical or invasive repair. It is also worth considering that the diagnosis of an incidental aneurysm does cause emotional angst in many patients.

Magnetic resonance imaging is another diagnostic modality in the diagnosis of SAH. MRI with proton density and FLAIR sequences may be as sensitive as head CT for the acute detection of SAH. MRI may provide a greater ability to evaluate other potential causes of headache, but its use is limited due to routine availability, motion artifact, longer study time, and cost.

Currently, the AHA/ASA guidelines advocate the use of noncontrast head CT followed by LP for the initial evaluation of suspected SAH. The ACEP Clinical Policy on the evaluation and management of acute headache states that in the adult ED patient who is still considered to be at risk for SAH after a negative noncontrast head CT, CTA of the head appears to be a reasonable alternative to LP and to use shared decision-making to select the best diagnostic testing modality after weighing potential pros and cons of LP versus CTA.

PEARLS

- A missed diagnosis of aneurysm bleed can result in re-rupture and associated significant increase in morbidity and mortality.
- Guidelines by AHA/ASA continue to recommend the combination of noncontrast CT head followed by LP to adequately rule out SAH.
- ACEP clinical policy recommends noncontrast head CT followed by LP or CTA after shared decision-making to adequately rule out SAH.
- A noncontrast head CT may rule out SAH when obtained within 6 hours of headache onset with the aforementioned caveats.

Suggested Readings

American College of Emergency Physicians Clinical Policies Subcommittee (Writing Committee) on Acute Headache; Godwin SA, Cherkas DS, Panagos PD, et al. Clinical policy: critical issues in the evaluation and management of adult patients presenting to the emergency department with acute headache. *Ann Emerg Med*. 2019;74(4), e41-e74.

Dubosh NM, Bellolio MF, Rabinstein AA, Edlow JA. Sensitivity of early brain computed tomography to exclude aneurysmal subarachnoid hemorrhage: a systematic review and meta-analysis. *Stroke*. 2016;47:750.

Edlow JA. What are the unintended consequences of changing the diagnostic paradigm for subarachnoid hemorrhage after brain computed tomography to computed tomographic angiography in place of lumbar puncture? *Acad Emerg Med*. 2010;17(9):991-995; discussion 996-997.

Perry JJ, Spacek A, Forbes M, et al. Is the combination of negative computed tomography result and negative lumbar puncture result sufficient to rule out subarachnoid hemorrhage? *Ann Emerg Med*. 2008;51(6):707-713.

Perry JJ, Stiell IG, Sivilotti ML, et al. Sensitivity of computed tomography performed within 6 hours of onset of headache for diagnosis of subarachnoid haemorrhage: prospective cohort study. *BMJ*. 2011;343:d4277.

176

LEAVE IT ALONE: BLOOD PRESSURE MEASUREMENT IN ISCHEMIC STROKE

AMIR A. ROUHANI, STEVEN LAI, AND KELLIE KITAMURA

Stroke is defined as any vascular injury that leads to a reduction of cerebral blood flow to an area of the brain, resulting in neurologic impairment. AIS accounts for approximately 85% of strokes and can result from thrombosis, embolism, or systemic hypoperfusion. Hemorrhagic stroke, which includes ICH and nontraumatic SAH, accounts for the remaining 15%.

After an acute stroke, blood flow and, therefore, oxygen transport are reduced locally, resulting in hypoxia of the areas near the location of the original insult. Within the ischemic cerebrovascular bed, there are two major zones of injury: the core ischemic zone and the ischemic "penumbra." The penumbra is the viable tissue immediately surrounding the irreversibly damaged ischemic core, where distal branches become dilated and perfusion pressure is low. The primary goal of acute stroke management is to salvage this penumbral tissue and optimize resultant brain function. This delicate balance between preserving cerebral perfusion and preventing further brain injury underscores the importance of BP management in the ED during the acute phase of stroke.

A central concept in the medical management of all acute strokes has focused on the maintenance of CPP in order to optimize perfusion to these zones of injury. CPP is derived by the following formula: CPP = MAP − ICP. Permissive hypertension involves the avoidance of aggressive lowering of BP to maintain an elevated MAP and thus preserve CPP.

In contrast to hemorrhagic stroke, where there may be a role for BP reduction in the ED phase of management, guidelines for AIS continue to emphasize *permissive hypertension*—the deliberate "hands-off" maintenance of BP in the ED. The goal of permissive hypertension is the avoidance of aggressive lowering of BP in order to maintain an elevated MAP and thus preserve CPP.

Elevated arterial BP is a common occurrence at the time of presentation among patients with AIS, occurring in up to three-quarters of cases. This may be due to underlying chronic hypertension, an acute sympathetic response, or other stroke-related mechanisms. This initial hypertensive response is most pronounced immediately following the acute stroke. BP will generally begin to decrease spontaneously within 90 minutes and steadily decline over the first 24 hours.

Multiple studies have found a U-shaped relationship between the admission BP and poor clinical outcomes. Extreme arterial hypertension can be detrimental because it may lead to worsening cerebral edema and hemorrhagic transformation, encephalopathy, cardiac complications, and renal insufficiency. Conversely, extreme arterial hypotension can lead to decreased perfusion to multiple organs, especially the ischemic brain. Finally, there may be certain situations where concomitant medical conditions, such as myocardial ischemia, aortic dissection, and heart failure, may accompany AIS and may be exacerbated by extreme changes in MAP. Therefore, moderate arterial hypertension might represent the best opportunity to optimize CPP while avoiding the harm of extreme hypertension.

The 2018 AHA/ASA guidelines for the early management of patients with AIS and the 2019 updated guidelines recommend that for patients who are not candidates for reperfusion therapy with fibrinolytic agents or mechanical thrombectomy, hypertension may be "permitted" unless it is *extremely* high (SBP > 220 mm Hg or DBP > 120 mm Hg) or if a concurrent medical condition warrants initiation of antihypertensive treatment. If BP-lowering strategies are initiated, a suggested target is a 15% reduction in SBP for the first 24 hours. In patients who are eligible for treatment with intravenous fibrinolytic agents or mechanical thrombectomy, BP should be carefully lowered so that SBP is less than 185 mm Hg and DBP less than 110 mm Hg. When present, hypotension and hypovolemia should also be corrected to maintain systemic perfusion levels necessary to support organ function.

First-line agents for BP management in AIS include labetalol, nicardipine, and clevidipine. These agents allow rapid and safe titration to the goal BP. Labetalol may be started at 10 to 20 mg intravenously over 1 to 2 minutes and may be repeated once before initiating a continuous infusion of 2 to 8 mg/min. Nicardipine may be started intravenously at 5 mg/h, titrating up by 2.5 mg/h every 5 to 15 minutes (maximum 15 mg/h). Clevidipine may be started at 1 to 2 mg/h, titrating up by doubling the dose every 2 to 5 min until the desired BP is reached (maximum 21 mg/h).

PEARLS

- The management of elevated BP in AIS should follow the principle of permissive hypertension. For those who are not treated with thrombolytic therapy or mechanical thrombectomy, antihypertensive therapy should only be considered if the hypertension is extreme (SBP > 220 mm Hg or DBP > 120 mm Hg) or if the patient has another clear indication (active myocardial ischemia, congestive heart failure, or aortic dissection).
- When treatment is indicated, the goal should be to lower BP by approximately 15% during the first 24 hours after stroke onset.
- For patients with AIS who are candidates for reperfusion therapy with thrombolytic therapy or mechanical thrombectomy, antihypertensive treatment may be initiated with a target SBP of less than 185 mm Hg and DBP less than 110 mm Hg. Labetalol, nicardipine, and clevidipine are the recommended first-line agents.

Suggested Readings

Fisher M. New approaches to neuroprotective drug development. *Stroke*. 2011;42(1 Suppl): S24-S27.

Peacock WF, Varon J, Baumann BM, et al. Clevidipine in acute hypertensive patients with intracerebral hemorrhage: a multicenter, randomized, double-blind, placebo-controlled trial. *Int J Stroke*. 2019;14(6):612-617.

Powers WJ, Rabinstein AA, Ackerson T, et al. Guidelines for the early management of patients with acute ischemic stroke: 2019 update to the 2018 guidelines for the early management of acute ischemic stroke: a guideline for healthcare professionals from the American Heart Association/American Stroke Association. *Stroke*. 2019;50:e344-e418.

Qureshi AI. Acute hypertensive response in patients with stroke: pathophysiology and management. *Circulation*. 2008;118(2):176-187.

Qureshi AI, Acosta FJ, Majidi S, et al. Effect of systolic blood pressure reduction on hematoma expansion, perihematomal edema, and 3-month outcome among patients with intracerebral hemorrhage: results from the antihypertensive treatment of acute cerebral hemorrhage study. *Arch Neurol*. 2011;68(5):570-576.

177

CEREBRAL VENOUS SINUS THROMBOSIS: A RARE DIAGNOSIS WITH A COMMON CHIEF COMPLAINT

STEVEN LAI, KELLIE KITAMURA, AND AMIR A. ROUHANI

CVST results in obstruction of the cerebral venous dural sinuses. It is a relatively uncommon phenomenon and frequently overlooked at initial presentation as it can mimic other acute neurologic conditions and requires a high index of suspicion. It is an important cause of stroke resulting from complete or partial occlusion of the major cerebral venous sinuses or smaller feeding cortical veins.

CVST generally occurs in younger adults, most commonly in their 30s to 50s, and is about 3 times as common in women than men, partially due to its association with pregnancy, the use of OCPs, and the puerperium period. A thorough investigation for underlying systemic inflammatory disease, malignancy, prothrombotic pathology, recent infections, or trauma will reveal at least one risk factor in 85% of patients (**Table 177.1**), but some patients, especially the older adult, may have no easily identifiable risk factors.

The clinical presentation of CVST is often variable and nonspecific, reflecting the location of the thrombus and the ability for a clot to extend or recanalize over time (**Table 177.2**). While a thrombus can result in specific clinical syndromes, it is often less linear clinically, especially if there are multiple sites of thrombosis simultaneously. If untreated, the thrombus may extend and lead to additional symptoms. As venous sinuses play a role in CSF drainage, sinus thrombosis can result in communicating hydrocephalus.

The majority of patients with CVST present with a general onset of headache. The headache is often the first symptom and is generally exacerbated by a supine position. The onset is typically gradual; however, a small subset of patients may present with a thunderclap headache, particularly if the CVST leads to a secondary subarachnoid hemorrhage. The headache may also be accompanied by localizing deficits, such as focal weakness or aphasia, focal seizures, encephalopathic behavior, or a combination of all. Headache with a seizure should prompt consideration of CVST as one-third of patients with CVST will have either focal or generalized seizure activity. Nonconvulsive seizures

TABLE 177.1 RISK FACTORS FOR CVST

Transient risk factors

- Infection—CNS (meningitis, cerebral abscess), ENT (mastoiditis, sinusitis, otitis media)
- Pregnancy and puerperium
- Head trauma (skull base fractures crossing venous sinuses)
- Lumbar puncture
- Neurosurgical procedures (external ventricular drain)
- Jugular and subclavian catheters (secondary thrombosis with intracranial extension)
- Drugs—OCPs, L-asparaginase, androgens, ecstasy, sildenafil, intrathecal methotrexate
- Diabetic ketoacidosis

Permanent risk factors

- Genetic—protein C/S, antithrombin deficiencies, factor V Leiden
- Acquired—antiphospholipid syndrome, nephrotic syndrome, HIT
- Malignancy—meningioma, leukemia, lymphoma
- Anemia—sickle cell disease, paroxysmal nocturnal hemoglobinuria, polycythemia, thrombocytopenia
- Inflammatory disease—systemic lupus erythematosus, Sjögren, granulomatosis with polyangiitis, inflammatory bowel disease, sarcoidosis

CNS, central nervous system; CVST, cerebral venous sinus thrombosis; ENT, ear, nose, throat; HIT, heparin-induced thrombocytopenia; OCPs, oral contraceptives.

may also occur, and physicians should have a low threshold for ordering EEGs among patients with altered mental status and suspicion of CVST. Deeper cerebral venous system occlusions in the straight sinus may present with more severe symptoms, such as alterations in mental status, motor deficits, and coma.

TABLE 177.2 CLINICAL MANIFESTATIONS OF CEREBRAL VENOUS THROMBOSIS ACCORDING TO SITE OF OCCLUSION

OCCLUDED VEIN/SINUS	CLINICAL PRESENTATION
Cavernous sinus	Headache, cranial nerve palsies (CN III, CN IV, CN V1, CN VI), ocular pain/chemosis/proptosis
Cortical veins	Seizures, focal neurologic signs depending on location
Deep venous system	Altered mentation, motor deficits (bilateral or fluctuating weakness)
Sigmoid sinus	Cranial nerve palsies, mastoid pain
Transverse sinus	Headache, seizures, contralateral pyramidal signs. Aphasia, cranial nerve palsies, ataxia can occur.
Superior sagittal sinus	Intracranial hypertension (eg, headache, papilledema, blurred vision, vomiting, seizures) and focal symptoms due to venous infarction (eg, cranial nerve palsies, aphasia, hemisensory loss, hemiparesis, hemianopia)

The diagnosis of CVST may fool even the most experienced clinicians as the onset may occur insidiously and the early clinical course is nonspecific. On average, it takes 7 days after symptom onset to establish a definitive diagnosis. Laboratory studies and lumbar puncture are not specifically indicated for the workup of CVST; however, they may be obtained as part of the broader workup to identify pathologies such as idiopathic intracranial hypertension, a condition with several overlapping clinical features. D-Dimer is of variable utility as the sensitivity varies between 80% and 90%, and in patients with moderate-to-high risk for CVST, imaging would be indicated regardless. If a lumbar puncture is performed, the opening pressure may be elevated and the CSF may be nonspecific (eg, elevated lymphocytes, erythrocytes, or elevated protein).

Appropriate neuroimaging can lead to definitive diagnosis and lifesaving treatment. CTV or MRV are both effective in diagnosing CVST. The combination of decreased blood flow with an abnormal signal in the sinus confirms the diagnosis. A non–contrast-enhanced head CT may show clues such as a "dense triangle sign," but the absence of findings does not exclude CVST as these can be normal in up to half of cases. Concurrent hemorrhage may be seen in up to one-third of patients and is generally not only parenchymal but may also be subarachnoid.

Although CVST can result in permanent disability or death, it generally has a favorable prognosis if the diagnosis is made early. The mainstay of treatment is anticoagulation, generally with parental heparin, with an aim of preventing thrombus propagation, facilitating recanalization, and improving venous outflow. Despite initiation of anticoagulation, patients may still deteriorate, particularly in the first 1 to 2 days, due to a range of complications. Patients who decompensate despite anticoagulation may benefit from endovascular procedures (eg, endovascular thrombolysis or thrombectomy) or neurosurgical interventions (eg, decompressive craniotomy).

PEARLS

- CVST is a heterogeneous process and can present in variable ways, making timely diagnosis difficult unless the provider maintains a high index of suspicion.
- CTV or MRV is the diagnostic imaging modality of choice.
- Neurologic deterioration can result from extension of thrombus, venous infarction, intracerebral hemorrhage, cerebral edema, and seizures. These patients may benefit from endovascular or neurosurgical interventions.

Suggested Readings

Alimohammadi A, Kim DJ, Field TS. Updates in cerebral venous thrombosis. *Curr Cardiol Rep*. 2022;24(1):43-50.

Idiculla PS, Gurala D, Palanisamy M, Vijayakumar R, Dhandapani S, Nagarajan E. Cerebral venous thrombosis: a comprehensive review. *Eur Neurol*. 2020;83(4):369-379.

Ropper AH, Klein JP. Cerebral venous thrombosis. *N Engl J Med*. 2021;385(1):59-64.

Spadaro A, Scott KR, Koyfman A, Long B. Cerebral venous thrombosis: diagnosis and management in the emergency department setting. *Am J Emerg Med*. 2021;47:24-29.

178

Blood Pressure in the Patient With Intracerebral Hemorrhage

Kellie Kitamura, Amir A. Rouhani, and Steven Lai

There are over 795,000 strokes per year in the United States with up to 10% of cases due to spontaneous ICH. The mortality and morbidity of ICH are high, and therefore early diagnosis and management are essential to optimize clinical outcomes. The mnemonic "ABCDS" can be used to remember the primary points of resuscitation of patients with ICH, as it includes Airway management, BP control, Coagulopathy correction, Diagnostic neuroimaging, and Surgical consultation. Optimal BP management in ICH is a complex and controversial topic that requires continued research, but in 2022, the AHA/ASA published new recommendations for management of patients with spontaneous ICH that help guide approach to BP management.

Chronic elevation of BP is thought to be the most common cause of ICH, and high BP is frequently noted upon patient presentation. It has been noted to contribute to hematoma expansion, continued bleeding, risk of rebleeding and is overall associated with greater neurologic deterioration with generally higher morbidity and mortality. **Table 178.1** summarizes the latest AHA/ASA guidelines based on the data from the INTERACT2 trial, ATACH-2 trial, several other smaller studies, and meta-analyses of the aforementioned studies.

The INTERACT2 trial attempted to investigate whether intensive, rapid, and maintained SBP lowering to a target of 140 mm Hg led to lower risk of death or severe disability at 90 days compared to SBP lowering to 180 mm Hg. Overall, findings did not demonstrate a significant difference in mortality or severe disability but did suggest aggressive BP control was safe and resulted in lower rates of hematoma expansion and improved functional outcomes.

The ATACH-2 trial used IV nicardipine and randomized groups with SBP goals of 110 to 139 mm Hg (intensive group) and 140 to 179 mm Hg (standard group) to

TABLE 178.1	Summarized Guidelines for BP Management in Acute ICH

RECOMMENDATION

Avoid large fluctuations in BP and aim for a continuous and smooth approach to reducing BP.

Initiate BP control within 2 h of ICH onset with goal to reach target BP within 1 h.

Patients with mild to moderate severity ICH with initial SBPs of 150-220 mm Hg should be lowered to goal SBP of 140, with a goal of maintaining 130-150 mm Hg.

Avoid lowering SBP to <130 mm Hg in patients with mild to moderate severity ICH with starting SBP >150 mm Hg as it may be harmful.

BP, blood pressure; ICH, intracerebral hemorrhage; SBP, systolic blood pressure.

determine whether there was decreased death or disability at 90 days in the intensive group. The study also found no significant differences in death or major disability but did find higher rate of renal failure within the intensive SBP group.

More recently, INTERACT3 trial looked at whether the implementation of a goal-directed care bundle that included protocols for lowering BP and managing hyperglycemia, coagulopathy, and temperature improved patient outcomes at 6 months. While the findings demonstrated better functional outcomes in the intervention group, it is not clear exactly which of these interventions was helpful in this unblinded trial.

Still, subsequent analyses of INTERACT2 and ATACH2 trials and several other smaller studies demonstrated that avoiding high SBP variability in the acute phase and early initiation of BP control may be beneficial but further research is needed to understand the optimal choice of BP-lowering agent. INTERACT2 used both oral and IV (including labetalol, nicardipine, hydralazine, diltiazem, and urapidil) whereas ATACH-2 trial used IV nicardipine. Overall, agents with rapid onset and short duration of action are preferred such as labetalol, clevidipine, and nicardipine. Clevidipine has demonstrated a shorter time-to-target BP with less variability and shorter half-life of elimination than both nicardipine and labetalol, though labetalol has an IV push formulation unlike the others.

BP management in ICH is an ongoing topic of research, and more investigation must be done to identify the safest magnitude and rate of SBP reduction in the early resuscitation of these patients. Further studies must also be done to determine the safety and efficacy of BP management for patients presenting with SBP greater than 220 mm Hg and for large or severe ICHs.

PEARLS

- ICH represents 10% of strokes and is associated with higher morbidity and mortality than ischemic strokes.
- BP reduction is safe and associated with improved clinical outcomes.
- In patients with ICH and elevated presenting SBP between 150 and 220 mm Hg, SBP should be lowered to a target of 140 mm Hg to maintain within 130 to 150 mm Hg with efforts to avoid large fluctuations in BP.
- Lowering SBP to less than 130 mm Hg may be harmful for those presenting with SBP greater than 150 mm Hg.
- Clevidipine, nicardipine, and labetalol are reasonable options for BP control.

SUGGESTED READINGS

Anderson CS, Heeley E, Huang Y, et al. Rapid blood-pressure lowering in patients with acute intracerebral hemorrhage. *N Engl J Med*. 2013;368(25):2355–2365.

Greenberg SM, Ziai WC, Cordonnier C, et al. 2022 guideline for the management of patients with spontaneous intracerebral hemorrhage: a guideline from the American Heart Association/American Stroke Association. *Stroke*. 2022;53(7):e282-e361.

Ma L, Hu X, Song L, et al. The third Intensive Care Bundle with Blood Pressure Reduction in Acute Cerebral Haemorrhage Trial (INTERACT3): an international, stepped wedge cluster randomised controlled trial. *Lancet (London, England)*. 2023;402(10395):27-40.

Qureshi AI, Palesch YY, Barsan WG, et al. Intensive blood-pressure lowering in patients with acute cerebral hemorrhage. *N Engl J Med*. 2016;375(11):1033–1043.

179

How to Disposition the Patient With Suspected TIA

Patricia Fermin

Transient ischemic attack (TIA) is a common life-threatening condition that occurs with an estimated annual incidence of 200,000 to 500,000 cases per year in the United States, accounting for 0.3% of all ED visits. In the not-so-distant past, TIA was described as a sudden-onset, focal neurologic event of vascular origin lasting less than 24 hours. However, as imaging studies evolved with greater sensitivity to detect tissue infarction, many presumed TIAs were more accurately diagnosed as strokes. In some cases, infarction can be found on diffusion-weighted MRI rapidly within 10 or 15 minutes of symptoms. The AHA/ASA currently defines TIA as a "transient episode of neurological dysfunction caused by focal brain, spinal cord, or retinal ischemia, without acute infarction." TIA is, therefore, an ischemic CNS disease on the same spectrum as stroke, which is differentiated by the presence of tissue infarction.

Patients with a suspected TIA must have rapid and accurate ED evaluation. Although many patients may have a benign course of disease, there is a considerable short-term risk for stroke. Large cohort and population-based studies have demonstrated a higher risk of early stroke after TIA than previously appreciated. Twelve to 30% of patients progress to having a stroke, with the highest risk in the first 48 hours. Therefore, disposition of the patient with TIA requires careful risk stratification.

The $ABCD^2$ score has been commonly used to risk stratify subsequent stroke; however, the score has not been externally validated and has demonstrated poor predictive value. Improved tools such as the $ABCD^2$-I and $ABCD^3$-I scores have limited use based on availability of advanced imaging. An alternative clinical decision tool is the Canadian TIA score, which stratifies patients to low, medium, and high risk of subsequent stroke within 7 days based on history, clinical data points, and neuroimaging (**Table 179.1**). This score has demonstrated a greater positive predictive value for stroke when compared to the $ABCD^2$ score.

In 2021, the Canadian TIA score was validated in a multicenter prospective cohort study. It includes nine components based on clinical history and examination and four components based on tests performed. The scores ranged from -3 to 23, with probability of subsequent stroke within 7 days ranging from 0.01% to more than 27.6%.

A national survey in Canada was performed to assess the anticipated use of the Canadian TIA score and risk stratification with actions recommended. Of the 131 surveys received from emergency physicians, 96% stated they would use the Canadian TIA score with definition of risks as minimal: less than 1%, low: 1% to 4.9%, high: 5% to 10%, and critical: more than 10% risk of subsequent stroke within 7 days. The proposed workup included further outpatient workup in minimal to low-risk patients, while high- to critical-risk patients included same-day imaging and cardiac monitoring. This includes obtaining an electrocardiogram to evaluate for atrial fibrillation, echocardiogram to evaluate for valvular abnormalities or thrombus, and Holter cardiac monitoring versus period of cardiac monitoring in the ED.

TABLE 179.1 CANADIAN TIA SCORE

ITEMS	POINTS
Clinical findings	
First TIA (in lifetime)	2
Symptoms ≥10 min	2
History of carotid stenosis	2
Already on antiplatelet therapy	3
History of gait disturbance	1
History of unilateral weakness	1
History of vertigo	−3
Initial triage diastolic blood pressure ≥110 mm Hg	3
Dysarthria or aphasia (history or examination)	1
Investigations in ED	
Atrial fibrillation on ECG	2
Infarction (new or old) on CT	1
Platelet count ≥400 × 10^9/L	2
Glucose ≥15 mmol/L	3
Total score (−3 to 23)	———

CT, computed tomography; ECG, electrocardiogram; TIA, transient ischemic attack.
From Perry JJ, Sharma M, Sivilotti ML, et al. A prospective cohort study of patients with transient ischemic attack to identify high-risk clinical characteristics. *Stroke*. 2013;45(1):92-100.

The TIA workup as recommended by the AHA/ASA includes neuroimaging within 24 hours of symptom onset (preferably with diffusion-weighted brain MR), noninvasive imaging of the cervical and intracranial vessels (with Doppler ultrasound, CT, or MR angiography), electrocardiogram, and routine blood tests. CT angiography may be used when assessing for large vessel occlusion. If negative, MRI with DWI is the gold standard for detection of ischemia distinguishing TIA versus stroke. However, even a DWI MRI may miss some early, small infarctions, most commonly in patients with posterior fossa infarcts.

Based on the ACEP TIA clinical policy, the disposition of post-TIA ED patients should be based not only on risk stratification but also on clinical judgment and local resource availability. Patients must have close and reliable follow-up to be considered for discharge, as a thorough workup should be completed as soon as possible, preferably within 48 hours. An alternative to admission may include workup in ED observation units or specialized TIA clinics.

PEARLS

- TIA is characterized by transient ischemia in the CNS that does not result in infarction (stroke) but portends an increased risk of stroke in the ensuing days and weeks.
- The validated Canadian TIA score shows greater predictability in subsequent stroke within 7 days.
- Risk stratification tools should be used in conjunction with clinical judgment and resource availability.

- The workup of a TIA should be preferably performed within 48 hours.
- Inpatient admission is strongly advised for moderate- and high-risk patients.

Suggested Readings

Easton JD, Saver JL, Albers GW, et al. Definition and evaluation of transient ischemic attack. A scientific statement for healthcare professionals from the American Heart Association/American Stroke Association Stroke Council; Council on Cardiovascular Surgery and Anesthesia; Council on Cardiovascular Radiology and Intervention; Council on Cardiovascular Nursing; and the Interdisciplinary Council on Peripheral Vascular Disease. *Stroke*. 2009;40(6):2276-2293.

Edlow JA, Kim S, Pelletier AJ, et al. National study on emergency department visits for transient ischemic attack, 1992–2001. *Acad Emerg Med*. 2006;13(6):666-672.

Giles MF, Rothwell PM. Risk of stroke early after transient ischaemic attack: a systematic review and meta-analysis. *Lancet Neurol*. 2007;6(12):1063-1072.

Lo BM, Carpenter CR, Hatten BW, et al. Clinical policy: critical issues in the evaluation of adult patients with suspected transient ischemic attack in the emergency department. *Ann Emerg Med*. 2016;68(3):354-370.e29.

Perry JJ, Losier JH, Stiell IG, Sharma M, Abdulaziz K. National survey of emergency physicians for transient ischemic attack (TIA) risk stratification consensus and appropriate treatment for a given level of risk. *CJEM*. 2016;18(1):10-18.

Perry JJ, Sharma M, Sivilotti ML, et al. A prospective cohort study of patients with transient ischemic attack to identify high-risk clinical characteristics. *Stroke*. 2013;45(1):92-100.

180

Know When to Use, and NOT to Use, the HINTS Examination

Laura Hemker Moles and Ryan Raam

Vertigo remains one of the most challenging patient presentations in the acute setting, due not only to the breadth of its differential but also to its propensity for pitfalls. The disparity in the morbidity and mortality of the benign versus dangerous diagnoses that present with vertigo makes the evaluation of these patients in a resource-conscious manner, paramount. Acute vestibular neuritis, a generally benign and self-limiting condition, is a diagnosis that has many similar clinical signs to a posterior cerebrovascular accident. A three-part bedside oculomotor test to assist in the diagnosis, the HINTS examination, has been cited as both highly sensitive (100%) and specific (96%) in differentiating between acute vestibular neuritis and cerebellar stroke. Subsequently, however, the utility of the examination came under question, as one study found that in the hands of emergency clinicians, the examination does not perform as well as when done by specially trained neurologists.

The effectiveness of the examination, as with any clinical procedure, is dependent on training and practice. The utility of the HINTS examination is closely tied to two key elements: appropriate patient selection and proper technique. One retrospective study demonstrated that the HINTS examination was inappropriately applied by emergency physicians 97% of the time. However, a subsequent study found that when trained appropriately, emergency physicians performed the examination with a sensitivity and specificity approaching that of neurologists.

The appropriate patient in which the HINTS examination should be used is one who has ongoing symptoms (hours to days), unsteady gait, and spontaneous nystagmus. Without these characteristics, the test becomes both unnecessary and misleading.

Any test performed in the ED should inform a subsequent clinical decision. In the case of the HINTS examination, that decision is whether or not to perform additional testing of a patient for a central cause of vertigo. Therefore, the HINTS examination can be excluded for patients who will receive additional testing based on a high level of clinical suspicion during the initial examination. High-risk features include focal neurologic deficits (including diplopia, dysarthria, dysmetria, dysdiadochokinesia), spontaneous vertical or torsional nystagmus, new onset of the inability to ambulate or truncal ataxia, severe headache, or severe neck pain. These patients should receive expedited advanced imaging with computed tomography and/or magnetic resonance imaging.

If the patient does not demonstrate any of the abovementioned high-risk features, the next point to evaluate is whether the symptoms have had a prolonged time course (hours to days). Importantly, the symptoms should be present at the time of the examination. Ongoing, prolonged symptoms are also a hallmark sign of cerebellar stroke. If a patient has vestibular symptoms that have resolved at the time of the encounter, a HINTS examination will be neither sensitive nor specific.

Many patients with both benign and concerning causes of vertigo will have some degree of gait instability. Again, this is true of both acute vestibular neuritis and cerebellar stroke. Except for gait instability, the patient with vestibular neuritis will have an otherwise intact neurologic examination without other signs of cerebellar dysfunction. Patients with posterior ischemic stroke may have abnormal cerebellar function tests, including rapid alternating movements, finger-to-nose, and heel-to-shin testing. However, these findings are not universal and can be absent in patients with a cerebellar stroke.

Spontaneously occurring nystagmus is another common feature shared by patients with both acute vestibular neuritis and cerebellar stroke. Cerebellar stroke can also manifest with horizontal nystagmus, which can mimic a benign peripheral vestibular syndrome. Other elements that are shared by vestibular neuritis and central pathology include sustained beating, short latency, and nonfatigable nystagmus. Vertical and unprovoked torsional nystagmus are highly suggestive of central etiologies of a patient's vertigo and should lead directly to advanced imaging studies for further evaluation. Another attribute that is specific to a central cause of vertigo is nystagmus that changes direction on eccentric gaze. Peripheral vestibulopathies are characterized by nystagmus that is exclusively unidirectional. If a patient has ongoing vertigo without visible nystagmus on examination, the HINTS examination will be unhelpful and alternative diagnoses should be considered.

If a patient presents with ongoing vertiginous symptoms lasting hours to days, unsteady gait, and spontaneous nystagmus, the HINTS examination is indicated as a decision-making tool to help differentiate acute vestibular neuritis from cerebellar stroke. Application of the test should be limited to this narrow indication. Inappropriate use of the test can lead to misdiagnosis and overutilization of resources. Like any other procedure, continued review of the examination and repeated practice is necessary to ensure it is performed accurately. It is beyond the scope of this chapter to explain in depth how to perform the maneuvers. However, there are many digital and written educational sources that can provide detailed explanations and instructions on how to perform each part of the HINTS examination. Each of these elements must result in the absence of central findings; otherwise, advanced imaging studies and/or neurology consult should be obtained for further evaluation. Taken together, appropriate patient selection and proper technique preserve the utility of the HINTS examination in the emergency setting.

PEARLS

- All initial evaluations of dizziness should begin with a careful and complete history and neurologic examination.
- Acute vestibular neuritis is characterized by ongoing symptoms for hours to days, gait instability, and nystagmus. These symptoms are shared by cerebellar stroke.
- The HINTS examination is a bedside diagnostic tool that can be used to help differentiate acute vestibular neuritis from central etiologies of vertigo.
- The effectiveness of the HINTS examination is predicated on appropriate selection of patients and proper performance of the test. It should not be used for patients who have episodic symptoms.
- With practice, a properly trained emergency clinician can achieve similar effectiveness as a neurologist in the use of the HINTS examination.

Suggested Readings

Dmitriew C, Regis A, Bodunde O, et al. Diagnostic accuracy of the HINTS exam in an emergency department: a retrospective chart review. *Acad Emerg Med*. 2021;28(4):387-393.

Gerlier C, Hoarau M, Fels A, et al. Differentiating central from peripheral causes of acute vertigo in an emergency setting with the HINTS, STANDING, and ABCD2 tests: a diagnostic cohort study. *Acad Emerg Med*. 2021;28(12):1368-1378.

Kattah JC, Talkad AV, Wang DZ, et al. HINTS to diagnose stroke in the acute vestibular syndrome: three-step bedside oculomotor examination more sensitive than early MRI diffusion-weighted imaging. *Stroke*. 2009;40(11):3504-3510.

Ohle R, Montpellier RA, Marchadier V, et al. Can emergency physicians accurately rule out a central cause of vertigo using the HINTS examination? A systematic review and meta-analysis. *Acad Emerg Med*. 2020;27(9):887-896.

181

Stop Asking Your Patient What They Mean by "Dizzy"

Beza Abebe and Ryan Raam

"Is the room spinning? Do you feel lightheaded?" Those are the questions emergency physicians have historically asked in an attempt to classify possible causes of the daunting chief complaint of "dizziness." However, the lack of efficacy of these past methods suggests that symptom quality is neither a reliable nor a valid discriminator.

Previous studies have shown that peripheral vestibular disorders have an estimated misdiagnosis rate of 74% to 81%, while 37% of acute posterior strokes were initially

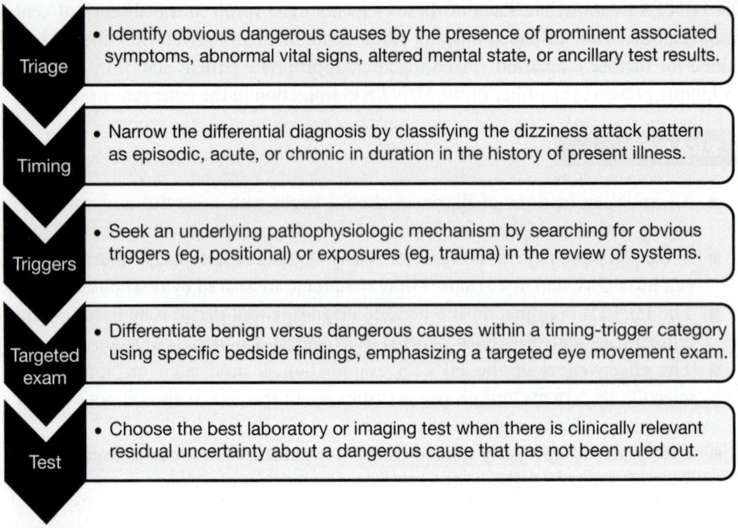

- **Triage**: Identify obvious dangerous causes by the presence of prominent associated symptoms, abnormal vital signs, altered mental state, or ancillary test results.

- **Timing**: Narrow the differential diagnosis by classifying the dizziness attack pattern as episodic, acute, or chronic in duration in the history of present illness.

- **Triggers**: Seek an underlying pathophysiologic mechanism by searching for obvious triggers (eg, positional) or exposures (eg, trauma) in the review of systems.

- **Targeted exam**: Differentiate benign versus dangerous causes within a timing-trigger category using specific bedside findings, emphasizing a targeted eye movement exam.

- **Test**: Choose the best laboratory or imaging test when there is clinically relevant residual uncertainty about a dangerous cause that has not been ruled out.

FIGURE 181.1 The "Triage-TiTrATE-Test" approach to diagnosing dizziness and vertigo. (Reprinted from Newman-Toker DE, Edlow JA. TiTrATE: a novel, evidence-based approach to diagnosing acute dizziness and vertigo. *Neurol Clin.* 2015;33(3): 577-599, viii, Figure 1, with permission from Elsevier.)

misdiagnosed in the ED. As a result, the acute care physician is tasked with using a better diagnostic approach for the undifferentiated dizzy patient.

Dizziness is a vague term used by patients to describe a general unwell feeling as well as a multitude of symptoms ranging from primary vestibular etiologies to secondary manifestations of toxidromes, arrhythmias, stroke, or hypotension. Rather than attempting to wade through an unreliable description of ambiguous symptoms, a thorough evaluation with an algorithmic approach (called TiTrATE) can help simplify the evaluation of these patients.

TiTrATE (**Figure 181.1**) provides a framework based on symptom **T**iming, **T**riggers, **A**nd **T**argeted bedside eye **E**xaminations that will improve the physician's ability to make a correct, timely diagnosis, with improved patient outcomes. These include better vestibular function as well as reduction of secondary injuries, anxiety, unnecessary prescriptions/testing, and long-term complications of missed TIA and stroke.

This framework revolves around the idea that there are two broad categories of vestibular syndromes (episodic/EVS and acute/AVS) that each contain two subcategories (triggered/spontaneous and postexposure/spontaneous) that should be considered in patients presenting to the ED with symptoms of dizziness. Important elements of the history and physical examination related to each of these categories guide the evaluation of these patients.

EVS

EVS involves intermittent dizziness that usually lasts seconds to minutes. This category of dizziness is characterized by the episodic nature of the symptoms, which is independent of the total duration of symptoms the patient has been experiencing. Typically, symptoms occur in discrete intermittent episodes spread out over time. This category is composed of two subcategories: triggered and spontaneous.

Triggered EVS

Triggered episodes are *precipitated* by a specific action or event that causes the vertigo symptoms. This should be distinguished from triggers that merely *exacerbate* continuous symptoms (which is a different phenomenon). Triggers can be common things like movement of the head or body or, less commonly, loud noises or Valsalva maneuvers. It is important to note that symptoms last for seconds to minutes. Symptoms lasting longer than this should be given special attention as to whether they fit under a different category of dizziness. One goal of the bedside encounter is to try and reproduce the symptoms by triggering the vertigo episode so that the physician can verify what the patient experiences. Important elements of the history and physical examination incorporate orthostatic signs and symptoms and the Dix-Hallpike maneuver. Examples of conditions that fit under this category include BPPV and orthostatic hypotension (which encompasses dangerous causes of this such as hemorrhage, sepsis, cardiac ischemia, or arrhythmia).

Spontaneous EVS

Spontaneous EVS symptoms can last from seconds to days, but mostly last minutes to hours. Patients often do not have symptoms at the time of presentation to the ED and cannot be provoked as with triggered episodic etiologies. Therefore, special attention should focus on the history to identify key causes. While conditions in this category may be exacerbated or triggered by certain precipitants, often, they are spontaneous and without apparent association with other contextual situations. Examples of conditions include vertebrobasilar insufficiency, TIA, cardiac arrhythmia, basilar migraine, and Ménière disease (characterized by episodic vertigo, hearing loss, and tinnitus).

AVS

AVS involves acute, persistent dizziness lasting days to weeks. Often, there are sequelae of disease after the underlying condition eventually resolves. AVS conditions consist of postexposure and spontaneous forms.

Postexposure AVS

Postexposure causes of AVS generally result from either trauma or toxic exposures. The exposure can be obvious or subtle. In cases of trauma, either direct or indirect trauma to the head can result in vertigo. Examples of this include blunt head trauma (concussion), blast injuries, and barotrauma. The mechanism of injury can be varied with these causes; however, careful attention should be made to evaluate for basilar skull fracture, intracranial hemorrhage, vertebral artery dissection, and ruptured tympanic membrane. There are myriad toxic exposures that can result in dizziness; however, the most commonly encountered are from supratherapeutic levels of anticonvulsants, especially phenytoin and carbamazepine. These exposures can often mimic signs and symptoms of posterior fossa strokes because of their spontaneous rotary nystagmus and other cerebellar findings on examination, including ataxia. Careful review of the patient's medications and environmental risks such as carbon monoxide poisoning and travel can help guide other causes of postexposure AVS.

Spontaneous AVS

This subcategory includes AVS characterized by spontaneous vertigo that is constant and unremitting for days to weeks, nystagmus at rest, and ataxic or unstable gait. Patients tend to be symptomatic at presentation in the ED, so a focused evaluation on physical examination can provide a significant amount of diagnostic information. An important point in the evaluation of these patients is distinguishing between symptoms that are *triggered* by head movement and relieved by rest, as opposed to *exacerbated* by movement and continues even when resting. The former is a hallmark of triggered EVS, and the latter is characteristic of spontaneous AVS. Beware of misinterpreting this point in the clinical encounter.

The diagnostic challenge of this category is distinguishing between vestibular neuritis and ischemic cerebellar stroke. These two diagnoses share much overlap in the abovementioned signs and symptoms, but with dramatically different dispositions, treatments, and outcomes. In the hands of an experienced and trained physician, the HINTS examination can help differentiate between vestibular neuritis and ischemic stroke. Like any other "procedure," if diligently studied, practiced, and appropriately applied, it can be a powerful tool to navigate a difficult clinical scenario.

Evaluating patients who are dizzy with consideration to the timing and triggers of their symptoms is a reliable method that will increase the sensitivity and accuracy of your history.

PEARLS

- Evidence researching the efficacy of past methods has shown that the type of dizziness is neither a reliable nor a valid discriminator as a diagnostic approach.
- A recommended pathway includes a thorough evaluation of dizziness with the TiTrATE method.
- Effort should also be heavily put forth to specify circumstances around the onset, duration, and evolution of symptoms in order to carefully classify symptom pattern acuity and episodic nature.

SUGGESTED READINGS

Gurley KL, Edlow JA. Diagnosis of patients with acute dizziness. *Emerg Med Clin North Am.* 2021;39(1):181-201.

Newman-Toker DE, Edlow JA. TiTrATE: a novel, evidence-based approach to diagnosing acute dizziness and vertigo. *Neurol Clin.* 2015;33(3):577-599, viii.

182

KNOW HOW TO PROPERLY PERFORM THE DIX-HALLPIKE AND EPLEY MANEUVERS

MADELEINE HELLER AND MARY CHEFFERS

Dizziness is a common yet challenging chief complaint in the ED. Emergency physicians justifiably focus the evaluation of dizzy patients on identifying critical diagnoses such as posterior-circulation stroke and teasing out true vertigo from other dizziness mimics. However, patients with BPPV experience significant distress due to symptoms and have a higher risk of residual dizziness with delayed diagnosis and incomplete treatment. BPPV is the most common vestibular cause of dizziness, with an estimated 2% lifetime prevalence. Busy ED physicians can use canalith repositioning maneuvers to provide patients with BPPV real symptomatic relief, avoiding extra time in the ED, unnecessary imaging studies, and medications that only symptomatically treat the patient (**Figure 182.1**).

In patients with BPPV, otoliths moving within one of the three semicircular canals simulate head movement, causing severe distress. A positive Dix-Hallpike (**Figure 182.2**) for posterior canal BPPV results in torsional nystagmus, sometimes with a short 5-second latency period, with the upper pole of the eyes beating toward the ear closest to the floor. Upward beating nystagmus toward the forehead may occur in the case of anterior canal BPPV and horizontal nystagmus in the case of horizontal canal BPPV. The test should be repeated with the head rotated left if previously to the right, or vice versa, to assess for canalolithiasis on either side.

A positive Dix-Hallpike test for posterior canalolithiasis should be followed immediately by the Epley maneuver, with each movement held for 30 to 60 seconds. A repeat attempt improves efficacy if partial improvement was obtained with the initial attempt and should be performed if the patient is able to tolerate it. If nystagmus is persistent, the otolith is likely lodged in place and a different maneuver will need to be used. If the maneuver appears successful, the patient's symptoms should be reassessed after several minutes. Improvement in symptoms and repeat negative testing further confirm the diagnosis of BPPV.

If the Dix-Hallpike test results in horizontal or no nystagmus in a patient with a history consistent with BPPV, clinical guidelines recommend testing for horizontal (lateral) canal BPPV, which is the most common type after posterior canal BPPV. Horizontal canal BPPV can be diagnosed with the supine roll test (**Figure 182.3**). Most commonly, rotation to the affected side will cause intense vertigo and nystagmus beating toward the bed and the affected ear. The patient's eyes should be observed for 30 seconds in each position to assess for nystagmus.

BPPV affecting the horizontal (lateral) semicircular canal can be categorized as geotropic (nystagmus beating toward the ground on the affected side) or apogeotropic (nystagmus beating toward the ceiling). To treat geotropic nystagmus, use the Gufoni maneuver, which has demonstrated both efficacy as well as ease for the patient and examiner. Like other maneuvers, position changes should be held for 30 to 60 seconds. Apogeotropic nystagmus can be treated using the modified Gufoni maneuver.

Anterior canal BPPV is uncommon and is characterized by vertical nystagmus with the Dix-Hallpike test. This should be treated with the Deep Head Hanging or Yacovino maneuver.

The Epley maneuver has demonstrated effectiveness while taking just a few minutes to complete. Unfortunately, canalith repositioning maneuvers for BPPV are underutilized by emergency physicians. Incorporating these maneuvers into your practice offers an opportunity for a positive outcome for your patient that may otherwise have been missed.

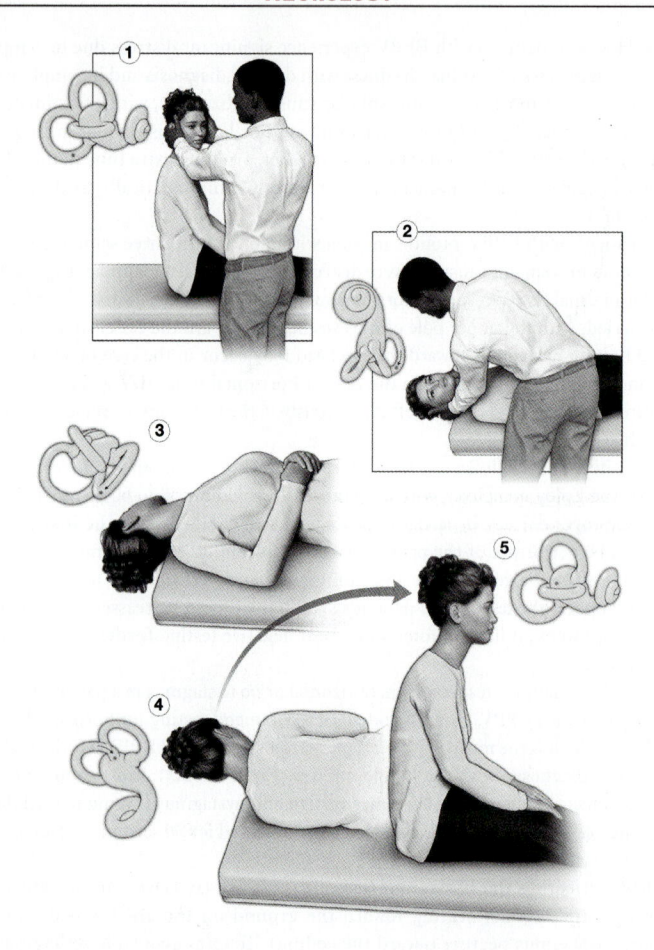

FIGURE 182.1 Canalith (Canalolith) repositioning maneuver for the right side. Steps: (1) Have the patient sit on a table positioned so that they may be laid back in the head-hanging position with the neck in slight extension. Stabilize the head and move it 45° toward the side to be tested. (2) Move the head, neck, and shoulders all together to avoid neck strain. Observe the eyes for nystagmus; hold them open, if necessary. If nystagmus is seen, wait for all nystagmus to abate and hold the position for another 15 seconds. (3) While the head is slightly hyperextended, turn the head 90° toward the opposite side, and wait 30 seconds. (4) Roll the body to the lateral body position, turn the patient's head toward the ground so that the patient is facing straight down, and hold for 15 seconds. (5) While maintaining the head position unchanged relative to the shoulders, have the patient sit up and hold on to the patient for 5 seconds or so to guard against momentary dizziness upon sitting up. This maneuver may be repeated several times or until symptoms and nystagmus cannot be reproduced. As an alternative, a clinician can use the Semont maneuver, where the patient is laid from side to side. (From Egan D. *Manual of Eye, Ear, Nose, and Throat Emergencies*. Wolters Kluwer; 2023. Figure 7.7.)

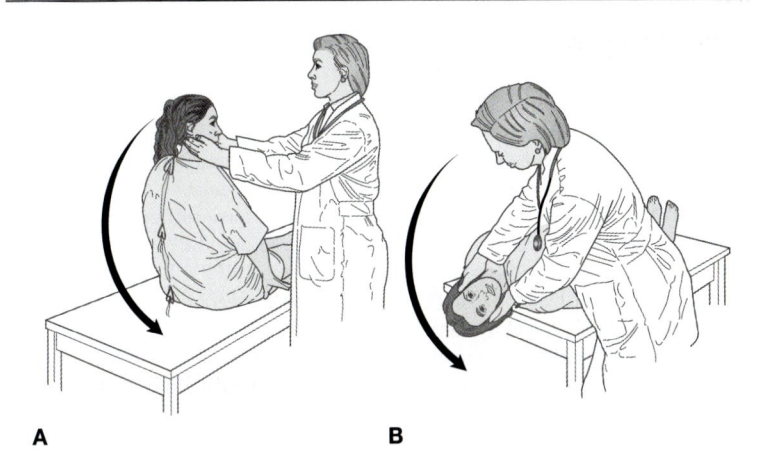

FIGURE 182.2 Dix-Hallpike to the right, going from the sitting position (**A**) to the head-hanging right position (**B**). (From Seffinger MA. *Foundations of Osteopathic Medicine*. 4th ed. Wolters Kluwer; 2019. Figure 48.5.)

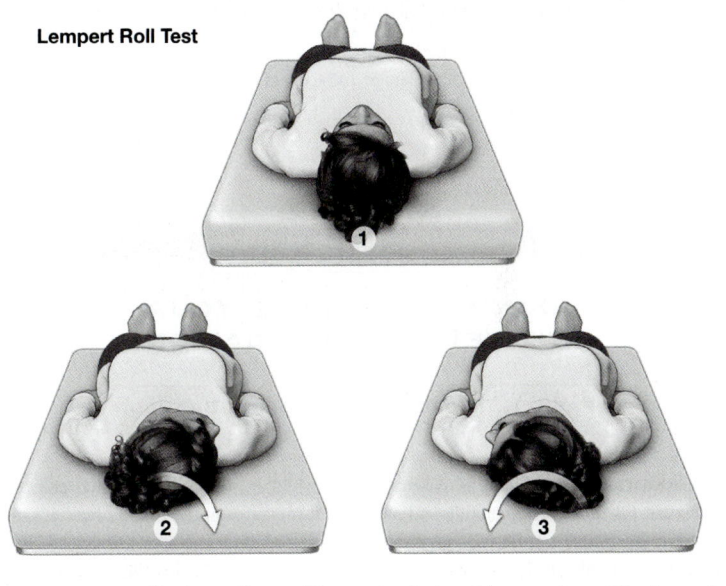

Lempert Roll Test

FIGURE 182.3 Supine roll test. The patient's head is moved rapidly from the straight supine position (1) to the right side (2). Observe for horizontal nystagmus and note the direction and intensity. Then move the patient's head back to the straight position (1) for 15 seconds. Then move the head from straight to the head-left position (3) and note any nystagmus and its direction and intensity. If the nystagmus is of the geotropic type, the side resulting in the strongest nystagmus is taken to be the affected side. (From Egan D. *Manual of Eye, Ear, Nose, and Throat Emergencies*. Wolters Kluwer; 2023. Figure 7.5.)

> **PEARLS**
>
> - Performing a canalith repositioning maneuver can save time in the evaluation and treatment of patients with BPPV and can effectively treat symptoms.
> - BPPV is caused by otoliths in any of the three semicircular canals, most commonly in the posterior canal, followed by the horizontal canal.
> - The Dix-Hallpike maneuver most commonly causes a torsional nystagmus, often after a brief latency period, in patients with posterior canal BPPV.
> - The Epley maneuver is used to treat posterior canal BPPV. Each step of the Epley should be held for 30 to 60 seconds to allow for therapeutic movement of causative otoliths out of the canal.
> - Alternative canalith repositioning maneuvers are the Gufoni maneuver for horizontal canal BPPV and the Deep Head Hanging/Yacovino maneuver for anterior canal BPPV.

SUGGESTED READINGS

Bhattacharyya N, Gubbels SP, Schwartz SR, et al. Clinical practice guideline: benign paroxysmal positional vertigo (update). *Otolaryngol Head Neck Surg.* 2017;156(3_suppl):S1-S47.

Edlow JA, Gurley KL, Newman-Toker DE. A new diagnostic approach to the adult patient with acute dizziness. *J Emerg Med.* 2018;54(4):469-483.

Kim J-S, Zee DS. Clinical practice. Benign paroxysmal positional vertigo. *N Engl J Med.* 2014;370(12):1138-1147.

183

DON'T UNDERDOSE YOUR ANTISEIZURE MEDICATIONS

FARID K. TADROS AND CAROLINE BRANDON

Approximately 1% to 2% of all patients in the ED will present with a chief complaint of seizure. Of those, between 3% and 30% will have status epilepticus. There are many different subtypes of epilepsy, but the focus of this chapter is the treatment of GCSE. Traditionally, only after seizure activity crossed the 30-minute threshold was it considered to be GCSE requiring pharmaceutical intervention. In 2015, national guidelines amended the definition to be any seizure lasting longer than 5 minutes (or more than one seizure within 5 minutes without return to baseline). This update was important because seizures lasting longer than 5 minutes become increasingly harder to terminate and are, therefore, associated with worsening neurologic disability, systemic complications, and mortality (~16% mortality in a first episode of GCSE in adults and 3.6% in children). For the purposes of the ED, it can be safely assumed that including transport time, anyone who arrives at the ED actively seizing, is likely to already be in status epilepticus.

Treating status not only involves medications but also focuses on evaluating and treating any underlying etiologies, as this is the main predictor of mortality in patients with GCSE. A treatment approach starts with the stabilization phase. First, address ABCDs, which includes placing the patient on the monitor. Then, obtain IV access and perform key blood tests, including a point-of-care glucose level, beta-hCG, and sodium level. Anticonvulsant drug levels can also be considered, if available, but treatment should not be delayed for these tests to result. Hypoglycemia is a known reversible cause of seizures with a straightforward treatment. In adult patients, if glucose is less than 60 mg/dL, give 50 mL IV push of D_{50}. For pediatric patients, the dose of glucose is 2 mL/kg of D_{25} for children, 5 mL/kg of D_{10} for infants, and 2 mL/kg of D_{25} for neonates. The goal blood glucose of a neonate under 48 hours is greater than 50 mg/dL.

Coincident with stabilizing the airway, breathing, and circulation (0-5 minutes), address the actively seizing patient by initiating antiseizure medications. There are several equivalent treatment options for the management of status, which includes a variety of medications, routes, and doses. This variability of options leads to a pervasive variability in physician dosing of antiseizure medications. The first dose of benzodiazepine for GCSE is underdosed in approximately 80% of cases. Despite having evidence-based, safe, and efficacious guidelines for the treatment of GCSE, underdosing exists in both out-of-hospital and in-hospital treatment.

According to the AES, the first-line treatment of GCSE is a benzodiazepine, and it advises selecting one of three equivalent options in **Table 183.1**. If seizing continues, there is no evidence-based preference, but the AES guidelines suggest moving to the second treatment phase and selecting one of the agents in **Table 183.1**. After 40 minutes without termination of the seizure, continue to the third treatment phase (**Table 183.1**). There is no clear evidence to guide therapy in this phase and whatever is chosen is less likely to be effective, given the refractory nature of the seizure at this point.

The most encountered reason for withholding what is considered "higher doses" of benzodiazepines in an actively seizing patient is the fear of respiratory depression, a known adverse effect of using benzodiazepines. However, numerous studies of patients in status epilepticus have shown less respiratory depression and fewer airway interventions in higher dose benzodiazepine treatment groups compared to those with lower dose benzodiazepines. This outcome is likely due to quicker seizure termination, obviating the need for airway intervention in patients with prolonged seizure activity. Another reason to use full-dose benzodiazepines is that the longer an episode of GCSE lasts, the less effective they are at controlling seizures because of synaptic internalization of GABA-A receptors. Finally, some outpatient antiepileptic medications (eg, carbamazepine, phenobarbital, phenytoin, oxcarbazepine) patients may be taking induce faster metabolization of benzodiazepines, requiring higher effective doses.

The potential for morbidity and mortality is quite high in GCSE, especially in cases of refractory GCSE. The most critical determinant of a patient's outcome is addressing any reversible etiologies and providing evidence-based pharmaceutical treatment as quickly as possible. Don't be afraid to give the correct dose of anticonvulsants.

TABLE 183.1	A Pharmaceutical Algorithm for Treating GCSE in Children and Adults		
MEDICATIONS	**ADULT**	**PEDS**	**COMMENT**
First line (*5-20 min*); select one			
Midazolam	IM 10 mg for >40 kg or 5 mg for 13-40 mg	IM 0.2 mg/kg, max 10 mg	Preferred over other agents in patients without IV access
Lorazepam	IV 0.1 mg/kg, max 4 mg/dose (may repeat dose once)	Same as adult	
Diazepam	IV 0.15-0.2 mg/kg, max 10 mg/dose (may repeat dose once)	Same as adult	
	If none of the above are available, can consider IV phenobarbital, PR diazepam, IN midazolam, buccal midazolam		
Second line (*20-40 min*); select one			
Fosphenytoin	IV 20 mg PE/kg, max 1,500 mg PE	Same as adults	Avoid in pregnancy, renal or hepatic failure, or alongside valproic acid (due to metabolic interactions)
Valproic acid	IV 40 mg/kg, max 3,000 mg	Same as adults	Avoid in pregnancy, or alongside fosphenytoin or phenytoin (due to metabolic interactions)
Levetiracetam	IV 60 mg/kg, max 4,500 mg	Same as adults	Preferred safety profile, especially in pregnant patients
Lacosamide	A newer agent that is not discussed in the 2016 AES guidelines		
Third line (*40-60 min*)			
Repeating second-line treatment phase medications *or*			
Anesthetic doses of thiopental, midazolam, pentobarbital, or propofol (all with continuous EEG monitoring)			

AES, American Epilepsy Society; EEG, electroencephalogram; GCSE, generalized convulsive status epilepticus; IM, intramuscular; IV, intravenous; PE, phenytoin sodium equivalents; PR, per rectum.

PEARLS

- Early cessation of GCSE is critical in improving prognosis.
- First-line treatment for GCSE is benzodiazepines (IM midazolam, IV lorazepam, or IV diazepam).
- Approximately 80% of patients in GCSE are underdosed with benzodiazepines.
- Higher doses of benzodiazepines in patients with GCSE result in decreased respiratory interventions and better clinical outcomes.

SUGGESTED READINGS

Burman RJ, Rosch RE, Wilmshurst JM, et al. Why won't it stop? The dynamics of benzodiazepine resistance in status epilepticus. *Nat Rev Neurol.* 2022;18(7):428-441.
Glauser T, Shinnar S, Gloss D, et al. Evidence-based guideline: treatment of convulsive status epilepticus in children and adults: report of the guideline committee of the American Epilepsy Society. *Epilepsy Curr.* 2016;16(1):48-61.
Honavar AG, Anuranjana A, Markose AP, et al. Profile of patients presenting with seizures as emergencies and immediate noncompliance to antiepileptic medications. *J Family Med Prim Care.* 2019;8(12):3977-3982.
Sathe AG, Underwood E, Coles LD, et al. Patterns of benzodiazepine underdosing in the established status epilepticus treatment trial. *Epilepsia.* 2021;62(3):795-806.

184

KNOW THE CAN'T MISS CAUSES OF HEADACHE

JORGE SERRANO AND RYAN RAAM

Headache comprises 2 to 3% of ED visits annually. About 98% of these presentations are benign and can be managed conservatively (primary headache). However, the remaining 2% of headache complaints presenting to the ED represent conditions with high morbidity and mortality (secondary headache), necessitating an expeditious diagnosis. It is imperative for the emergency clinician to be able to identify the often subtle differences, or "red flags," in the history and clinical examination that differentiate between primary and secondary headache. A common pitfall in the evaluation of headache is dismissing the presence of a secondary headache because of resolution with analgesics. Of note, age is a significant contributor to the development of a secondary headache. Patients presenting with headache under the age of 50 years have a 1% incidence of a significant secondary headache. However, this incidence jumps to 11% if the patient is at least 75 years old.

SAH

Classically, patients present with a severe, sudden, and maximal at onset headache. Approximately 8% of patients presenting with this "thunderclap" headache will be diagnosed with SAH. SAH is often associated with altered mental status, vomiting, neck stiffness, syncope, seizure, and neurologic deficits. However, more than half of SAHs will present with a nonfocal neurologic examination. History of a "sudden-onset" headache is 97% sensitive for SAH, but characterization as "worst headache of my life" has not been shown to be a significant predictor. The Ottawa SAH rule has been validated with a sensitivity of 100% for the evaluation of SAH, but the specificity is very low and its use may result in the overuse of CT imaging. In addition, CT imaging within 6 hours of symptom onset has also been shown to have 100% sensitivity in a recent study, although it has many caveats to its application. CTA can be a reasonable alternative to performing an LP to evaluate for a cerebral aneurysm, but physicians must be aware of its limitations. The CTA is not sensitive for aneurysms less than 3 mm and may show false-positive findings.

BACTERIAL MENINGITIS

Consider meningitis especially in the immunocompromised or unvaccinated, especially pediatric patients or those with a history of HIV. 95% of patients will present with at least two of the following: headache, fever, altered mental status, or neck stiffness. However, most (77%) patients will present with a nonfocal neurologic examination. Kernig and Brudzinski signs have both been found to be highly specific (98%) for meningitis, but not sensitive. LP remains the gold standard for the diagnosis of meningitis. In patients infected with known HIV, remember to measure the opening ICP during the LP when assessing for cryptococcal infection. Initiation of antibiotics should not be delayed for any part of the diagnostic workup!

ACUTE ANGLE-CLOSURE GLAUCOMA

These patients will present with acute unilateral eye pain, blurred vision, and headache. Nausea and vomiting are common as well. It can be precipitated by pupillary dilation, for example, when walking from a bright to dark room. On examination, you will commonly see an injected conjunctiva with a fixed mid-dilated pupil. An intraocular pressure of 60 to 90 mm Hg is diagnostic, but any reading above 30 mm Hg should raise concern for the diagnosis.

CVT/CVST

The headache in these patients will commonly present as slowly progressive, but a minority of patients with CVT will have an abrupt "thunderclap" headache. This condition presents with a wide array of neurologic symptoms, including altered level of consciousness, CN VI abducens palsy, aphasia, coma, or seizure. Have high suspicion in patients with hypercoagulable disorders, OCP use, pregnancy, or recent infections involving the head and neck. Also, signs of increased ICP such as papilledema, caused by occluded CSF outflow, may be present. CT or MR venography is the study of choice in the evaluation of these patients.

CAD

Two subtypes of CAD exist: ICAD and VAD. ICAD will commonly present with anterior circulation deficits, such as Horner syndrome, CN XII palsy, or pulsatile tinnitus. VAD will commonly present with posterior circulations symptoms, such as vertigo, diplopia, and dysarthria. Patients will often describe having sudden-onset headache or neck pain with CADs. Both may present with delayed onset of key neurologic findings (ICAD ~4 days, VAD ~14.5 hours), making the diagnosis more difficult. Pediatric patients with recent neck trauma who exhibit any of the aforementioned neurologic findings are at high risk for CAD.

GCA

GCA almost never develops in a patient younger than 50 years and typically occurs in patients older than 70 years. The most common symptom is headache, but patients can also present with vision disturbances, decreased temporal artery pulse, and temporal artery tenderness. Classically, the ESR and CRP will be elevated, but a small portion of patients will have normal labs. If there is a high suspicion for GCA, corticosteroids should be started immediately to mitigate permanent vision loss.

This list is not exhaustive, and it is important to remember that there are other "can't miss" causes of headache. Consider preeclampsia in the pregnant or postpartum

TABLE 184.1	FACTORS TO BE CONSIDERED IN APPLYING THE 6-HOUR RULE FOR CT IN SAH

Patient factors

- The time of onset of the headache is defined unambiguously
- The CT is performed within 6 hours of headache onset
- The presentation is an isolated thunderclap headache (no primary neck pain, seizure, or syncope at onset, etc)
- There is no meningismus, and the neurologic examination is normal

Radiologic factors

- The CT scanner is a modem, third-generation, or newer machine
- The CT is technically adequate without significant motion artifact
- Thin cuts 5 mm or more are done through the base of the brain
- The hematocrit is greater than 30%
- The physician interpreting the scan is an attending level radiologist (or has equivalent experience in reading brain CT scans)
- Radiologists should specifically examine brain CTs for thunderclap headache for subtle hydrocephalus, small amounts of blood in the dependent portions of the ventricles, and small amounts of isodense or hyperdense material in the basal cisterns

Communication factors

- The clinician should communicate the specific concern to the radiologist (eg, "severe acute headache, rule-out SAH")
- After a negative CT, the clinician should communicate to the patient the post-test risk of SAH that persists (1-2/1,000)

CT, computed tomography; SAH, subarachnoid hemorrhage.
From Dubosh NM, Bellolio MF, Rabinstein AA, Edlow JA. Sensitivity of early brain computed tomography to exclude aneurysmal subarachnoid hemorrhage: a systematic review and meta-analysis. *Stroke*. 2016;47(3):750-755.

patient. Think about carbon monoxide poisoning in the patient who presents with other sick family members in the middle of the winter—their carboxyhemoglobin levels will be elevated. A space-occupying lesion should be considered in anyone with a history of malignancy or prolonged symptoms.

Headache is a common complaint, and most of the time, the etiology is benign. However, a thorough history and physical examination tailored to the patient's presentation, and risk factors will provide you with the information needed to make the life-threatening diagnoses. If you don't look for them every time, you *will* miss them.

PEARLS

- Age is a significant predictor of a dangerous secondary headache, with incidence increasing to approximately 11% after the age of 75.
- When obtained within 6 hours of headache onset, a noncontrast head CT can reliably rule-out SAH, with the appropriate caveats (see **Table 184.1**).
- Obtaining a good history and physical examination is crucial to identify risk factors and "red flags" for dangerous causes of headache.
- A patient presenting with headache and new neurologic deficits should heighten your suspicion for a "can't miss" headache, especially in high-risk patients.

Suggested Readings

American College of Emergency Physicians Clinical Policies Subcommittee (Writing Committee) on Acute Headache; Godwin SA, Cherkas DS, et al. Clinical policy: critical issues in the evaluation and management of adult patients presenting to the emergency department with acute headache. *Ann Emerg Med.* 2019;74(4):e41-e74.

Dubosh NM, Bellolio MF, Rabinstein AA, Edlow JA. Sensitivity of early brain computed tomography to exclude aneurysmal subarachnoid hemorrhage: a systematic review and meta-analysis. *Stroke.* 2016;47(3):750-755. PMID: 26797666.

Raam R, Tabatabai RR. Headache in the emergency department: avoiding misdiagnosis of dangerous secondary causes, an update. *Emerg Med Clin North Am.* 2021;39(1):67-85.

185

Don't Miss the Myasthenic

Ashley Rebekah Allen and Anna Darby

MG is an autoimmune disease that causes musculoskeletal weakness and can lead to life-threatening symptoms such as respiratory failure in the setting of a myasthenic crisis. A typical clinical presentation can involve ocular symptoms such as ptosis and diplopia, bulbar symptoms such as dysarthria and dysphagia, or neck extensor and proximal muscle weakness. An ice pack test can aid in the diagnosis of ocular myasthenia gravis. Known patients with myasthenia can be treated with an AChEI such as pyridostigmine.

The EP's most important role in the care of the patient with myasthenia is the awareness of its most extreme clinical presentation, the acute myasthenic crisis. Myasthenic crisis is commonly defined as an episode of profound weakness that leads to respiratory failure and requires mechanical or noninvasive ventilatory assistance to avoid imminent respiratory collapse and death. The diagnosis and appropriate management of a patient with myasthenic crisis is a critical skill for the EP as a myasthenic crisis is the very first presentation of the disease in approximately 20% of patients and 1 in 5 patients with myasthenia will experience a myasthenic crisis during their lifetime.

Common causes of a myasthenic crisis include infection, surgery, pregnancy, and medication changes. Given the potential of causing worsening myasthenia, the EP must avoid administration of high-risk medications such as aminoglycosides, fluoroquinolones, and class IA antiarrhythmics that can all lead to worsening symptoms. Notably, a cholinergic crisis, from overmedication with an AChEI, can present similar to a myasthenic crisis with respiratory symptoms. A cholinergic crisis is rarely seen in the absence of high, escalating doses of AChEI and typically presents with other signs of cholinergic toxicity such as increased salivation, lacrimation, and diarrhea.

A thorough history and physical examination, while paramount in any patient presenting with complaints of weakness, can be deceptive in the myasthenic. Respiratory symptoms develop as a result of profound accessory muscle and diaphragmatic weakness. Rather than presenting with traditional signs of respiratory failure, patients may present with more subtle signs including a weak cough, difficulty controlling secretions, or difficulty speaking full sentences. The potential subtlety of respiratory compromise contributes to the high rate of death in patients in myasthenic crisis (4%-12%). The "single-breath counting test" asking the patient to count to 20 in a single breath can be a useful bedside tool for the EP in assessing early respiratory compromise. Other adjuncts for evaluating respiratory function include abnormal respiratory tests such as a low NIF (<20 cm H_2O), low VC (<1 L or 20-25 mL/kg), and/or presence of respiratory acidosis. These findings are suggestive of severe respiratory weakness and support the decision for emergent intervention with mechanical ventilation.

Early use of noninvasive ventilation such as BiPAP can stave off intubation in myasthenic crisis, but these patients need to be closely monitored for persistent signs of clinical worsening. Worsening respiratory, mental status, or progressive respiratory acidosis can be deadly, as these patients have poor respiratory reserve, and patients develop a higher risk for aspiration as bulbar weakness worsens. Thus, early intubation is commonly used for management of myasthenic crisis, especially if any of the aforementioned adjuncts show worsening respiratory function.

When considering medications for RSI, the EP must consider that succinylcholine is less effective since the myasthenic's postsynaptic ACh receptors are downregulated. Physicians should use rocuronium or other nondepolarizing paralytic agents instead. It is recommended to reduce the dose of paralytic by approximately 50% (eg, using ~0.6 mg/kg rocuronium rather than the normal 1 mg/kg dosing) to avoid prolonged paralysis. Etomidate dosing can remain unchanged without untoward effects, as can ketamine and opioids. Propofol is a safe choice for post-sedation analgesia.

In addition to airway management during a myasthenic crisis, the EP should consult with their neurology colleagues early to initiate other potential interventions including plasmapheresis and IVIG. Patients with high suspicion for myasthenic crisis should be admitted to the intensive care unit.

Drugs to Avoid

- Antiarrhythmics: beta-blockers, procainamide, quinidine
- Antibiotics: aminoglycosides, macrolides, fluoroquinolone, tetracyclines
- Anticonvulsants: phenytoin, gabapentin, barbiturates
  Antipsychotics/mood stabilizers: amitriptyline, amphetamines, haldol, lithium
- Botulinum toxin (Botox)
- Corticosteroids** rate/titration matter
  Magnesium (parenteral> enteral)
- Statins
- Succinylcholine

PEARLS

- MG is the most common NMJ disorder, and 1 in 5 patients with MG will experience myasthenic crisis.
- Single-breath counting test less than 20, NIF less than 20, VC less than 1 L or CO_2 greater than 45 mm Hg are indications for respiratory support.
- Early NIV (BiPAP) and intubation in those with myasthenic crisis/respiratory failure is lifesaving.

- IVIG/plasmapheresis and steroids are the pharmacologic mainstays; consider antibiotics for concomitant infection.
- Diagnostic testing should never delay emergent interventions.

SUGGESTED READINGS

Abel M, Eisenkraft J. Anesthetic implications of myasthenia gravis. *Mt Sinai J Med*. 2002; 69(1,2):31-37.

Adeyinka A, Kondamudi N. Cholinergic crisis. *StatPearls [Internet]*. StatPearls Publishing; 2023. PMID: 29494040.

Aguirre F, Fernández RN, Arrejoría RM, et al. Peak expiratory flow and the single-breath counting test as markers of respiratory function in patients with myasthenia gravis. *Neurologia (Engl Ed)*. 2020:S0213-4853(20)30432-1. PMID: 33317968.

Juel V. Myasthenia gravis: management of the myasthenic crisis and perioperative care. *Semin Neurol*. 2004;24(1):75-81.

Wendell L, Levine J. Myasthenic crisis. *Neurohospitalist*. 2011;1(1):16-22.

186

WHAT DO I DO WITH WAKE-UP STROKE?

DAVID ALEXANDER GREGOR AND MICHAEL SHAMOON

It is a vexing clinical scenario when a patient presents to the ED with a clear stroke syndrome but an unclear last known well time (LKWT). Patients with stroke who wake up from sleep with new neurologic deficits are said to have had a "wake-up" stroke. It is difficult or impossible to tell the exact time of onset in such cases. This presents a dilemma for patients and clinicians, given that timing is critical for effective stroke evaluation and treatment.

Improving stroke outcomes is important because stroke causes widespread morbidity and mortality: one in four people experience stroke, and stroke is the second leading cause of death worldwide. In the United States, approximately 85% of acute strokes are ischemic and one in five ischemic strokes is wake-up. Evidence suggests that wake-up and awake-onset strokes have similar pathophysiology, raising the question of whether patients with wake-up stroke might benefit from the same treatment offered for awake-onset stroke, including thrombolysis with tPA and EVT.

EVALUATING WAKE-UP STROKE

Evaluation of a patient with stroke in the ED begins with rapid assessment of neurologic deficits via history, physical examination, and neuroimaging. The standard initial diagnostic study is noncontrast CT head (NCCTH). If this shows ICH or suggests a stroke mimic, patients should be treated accordingly. If not, patients are typically treated empirically for AIS. Some centers also utilize additional imaging modalities, either as part of initial workup or following NCCTH. These include CT or MR angiography to identify LVO strokes amenable to EVT. Some centers also utilize CT perfusion studies or MR diffusion-weighted imaging (DWI)-fluid-attenuated inversion recovery (FLAIR) mismatch to identify early ischemia and guide management.

Evidence for Treating Wake-Up Stroke With tPA or EVT

Intravenous thrombolysis with tPA has been the cornerstone AIS treatment since the mid-1990s (using alteplase and, more recently, tenecteplase). Historically, patients with wake-up stroke were not offered tPA, as their LKWT could not be determined to fall within the indication window. Risk of iatrogenic ICH increased significantly with tPA given outside this time frame.

Treatment options have expanded for some patients based on recent evidence. Ongoing research has attempted to determine whether tPA and EVT are safe and effective for patients with wake-up stroke. Recent trials suggest substantial benefits of treating LVO strokes with EVT, including DAWN and DEFUSE 3, which showed that EVT can be beneficial and safe up to 24 hours after LKWT. Meta-analyses analyzing pooled results specifically for patients with wake-up stroke with an LVO of the carotid artery or middle cerebral artery suggest benefit from EVT up to 24 hours from symptom onset.

The benefit of thrombolytics for wake-up stroke is less clear. While there is no strong evidence supporting the safety or efficacy of routinely offering tPA to all patients with wake-up stroke, there may be a subset of patients with wake-up stroke or unknown LKWT who could benefit from thrombolysis. The latest American Heart Association/American Stroke Association guidelines for AIS management (2019) note that giving tPA within 4.5 hours of stroke symptom recognition can be beneficial for some patients with AIS with wake-up stroke or unclear LKWT, if they have DWI-FLAIR findings consistent with criteria found to be beneficial in the WAKE-UP trial discussed later. Patients should be evaluated on a case-by-case basis. Further research is needed to determine standard of care.

Searching for a Subset of Patients With Wake-Up Stroke Who Might Benefit From tPA

Overall, recent data do not suggest that the benefits of routine tPA administration outweigh the risks for non-LVO wake-up strokes. Routine tPA for all wake-up strokes is of questionable benefit. Notable studies include the following:

The 2018 WAKE-UP trial investigated whether patients with AIS with unknown LKWT whose strokes appeared less than 4.5 hours old on DWI-FLAIR could benefit from tPA. The study found an 11% benefit (mRS 0 to 1) with thrombolysis, but an increase in deaths, although it did not reach statistical significance. There was no difference in "death or dependence" (14% vs 18%). While the authors concluded that thrombolytics increased favorable outcomes, thrombolytics increased deaths, did not change patient-oriented outcomes, and trial results were suspect because the trial was stopped early after enrolling only 503 of 800 planned patients.

In 2019, the EXTEND trial examined treating patients with AIS who presented 4.5 to 9 hours after LKWT with thrombolytics. The trial enrolled 225 of 400 planned patients, roughly 66% with wake-up strokes. Patients had CT or MR perfusion imaging and received alteplase or placebo if their studies showed salvageable lesions. EXTEND was stopped early based on the researchers' view that WAKE-UP showed clear benefit with tPA, eliminating "equipoise" in the study groups. Favorable outcome was mRS of 0 to 1, 35% versus 30% in treatment versus control groups, but with an unadjusted analysis suggesting no benefit. The authors claimed statistical significance using adjusted analysis methods that were not planned before the study was started. Mortality and ICH were higher with alteplase but again not statistically significant.

A systematic review and meta-analysis in 2020 examined patient data for WAKE-UP, EXTEND, and related studies THAWS and ECASS-4, pooling 843 patients' results. It found an 8% increase in favorable outcomes using tPA but a 3% increase in mortality. Subgroup analysis showed no benefit with thrombolytics for patients with non-LVO strokes or with no clearly implicated vessel.

Conclusion

Hopefully, treatment options will continue to improve for patients with wake-up stroke and stroke with uncertain LKWT. Patients with wake-up stroke need rapid diagnosis of their condition and aggressive supportive care, regardless of attempts at revascularization. This includes careful management of blood pressure, blood glucose, body temperature, and oxygenation; minimizing the risk of further neurologic insults; and optimizing recovery. Patients should be transferred to primary or comprehensive stroke centers as needed, depending on the clinical scenario and local resources.

PEARLS

- Wake-up stroke is common. Although its pathophysiology is like that of awake-onset stroke, efficacy and safety of reperfusion strategies differ.
- Evidence does not support routine administration of tPA for wake-up stroke.
- CT or MR perfusion imaging may help identify patients with wake-up stroke who could benefit from tPA, with the acknowledged potential increased risk of ICH.
- EVT can be beneficial and safe for patients with LVO stroke 0 to 24 hours after LKWT.

Suggested Readings

Biggs D, Silverman ME, Chen F, et al. How should we treat patients who wake up with a stroke? A review of recent advances in management of acute ischemic stroke. *Am J Emerg Med.* 2019;37(5):954-959.

Feigin VL, Brainin M, Norrving B, et al. World Stroke Organization (WSO): global stroke fact sheet 2022 [published correction appears in *Int J Stroke.* 2022;17(4):478]. *Int J Stroke.* 2022;17(1):18-29.

Gottlieb M, Meissner H, Kalina M. What is the efficacy and safety of intravenous thrombolysis and thrombectomy among patients with a wake-up stroke? *Ann Emerg Med.* 2022; 80(2):165-167.

Ma H, Campbell BCV, Parsons MW, et al. Thrombolysis guided by perfusion imaging up to 9 hours after onset of stroke. *N Engl J Med.* 2019;380(19):1795-1803.

Powers WJ, Rabinstein AA, Ackerson T, et al. Guidelines for the early management of patients with acute ischemic stroke: 2019 update to the 2018 guidelines for the early management of acute ischemic stroke: a guideline for healthcare professionals from the American Heart Association/American Stroke Association [published correction appears in *Stroke.* 2019;50(12):e440-e441. PMID: 31662037]. *Stroke.* 2019;50(12):e344-e418.

Roaldsen MB, Lindekleiv H, Mathiesen EB. Intravenous thrombolytic treatment and endo-vascular thrombectomy for ischaemic wake-up stroke. *Cochrane Database Syst Rev.* 2021;12(12):CD010995.

Thomalla G, Boutitie F, Ma H, et al. Intravenous alteplase for stroke with unknown time of onset guided by advanced imaging: systematic review and meta-analysis of individual patient data. *Lancet.* 2020;396(10262):1574-1584.

187

It's Not All in My Head! Evaluation of the Patient With Suspected Psychogenic Nonepileptiform Seizures

Vian Zada and Ramin Tabatabai

If you were to measure the electrical activity of PNES, you would find no abnormalities. And so, at first glance, PNES might not seem like a medical emergency—and certainly not one you would test in the ED. However, failing to quickly recognize PNES can lead to inappropriate interventions and significant iatrogenic harm.

Background

PNES appear outwardly like generalized tonic-clonic seizures, with involuntary changes in movement and consciousness. Psychogenic seizures have been postulated to be a maladaptive defense mechanism, in which reduced awareness or disinhibition during distress leads to a dissociative effect. The pathophysiology of this neural sensorimotor response to stress remains unclear. Importantly, episodes of PNES are not conscious or staged. There are many other causes of nonepileptic seizures, such as metabolic abnormalities, toxic ingestion, substance withdrawal, and infection.

PNES is widely accepted as a biopsychosocial disorder. Most patients have psychiatric comorbidities or a history of trauma. Women and individuals from lower socioeconomic groups are at higher risk.

Diagnosis

Some clinical signs may be more suggestive of PNES; however, no one feature alone can diagnose it (**Table 187.1**). Unlike epileptiform seizures, in PNES, patients can sometimes be responsive to stimuli. Jaw clenching or tightly closed eyes also point to nonepileptiform seizures. Patients may also lack the postictal period typically seen in epileptic convulsions.

TABLE 187.1 DISTINGUISHING FEATURES OF PNES

Nonepileptiform Seizure Clues	Historical Clues
Distractibility	PTSD
Crying	Sexual, emotional, or physical trauma
Stuttering	Depression, anxiety
Retained or partially retained awareness	Adverse childhood events
Eye closure	Grief
Jaw clenching	Traumatic brain injury
Side-to-side head shaking	High frequency
Waxing and waning consciousness	Later age of onset
Asynchronous jerking of the left and right extremities	
Absent postictal state	
Absent physical injury	

PNES, psychogenic nonepileptiform seizures; PTSD, posttraumatic stress disorder.

Evaluating PNES in the ED requires a careful history and examination. PNES can occur at any age, but typically emerge in the second and third decades of life. Circumstances of onset and a brief social history can point to the psychological underpinnings of PNES. Quickly screen for any past neurologic workup, employment status, history of trauma, recent stress, or adverse childhood effects. As with all seizures, witness information can further the diagnostic process. Importantly, do not administer noxious stimuli in order to "test" the veracity of a patient's examination. This can cause harm and break down trust that will be necessary for effective treatment in the longer term.

Even as retrospective data points, laboratory values may not be helpful in forming your differential. Lactate levels are not specific for epileptic convulsions. Elevated CK levels correlate strongly with generalized convulsive status epilepticus but have only moderate sensitivity. CK levels are more likely to be normal in PNES but may also be normal in focal epileptic seizures.

The only way to accurately diagnose PNES is an EEG, showing no abnormal activity during an event. One in 10 patients have a comorbid epileptic seizure disorder, which can further complicate the differential. Whether the patient requires an admission for a diagnostic EEG will depend on the clinical picture. A neurologist, if available, can help guide appropriate next steps.

TREATMENT

If PNES can be clinically diagnosed in the ED, the first step after diagnosis is to avoid invasive medical procedures and ASMs. Administering or prescribing ASM to patients with PNES may condemn them to years of unnecessary medication. For patients already diagnosed with PNES, weaning them off ASMs may be dangerous in the outpatient setting. The most efficacious treatment for PNES is thought to be cognitive behavioral therapy, which has been shown to reduce PNES frequency and improve quality of life. This is often resisted by patients due to the stigma of psychiatric diseases and the lack of recognition that PNES is a neurologic disease with a psychiatric/behavioral treatment.

Recognize that this is a complex disease associated with stigma. There is also the misconception that the patient is "faking" their presentation. Some patients may find the diagnosis confusing or upsetting. As such, diagnosis should be delivered with thoughtfulness and compassion. Patients may be started on medications for anxiety or depression in the outpatient setting. A focus on the psychogenic underpinnings and ultimately a referral to mental health resources should lead therapy.

PEARLS

- PNES is important to recognize in the ED. PNES can appear outwardly like epileptic seizure. They are not intentional or staged.
- Evaluating PNES in the ED requires a careful history and examination. As with any seizure, CK and lactate levels will likely not provide sufficient diagnostic value.
- Avoid inappropriate interventions and ASMs in PNES.
- PNES is a biopsychosocial disorder, and therapeutic success will require a multidisciplinary approach.

Suggested Readings

Asadi-Pooya AA, Myers L, Valente K, et al. Sex differences in demographic and clinical characteristics of psychogenic nonepileptic seizures: a retrospective multicenter international study. *Epilepsy Behav*. 2019; 97:154–157.

Balachandran N, Goodman AM, Allendorfer JB, et al. Relationship between neural responses to stress and mental health symptoms in psychogenic nonepileptic seizures after traumatic brain injury. *Epilepsia*. 2021;62(1):107-119.

Hoerth MT, Wellik KE, Demaerschalk BM, et al. Clinical predictors of psychogenic nonepileptic seizures: a critically appraised topic. *Neurologist*. 2008;14(4):266-270. PMID: 18617856.

Huff JS, Murr N. *Psychogenic nonepileptic seizures*. In: *StatPearls* [Internet]. StatPearls Publishing; 2022. https://www.ncbi.nlm.nih.gov/books/NBK441871/

Javali M, Acharya P, Shah S, Mahale R, Shetty P, Rangasetty S. Role of biomarkers in differentiating new-onset seizures from psychogenic nonepileptic seizures. *J Neurosci Rural Pract*. 2017;8(4):581-584. PMID: 29204018.

Tilahun BBS, Bautista JF. Psychogenic nonepileptic seizure: an empathetic, practical approach. *Cleve Clin J Med*. 2022;89(5):252-259. PMID: 35500924.

Tolchin B, Martino S, Hirsch LJ. Treatment of patients with psychogenic nonepileptic attacks. *JAMA*. 2019;321(20):1967-1968. PMID: 31026015.

van Ool JS, Haenen AI, Snoeijen-Schouwenaars FM, et al. Psychogenic nonepileptic seizures in adults with epilepsy and intellectual disability: a neglected area. *Seizure*. 2018;59:67-71.

188

Can't Miss Moves in the Patient with TBI

Chase Luther and Ryan Raam

Traumatic brain injury (TBI) is regularly encountered in the ED, often associated with high morbidity and mortality. Actions taken in the ED should focus on identifying, preventing, and treating elevations of ICP as well as preventing secondary insults to the brain. Though this chapter is focused on the management of TBI specifically, all patients with trauma should have a comprehensive trauma evaluation, including vital signs, performing a trauma survey, and establishing adequate IV access upon arrival to the ED. Patients with a depressed GCS suggesting severe TBI, respiratory distress, or with a rapid decline in mental status attributed to their TBI should be intubated for airway protection after adequate resuscitation.

Intracranial Pressure

When the cranial vault is intact, the total volume within this space is a fixed constant and is composed of three separate components: brain parenchyma, CSF, and intravascular blood. The total volume of these components determines the ICP, and an increase in one component necessitates a decrease in the other components if the ICP is to remain physiologic. Neurotrauma can lead to elevations in ICP in a variety of ways, including hemorrhagic lesions, cerebral edema, or lesions causing obstructive hydrocephalus. Pathologic elevations to ICP can result in poor cerebral perfusion and eventually herniation.

Direct measurement of ICP requires invasive monitoring placed by a neurosurgeon and is rarely immediately available in the ED. Emergency physicians must rely on other methods to determine when patients may have an elevated ICP, namely, an adequate neurologic examination as well as CT imaging of the head. An adequate neurologic examination should be performed before administration of paralytics or sedatives and should include monitoring of vital signs, a GCS assessment, and a pupillary examination. Clinical evidence suggestive of severe TBI and elevated ICP may include a Cushing reflex (hypertension, bradycardia, irregular respirations), GCS less than 9, decorticate or decerebrate posturing, unilateral weakness, or an abnormal pupillary examination. CT evidence of elevated ICP may include midline shift, effacement of the ventricles, or imaging evidence of herniation.

When pathologic ICP is suspected, there are several options for empiric treatment. Start with elevation of the head of the bed to 30° in order to increase cerebral venous outflow and decrease CSF volume. Other initial steps in management include adequate analgesia and adequate sedation in the setting of agitation/endotracheal intubation. Intubation should be done with strict cervical spine precautions and close attention to maintaining adequate blood pressure. Although therapeutic hyperventilation was performed in the past, it is no longer regularly recommended as its therapeutic effects are transient and can ultimately lead to worsened cerebral perfusion.

An additional measure to reduce ICP is administration of hyperosmotic agents to reduce cerebral edema. The agents most commonly used are HTS and mannitol. Though both work well in reducing ICP, HTS is often preferred, given that it can act as a volume expander where mannitol is a powerful diuretic that can cause hypotension and/or kidney injury. HTS at 3% concentration is common with boluses of 150 to 250 mL. Ultimately, neurosurgical consultation is needed, and the patient may require surgical management, such as ventriculostomy or craniectomy, to measure and manage ICP.

Secondary Insults

Secondary insults are those that occur after the initial neurotrauma and may lead to worse outcomes. Some of these insults include, but are not limited to, coagulopathy, hypotension, oxygen derangement, glucose derangement, and seizure. These secondary insults may be prevented or minimized with diligent monitoring and management of these conditions in the ED.

Coagulopathy may be iatrogenic, secondary to preexisting medical conditions, or may develop secondary to systemic responses to severe injury and TBI. It may be identified based on patient history as well as lab testing. Treatment for coagulopathy will often depend on the etiology and may include specific antidotes or reversal agents, blood product transfusions, or desmopressin. Coagulopathy should be reversed or treated in patients with severe TBI. Consider discussing this aspect of management with your neurosurgical colleagues in patients with minor TBI.

Hypotension and decreased MAP can lead to worse CPP (CPP = MAP − ICP) and ultimately worse patient outcomes. All efforts should be made to address hypotension in the ED, and maintaining adequate MAP (70-80 mm Hg) often takes precedence over permissive hypotension that may be tolerated in patients with other traumatic injuries. The BTF recommends maintaining SBP greater than 100 mm Hg for patients aged 50 to

69 years and greater than 110 mm Hg for those 15 to 49 or older than 70 years. Treatments for hypotension may include crystalloid volume expanders, vasopressors, or transfusion of blood products.

Oxygen derangements include both hypoxia and hyperoxia. Hypoxia can lead to worsened ischemia and increased mortality. All efforts should be made to prevent hypoxia, starting from the prehospital phase and throughout the ED stay. If PaO_2 is available, note that levels greater than 300 have been shown to be associated with worse outcomes.

Brain tissue is highly dependent on glucose for normal cellular function, and hypoglycemia can cause worsened ischemia. Treatment with D_{50} is preferred over hypoosmotic agents such as D_5, which may lead to worsened cerebral edema. Conversely, hyperglycemia has also been shown to be associated with worse outcomes in patients.

Finally, post-traumatic seizures are common and should be addressed. Seizures may have a negative impact on brain healing, and status epilepticus has been associated with a worse prognosis in patients with TBI. The BTF currently recommends routine use of phenytoin to prevent early post-traumatic seizures. However, levetiracetam is more commonly being used due to its lower risk of adverse effects and may be a reasonable alternative.

PEARLS

- Diligently monitor patients for clinical evidence of elevated ICP.
- Perform a thorough neurologic examination before sedation and/or paralytics before placement of an endotracheal tube.
- Reverse any anticoagulation.
- Elevate the head of the bed, consider osmotic therapy, and prevent secondary insults in patients with elevated ICP.
- Consult a neurosurgeon early in the care of the patient with traumatic brain injuries.

Suggested Readings

Carney N, Totten AM, O'Reilly C, et al. Guidelines for the management of severe traumatic brain injury, Fourth edition. *Neurosurgery*. 2017;80(1):6-15.

Long B, Koyfman A. Secondary gains: advances in neurotrauma management. *Emerg Med Clin North Am*. 2018;36(1):107-133.

Swadron SP, LeRoux P, Smith WS, et al. Emergency neurological life support: traumatic brain injury. *Neurocrit Care*. 2012;17(suppl 1):S112–S121.

Vespa PM, Nuwer MR, Nenov V, et al. Increased incidence and impact of nonconvulsive and convulsive seizures after traumatic brain injury as detected by continuous electroencephalographic monitoring. *J Neurosurg*. 1999;91(5):750-760.

SECTION XV
OBSTETRICS/GYNECOLOGY

189

PITFALLS IN THE PURSUIT OF OVARIAN TORSION

MATTHEW C. DELANEY

While the overall incidence of ovarian torsion is fairly low, cases of ovarian torsion that present to the ED have a high rate of misdiagnosis on the initial visit, have significant associated morbidity, and can be a source of significant medico-legal risk to the provider. Ovarian torsion should, therefore, be a part of the differential diagnosis when evaluating any female with abdominal pain. Being aware of several persistent myths and misconceptions that exist may allow providers to refine their workups and more accurately estimate pre- and post-test probability of torsion.

CLASSIC DOESN'T MEAN COMMON

Classically, pain from ovarian torsion has been described as sharp, sudden, unilateral pain occurring in women of reproductive age. In practice, the patient's demographics and symptoms have significant variability; however, several features may increase the pretest probability of ovarian torsion. In a retrospective review, 70% of patients reported "sharp or stabbing" pain, symptoms had an abrupt onset in only 59% of cases, and 70% of patients reported associated nausea and vomiting. The majority of cases of torsion occur after the onset of menarche; however, up to 15% of cases occur in the pediatric population with a similar percentage of cases occurring in patients who are postmenopausal, and roughly 20% of cases of ovarian torsion occur during pregnancy. While most patients with ovarian torsion have a structurally abnormal ovary, patients commonly have no preceding history, with only 25% of patients reporting a previous history of ovarian cyst or mass. In pediatric cases, up to 58% of patients had no obvious ovarian pathology. Features such as a history of previous pelvic surgery or pelvic inflammatory disease may increase the likelihood of a patient developing torsion; however, these historical elements are present in a minority of the reported cases.

DON'T RELY ON YOUR BEDSIDE EXAMINATION

Bedside examination is rarely helpful when trying to make the diagnosis of ovarian torsion. The presence of abdominal pain, pelvic mass, or significant adnexal tenderness may increase the likelihood of ovarian torsion, yet in practice, the bedside examination suffers from poor sensitivity and specificity and should not be used to rule out cases of torsion. In addition, the sensitivity of the pelvic examination for detecting adnexal masses ranged from 15% to 36% despite being performed under near-ideal circumstances by gynecology attendings in an operative setting.

CT May Be an Adequate Study

For patients with a convincing story for possible torsion, ultrasound is the most reasonable first-line imaging study. Given the variable presentations of torsion, providers may instead order a CT of the abdomen/pelvis when patients present with a complaint of nonspecific abdominal pain. When faced with a nondiagnostic CT scan, providers will order an ultrasound to more fully evaluate for ovarian pathology, including torsion. Recent studies have suggested that CT may be a reasonable imaging modality and have questioned the added utility of ultrasound with reported sensitivities and specificities of 80% to 100% for both CT and ultrasound when diagnosing ovarian torsion. Given this diagnostic accuracy, when torsion is seen on the CT scan, patients do not need further imaging.

More commonly, providers have a patient with ongoing pain and a CT scan that does not show torsion. In this scenario, CT scan may be helpful in terms of identifying other ovarian pathology that could lead to the patient developing torsion. The incidence of ovarian torsion occurring in patients with completely normal imaging is extremely low. When compared to ultrasound, CT has been shown to be more likely to detect abnormal ovarian pathology. Given the high sensitivity of CT scan for detecting ovarian pathology and the rare incidence of torsion in patients with normal ovarian anatomy, a truly negative CT scan in a patient with abdominal pain may effectively rule out ovarian torsion in a large majority of patients.

Ultrasound Has Significant Limitations

Ultrasound has a wide range of reported sensitivities (~36%-85%) in the evaluation of patients with potential ovarian torsion. When present, features such as a lack of blood flow or obvious ovarian edema have a high degree of diagnostic accuracy. While Doppler ultrasound can be diagnostic when used to identify a lack of blood flow, normal Doppler scans are seen in up to one-third of patients with surgically proven ovarian torsion. As with CT scans, cases of torsion in a patient with normal ovarian anatomy on ultrasound do occur but are exceedingly rare. MRI has good reported diagnostic characteristics; however, logistically, it may be difficult to obtain in a timely manner when evaluating a case of acute abdominal pain.

Given the limitations associated with patient history, examination, and imaging, providers should remain vigilant for patients who present with a concerning story for ovarian torsion. In any scenario where the patient has a high pretest probability of ovarian torsion, providers should have a low threshold to consult OB/GYN despite negative imaging studies if there is ongoing clinical concern for ovarian torsion.

PEARLS

- History and examination cannot be used to reliably rule out ovarian torsion.
- CT scan can reliably identify torsion in the majority of cases.
- Ultrasound may be normal in the setting of intermittent torsion.
- Torsion is exceedingly rare in patients who have completely normal ovarian anatomy.
- If concerned for intermittent torsion, providers should consult OB/GYN.

SUGGESTED READINGS

Houry D, Abbott JT. Ovarian torsion: a fifteen-year review. *Ann Emerg Med.* 2001;38(2): 156-159.
Mashiach R, Melamed N, Gilad N, et al. Sonographic diagnosis of ovarian torsion: accuracy and predictive factors. *J Ultrasound Med.* 2011;30(9):1205-1210.
Padilla LA, Radosevich DM, Milad MP. Accuracy of the pelvic examination in detecting adnexal masses. *Obstet Gynecol.* 2000;96(4):593-598. PMID: 11004365.
Schmitt ER, Ngai SS, Gausche-Hill M, et al. Twist and shout! Pediatric ovarian torsion clinical update and case discussion. *Pediatr Emerg Care.* 2013;29(4):518-523, quiz 524-526.
Swenson DW, Lourenco AP, Beaudoin FL, et al. Ovarian torsion: case–control study comparing the sensitivity and specificity of ultrasonography and computed tomography for diagnosis in the emergency department. *Eur J Radiol.* 2014;83(4):733-738.198

190

SEIZING YOUNG FEMALE? THINK ECLAMPSIA. THINKING ECLAMPSIA? THINK AGAIN

KENNETH D. MARSHALL AND ALLYSON M. BRIGGS

Patients actively experiencing seizures or in the postictal phase are a common presentation in the ED. One particular cause of seizure is worth special consideration: eclampsia. Eclampsia's pathophysiology and treatment are unique, the diagnostic clues are sometimes subtle, and mismanagement may lead to greater morbidity or even death. It must be a primary consideration in all female patients of childbearing age experiencing seizures.

The incidence of eclampsia is estimated to range from 1 in 1,000 to 1 in 5,000. It is classically defined as new-onset seizures in a pregnant patient with clinical features of preeclampsia, not clearly attributable to other causes. However, presentations may vary widely, and there are three special scenarios that require vigilance to correctly recognize, diagnose, and treat eclampsia.

The first scenario is the pregnant patient with first-time seizures without typical features of preeclampsia, in particular, lacking proteinuria or hypertension. This occurs in 15% to 40% of patients experiencing eclampsia. Subsequent investigation often reveals signs or symptoms of preeclampsia (headache, visual changes, right upper quadrant pain) antecedent to the seizure. However, up to 25% of patients experiencing eclampsia present without premonitory signs or symptoms. Therefore, absence of the hallmark features of preeclampsia should not deter workup (or even initiating treatment) for eclampsia.

The second scenario is postpartum eclampsia. The majority of cases of eclampsia occur ante- or intrapartum, but 20% to 25% occur postpartum. Most eclamptic seizures occur within 48 hours of delivery but may occur up to 6 weeks postpartum. Despite effective management reducing the incidence of ante- and intrapartum eclampsia, the relative incidence of postpartum eclampsia has risen. It is possible that a nongravid female patient experiencing seizures or in the postictal phase, unable to provide a history of recent delivery, is presenting with eclampsia.

The third scenario is that of eclampsia in an unrecognized pregnancy. Preeclampsia and eclampsia may be the initial presentation of a previously undiagnosed late pregnancy. Molar pregnancies may cause severe preeclampsia and eclampsia as early as 15 to 20 weeks of gestation.

There is a critical counterpoint to the earlier discussion. While eclampsia can be an elusive diagnosis, it also remains a diagnosis of exclusion. Even when eclampsia is a likely explanation for a patient experiencing seizure, failure to exclude other causes is folly. Ischemic or hemorrhagic strokes, as well as cerebral venous sinus thrombosis and arterial dissection, can produce seizures and altered sensorium. To make it even more complex, strokes may be caused by eclampsia. Thrombotic thrombocytopenic purpura is another potentially grave condition precipitated by pregnancy, may also cause convulsions and altered mental status, and its defining laboratory features can mimic the HELLP syndrome of severe preeclampsia.

A structured approach to the diagnosis of new-onset seizures in a young patient capable of pregnancy should be undertaken. Diagnostic laboratory testing generally includes a complete blood count, renal and hepatic profiles, coagulation profile, toxicology screen, and beta-HCG level. If the beta-HCG is positive, an LDH, magnesium level, and urinalysis for proteinuria should also be obtained. Advanced imaging includes a noncontrast CT of the head.

If the patient experiencing seizure is pregnant with features typical of uncomplicated eclampsia (hypertensive, laboratory features of preeclampsia, return to baseline mental status after brief seizure), treatment for eclampsia should be initiated and no further diagnostic testing is generally necessary. However, if eclampsia is considered but the presentation is atypical (focal neurologic deficits, persistent visual disturbances, symptoms refractory to magnesium and antihypertensives), expanded diagnostic testing, including MRI/MRA, is recommended.

Management goals of eclampsia are to prevent secondary injury from seizures (hypoxia, trauma), prevent recurrent seizures, control marked hypertension, and arrange prompt evaluation for delivery. Delivery is the definitive treatment for preeclampsia and eclampsia. Clinicians need to remain aware of these varied presentations of eclampsia, standing ready to diagnose and manage them correctly.

PEARLS

- Eclampsia can occur without preceding symptoms.
- Eclampsia can occur without hypertension or proteinuria.
- Eclampsia can occur up to 6 weeks postpartum.
- Eclampsia that is atypical (focal neurologic deficits, persistent visual changes, seizures, or altered mental status refractory to treatment) needs comprehensive neurologic workup, likely including MRI/MRA.

Suggested Readings

Berhan Y, Berhan A. Should magnesium sulfate be administered to women with mild preeclampsia? A systematic review of published reports on eclampsia. *J Obstet Gynaecol Res*. 2015;41(6):831-842.

Douglas KA, Redman CW. Eclampsia in the United Kingdom. *BMJ*. 1994;309(6966): 1395-1400.

Edlow JA, Caplan LR, O'Brien K, et al. Diagnosis of acute neurological emergencies in pregnant and post-partum women. *Lancet Neurol*. 2013;12(2):175-185.

Fong A, Chau CT, Pan D, et al. Clinical morbidities, trends, and demographics of eclampsia: a population-based study. *Am J Obstet Gynecol*. 2013;209(3):229.e1-229.e7.

191

TIME'S A WASTIN': PERIMORTEM CESAREAN DELIVERY

VIVIENNE NG

Greek God Apollo performed the first cesarean delivery on his wife, Coronis, while on the funeral pyre birthing their son, Asclepius, the demigod of medicine and healing. Rome's second king, Numa Pompilius, decreed that a child be excised from any woman who died in late pregnancy, to allow proper religious burial of both. Known as *lex regis de inferendo mortus*, the "perimortem cesarean delivery" first appears in 715 BC.

Historically, PMCD was performed for last minute fetal salvage when maternal mortality was inevitable. The medical literature describes just over 300 PMCDs, with few in the past decade due to an increase in preventable maternal deaths and improved maternal health. In 1986, a published case series noted a surprising increase in the survival of moribund mothers who underwent timely PMCD with concurrent maternal CPR, leading to the current recommendations of the procedure. Today, the purpose of PMCD is 2-fold: to facilitate maternal resuscitation by relieving aortocaval compression and to deliver early a neurologically intact neonate. While some argue for a terminology change to resuscitative hysterotomy, the American Heart Association and Society for Obstetric Anesthesiology and Perinatology both use PMCD for consistent guidance across fields. Most would agree that the initial call for help must convey the potential for cesarean delivery and reduce confusion among multidisciplinary teams in an already chaotic situation, which resuscitative hysterotomy does not necessarily.

Key features of a successful PMCD include expeditious procedural performance and adequate resuscitation of the pregnant woman. As such, an appreciation of the changes in cardiopulmonary physiology during pregnancy is essential. While cardiac output is increased overall, approximately 30% is diverted to perfuse the gravid uterus. In addition, around 20 weeks of gestation, the gravid uterus reduces venous return and distal aortic flow due to aortocaval compression. Oxygen consumption is higher in pregnancy, complicated by a reduced functional residual capacity and decreased oxygen-carrying capacity from dilutional anemia. Finally, external cardiopulmonary compressions only provide about one-third of normal cardiac output, and is only 80% efficient, at best. Progesterone causes mucosal edema, while estrogen makes tissues friable and hyperemic. Added to a laxity of connective tissues, a tougher intubation ensues. Therefore, early difficult airway management and manual left lateral uterine displacement without downward pressure enhance resuscitation efforts. Evacuation of the uterus—the cesarean delivery—optimizes maternal resuscitation in multiple ways and must be considered early in the course.

The two most important factors to consider in performing a PMCD are fetal viability and timing. Fetal survival with good neurologic outcomes is directly related to the time between maternal death and fetal delivery, with the best outcomes in those delivered within 5 minutes of maternal cardiac arrest. Current recommendations are to begin the PMCD by minute 4 of maternal pulselessness, completing fetal delivery within 1 minute of incision. Of note, successful deliveries up to 30 minutes or more of cardiac arrest have been reported. First, PMCD should still be considered if patients present late in their arrest. Second, PMCD should only be attempted on fetuses 24 weeks or more of gestational age. Time is of the essence; thus, dating by ultrasound is not recommended. A uterine fundus extending to the umbilicus is approximately 20 weeks of gestation. Therefore, a quick and easy way to determine fetal viability of 24 weeks is the ability to palpate the fundus approximately four fingerbreadths above the umbilicus.

Ongoing resuscitation efforts must occur concurrently with the PMCD for greatest success. Optimally, two teams of clinicians should be arranged, one each for the mother and neonate. Ideally, the assistance and expertise of an obstetrician and neonatologist should also be sought. The most experienced person available should perform the PMCD. If time permits, obtain vascular access above the uterus, prepare the abdomen, and decompress the bladder with a Foley catheter; however, do not delay for these.

Maximal exposure is *key* to rapidly access the fetus. Start with a vertical midline incision beginning from the xiphoid process extending to the pubic symphysis (cut around the umbilicus), using the linea nigra as a guide. Carry the incision through all the abdominal layers to the peritoneal cavity or bluntly dissect to the peritoneum, which is incised vertically with scissors. To expose the uterus, retract any bowel and the bladder inferiorly from the visual field. Extract the uterus and vertically incise 5 cm through the lower uterine wall until amniotic fluid is obtained or the uterine cavity is clearly entered. With the other hand, elevate the uterine wall away from the fetus and extend the incision vertically toward the fundus with bandage scissors. Cutting through an anteriorly placed placenta causes little harm. Find the fetal head and disengage it from the pelvis if necessary. As in a spontaneous vaginal delivery, deliver the body, and clamp and cut the umbilical cord, ideally retaining a segment for a cord gas. Premature infants are more likely to present in breech position, in which case, deliver the feet first. Separate and remove the placenta, ensuring the uterus is wiped out to prevent retention of placental products. Close the uterus with large, locking, absorbable sutures starting in the lower segment working cephalad and with layers as needed; avoid staples as these are unlikely to hold. The mother has the highest chance of return of spontaneous circulation at the moment of fetal delivery but anticipate an increase in bleeding. Apply fundal massage and consider a slow infusion of the smallest effective dose of oxytocin, a potent systemic vasodilator and negative inotrope, as bolus administration may precipitate rearrest. Now, take a breath; you may have just saved a life, perhaps even two.

PEARLS

- Don't be caught off guard.
- Identify the right situation for PMCD; obtain specialty assistance whenever possible.

- 24/4/4: 24 weeks or more of gestation, four fingerbreadths above the umbilicus, begin by 4 minutes.
- Continue CPR throughout the entire resuscitation, before and after delivery of the fetus.
- Know your policies; prepare and practice.

SUGGESTED READINGS

Bennett TA, Zealot CM. Cardiopulmonary resuscitation (CPR) in pregnancy. In: Phelan JP, Pacheco LD, Foley MR, Saade GR, Dildy GA, Belfort MA, eds. *Critical Care Obstetrics*. 6th ed. Wiley-Blackwell; 2019.

Jeejeebhoy FM, Zelop CM, Lipman S, et al. Cardiac arrest in pregnancy: a scientific statement from the American Heart Association. *Circulation*. 2015;132(18):1747-1773.

Lipman SS, Cohen S, Mhyre J, et al. Challenging the 4- to 5-minute rule: from perimortem cesarean to resuscitative hysterotomy. *Am J Obstet Gynecol*. 2016;215(1):129-131.

192

DYSPNEA IN PREGNANCY

TINA GODINHO ROSENBAUM AND NAM TRINH

Dyspnea is a common complaint in pregnancy, with up to 60% to 75% of pregnant patients experiencing this symptom at some point during their pregnancy. The differential is broad and includes not only benign etiologies but also life-threatening diagnoses, including PE and cardiomyopathy.

Normal physiologic changes can lead to the sensation of dyspnea in the second half of pregnancy. Progesterone-driven changes cause a 30% to 40% increase in tidal volume and minute ventilation, leading to mild respiratory alkalosis with a 10% to 15% decrease in functional residual capacity. Furthermore, pregnancy causes dilutional anemia, increased cardiac output, and an approximately 20% rise in oxygen consumption with shunting of up to 25% of circulating blood to the fetus. Taken together, these changes make the sensation of dyspnea common.

DIFFERENTIAL DIAGNOSIS

Thorough clinical history and physical examination help differentiate physiologic dyspnea of pregnancy from disease states. Physiologic dyspnea of pregnancy presents as an isolated finding without associated symptoms, such as cough, wheezing, fever, sputum, tachypnea, chest pain, hemoptysis, isolated leg swelling, signs of fluid overload, or urticaria. Vital signs typically remain within normal ranges, so unexplained tachypnea, tachycardia, and hypoxia warrant further investigation.

The differential diagnosis of dyspnea up to 20 weeks of gestation is similar to nonpregnant patients. After 20 weeks and postpartum, preeclampsia, peripartum cardiomyopathy, pulmonary or amniotic fluid embolism, and sepsis must be included in the differential.

Increased Risk of PE

The risk of PE in pregnancy is 4- to 5-fold higher compared to nonpregnant patients and has a 30% fatality rate if left untreated. Virchow triad of endothelial injury, hypercoagulability, and stasis of blood flow is mimicked in pregnancy due to hormonal, vascular, and mechanical changes, which increase the risk of DVT. Pregnant patients experience more venous stasis secondary to IVC compression by the uterus and decreased physical movement. Hormonal changes induce a hypercoagulable state due to changes in multiple clotting factors, including increased fibrinogen levels and decreased protein S. The risk increases even further for patients undergoing a cesarean section delivery and extends into the postpartum period for up to 12 weeks.

Presentation and Diagnosis

Patients with PE may present with tachypnea, tachycardia, chest pain, and dyspnea. Massive PE may be associated with syncope and hypotension, or cardiac arrest. An ECG may show sinus tachycardia or signs of right heart strain ($S_I Q_{III} T_{III}$, pattern, T-wave inversions in the right precordial leads, and right bundle branch block patterns).

As in nonpregnant patients, diagnosing PE in pregnancy may include using a D-dimer and pretest probability calculations with established clinical decision rules. Data support the use of D-dimer in a low suspicion group but at a higher cutoff. A study published in 2022 demonstrates that the application of YEARS criteria successfully excluded PE. For YEARS, the three criteria include clinical signs of DVT, hemoptysis, and PE as the most likely diagnosis. If 0 YEARS criteria plus a D-dimer less than 1,000 ng/mL, then PE can be excluded. In patients with greater than 1 YEARS criteria, a D-dimer less than the age-adjusted threshold suffices to rule out PE. Another 2022 study further supports the YEARS criteria in pregnancy and also found that the Wells and modified Geneva criteria have 100% sensitivity and negative predictive value when applied to pregnant women. If the D-dimer is positive, or if PE is highly suspected on clinical gestalt or using the Wells or modified Geneva criteria, proceed straight to imaging.

Ultrasound, $\dot{V}/\dot{Q}$ scanning, and helical pulmonary CTA all may play a role in diagnosing PE. CTA and $\dot{V}/\dot{Q}$ are both acceptable studies as both have low radiation risk to the fetus. $\dot{V}/\dot{Q}$ is most useful in patients with normal chest x-rays; results in patients with abnormal chest x-rays may be nondiagnostic. CTA may be easier to obtain around the clock and faster to complete. Some authors recommend starting with ultrasound of the lower extremities, particularly in patients presenting with symptoms of lower extremity DVT. However, compression ultrasonography may miss pelvic DVT. If ultrasound is negative in a patient with high suspicion for PE, the patient should still undergo CTA or $\dot{V}/\dot{Q}$.

Treatment

PE in pregnancy is treated with LMWH or unfractionated heparin dosed based upon the patient's pre-/early pregnancy weight. Warfarin is contraindicated in pregnancy as it crosses the placenta and has teratogenic effects. DOACs have limited evidence to support their use in pregnancy. If signs of cardiovascular collapse, thrombolysis should be considered either via mechanical or using thrombolytic agents. IVC filters have a role in the management of recurrent DVT/PE despite anticoagulation or in patients who cannot use heparin products.

PEARLS

- Dyspnea in pregnancy occurs frequently ranging from benign physiologic changes to life-threatening conditions.
- In physiologic dyspnea in pregnancy, vital signs should remain within normal limits.
- Venous thrombosis risk is 4- to 5-fold higher in pregnancy and postpartum.
- There is a role for D-dimer in the evaluation of PE in pregnancy.
- Treatment for PE is with unfractionated heparin or LMWH.

Suggested Readings

Eddy M, Robert-Ebadi H, Richardson L, et al. External validation of the YEARS diagnostic algorithm for suspected pulmonary embolism. *J Thromb Haemost.* 2020;18(12):3289-3295. PMID: 32869501.

LoMauro A, Aliverti A. Respiratory physiology of pregnancy: physiology masterclass. *Breathe (Sheff).* 2015;11(4):297-301.

Potgieter R, Becker P, Suleman F. The effectiveness of the pregnancy adapted YEARS algorithm to safely identify patients for CT pulmonary angiogram in pregnant and puerperal patients suspected of having pulmonary embolism. *SA J Radiol.* 2022;26(1):2454.

Sadeghi S, Bahrami P, Kimiyaee Far S, Arabi Z. Determining the diagnostic value of three clinical criteria Wells', YEARS and modified Geneva in pregnant women with suspected pulmonary thromboembolism. *Am J Cardiovasc Dis.* 2022;12(4):240-246.

193

Peripartum Cardiomyopathy Pearls

Glennette Castillo and Diana Ladkany

A patient presents to your ED with complaints of mild chest discomfort, difficulty breathing, and leg swelling. The patient is 38 weeks' pregnant and had been doing well until recently. These symptoms have progressively worsened, and now the patient is struggling to walk due to worsening leg swelling and shortness of breath while walking or laying down flat. On physical examination, you note significant pitting edema and fine inspiratory crackles on auscultation.

What Do You Do Next?

The differential diagnosis for peripartum chest pain, dyspnea, and peripheral edema is broad but must include new-onset heart failure as early recognition and appropriate management can improve outcomes and prevent maternal morbidity and mortality. PPCM has been defined as a new diagnosis of cardiomyopathy during pregnancy or postpartum in patients with no previously diagnosed heart conditions. Pertinent findings on physical examination include respiratory distress and signs of volume overload within the last month of pregnancy and up to 5 months postpartum.

PPCM is a diagnosis of exclusion and requires the criteria of LVEF of less than 45% on echocardiogram, with or without associated ventricular dilation, and no other cause of cardiomyopathy. Therefore, ED evaluation hinges on the assessment of LV function on echocardiogram, as well as additional diagnostic tests such as labs to rule out other causes of dyspnea in the peripartum period (**Table 193.1**). Imaging studies include chest x-ray or point-of-care ultrasound to evaluate for pulmonary venous congestion and ECG for evidence of peri/myocarditis or ACS. Given a similar presentation of PPCM to pulmonary embolism, imaging such as pulmonary CTA or V̇/Q̇ scan may be indicated.

Management starts with supporting the ABCs. PPCM can present on a spectrum from minimally symptomatic to severe respiratory distress or fulminate cardiogenic

| TABLE 193.1 | \multicolumn{5}{c}{LAB AND DIAGNOSTIC COMPARISON OF PPCM TO OTHER PERIPARTUM DISORDERS} |

	PPCM	PREECLAMPSIA/ HELLP*	PULMONARY EMBOLISM	ACS	THYROID STORM
CBC	Normal	Anemia* Thrombocytopenia*	Normal	Normal	Normal
TSH/T$_4$/T$_3$	Normal	Normal	Normal	Normal	Low TSH Elevated T$_4$/T$_3$
Pro-BNP	Elevated	Normal	+/− Elevated	+/− Elevated	+/− Elevated
Troponin	Elevated	Normal	+/− Elevated	Elevated	Normal
Liver function tests	Normal	Elevated*	Normal	Normal	Normal
LDH	Normal	Elevated	Normal	Normal	Normal
Uric acid	Normal	Elevated	Normal	Normal	Normal
Fibrinogen	Normal	Normal	Normal	Normal	Normal
Urinalysis	Normal	Proteinuria >0.3 g/d	Normal	Normal	Normal
Urine protein/creatine ratio	Normal	>0.3 mg/mg	Normal	Normal	Normal
ECG	Normal, sinus tachycardia	Normal	Sinus tachycardia, right-axis deviation	ST-segment changes	Sinus tachycardia
Echo	Systolic dysfunction with or without dilated LV	Diastolic dysfunction	Right heart strain, RV dilated	Wall motion abnormalities	+/− Dilated cardiomyopathy, systolic dysfunction

ACS, acute chest syndrome; CBC, complete blood count; ECG, electrocardiogram; LDH, lactate dehydrogenase; LV, left ventricle; PPCM, peripartum cardiomyopathy; pro-BNP, pro-brain natriuretic peptide; RV, right ventricle; TSH, thyroid-stimulating hormone.

shock. Patients may need oxygen support including NPPV, which will help assist with preload reduction. In severe cases, patients may require endotracheal intubation. Antihypertensives such as hydralazine or nitroglycerin in patients not in cardiogenic shock will assist with afterload reduction. Both are considered safe during pregnancy. There are current recommendations against using nitroprusside during pregnancy due to the risk of cyanide toxicity to the fetus.

Patients presenting with hypotension and signs of poor perfusion, such as altered mental status or cool skin, are likely in cardiogenic shock due to poor cardiac contractility. Inotropic support includes dobutamine or milrinone drips, with a preference toward dobutamine over milrinone if the patient is hypotensive. Norepinephrine may assist in improving blood pressure but used with caution in the antepartum period due to vasoconstricting effects on the placenta and risk of fetal hypoperfusion. Dopamine is an alternative as well. Coordinating with intensivists, cardiologists, maternal fetal medicine specialists, and neonatologists is critical as patients who are clinically deteriorating may require further interventions, such as ECMO or intra-aortic balloon pumps.

For patients with overt signs of volume overload, such as jugular venous distension, peripheral edema, or crackles on respiratory examination, diuresis with hydrochlorothiazide and furosemide are safe to use in pregnancy and lactation in small doses. ACE inhibitors and ARBs are contraindicated in pregnancy due to teratogenic effects on the fetus and are excreted in breastmilk. Admission with telemetry is indicated in all patients who are being evaluated for PPCM as there is a risk of arrhythmias, in particular if there is an EF of less than 30%. Currently, there are no guidelines on implementation of cardioverter defibrillators, but beta-blockers and calcium channel blockers are indicated as rate control agents and for long-term management of heart failure in patients not in acute decompensated heart failure. Beta-1 selective blockers, such as carvedilol, are preferred to nonselective beta-blockers during pregnancy to avoid antitocolytic action through beta-2 receptor pathways. In the postpartum period, metoprolol is preferred during breastfeeding to carvedilol, with caution and infant monitoring. Dihydropyridine calcium channel blockers, such as amlodipine, may be used in postpartum heart failure management but requires caution during pregnancy due to possible uterine hypoperfusion and is not compatible with breastfeeding (**Table 193.2**).

TABLE 193.2 PHARMACOLOGIC MANAGEMENT OF PPCM

MEDICATION	DURING PREGNANCY	DURING BREASTFEEDING	STARTING DOSE
Antihypertensives			
Hydralazine	C	Ok to breastfeed	10 mg TID
Nitroglycerin drip	C	Unknown	5-200 mcg/min
Nitroprusside drip	X	Unknown	0.1-5 mcg/min
Inotropes/vasopressor continuous drips			
Dobutamine	B	Unknown	2-10 mcg/kg/min
Milrinone	C	Unknown	0.125 mcg/kg/min
Norepinephrine	C	Unknown	2-10 mcg/min
Dopamine	C	Unknown	1-20 mcg/kg/min
Epinephrine	C	Unknown	0.01-0.5 mcg/kg/min

(continued)

TABLE 193.2	PHARMACOLOGIC MANAGEMENT OF PPCM (CONTINUED)		
Diuretics			
Hydrochlorothiazide	B	Ok to breastfeed	12.5 mg daily
Furosemide	C	Ok to breastfeed	20 mg daily
Other cardiac medicines			
Digoxin	C	Ok to breastfeed	0.5 mg load once
ACE inhibitors and ARBs			
Captopril	D	Ok to breastfeed	6.25 mg TID
Enalapril	D	Stop breastfeeding	1.25 mg BID
Lisinopril	D	Stop breastfeeding	2.5 mg daily
Candesartan	D	Stop breastfeeding	2 mg daily
Valsartan	D	Stop breastfeeding	40 mg BID
Spironolactone	D	Ok to breastfeed	12.5 mg daily
Beta-blockers and calcium channel blockers			
Carvedilol	C	Caution	3.125 mg BID
Metoprolol	C	Ok to breastfeed	0.125 mg daily
Amlodipine	C	Stop breastfeeding	5 mg daily

Class B = Animal reproduction studies failed to show risk to the fetus, or adequate and well-controlled studies in pregnant patients failed to demonstrate a risk to the fetus in any trimester.

Class C = Animal reproduction studies show an adverse effect to the fetus, and there are no adequate and well-controlled human studies, but potential benefits may warrant the use of the drug in pregnant patients despite risks.

Class D = Positive evidence of human fetal risk has been shown, but potential benefits may warrant the use other drug in pregnant patients despite risks.

Class X = Studies in animals or humans have shown fetal abnormalities and positive evidence of human fetal risk, risks involved in use of the drug in pregnant patients outweigh potential benefits.

ACE, angiotensin-converting enzyme; ARBs, angiotensin receptor blockers; BID, twice daily; TID, three times daily.

The majority of patients (50%-70%) will achieve full recovery of their heart function within 3 to 6 months postpartum, though studies have shown it may take up to 48 months. Patients are closely followed by cardiologists, and if there are concerns for recovery, they undergo evaluation for an LV assist device or heart transplants. Patients should be counseled at high risk of recurrence of PPCM in subsequent pregnancies.

PEARLS

- PPCM is a diagnosis of exclusion.
- Criteria include LVEF less than 45% without other etiologies within the last month of pregnancy up to 5 months postpartum and no prior cardiac history.

- The initial resuscitative measures will focus on respiratory and cardiac support.
- Evaluation includes ruling out other conditions, such as pulmonary embolism, HELLP, and preeclampsia with severe features.
- Diagnosis and management will require a multidisciplinary approach with the cardiology and obstetrics/maternal fetal medicine teams, as well as possibly intensivists and neonatologists.

SUGGESTED READINGS

Azibani F, Sliwa K. Peripartum cardiomyopathy: an update. *Curr Heart Fail Rep*. 2018;15(5): 297-306. PMID: 30051292.

Davis MB, Arany Z, McNamara DM, Goland S, Elkayam U. Peripartum cardiomyopathy: JACC state-of-the-art review. *J Am Coll Cardiol*. 2020;75(2):207-221. PMID: 31948651.

194

KNOW THESE POSTABORTION COMPLICATIONS

MARIA MAGDALENA LAWRYNOWICZ AND JEFFREY URIBE

Induced abortions performed under the supervision of a physician are safe outpatient procedures. In the United States in 2020, there were approximately 11.2 abortions per 1,000 women aged 15 to 44 years, with major complications rates between 0.11% and 0.16% and mortality rates of 0.62 per 100,000 in the United States. The majority were medical abortions (51.0%) performed 9 or less weeks of gestation, followed by surgical abortions (40.0%) at 13 or less weeks of gestation.

Medication-assisted abortions in the United States are primarily performed before 11 weeks of gestation with an initial dose of mifepristone 200 mg, a synthetic progesterone antagonist that disrupts pregnancy growth, followed by self-administration of misoprostol 800 mcg sublingually or vaginally, a synthetic prostaglandin analogue that induces myometrial contraction 24 to 48 hours later.

Vaginal bleeding begins 1 to 4 hours after misoprostol administration, with fetal tissue passage occurring in 3 to 8 hours. Median duration of bleeding most patients experience is 11 to 13 days. While bleeding is heavier with medication-assisted abortions, the need for blood transfusion is exceedingly rare (<0.1%). Additional side effects including cramping, low-grade fevers, flushing, and gastrointestinal symptoms occur and are usually self-limited.

Surgical abortions are considered more effective for pregnancy termination; however, they are more invasive and pose different risks depending on timing of the procedure.

First-trimester uterine aspiration involves cervical dilation, insertion of a cannula into the uterine cavity, and vacuum aspiration of fetal tissue. Patients may be treated with misoprostol, a cervical ripening agent, before the procedure. Second-trimester D&E is a short procedure (<30 minutes) with procedural sedation or general anesthesia. This involves preparation of the cervix with osmotic dilators, medications, or mechanical dilation, followed by uterine evacuation using aspiration, extraction with forceps, or curettage.

With the increase in abortion restrictions, physicians may encounter more patients with self-managed abortions.

OVERALL EVALUATION

When evaluating postabortion complications, obtain gestational history, estimated gestational age at the time of abortion, details of the procedure (date, medical vs surgical, medications used, and complications), current symptoms, and comorbidities. If available, contact the facility that performed the abortion for pertinent details.

Workup includes laboratories (CBC, CMP, type/screen, coagulation factors, hCG level), pelvic examination, and initial point-of-care ultrasound to assess for intrauterine pregnancy or free fluid. Advanced radiologic ultrasound may be required to assess for more complex findings.

On speculum examination, bleeding from small lacerations may resolve with direct pressure or silver nitrate. Extensive lacerations often require absorbable sutures and GYN consultation. Ultrasound helps determine whether RPOC, uterine blood, or hematoma is present. It may also show free fluid or air in the pelvis from uterine perforation. **RPOC or hematometra** will necessitate vacuum aspiration or D&E. In resource-limited settings, manual vacuum aspiration in the ED may be necessary with bleeding unresponsive to medications.

If there is ongoing hemorrhage, and speculum examination and ultrasound are unrevealing, consider **uterine atony** management. Perform bimanual massage, administer uterotonic agents, and consider early IV TXA, blood products, or activation of massive transfusion protocols. If not effective, intrauterine tamponade may be placed under ultrasound guidance using Bakri balloon, Sengstaken-Blakemore tube, or a latex condom secured to a Foley catheter and inflated to approximately 250 to 300 mL of water. If heavy bleeding continues and is refractory to all therapies, or in cases of abnormal placentation or uterine artery pseudoaneurysm, **uterine artery embolization** may be required in consultation with interventional radiology. If diagnosis is unclear or in cases of heterotopic pregnancy, surgical management including laparotomy or laparoscopy is required. Definitive treatment is emergency hysterectomy.

Ectopic pregnancies present in less than 1% of patients presenting for abortion and are most likely to occur in a pregnancy of unknown location (ie, no yolk sac or fetal pole present on ultrasound), again highlighting the importance of gestational history.

Ultrasound should be sufficient to visualize any complicated **uterine perforation**; however, in cases of equivocal imaging, CT or MRI is necessary. Such patients often require operative management with gynecology and general surgery.

Cervical dilators placed before D&E may cause bleeding, rupture of membranes, preterm labor, or allergic reaction. Although rare, if found, such retained surgical bodies require removal.

Infection may be due to RPOC or instrumentation, and sanguinopurulent vaginal discharge is often seen on pelvic examination. In addition to sepsis labs, obtain cervical cultures and start broad-spectrum antibiotics. Infections with group A *Streptococcus* and *Clostridium* species can result in rapid deterioration and lead to **toxic shock syndrome**. Most patients are afebrile with massive, rapidly increasing leukocytosis, usually greater than 100,000 cell/mcL. Ultrasound may demonstrate hydrosalpinges or adnexal mass to suggest a pelvic abscess. CT can be obtained if intra-abdominal mass is suspected or another condition/complication.

Consider the diagnosis of AFE in afebrile patients with sudden cardiopulmonary collapse and DIC with symptoms developing during labor or delivery of products of conception. Immediate evacuation of RPOC and aggressive resuscitation is key. Consider venoarterial ECMO in severe cases.

SELF-MANAGED ABORTIONS

Complications from self-managed abortions can be difficult to predict. Oral medications obtained online may contain unregulated substances. **Misoprostol toxicity**, typically in the 3 to 8 mg range, results in severe fever, rigors, abdominal cramping, vomiting, diarrhea, agitation, altered mental status, hypotension, hypoxemia, and rhabdomyolysis. Treatment is supportive and can include gastric lavage. Ingestions greater than 12 mg may result in multiorgan failure and death. Instrumentation increases the risk of infection, and procedures using vaginal douches/preparations can cause trauma to the pelvic or abdominal organs. Patients may also attempt self-inflicted blows/falls, causing trauma to the abdominal organs or uterine rupture.

PEARLS

- Involve obstetrical colleagues early, especially if the patient will require transfer.
- Be prepared for the patient with heavy vaginal bleeding (medications, blood products, and tamponade).
- Consider AFE in patients with sudden and refractory circulatory collapse or DIC.
- Treat potential septic abortions aggressively and watch for toxic shock syndrome.
- Be aware of self-induced abortion as patients may not disclose this information.

SUGGESTED READINGS

Bridwell RE, Long B, Montrief T, Gottlieb M. Post-abortion complications: a narrative review for emergency clinicians. *West J Emerg Med*. 2022;23(6):919-925. PMID: 36409940.

Cleland K, Creinin MD, Nucatola D, Nshom M, Trussell J. Significant adverse events and outcomes after medical abortion. *Obstet Gynecol*. 2013;121(1):166-171. PMID: 23262942.

Orlowski MH, Soares WE, Kerrigan KA, Zerden ML. Management of postabortion complications for the emergency medicine clinician. *Ann Emerg Med*. 2021;77(2):221-232. PMID: 33341294.

195

EVALUATING THE PREGNANT PATIENT AFTER A MOTOR VEHICLE CRASH

KAYTLIN E. HACK AND JENNIFER YU

MVCs are the most commonly encountered form of unintentional trauma in pregnancy. One population-based cohort study in 2008 in Sweden found that MVCs occur in approximately 207 out of 100,000 pregnancies. MVCs account for approximately 49% of all traumatic injuries sustained during pregnancy and are one of the leading causes of both maternal and fetal mortality.

ED EVALUATION

The evaluation in the ED for a pregnant patient who has been involved in an MVC should follow the ATLS algorithm. Optimal resuscitation of the mother will also improve outcomes for the fetus; thus, maternal stabilization takes priority. A primary survey of the mother to assess airway, breathing, circulation, disability, and exposure should be followed by assessment of the fetus using ultrasonography, followed by a secondary survey of the mother for additional injuries.

AIRWAY AND BREATHING

The hormonal changes in pregnancy stimulate the respiratory center by increasing minute ventilation and oxygen consumption (manifested as dyspnea) and hyperemia and edema of the upper airway mucosa. The gravid uterus also causes diaphragm elevation and decreased total lung capacity. Intubation of the pregnant patient may be challenging, as they are more prone to desaturation and a difficult airway. If a thoracostomy tube is required, consider placing it in one or two intercostal spaces above the usual landmarks.

CIRCULATION

The physiologic changes in pregnancy resulting in an increased circulating blood volume and baseline mild tachycardia may make the detection of shock more challenging. A pregnant patient is able to lose a significant amount of blood before tachycardia, hypotension, and other signs of hypovolemia occur. IV access should be established using two large-bore IVs. Positioning of the patient by manual displacement of the gravid uterus to the left helps to reduce compression of the IVC and improve venous return. Spinal motion restriction can be maintained by logrolling the patient to the left lateral decubitus position and providing support using a wedge or blanket rolls. Any pregnant patient with massive uncontrolled bleeding from the perineum should prompt emergent consultation with obstetrics and the trauma surgery teams to assist with resuscitation and management of possible placental abruption or uterine rupture and associated hypovolemic shock. However, placental abruption can result in occult bleeding in up to approximately one-third of cases.

DISABILITY AND FETAL CONSIDERATIONS

The fetus may be in distress from placental hypoperfusion, while the mother's vital signs appear "stable." Prompt assessment of the fetus using ultrasonography is critical.

In gravid patients with fetuses greater than 20 to 24 weeks of gestational age, utilize point-of-care ultrasonography to perform a FAST as well as to confirm the presence of fetal heart activity and the orientation of the fetus.

SECONDARY SURVEY

The secondary survey should pay special attention to the abdominal region searching for uterine contractions, which suggest early labor, and uterine tetany, which is concerning for placental abruption. In addition, a pelvic examination to assess for the presence of amniotic fluid (using pH or nitrazine paper) in the vagina, which suggests rupture of membranes, as well as the condition of the cervix (presence of effacement or dilation), and fetal presentation is essential.

ADDITIONAL CONSIDERATIONS

Radiologic exposure using CT is a concern of many pregnant patients. It is important to note that there is unlikely any fetal harm after 15 weeks of gestation and that the dose of exposure of a single abdominopelvic CT is approximately half the lowest reported cumulative dose that is associated with fetal loss or anomalies. In the stable patient, alternative imaging modalities such as magnetic resonance and ultrasonography can be utilized to assess for occult injury.

Fetomaternal hemorrhage can occur in up to 30% of pregnant patients with trauma. Obtain a type and screen and administer 300-mcg anti-D immunoglobulin IM to all Rh-negative pregnant patients within 72 hours after trauma.

Any pregnant patient who has sustained a significant injury after an MVC or is experiencing symptoms such as vaginal bleeding, uterine irritability, abdominal tenderness, cramping, changes in or absence of fetal heart tones, or leakage of amniotic fluid should be emergently evaluated by obstetrics and admitted for continuous fetal monitoring. Patients who have been in a low-velocity MVC and do not have any pain, cramping, vaginal bleeding, rupture of membranes, uterine contractions, or changes in maternal or fetal vital signs should be monitored for 4 hours with continuous fetal monitoring and tocometry. If no changes occur in this 4-hour period, patients are generally considered at low risk for discharge from the ED or labor and delivery.

PEARLS

- Resuscitation of the mother provides the best outcome for the fetus.
- Place the patient in left lateral decubitus position or manually displace the uterus to the left to avoid IVC compression and improve cardiac output.
- Do not delay critical imaging modalities, including CT scan.
- Obtain a type and screen and give Rh immunoglobulin therapy to Rh-negative patients.
- Bleeding from placental abruption can be occult in up to one-third of cases.

SUGGESTED READINGS

Mendez-Figueroa H, Dahlke JD, Vrees RA, Rouse DJ. Trauma in pregnancy: an updated systematic review. *Am J Obstet Gynecol*. 2013;209(1):1-10.

Trauma in pregnancy and intimate partner violence. In: *ATLS: Advanced Trauma Life Support Student Course Manual*. 10th ed. American College of Surgeons; 2018:279-292.

196

Do You Need to Do a Pelvic Exam in the ED Anymore?

Amanda L. Joy and Alex Y. Koo

Abdominal pain comprises about 7% of annual ED visits. For female patients, it's important for clinicians to differentiate genitourinary and pelvic etiologies from other intra-abdominal etiologies. Traditionally, this has included performing a pelvic exam; however, as diagnostic tests and imaging have improved, the utility of the pelvic exam has been questioned. The most common reasons for performing a pelvic exam in the ED are to assess for adnexal and cervical motion tenderness, followed by checking for adnexal masses, vaginal discharge, and bleeding.

Patient Considerations

The pelvic exam can be invasive, uncomfortable, and logistically challenging. In several studies, pelvic exams were found to be painful, discomforting, anxiety provoking, and/or embarrassing for patients, especially those who had reported a history of sexual violence and post-traumatic stress disorder. Linden et al found that pregnant patients presenting to the ED with abdominal pain or vaginal bleeding randomized to pelvic exam or no pelvic exam had similar perceptions of the thoroughness of their ED care; however, patients who received a pelvic exam were more likely to report feeling "uncomfortable" or "very uncomfortable." Not only is patient discomfort a consideration, but the logistical needs of staff, chaperone, equipment, and private room procurement can also make setting up for a pelvic exam labor intensive and time-consuming.

Accuracy and Interexaminer Reliability

The pelvic exam is taught as necessary to gain valuable clinical information, but how accurate is the information obtained from the exam? One study found that attending gynecologist performing bimanual exams on anesthetized patients—ideal circumstances for accuracy—were correct in assessing the uterus and adnexa in only 70% of cases. For emergent conditions such as ectopic pregnancy, there is no combination of exam findings that can confirm or exclude this diagnosis with a high degree of reliability, and the ACEP Clinical Policy recommends obtaining a pelvic ultrasound on all symptomatic patients with concern for ectopic pregnancy. With respect to ovarian torsion, a 15-year review of 87 patients diagnosed with torsion found that 29% of patients had no tenderness on pelvic exam and that an adnexal mass was palpable in only 47% of patients, suggesting that a pelvic exam alone is not sufficient to confirm the diagnosis. A 2011 study by Brown et al studied 183 female (pregnant and nonpregnant) patients presenting to the ED with abdominal pain and/or vaginal bleeding. This prospective trial found that the pelvic exam changed clinical management in only 6% of cases.

Interexaminer reliability of bimanual pelvic exams performed by emergency physicians appears to be poor. One study found that when pelvic exams were performed by both an ED attending and a senior ED resident on the same patient, the two physicians agreed on the presence of an abnormal finding only 17% to 33% of the time. With the increasing accessibility and superior sensitivity that imaging modalities, including ultrasound, computed tomography, and magnetic resonance imaging, have compared to physical exam, it can be argued the pelvic exam may not add significant diagnostic value and with detrimental to the patient.

Pelvic Exams for STI Testing

Another common reason for performing an ED pelvic exam is to collect endocervical samples for STI testing. For both gonorrhea and chlamydia, vulvovaginal self-swabs for PCR testing are equivalent to endocervical swabs in patients with and without symptoms suggestive of STIs. These data suggest patients requesting STI screening or with vaginal discharge with the absence of abdominal pain do not warrant a pelvic exam.

When Are ED Pelvic Exams Warranted?

ED pelvic exams are warranted in certain situations. Any hemodynamic instability and active vaginal bleeding warrant a pelvic exam to determine a source of bleeding and possible source control. Survivors of sexual assault with vaginal or anal penetration should be offered a pelvic exam by a trained SAFE for evidence collection, legal documentation, and trauma—10% of sexual assault survivors will have genital trauma. Patients requiring removal of a vaginal foreign body will need a pelvic exam. Children, in particular, ages 3 to 10, are at risk for missed retained vaginal foreign bodies. In addition, up to 10% of children with persistent vaginal discharge had a retained vaginal foreign body.

Pregnant patients presenting in active labor or possible labor require a sterile speculum exam to determine whether membranes have ruptured or if delivery is imminent.

The diagnosis of PID technically requires a bimanual exam to assess for one of the three minimum clinical criteria: cervical motion tenderness, uterine tenderness, or adnexal tenderness. However, studies suggest poor inter-rater reliability, and it is reasonable to begin empiric treatment for PID without a pelvic exam.

Finally, deferring a pelvic exam may lead to missed cervical or vaginal lesions, fistulas, and cysts.

When deciding whether or not to perform a pelvic exam, it is important to account for the patient's severity of symptoms, their wishes, and the ability for follow-up for a timely outpatient evaluation. It is reasonable to offer a pelvic exam and engage in shared decision-making with the patient, recognizing the benefits and limitations of the pelvic exam.

PEARLS

- Pelvic exams are uncomfortable for a proportion of patients.
- The pelvic exam is inaccurate, and imaging should be obtained if there is concern for emergent conditions, such as ectopic pregnancy, ovarian torsion, tubo-ovarian abscess, and threatened abortion.
- Vulvovaginal self-swabs for testing for STIs are sufficient—pelvic exam is not needed for collection.
- While technical criteria for diagnosis of PID require a pelvic exam, empiric treatment for PID without a pelvic exam is reasonable.
- Pelvic exam should be performed in patients following sexual assault, with retained foreign bodies or life-threatening vaginal bleeding, and to rule out labor or rupture of membranes.

Suggested Readings

Brown J, Fleming R, Aristzabel J, et al. Does pelvic exam in the emergency department add useful information? *West J Emerg Med*. 2011;12(2):208-212. PMID: 21691528.

Linden JA, Grimmnitz B, Hagopian L, et al. Is the pelvic examination still crucial in patients presenting to the emergency department with vaginal bleeding or abdominal pain when an intrauterine pregnancy is identified on ultrasonography? A randomized controlled trial. *Ann Emerg Med*. 2017;70(6):825-834. PMID: 28935285.

Lunny C, Taylor D, Hoang L, et al. Self-collected versus clinician-collected sampling for chlamydia and gonorrhea screening: a systemic review and meta-analysis. *PLoS One*. 2015;10(7):e0132776. PMID: 26168051.

Weitlauf JC, Frayne SM, Finney JW, et al. Sexual violence, posttraumatic stress disorder, and the pelvic examination: how do beliefs about the safety, necessity, and utility of the examination influence patient experiences? *J Womens Health (Larchmt)*. 2010;19(7):1271-1280. PMID: 20509787.

197

Caring for the Sexual Assault Survivor

Deanna Bridge Najera and Maryann Mazer-Amirshahi

Sexual assault remains a common occurrence, with a broad spectrum of presentations. While stabilization of injuries and prevention of pregnancy and STIs take priority, any individual who presents to the ED reporting sexual trauma should be considered a person with potential legal involvement, which requires specific documentation and psychosocial considerations.

Prioritize Stabilization and Evaluation

The initial approach to the sexual assault patient is the same as any ED interaction: Evaluate and stabilize any emergent medical conditions and traumatic injuries. In addition, for the sexual assault patient, health care members should try to preserve evidence whenever possible. If the patient must undress, place each article of clothing in a separate brown paper bag and leave the bag open to the air. Clinicians should also consider potential human trafficking, which is grossly underestimated, and ensure patient safety while in the ED.

The Sexual Assault Forensic Examination

When available, activate a sexual assault response team as soon as possible. These often include a forensic examiner and, in some cases, a patient advocate. Forensic examinations may be conducted by anyone with the necessary forensic training and may include RNs or any licensed health care provider. Generally, the longest window for forensic DNA specimen collection is 120 hours from the time of the assault; adult patients must be clinically sober and consent to forensic examination collection.

Diagnostic Evaluation

Diagnostic imaging should be performed based on suspected injuries; particular care should be taken to assess for strangulation injuries, and if there is concern, a CT angiography of the neck should be obtained. Laboratory evaluation depends on the need for assessment of associated injuries and nPEP. A complete blood count and complete metabolic panel can be obtained if the patient will be taking nPEP for HIV. In addition, baseline testing of HIV, syphilis, and hepatitis B and C is recommended. Pregnancy determination should be performed in people of childbearing age. If drug-facilitated sexual assault is suspected, toxicology specimens may be obtained by the forensics team, so patients should be encouraged to avoid urinating. Of note, measurement of a blood alcohol concentration and urine toxicology is rarely indicated and should be deferred as there may be disagreement between forensic samples and routine clinical samples.

Avoid Secondary Trauma

It is important to minimize additional trauma during the ED encounter. This could be caused by the use of judgmental language, incorrect use of pronouns or names for sexual- and gender-diverse people, or asking the patient to repeatedly recount the event. Close working relationships with community organizations that are experienced with assisting sexual assault survivors can provide real-time help and follow-up support in addition to training for ED staff.

Know Your Local Laws and Protocols

Emergency clinicians must be cognizant of state and hospital protocols for sexual assault survivors. Significant variability exists between jurisdictions for when forensic evidence collected is considered valid from a legal perspective. In addition, patients may decline a forensics examination or may choose to report anonymously.

Avoid Documentation Pitfalls

When documenting the patient's assault, clinicians must be clear about what the patient says, while avoiding verbiage that may be disparaging. For example, do not say "patient alleges"; instead, describe exactly what the patient reports, even if they are unclear about certain events. This extends to the physical examination, and photographs of injuries are preferred when possible, with patient consent and entered into the medical and forensic record. One must document carefully to avoid creating avenues for disagreement between the clinician chart and other records. Documenting "multiple areas of bruising" is better than incorrectly counting the number of areas with injuries. A body map diagram is an excellent alternative to written descriptors of injuries. It is also acceptable to reference the forensics examination, such as "see SAFE notes for full description of injuries."

Provide the Appropriate Postexposure Prophylaxis

Empiric antimicrobial therapy for the prevention of chlamydia and gonorrhea is recommended for all patients; medication for the prevention of trichomonas is recommended for biologically female patients (**Table 197.1**). For encounters that carry a substantial risk of HIV infection, a 28-day course of nPEP is indicated and should be started within 72 hours of the assault. If the patient has not been vaccinated against hepatitis B and the status of the assailant is unknown, the hepatitis B vaccine series can be initiated. Patients can also be referred for vaccination against human papillomavirus if they have not been previously vaccinated. For encounters that may result in pregnancy, emergency contraception is indicated with considerations based on the patient's BMI and time since the encounter (**Table 197.2**). The initial dose of all medications should be administered in the ED, and barriers to obtaining postexposure prophylaxis should be addressed before discharge, including any state or hospital requirement for dispensing the extended treatment regimens.

TABLE 197.1	Postexposure prophylaxis for sexually transmitted infections
Medication	**Comments**
Ceftriaxone 500 mg intramuscularly × 1 dose	Administer 1 g in patients >150 kg
Doxycycline 100 mg PO twice daily × 7 d	Avoid in pregnant patients, instead provide azithromycin 1 g PO once
Metronidazole 500 mg PO twice daily × 7 d	Not necessary in cis-male patients

Information from https://www.cdc.gov/std/treatment-guidelines/sexual-assault.htm
PO, orally.

TABLE 197.2	Emergency contraception		
Product	**Ulipristal**	**Levonorgestrel**	**Copper IUD**
Dose	30 mg PO × 1 dose	1.5 mg PO × 1 dose	Not applicable
Time to dose (after intercourse)	Sustained efficacy up to 120 h	Efficacy decreases over time; administer within 72 h	Sustained efficacy for up to 120 h
Availability	Prescription	Over the counter	Requires provider insertion
Weight considerations	Effective for BMI >25	Decreased efficacy BMI >25	Effective regardless of BMI

BMI, body mass index; IUD, intrauterine device; PO, orally.

Discharge Instructions

Connecting the patient with community resources at the time of discharge is another important aspect of healing. These resources may include a local rape crisis center, state attorney's victim advocacy center, or local health department. It is of particular importance that the survivor understands the need for repeat testing for STIs and HIV at 6 weeks and 3 months after the incident.

PEARLS

- Activate a sexual assault response team as soon as possible.
- Stabilize the patient and assess for any traumatic injuries or emergent medical conditions before proceeding with a forensic examination.
- Avoid language and practices that may further traumatize the patient.
- Use ulipristal or a copper IUD for patients with a BMI greater than 25 and those who present between 72 and 120 hours after the assault that requires emergency contraception.
- Engage support services during the initial evaluation and for ongoing psychosocial support and provide instructions for follow-up testing.

Suggested Readings

American College of Emergency Physicians Evaluation and management of the sexually assaulted or sexually abused patient. 2013. https://www.acep.org/globalassets/new-pdfs/sexual-assault-e-book.pdf

Centers for Disease Control and Prevention. Sexual assault and abuse and STIs—adolescents and adults. 2021. https://www.cdc.gov/std/treatment-guidelines/sexual-assault.htm

National Clinician Consultation Center. PEP: Post-Exposure Prophylaxis. https://nccc.ucsf.edu/clinician-consultation/pep-post-exposure-prophylaxis/

US Department of Justice. National best practices for sexual assault kits: a multidisciplinary approach. 2017. https://www.ojp.gov/pdffiles1/nij/250384.pdf

Additional Resources

National Human Trafficking Hotline 888-3737-888
National Sexual Violence Resource Center https://www.nsvrc.org/
Rape Abuse Incent National Network (RAINN.org) 800-656-4673
Sexual assault and the LGBT community https://www.hrc.org/resources/sexual-assault-and-the-lgbt-community

198

Hyperemesis Gravidarum

Lindsey DeGeorge and Kelly Lew

HG is defined as severe intractable nausea and vomiting that results in clinical signs of dehydration or weight loss. While nausea and vomiting affect about 70% of pregnancies, HG is estimated to occur in only 0.3% to 3% of pregnancies.

The pathogenesis of HG has not been fully elucidated and is thought to be multifactorial. Elevated levels of estrogen and progesterone may play a role as they act by relaxing smooth muscle in the GI tract, slowing GI motility. hCG has also been suggested to contribute, given that the timing of peak hCG levels coincides with peak symptoms of nausea and vomiting. Risk factors for HG include multiple gestations, hydatidiform molar pregnancy, family history of HG, personal history of HG, and a history of acid reflux. Complications include maternal Wernicke encephalopathy, acute tubular necrosis, Mallory-Weiss tear, and low birth weight in the fetus.

Initial ED Evaluation

In the ED, it is important to promptly diagnose HG, provide symptomatic management, adequately resuscitate, and to consider admission for severe cases. Early vital sign changes include tachycardia, hypotension, and orthostatic hypotension. Patients may have presyncope, postural dizziness, dry mucous membranes, or poor skin turgor.

HG is a clinical diagnosis without definitive diagnostic criteria. The following symptoms are associated with HG: persistent vomiting in the setting of pregnancy, weight loss exceeding 5% of prepregnancy body weight, ketonuria, and inability to tolerate food or maintain adequate hydration.

Labs including a BMP, urinalysis, and liver function tests are frequently obtained in the ED to aid in quantifying disease severity and guide resuscitation. A BMP can identify electrolyte abnormalities, including hypochloremia, hyponatremia, and hypokalemia with a metabolic alkalosis due to the loss of gastric secretions. Acute kidney injury as seen by elevated creatine can occur. Urinalysis may reveal ketones and elevated specific gravity. Liver function tests, lipase, a complete blood count, magnesium, and phosphorus may be helpful to evaluate for other possible etiologies for HG, including infection, diabetes mellitus, gastroenteritis, hepatitis, pancreatitis, or HELLP.

Pelvic ultrasound is recommended if there is no previous imaging to confirm a viable intrauterine pregnancy. This will also assist in a differential diagnosis for HG including multiple gestation as well as trophoblastic disease.

MANAGEMENT

Fluid resuscitation should target euvolemic state through IV administration of dextrose-containing solution, such as D5½ normal saline. Patients may have chronic hyponatremia, and repletion of sodium should be performed slowly in order to prevent central pontine myelinolysis. Electrolytes including magnesium, potassium, calcium, and phosphorus should be repleted as needed. In severe cases of HG, thiamine 100 mg IV should be given before dextrose-containing fluids to avoid Wernicke encephalopathy.

Treatment of HG is primarily administered IV due to the inability to tolerate oral fluids. There are three categories of antiemetics used: dopamine antagonists, H_1 antagonists, and selective serotonin antagonists.

Metoclopramide is a dopamine antagonist that is administered 5 to 10 mg IV every 8 hours. A large meta-analysis of six cohort studies evaluating metoclopramide exposure did not reveal significant congenital anomalies in exposed infants. If maternal side effects such as dystonia and tardive dyskinesia occur, an alternative treatment should be initiated.

Promethazine is a weak dopamine antagonist and an H_1 receptor blocker that can be prescribed PO or as a rectal suppository as 12.5 to 25 mg every 4 hours. Prochlorperazine acts similarly to promethazine and can be given as 5 to 10 mg IV or intramuscularly every 6 hours or rectally twice a day. Antihistamines such as diphenhydramine taken 25 to 50 mg PO every 4 to 6 hours as needed can be used as an adjunct. Main side effects of these agents include sedation and QT prolongation.

Serotonin antagonists such as ondansetron 4 to 8 mg IV every 8 hours have been shown to be as effective as metoclopramide in HG. In the past, ondansetron use during first-trimester pregnancy was controversial due to the risk for congenital anomalies, particularly a concern for cardiac malformations. The largest retrospective cohort study to date looking at this issue published in 2018 concluded that first-trimester ondansetron exposure did not cause increased risk of congenital or cardiac malformation; however, there was a slightly increased risk of fetal oral clefts (absolute risk difference 11.1 vs 14 per 10,000).

Glucocorticoids are considered last-line therapy for refractory symptoms due to contradicting placebo-controlled trials and systematic reviews. The decision to start steroids should be made in conjunction with obstetrics as the use of steroids is associated with an increased risk of fetal oral cleft before 10 weeks of gestation. In addition, glucocorticoids may cause hyperglycemia.

Disposition

All patients discharged from the ED should have close follow-up with obstetrics and be encouraged to make lifestyle and diet modification. Small portions and eating slowly can minimize overdistension of the stomach. Elimination of coffee, spicy, or acidic foods while adding ginger can reduce nausea. For nausea without hypovolemia, pyridoxine (vitamin B_6) can be taken at a recommended dose of 10 to 25 mg PO every 6 to 8 hours. Second line is a doxylamine-pyridoxine combination that can be taken up to 4 times a day. HG with symptomatic control and resolution of ketonuria and electrolyte abnormalities should be prescribed both PO and PR medications similar to agents used in the ED with close obstetric follow-up.

HG with persistent vomiting despite resuscitation and treatment or with persistent ketonuria requires hospitalization. Severe electrolyte abnormalities are indicative of malnutrition and often require admission for further parenteral therapy.

PEARLS

- Prevention of HG with early treatment of nausea/vomiting includes lifestyle and diet modifications as well as pyridoxine course.
- Initial ED evaluation includes BMP, urinalysis, and pelvic ultrasound if no previous imaging has been performed for this pregnancy.
- Recent studies show ondansetron can be safely used in HG during the first trimester.
- Dopamine antagonists such as metoclopramide, H_1 blockers such as promethazine and prochlorperazine, and ondansetron should be used in acute treatment of HG.
- Refractory HG with persistent vomiting, persistent ketonuria, *or* severe electrolyte derangements are indications for admission.

Suggested Readings

Committee on Practice Bulletins-Obstetrics. ACOG practice bulletin no. 189: nausea and vomiting of pregnancy. *Obstet Gynecol*. 2018;131:e15. Reaffirmed 2020.

Matthews A, Haas DM, O'Mantuna DP, Dowswell T. Interventions for nausea and vomiting in early pregnancy. *Cochrane Database Syst Rev*. 2015;(9):CD007575.

199

CRITICAL CONSIDERATIONS IN POSTMENOPAUSAL BLEEDING

SARAH B. DUBBS AND MIMI LU

Postmenopausal bleeding refers to any vaginal bleeding that occurs after a woman has gone through menopause, defined as 12 consecutive months without menstruation. Presentations can range from mild and bothersome to life-threatening hemorrhage. It is essential for emergency clinicians to understand the critical considerations in postmenopausal bleeding and recognize common errors to avoid to optimize patient outcomes.

STABILIZATION

Though rare, vaginal bleeding in a postmenopausal patient can be severe and present as hemorrhagic shock. Patients who are unstable should be resuscitated with blood products. A critical action in this patient population, who are older and have more comorbidities, is to administer anticoagulant reversal agents if applicable. Early source identification and control should be pursued through examination and, if possible, imaging. Consultation with OB/GYN and possibly IR should also be initiated emergently for patients who are unstable. Options for early temporizing interventions include vaginal packing or tamponade device such as a Foley catheter balloon. REBOA has also been employed as a temporizing measure for obstetric and gynecologic hemorrhage for postpartum hemorrhage and uterine rupture. It is limited to patients at a REBOA-capable center and for those below 70 years of age (relative contraindication). Progestins and tranexamic acid may be considered as pharmacologic adjuncts to help reverse uterine bleeding. Patients in hemorrhagic shock from uterine or vaginal bleeding are likely to require definitive bleeding control in the operating theater with OB/GYN or interventional suite with IR.

CRITICAL CONSIDERATIONS FOR STABLE PATIENTS

Most patients with postpartum bleeding are stable, but there are critical steps that must not be missed in their management. The foremost concern in all of these patients should be endometrial cancer, consistent with the adage "post-menopausal bleeding is endometrial cancer until proven otherwise." Among women presenting to the ED with postmenopausal bleeding, 10% are ultimately diagnosed with endometrial cancer. The remaining differential diagnosis list includes vaginal laceration or other trauma, STIs, benign masses, pseudoaneurysm, other malignancies, and endometrial atrophy (most common and a diagnosis of exclusion for the ED). When a definitive diagnosis is not identified, the emergency clinician must ensure that the patient understands the need for prompt follow-up with gynecology to investigate the possibility of cancer.

A comprehensive history should be obtained, including details about the onset, duration, frequency, and severity of bleeding. Any associated symptoms such as pelvic pain, weight loss, or vaginal discharge should be noted. In addition, inquire about prior gynecologic history, including previous menstrual patterns, pregnancies, and hormonal therapies. Asking about a family history of malignancies of breast or gynecologic origins may offer additional insight. A hematologic ROS should also be obtained to identify other symptoms of a more general bleeding disorder. The clinician should inquire about epistaxis, gum bleeding, hemoptysis, hematuria, hematochezia, melena, bruising, or petechial rash.

An assessment of risk factors is also crucial to guide the evaluation of postmenopausal bleeding. Advanced age, obesity, nulliparity, tamoxifen use, and unopposed estrogen therapy are risk factors associated with endometrial cancer. Other factors such as smoking, diabetes, and hypertension may also increase the risk of endometrial pathology.

In any patient with vaginal bleeding, a pelvic examination is essential to assess for any abnormalities such as vaginal or cervical lesions, uterine enlargement, masses, or cervical motion tenderness. Vaginal or endocervical samples can be obtained during examination for STI testing and vaginal pathogens (NAAT or wet mount). It is important to consider other sources that may be misidentified as vaginal bleeding such as hematuria or gastrointestinal bleeding.

Other laboratory testing should include CBC, TSH, BMP, and basic coagulation tests. An HCG is valuable in patients who are perimenopausal. A blood type and crossmatch should be performed in all patients who are unstable or when transfusion is anticipated by history or examination.

TVUS is the initial imaging modality of choice for evaluating postmenopausal bleeding. It helps visualize the endometrial thickness, presence of polyps or fibroids, and assesses the ovaries for any abnormalities. In cases where TVUS findings are inconclusive or further evaluation is needed, nonemergent MRI may provide additional details, particularly for assessing myometrial invasion in cases suspicious for malignancy.

Endometrial biopsy is the gold standard for diagnosing endometrial pathology, particularly endometrial cancer. It is crucial to obtain tissue samples for histologic examination to confirm or rule out malignancy, but it is also important to note that obtaining the biopsy in the ED is neither expected nor the standard of care. Patients should be advised and referred for timely outpatient evaluation. Delaying referral or inadequate follow-up may result in delays in treatment initiation and compromise patient outcomes.

Conclusion

Postmenopausal bleeding is a concerning symptom that requires a thorough evaluation to identify its underlying cause. Common errors to avoid include attributing bleeding solely to perimenopause, failing to consider a wide differential including generalized bleeding disorder, and inadequate follow-up and referral. By adopting a systematic approach and avoiding these errors, clinicians can ensure timely diagnosis and appropriate management, ultimately improving patient outcomes and quality of care.

PEARLS

- Hemorrhagic shock from vaginal bleeding requires prompt resuscitation with blood products, reversal of anticoagulation if applicable, early OB/GYN ± IR consultation, while temporizing bleeding source with packing or tamponade.
- All postmenopausal bleeding is endometrial cancer until proven otherwise, but a thorough workup with a history and examination, labs, and TVUS is important to narrow the differential.
- Patients with postmenopausal vaginal bleeding should be counseled and referred for timely outpatient evaluation by a gynecologic specialist.

SUGGESTED READINGS

Abbas T, Husain A. Emergency department management of abnormal uterine bleeding in the nonpregnant patient. *Emerg Med Pract*. 2021;23(8):1-20. PMID: 34310092.

Hurtado S, Shetty MK. Post-menopausal bleeding: role of imaging. *Semin Ultrasound CT MR*. 2023;44(6):519-527. PMID: 37832697.

Sung S, Carlson K, Abramovitz A. Postmenopausal bleeding. In *StatPearls* [Internet]. **StatPearls Publishing**; 2024. https://www.ncbi.nlm.nih.gov/books/NBK562188/

200

PITFALLS IN THE CARE OF PATIENTS WHO HAVE HAD IVF

DIANA LADKANY AND HANIA HABEEB

ART includes all fertility treatments in which either eggs or embryos are handled. Use of ART is becoming more common, and emergency clinicians must be familiar with its potential complications. Complications from ART are predominantly due to hormonal ovarian stimulation and egg retrieval. The patient's reproductive specialist should be engaged early in the patient's ED course.

OVARIAN HYPERSTIMULATION SYNDROME

One of the most serious complications is OHSS. OHSS is a complex disease characterized by fluid retention and capillary leakage and can range from mild to life-threatening. Patients undergoing IVF are at the highest risk for OHSS, which most commonly occurs during the ovarian stimulation phase before egg retrieval.

The pathophysiology of OHSS is thought to be related to arteriolar vasodilation and increased capillary permeability, resulting in fluid shifts into the extravascular space or "third spacing." This ultimately leads to a severe state of hypovolemia and hypovolemic hyponatremia often with critical hyperkalemia. It is also associated with the other complications of shock and fluid overload, including renal failure, ascites, pulmonary edema, pericardial and pleural effusions, severe electrolyte abnormalities, hemoconcentration, and hypercoagulability.

Mild OHSS, which does not require any treatment, is associated with abdominal pain/distension, nausea, vomiting, diarrhea, and enlarged ovaries on ultrasound. There are no significant laboratory abnormalities. Moderate OHSS is characterized by evidence of ascites and hemoconcentration, while severe OHSS has more extreme laboratory abnormalities (electrolyte disturbances, renal failure, and liver failure), along with symptoms of dyspnea, severe abdominal pain and nausea and vomiting, anuria, and even altered mental status. Moderate-to-severe OHSS occurs in about 1% to 5% of ovarian stimulation cycles.

Lab work should include a complete blood count to assess for hemoconcentration, a complete metabolic panel to assess renal and liver function as well as electrolytes, and coagulation studies. Emergency imaging should include ultrasound of the enlarged ovaries and the abdominal cavity looking for ascites. Other imaging may be required to rule out thromboembolism, pericardial effusions, pleural effusions or hydrothorax, and neurologic complications such as ischemic stroke due to a hypercoagulable state.

In addition to OHSS, enlarged ovaries with numerous luteal cysts place the patient at higher risk for ovarian torsion; therefore, ultrasound should include Doppler studies to confirm ovarian blood flow. Furthermore, enlarged ovarian follicles are fragile and are at higher risk of rupture, so a pelvic examination may be deferred until gynecology has been consulted.

Procedural Complications of IVF

Complications due to egg retrieval include bleeding, infection, allergic reactions, and anesthetic complications. Ultrasound-guided transvaginal approach has become the gold standard for egg retrieval, reducing the risk of injury to nearby organs compared to laparoscopic or transabdominal routes. Levi-Setti et al reviewed 23,827 oocyte retrievals and found that the overall complication rate was 0.4% per retrieval. Risk factors associated with the occurrence of complications were a high number of oocytes retrieved, long duration of the procedure and mean time per oocyte retrieved, inexperience of the surgeon, younger patients with a low BMI, and a history of prior abdominopelvic surgery or pelvic inflammatory disease.

Minor vaginal bleeding or spotting for 1 to 2 days after egg retrieval is common and generally stops spontaneously. A rare but serious complication is peritoneal bleeding. Ovarian bleeding may result from injury to ovarian vessels or bleeding from ruptured follicles and rarely can lead to severe hemoperitoneum. Additional complications that have been reported include ureterovaginal fistulas, pseudoaneurysm of the iliac artery, perforated appendix, ureteral injury, bladder injury with hematuria, ovarian torsion, and ovarian abscess.

The risk of pelvic infection after egg retrieval or embryo transfer is less common, secondary to the use of prophylactic antibiotic administration. Patients with a history of pelvic infections or endometriosis are at higher risk of developing a pelvic infection following egg retrieval. Clinicians should consider that pelvic abscesses can develop long after the completion of the IVF cycle. Complications related to anesthetic agents may require emergency management, including nausea/vomiting, arrhythmia, hypotension, or agitation.

Pregnancy-Related Risks of IVF

Pregnancy-related risks that may be associated with ART include multifetal pregnancies, prematurity, low birth weight, small for gestational age, perinatal mortality, cesarean delivery, placenta previa, placental abruption, preeclampsia, and birth defects. Although these risks are higher in multifetal pregnancies, the ACOG reports that even singleton pregnancies achieved with ART and ovulation induction may be at higher risk than singletons from naturally occurring pregnancies.

IVF has been associated with increased risk of ectopic and heterotopic pregnancy. The incidence of ectopic pregnancy following ART is 2% to 4%, which is 2 to 3 times greater than the background incidence. The incidence of heterotopic pregnancy is also increased after IVF related to multiple embryo transfer. Clinicians should inquire if a pregnant patient has undergone ART and consider obtaining a formal radiology ultrasound (as opposed to performing their own point-of-care study) if there is concern for ectopic or heterotopic pregnancy.

PEARLS

- OHSS is a potentially life-threatening condition in patients undergoing ART that is characterized by third spacing of fluid.
- Important complications of OHSS include hypovolemia, hyponatremia, hyperkalemia, fluid overload, and thromboembolic events including stroke.
- Enlarged ovaries during the stimulation phase of IVF can result in ovarian torsion or even follicular rupture.
- Hemoperitoneum is a rare but life-threatening complication after egg retrieval.
- IVF has been associated with increased risk of ectopic and heterotopic pregnancy; consider formal radiology ultrasound for these patients.

SUGGESTED READINGS

Binz NM. Complications of gynecologic procedures. In: Tintinalli JE, Ma O, Yealy DM, et al, eds. *Tintinalli's Emergency Medicine: A Comprehensive Study Guide*. 9th ed. McGraw-Hill Education; 2020.

Delvigne, A. Review of clinical course and treatment of ovarian hyperstimulation syndrome (OHSS). *Hum Reprod Update*. 2003;9(1):77-96.

Levi-Setti PE, Cirillo F, Scolaro V, et al. Appraisal of clinical complications after 23,827 oocyte retrievals in a large assisted reproductive technology program. *Fertil Steril*. 2018;109(6):1038-1043.e1. PMID: 29871795.

The American College of Obstetricians and Gynecologists. Perinatal risks associated with assisted reproductive technology. Committee Opinion No. 671, September 2016 (Reaffirmed 2020). https://www.acog.org/-/media/project/acog/acogorg/clinical/files/committee-opinion/articles/2016/09/perinatal-risks-associated-with-assisted-reproductive-technology.pdf

201

HOW DO I EVALUATE A BREAST MASS IN THE EMERGENCY DEPARTMENT?

JANET ANNE SMERECK AND GAVIN K. CLARK

A patient presenting to the ED with a chief complaint of breast mass may harbor one of a number of clinical entities, including infection, neoplasm, or post-traumatic complication. Appropriate ED evaluation is based upon recognition of potential time-sensitive complaints, use of available imaging modalities including POCUS, and urgent referral when indicated for specialized imaging, potential surgical intervention, and tissue sampling.

Infectious Conditions Presenting as Breast Mass

Infectious mastitis is most commonly associated with breastfeeding (lactational or puerperal mastitis) due to ductal stasis and bacterial entry of skin flora into the glandular tissue; most common pathogens are staph and strep, although polymicrobial infection is also reported. Mastitis may occur in up to 10% of breastfeeding patients; it is also seen less commonly in non-lactational states and also in the neonatal period. Neonatal mastitis is uncommon but potentially serious and is complicated by bacteremia in 3% to 4% of cases as well as potential for abscess formation. Treatment of mastitis includes anti-staphylococcal antimicrobial therapy, including amoxicillin-clavulanate or cefalexin. Clindamycin is often prescribed when there is concern for methicillin resistance and for cases of penicillin or cephalosporin allergy; clindamycin may lead to diarrhea in the nursing infant. Trimethoprim-sulfamethoxazole should be avoided if the breastfeeding infant is less than 2 months of age. Vancomycin intravenously is given to patients requiring hospitalization. Breastfeeding or pumping should be continued in the case of lactational mastitis; relief of ductal stasis is important to help prevent abscess formation and the patient should be reassured that the breastfeeding infant is not at risk of acquiring infection from consuming milk from the infected breast.

Mastitis may be complicated by breast abscess formation in 3% to 11% of cases, which can lead to ductal scarring and fistula formation. POCUS is useful for differentiating cellulitis from abscess, distinguished by a distinct, circumscribed fluid collection. Management of breast abscesses in the ED is subject to practice variation; drainage procedures carry risk for complications that stem from the glandular nature of breast tissue, including ductal scarring and fistula formation. Milk fistula is reported to occur in 1.4% of drained lactational breast abscesses. Massive milk fistula is a rare but troublesome complication and both impairs quality of life for the patient and may lead to discontinuation of breastfeeding. Needle aspiration of small superficial abscesses (<2-3 cm) under ultrasound guidance may relieve symptoms and allow for microbial analysis and potential cytology. Depending on institutional practice, this procedure may be performed by an emergency physician or a breast surgeon.

Neoplastic Conditions Presenting Acutely with Breast Mass

A complete discussion of neoplastic disease of the breast is beyond the scope of this chapter as well as beyond the scope of ED evaluation. It is important to note that breast malignancy may mimic other conditions such as infectious and granulomatous mastitis and breast abscess, stressing the importance of imaging in evaluation of breast complaints. An estimated 5% of breast cancer diagnoses were found to be ED mediated in one large study of older women utilizing a Medicare-linked database. Ultrasonography performed in the ED can help identify a solid mass so as to guide therapy and facilitate expedited breast surgery follow-up. Breast T-lymphoblastic lymphoma is a rare condition that has been reported as presenting as a solitary breast mass. Inflammatory breast cancer, the most aggressive form of breast malignancy, may be initially misdiagnosed as mastitis; absence of constitutional symptoms such as fever and lack of response to antibiotic therapy should prompt the emergency physician to facilitate expedited follow-up for mammography and formal radiology-performed breast ultrasonography as well as surgical referral for tissue sampling when malignancy is under consideration.

Post-traumatic Conditions Presenting as Localized Breast Mass

Post-traumatic conditions such as hematoma, fat necrosis, and implant rupture after blunt chest wall trauma may present as a localized, painful breast mass and can be a feature of the "seat belt sign" sometimes observed following a motor vehicle collision. POCUS can be utilized to screen for breast implant rupture but is reported to have low sensitivity, stressing the need for radiology-performed ultrasound to confirm the diagnosis. Mondor's disease, an uncommonly seen thrombophlebitis of a superficial vein in the breast, appears as a subcutaneous cordlike mass and may follow localized trauma or use of a tight-fitting, rigid underwire bra. Sequelae of breast trauma generally resolve within 4 to 6 weeks of injury and persistence of a palpable mass after minimal trauma, in the absence of ecchymosis, should raise suspicion for malignancy.

Benign Inflammatory and Cystic Conditions Presenting as Breast Mass

Idiopathic granulomatous mastitis is a rare, biopsy-identified condition that usually presents as a tender palpable breast mass. Topical steroids have been efficacious in management. Fibrocystic mastalgia is a common cause of breast pain and diffuse thickening of breast tissue which is often cyclic; rarely this can present as a solitary breast mass mimicking malignancy.

PEARLS

- Maintain a broad differential for new-onset breast swelling, tenderness, or erythema, including lactational and non-lactational mastitis, abscess, and inflammatory breast cancer.
- POCUS is a useful tool for evaluation of a breast mass to help distinguish cellulitis from abscess as well as identify a solid neoplasm.
- Lactational mastitis is managed with continued breast milk extraction when feasible (pumping or direct feeding) and antimicrobial agents with activity against staph spp.; amoxicillin-clavulanate or cefalexin are generally given as first-line therapy.
- Percutaneous or surgical drainage of a suspected breast abscess carries potential complications including scarring, fistula formation, and delayed diagnosis of a cavitating malignancy.

Suggested Readings

Acuna J, Pierre C, Sorenson J, Adhikari S. Point of care ultrasound to evaluate breast pathology in the emergency department. *West J Emerg Med.* 2020;22(2):284-290.

Boakes E, Woods A, Johnson N, Kadoglou N. Breast infection: a review of diagnosis and management practices. *Eur J Breast Health.* 2018;14:136-143.

Roberts J, Digiacinto W, Nguyen Q. Pitfalls of breast evaluation in the emergency department. *Cureus.* 2020;12(9):e10612.

Sheridan P, Lyratzopoulous G, Murphy J, Thompson C. Emergency department-mediated cancer diagnosis among older adults in the United States. *J Clin Oncol.* 2019;37(27 suppl):139.

202

ERRORS IN ECTOPIC PREGNANCY EVALUATION AND MANAGEMENT

SUPRIYA J. DAVIS AND KERRI LAYMAN

Ectopic pregnancy is a critical diagnosis in emergency medicine. Though relatively uncommon in the general population (estimated to occur in <1%-2% of all pregnancies), the prevalence of ectopic pregnancy in symptomatic ED patients is as high as 13% in some series. Ruptured ectopic pregnancy is the leading cause of maternal mortality in the first trimester and accounts for 2% to 3% of all pregnancy-related deaths. The presentation of ectopic pregnancy is variable and can be asymptomatic. Most patients will present with abdominal or pelvic pain with or without vaginal bleeding, and some will have hemodynamic collapse. Several factors, highlighted later, can lead to errors in both the evaluation and management of this emergency condition.

DO NOT RELY ON RISK FACTORS

The risk factors classically associated with increased incidence of ectopic pregnancy include a history of prior ectopic pregnancy, prior tubal surgery, IUD in place at the time of pregnancy, cigarette smoking, prior pelvic/abdominal surgery, and prior spontaneous abortion. Additional risk factors include prior sexually transmitted infections and infertility treatments.

Despite these well-known risk factors, nearly half of patients diagnosed with an ectopic pregnancy have no identifiable risk factors. As a result, any patient presenting with a first-trimester pregnancy without a sonographically identified IUP should be evaluated for a potential ectopic pregnancy.

BETA-hCG TRENDS CAN BE DECEIVING

Often, patients in the ED are diagnosed with a PUL when the beta-hCG is positive but no IUP is visualized on pelvic ultrasound. The incidence of PUL has been reported to be anywhere between 5% and 42%. Following this diagnosis, patients are typically instructed to follow up in 48 hours for a repeat beta-hCG level. An increase of 35% over 2 days suggests a possible viable IUP, whereas an increase of less than 35% suggests a nonviable pregnancy, such as a failed pregnancy, spontaneous abortion, or an ectopic pregnancy. However, it is critical to note that an ectopic pregnancy can be present at any beta-hCG level, and a downtrending, stable, or even rising beta-hCG level does not rule out ectopic pregnancy. Beta-hCG levels need to be followed until they fall below the threshold of pregnancy before excluding the possibility of an ectopic pregnancy, and a clinician's judgment with respect to the presentation of the patient must guide the workup.

ULTRASOUND FEATURES OF ECTOPIC PREGNANCY CAN VARY

Pelvic ultrasound is key to the diagnosis of ectopic pregnancy and should be obtained for symptomatic pregnant patients with any beta-hCG level. Features of ectopic pregnancy that can be visualized on ultrasound include an empty uterus, free fluid in the pelvis, suspicious adnexal mass, and, occasionally, an adnexal gestational sac/yolk sac. It is possible, however, that none of these features will be identified and/or one of these features may be misinterpreted, resulting in a diagnosis of PUL. In particular, inability to visualize a yolk sac at a beta-hCG level of greater than 3,500 mIU/mL should raise suspicion for a nonviable pregnancy, and 50% to 70% of cases represent an ectopic pregnancy. Studies suggest that the sensitivity of initial ultrasound for the diagnosis of ectopic pregnancy ranges from 74% to 88%. Failure to identify the aforementioned features should not lead to premature closure of the consideration of ectopic pregnancy.

New Technologies and Treatments

Heterotopic pregnancy, in general, is a rare occurrence, accounting for 1 per 30,000 pregnancies. With the increased utilization of ARTs, the incidence of heterotopic pregnancies is increasing and approaches 1 to 3 per 100 pregnancies when ART has been utilized. Maintain a high index of suspicion for heterotopic pregnancy in patients presenting after the use of ART, particularly in the presence of symptoms such as vaginal bleeding and/or abdominal pain.

An additional confounding factor could be the use of emergency contraceptives. While there is no link to increased ectopic pregnancy rates identified in patients who utilize emergency contraceptives, failure of these medications may lead to an ectopic pregnancy progressing.

So You've Diagnosed an Ectopic. Now What?

When there is significant concern for ectopic pregnancy or a confirmed ectopic, lab work including a complete blood count, renal function, liver function, and a type and screen should be ordered. Rho(D) immunoglobulin should be administered for all RhD-negative patients.

The decision between medical versus surgical management will ultimately be determined in conjunction with obstetric colleagues. Surgical management is indicated in patients who are hemodynamically unstable or who have a ruptured ectopic pregnancy. Medical management with methotrexate can be considered when patients are hemodynamically stable, have a nonruptured ectopic, and do not have any contraindications to methotrexate therapy. Relative contraindications to methotrexate include hCG level greater than 5,000 mIU/mL, fetal cardiac activity, and ectopic pregnancy greater than 4 cm in size on transvaginal ultrasound due to higher failure rates of medical management. Single-dose methotrexate has a failure rate of around 10%, so patients should have a reliable follow-up plan in place before being offered methotrexate treatment. Protocols recommend follow-up hCG testing at days 4 and 7 after initial methotrexate dose to ensure adequate decrease in hormone level or identify the need for subsequent methotrexate dosing versus transition to surgical intervention.

Methotrexate is toxic to hepatocytes and cleared renally, so it should not be used in patients with elevated creatinine or elevated aminotransferase levels. It preferentially impacts rapidly dividing cells, such as the bone marrow, buccal mucosa, intestinal mucosa, and respiratory epithelium. For this reason, methotrexate treatment should also be avoided in patients with immunodeficiency, anemia, leukopenia, thrombocytopenia, active peptic ulcer disease, and active respiratory disease.

Patients should be counseled on the side effects of methotrexate, which include nausea, vomiting, abdominal pain, and spotting. They should also be advised to avoid consuming folic acid supplements, foods with folic acid, and NSAIDs and to avoid excessive sun exposure due to the risk of dermatitis.

PEARLS

- An ectopic pregnancy can be present at any beta-hCG level; pelvic ultrasound should be obtained for symptomatic pregnant patients, regardless of the beta-hCG level.
- Maintain a high level of suspicion for ectopic pregnancy in any patient diagnosed with a PUL, regardless of the beta-hCG trend, until a definitive diagnosis is made.
- Consider heterotopic pregnancy in patients with a history of in vitro fertilization or other use of ART.
- Consider ectopic pregnancy even in patients who may have utilized emergency contraceptives.
- Understand the indications and contraindications of ectopic management, and work with your obstetric colleagues to ensure the appropriate method is selected.

Suggested Readings

American College of Obstetricians and Gynecologists' Committee on Practice Bulletins—Gynecology. ACOG practice Bulletin No. 193: tubal ectopic pregnancy. *Obstet Gynecol*. 2018;131(3):e91-e103.

Hahn SA, Promes SB, Brown MD. Clinical policy: critical issues in the initial evaluation and management of patients presenting to the emergency department in early pregnancy. *Ann Emerg Med*. 2017;69(2):241-250.e20.

Young L, Barnard C, Lewis E, et al. The diagnostic performance of ultrasound in the detection of ectopic pregnancy. *N Z Med J*. 2017;130(1452):17-22.

SECTION XVI
PSYCHOLOGY

203

DIFFERENTIATING DEMENTIA VERSUS DELIRIUM

CASEY CARR AND MEGAN RIVERA

Disruptions in cognition and behavior are frequent complaints among patients presenting to the ED. The first step in assessing a patient presenting with a cognitive complaint is to determine whether the patient has delirium, dementia, or both. Dementia and delirium are similar disorders affecting cognitive processing, with subtle differences that can be difficult to distinguish in the acute setting. Both disorders are common, with a predilection toward the older patients and medically fragile.

Less commonly, critically ill children presenting to the ED may develop delirium, whereas dementia is exceptionally rare in the pediatric population. Traditionally, dementia is classified as progressive cognitive dysfunction with loss of functional ability. *Dementia* is commonly thought of as an umbrella term for various progressive cognitive disorders. Few causes of dementia are reversible, and with limited treatment options. Risk factors for dementia include older age, family history, cardiovascular disease, diabetes, the use of anticholinergic medications, and lower education level. Approximately 50 million people have dementia worldwide, with this number projected to triple by 2050. The pathophysiology of dementia is broad, depending greatly on the underlying cause.

Delirium, however, is defined as an acute change in cognitive functioning and sensorium, typically secondary to an underlying medical condition. Unlike dementia, delirium is often accompanied by abnormal vital signs or physical examination findings. Risk factors for delirium include age, poor cognitive function, poor functional status, sensory impairment, coexisting medical illness, and polypharmacy. Approximately 30% of hospitalized patients develop delirium. The pathophysiology behind the mechanism of how medical illness causes delirium is poorly understood. Theories include neurotransmitter abnormalities in response to systemic insult and transient occult brain injury. It has been estimated that emergency physicians recognize the diagnosis of delirium or cognitive impairment only 28% to 38% of the time. The predilection of both these disorders in the older patients creates the potential for diagnostic confusion and increased morbidity and mortality risk.

DIAGNOSIS

The most common existing tools to assess an adult patient's mental status are the MMSE and the CAM. In children, the pCAM and the CAPD exist to screen for delirium.

Definitive diagnosis of cognitive disorders can be time-intensive in the ED, but certain characteristics that are more indicative of one disease process or the other another can aid in differentiating the two.

Dementia is insidious, with a progressive decline in functioning and behavior over time. Patients who suffer from dementia often have personality and mood changes, normal to fluctuating alertness, and word-finding difficulty. Patients who are delirious, however, have abrupt changes in their memory and attention, altered behavior, and incoherent speech. Common features of dementia and delirium are shown in **Table 203.1**.

Both dementia and delirium have a wide range of underlying causes (**Table 203.2, Table 203.3**). Diagnostic interventions should aggressively search out for underlying cause as treatment can improve delirium or unmask an irreversible dementia. There should be a low threshold for cross-sectional imaging, especially in patients who are at high risk for structural CNS disease, such as the older patients, patients at high risk of bleeding, or those who have a history of malignancy.

TREATMENT

If a reversible cause of dementia is identified, such as hypothyroidism or depression, efforts should be made toward treating this underlying cause. Similarly, treatment of delirium should be focused on treating emergent etiologies. Differentiation between the two disease processes leads to vastly different treatment plans and patient disposition.

A commonly encountered challenge, however, is the decision to intervene when a patient becomes increasingly combative and agitated. Nonpharmacologic interventions are preferred in both patients with dementia and delirium. Attention should be placed on decreasing stimulation, treating pain, frequent communication, and minimal sleep disruptions. Optimization of their environment, such as providing the patient with their own glasses, hearing aids, and reorientation, is the cornerstone of management. For both adults and children, having blankets, home photos, or a familiar person at their bedside is beneficial. Physical and chemical restraints should be kept to a minimum and only considered if a patient poses a risk to themself or staff. Benzodiazepines should be avoided, as benzodiazepines and polypharmacy increase the risk of delirium. If medications are needed, atypical antipsychotics are preferred and dexmedetomidine can be considered.

TABLE 203.1 FEATURES OF DEMENTIA AND DELIRIUM

FEATURES	DEMENTIA	DELIRIUM
Description	Memory impairment, decline of cognitive ability, mood, and personality changes	Impairment of immediate memory, abrupt inattention
Onset	Insidious and gradual	Acute and episodic
Duration	Months to years	Hours
Course	Chronic, progressive	Fluctuating
Reversibility	No	Frequently
Agitation	Common to variable	Common to variable
Alertness	Normal to fluctuating	Altered
Speech	Word-finding difficulty, hypophonic, or altered speech output	Incoherent

TABLE 203.2	COMMON ETIOLOGIES OF DEMENTIA
Vascular causes	Vascular insults, vasculitis
Vitamin causes	B_1, B_6, B_{12}, folate
Neurologic disorders	Alzheimer disease, normal pressure hydrocephalus, neoplasia, Lewy body dementia, epilepsy
Systemic disorders	Systemic lupus erythematosus, Wilson disease, Parkinson disease
Infection	Creutzfeldt-Jakob disease, tertiary syphilis, HIV/AIDS, PML, HSV encephalitis, prion diseases
Hormonal disorders	Hypothyroidism, hyperparathyroidism
Electrolyte disorders	Hyponatremia, hypocalcemia, hypercalcemia
Miscellaneous	Cerumen impaction, medication adverse effect, depression

HIV, human immunodeficiency virus; AIDS, acquired immunodeficiency syndrome; PML, progressive multifocal leukoencephalopathy; HSV, herpes simplex virus.

TABLE 203.3	COMMON ETIOLOGIES OF DELIRIUM
CNS disorders	Vascular abnormalities, compressive lesions, postictal state, intracranial hemorrhage
Metabolic disorders	Electrolyte abnormalities, ammonia, hepatic encephalopathy, hypoxia, hypoglycemia, Wernicke encephalopathy
Infection	Urinary tract infection, pneumonia, meningitis, sepsis
Environmental causes	Sensory deprivation, postoperative state, polypharmacy, substance abuse, substance withdrawal
Systemic illness	Myocardial infarction, pulmonary embolism, toxic ingestions, heavy metal poisoning

CNS, central nervous system.

PEARLS

- Dementia is a progressive loss of cognitive processing and functional ability, whereas delirium is the rapid loss of cognitive functioning secondary to an underlying acute medical condition.
- Risk factors for dementia include older age, family history, cardiovascular disease, diabetes, the use of anticholinergic medications, and lower education level. Risk factors for delirium include age, poor cognitive function, poor functional status, sensory impairment, coexisting medical illness, and polypharmacy.
- MMSE and CAM are screening tools to help detect dementia and delirium in the adult population, whereas pCAM and CAPD are used in the pediatric population.
- Know the common etiologies of dementia and delirium and those who require immediate intervention in the ED.
- Implement environmental interventions for behavioral control in the ED—avoid using chemical and physical restraints.

Suggested Readings

Falk N, Cole A, Meredith TJ. Evaluation of suspected dementia. *Am Fam Physician.* 2018; 97(6):398-405.

Inouye SK. Delirium in older persons. *N Engl J Med.* 2006;354:1157-1165.

Mutter MK, Snustad D. Evaluating dementia and delirium in the emergency department. *Emerg Med Rep.* 2015;36(19):217-231.

Patel AK, Bell MJ, Traube C. Delirium in pediatric critical care. *Pediatr Clin North Am.* 2017;64(5):1117-1132.

204

Ask About Suicide Risk

Arsam Nadeem and Trent R. Malcolm

Evaluation of the suicidal patient to determine imminent risk or the ability to safely discharge can be challenging, especially for a patient with whom you have no prior relationship or when working in a busy department with limited mental health resources. There is no way to completely safeguard against ultimate death by suicide, but employing a rational, standardized approach to suicidal risk assessment will help minimize risk and improve patient care.

Suicidal risk assessment is a subjective task that demands a thorough history. All suicidal patients should be asked about past psychiatric history, which includes psychiatric hospitalizations, ongoing psychiatric treatment (eg, counseling, medications, and adherence), and details related to prior suicide attempts. In addition, all patients should be asked about recent life stressors, feelings of depression or hopelessness, and protective factors, such as family and social support networks. There is no evidence that asking direct questions about suicide will introduce or worsen suicidal thoughts. It is, therefore, essential to ask specifically about recent or ongoing suicidal ideation, plans, and intent. Lastly, every patient should be asked about access to firearms or other lethal means to carry out the stated plan. Responses may provide considerable insight into a patient's thought process, protective factors, and potential lethality of any stated plan.

Severe depression, feelings of hopelessness, and prior suicide attempts are the strongest predictors of suicidal behavior. Additional risk factors include age (adolescents and older), biological sex (females are more likely to attempt suicide, but males are more likely to complete suicide), sexual and gender diverse status (LGBTQI+ youth have higher rates of suicidal ideation), substance and alcohol use, organized plan, comorbid psychiatric illness, family history of suicide, impulsivity, recent unemployment, recent incarceration, recent initiation of antidepressant medication, social isolation, and chronic illness. Although many suicide risk factors are well established, our understanding of patient demographics and personal risk factors continues to evolve. For example, recent data show dramatic increases in ED visits for suicidal ideation or suicide attempts in young people and older adults over the past two decades. Pediatric and geriatric patients with suicidal ideation pose unique challenges to ED clinicians, such as increased emotional burden and increased ED boarding due to the lack of pediatric and geriatric inpatient psychiatric bed availability.

Alcohol use disorder is a major lifetime risk factor for suicide, and acute alcohol intoxication increases the immediate probability of suicide in at-risk patients. In one study, one-third of completed suicides had elevated blood alcohol levels at autopsy. Yet, patients expressing suicidal ideation while intoxicated frequently recant these feelings when sober. Consequently, mental health consultants often insist on patient sobriety before initiating an evaluation. Some institutions require that the blood alcohol level be below a specific cutoff (eg, 0.1 g/dL) before assessment. Such requirements may unnecessarily delay assessment and disposition. The decision to commence a psychiatric assessment should be based on the patient's cognitive function and decision-making capacity, not on their blood alcohol level. This is especially important in patients with physiologic dependence on alcohol for whom delaying evaluation until the blood alcohol level falls below a cutoff only invites the onset of acute alcohol withdrawal.

It is essential for ED clinicians to be able to conduct a thorough suicide risk assessment based on the patient's history and suicide risk factors. Several clinical decision support tools, including the C-SSRS, Suicide Prevention Resource Center ED Guide, and the SAFE-T, are available to aid in suicide screening and risk assessment. C-SSRS has multiple versions, including a truncated screening tool that is widely used in ED triage to identify patients requiring more comprehensive risk assessment. The Suicide Prevention Resource Center ED Guide is a simple six-question decision support tool meant to aid clinicians to distinguish high-risk patients requiring comprehensive risk assessment from low-risk patients who may be discharged with outpatient follow-up after a brief ED intervention. SAFE-T provides a stepwise guide to a more comprehensive evaluation of suicidal risk factors, protective factors, suicidal thoughts, and plans to aid in the determination of overall suicide risk. Such clinical decision support tools are valuable in guiding the assessment of the suicidal patient, but ED clinicians should not rely solely on such decision tools as few are validated for use in the ED. ED clinicians may consider discharging the lowest risk patients without a mental health consultation, but many will require a comprehensive risk assessment by a mental health specialist.

When working with a mental health consultant, it is essential to remember that the decision to admit or discharge rests with the primary physician. Therefore, it is essential to have detailed conversations with consultants to understand the reasoning behind their recommendations. When opinions differ, never discharge a patient you feel will be unsafe. In high-risk patients, voluntary admission is preferred. However, if the patient refuses admission, involuntary admission may be justified. The decision to pursue involuntary admission involves a careful deliberation of the risks and benefits of admission, including the potential harms of coercive treatment including the potential for involuntary chemical or physical restraint. Given the inherent risks of evaluating the suicidal patient, it is critical to document all pertinent aspects of the patient history, ED course including changes in mood and suicidal ideation, evidence of intoxication or sobriety, discussions with consultants, and the rationale underpinning the overall risk assessment.

PEARLS

- Perform a suicide risk assessment in every patient expressing suicidal ideation.
- Ask direct questions about suicidal thoughts—there is no evidence that these questions worsen suicidality.

- An appropriate suicide risk assessment depends on the patient's cognitive function, not on their blood alcohol level.
- Clinical decision support tools such as C-SSRS, Suicide Prevention Resource Center ED Guide, and SAFE-T may guide risk assessment.

SUGGESTED READINGS

Betz ME, Boudreaux ED. Managing suicidal patients in the emergency department. *Ann Emerg Med*. 2016;67(2):276-282.

Bowden CF, True G, Cullen SW, et al. Treating pediatric and geriatric patients at risk of suicide in general emergency departments: perspectives from emergency department clinical leaders. *Ann Emerg Med*. 2021;78(5):628-636.

Brenner JM, Marco CA, Kluesner NH, et al. Assessing psychiatric safety in suicidal emergency department patients. *JACEP Open*. 2020;1:30-37.

205

ANXIETY IN THE EMERGENCY DEPARTMENT

AFRAH A. ALI

Anxiety is the most common mental health disorder worldwide. It is the state of heightened arousal that can range from excessive worrying to extreme somatic symptoms, which usually prompts patients to seek medical care in the ED. Emergency physicians may not definitively diagnose patients with primary anxiety but should be able to differentiate between types of anxiety disorders: mild phobias, GADs, ASDs, PTSDs, and PD.

Patients with GAD are defined as having chronic excessive anxiety and worry about real or imagined events, occurring more days than not, for at least 6 months. This often leads to disruption in patients' daily life activities and is associated with at least three of the following symptoms: restlessness or feeling on edge, easily fatigued, difficulty concentrating or mind going blank, irritability, muscle tension, and sleep disturbances. In contrast, patients with PD present with short, acute episodes of anxiety often coupled with somatic symptoms, such as chest pain, palpitations, shortness of breath, lightheadedness, paresthesia, fatigue, and gastrointestinal discomfort. Patients with ASD and PTSD have symptoms of reexperiencing prior traumatic events, hypervigilance, and avoidance of triggers that relate to the prior event.

Signs and symptoms of anxiety disorders may mimic an acute life-threatening condition, such as MI, PE, hypoglycemia, thyroid conditions, and stroke (see **Table 205.1**). A comprehensive history and physical examination is required to rule out any serious underlying medical conditions. Although it may be tempting to diagnose primary anxiety to arrive at a quick disposition, it is important to address the patient's symptoms diligently. This helps to establish a relationship of trust and ensures no medical conditions will be overlooked.

TABLE 205.1	MEDICAL CONDITIONS WITH ANXIETY AS A COMMON SYMPTOM	
	CONDITIONS	**TESTS TO CONSIDER**
Cardiovascular	MI, angina, ADHF, dysrhythmia, mitral valve prolapse	ECG, cardiac enzymes, stress testing, pro-BNP, echocardiography
Pulmonary	PE, asthma, COPD, spontaneous pneumothorax	CXR, D-dimer, $\dot{V}/\dot{Q}$ scan, CTA of the chest
Endocrine	Hyperthyroidism/hypothyroidism, hypoparathyroidism, hyperglycemia/hypoglycemia, pheochromocytoma, hypercortisolism	Glucose, TSH, free T_4, calcium, PTH, cortisol
Neurologic	CVA, TIA, seizure, epilepsy, multiple sclerosis, Huntington, Alzheimer, Parkinson, TBI, concussion	CT of the head, MRI, EEG, CSF studies

Common toxicologic causes
Intoxication: amphetamines, caffeine, cocaine, cannabis, LSD, PCP, MDMA, nicotine.
Withdrawal: alcohol, benzodiazepines, barbiturates, opioids, nicotine.

ADHF; COPD, chronic obstructive pulmonary disease; CSF, cerebrospinal fluid; CT, computed tomography; CTA, computed tomography angiography; CVA, costovertebral angle; CXR, chest x-ray; ECG, electrocardiogram; EEG, electroencephalogram; LSD; MDMA; MI, myocardial infarction; MRI, magnetic resonance imaging; PCP; PE, pulmonary embolism; PRO-BNP, PRO-brain natriuretic protein; PTH, parathyroid hormone; TBI, traumatic brain injury; TIA, transient ischemic attack; TSH, thyroid-stimulating hormone; $\dot{V}/\dot{Q}$, ventilation/perfusion.
Reprinted from Craven P, Cinar O, Madsen T. Patient anxiety may influence the efficacy of ED pain management. *Am J Emerg Med*. 2013;31(2):313-318, with permission from Elsevier.

Engaging the patient with anxiety with open-ended questions and listening calmly can help limit distress and may be therapeutic. Determine the timing of events, environmental factors, and recent life stressors that may have triggered the episode of anxiety. Exacerbations often occur without an identifiable trigger, and patients may have a history of recurrent attacks. Suicidal or homicidal ideation must be addressed in any severely patients with anxiety, leading to consideration for emergent psychiatric evaluation and admission. It is important to assess drug and alcohol use in all patients with anxiety. Substance use including marijuana and withdrawal, as well as opioid and alcohol withdrawal, are the common causes of anxiety. Stimulants, including caffeine and nicotine, can worsen anxiety and should be avoided by these patients.

Patients with abnormal vital signs, such as hypoxia, tachycardia, tachypnea, and hypertension, should be immediately placed on cardiac and pulse oximetry monitoring; these vitals should prompt further workup for secondary causes of symptoms. Even though these signs may be present with a psychiatric etiology, the workup must address the possibility of an underlying medical condition. Patients with advanced age and significant comorbidities may require more extensive workup when compared to young adult and pediatric population in whom a thorough history and physical examination may be sufficient.

MANAGEMENT

The ED can be a distressing environment for the patient with anxiety. If available, patient should be roomed in a quiet environment. If medical causes are suspected, primary treatment should be based on the underlying cause. Patients with symptoms and examination consistent with primary anxiety disorder should be referred for psychotherapies, such as CBT, behavioral therapy, and counseling. The therapeutic process may be initiated with calm reassurance during the patient interview. Multiple studies have found the existence of racial disparities in prescribing outpatient benzodiazepines. Non-Hispanic White patients were more likely to be prescribed benzodiazepines when compared to Hispanic and non-Hispanic Black patients. A multidisciplinary team approach, involving a social worker and licensed therapist, will help in achieving patient-centered care.

Anxiolytics such as diphenhydramine or, in select cases, low-dose short- or long-acting benzodiazepines should be considered for patients in the ED to help relieve acute anxiety symptoms. A one-time dose of benzodiazepines, such as lorazepam 0.5 to 1 mg, clonazepam 0.25 to 0.5 mg, or diazepam 2.5 to 5 mg, may calm the patient with anxiety enough to get a more reliable history and examination. The patient's medication list should be reviewed before administering anxiolytics to avoid drug interactions due to polypharmacy. Benzodiazepines may be less effective in patients who have developed a tolerance through chronic use. Caution is advised when considering prescribing benzodiazepines for outpatient management; it is best to restrict benzodiazepine anxiolytics to a limited prescription for breakthrough anxiety to avoid complications of tolerance and dependence. SSRIs are first-line chronic pharmacologic treatment that are typically prescribed by psychiatrist or primary care physician after establishing diagnosis, since doses need to be titrated while monitoring for therapeutic and adverse effects.

SPECIAL POPULATION

Pediatric

Children experience anxiety in the ED due to its chaotic environment and anticipation of painful procedures, such as intravenous access. Nonpharmacologic management, such as the use of child life services, parental coaching, and toys, may help relieve patients' symptoms. First line of treatment for mild-to-moderate anxiety remains CBT; medications such as SSRI can be considered in conjunction with a psychiatrist for severe cases.

Older Patients

Age, risk factors, and comorbidities should prompt a comprehensive workup to rule out any underlying medical conditions, with a low threshold to admit for medical conditions. Antipsychotics are preferred in this population—Benzodiazepines should be avoided due to the risk of falls, cognitive impairment, worsening dementia, paradoxical agitation, and polypharmacy.

Pregnancy

Pregnant patients are at increased risk of PE, which can mimic symptoms of a PD. Benzodiazepines and diphenhydramine are safe in pregnancy in the acute setting, although diphenhydramine should be avoided in lactating patients as it can affect breastmilk production. SSRIs are also safe in pregnancy and can be prescribed by a primary care physician or psychiatrist.

Disposition

After medical causes are ruled out, most patients presenting to the ED with anxiety are discharged home. Reassurance is the mainstay of treatment of patients presenting with an exacerbation of a primary anxiety disorder. Breathing exercises can be described and practiced with the patient. Encourage mindfulness-based stress reduction strategies, exercise, and healthy nutrition. Ensure that the patient has an emotional support system, and offer to involve family members in treatment plans with patient permission. Counsel patients to avoid stimulants, such as caffeine and nicotine. Provide referral to substance abuse counseling and detox centers for patients with substance use disorders. Prompt follow-up with primary care physician or referral for a psychiatrist should be recommended to all patients.

PEARLS

- A thorough history and physical examination is required to rule out acute life-threatening conditions.
- Older patients with comorbidities require a comprehensive workup to rule out cardiac-, pulmonary-, neurologic-, and endocrine-related etiologies.
- Provide patient with a quiet area, and carefully listen to their concerns.
- Low-dose benzodiazepines can be offered to help patients in distress.
- Avoid benzodiazepines in older patients as they are prone to falls, polypharmacy, and cognitive impairment.

SUGGESTED READINGS

American Psychiatric Association, American Psychiatric Association, DSM-5 Task Force. *Diagnostic and Statistical Manual of Mental Disorders: DSM-5.* 5th ed. American Psychiatric Association; 2013:947.

DeSelm TM. Mood and anxiety disorders. In: Tintinalli JE, Ma O, Yealy DM, et al., eds. *Tintinalli's Emergency Medicine: A Comprehensive Study Guide*. 9th ed. McGraw Hill; 2020.

Zun L, Chepenik L, Mallory M. Behavioral emergencies for the emergency physician. In: Chepenik L, Mallory M, Zun L, eds. *Behavioral Emergencies for the Emergency Physician*. Cambridge University Press; 2013:iii.

206

SUBSTANCE USE DISORDERS IN THE EMERGENCY DEPARTMENT

LAURA JANNECK AND DEREK MARTINEZ

As emergency physicians, our role in the care of patients with substance use disorders frequently amounts to stabilization and supportive care during episodes of intoxication, overdose, or withdrawal. Substance use has high rates of morbidity and mortality, and addressing patients' substance use when they are in the ED can have a significant health impact. As of 2020, opioid overdose is the leading cause of unintentional death for adults under age 50 years in the United States. Emergency physicians are in a unique position to initiate interventions aimed toward treatment and harm reduction.

SCREENING IN THE ED

Screening ED patients for drug and alcohol use can identify potential complications to medical treatment as well as those patients most likely to benefit from harm reduction interventions. It is important to avoid accusatory or stigmatizing language when talking with patients struggling with substance use. Screening for substance use should include amount and frequency of consumption, including the number of days of use per week, amount consumed per episode, and amount consumed per week. Screening questions should also be directed toward the social, health, and economic consequences of a patient's substance use. In patients presenting with intoxication or overdose, physicians should consider and ask about possible coingestions and polysubstance use. Any ED staff member can ask the abbreviated National Institute on Drug Abuse Quick Screen: "How many times in the past year have you used an illegal drug or used a prescription medication for nonmedical reasons?" The CAGE-AID Questionnaire (see **Table 206.1**) is another tool used to screen for both substance and alcohol use. Positive screening using formal screening tools or high clinical suspicion of substance use should prompt the emergency physician to employ a brief intervention.

If patients screen positive for substance use, consider withdrawal prophylaxis utilizing benzodiazepines or phenobarbital in patients at risk of alcohol withdrawal, ordering opioid maintenance therapy if a patient is already on it, or administering nicotine patches as appropriate.

INTERVENTION IN THE ED

Feeling constrained by time pressures, ED physicians frequently treat and disposition patients with substance use disorders without directly discussing substance use treatment. Yet, there is a growing body of evidence to suggest that intervention in the ED significantly increases engagement in formal treatment.

There is now broad consensus discouraging abstinence-based therapy for opioid use disorder in favor of medical-assisted therapy (MAT) (see **Figure 206.1**). If a patient presents with opioid-withdrawal syndrome with a COWS score at least 8-13, they should be offered initiation of MAT, generally with buprenorphine. As a partial agonist, buprenorphine evokes limited effects, and even at high doses, euphoria and respiratory depression are minimal. In patients with abstinence-induced opioid withdrawal, buprenorphine is generally sufficient to quell the symptoms of withdrawal. Buprenorphine also has high-receptor affinity, so it is protective against overdose and limits euphoria during subsequent administration of full opioid agonists, such as heroin. Of note, in an opioid-dependent patient not in withdrawal, buprenorphine can precipitate opioid withdrawal since its high-receptor affinity will displace other opioids from the mu receptors, so it is important to

TABLE 206.1 CAGE-AID QUESTIONNAIRE

C	Have you ever felt the need to **cut** down on your drinking or drug use?	Yes No
A	Have people **annoyed** you by criticizing your drinking or drug use?	Yes No
G	Have you ever felt **guilty** about drinking or drug use?	Yes No
E	Have you ever felt you needed a drink or used drugs first thing in the morning to steady your nerves or to get rid of a hangover (**Eye-Opener**)?	Yes No

Scoring: A "yes" answer to one item indicates a possible substance use disorder and a need for further testing.
Reprinted from Brown RL, Leonard T, Saunders LA, Papasouliotis O. The prevalence and detection of substance use disorders among inpatients ages 18 to 49: an opportunity for prevention. *Prev Med.* 1998;27(1):101-101, with permission from Elsevier. Copyright © 1998 American Health Foundation and Academic Press. All rights reserved.

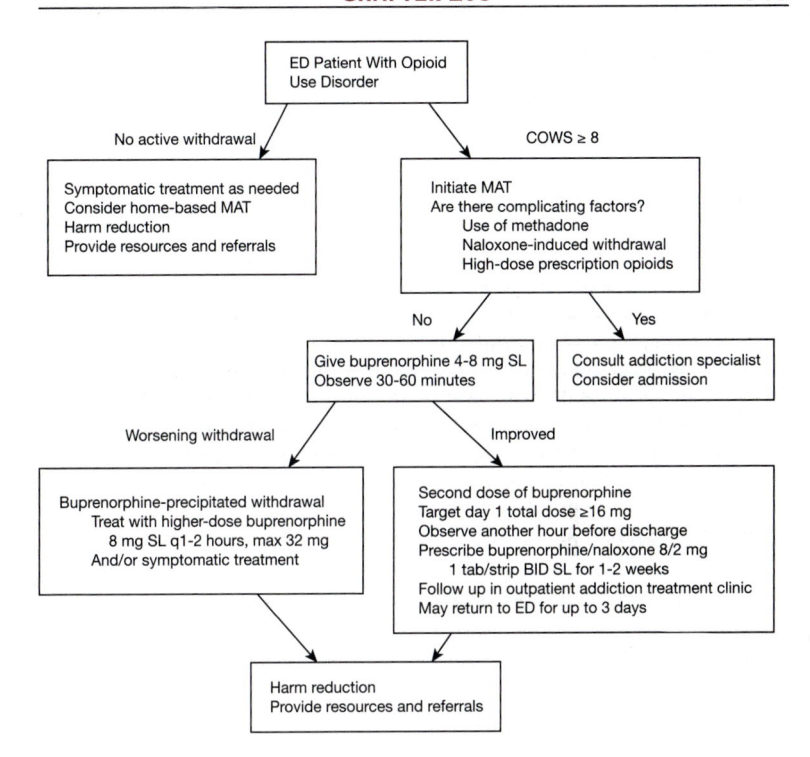

```
                    ┌─────────────────────┐
                    │ ED Patient With Opioid│
                    │ Use Disorder         │
                    └─────────────────────┘
              No active withdrawal    COWS ≥ 8
              ↓                                ↓
    ┌──────────────────────────┐   ┌──────────────────────────┐
    │ Symptomatic treatment as needed │ Initiate MAT                │
    │ Consider home-based MAT         │ Are there complicating factors? │
    │ Harm reduction                  │   Use of methadone            │
    │ Provide resources and referrals │   Naloxone-induced withdrawal │
    └──────────────────────────┘   │   High-dose prescription opioids │
                                    └──────────────────────────┘
```

Figure 206.1 Treatment algorithm for opioid use disorder. BID, twice daily; COWS, Clinical Opiate Withdrawal Scale; ED, emergency department; MAT, medical-assisted therapy; SL, sub-lingual.

only initiate buprenorphine after the patient has begun to experience symptoms of mild-to-moderate opioid withdrawal. ACEP provides physicians with a tool (https://www.acep.org/patient-care/bupe) to help initiate buprenorphine in the ED.

If opiate agonist therapy is not available, patients with opioid withdrawal should be treated with medications tailored to their symptoms, such as antiemetics for vomiting, antispasmodics for abdominal cramping, NSAIDs and acetaminophen for pain, and clonidine for autonomic dysfunction, including hypertension, diaphoresis, and irritability.

ED visits may be the most effective time to initiate intervention. To help patients decide to seek treatment for substance use, use a brief negotiated interview, which relies on four key strategies: (1) establishing rapport, (2) providing feedback on the consequences of substance use, (3) enhancing motivation to seek assistance, and (4) negotiating a goal and course for follow-up.

REFERRAL FOR TREATMENT

ED interventions for substance use should bridge to longitudinal treatment. EDs should be able to provide a list of local resources and preferably have a referral set up with those organizations. When available, ED social workers and case managers can assist with these referrals. Many EDs employ peer recovery counselors who can support patients during their ED stay and follow up with them to connect them to resources and act as advocates. Patients who are not yet ready to commit to treatment for their substance use disorder should be advised to closely follow up with a primary care physician and encouraged to return to the ED at any time when they are ready.

HARM REDUCTION

ED physicians can also help reduce the harms associated with substance use. This includes discussing safe injection practices and how to access clean needles, offering or advising outpatient screening for hepatitis C and HIV, and advising against driving while intoxicated. Naloxone should be provided to all patients at risk of opiate overdose, which includes any patient using opioids or other drugs that may be contaminated with opioids such as methamphetamine and benzodiazepines. These patients should be educated on the risk of opioid exposure and overdose, be given naloxone, and educated on how to use it. As physicians on the front lines, we should strive to reduce the stigma around substance use disorders and promote evidence-based treatment and referral services. Numerous interventions and strategies can be employed in the ED to reduce negative consequences for patients with substance use.

PEARLS

- Avoid accusatory statements regarding substance use and establish rapport with patients before initiating a conversation.
- Any suspicion of drug or alcohol use should prompt physicians to screen for clinically significant substance use disorders.
- MAT programs should be implemented widely with connection to outpatient treatment programs.
- Provide follow-up with a referral to a treatment program or, if the patient is unwilling, health-focused outpatient care.
- Provide resources and prescriptions to reduce harm, even if a patient is unwilling to abstain from or reduce substance use.

SUGGESTED READINGS

ACEP BUPE tool. Accessed May 2, 2023. https://www.acep.org/patient-care/bupe

Center for Substance Abuse Treatment. Enhancing Motivation for Change in Substance Abuse Treatment. Revised 2014 ed. U.S. Department of Health and Human Services, Substance Abuse and Mental Health Services Administration; 2014. Publication No. (SMA) 13-4212.

D'Onofrio G, O'Connor PG, Pantalon MV, et al. Emergency department-initiated buprenorphine/naloxone treatment for opioid dependence: a randomized clinical trial. *JAMA*. 2015;313(16):1636-1644. PMID: 25919527.

Hawk K, D'Onofrio G. Emergency department screening and interventions for substance use disorders [published correction appears in *Addict Sci Clin Pract*. 2019;14(1):26]. *Addict Sci Clin Pract*. 2018;13(1):18. PMID: 30078375.

Strayer RJ, Hawk K, Hayes BD, et al. Management of opioid use disorder in the emergency department: a white paper prepared for the American Academy of Emergency Medicine. *J Emerg Med*. 2020;58(3):522-546. PMID: 32234267.

Wheeler E, Burk K, McQuie H, et al. Guide to Developing and Managing Overdose Prevention and Take-Home Naloxone Projects. Harm Reduction Coalition; 2012.

207

Mastering Management of the Acutely Agitated Patient

Kyle Fischer and Rachel Wiltjer

Agitated patients are commonly seen in the ED, with presentations ranging from restlessness and pacing to physical aggression or self-harm. Early recognition of escalating behaviors provides the opportunity to intervene with de-escalation techniques, creating a safer environment for patients, staff, and clinicians. Importantly, agitation can be secondary to a variety of causes; thus, delirium and the workup of altered mental status are covered elsewhere (see Chapters 203 and 211).

When a patient displays agitation, clinicians should rapidly assess scene safety and in the absence of physical aggression or violence should attempt verbal de-escalation. While verbal de-escalation is not always successful, it is an important starting point for the management of acutely agitated patient. Becoming skilled in its use may prevent the need for emergent medication or restraint—improving patient and staff safety as well as satisfaction. When verbal de-escalation fails, emergent medication may be needed. If the patient is cooperative, consider offering oral medications to prevent escalating behavior and obviate the need for involuntary medication.

Clinicians can maximize their opportunity for successful verbal de-escalation by initiating it at the first signs of agitation. These signs can include repetitive and non–goal-oriented physical activity, vocalizations of repetitive thoughts, reported anxiety, or threatening gestures. Early recognition of risk factors for agitation and signs of impending escalation provides an opportunity to intervene before violence. Agitation and aggression are not synonymous but may coexist, with aggression being one extreme on the continuum of agitation. Treatment of pain and physical symptoms may help preempt agitation.

Previously termed "the 10 commandments of de-escalation," there exists a set of strategies described in the literature as techniques to utilize for de-escalation (**Table 207.1**). Adjunctive measures to these strategies include environmental alterations, such as providing patients with food or drink (when medically appropriate), providing

---

TABLE 207.1 TEN STRATEGIES FOR VERBAL DE-ESCALATION

1. Respect the patient's personal space
2. Do not provoke the patient
3. Have one person interact verbally with the patient
4. Be concise and utilize repetition
5. Identify wants and feelings
6. Use active listening skills
7. Either find a point of agreement with the patient or agree to disagree
8. Respectful establishment of reasonable boundaries/limits
9. Offer choices
10. Debrief the patient and staff

blankets, utilizing larger/less cramped spaces (to make the patient feel less trapped), and decreasing stimuli (dimming lights, decreasing noise level).

Implicit in this approach is the importance of not worsening the situation. One unconscious way the situation may be further escalated is through body language that is perceived by the patient as threatening. Gestures and positioning that may be adopted naturally when feeling defensive—such as clenched fists, crossed arms, concealed hands (in pockets or behind the back), and standing in the doorway—may be read as hostile or confrontational by patients.

When attempting verbal de-escalation, it is critical to ensure the physical safety of the patient, physician, and staff. Clinicians should be cognizant of the physical environment and utilize appropriate distancing techniques. Exits should be easily accessible to both staff and patients, furniture should be moved when necessary, and objects that could become projectiles removed. Ideally, there should be two arm's length of space between the primary communicator and the patient to respect the patient's personal space as well as to promote safety in the case of unexpected physicality.

Trauma-informed care (TIC) is increasingly described in the literature as an approach pertinent to emergency physicians. At its core, TIC aims to recognize the experiences of patient, acknowledging that trauma is not only physical but also emotional, psychological, and societal/structural, then delivering care that is sensitive to individual needs arising from prior traumatic experiences. Prior traumatic experiences are common in agitated patients, especially those with a history of mental illness, substance use disorders, or who have experienced physical or sexual violence.

The experience of trauma is associated with physiologic changes and may manifest outwardly with hyperarousal, hypervigilance, emotional dysregulation, and difficulty with attention. There are general principles for providing TIC, but from a practical standpoint, many described strategies for verbal de-escalation fit well within TIC. There is no one correct way to utilize TIC but being aware of and accounting for personal biases (explicit and implicit), utilizing neutral, patient-centric language, allowing physical and emotional space when appropriate, and returning agency to the patient can all help in preventing retraumatization.

Certain populations require special attention to optimize care. This includes both geriatric and pediatric patients. For both these populations, the presence of family at the bedside may help calm patients (or can further escalate agitation depending on the demeanor of the family member). Developmental delay and autism spectrum disorder can also present challenges in the recognition and management of agitation. It is important to take developmental level and developmental appropriateness into account when assessing and interacting with the patient. Recognizing triggers for agitation and escalation, such as sensory issues and overstimulation, may help in mitigating these issues. Consider the patient's usual means of communication and try to utilize this. Patients with prior trauma (specifically sexual or gun violence) and post-traumatic stress disorder may respond unexpectedly, as the ED itself can precipitate symptoms of traumatic stress; thus, TIC approaches are critical.

PEARLS

- Recognize early signs of agitation and intervene early to preempt escalation.
- Have a single primary communicator with the patient.

- Refer to the "10 commandments" of de-escalation.
- Consider offering voluntary oral medications before emergent, involuntary administration of medications.
- Practice TIC, recognizing that patients commonly have prior traumatic experiences.

Suggested Readings

Fischer KR, Bakes KM, Corbin TJ, et al. Trauma-informed care for violently injured patients in the emergency department. *Ann Emerg Med*. 2019;73(2):193-202.

Gerson R, Malas N, Feuer V, et al. Best practices for evaluation and treatment of agitated children and adolescents (BETA) in the emergency department: consensus statement of the American Association for Emergency Psychiatry. *West J Emerg Med*. 2019;20(2):409-418.

Gottlieb M, Long B, Koyfman A. Approach to the agitated emergency department patient. *J Emerg Med*. 2018;54(4):447-457.

Richmond JS, Berlin JS, Fishkind AB, et al. Verbal de-escalation of the agitated patient: consensus statement of the American Association for Emergency Psychiatry Project BETA De-escalation Workgroup. *West J Emerg Med*. 2012;13(1):17-25.

208

Droperidol Is Back

Ashley N. Martinelli and Daniel B. Gingold

Droperidol was once used with regularity in emergency medicine but has been absent in recent years. It has a unique mechanism as an antagonist of dopamine, serotonin, alpha-2, and histamine. This versatile activity makes droperidol a useful treatment modality for acute agitation as well as migraines, nausea, and pain.

Since coming to the market in 1967, droperidol was widely available and used until 2001. At that time, the FDA listed a new black box warning on droperidol due to its effects on QT prolongation, a known adverse event, and the risk of developing torsades de pointes. This warning was added after review of a postmarketing studies and safety reports from across the world despite decades of studies documenting safe use. Interestingly, many patients who experienced torsades de pointes had utilized supratherapeutic doses (25-600 mg IV) predominantly in countries outside the United States. There were also concerns over inappropriate or irregular reporting of these cases. Droperidol was not removed from the market, but the supply was unavailable for many years following the black box warning due to reduced manufacturing and lack of demand. In its absence, haloperidol was the only similar medication available.

In 2019, a new generic manufacturer resumed the production of droperidol for injection. This in combination with the renewed interest in multimodal treatment and opioid avoidance has increased interest in droperidol. Now that droperidol is back in the supply chain, it is important to understand how to appropriately utilize it and how it differs from haloperidol, which most clinicians are more accustomed to using. Both droperidol and haloperidol should be avoided in patients with a prolonged QTc interval (>440 msec in males, >450 msec in females). It may not always be possible to obtain an ECG, especially in an acutely agitated patient; therefore, a review of concomitant medications should be performed to ensure that multiple QT prolonging medications are not on board. If multiple doses of droperidol, haloperidol, or other QT prolonging medications are required, ECG monitoring is recommended. The EPS for droperidol are similar to other antipsychotic medications, which include drowsiness, akathisia, dysphoria, and hyperactivity. In very rare instances, neuroleptic malignant syndrome has been reported.

To address these safety concerns, ACEP published a policy statement on the use of droperidol in the ED in 2021. Specifically, ACEP and FDA recommend that droperidol doses less than 2.5 mg given IV do not require telemetry monitoring or ECG before or after administration. ACEP further states that higher doses of droperidol should also not have restrictions, provided that cardiac monitoring is available soon after drug administration for high-risk patients: age above 65 years, female, hypokalemia, and those taking concomitant QT prolonging medications. When treating acute agitation, doses of 5 to 10 mg IM or IV can be given without initial ECG in the emergency or prehospital setting. ACEP also recommended a revision to the current black box warning that has not occurred. In 2013, the AAEM published a position statement with similar recommendations.

Acute agitation in the patient presenting with psychiatric complaints should always be managed with de-escalation techniques before medication administration. This builds patient trust and can reduce aggressive behaviors (see Chapter 207). If this fails, medication therapy is often required to protect patients and staff and to facilitate any indicated medical workup.

Droperidol is only available as a solution for injection by the IV or IM route. In contrast, haloperidol and several second-generation antipsychotics can be administered PO, which can be helpful in cases of mild or anticipated agitation. If patient is amenable, using oral medications can be simpler and less painful to administer as well as less sedating than drugs given by parental routes. Consider offering alternative medications available in oral formulation before IM injection of droperidol, or if an IV line is not otherwise necessary. Droperidol has a significantly faster onset of action compared to haloperidol, especially when administered IM (see **Table 208.1**). Since this is potentially the safest or only available route in an acute situation, this is a highly desirable property. A pitfall with

TABLE 208.1 COMPARISON OF PHARMACOLOGIC CHARACTERISTICS OF ANTIPSYCHOTICS COMMONLY USED FOR AGITATION IN THE ED

ANTIPSYCHOTIC	DOSE (MG)	ONSET (PO)	ONSET (IM)	DURATION (IM)
Haloperidol	5	30-60 min	25-45 min	4-6 h
Droperidol	5	-	5-15 min	2-4 h
Risperidone	2	60 min	-	-
Ziprasidone	10	6-8 h	15-60 min	2-5 h
Olanzapine	10	4-6 h	15-45 min	24 h

ED, emergency department; IM, intramuscularly; PO, by mouth.

TABLE 208.2	RECOMMENDED DROPERIDOL DOSING FOR COMMON ED INDICATIONS
INDICATION	RECOMMENDED DOSING
Acute agitation	5 mg IV or IM; can repeat up to a total of 10 mg
Migraine	2.5 mg IV or IM
Analgesia	2.5 mg IV or IM
Nausea	0.625-1.25 mg IV or IM

IM, intramuscularly; IV, intravenously.
Adapted Mattson A, Friend K, Brown CS, Cabrera D. Reintegrating droperidol into emergency medicine practice. *Am J Health Syst Pharm*. 2020;77:1838-1845.

using a medication with a slower onset is that the clinician may be unsure if the medication worked, or if clinical effect has yet to peak. This can lead to earlier repeat dosing and a longer cumulative effect of the medication, resulting in oversedation due to dose stacking. In addition, droperidol has a shorter duration of action than alternative agents (see **Table 208.1**). This makes droperidol ideal for treating agitated patients intoxicated with drugs or alcohol—rapid onset quickly resolves agitation, while shorter duration allows for earlier reassessment for sobriety and final disposition.

In cases of severe agitation, an antipsychotic and a benzodiazepine may need to be coadministered. Since midazolam has a faster onset of action and shorter duration of action than lorazepam, consider using midazolam and droperidol in place of the traditional combination of haloperidol, lorazepam, and diphenhydramine. There is data to suggest droperidol with midazolam is superior to the combination of midazolam and haloperidol, in achieving sedation faster and reducing the need for rescue sedation without an increased risk of EPS or prolonged sedation. EPS are rare after droperidol administration and can be managed with diphenhydramine or benztropine should it occur, in lieu of prophylaxis.

The safety profile of droperidol is comparable to alternative medications used for similar indications. Being mindful of modest safety considerations and anticipated adverse effects, the use of droperidol within the recommended indication-specific dosing can provide safe, evidence-based, and effective symptom control for numerous common conditions in the ED (see **Table 208.2**).

PEARLS

- Droperidol is a safe and effective medication to use in the ED for a variety of indications if dosed within the recommended ranges.
- Patients at high risk for QT prolongation should have cardiac monitoring after droperidol administration.
- In cases of severe agitation, the combination of droperidol and midazolam can be utilized due to a shorter onset of action, reduced need for rescue medication, and lower risk of prolonged sedation.
- Prophylactic coadministration of an antihistamine is not routinely recommended to prevent EPS as it increases the incidence and duration of drowsiness.

Suggested Readings

American College of Emergency Physicians. *Clinical policy: use of droperidol in the emergency department*. Approved January 2021. https://www.acep.org/globalassets/new-pdfs/policy-statements/use-of-droperidol-in-the-emergency-department.pdf

Mattson A, Friend K, Brown CS, Cabrera D. Reintegrating droperidol into emergency medicine practice. *Am J Health Syst Pharm*. 2020;77:1838-1845.

Roppolo LP, Morris DW, Khan F, et al. Improving the management of acutely agitated patients in the emergency department through implementation of Project BETA (Best Practices in the Evaluation and Treatment of Agitation). *JACEP Open*. 2020;1:898-907.

Thiemann P, Roy D, Huecker M, et al. Prospective study of haloperidol plus lorazepam versus droperidol plus midazolam for the treatment of acute agitation in the emergency department. *Am J Emerg Med*. 2022;55:76-81.

209

Do Not Forget About Me: The Psych Boarder in Your ED

Kelli Robinson

Patient boarding is a challenge prevalent in the EDs across the nation. Boarding patients are defined as having completed their initial medical evaluation and are awaiting transport to an inpatient hospital bed or transfer to another facility. Patients awaiting psychiatric inpatient admission may board for several hours or even days, especially while awaiting transfer to an outside psychiatry facility. Prolonged length of stay in the ED puts this population at an increased risk for oversight and error. Furthermore, ED boarding can delay stabilization of acute psychiatric illness. Optimizing care of the boarding psychiatric patient in the ED can improve mental health care and avoid decompensation in advance of transfer to definitive care.

Monitoring psychiatric patients boarding in the ED requires a team effort between emergency physicians, mental health professionals, nursing staff, patient technicians, pharmacists, social workers, and administration. Early psychiatric evaluation is essential to develop a care plan for patients. Psychiatric consultation should be obtained as early in the clinical care course as is feasible, either in person or via telemedicine. Psychiatric recommendations should be initiated in addition to any established protocols for boarding patients. During this time, a 1:1 sitter should be instituted for patients with elevated risk for elopement, suicide, or violence. Close observation by a sitter ensures the safety of the patient and others in the ED. Guidelines for boarding psychiatric patients should include frequency of nursing assessments, medication regimen, establishing a calming and safe environment, and substance-withdrawal assessments as applicable, such as Alcohol Withdrawal Scale and Clinical Opiate Withdrawal Scale.

Home medications are ideally initiated promptly in the ED. Consider an initial electrocardiogram for patients being given multiple doses of QTc prolonging medications, although this is not necessary before initial antipsychotic administration. Medication reconciliation should be performed early. Ancillary staff can assist with the medication reconciliation. Moreover, family, caretakers, roommates, and pharmacists can provide collateral information to confirm dosages and time medications were last taken. Patients experiencing mental health crisis have frequently not been fully adherent to their psychiatric medication plan. Reinstituting voluntary oral home medications, especially antipsychotics, can begin to stabilize the patient's symptoms and avoid escalation of behavior or decompensation of psychiatric or chronic medical illnesses. Improving comfort by treating physical symptoms such as nausea and pain can improve patient experience, decrease distress, improve mood, and avoid behavioral escalation. If anxiety symptoms or behavioral escalation persist, second-line treatment includes medications such as benzodiazepines or antihistamines. Care should be taken to avoid drug interactions between reconciled and new medical and psychiatric medications. Psychiatric patients, especially geriatric patients, are at an increased risk for polypharmacy. Sleep aids and nicotine patches can be provided preemptively.

Assuming no medical or safety contraindications, psychiatric patients should be given food and drink and placed in calming spaces with minimal noise, light, and stimulation. Wearing an easily identifiable gown and removing patient belongings and other potentially harmful objects are necessary for safety. Patients should be informed that this is a process for all patients under psychiatric evaluation to alleviate any stigma felt in doing so. Access to a telephone and an allotment of phone calls (with a mutual understanding of restrictions) are reassuring for patients, family, and caretakers. Consider placing patients of similar age groups in waiting areas together. This space is particularly important for pediatric psychiatric patients whose response to isolation may differ greatly than adult patients. While space is limited in most EDs, arrangements can be made with available space and as resources allow. Creating a comfortable environment facilitates patience and calmness while awaiting an inpatient bed.

Psychiatric patients should be included in the ED physician sign-out report and nursing staff patient handoff reports. These communications should include documentation of voluntary or involuntary status, plan for administration of emergent medication for agitation or decompensation, active medications, reason for inpatient admission, working diagnosis, planned destination, and any additional pertinent medical information. Reassessment of patients at shift change is critical. Frequent reassessments are needed for patients who received sedating medications, physical restraints, on withdrawal protocols, or who require close monitoring of chronic illness, such as point-of-care glucose testing for patients with diabetes. Communication between physicians and staff is a necessity, and physicians should be informed of any development or alteration in symptoms or patient condition. The status of the pending admission or transfer should also be discussed and barriers to the process addressed when feasible.

On an institutional level, dedicated psychiatric social workers and case management may facilitate and expedite the admission and transfer process for psychiatric patients boarding in the ED. Some hospital and government programs have implemented mobile crisis unit teams to route patients experiencing a mental health crisis directly to psychiatric facilities, bypassing EDs. Psychiatric Emergency Services situated within or adjacent to EDs are another resource that aids in reducing the number of boarding psychiatric patients. Reducing psychiatric boarding will require substantial policy change to increase community and inpatient mental health care capacity and coordination. In the meantime, EDs can implement simple but effective practices to optimize the treatment of patients under their care awaiting definitive psychiatric disposition.

> **PEARLS**
>
> - Early psychiatric evaluation is recommended to formulate an initial care plan for patients.
> - Implement guidelines to standardized care for boarding patients and maintain safety of individuals within the ED.
> - Perform medication reconciliation and reinitiate medical and psychiatric home medications.
> - Create a comfortable environment for boarding psychiatric patients as resources allow.
> - Include psychiatric patients in the ED sign-out process to ensure consistent reassessment.

SUGGESTED READINGS

Bender D, Pande N, Ludwig M. Psychiatric boarding interview summary. United States Department of Health and Human Services; 2009. Accessed January 9, 2023. https://aspe.hhs.gov/system/files/pdf/75756/PsyBdInt.pdf

Chang B. Keep safe while boarding psychiatric patients in the emergency department. *ACEP Now;* 2021. acepnow.com

Nordstrom K, Berlin JS, Nash SS, Shah SB, Schmelzer NA, Worley LLM. Boarding of mentally ill patients in emergency departments: American Psychiatric Association resource document. *West J Emerg Med*. 2019;20(5):690-695. PMID: 31539324.

Simon J, Kraus C, Basford J, Clayborne E, Kluesner N, Bookman K. In: ACEP Board of Directors, ed. *The Impact of Boarding Psychiatric Patients on the Emergency Department: Scope, Impact and Proposed Solutions*. An Information Paper. American College of Emergency Physicians; 2019.

210

DO YOU HAVE THE CAPACITY TO ASSESS CAPACITY?

BOBBI-JO LOWIE AND CHRISTINA SAJAK

Emergency physicians assess patient capacity almost daily throughout their careers. We often think to assess capacity when patients want to leave "against medical advice" or refuse a necessary procedure, when truthfully, it should be completed for any encounter that requires patient consent or decision-making. Luckily, capacity is usually ascertained by the emergency physician simultaneously as the patient is being evaluated for their clinical complaint. In most cases, the patient can easily be deemed to have capacity unless they show obvious signs of impairment.

Assessing capacity consists of four components, which must be evaluated by the emergency physician. The four components are understanding, appreciation or application, reasoning, and expression (**Table 210.1**). For understanding, the patient must be able to understand the medical information relevant to their situation. *Is the patient engaged in your conversation? Are they asking appropriate questions? Are they showing reasonable insight regarding the matter you are discussing?* The teach-back method can help evaluate how much information they have understood. For example: *I know that was a lot to digest—can you tell me your understanding of what is going on?* This allows the patient to paraphrase what you have told them in their own words to demonstrate understanding. Assuming patient understanding without assessment could miss a patient who may have poor understanding of information related to their condition, proposed procedure, or management decision.

The second component of capacity is appreciation, which is the application of relevant information, particularly risks or consequences of treatment plans, to their own specific situation. The patient should be able to acknowledge their condition and describe what is likely to happen to them when pursuing different treatment courses. This can be elicited by simply asking patients what medical conditions they believe they have or what therapies they believe they might need. A patient with cancer who is alert and oriented but who cannot acknowledge that they have cancer is unlikely to be able to make informed decisions on therapy even if they are "of sound mind."

The third component of capacity is reasoning, which refers to a patient's ability to manipulate information in a rational way when making a choice. If the patient is declining a recommended intervention, they will often be upfront about their reasoning when asked in a nonjudgmental way. Try asking, *"I understand you do not want to undergo the procedure we are recommending. May I ask why?"* and *"Are there any specific concerns I could address for you or questions I could answer?"* Note that a patient may have priorities that differ from that of the physician but have sound reasoning and still have capacity. A common example is a patient who wishes to forego therapeutic treatment or admission to adhere to other social, familial, or religious obligations.

Finally, the patient should be able to express a clear and consistent choice. This can be elicited by simply asking the patient to express their choice. Commonly, the patient's ability to do so is documented by verbal conversation and, in many cases, by way of consent forms as well. If a decision is made by the patient but followed by frequent reversals or changes, it may indicate a lack of capacity.

Patients must have all four of these components to have capacity. Missing one aspect is sufficient to identify a patient as lacking capacity. Accommodations should be made for the entirety of the capacity assessment, including the expression component,

TABLE 210.1 THE FOUR COMPONENTS OF CAPACITY ASSESSMENT

COMPONENT	EXAMPLE QUESTIONS
Understanding	I know this has been a lot of information; can you tell me your understanding of what is going on?
Appreciation (application)	What medical conditions do you have, and what therapies do you believe you need for your current condition? What could happen if we do not do the procedure?
Reasoning	I understand you do not want to undergo the procedure we are recommending. May I ask why?
Expression	Can you tell me what your decision is?

for patients with language or other barriers to communication. Be careful not to assume that a patient has full understanding of their medical situation if it is presented to them in a language that is not their first learned language. Finally, all patients should be addressed at their level of education, which is most likely to foster mutual understanding between patient and clinician.

Capacity is dynamic and can change over time and situation. A patient who is intoxicated with drugs or alcohol may not have decision-making capacity at the time of their arrival in the ED, but very well may have capacity once reaching clinical sobriety. The reverse is true in a patient who arrives with capacity but, through worsening of their disease process, develops significantly altered mental status. In addition, patients may demonstrate capacity to make some decisions and not others; capacity can, therefore, be assessed separately for individual decisions and is not a binary or absolute determination. These examples reinforce the importance of reassessment and documentation of capacity during patient encounters.

Minors in the ED present a unique situation as they alone cannot provide consent, except in certain circumstances. When minors can provide consent varies by state, it is crucial to be aware of the laws in your area of practice. In general, minors who are married, a parent of a child, or legally emancipated can provide consent. In addition, minors seeking care for pregnancy, sexually transmitted infections, or some forms of psychiatric care or substance use are considered to have medical decision-making capacity and can give consent in certain states.

Finally, assessing capacity in patients with psychiatric illness can be challenging due to waxing and waning decision-making capacity. The emergency physician can, in principle, determine the capacity of a patient with psychiatric illness on their own but should consider obtaining psychiatric consultation for assistance with complex cases or when capacity is unclear.

PEARLS

- Remember to assess capacity, even when your patient agrees to your plan of care.
- Reassess capacity for each procedure or decision, or when there is a change in clinical status.
- Fully document all capacity discussions.
- Educate yourself on state and local laws for pediatric consent.
- Have confidence in your ability to assess capacity but utilize your consultants when necessary!

Suggested Readings

Ganzini L, Volicer L, Nelson WA, Fox E, Derse AR. Ten myths about decision-making capacity. *J Am Med Dir Assoc*. 2005;6(3 Suppl):S100-S104. PMID: 15890283.

Goldfrank LR, Wittman I. Capacity? Informed consent; informed discharge? Uncertainty! *Ann Emerg Med*. 2017;70(5):704-706.

Larkin GL, Marco CA, Abbott JT. Emergency determination of decision-making capacity: balancing autonomy and beneficence in the emergency department. *Acad Emerg Med*. 2001;8(3):282-284.

Magauran BG. Risk management for the emergency physician: competency and decision-making capacity, informed consent, and refusal of care against medical advice. *Emerg Med Clin North Am*. 2009;27(4):605-614.
Marco CA, Brenner JM, Kraus CK, McGrath NA, Derse AR. Refusal of emergency medical treatment: case studies and ethical foundations. *Ann Emerg Med*. 2017;70(5):696-703.
Simon JR. Refusal of care: the physician-patient relationship and decisionmaking capacity. *Ann Emerg Med*. 2007;50(4):456-461.

211

DO YOU REALLY NEED THOSE LABS FOR MEDICAL CLEARANCE?

SPENCER LOVEGROVE AND GABRIELLA MILLER

Emergency physicians are frequently asked to order "screening labs" for patients presenting with psychiatric complaints to "medically clear" patients for mental health evaluation. The goal is to identify any medical mimics of psychiatric symptoms and stabilize concomitant medical issues that may not be safely managed at a psychiatric treatment facility with limited resources. Tests are often ordered based on institutional policy rather than tailored to individual patients. These tests can incur excess costs and may delay appropriate psychiatric evaluation, admission, or transfer. Determining which patients benefit from additional workup before evaluation by a mental health professional is critical to providing quality care to patients and allowing for efficient ED throughput.

For patients who can participate in a history and physical examination, diagnostic testing may not be necessary before evaluation by a mental health professional. Clinical practice guidelines from ACEP clearly state that diagnostics such as labs and imaging should not be routinely performed in alert, cooperative patients presenting to the ED with psychiatric symptoms. Instead, testing should be guided by history and physical examination. The American Academy of Pediatrics states agreement with the ACEP regarding tailoring workup to needs of individual pediatric patients. If a patient reports a history concerning a life-threatening medical complaint, or has abnormal vital signs or physical examination findings, further diagnostics should be pursued.

If a patient has both an acute medical and psychiatric complaint, their medical complaint should be evaluated with appropriate workup, including any relevant diagnostics. It may be appropriate to defer evaluation of a non–life-threatening or chronic medical complaint to facilitate definitive psychiatric care for their life-threatening psychiatric illness.

Some patient presentations, such as delirium and substance-induced psychosis, are frequently confused with a primary psychiatric illness. Patients who are older, immunocompromised, or presenting with new-onset psychosis in the absence of prior history of mental health disorder or substance use may benefit from a tailored workup to determine whether there is a reversible medical cause for a patient's symptoms (**Table 211.1**).

Two of the most controversial screening labs are the UDS and the serum ethanol level. A UDS may assist disposition when leaving the hospital (ie, to a dual

TABLE 211.1	SCREENING TESTS FOR CONSIDERATION

Basic screening labs
CBC
CMP
Urinalysis
Urine pregnancy test
Additional studies to consider
TSH and free T_4
B_{12}/folate
ECG
Cerebrospinal fluid studies
UDS
Ethanol level
Head CT

CBC, complete blood count; CMP, complete metabolic panel; CT, computed tomography; ECG, electrocardiogram; TSH, thyroid-stimulating hormone; UDS, urine drug screen.

diagnosis program or substance use program). Since UDSs are notoriously inaccurate, rarely change ED management, and may take hours to collect, the ACEP clinical policy cautions that a UDS should not delay a patient's evaluation by a mental health professional. Both medical and psychiatric complaints are unreliable in patients who are under the influence of alcohol. There are no data to suggest that a specific serum ethanol level should be used as a cutoff to decide when it is appropriate for a patient to be evaluated by a mental health professional. Rather, patients who report psychiatric symptoms while intoxicated with alcohol should be reassessed when they are clinically sober.

Head CT should be avoided for patients with isolated psychiatric complaints unless there is a focal neurologic deficit present on examination, or a suspicion for head trauma.

Testing that is unlikely to change ED management should be deferred. But just because "screening labs" or additional tests aren't ordered in the ED, it doesn't mean that a patient's medical workup is completed. Further evaluation may certainly be pursued by the service admitting the patient or by the facility accepting patient for transfer (such as obtaining drug or ethanol levels, evaluating baseline renal/hepatic function for safe drug dosing), but this should not delay the patient's disposition. This is supported by two studies demonstrating that when laboratory testing is conducted after admission to a psychiatric service, an exceedingly low percentage of findings would have resulted in a change in ED management or disposition (0.19%-0.5%) if they had been identified while the patient was still in the ED.

In summary, for patients presenting to the ED with a psychiatric complaint, no additional life-threatening medical complaints, and no red flags on history, vital signs, or physical examination, "screening labs" or other tests are not indicated as part of an ED evaluation. If testing must be ordered, careful consideration should be given to which tests should be obtained to tailor a medical workup to the patient's specific presentation and risk factors, or which testing can be safely deferred until the patient has reached their next phase of care.

PEARLS

- Adult and pediatric patients presenting with psychiatric complaints who can participate in history and physical examination do not need routine labs if there are no red flags during history and physical examination.
- Special populations that should prompt consideration of a more thorough medical workup for psychiatric complaints include patients with new-onset psychosis, those with immunocompromised status, and older patients.
- Collection of a UDS provides little benefit in ED management of psychiatric complaints.
- Timing of assessment by the psychiatric consultants should be based on clinical sobriety, not an arbitrary ethanol level.
- Unless there is a suspicion of head trauma or a focal neurologic deficit on examination, head CTs are of limited utility in patients with isolated psychiatric complaints.

Suggested Readings

Anderson EL, Nordstrom K, Wilson MP, et al. American association for emergency psychiatry task force on medical clearance of adults part I: introduction, review and evidence-based guidelines. *West J Emerg Med*. 2017;18(2):235-242.

Bagøien G, Morken G, Zahlsen K, Aamo T, Spigset O. Evaluation of a urine on-site drugs of abuse screening test in patients admitted to a psychiatric emergency unit. *J Clin Psychopharmacol*. 2009;29(3):248-254.

Brown MD, Byyny R, Diercks DB, et al. Clinical policy: critical issues in the diagnosis and management of the adult psychiatric patient in the emergency department. *Ann Emerg Med*. 2017;69(4):480-498.

Chun TH, Mace SE, Katz ER, et al. Executive summary: evaluation and management of children and adolescents with acute mental health or behavioral problems. Part I: common clinical challenges of patients with mental health and/or behavioral emergencies. *Pediatrics*. 2016;138(3):e20161570.

Janiak BD, Atteberry S. Medical clearance of the psychiatric patient in the emergency department. *J Emerg Med*. 2012;43:866-870.

Parmar P, Goolsby CA, Udompanyanan K, Matesick LD, Burgamy KP, Mower WR. Value of mandatory screening studies in emergency department patients cleared for psychiatric admission. *West J EmergMed*. 2012;13(5):388-393.

Wilson MP, Nordstrom K, Anderson EL, et al. American Association for Emergency Psychiatry task force on medical clearance of adult psychiatric patients. Part II: controversies over medical assessment, and consensus recommendations. *West J Emerg Med*. 2017;18:640-646.

SECTION XVII
GENITOURINARY

212

CARING FOR THE PATIENT WHO HAS HAD GENDER AFFIRMING SURGERY

MATTHEW J. GRANT

According to recent estimates, approximately 1,000,000 Americans identify as transgender. Historically, this group of people have experienced neglect through systematic discrimination and prejudice, from lack of provider knowledge to deliberate refusal of care based on gender identity. To treat patients effectively and holistically, health-care providers must acknowledge the additional health-care disparities affecting this unique patient population. This starts with establishing mutual respect between the patient and health-care team.

Clinicians must also familiarize themselves with terminology specific to this group of people to promote open communication and demonstrate cultural safety. Important terminology includes surgical and nonsurgical interventions that patients may use to support their gender identity. Nonsurgical interventions may include such measures as binding or tucking, in which a patient compresses their breast and penis, respectively, to minimize their appearance and related gender dysphoria.

Gender affirming surgeries (GAS) describe a group of procedures that change a patient's appearance and/or bodily functions to transition toward their self-identified gender. The process of transitioning is not limited to surgery. Before undergoing GAS, patients have often already undergone rigorous physical, mental, and social transitions.

When caring for patients who have undergone GAS, it is important to familiarize yourself with common procedures to provide comprehensive care.

FEMINIZING PROCEDURES

"Bottom surgery" in transfeminine patients typically refers to manipulation of male genitalia to appear female. This may include penectomy and orchiectomy with vaginoplasty, clitoroplasty, and/or vulvoplasty. Patients may choose to have all or only some of these procedures, with each serving cosmetic and functional purposes.

Facial feminization surgery is a group of procedures to soften traditionally masculine bone structures. These procedures may include brow lift, rhinoplasty, frontal cranioplasty, and more. Nonsurgical interventions include the use of injections including Botox, fillers, silicone, and more. These injections help define and mold facial features toward a more traditionally feminine appearance.

Masculinizing Procedures

"Top surgery," also known as mastectomy, involves removal of breast tissue and relocation of the nipples to provide a more gender-congruent appearance.

"Bottom surgery" in transmasculine patients may include hysterectomy with or without salpingo-oophorectomy (removal of the uterus, ovaries, and fallopian tubes which prevents menstruation and prevent pregnancy). This may be additionally followed by one of the following:

- Phalloplasty and scrotoplasty involve manipulation of tissue to create traditional male genitalia. Again, this serves both a cosmetic as well as functional purpose.
- Metoidioplasty involves using native clitoral tissue following growth of the clitoris with long-term testosterone to create a small phallus.

General Considerations

Transgender persons are often misgendered during hospital registration process. This can be triggering for patients and studies suggest that using a transgender person's preferred name is linked to reduced depressive symptoms and increased patient-provider confidence. Standardizing the collection of SOGI information from all patients is recommended and has shown high acceptability among patients.

Though patients may have undergone GAS, they remain at risk for certain pathologies based on their assigned sex at birth that requires appropriate screening and surveillance. For example, a transfeminine patient with retained prostate may still be at risk for benign prostate hypertrophy and even prostate cancer. When considering cancer risk, or evaluating nonspecific abdominal pain in transgender patients, a full organ inventory is an essential step to ensuring comprehensive care. Reviewing medical and surgical history is critical. Viewing operative reports may be necessary for increased accuracy.

Health-care workers must also be aware that physical exams can be very uncomfortable for transgender patients, especially those who have undergone GAS. Using gender-neutral language, limiting observers, and using appropriately sized equipment can minimize patient discomfort. For example, to understand post-op complications in patients following vaginoplasty and the need for staged dilation, providers may opt to offer a pediatric speculum or even an anoscope to perform a pelvic exam. The use of smaller speculums may also increase tolerance of the procedure for patients who experience dysphoria related to vaginal examination and should be considered on a patient-by-patient basis.

Sexually transmitted disease/infection screening should be completed based on risk factors, exposures, and sexual activities. Risk assessment should be based on current anatomy and sexual behaviors.

It is also very important to recognize that transgender patients are at a significantly higher risk for depression, suicide, and intimate partner violence than the general population. Regularly screening patients for depression and suicidality is essential to their care.

Finally, due to the high demand for gender-affirming procedures and lack of insurance coverage, some patients may seek procedures outside of licensed medical centers. There may be a higher risk of serious complications including infection, allergic reaction, silicone pulmonary embolism, and organ damage. Providers must be aware that these complications can evolve over time.

Considerations for the Transfeminine Patient

It is important to recognize both acute and chronic postoperative complications from feminizing GAS. Acute complications can vary from infection and bleeding to necrosis and fistulation of the neovagina, all of which may require surgical consultation.

Chronic complications include scarring, urethral stenosis, dyspareunia, and in rare cases bowel obstruction from intestinal vaginoplasty. Following GAS, patients are also at an increased risk of UTI as the postsurgical urethra is considerably shorter. There is also an increased risk of intraneovaginal infections due to regular dilator use.

Depending on the type of GAS performed, transfeminine patients who have undergone vaginoplasty may have an increased susceptibility to certain STIs. While neovaginal STIs have not been extensively reported, HSV and HPV have been reported in neovaginas constructed from penile or scrotal tissue. *Chlamydia trachomatis* and *Neisseria gonorrhoeae* have been noted in both urethral and intestinal grafts. Recommendations for testing should take surgical history into consideration along with sexual practices and risk factors.

It is important to be aware that transgender women are often taking exogenous estrogen. Though the risk of VTE is lower with the new estrogen formulations, there is still a higher risk when compared to cisgender women, not on estrogen.

Considerations for the Transmasculine Patient

Post-op complications from transmasculine patients following GAS involve risk for infection and necrosis but are at a particularly higher risk for UTI, urinary catheter, and prosthetic malfunction when GAS include phalloplasty. In these cases, it is advised to involve surgical services such as urology and plastic surgery.

PEARLS

- Ask for and use appropriate pronouns, names, and genders to create a safe space and establish mutual respect.
- Screen for depression, suicidality, and intimate partner violence.
- Understand common GAS procedures and terminology.
- Recognize the acute and chronic postsurgical complications from GAS.
- Using gender-neutral language, limiting observers, and using appropriately sized equipment can minimize patient discomfort when performing physical exams.

Suggested Readings

James SE, Herman JL, Rankin S, Keisling M, Mottet L, Anafi M. (2016). *The Report of the 2015 U.S. Transgender Survey*. National Center for Transgender Equality; 2016.

Russell ST, Pollitt AM, Li G, Grossman AH. Chosen name use is linked to reduced depressive symptoms, suicidal ideation, and suicidal behavior among transgender youth. *J Adolesc Health*. 2018;63(4):503-505. PMID: 29609917.

213

Fournier Gangrene: A Lethal Infection You Can't Sit On!

Bobbi-Jo Lowie

With an average mortality rate of 20% to 30%, FG is a true emergency requiring prompt diagnosis and aggressive treatment. Named after Jean-Alfred Fournier, it is defined as a fulminant, necrotizing fasciitis of the perineal, genital, and/or perianal regions. FG is a rare disease but one with devastating effects if missed. Classically, sources of this soft tissue infection include the gastrointestinal tract (eg, perianal abscess, colonic perforation, malignancy), the genitourinary tract (eg, indwelling catheters, urethral calculi, urethral stricture), and local cutaneous disease (eg, hidradenitis suppurativa, skin ulcers). Local trauma, in the form of piercings, penile implants, drug injections, and rectal foreign bodies, is also a recognized factor in some cases. FG most frequently targets the scrotum and penis or anorectal region; however, advanced cases may involve the anterior abdominal wall, chest wall, or thighs. Classically, this necrotizing soft tissue infection spares deeper muscular structures.

Since survival hinges on early diagnosis, the clinician must be aware of its range of clinical symptoms and signs. A classic presentation of FG involves a diabetic male with rapidly progressing perineal pain, redness, and swelling. One may note crepitus upon palpation (due to bacterial gas formation) and pain out of proportion to examination. In more advanced stages, a dusky appearance and frankly necrotic tissue will appear. However, less classic patients, those who present very early, subtle skin changes on darker skin tones, or those with atypical presentations can easily be missed.

Most importantly, not all cases of FG are clinically overt. Early in the course, an inspection of the skin may be relatively benign or even normal, disguising severe damage to deeper tissue. In addition, this necrotizing soft tissue infection can fool the clinician with an insidious onset and slow progression. In these patients, systemic signs may tip the emergency provider off. Patients frequently present with SIRS, vomiting, lethargy, or, in advanced cases, septic shock with multiorgan failure. Typically, FG is associated with pain, but late-presenting infections may have relatively little pain due to destruction of nervous tissue.

FG is seen in women and children, though less commonly. Gynecologic sources of infection may include Bartholin gland abscess, septic abortions, and pelvic surgery. Pediatric variants may arise from circumcision, omphalitis, or a strangulated inguinal hernia. In addition, while the majority of patients are diabetic, several chronic conditions that impair immunity have been described as risk factors for this disease. These comorbidities include hypertension, obesity, cirrhosis, alcohol abuse, HIV, systemic lupus erythematosus, malignancy, and chronic steroid use. There has also been a recently identified association between the use of SGLT2 inhibitors and the development of FG, resulting in an FDA warning issued in 2018. The mechanism of action related to FG development is not fully understood, but it is important to recognize this association as these medications have become popular in the treatment of diabetes due to their favorable cardiac and renal profiles.

Because the clinical presentation does not always reveal the true extent of the infection, diagnostic imaging may be necessary to solidify the diagnosis. Because early diagnosis is critical to management, it is still important that the process of obtaining advanced imaging never delays surgical consultation. Plain radiography may show air along the fascial planes, but its absence does not exclude the diagnosis. Ultrasound may show an edematous scrotal wall with gas artifact and is useful to rule out other causes of acute scrotal pain, such as testicular torsion. CT and, less commonly, MRI are obtained to look for subcutaneous air, thickened fascia, and fat stranding. Of note, the testes are classically spared due to their direct blood supply from the aorta via the testicular arteries; therefore, any testicular involvement (ie, orchitis) points to a retroperitoneal or intra-abdominal source of infection. This may be delineated by advanced imaging (ie, CT or MRI).

Once the diagnosis of FG is entertained, an aggressive management plan should be instituted. Hemodynamic stabilization and early antibiotics are key components of treatment. Since the pathogenesis of this necrotizing fasciitis is polymicrobial, involving both aerobic and anaerobic bacteria, broad-spectrum antibiotics should be administered. Bacterial culprits include coliforms (most commonly *Escherichia coli*), *Streptococci*, *Staphylococci*, *Clostridia*, *Bacteroides*, and *Pseudomonas* spp. Rarely, fungus may be involved, such as *Candida albicans*. The standard regimen involves triple therapy, usually a combination of clindamycin, a beta-lactam antimicrobial, and metronidazole. Vancomycin may be added for extended gram-positive coverage. Amphotericin B may be used in the case of fungal infection. Most importantly, however, early aggressive surgical debridement is associated with a reduced mortality rate and is the mainstay of treatment. A multidisciplinary approach, involving emergent consultation with general surgery and urology or gynecology, is optimal. In surgery, purulent discharge described vividly as "dirty dishwater fluid" may be seen and necrotic tissue must be removed. Patients may require several surgical procedures to control the infection, with one study reporting 3.5 surgical procedures per patient on average.

The consequences of delayed diagnosis and/or surgical management are numerous, debilitating, and often life-threatening. In the short term, death may result from diabetic ketoacidosis, septic shock, coagulopathy, acute renal failure, or multiorgan failure. Those who survive may suffer from lifelong pain, sexual dysfunction, bowel incontinence, disfiguring scars, and/or lymphedema.

PEARLS

- FG may present atypically and requires a high index of suspicion, paying attention to systemic signs, the presence of crepitus, and pain out of proportion to examination.
- Complete thorough examinations in all patients with signs of infection, especially those with altered mental status.
- FG can be seen in women and children and in patients using SGLT2 inhibitors.
- Once suspected, resuscitative efforts, early antibiotics, and emergent surgical consultation are critical to saving the patient's life.
- Surgical consult should be initiated without awaiting imaging in patients whom this diagnosis is suspected.

SUGGESTED READINGS

Bourke MM, Silverberg JZ. Acute scrotal emergencies. *Emerg Med Clin North Am*. 2019; 37(4):593-610.

Chawla SN, Gallop C, Mydlo JH. Fournier's gangrene: an analysis of repeated surgical debridement. *Eur Urol*. 2003;43(5):572-575.

Eke N. Fournier's gangrene: a review of 1726 cases. *Br J Surg*. 2000;87(6):718-728.

Huayllani MT, Cheema AS, McGuire MJ, Janis JE. Practical review of the current management of Fournier's gangrene. *Plast Reconstr Surg Glob Open*. 2022;10(3):4191.

Montrief T, Long B, Koyfman A, Auerbach J. Fournier gangrene: a review for emergency clinicians. *J Emerg Med*. 2019;57(4):488-500.

Serrano OA, Bueno Moral AI, Martínez Bañón C, González Mesa E, Jiménez López JS. Fournier's gangrene under sodium-glucose cotransporter-2 inhibitors therapy in gynecological patients. *Int J Environ Res Public Health*. 2022;19(10):6261.

214

TESTICULAR TORSION TRICKERY

JEREMY ST. THOMAS AND KATHLEEN STEPHANOS

Testicular torsion occurs when the testis twists on itself, cutting off arterial blood supply to the affected testicle and resulting in ischemia. Without prompt recognition and intervention, complications such as infertility, diminished exocrine and endocrine function, infection, cosmetic deformity, and loss of the testis can occur. While it can occur at any age, there are two age peaks of testicular torsion—infancy and early adolescence. Normally, the testicle is fixed to the tunica vaginalis posteriorly and superiorly. Patients with congenital anatomic variants such as the "bell clapper" deformity, where the testicle is not attached posteriorly but instead 360° around the tunica vaginalis superiorly, are at increased risk for testicular torsion. This variant is estimated to occur in 12% of all males. Testicular torsion is the cause of acute scrotal pain in 15% to 30% of cases.

Symptoms of testicular torsion include sudden onset of pain, vomiting, redness, and swelling of the affected testicle. It is important to note that while trauma and vigorous physical activity can precipitate torsion, most cases occur in the absence of mechanical injury. On examination, typical findings include erythema, swelling, and a change in position of the testicle from a vertical to horizontal lie. An absent cremasteric reflex may occur during testicular torsion, but its presence does not rule out the diagnosis of torsion. Be wary of the adolescent male who complains of "abdominal pain" and always include a testicular examination in your evaluation of these patients, who may not readily admit to having pain in their genital area. In addition, abdominal pain and vomiting may be the only presenting symptoms—in one study, 11% of patients did not report other complaints.

Patients who have testicular torsion often have a history of testicular pain, having a pattern of intermittent pain, or "torsion/detorsion." Do not forego evaluation by ultrasound of a patient who presents with worsening testicular pain, simply because they had a recent negative ultrasound. Return precautions in the patient who is pain free and has a reassuring ultrasound should include a documented discussion of the torsion/detorsion phenomenon.

Another high-risk group is the nonverbal or preverbal patient who presents with acute pain or crying of unknown origin. These patients may present with vague complaints of agitation, irritability, or simply fussiness. Always do a GU examination to look for the cardinal signs of torsion in the male infant presenting with crying as a chief complaint. Nonpalpable testes should raise suspicion for torsion, as patients with undescended testicles are at increased risk for testicular torsion. With no obvious outward physical examination findings to suggest torsion of an intra-abdominal testicle, one must remember to consider it. Ultrasound findings of torsion of the intra-abdominal testicle can also be challenging to interpret compared with that of the testis in the scrotal sac. If clinical suspicion is high, surgical evaluation should still be pursued, regardless of ultrasound results.

Ultrasound is the test of choice for evaluation of torsion, with a specificity of 75% to 100% and a sensitivity of 85% to 100% depending on the sonographer; however, there is a risk of false-negative testing in patients with the twist high in the spermatic cord, or those with torsion-detorsion. In patients where there is high clinical suspicion for torsion, the appropriate surgical consultant should be contacted—typically urology or pediatric surgery. This should be done as soon as possible, regardless of ultrasound results.

Treatment consists of detorsion, either manually or surgically, as soon as possible. Salvage rates of testicular torsion plummet after 12 hours of symptoms, and ideally, torsion should be definitively fixed before 6 hours of symptoms. Manual detorsion should be tried if surgical resources are not available promptly. When performing manual detorsion, classic teaching is rotation of the testicle outward in a medial-to-lateral direction (like you are "opening a book"). Approximately one-third of cases will have the opposite rotation, so clinical symptom improvement and restoration of blood flow on ultrasound (if available) should be noted when performing manual detorsion. Remember, the testis may be twisted more than 360°, so continue detorsion until the patient expresses pain relief or a bedside ultrasound shows return of blood flow to the affected testicle. Even after manual detorsion, exploratory surgery must be done as soon as possible, as residual torsion may exist in up to one-third of patients.

PEARLS

- Consider testicular torsion in a preverbal or nonverbal patient who presents with crying, fussing, or irritability as the chief complaint.
- Do not hesitate to order an ultrasound in a patient with a history of testicle pain and a normal prior ultrasound—they may be experiencing torsion/detorsion.
- Consult your appropriate local surgeon for the management of torsion if symptoms are suspicious for torsion.
- To maximize salvage of the affected testicle, repair should ideally occur before 6 hours from the onset of pain.
- Manual detorsion should be attempted if a prolonged time to definitive repair is expected.

SUGGESTED READINGS

Anthony T, D'Arcy FT, Lawrentschuk N, et al. Testicular torsion and the acute scrotum: current emergency management. *Eur J Emerg Med*. 2016;23:160-165.

Gupta A, Croake A, Rubens D, Dogra V. Do not get it twisted: common and uncommon manifestations of testicular torsion. *J Ultrasound Med*. 2022;41(2):271-283. PMID: 33885184.

Keays M, Rosenberg H. Testicular torsion. *CMAJ*. 2019;191(28):E792. PMID: 31308008.

Ramos-Fernandez MR, Medero-Colon R, Mendez-Carreno L, et al. Critical urologic skills and procedures in the emergency department. *Emerg Med Clin North Am*. 2013;31(1):237-260.

215

PYELONEPHRITIS: WHEN IT'S COMPLICATED URINE TROUBLE

DEVANG PATEL AND DREW CHARLES

Pyelonephritis is a UTI of the upper urinary tract including the kidneys and ureter, typically resulting from an ascending lower cystitis, which is a lower UTI. Rarely, descending infections may result from hematogenous spread due to bacteremia. Clinical symptoms of pyelonephritis include fever, flank pain, nausea, vomiting, malaise, confusion (especially in the older patients), as well as dysuria or hematuria and urinary frequency. Patients suspected of having pyelonephritis should obtain a urinalysis with urine culture and sensitivity. Empiric treatment should be initiated based on risk factors, prior urine cultures, and common pathogens. *Escherichia coli* is the pathogen responsible for 75% to 95% of UTIs. Antibiotic resistance patterns vary considerably between regions, and treatment selection should reflect patient allergies, medication interactions, and local resistance patterns. Without prompt and appropriate treatment, pyelonephritis may be associated with significant morbidity with progression to sepsis in many cases. Providers can optimize care of patients with pyelonephritis in the ED by avoiding the common management errors described later.

One common error in the ED management of pyelonephritis is the use of antibiotics with poor renal tissue penetration. Although frequently used to treat cystitis, nitrofurantoin should not be used for patients with pyelonephritis because adequate renal tissue levels are not achieved. When cystitis symptoms are accompanied by fever, flank pain, costovertebral angle tenderness, or a prolonged duration of symptoms (>5-7 days), early pyelonephritis should be considered. When cystitis cannot clearly be distinguished from early pyelonephritis, nitrofurantoin and other medications with poor renal penetration such as fosfomycin should be avoided.

A second common error in ED management is failure to appropriately distinguish between uncomplicated and complicated pyelonephritis. ED disposition often depends upon whether the infection is uncomplicated or complicated. Uncomplicated pyelonephritis occurs in young, healthy, immunocompetent, nonpregnant females without known structural or functional abnormalities of the urinary tract.

Most patients with uncomplicated pyelonephritis who are not septic and able to tolerate oral medications can be managed as outpatients with oral antibiotics and follow-up of urine culture results. Common outpatient antibiotic regimens for uncomplicated pyelonephritis include ciprofloxacin 500 mg twice daily for 7 days, levofloxacin 750 mg daily for 5 days, or trimethoprim-sulfamethoxazole 160/800 mg twice daily for 14 days. There is a trend toward shorter treatment courses in recent years—consult up-to-date guidelines when prescribing.

Any case of pyelonephritis occurring in a male or someone who is pregnant, has diabetes, immunosuppressed (eg, transplant recipient), has a genitourinary abnormality whether functional (eg, neurogenic bladder) or structural (eg, nephrolithiasis), or has any underlying medical condition that increases the risk of infection is classified as complicated. In these patients, the risk of disease progression is greatly increased.

216

What Goes Up Must Come Down

Jessica Lange Osterman

Priapism is defined as a sustained erection, lasting longer than 4 hours, in the absence of sexual stimulation or persisting after the cessation of sexual stimulation. It is a rare but potentially devastating condition that can result in permanent erectile dysfunction for the patient and should be considered a urologic emergency when it presents to the ED.

Perhaps, the most common error in the management of priapism is the physician's failure to establish the etiology of priapism. There are two main types of priapism, ischemic and nonischemic, and their treatment differs significantly. Therefore, it is important for the treating physician to identify the type expediently to facilitate treatment. Ischemic, or low-flow, priapism is far more common and is a true urologic emergency that must be treated emergently to avoid permanent structural damage to the penis and permanent erectile dysfunction. In ischemic priapism, there is an accumulation of venous blood in the corpora, which leads to venous congestion, pain, ischemia, and, eventually, fibrosis. Ischemic priapism is essentially a compartment syndrome of the penis, and if it lasts longer than 24 hours, it is associated with up to a 90% rate of subsequent erectile dysfunction. The ischemic form is most often due to medication usage but can also be related to underlying conditions, such as sickle cell disease, hyperviscosity syndromes, or malignancy. Nonischemic, or high-flow, priapism is the rarer of the two forms and is caused by abnormal arterial inflow into the cavernosa. Nonischemic priapism is often associated with trauma and is typically either pain free or significantly less painful than the ischemic form. Aspiration and blood gas analysis of corporal blood are reliable methods for determining the category of priapism and can be performed if there is any clinical question of which type is present. If ischemic, corporal blood should be hypoxic, hypercarbic, and acidotic (generally Po_2 <30 mm Hg, Pco_2 >60 mm Hg, pH <7.25). In the nonischemic form, the cavernous blood gas should reflect normal arterial blood.

Treatment should be initiated expediently after determining the type of priapism present in the patient.

After establishing the type of priapism, another possible error is the failure to evaluate the underlying etiology for the condition when no obvious cause exists. In cases of ischemic priapism without a distinct history of contributory medications or drugs, a thorough workup should be done to rule out other associated conditions. Ischemic priapism may be the presenting symptom of a new malignancy such as lymphoma or be associated with hyperviscosity syndrome from another underlying malignancy. Likewise, in children, it can be the first presentation of sickle cell disease. In these situations, laboratory studies such as a complete blood count or hemoglobin electrophoresis may be helpful in establishing an underlying condition or cause.

Finally, the successful and emergent treatment of ischemic priapism is essential for restoring normal erectile function and avoiding significant morbidity. First-line therapy in the treatment of ischemic priapism focuses on corporal aspiration of venous blood as well as the instillation of alpha-adrenergic agonists, such as phenylephrine, into the corpora. The key to successful treatment is appropriate anesthesia to facilitate corporal drainage and detumescence; don't make the error of inadequately anesthetizing the patient. Anesthesia should be attained through performance of a dorsal penile block or a local penile shaft block. The dorsal penile block targets the left and right dorsal penile nerves that run at approximately 2 and 10 o'clock positions at the base of the penis. After cleansing, the physician should start by anesthetizing the skin over the 2 and 10 o'clock with superficial wheals of lidocaine without epinephrine (although some controversy exists about the use of epinephrine in these penile blocks, literature supporting its use is lacking). The needle should then be inserted about 0.5 cm into the skin or until the needle enters Buck fascia at the 2 and 10 o'clock positions. After aspirating to ensure the needle is not in a vessel, approximately 2 mL of lidocaine should be instilled at each location. A complete block will greatly facilitate the ease of aspiration and instillation of medications to achieve detumescence and restore normal penile function. If the patient is unable to tolerate one of the local penile blocks, moderate or conscious sedation should be considered to facilitate drainage. Aspiration alone resolves approximately 20% to 30% of cases of nonischemic priapism. For patients failing to detumesce after aspiration, the American Urological Association guidelines recommend starting with 300 mcg injections of phenylephrine into the corpora every 3 to 5 minutes. Patients receiving intracavernosal phenylephrine should have their blood pressure and heart rate monitored during and after instillation of the drug.

Treatment of nonischemic priapism is completely different. Since the nonischemic form is associated with the flow of well-oxygenated blood, there is no indication for removal of blood from the corpora or instillation of vasoconstrictors. This type generally does not necessarily represent an emergency, as outcomes do not worsen over time. Nonischemic priapism may actually improve spontaneously; thus, it may be treated with a period of observation after urgent referral to urology.

PEARLS

- First identify the subtype of priapism present.
- Investigation into the underlying cause can help guide treatment and the urgency of urologic intervention.

- Adequate anesthesia with a dorsal penile block will facilitate successful aspiration and aid in the restoration of normal penile function.
- If aspiration alone does not result in detumescence, consider intracavernosal phenylephrine administration.

Suggested Readings

Bivalacqua TJ, Allen BK, Brock GB, et al. The diagnosis and management of recurrent ischemic priapism in sickle cell patients, and non-ischemic priapism: an AUA/SMSNA guideline. *J Urol.* 2022;208(1):43-52.

Burnett AL, Bivalacqua TJ. Priapism: current principles and practice. *Urol Clin North Am.* 2007;24:631-642.

Levey HR, Segal RL, Bivalacqua TJ. Management of priapism: an update for clinicians. *Ther Adv Urol.* 2014;6(6):230-244.

Shlamovitz GZ. Dorsal penile nerve block. *Medscape.* October 8, 2015. http://emedicine.medscape.com/article/81077-overview

Vilke GM, Harrigan RA, Ufberg JW, Chan TC. Emergency evaluation and treatment of priapism. *J Emerg Med.* 2004;26(3):325-329.

217

The Bleeding Dialysis Fistula

Christina Sajak

Bleeding is a common reason for presentation to the ED, and as such, we as emergency physicians are well prepared to handle hemorrhage, regardless of the location of origin. Some sites, however, have increased potential for fatal hemorrhage, such as bleeding from a hemodialysis fistula. These fistulas are created by surgical anastomosis between an artery and a vein, and after maturation, are considered the preferred access site for patients with end-stage renal disease requiring hemodialysis, making them common among ED patients. Their purpose is to create a large caliber vessel capable of undergoing repetitive blood draws and withstanding high-volume flow during hemodialysis, which also makes them susceptible to high-volume bleeding.

In the case of dialysis fistula hemorrhage, as with all compressible sites of bleeding, after initial assessment, direct pressure should first be applied. This pressure must be constant and uninterrupted, with the minimum amount of surface area in contact. For example, if the wound would be covered by two fingers, do not place the entire palm of the hand down, as this spreads the force over a larger area, effectively decreasing pressure. Using folded gauze or an upside-down (small) bottle cap can aid with this. Patients who present from a hemodialysis center or via EMS may already have had attempted direct pressure. However, it is reasonable to attempt once in the ED to ensure uninterrupted pressure. If direct pressure alone for 10 minutes is unsuccessful, a hemostatic dressing can be considered in addition, such as gelatin sponges or topical thrombin.

In addition, the emergency physician must consider timing of the patient's last dialysis session, as heparin is used for anticoagulation around the time of access. If dialysis access occurred within the last few hours before hemorrhage, consider protamine administration for reversal of heparin. Evaluation of the patient's medication list may also elicit other reversible anticoagulants. Similarly, patients with end-stage renal disease are often considered to have platelet dysfunction and uremia. Thus, many emergency physicians consider the addition of desmopressin, or DDAVP in this instance, with mindfulness to its contraindications and lack of literature on this particular use. Maximum effect of DDAVP is usually seen in approximately 30 minutes.

If a physician has attempted direct pressure, topical hemostasis agents, and considered the addition of systemic medications and yet the bleeding continues, the patient may require additional intervention. If inspection of the fistula demonstrates a laceration, a suture can be placed in an attempt to repair it. Finally, if all other measures have failed, hemostasis can be achieved by placing a figure of eight stitches or purse string suture on the fistula.

If all else fails, or in cases of severe rapid hemorrhage, placing a tourniquet above and below the fistula site can aid in achieving a bloodless field to facilitate this bedside procedure. Because the graft has both arterial and venous flow, both tourniquets are required for hemostasis. If the sutures do not maintain hemostasis after the tourniquets have been released, consider reinitiating the tourniquets as a temporizing measure in severe hemorrhage. This is considered a last resort, as it holds the risk of thrombosing off the access site.

Of course, all life-threatening bleeding from a dialysis fistula should prompt an emergent vascular surgery consult concurrently with the measures above. As with all major bleeding, resuscitate these patients as indicated based on volume of blood loss, vital signs, and clinical stability, considering massive transfusion event activation if necessary. In addition, it is important to remember that even if hemostasis is achieved with one of the earlier mentioned methods, the patient will likely require monitoring to watch for rebleeding, and possibly further vascular studies to determine patency of the fistula after these interventions.

PEARLS

- As with all major bleeding, resuscitate appropriately with blood products based on clinical scenario and stability.
- Direct pressure should be applied with the minimum amount of surface area in contact with the area of hemorrhage.
- Consider reversal of any anticoagulation, particularly with protamine if patient has had a recent dialysis session, and consider DDAVP to counteract potential platelet dysfunction in patients with ESRD.
- Tourniquets should be applied both above and below the fistula for life-threatening hemorrhage.
- Consider the need for observation/further studies even in bleeding that achieves ED hemostasis, and consult vascular surgery emergently for severe or life-threatening bleeding or complication management.

Suggested Readings

ACEP Now. *Dialysis Access Emergencies*. ACEP Now. Accessed August 15, 2023. https://www.acepnow.com/article/dialysis-access-emergencies/?singlepage=1#:~:text=Any%20bleeding%20that%20warrants%20an

EM:RAP. *Suturing a Bleeding Dialysis Fistula*. EM:RAP. Accessed August 15, 2023. https://www.emrap.org/episode/suturinga/suturinga

Marsh AM, Genova R, Buicko Lopez JL. Dialysis fistula. [Updated May 23, 2023.] In: *StatPearls* [Internet]. StatPearls Publishing; 2023. https://www.ncbi.nlm.nih.gov/books/NBK559085/

218

What Are We Doing With Stones These Days?

Alvin Varghese and Ryan Spangler

Renal stone disease, and more specifically ureteral colic, is a common, bread-and-butter emergency medicine diagnosis. Nearly 2% of adult visits to the ED are for suspected renal colic. Despite this, the breadth of the disease, imaging options, and optimal treatments can seem to be a moving target.

Clinical Manifestations

The classic presentation of kidney stone is sudden-onset, episodic, severe flank pain that radiates to the ipsilateral groin associated with dysuria, urgency, and frequency. The renal capsule shares splanchnic innervation with the intestine, leading patients to also experience nausea and vomiting. Fever is generally not seen unless associated with infection.

The Best Diagnostic Study Should be Ordered to Assess Patients With Suspected Kidney Stones

Imaging is currently used for two purposes: to obtain information about the stone size and location and to confirm the diagnosis or rule out other diagnoses.

Noncontrast CT of the abdomen and pelvis is considered the gold standard imaging study, with the highest specificity and sensitivity for ureteral stone disease (almost 100%). However, comparing the negative predictive value of noncontrast CT versus contrast-enhanced CT showed that contrast-enhanced CT can safely exclude obstructing ureteral stones. This is important because of the benefit of the IV contrast in diagnosing other abdominopelvic pathology, such as aortic disease and appendicitis.

Ultrasound can also be used in evaluating renal or ureteral stones. Ultrasound is quick, inexpensive, and noninvasive and does not expose patients to radiation. In patients with high clinical suspicion for stone disease, using ultrasound as the primary and only imaging modality has shown to be both safe and effective in appropriately identifying stone disease, without missing alternate diagnoses. The sensitivity and specificity, however, vary depending on the performer's skill, the patient's body habitus, as well as the equipment.

KUB x-ray has poor sensitivity and specificity for identifying stones and cannot accurately size a stone. It has very limited utility in an emergency setting.

MEDICAL MANAGEMENT FOR KIDNEY STONES?

Pain. In these patients, one of the main goals of care is pain control. Due to prostaglandin's role in renal colic pain, NSAIDs are the preferred treatment. Narcotics, in comparison, do not inhibit prostaglandins and, in some studies, have shown to increase ureteric muscle tone. In patients with GI bleeds and impaired renal function, narcotics are helpful in the treatment of renal colic pain and can also be used concurrently with NSAIDs for patients with severe pain.

IV Hydration. Although a 2010 Cochrane review did not find any benefit for aggressive fluid resuscitation in stone passage in acute ureteral colic, it is important to consider IV hydration for individuals who are dehydrated from vomiting or a decrease in oral intake secondary to the pain. Antiemetics may be needed to transition to oral fluids for discharge.

MET. Most stones less than 5 mm in diameter pass spontaneously. There is a progressive decrease in stone passage when larger than 4.5 mm in diameter is very unlikely for stones larger than 10 mm in diameter. The more distally in the ureter the stone is located, the greater the likelihood of spontaneous passage (84% below sacroiliac joint vs 52% above). For the stones that do not pass spontaneously, MET initiation, such as tamsulosin 0.4 mg daily, an alpha-blocker, can also be considered to assist stone passage. Alpha-blockade inhibits the smooth muscle contraction in the ureter, theoretically facilitating the stone passage. Study outcomes are mixed regarding the efficacy of MET. Some studies suggest that it is only beneficial for patients with 5- to 10-mm stones and not in patients whose stones measure less than 5 mm. In many cases, the risks of starting alpha-blockers are relatively low, but in patients at risk for hypotension and falls, careful consideration in use is warranted.

WHEN SHOULD PATIENTS GET ANTIBIOTICS?

In patients with evidence of urinary tract infection based on urinalysis in the setting of kidney stones, they should be prescribed antibiotics. Studies suggest that pyuria as low as 5 WBC/hpf has 86% sensitivity and 79% specificity for a positive culture, and the likelihood increases as the concentration of WBCs increases. A urine culture should always be sent if there are signs of infection to help guide antibiotic therapy. Generally, the antibiotics should target urinary pathogens, including *Escherichia coli*, *Klebsiella*, and *Proteus*. Options include a fluoroquinolone such as ciprofloxacin or levofloxacin. If, however, there is a concern for fluoroquinolone resistance, interaction, or side effect, patients can get a dose of long-acting parenteral agent such as IV ceftriaxone and be sent home with oral TMP-SMX, amoxicillin-clavulanate, or cefpodoxime.

Patients with recent urologic procedures or hospitalization should also get pseudomonal coverage, such as a carbapenem if admitted or oral fluoroquinolone if outpatient treatment. Although most patients can be discharged home with PO antibiotics, admission for IV antibiotics and decompressive surgery for patients with obstructive stones and UTI are a urologic emergency.

Disposition. Patients can be discharged home in many cases. If the patient has their pain well controlled, does not have renal dysfunction, and is tolerating oral, discharge is often possible. Patients with uncontrolled pain, intractable vomiting, systemic symptoms of infection, single kidney, or significant obstruction should be admitted for further observation and consideration for surgical procedure. Patients with obstruction AND infection should have urgent urologic consultation to prevent progression to sepsis and septic shock.

Renal stone disease frequently presents in a typical, predictable manner as the cause of flank pain. However, the risk of misdiagnosis exists due to similar presentations of other common, sometimes deadly illnesses. Using a well-thought-out plan for imaging in the appropriate situations can help expedite patient care and ensure safe evaluation. Knowledge of the complications of renal stone disease, particularly infection and acute kidney injury, will help the emergency physician provide optimal treatment for patients with renal stone disease.

PEARLS

- UTI along with obstructed stone is a urologic emergency.
- Poor outcomes are seen in patients with kidney stones combined with decreased renal function, previous urologic interventions, and symptoms of infections.
- MET initiation is best used for stones between 5 and 10 mm.
- Obtain CT with contrast when considering other pathologies as it can safely exclude stones.
- A urine culture should always be sent if there are signs of infection to help guide antibiotic therapy.

SUGGESTED READINGS

Jennings CA, Khan Z, Sidhu P, et al. Management and outcome of obstructive ureteral stones in the emergency department: emphasis on urine tests and antibiotics usage. *Am J Emerg Med*. 2019;37(10):1855-1859.

Raskolnikov D, Hall MK, Ngo SD, et al. Strategies to optimize nephrolithiasis emergency care (STONE): prospective evaluation of an emergency department clinical pathway. *Urology*. 2022;160:60-68.

219

Don't Get Left Behind: New STI Treatment Guidelines

Bobbi-Jo Lowie and Matthew Poremba

Many ED visits are accounted for by patient's seeking management of STIs. Appropriate management of STIs is a critical public health issue, with an all-time high of over 2.5 million sexually transmitted infections reported in 2019. The Centers for Disease Control and Prevention most recently published updated guidance for the treatment of sexually transmitted infections in 2021. This chapter will focus on key updates and antimicrobial pearls from this guidance.

NEISSERIA GONORRHOEAE
The first-line treatment for uncomplicated infections is now ceftriaxone 500 mg IM × 1 dose for adult patients. For patients weighing 150 kg or more, the recommended dose is ceftriaxone 1 g IM × 1 dose. Previously, the recommended treatment was ceftriaxone 250 mg IM plus azithromycin 1 g po × 1 dose. Azithromycin is no longer recommended as resistance rates have increased almost 10-fold from 2013 to 2019. Uncomplicated infections for infants and children weighing less than or equal to 45 kg is 25 to 50 mg/kg of ceftriaxone IM once (up to a max dose of 250 mg).

CHLAMYDIA TRACHOMATIS
The first-line treatment for infection is now doxycycline 100 mg po every 12 hours for 7 days. Multiple observational studies and a Cochrane systematic review found treatment failure rates to be higher with azithromycin when compared to doxycycline. In patients where adherence to a 7-day regimen may be a concern, azithromycin 1 g × 1 dose may be a reasonable alternative regimen. If azithromycin is used, it may warrant posttreatment evaluation and testing, as a randomized trial comparing doxycycline to azithromycin for treatment for rectal chlamydia infection showed a 100% cure rate with doxycycline versus 74% cure rate with azithromycin. For infants and children weighing less than 45 kg, the preferred regimen is erythromycin base or ethyl succinate 50 mg/kg body weight/day orally divided into four doses daily for 14 days. For infants and children weighing 45 kg or more but less than 8 years old, the preferred treatment is azithromycin 1 g orally once. Doxycycline is avoided in patients younger than 8 years due to the risk of tooth staining.

TRICHOMONAS VAGINALIS
Trichomoniasis is estimated to be the most prevalent nonviral STI worldwide, and prevalence in the United States is 2.1% among females and 0.5% among males. Recommended treatment for vaginal trichomoniasis is metronidazole 500 mg po twice daily for 7 days. This is supported by a study which demonstrated a lower proportion of women with positive results at 1-month test of cure with a 7-day regimen versus a single dose of metronidazole 2 g. There is no published trial comparing these dosing strategies in male patients, and the recommended dose for men is metronidazole 2 g po once.

PELVIC INFLAMMATORY DISEASE
First-line treatment for PID is ceftriaxone 500 mg IM once (or 1 g for patient's weighing 150 kg or more) and doxycycline 100 mg po every 12 hours plus metronidazole 500 mg po every 12 hours for 14 days. This regimen covers vaginal microflora as well as *N. gonorrhoeae* and *C. trachomatis*. Even if endocervical screening is negative for *N. gonorrhoeae* and *C. trachomatis*, this does not rule out upper genital tract infections, and all PID regimens should still include coverage of these pathogens.

Both PID and trichomoniasis treatment regimens contain metronidazole. Patients have historically been advised to avoid alcohol while taking metronidazole out of concern that they may develop a disulfiram-like reaction. However, unlike disulfiram, metronidazole does not inhibit acetaldehyde dehydrogenase. A review found no trials, in vitro studies, or adverse event reports that provided evidence of this reaction. Thus, it is not required for patients to abstain from alcohol use while taking metronidazole.

MYCOPLASMA GENITALIUM
Resistance-guided therapy is preferred if testing is available. For macrolide-sensitive *Mycoplasma genitalium*, the preferred treatment is doxycycline 100 mg po every 12 hours for 7 days followed by azithromycin 1 g po once plus 500 mg po daily for 3 additional

days. For macrolide-resistant *M. genitalium* and in cases where resistance testing is not available, the preferred treatment is doxycycline 100 mg po every 12 hours for 7 days followed by moxifloxacin 400 mg po daily for 7 days. Azithromycin monotherapy is not an appropriate treatment due to high rates of macrolide resistance and treatment failures associated with this regimen.

PENICILLIN AND BETA-LACTAM ALLERGIES

Penicillin allergies are frequently over reported. The updated STI guidelines place a new emphasis on validation of patient-reported penicillin and beta-lactam antibiotic allergies documented. These medications have a vital role in management of STIs, and in some situations, might be the only appropriate option. Practitioners should take care to clarify true hypersensitivity reactions from drug intolerances and idiosyncratic reactions. Skin testing for penicillin allergy is recommended if there is any indication of a prior IgE-mediated hypersensitivity reaction, or to definitively remove a documented allergy from the medical record. The Penicillin Allergy Decision Rule (PEN-FAST) is a clinical tool that can be used to guide risk assessment and treatment and need for formal allergy testing. The use of third- and fourth-generation cephalosporins, such as ceftriaxone, is generally appropriate due to low rates of cross-reactivity with patients who are allergic to penicillin (<1%).

PEARLS

- Ceftriaxone 500 mg IM for patients weighing less than 150 kg and ceftriaxone 1 g IM for patients weighing 150 kg or more are the first-line treatments for gonorrhea in adults.
- Doxycycline 100 mg po for 7 days is the first-line treatment for chlamydia in adults, or azithromycin 100 mg once po if adherence is a concern.
- Recommended trichomonas treatment is metronidazole 2 g × 1 dose for male patients and metronidazole 500 mg twice daily for 7 days for female patients.
- First-line PID treatment is a three-drug regimen consisting of ceftriaxone 500 mg IM × 1 dose, doxycycline 100 mg po bid × 14 days, and metronidazole 500 mg po bid × 14 days.
- Metronidazole does not inhibit acetaldehyde dehydrogenase, and avoiding alcohol consumption while taking metronidazole is unnecessary.

SUGGESTED READINGS

Dombrowski JC, Wierzbicki MR, Newman LM, et al. Doxycycline versus azithromycin for the treatment of rectal chlamydia in men who have sex with men: a randomized controlled trial. *Clin Infect Dis*. 2021;73(5):824-831.

Fjeld H, Raknes G. Er det virkelig farlig å kombinere metronidazol og alkohol? [Is combining metronidazole and alcohol really hazardous?]. *Tidsskr Nor Laegeforen*. 2014; 134(17):1661-1663.

Páez-Canro C, Alzate JP, González LM, Rubio-Romero JA, Lethaby A, Gaitán HG. Antibiotics for treating urogenital chlamydia trachomatis infection in men and non-pregnant women. *Cochrane Database Syst Rev*. 2019;1(1):CD010871.

Trubiano JA, Vogrin S, Chua KYL, et al. Development and validation of a penicillin allergy clinical decision rule. *JAMA Intern Med*. 2020;180(5):745-752.

Workowski KA, Bachmann LH, Chan PA, et al. Sexually transmitted infections treatment guidelines, 2021. *MMWR Recomm Rep*. 2021;70(4):1-187. PMID: 34292926.

220

Pitfalls in Prostatitis

Meghin Moynihan and Ryan Spangler

Prostatitis is a common urinary tract syndrome characterized by voiding symptoms, genitourinary pain, and potentially sexual dysfunction. Unfortunately, it is frequently misdiagnosed in the ED but continues to be the most common urologic diagnosis in men younger than 50 years and third most common diagnosis in men 50 years and older in the outpatient setting.

Prostatitis is further classified into four separate groups: ABP, CBP, CP/CPPS, and asymptomatic inflammatory prostatitis. Though only a small percentage of men with prostatitis have bacterial infections—ABP approximately 4% and CBP 10% of all cases—clinicians should keep prostatitis on their differential when urologic symptoms are present upon arrival to the ED.

An appropriate diagnosis of prostatitis includes a detailed patient history, as this can differentiate acute versus chronic presentation and will affect the duration of treatment. Most patients, regardless of classification, will experience voiding symptoms, testicular, low back or perineal pain, and potentially ejaculatory symptoms.

Patients with ABP typically present with fever, chills, malaise, and myalgias in addition to dysuria and pain. Physical exam findings are pertinent to diagnose ABP. The prostate will be tender, warm, swollen, and firm. In the setting of ABP, do not attempt to massage the acutely inflamed prostate as this has potential to spread infectious organisms. Complications to be aware of in ABP include bacteremia, epididymitis, prostatic abscess, and potential conversion to chronic prostatitis. To rule out prostatic abscess, a transrectal ultrasound or CT of the abdomen and pelvis should be considered.

CBP and CP/CPPS may prove more difficult to diagnose in the ED as physical exams are typically normal, but there may be prostate tenderness, firm induration, or softening present. Patients may experience more-prolonged urogenital symptoms such as relapsing dysuria, urgency, and frequency as well as perineal discomfort. A low-grade fever may also be present. This "prolonged period" is considered 3 or more months.

In any case of prostatitis, a urinalysis and urine culture should be collected. Although prostatic massage is not recommended in ABP, it is recommended to collect urine directly after a prostatic massage is performed in patients with CBP for best results. Screening for sexually transmitted infections is also warranted for those who may be at risk.

Treatment of prostatitis should be tailored to the specific classification of prostatitis and can be further categorized by age and complications of presentation (Table 220.1).

An area of controversy in prostatitis management is often how long to continue antibiotic treatment courses. An extended course of therapy for 4 to 6 weeks is no longer indicated for every patient. In fact, patients with ABP who are uncomplicated should only be treated for 14 days. If the presence of a prostatic abscess, bacteremia, or any other complications in ABP, treatment should be extended to a 4-week course. Those being treated for CBP should also receive an entire course of treatment for 4 weeks duration.

TABLE 220.1

CLASSIFICATION	LIKELY PATHOGEN	TREATMENT
ABP	Age <35 yr: - *Neisseria gonorrhoeae* - *Chlamydia trachomatis* Age >35 yr: - Enterobacteriaceae or *Escherichia coli (most common)* - *Enterococcus* sp. - *Pseudomonas aeruginosa*	Complicated[a] (by bacteremia or prostatic abscess): - Levofloxacin 750 IV q24h - Ciprofloxacin 400 mg IV q12h - Piperacillin/tazobactam 3.375 g IV q6h or 4.5 g IV q8h - Ceftriaxone 2 g IV q24h - Cefotaxime 2 g IV q8h Uncomplicated (<35 yr old): - Ceftriaxone 500 mg IM × 1 dose OR cefixime 400 mg PO × 1 dose followed by doxycycline 100 mg PO bid for 14 d Uncomplicated (>35 yr old): - Levofloxacin 750 mg PO daily - Ciprofloxacin 500 mg PO bid - Trimethoprim/sulfamethoxazole 1 double-strength tablet PO bid
CBP	- Enterobacteriaceae (80%) - *Enterococci* (15%) - *P. aeruginosa*	Preferred: - Ciprofloxacin 500 mg PO bid - Levofloxacin 750 mg PO daily Alternative: - Trimethoprim/sulfamethoxazole 1 double-strength tablet PO bid - If *C. trachomatis* suspected: azithromycin - If no other PO alternatives, may consider Fosfomycin (ESBL-producing organism)
CP/CPPS	Consider atypical pathogens: - *Mycoplasma hominis* - *C. trachomatis* - *Trichomonas vaginalis* - *Ureaplasma urealyticum*	Utilize the 5 As: - Avoid dietary or physical activities that exacerbate symptoms. - Antibiotics: if 4-wk treatment fails, no further antibiotics recommended unless confirmed UTI. - Alpha blockers: tamsulosin 0.4 mg PO daily OR doxazosin 1 mg PO daily OR prazosin 1 mg PO bid/tid OR terazosin 1 mg PO qhs - Anti-inflammatory agents - 5-Alpha reductase inhibitor (men >50 with enlarged prostate): tamsulosin 0.4 mg PO daily

ABP, acute bacterial prostatitis; CBP, chronic bacterial prostatitis; CP/CPPS, chronic prostatitis/chronic pelvic pain syndrome; ESBL, extended-spectrum beta-lactamase; IV, intravenous; IM, intramuscular; PO, by mouth; UTI, urinary tract infection.

[a]Ertapenem for resistant Enterobacteriaceae; Imipenem or meropenem for resistant PsA.

Antibiotic Selection Pearls

Fluoroquinolones remain the mainstay of antibiotic therapy for bacterial prostatitis treatment—unless bacterial prostatitis is presumed to be STI related—due to their favorable pharmacokinetics such as good bioavailability and excellent penetration into the prostate. Unfortunately, resistance rates continue to rise for their efficacy in treating *Escherichia coli*. Due to this, local resistance rates should be considered and assessed before initiating therapy with these agents. Fluoroquinolones are no longer considered appropriate therapy for gonococcal infections due to their resistance rates. Patient-specific factors should also be considered when prescribing prolonged courses of fluoroquinolones, including older age, concomitant therapy with QT-prolonging agents, or a history of *Clostridium difficile*. In these instances, other agents should be considered and risks and benefits should be weighed.

If levofloxacin is selected for treatment, be sure to prescribe 750 mg daily due to treatment failures with the 500 mg dose, even though 500 mg daily is the FDA-approved dosing regimen. If selecting trimethoprim/sulfamethoxazole, keep in mind this agent has no activity against pseudomonas.

PEARLS

- A thorough patient history is pertinent to determine and classify a proper diagnosis of acute versus chronic prostatitis which ultimately influences treatment decisions.
- Examination of prostate should be considered to aid in diagnosis, and imaging to evaluate for abscess can guide management.
- For ABP, only 14 days of antibiotic therapy when no other complications are present
- Before selecting antibiotic therapy, be sure to check resistance rates in your area of practice as fluoroquinolone resistance continues to rise.

Suggested Readings

Campos SC, Elkins JM, Sheele JM. Descriptive analysis of prostatitis in the emergency department. *Am J Emerg Med*. 2021;44:143-147.

Lipsky BA, Byren I, Hoey CT. Treatment of bacterial prostatitis, clinical infectious diseases. *Clin Inf Dis*. 2010;50(12):1641-1652.

Polackwich AS, Shoskes DA. Chronic prostatitis/chronic pelvic pain syndrome: a review of evaluation and therapy. *Prostate Cancer Prostatic Dis*. 2016;19(2):132-138.

Rees J, Abrahams M, Doble A, Cooper A; Prostatitis Expert Reference Group (PERG). Diagnosis and treatment of chronic bacterial prostatitis and chronic prostatitis/chronic pelvic pain syndrome: a consensus guideline. *BJU Int*. 2015;116(4):509-525.

221

Chronic Catheters—Do I Treat That UA?

Arthur J. Pope and Chinezimuzo Ihenatu

UTIs make up approximately 30% of all hospital-related infections, of which 70% to 80% are related to indwelling catheterization. Because a sizable portion of these can be preventable, recent literature and interventions regarding urethral catheterization aim to reduce and prevent morbidity associated with Foley catheter placement. The best way to do so is to minimize initial urethral catheterization, maintain sterile technique if insertion is deemed appropriate, and promptly identify the time for removal. In this chapter, we identify the common types of bacteria associated with CAUTIs, detail how to properly obtain a urine sample for testing, and identify when it is appropriate to treat a positive UA in a patient with an indwelling catheter.

Contributing Factors

Bacteria can be introduced to the urinary system by contamination of the Foley during insertion or from ascension of bacteria colonized at the distal urethra. There are several risk factors associated with CAUTIs, even when sterile technique is used, the chief of which is prolonged catheterization. The daily risk of getting a CAUTI is 3% to 7% with indwelling catheters. Female sex, diabetes mellitus, old age, history of previous catheterization, and prolonged hospital stay all contribute to additional risk of developing CAUTI. The best way to avoid CAUTIs is to avoid unnecessary insertion of Foley altogether.

Types of Bacteria

Sixty percent to 80% of CAUTIs are due to gram-negative bacteria. The most common bacterial etiology of CAUTIs is *Escherichia coli*. Other offending organisms include *Klebsiella*, coagulase-negative staph, *Pseudomonas aeruginosa*, and *Enterococci* spp. *Proteus mirabilis* is more common among patients with chronic catheters and is rarely seen in patients with short-term catheters.

Obtaining the Sample

It is important to properly obtain the sample to get the most accurate results, so do not forget to use a sterile technique. In addition, the sample should not be taken directly from the Foley bag—instead, it should be taken from the port. Some patients with chronic indwelling catheters may have a biofilm or colonization, while others may have an active infection. The Foley should be exchanged entirely if the patient has a long-term indwelling catheter in order to avoid contamination with biofilm or colonization. However, don't remove the Foley if there is prior history of difficult insertion or recent urologic surgery. Consider reaching out to urology instead. If Foley catheter exchange is not possible, the clinician should treat the patient while advising early catheter exchange in the treatment course.

Symptomatology and When to Treat

Many chronic indwelling catheter patients with bacteriuria will be asymptomatic. Just as in patients without catheters, CA-ASB should not be treated or even screened for infection as this leads to unnecessary treatment and increased antibiotic resistance. However, chronically catheterized patients with CA-ASB should be treated in the case of pregnancy and patients undergoing urologic surgery.

Antibiotic selection should be guided by culture results; however, that can take time and is usually not possible in the ED setting. It is appropriate to use UA, but ensure that a urine culture is sent to the lab for testing. Presenting symptoms typically guide empiric treatment with assistance from local antibiograms. For patients who complain of dysuria, urgency, or frequency, treatment can follow that of acute cystitis. Treat empirically as acute complicated UTI for patients with fever, flank pain, and other symptoms showing evidence of disease beyond the bladder. For patients with chronic catheters and a history of UTIs, it is helpful to look at prior urine cultures and sensitivities to help with antibiotic selection. Hemodynamically unstable patients warrant broad-spectrum antibiotics, such as cefepime and piperacillin-tazobactam, as simple CAUTIs can lead to sepsis and bacteremia. Once CAUTI is suspected, Foley exchange should occur as noted earlier. Ultimately, the best way to treat is to remove the catheter entirely or transition to intermittent catheterization, a decision not typically made by ED providers, as most patients presenting have chronic catheters.

PEARLS

- Prevention is key in the management of CAUTIs. Know the indications for Foley catheterization to avoid CAUTIs.
- It is best to obtain urine samples for culture testing after the Foley has been exchanged in patients with chronic indwelling catheters who are suspected to have CAUTIs to prevent contamination from biofilm and colonization. However, perform a thorough history to ensure the Foley can be removed safely.
- Evaluate and treat for asymptomatic bacteriuria only in the cases of pregnancy and urologic procedures.
- Look at prior culture data to help guide treatment in symptomatic patients with evidence of a UTI on UA.

Suggested Readings

Klevens RM, Edwards JR, Richards CL Jr, et al. Estimating health care-associated infections and deaths in U.S. Hospitals, 2002. *Public Health Rep.* 2007;122(2):160-166. PMID: 17357358.

Li F, Song M, Xu L, Deng B, Zhu S, Li X. Risk factors for catheter-associated urinary tract infection among hospitalized patients: a systematic review and meta-analysis of observational studies. *J Adv Nurs.* 2019;75(3):517-527. PMID: 30259542.

Raz R, Schiller D, Nicolle LE. Chronic indwelling catheter replacement before antimicrobial therapy for symptomatic urinary tract infection. *J Urol.* 2000;164(4):1254-1258. PMID: 10992375.

Trautner BW. Management of catheter-associated urinary tract infection. *Curr Opin Infect Dis.* 2010;23(1):76-82. PMID: 19926986.

SECTION XVIII
THORACIC

222

PROPERLY RISK STRATIFY THE PATIENT WITH SUSPECTED PULMONARY EMBOLISM

KELLY WILLIAMSON

VTE is a common cardiovascular disease with an annual incidence of 100 to 200 per 100,000. PE is the most serious VTE, as it interferes with both circulation and gas exchange and can lead to significant right heart strain and death from RV failure. The diagnosis of PE can be challenging, as presenting signs and symptoms are nonspecific, including dyspnea, chest pain, or syncope. Commonly obtained studies used in the evaluation of these complaints, such as laboratory tests, an electrocardiogram, and chest x-ray, do not confirm the diagnosis of PE. To further complicate the diagnosis, 30% of patients with a confirmed PE have no determinable risk factor and 40% have normal oxygen saturation readings.

To properly risk stratify patients undergoing evaluation for PE, it is essential to determine a clinical pretest probability. The PIOPED investigators confirmed the accuracy of a provider's "gestalt" or global clinical judgment. However, as one must have adequate experience to form an appropriate clinical judgment, there are also several clinical decision instruments that can be applied. The Wells score evaluates the presence or absence of specific clinical factors to determine the likelihood that a PE exists: signs and symptoms of DVT (3 points), an alternative diagnosis that is less likely than PE (3 points), heart rate greater than 100 beats/min (1.5 points), immobilization or surgery in the previous 4 weeks (1.5 points), previous DVT/PE (1.5 points), hemoptysis (1 point), and malignancy (1 point). Application of a provider's clinical judgment in conjunction with an established prediction rule such as the Wells score allows one to classify patients with suspected PE into categories of probability.

In patients with a low pretest probability of PE (Wells score <2), it is appropriate to apply the PERC rule. Developed by Kline and colleagues, the PERC rule advocates that PE can be excluded if all of the following eight criteria are present: age less than 50 years, pulse less than 100 beats/min, oxygen saturation readings greater than 95%, no hemoptysis, no estrogen use, no surgery or trauma requiring hospitalization within 4 weeks, no prior VTE, and no unilateral leg swelling. In patients with a low pretest probability of PE, the PERC rule has a sensitivity of 96% and a specificity of 27%. There are three common pitfalls that must be avoided when applying the PERC rule.

First, a patient must meet all eight criteria or the sensitivity of its application decreases. In addition, this rule is only valid in patients with a low pretest probability of PE and should not be applied in the moderate- and high-probability groups. Finally, there were patients excluded from the initial PERC trial, including patients with cancer and those with personal or a family history of thrombophilia, so its application may be unreliable in these patient populations.

If a patient has a moderate pretest probability of PE or does not meet the PERC exclusion criteria in the low probability group, then it is appropriate to order a D-dimer assay. D-dimer is a degradation product of cross-linked fibrin that is elevated in PE because of the concurrent activation of coagulation and fibrinolysis. While the D-dimer has a high sensitivity and negative predictive value for the diagnosis of PE, its specificity is poor as fibrin is also produced in other inflammatory states. The D-dimer should not be used in patients with a high pretest probability of PE given its low negative predictive value in that population. In addition, a negative D-dimer may also not exclude PE in patients with symptoms over 14 days or those already on anticoagulation. As D-dimer concentration also typically increases with age, Douma and colleagues instituted an "age-adjusted" D-dimer cutoff value of patient's age $\times$ 10 mcg/L. In patients aged 50 years or older with a low to moderate pretest probability, this modified cutoff greatly increased the proportion of patients in whom PE could be safely excluded.

In patients with a high pretest probability of PE or those in the low or moderate groups with a positive D-dimer, a CTA of the chest is the next step in the diagnostic workup. The PIOPED II trial established that CTA has 83% sensitivity and 96% specificity for the diagnosis of PE. The addition of venous compression ultrasonography of the lower extremities does not significantly alter the posttest probability of PE in patients with a negative CTA, though may be helpful in proceeding to treatment without obtaining a CTA in certain patient populations, such as those whose renal function precludes contrast administration and in pregnant patients. Given the negligible utility of repeat CTA after an initial negative study, Kline and colleagues published a clinical decision rule recommending that patients with dyspnea and a normal CTA undergo echocardiography given the high probability of isolated RV dysfunction or overload. If patients are unable to undergo CTA testing, then ventilation-perfusion scintigraphy ($\dot{V}/\dot{Q}$ scan) is also an option; the sensitivity of a high-probability scan was 77.4% and the specificity for a very low probability or normal scan was 97.7%.

For patients with a positive CTA, the PESI can be applied to determine the risk of a 30-day mortality using 11 clinical criteria that are assigned varying point values: age, sex, history of cancer, history of heart failure, history of chronic lung disease, heart rate greater than 110 bpm, systolic blood pressure less than 100 mm Hg, respiratory rate greater than 30 breaths per minute, temperature less than 36 °C, altered mental status, and oxygen saturation less than 90%. For those patients with very low risk (score <65), all studies showed a 30-day mortality of less than 2%, and low-risk (66-85) patients had a 90-day mortality of 1.1%. A noninferiority trial further demonstrated that very-low-risk and low-risk patients could have been treated as outpatients in the appropriate clinical setting.

The prevalence of confirmed PE in patients undergoing diagnostic workup is low (10%-35%). It therefore becomes necessary to utilize these diagnostic strategies to achieve a balance between appropriate diagnosis and avoidance of unnecessary testing. A diagnostic algorithm is provided in **Figure 222.1**.

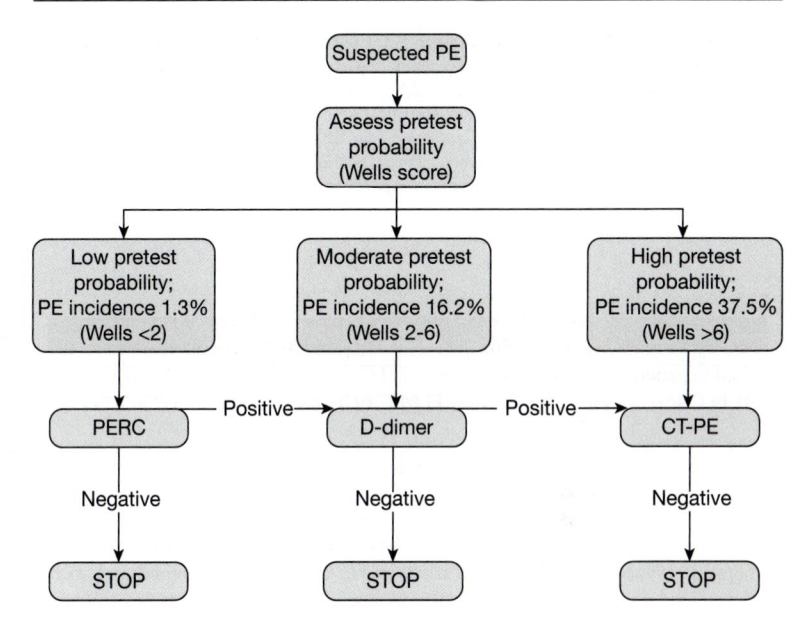

```
                    ┌──────────────┐
                    │ Suspected PE │
                    └──────┬───────┘
                           │
                    ┌──────▼───────┐
                    │ Assess pretest│
                    │  probability  │
                    │ (Wells score) │
                    └──────┬───────┘
           ┌───────────────┼───────────────┐
           ▼               ▼               ▼
   Low pretest      Moderate pretest   High pretest
   probability;    probability;        probability;
   PE incidence 1.3%  PE incidence 16.2%  PE incidence 37.5%
   (Wells <2)      (Wells 2-6)         (Wells >6)
        │                  │                  │
        ▼   —Positive—▶    ▼   —Positive—▶    ▼
      PERC              D-dimer            CT-PE
        │                  │                  │
     Negative           Negative           Negative
        ▼                  ▼                  ▼
       STOP               STOP               STOP
```

FIGURE 222.1 Risk stratification algorithm. CT, computed tomography; PE, pulmonary embolism; PERC, pulmonary embolism rule-out criteria.

PEARLS

- Determination of clinical pretest probability is the foundation of any diagnostic strategy and may be established by clinical gestalt or application of the Wells score.
- In patients with a low pretest probability of PE, one may apply the PERC rule. A PE can be ruled out if all eight criteria are present.
- If a patient has a moderate pretest probability of PE or does not meet the PERC exclusion criteria in the low probability group, order a D-dimer assay.
- In patients with a high pretest probability or those in the low to moderate groups with a positive D-dimer, a CTA is the next step in the diagnostic workup.

SUGGESTED READINGS

Douma RA, le Gal G, Sohne M, Righini M, Kamphuisen PW, Perrier A et al. Potential of an age adjusted D-dimer cut-off value to improve the exclusion of pulmonary embolism in older patients: a retrospective analysis of three large cohorts. *BMJ*. 2010; 340:c1475.

Jaff MR, McMurtry MS, Archer SL, et al. Management of massive and submassive pulmonary embolism, iliofemoral deep vein thrombosis, and chronic thromboembolic pulmonary hypertension: a scientific statement from the American Heart Association [published correction appears in *Circulation*. 2012;126(7):e104] [published correction appears in *Circulation*. 2012;125(11):e495]. *Circulation*. 2011;123(16):1788-1830.

Kline JA, Mitchell AM, Kabrhel C, Richman PB. Courtney DM. Clinical criteria to prevent unnecessary diagnostic testing in emergency department patients with suspected pulmonary embolism. *J Thromb Haemost*. 2004;2(8):1247-55.

Maraziti G, Cimini LA, Becattini C. Risk stratification to optimize the management of acute pulmonary embolism. *Expert Rev Cardiovasc Ther*. 2022;20(5):377-387. PMID: 35544707.

Triantafyllou GA, O'Corragain O, Rivera-Lebron B, Rali P. Risk stratification in acute pulmonary embolism: the latest algorithms. *Semin Respir Crit Care Med*. 2021;42(2):183-198.

223

KNOW THE MANAGEMENT OF HEMOPTYSIS

DANIEL CALICK AND MATTHEW P. BORLOZ

Hemoptysis describes "the spitting up of blood" from a subglottic source. Massive hemoptysis is inconsistently defined as a variable volume of blood produced within 24 hours; however, a more practical definition of massive hemoptysis is a sufficient volume of blood to impair gas exchange or result in hemodynamic instability. Pitfalls in the evaluation of hemoptysis include failure to identify the true source of bleeding (ie, pulmonary vs gastrointestinal), a lack of appreciation for the danger posed by the underlying cause (eg, pulmonary embolism, bioterrorism agents), and underestimation of the volume or rate of hemorrhage. The alveoli can harbor several hundred milliliters of blood before gas exchange is measurably impaired.

CAUSES

Determining the precise etiology of hemoptysis is often not possible in the ED, and admission for further investigations is frequently necessary (**Table 223.1**). The bronchial arteries account for 90% of cases of massive hemoptysis, with the balance from pulmonary or systemic arteries. Bronchitis, bronchiectasis, pneumonia, and tuberculosis are responsible for approximately 80% of cases of hemoptysis; the latter three and bronchogenic carcinoma most commonly cause massive hemoptysis. Though rare in pediatrics, hemoptysis is often secondary to an infectious etiology or foreign body aspiration.

A directed history should focus on risk factors for VTE and tuberculosis; a history of tobacco use, immunosuppression, vasculitis, coagulopathy, or chronic bronchopulmonary disease; the use of antithrombotic agents; exposure to toxins; signs and symptoms of acute infection; and recent chest trauma or procedures. Attempts should be made to quantify the volume of blood expectorated (though often inaccurate) and describe its composition (ie, gross blood, clots, blood-streaked sputum).

Helpful findings on physical examination include evidence of DVT; petechiae or ecchymosis to suggest thrombocytopenia, platelet dysfunction, or coagulopathy; a diastolic murmur of mitral stenosis; abnormal lung sounds; and any new murmur that might suggest endocarditis, particularly in patients who are febrile. For patients of darker complexion, the identification of petechiae may be difficult but is aided by checking for blanching of the skin (petechiae will not blanch) and searching for lesions of the buccal mucosa or conjunctivae. Bedside ultrasound may identify signs of VTE, particularly

TABLE 223.1 CAUSES OF HEMOPTYSIS

Bioterrorism agents
- Anthrax
- Plague
- Tularemia

Cardiac disease
- Congenital heart disease
- Congestive heart failure
- Endocarditis
- Mitral stenosis

Chronic lung conditions
- **Bronchiectasis**
- Chronic obstructive pulmonary disease

Coagulopathy or platelet dysfunction (drug induced or endogenous)

Infectious
- **Bronchitis**
- Fungal or parasitic infection
- Lung abscess
- **Pneumonia**
- **Tuberculosis**

Inflammatory/autoimmune disease
- Goodpasture disease
- Systemic lupus erythematosus
- Wegener granulomatosis

Malignancy (primary or metastatic)

Toxins
- Cocaine abuse
- Nitrogen dioxide inhalation

Trauma
- Blunt or penetrating chest trauma
- Foreign body aspiration
- Iatrogenic

Vascular
- Bronchovascular fistula
- Collagen vascular disease
- Dieulafoy lesion
- Pulmonary arteriovenous malformation
- **Pulmonary embolism**

Other
- Catamenial hemoptysis (pulmonary endometriosis)
- Cryptogenic (no cause identified despite thorough evaluation, up to one-third of patients)
- Pseudohemoptysis (upper gastrointestinal or upper airway source of bleeding)

Bolded items are either particularly common causes of hemoptysis or those that would be unfortunate to miss due to patient or public health implications.

right heart strain or DVT. The oral and nasal cavities should be inspected for an upper airway source of bleeding, and if the history is insufficient to confirm hemoptysis instead of hematemesis, a nasogastric aspirate can be tested for the presence of blood. Testing the pH of the bloody material may be illuminating (acidic = gastrointestinal source, alkaline = pulmonary source).

CXR will be abnormal in more than 50% of patients with hemoptysis. Stable patients with nondiagnostic CXR should undergo chest CT with IV contrast. If suspicion is high for pulmonary embolism, the IV contrast bolus should be timed for CT pulmonary angiography. Results of CT will determine the need for bronchoscopy, as well as subsequent management. Laboratory testing depends on patient specifics but may include markers of bleeding severity and respiratory failure (hemoglobin, arterial blood gas), studies to diagnose the underlying cause (creatinine, coagulation studies, sputum Gram stain, acid-fast bacillus, urinalysis, D-dimer), as well as tests to facilitate treatment (crossmatch, thromboelastography).

MANAGEMENT

Patients with massive hemoptysis are ideally managed at a facility with interventional pulmonologists (for balloon tamponade, topical hemostatic application, or iced saline lavage, among other options), interventional radiologists (for bronchial artery embolization if bronchoscopic interventions are unsuccessful), and thoracic surgeons (for lobectomy or pneumonectomy if other measures fail). Transfer should be pursued if these services are not available at the presenting facility. Unstable patients will benefit from measures to optimize oxygenation and ventilation and efforts to avoid asphyxiation from blood filling the airways and rapidly eliminating interfaces for gas exchange. Blood products are transfused to correct anemia, optimize hemodynamics, and correct coagulopathy. If the side of bleeding can be determined based on history, examination, or imaging, the patient should be placed in a bleeding-lung-down position to exploit gravity and keep blood from spilling into the nonhemorrhagic lung. In recent years, TXA has been studied as an adjunct to managing hemoptysis. Though data are limited, nebulized TXA in stable adults with nonmassive hemoptysis has resulted in quicker resolution of hemoptysis and shorter hospital length of stay. Existing studies relied on a dose of 500 mg every 8 hours.

When massive hemoptysis results in frank or impending respiratory failure, endotracheal or endobronchial intubation should be performed. The use of a size 8.0 tube, or larger, is desirable to facilitate clot removal and introduction of a flexible bronchoscope. If the side of bleeding has been determined, and the bleeding is imminently life-threatening, the unaffected lung may be isolated by intubation of the main bronchus (eg, if right lung bleeding, intubate left main bronchus). This is ideally performed with bronchoscopic guidance. Intubating the right main bronchus is complicated by occlusion of the right upper lobe bronchus. If performed blindly, rotating the tube 90° in the direction of the desired side may aide in correct placement. Tube position should be confirmed by CXR. If this fails, placement of a double-lumen tube by an anesthesiologist may be considered when available.

Most hemoptysis will be "nonmassive," and many patients with minimal hemoptysis (<30 mL in 24 hours) are ultimately discharged pending normal vital signs, a stable ED course, a workup that has reasonably excluded acute life threats (eg, pulmonary embolism, anemia), the absence of comorbid cardiopulmonary conditions or known malignancy, and reliable outpatient follow-up. In other words, hemoptysis alone does not mandate hospital admission.

> **PEARLS**
>
> - Carefully inspect the oral and nasal cavities to evaluate for an upper airway source of bleeding.
> - Patients with massive hemoptysis should ideally be managed at a facility with interventional pulmonologists and radiologists, as well as thoracic surgeons.
> - If identified, the bleeding lung should be placed in a dependent position.
> - In cases of life-threatening massive hemoptysis, intubation of the main bronchus of the nonbleeding lung with a size 8.0 or larger tube should be attempted.
> - Nebulized TXA may prove beneficial in the management of hemoptysis.

Suggested Readings

Atchinson PRA, Hatton CJ, Roginski MA, Backer ED, Long B, Lentz SA. The emergency department evaluation and management of massive hemoptysis. *Am J Emerg Med*. 2021; 50:148-155. PMID: 34365064.

Davidson K, Shojaee S. Managing massive hemoptysis. *Chest*. 2020;157(1):77-88. PMID: 31374211.

Hurt K, Bilton D. Haemoptysis: diagnosis and treatment. *Acute Med*. 2012;11(1):39-45.

Simon DR, Aronoff SC, Del Vecchio MT. Etiologies of hemoptysis in children: a systematic review of 171 patients. *Pediatr Pulmonol*. 2017;52(2):255-259. PMID: 27575742.

Wand O, Guber E, Guber A, Epstein Shochet G, Israeli-Shani L, Shitrit D. Inhaled tranexamic acid for hemoptysis treatment: a randomized controlled trial. *Chest*. 2018;154(6):1379-1384. PMID: 30321510.

Yendamuri S. Massive airway hemorrhage. *Thorac Surg Clin*. 2015;25:255-260.

224

Use High-Flow Nasal Cannula in Patients With Mild-to-Moderate Respiratory Distress From Hypoxemia

Matthew Welles and Neil K. Dasgupta

Emergency physicians often classify patients with respiratory distress into select categories based on the severity of illness. Patients with mild-to-moderate respiratory distress generally have the ability to phonate and do not demonstrate significant hypoxemia, as measured by pulse oximetry. In contrast, patients with severe respiratory distress may have significant hypoxemia, hypercarbia and altered mental status, or signs of imminent respiratory failure (ie, severe tachypnea, cyanosis). Some patients may even present with a mixture of hypoxemia and hypercarbia. HFNC has been established as a therapy for patients with mild-to-moderate hypoxemic respiratory failure and rescue therapy for patients not tolerating other oxygen delivery methods.

HFNC devices can deliver up to 70 L/min of heated, humidified oxygen to an adult patient. In contrast to the traditional nonrebreather mask that entrains room air through side-port 'holes, HFNC devices can deliver an FiO_2 close to 100% because of flow rates that exceed the patient's intrinsic peak inspiratory flow. HFNC devices decrease upper airway dead space by washing out carbon dioxide, thus optimizing minute ventilation. In addition, the high flow decreases respiratory effort and respiratory rate while maintaining alveolar ventilation while increasing end-expiratory lung volume. HFNC devices may provide a small amount of PEEP, though this remains controversial. Several studies have suggested that HFNC devices can generate approximately 5 to 8 cm H_2O of PEEP. The amount of PEEP generated is dependent upon nasal prong position and whether the patient's mouth is open or closed. Finally, the heated and humidified air improves patient tolerance of the device and may enhance mucociliary clearance.

At present, the best evidence for the use of HFNC is in the patient with isolated hypoxemia due to pneumonia that does not require immediate airway management and mechanical ventilation. A prospective, multicenter, randomized controlled trial in patients with hypoxemic respiratory failure and normal work of breathing demonstrated decreased mortality with the use of HFNC compared with NIV. Importantly, mortality was a secondary outcome, and the benefit was primarily seen in patients with pneumonia. Patients with chronic lung disease were excluded from this trial. HFNC may also be used in patients with hypoxemia due to other etiologies (ie, congestive heart failure); however, the evidence that supports its use is less robust.

Several ICU studies before and during the COVID-19 pandemic have shown that the use of early HFNC in patients with hypoxia can reduce rates of intubation. These findings were not replicated in ED-based studies or a meta-analysis of such. However, given the shorter length of therapy in the ED, it could be due to lower incidence of therapy failure and need for greater sample sizes to detect such a difference.

The use of HFNC for patients with hypercapnic respiratory failure is limited to case reports. It is important to note that HFNC devices do not have a direct effect on tidal volume or respiratory rate, the two primary determinants of ventilation and carbon dioxide exchange. Risks of HFNC use in this specific patient population include the administration of high levels of oxygen that may mask worsened pulmonary function and delayed intubation. Studies have shown to delayed intubation, especially greater than 48 hours from initiation of HFNC has worse outcomes.

HFNC has also been used for preoxygenation and to provide apneic oxygenation for patients undergoing RSI. The evidence for this is mixed, and no study formally demonstrates the superiority of HFNC to conventional preoxygenation; however, HFNC may extend the safe apneic period during intubation. Some evidence shows that NIV is superior for preoxygenation in patients with severe hypoxemia. Emergency physicians should consider each strategy on a case-by-case basis.

PEARLS

- HFNC is a safe, effective oxygenation method that may be more effective for patients in extremis for a variety of reasons.
- HFNC delivers heated, humidified oxygen at a high concentration and washes out dead space from the upper airway while reducing work of breathing.
- HFNC has been proven to reduce rates of intubation in hypoxic respiratory failure.

- HFNC should not be routinely used for patients with hypercapnic respiratory failure. NIV is a better choice.
- Despite mixed evidence, HFNC is an effective method of preoxygenation for RSI and may extend the safe apneic time during intubation.

Acknowledgments

We gratefully acknowledge the contributions of previous edition authors, Ross McCormack and Jonathan Elmer, as portions of their chapter have been retained in this revision.

Suggested Readings

Chua MT, Ng WM, Lu Q, et al. Pre- and apnoeic high-flow oxygenation for rapid sequence intubation in the emergency department (the Pre-AeRATE trial): a multicentre randomised controlled trial. *Ann Acad Med Singap*. 2022;51(3):149-160.

Frat JP, Quenot JP, Badie J, et al. Effect of high-flow nasal cannula oxygen vs standard oxygen therapy on mortality in patients with respiratory failure due to COVID-19: the SOHO-COVID randomized clinical trial. *JAMA*. 2022;328(12):1212-1222.

Frat JP, Thille AW, Mercat A, et al. High-flow oxygen through nasal cannula in acute hypoxemic respiratory failure. *N Engl J Med*. 2015;372:2185-2196.

Miguel-Montanes R, Hajage D, Messika J, et al. Use of high-flow nasal cannula oxygen therapy to prevent desaturation during tracheal intubation of intensive care patients with mild-to-moderate hypoxemia. *Crit Care Med*. 2015;43(3):574-583.

Ricard JD, Roca O, Lemiale V, et al. Use of nasal high flow oxygen during acute respiratory failure. *Intensive Care Med*. 2020;46(12):2238-2247.

Vourc'h M, Asfar P, Volteau C, et al. High-flow nasal cannula oxygen during endotracheal intubation in hypoxemic patients: a randomized controlled clinical trial. *Intensive Care Med*. 2015;41(9):1538-1548.

225

Know Which Patients With Submassive Pulmonary Embolism May Benefit From Thrombolytic Therapy

Curtis Dickey and Joseph Schramski

A general understanding of the different classifications of PE is crucial to appropriately care for patients with acute PE. Treatment options for patients with massive PE and low-risk PE are straightforward. For massive PE, the severe afterload on the RV must be emergently unburdened either with thrombolysis or surgical embolectomy. For low-risk PE, standard anticoagulation is adequate. For patients with submassive PE (also

Hemodynamics	Classification	Risk	Imaging Evidence of RV Dysfunction	Biochemical Markers of RV Dysfunction
Stable	Non-massive	Low risk	No	No
	Sub-massive	Intermediate-low risk	Yes -OR-	Yes
	Sub-massive	Intermediate-high risk	Yes -AND-	Yes
Unstable*	Massive	High risk		

* Hypotension with systolic blood pressure <90, drop in systolic blood pressure >40 for >15 min, or requires vasopressor/ionotropic support and is not explained by other causes.

FIGURE 225.1 Classifications of pulmonary embolism. RV, right ventricle.

referred to as intermediate risk), the selection of the right therapeutic intervention remains controversial. For this group of patients, the benefits of thrombolysis (ie, decrease in death, pulmonary hypertension, and recurrent PE) may be offset by the risk of major bleeding events, such as ICH. Further classifying this heterogeneous group into intermediate-low risk and intermediate-high risk may support a better benefit-to-risk ratio (**Figure 225.1**).

For patients with a newly diagnosed PE, evidence of RV dysfunction can be detected on the CTA of the chest, ECHO, and biochemical markers. RV dysfunction is indicated on CTA of the chest if the ratio of the internal diameter of the RV to the left ventricle is greater than 0.9 in the transverse plane. On ECHO, RV dysfunction is defined as any one of the following findings:

- RV end-diastolic diameter greater than 30 mm (parasternal long-axis or short-axis view)
- Right-to-left ventricular end-diastolic diameter greater than 0.9 (apical or subcostal four-chamber view)
- Hypokinesis of the right ventricular free wall (any view)
- Tricuspid systolic velocity greater than 2.6 m/s (apical or subcostal four-chamber view)

Biochemical markers of RV dysfunction include the following lab abnormalities:

- BNP greater than 90 pg/mL or NT-proBNP greater than 900 pg/mL.
- Troponin I greater than 0.06 mcg/L or troponin T greater than 0.01 mcg/L.

Other clinical findings not included in categorizing PE that may encourage escalation of treatment:

- Tachycardia, bradycardia, hypoxemia, signs of respiratory distress, patient feeling of impending doom, extensive clot burden, lactate greater than 2, shock index greater than 1, diaphoresis, large clot in transit, syncope, cool extremities, mottling, changes on electrocardiogram suggestive of right heart strain, extensive DVT, and deterioration despite current treatment

The use of systemic thrombolysis in patients with a submassive PE might be considered for hemodynamically stable individuals who have objective radiographic and biochemical evidence of RV dysfunction (intermediate to high risk) without absolute contraindication for thrombolysis. However, the evidence for systemic thrombolysis, even in this specific patient population, remains uncertain because of the lack of standardization on the type, dose, or route of thrombolytic administration used in recent studies. Equally important is the timing of initiating anticoagulation after administration of the thrombolytic agent. Major bleeding in various trials is loosely defined as intracranial hemorrhage, a decrease in hemoglobin of 2 g/dL within 24 hours that requires a transfusion, or the need for endoscopic, radiologic, or surgical intervention. For patients older than 65 years, the risk of bleeding with thrombolysis is too high to provide therapeutic benefit. A common criticism of the studies evaluating this relationship is often critiqued for overly aggressive anticoagulation with heparin while giving thrombolytics.

CDT, where thrombolytic medications are administered via a catheter placed directly into the pulmonary arteries, has shown promise for carefully selected intermediate-high-risk patients. While recent studies have demonstrated the benefit of a lower dose of thrombolytic therapy with ultrasound guidance when compared to anticoagulation alone, it has not been compared to systemic administration of thrombolytic agents. However, the first clinical trial comparing the two (NCT03581877) will hopefully give us better insight. Until then it would seem reasonable to prefer CDT in any patient with increased risk of bleeding who needs thrombolytics. Because the pulmonary circulation receives 100% of the cardiac output in comparison with cerebral or coronary circulations, it can be hypothesized that the systemic dose required to lyse the clot may not need to be as high as that for a stroke or a STEMI nor should it necessitate a special catheter to deliver it to the pulmonary circulation to mitigate risk of bleeding. Until further trials are done, the optimal dose of thrombolytic therapy for patients with intermediate-high-risk submassive PE is one that causes the least harm and provides the most economic benefit. **Figure 225.2** illustrates a PE algorithm.

PEARLS

- Submassive PE is a heterogeneous group that is defined as hemodynamically stable with evidence of RV dysfunction but can further be broken down into intermediate-low-risk and intermediate-high-risk populations.
- RV dysfunction can be detected on CTA of the chest, ECHO, BNP, or troponin.
- There are currently many ongoing trials evaluating lower-dose systemic thrombolytics and effectiveness of CDT.
- If above 65 years old, high risk of bleeding, or relative/absolute contraindications to systemic thrombolytics may consider CDT, surgical intervention, IR intervention, or reduced dose in those with intermediate-high-risk PE. The risk of bleeding with thrombolysis likely outweighs the benefit in patients older than 65 years.
- The optimal dose of thrombolytic therapy for patients with intermediate-high-risk submassive PE is one that causes the least harm and provides the most economic benefit.

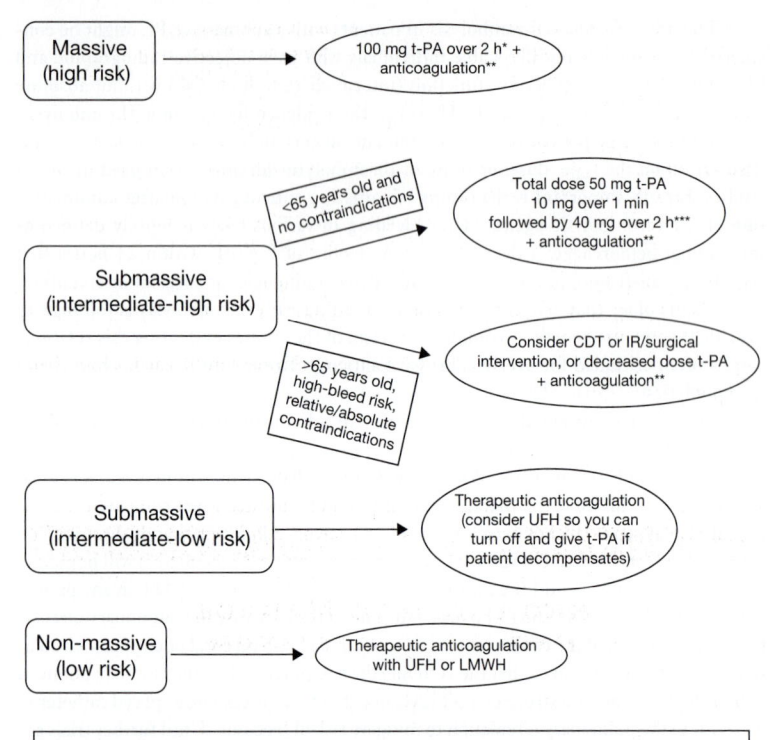

Decision-making algorithm for pulmonary embolism

Massive (high risk) → 100 mg t-PA over 2 h* + anticoagulation**

Submassive (intermediate-high risk)
- <65 years old and no contraindications → Total dose 50 mg t-PA, 10 mg over 1 min followed by 40 mg over 2 h*** + anticoagulation**
- >65 years old, high-bleed risk, relative/absolute contraindications → Consider CDT or IR/surgical intervention, or decreased dose t-PA + anticoagulation**

Submassive (intermediate-low risk) → Therapeutic anticoagulation (consider UFH so you can turn off and give t-PA if patient decompensates)

Non-massive (low risk) → Therapeutic anticoagulation with UFH or LMWH

*If crashing patient then can bolus over 15 min. If cardiac arrest due to PE then can bolus 50 mg.

**UFH likely preferred since you can turn it off. Can start before or after t-PA given. Common practice to hold while actively receiving thrombolytics. Restart when aPTT back to <2 times normal. Some may also wait to see if fibrinogen is at least 150-200 after t-PA to start anticoagulation.

***Dosing adapted from MOPETT trial. (if <50 kg patient then total dose 0.5 mg/kg of t-PA, 10 mg administered in 1 min, followed by rest over 2 h)

FIGURE 225.2 Decision-making algorithm for pulmonary embolism. aPTT, activated partial thromboplastin time; CDT, catheter-directed thrombolysis; IR, interventional radiology; LMWH, low-molecular-weight heparin; PE, pulmonary embolism; t-PA, tissue plasminogen activator; UFH, unfractionated heparin.

Suggested Readings

Avgerinos ED, Jaber W, Lacomis J, et al. Randomized trial comparing standard versus ultrasound-assisted thrombolysis for submassive pulmonary embolism: the SUNSET sPE trial. *JACC Cardiovasc Interv*. 2021;14(12):1364-1373.

Chatterjee S, Chakraborty A, Weinberg I, et al. Thrombolysis for pulmonary embolism and risk of all-cause mortality, major bleeding, and intracranial hemorrhage: a meta-analysis. *JAMA*. 2014;311(23):2414-2421.

Engelberger RP, Moschovitis A, Fahrni J, et al. Fixed low-dose ultrasound-assisted catheter-directed thrombolysis for intermediate and high-risk pulmonary embolism. *Eur Heart J*. 2015;36(10):597-604.

Kline J, Nordenholz KE, Courtney DM, et al. Treatment of submassive pulmonary embolism with tenecteplase or placebo: cardiopulmonary outcomes at 3 months: multicenter double-blind, placebo-controlled randomized trial. *J Thromb Haemost*. 2014;12(4):459-468.

Kucher N, Boekstegers P, Muller OJ, et al. Randomized controlled trial of ultrasound-assisted catheter directed thrombolysis for acute intermediate-risk pulmonary embolism. *Circulation*. 2014;129(4):479-486.

Meyer G, Vicaut E, Danays T, et al. Fibrinolysis for patients with intermediate-risk pulmonary embolism. *N Engl J Med*. 2014;10(370):1402-1411.

Sharifi M, Bay C, Skrocki L, Rahimi F, Mehdipour M; "MOPETT" Investigators. Moderate pulmonary embolism treated with thrombolysis (from the "MOPETT" *Trial*). *Am J Cardiol*. 2013;111(2):273-277.

Triantafyllou GA, O'Corragain O, Rivera-Lebron B, Rali P. Risk stratification in acute pulmonary embolism: the latest algorithms. *Semin Respir Crit Care Med*. 2021;42(2):183-198. PMID: 33548934.

Zuo Z, Yue J, Dong BR, et al. Thrombolytic therapy for pulmonary embolism. *Cochrane Database Syst Rev*. 2021;4:CD004437.

226

Know How to Manage Pneumomediastinum

Ani Aydin

A pneumomediastinum, or mediastinal emphysema, occurs secondary to a sudden increase in intrathoracic pressure, causing free air to surround the mediastinal structures. The origin of the free air can be disruptions in the pharynx, the tracheobronchial tree including the alveoli, or the esophagus.

Regardless of the etiology of the free air, once it dissects the perivascular connective tissue, it leads to air in the mediastinal space. With superior extension, the air can further dissect into the neck's subcutaneous, retropharyngeal, and visceral spaces. The subcutaneous space in the neck is contiguous with other subcutaneous spaces in the body, which can lead to diffuse spread of emphysema. Inferior extension of the free air can cause invasion of the retroperitoneum and extraperitoneal spaces.

Free air secondary to alveolar rupture will also result in a pneumothorax. Dissection of the alveolar free air along the bronchovascular sheaths and extension into the mediastinum is known as the *Macklin effect*. Extension of the free air into the pericardium can cause a pneumopericardium. Rupture of the esophagus can lead to mediastinitis. While a spontaneous pneumomediastinum is usually benign, ultimately, the prognosis and treatment of this disease depend on the etiology and severity of the disease.

Pathophysiology

Spontaneous Pneumomediastinum

A spontaneous pneumomediastinum is a rare event with a low rate of recurrence. This entity can result from increased intrathoracic pressure due to forced expiration against a closed epiglottis, or Valsalva maneuver, as can occur with forceful coughing, vomiting, sneezing, or strenuous activity. In the literature, this is most often described in young men or pregnant women, with risk factors that predispose to the development of spontaneous pneumomediastinum, including smoking, asthma, idiopathic pulmonary fibrosis, and chronic obstructive lung disease.

Secondary Pneumomediastinum

Air in the mediastinum is classified as a secondary pneumomediastinum when the etiology of the free air can be identified and can result from iatrogenic, traumatic, or nontraumatic injuries. An iatrogenic pneumomediastinum can occur after a procedure or instrumentation of the aerodigestive systems, such as traumatic intubations, tracheostomy placements, bronchoscopies, or endoscopies. This can also result from operative interventions of the tracheobronchial tree or esophagus. A traumatic pneumomediastinum can occur after blunt chest trauma or after penetrating injuries to the chest or abdomen.

There are several causes of a nontraumatic pneumomediastinum, including acute severe exacerbation of obstructive diseases, such as asthma or COPD exacerbations, which can result in ruptured alveoli or pulmonary blebs. Other causes include complicated childbirth with severe straining or inhalation of toxic fumes or recreational drugs. Strenuous activity or sports, especially those associated with changes in altitude, such as skydiving or scuba diving, have also been known to cause a pneumomediastinum. Finally, positive pressure ventilation, especially when associated with high airway pressures, could lead to a secondary pneumomediastinum.

Tension Pneumomediastinum

A tension pneumomediastinum, also known as a *malignant pneumomediastinum*, is a rare and life-threatening condition. Similar to other forms of obstructive shock, a tension pneumomediastinum can exert excess pressure in the mediastinal space, leading to cardiovascular collapse, and requires immediate treatment with surgical exploration.

SIGNS, SYMPTOMS, AND DIAGNOSIS

A pneumomediastinum can present with a wide range of symptoms. While some patients may be asymptomatic, most will present with severe chest pain with radiation to the face, neck, or upper extremities, dyspnea, cough, subcutaneous emphysema, odynophagia, dysphagia, changes in their voice, chest or neck swelling, and in some cases, pneumothorax.

Signs of a pneumomediastinum can also be subtle and vague. Patients may be noted to have subcutaneous emphysema, dyspnea, chest wall pain, and increased work of breathing. Hamman crunch may be noted on physical examination about 20% of the time, characterized by a precordial "crunching" noise associated with the cardiac cycle on auscultation examination. Patients with a tension pneumomediastinum may be hypotensive with distended neck veins, dyspnea, and cyanosis.

A pneumomediastinum can be diagnosed on a chest x-ray, with air noted adjacent to the mediastinal structures along the fascial planes, or on CT scan imaging. Once diagnosed, the clinician should evaluate for the etiology of the free air or causes of a secondary pneumomediastinum. This can include a contrast study of the chest, a bronchoscopy, an endoscopy, and an upper gastrointestinal swallow study. In rare instances, if no etiology is found, the patient can then be diagnosed with a spontaneous pneumomediastinum.

MANAGEMENT

The management of a pneumomediastinum involves searching for the underlying etiology of the disease and decreasing the risk of expansion or recurrence. For example, if caused by high airway pressures on mechanical ventilation, the goal should be to minimize the excess pressures. While most cases can be managed by minimizing additional stressors and symptom management, cases of tension pneumomediastinum may require percutaneous or operative interventions, including placement of a tube thoracostomy or a thoracostomy with progression of the disease. Those with associated pneumothoraxes, pneumocardia, or mediastinitis may require additional targeted treatment. Most patients should be observed in the hospital for 24 to 48 hours for disease progression.

PEARLS

- A pneumomediastinum occurs secondary to a sudden increase in intrathoracic pressure, causing free air to surround the mediastinal structures.
- The origin of the free air can be the pharynx, the tracheobronchial tree, or the esophagus.
- The prognosis of the pneumomediastinum depends on the etiology and severity of the disease.
- A pneumomediastinum can be spontaneous or classified as a secondary pneumomediastinum when it occurs secondary to an iatrogenic, traumatic, or nontraumatic etiology.
- A tension pneumopericardium is a rare and life-threatening complication associated with cardiovascular collapse and obstructive shock physiology of cardiac tamponade, requiring immediate treatment by thoracotomy or pericardial window.

SUGGESTED READINGS

Cerolio RJ. Pneumothorax and pneumomediastinum. In: Sugarbaker DJ, Bueno R, Burt BM, et al, eds. *Sugarbaker's Adult Chest Surgery*. 3rd ed. McGraw-Hill Education; 2020.

Clancy DJ, Lande AS, Flynn PW, et al. Tension pneumomediastinum: a literal form of chest tightness. *J Intensive Care Soc.* 2017;18:52-56.

Farkas J. Pneumomediastinum. *The Internet Book of Critical Care*. 2024. Last accessed February 25, 2024. https://emcrit.org/ibcc/pneumomediastinum/

Kouritaas VK, Papagiannopoulos K, Lazaridis G, et al. Pneumomediastinum. *J Thorac Dis.* 2015;7:S44-S49.

Morgan CT. Putting on airs again: new insights and questions about spontaneous pneumomediastinum recurrence. *J Thorac Dis.* 2023;15:2890-2892.

Susai CJ, Banks KC, Alcasid NJ, Velotta JB. A clinical review of spontaneous pneumomediastinum. *Mediastinum*. 2023;8:4.

227

DOES MAGNESIUM WORK IN ACUTE ASTHMA EXACERBATION?

MARINA BOUSHRA AND LAUREN MOORE

Acute asthma exacerbations carry a significant burden of morbidity, mortality, and socioeconomic cost. Many society guidelines exist for their management, with inhaled beta-antagonists and steroids being the cornerstones of care. Magnesium sulfate is a safe and low-cost intervention that has been recommended as an adjunctive treatment in patients with severe exacerbations but its role and efficacy remain debated.

MECHANISM

The mechanism of action of magnesium in asthma has not been fully elucidated but is suspected to be multimodal relief of airflow obstruction. First, magnesium may play a direct role in bronchial smooth muscle relaxation while inhibiting smooth muscle contraction through competitive antagonism of voltage-gated calcium channels. Additionally, magnesium may contribute to reducing inflammation by inhibiting the release of reactive oxygen species as well as acetylcholine and histamine. Serious adverse reactions with IV magnesium such as hypotension or muscle weakness are rare and typically occur with high doses or rapid IV infusions. Because of this, extra caution must be taken in patients with renal insufficiency due to the possibility of rapid accumulation.

DATA

Several studies have investigated the efficacy of magnesium sulfate in both its inhaled and IV forms for asthma exacerbation, and ultimately the data are somewhat conflicting. The MAGNETIC is a randomized and placebo-controlled multicenter pediatric trial which compares efficacy of three adjunctive nebulized magnesium treatments to nebulized saline placebo every 20 minutes. The inhaled magnesium group had lower asthma scores at 60 minutes in the subgroups that included patients with the most severe exacerbations and those with symptoms starting within 6 hours of presentation. In contrast, a larger randomized double-blind controlled trial by Schuh et al. evaluating the efficacy of adjunctive nebulized magnesium in pediatric patients with moderate-to-severe asthma exacerbations found no difference between groups in asthma score, respiratory rate, oxygen saturation, or blood pressure within 4 hours of administration. Furthermore, there were no differences between the groups in these or in several other studies comparing inhaled magnesium and placebo in important outcomes, such as hospital admission, IV bronchodilator use, or length of inpatient stay in pediatric or adult patients.

Evidence for the use of IV magnesium as an adjunctive therapy in asthma exacerbation is similarly conflicting. 3Mg is a randomized controlled trial comparing the effects of adjunctive IV magnesium or inhaled magnesium to standard care in severe acute exacerbations. Patients in all groups received nebulized short-acting beta agonists and anticholinergics along with systemic steroids for severe acute asthma exacerbations. In this study, IV magnesium was associated with a lower breathlessness score when compared to inhaled magnesium, but there was no significant clinical benefit to using magnesium in either form for exacerbation compared with standard care. Conversely, a 2016 Cochrane review of three small pediatric studies noted a reduction in the rate of admissions to the hospital by 68% in the group that received IV magnesium. This supported evidence from a 2014 Cochrane review, in which 14 studies with a total of 2,300 patients with asthma exacerbations of all severities indicated that a single infusion of 1.2 or 2 g IV magnesium over 15 to 30 minutes also reduced hospital admission and possibly improved lung function.

Patient Selection

All in all, while the reviewed data surrounding magnesium in asthma exacerbation are limited and conflicting, the data better support a role for IV magnesium infusion in any asthmatic exacerbation more so than inhaled magnesium. It should be noted, however, that there may be a limited role for inhaled magnesium in very severe pediatric exacerbations only. Furthermore, the data more strongly support the benefit of IV magnesium in pediatric patients rather than adult patients, and also in those with severe exacerbations rather than all comers. Fortunately, magnesium is a relatively safe medication when administered at the proper dose and rate. Therefore, the harm of giving it in most cases is low, and it may be beneficial in some patient populations as discussed above.

PEARLS

- Data informing the use of magnesium as an adjunct in asthma exacerbations are limited and conflicting.
- Data do not support the use of inhaled magnesium in asthma exacerbations, although it may have a limited role in the subset of very severe pediatric asthma exacerbations.
- IV magnesium is a safe medication and can be considered as an adjunct in asthma exacerbations. Its use is best supported in pediatric patients and in patients with severe exacerbation.
- IV magnesium should be used with caution in patients with known or suspected renal impairment due to risk of accumulation and subsequent adverse effects.

Suggested Readings

Goodacre S, Cohen J, Bradburn M, et al. The 3Mg trial: a randomised controlled trial of intravenous or nebulised magnesium sulphate versus placebo in adults with acute severe asthma. *Health Technol Assess*. 2014;18(22):1-168. PMID: 24731521.

Griffiths B, Kew KM. Intravenous magnesium sulfate for treating children with acute asthma in the emergency department. *Cochrane Database Syst Rev*. 2016;4(4):CD011050.

Kew KM, Kirtchuk L, Michell CI. Intravenous magnesium sulfate for treating adults with acute asthma in the emergency department. *Cochrane Database Syst Rev*. 2014;(5):CD010909. PMID: 24865567.

Powell C, Kolamunnage-Dona R, Lowe J, et al. Magnesium sulphate in acute severe asthma in children (MAGNETIC): a randomised, placebo-controlled trial. *Lancet Respir Med*. 2013;1(4):301-308.

Schuh S, Sweeney J, Rumantir M, et al. Effect of nebulized magnesium vs placebo added to albuterol on hospitalization among children with refractory acute asthma treated in the emergency department: a randomized clinical trial. *JAMA*. 2020;324(20):2038-2047.

228

Be Careful With Fluids in Pulmonary Hypertension

Andrea Alvarado

PH can be caused by a variety of conditions including vascular, cardiac, rheumatologic, and thromboembolic diseases. PH is diagnosed by measuring pulmonary artery pressures with a right heart catheterization. The prior criterion of PH was an mPAP of 25 mm Hg or more. The most recent definition of PH is an mPAP greater than 20 mm Hg to include the cohort of patients that were previously excluded from the diagnosis but have high risk of mortality. Furthermore, in 1998, the WHO introduced the five classifications of PH based on the underlying etiologies (**Table 228.1**).

Pathophysiology

The pathophysiology of PH is complex and varies based on the etiology. WHO Class 1 PH is characterized by pulmonary arterial wall thickening and narrowing of the vascular lumen. Class 2 PH occurs when elevated filling pressures are transmitted from the left heart into the pulmonary vasculature inducing vasoconstriction and vascular remodeling. PH secondary to left heart failure is the most common of the classifications. WHO Class 3 is characterized by hypoxic vasoconstriction and capillary bed damage in the setting of underlying pulmonary disease. WHO Class 4 is characterized by both acute and chronic thromboembolic disease leading to inflammation-mediated endovascular remodeling and vasculopathy. WHO Class 5 represents idiopathic and multifactorial etiologies of PH that do not fit into the other categories.

These pathologies lead to increased PVR and consequently increased right heart afterload. RV remodeling has a profound effect on the hemodynamics of the LV due to the ventricular interdependence between the left and right heart. Patients with PH

TABLE 228.1 WHO CLASSIFICATION OF PH BASED ON PATHOPHYSIOLOGY AND UNDERLYING ETIOLOGIES

WHO Class	Classification	Etiologies/Examples
1	Pulmonary arterial hypertension	Drug induced, idiopathy, genetic, connective tissue disease, inflammatory conditions, HIV
2	PH secondary to left heart disease	Left heart failure, left heart valvular disease
3	PH secondary to pulmonary disease	Chronic obstructive lung disease, interstitial lung disease, sleep apnea, developmental abnormalities
4	PH secondary to thromboembolic disease	Pulmonary embolism
5	Multifactorial	Hematologic conditions, vasculitis, congenital shunts, metabolic disorders

PH, pulmonary hypertension; WHO, World Health Organization.

may present to the ED with RV dysfunction or RV failure. Acute elevations in PVR will increase RV afterload leading to increased RVEDV, which leads to an increase in RV diameter and increased wall stress on the RV. Due to the ventricular interdependence, an increase in RVEDV and, consequently, increased RVEDP cause paradoxical movement of the interventricular septum toward the LV. This abnormal septal motion will impair LV filling and lead to a drop in cardiac output. In the acute setting, hypoxia, hypercapnia, and acidosis are potent pulmonary vasoconstrictors. Therefore, optimizing a patient's oxygenation, ventilation, and metabolic derangements is critical to prevent further increases in PVR and worsening RV failure.

Consequences of Volume Overload

The right heart is made of a thin-walled muscle that is more susceptible to afterload changes than the LV. Any increase in PVR can negatively affect RV hemodynamics because RV function is greatly susceptible to volume changes. When resuscitating patients with PH, it is challenging to determine the right amount of preload necessary to optimize CO without overloading the RV, which in turn will affect the LVEDV. Hypovolemia can lead to poor RV preload, poor LVEDV, and low CO. On the other hand, hypervolemia and excessive fluid resuscitation lead to RV myocardial wall stress and dilation leading to tricuspid regurgitation and RV dysfunction. Poor diastolic RV function leads to systemic venous congestion, which presents clinically with anasarca and jugular venous distention. Laboratory results may show acute kidney injury from renal congestion and transaminitis from congestive hepatopathy.

Patients with chronic PH can have ultrasound findings suggestive of RV hypertrophy due to compensatory changes in the setting of chronically elevated PVR. These patients may also have LV atrophy due to remodeling secondary to LV deconditioning. Despite these compensatory changes, the RV is still susceptible to dilation and dysfunction if the volume and pressure overload is consistent. RV dilation, paradoxical septal motion, LV compression, poor LV filling, and decreased SV eventually lead to LV failure, poor CO, and end-organ hypoperfusion. This is why acute changes in volume status can have profound effects on systemic circulation. Acute PH (eg, rebound PH from vasodilatory medication withdrawal, acute PE) leads to acute elevation in LV filling pressures and systemic low-output heart failure. These hemodynamic changes can cause acute ischemic hepatitis and poor renal perfusion.

While there is no standardized modality to evaluate volume status in patients with PH, it is important to consider a multidisciplinary approach for fluid assessment in patients with PH and right heart failure. Ultrasound can be used to look for static and dynamic measures of RV function. RV dilation is assessed by looking at the ratio of RV diameter to LV diameter. A ratio more than 1.0 is indicative of RV dilation. A plethoric IVC with minimal or no respiratory variation is also indicative of elevated right heart pressures. Septal flattening or paradoxical septal motion during systole is characterized by the "D sign." RV systolic function can be assessed by measuring the TAPSE, which quantifies the movement of the tricuspid annulus toward the apex of the heart during systole and diastole. A TAPSE less than 1.7 cm is considered abnormal. One can also derive a patient's PASP by measuring the tricuspid regurgitant jet, estimating CVP from IVC diameter and collapsibility and inserting these variables into Bernoulli equation. Assessment of the TAPSE:PASP has been used for prognostication in patients with a diagnosis of PH. The TAPSE:PASP ratio is representative of RV contractile function and smaller ratios (defined in mm/mm Hg) are associated with greater mortality. Other more invasive methods, including right heart catheterization and pulmonary artery catheter placement, provide dynamic data of right and left heart filling pressures and can help guide resuscitation.

Patients with PH presenting with concern for right heart failure should undergo thorough examination and reversal of any factors contributing to elevated PVR. Patients with right heart failure without clinical or echocardiographic signs of volume overload may undergo resuscitation with small aliquots of intravenous fluids while repeatedly assessing volume status, RV function via ultrasound, CO, and end-organ function. Patients with concerns for volume overload, RV dilation, and poor CO should be evaluated for the institution of inotropes as a means of providing RV support. In patients with PH presenting to the ED, it is important to collect objective data regarding volume status before administration of fluids as volume overload can precipitate cardiogenic shock and eventual cardiac arrest.

PEARLS

- Acute PH can be precipitated by PH medication withdrawal and acute PE.
- Volume overload leads to RV dilation and LV compression leading to poor CO.
- Ultrasound is an unreliable method to assess volume status in right heart failure.
- TAPSE:PASP ratio can be used as a prognostic indicator in patients with PH.
- The resuscitation of patients with PH should focus on optimizing preload, preventing RV dilation, and decreasing PVR by reversing hypoxia, hypercapnia, and acidosis.

SUGGESTED READINGS

Aryal S, King CS. Critical care of patients with pulmonary arterial hypertension. *Curr Opin Pulm Med*. 2020;26(5):414-421. PMID: 32740380.

Maron BA. Revised Definition of Pulmonary Hypertension and Approach to Management: A clinical primer. *J Am Heart Assoc*. 2023 Apr 18;12(8):e029024. PMID: 37026538.

Mullin CJ, Ventetuolo CE. Critical care management of the patient with pulmonary hypertension. *Clin Chest Med*. 2021;42(1):155-165. PMID: 33541609.

Price LC, Martinez G, Brame A, et al. Perioperative management of patients with pulmonary hypertension undergoing non-cardiothoracic, non-obstetric surgery: a systematic review and expert consensus statement. *Br J Anaesth*. 2021;126(4):774-790.

Tello K, Axmann J, Ghofrani HA, et al. Relevance of the TAPSE/PASP ratio in pulmonary arterial hypertension. *Int J Cardiol*. 2018;266:229-235.

Wilcox SR, Kabrhel C, Channick RN. Pulmonary hypertension and right ventricular failure in emergency medicine. *Ann Emerg Med*. 2015;66(6):619-628.

229

Know the Causes of Shortness of Breath—It's Not All in the Lungs

Chloe Renshaw

Shortness of breath is a frequent presenting complaint, accounting for approximately 8% of emergency room visits. Dyspnea, or the sensation of not getting adequate breath, is affected by multiple physiologic, environmental, and psychological factors. Developing a comprehensive differential beyond pulmonary pathology is imperative for landing the appropriate diagnoses and management.

Cardiovascular

Adequate oxygenation is dependent on sufficient cardiac output, and dyspnea develops as a compensatory mechanism to cardiac dysfunction. Two-thirds of atrial fibrillation patients will present with dyspnea. Heart blocks often present with fatigue, and acute coronary syndromes can present with isolated shortness of breath. Aortic stenosis and mitral insufficiency are the two most common valvular disorders to cause dyspnea. Consider pericardial tamponade, myocarditis, and decompensated heart failure. A bedside echocardiogram can reveal pericardial effusion, ventricular strain, and valvular dysfunction. Obtain an ECG in undifferentiated dyspneic patients to evaluate for dysrhythmias, heart strain, and ischemic changes, and cardiac biomarkers in patients with risk factors for coronary disease and cardiac strain.

ENT

Conditions that cause airway obstruction and impair patency often result in stridor and dyspnea is often reported once tidal volume has been reduced by 30%. Acute stridor due to aspiration of a foreign body is common in children. Infectious processes such as croup, bacterial tracheitis, or epiglottitis can cause rapidly progressive airway edema and respiratory compromise. Noninfectious edema can develop due to allergic reaction, angioedema, smoke inhalation, or caustic ingestion. Early identification and airway intervention are imperative for an acutely worsening or unpredictable clinical course.

Laryngeal neoplasms and goiters typically have a more indolent and progressive timeline. Patients may have waxing and waning airway obstruction from vocal cord paralysis or spasm. Both blunt and penetrating injuries can lead to edema, hematoma, and cartilaginous disruption of the trachea rings. In stable patients, evaluation with flexible fiberoptic laryngoscopy can be performed at bedside to identify suspicious lesions and injuries.

Endocrine-Metabolic

Hypoglycemia leads to a sympathetic surge, which results in increased cardiac output, metabolic demand, and shortness of breath. Hyperglycemia can evolve into diabetic ketoacidosis, causing a buildup of ketones and lactic acid, decreasing pH, and triggering a compensatory respiratory alkalosis. Consider a POC when patients present with increased work of breathing.

Hypothyroidism results in weakened respiratory muscles. It can cause pleural and pericardial effusion and pulmonary fibrosis. Hyperthyroidism, in turn, causes an increased respiratory drive and can be associated with pulmonary hypertension. Evaluate for stigmata of thyroid disease and consider sending thyroid studies.

Any conditions that increase metabolic demand will cause an increase in oxygen consumption. Compensatory increases in respiratory effort, gas exchange, cardiac output, and oxygen delivery utilize aerobic metabolization. If metabolic need exceeds what can be provided through aerobic processes, then anaerobic metabolization is utilized. The by-product is lactate, which causes metabolic acidosis and contributes to dyspnea from compensatory respiratory alkalosis. The differential is broad and includes crush injury, thyrotoxicosis, heat stroke, tissue ischemia, sepsis, and acute renal failure.

HEMATOLOGIC

Individuals who experience chronic anemia compensate through a rightward shift of the oxygen dissociation curve. Anemia becomes symptomatic, with dyspnea as a common manifestation, during periods of acute loss or when the body is no longer able to compensate for the deficiency. Up to 30% of premenopausal, nonpregnant females live with anemia secondary to menstruation. Gastrointestinal bleeds can cause both chronic and acute anemia related to peptic or duodenal ulcers, neoplasms, gastropathy or varices, and inflammatory bowel disease. Management is largely dependent on the rate and degree of blood loss and the need for transfusion or endoscopy. Patients may be symptomatic without requiring transfusion, with iron replacement being a mainstay of management.

Other special populations to consider are those with underlying hemoglobinopathy, such as sickle cell, who are prone to severe anemia when sick or under stress. Acquired conditions that affect hemoglobin-binding affinity include carbon monoxide poisoning, methemoglobinemia, and changes in altitude. Consider blood gas analysis to evaluate for heme toxicity.

NEUROMUSCULAR

Disease processes that cause bulbar weakness, such as stroke, amyotrophic lateral sclerosis, or botulism, disrupt the coordination of oropharyngeal muscles, leading to chronic aspiration, impaired cough, and decreased air delivery. Myasthenia gravis can cause progressive bulbar fatigue and diaphragmatic exhaustion. Guillain-Barré presents with ascending weakness and decreased deep tendon reflexes, with weakness classically progressing cranially. To evaluate for diaphragmatic weakness, measuring respiratory parameters with maximal inspiratory pressure can assist in guiding management.

MUSCULOSKELETAL

External compression from obesity, pregnancy, or large-volume ascites decreases tidal volume and increases respiratory rate. People with scoliosis or kyphosis may have limited chest wall flexibility and impaired lung expansion. Pain also limits chest wall expansion. Rib fractures or contusions lead to splinting, decreased lung expansion, and atelectasis.

TOXINS

Salicylate poisoning is unique as it activates the medullary respiratory center, leading to tachypnea and hyperventilation in the early stages after ingestion. Sympathomimetics, such as PCP, MDMA, and cocaine, excite the CNS and lead to increased respiratory rate. Withdrawal from CNS depressants, such as alcohol, benzodiazepines, and opioids, causes rebound tachypnea and anxiety. Ingestion of methanol and ethylene glycol causes a metabolic acidosis, which in turn triggers a respiratory alkalosis. Most recreational intoxications and withdrawal are treated supportively, with specific antidotes and dialysis considered for more high risk and refractory poisonings.

PSYCHOLOGIC

Stress and anxiety can lead to hyperventilation and the experience of dyspnea. Patients who experience panic attacks are often able to identify their dyspnea as their typical stress response. However, dyspnea due to psychological stress should be a diagnosis of exclusion once other etiologies are considered and evaluated.

	CONSIDERATIONS	EVALUATION
Cardiovascular	Dysrhythmia, valvular stenosis or insufficiency, ACS, pericardial tamponade, heart failure	ECG, telemetry, echo, troponin, BNP
ENT	Aspiration, infection, angioedema, inhalation injury or caustic ingestion, goiter, trauma, tumor	Auscultate, flexible fiberoptic laryngoscopy, early airway intervention
Endocrine	Hypoglycemia, DKA, hyperthyroidism, hypothyroidism	POC glucose, BMP, VBG, TSH/T4/T3
Hemoglobin	Anemia, hemoglobinopathies, carbon monoxide, methemoglobinemia, altitude	Hemoglobin/hematocrit, T&S, carboxyhemoglobin, blood gas and co-oximetry
Metabolic	Crush injury, sepsis, heatstroke, tissue ischemia, acute renal failure	Temperature, BMP, CK, lactate, infectious studies
Neuromuscular	CVA, ALS, Guillain-Barré, botulism, myasthenia gravis	CT/MR, MIP
Toxins	Sympathomimetics: amphetamine, PCP, MDMA, cocaine, etc. Withdrawal: alcohol, benzodiazepine, opioids	Supportive care, antidotes, dialysis
Psych	Panic disorder, anxiety disorder, PTSD	Anxiolytics

ACS, acute coronary syndrome; ALS, amyotrophic lateral sclerosis; BMP, basic metabolic panel; BNP, brain natriuretic peptide; CK, creatine kinase; CT/MR, computed tomography/magnetic resonance; CVA, cerebrovascular accident; DKA, diabetic ketoacidosis; ECG, electrocardiogram; ENT, ear, nose, throat; MDMA, 3,4-methylenedioxymethamphetamine; MIP, maximum inspiratory pressure; PCP, phencyclidine; POC, point-of-care; PTSD, posttraumatic stress disorder; TSH/T4/T3, thyroid-stimulating hormone/thyroxine/triiodothyronine; T&S, type and screen; VBG, venous blood gas.

PEARLS

- Dyspnea is based on subjective patient experience and not respiratory parameters.
- Consider an ECG in all dyspneic patients and a POC glucose for those in respiratory distress.
- Hyperventilation is the primary acute compensatory mechanism for metabolic acidosis—identify and treat the underlying cause.
- Always consider toxic exposures or ingestions.

SUGGESTED READINGS

Guttikonda SNR, Vadapalli K. Approach to undifferentiated dyspnea in emergency department: aids in rapid clinical decision-making. *Int J Emerg Med*. 2018;11(1):21.
Hale ZE, Singhal A, Hsia RY. Causes of shortness of breath in the acute patient: a national study. *Acad Emerg Med*. 2018;25(11):1227-1234. PMID: 29738108.

230

Ventilator Management for the Boarded ED Patient

Erika Danelski and Nicholas Goodmanson

Critically ill patients, and specifically those requiring invasive mechanical ventilation, constitute an increasing percentage of ED presentations. A rising number of patients admitted to the hospital remain in EDs due to inpatient bed constraints, a phenomenon often termed boarding. As time spent in the ED increases, a patient's time spent on the ventilator, intensive care unit stay duration, and risk of mortality also increase. As such, EPs must optimize care of patients who are critically ill and on mechanical ventilator during their ED stays.

Common conditions requiring mechanical ventilation include ventilatory failure, oxygenation failure, increased work of breathing, and inadequate airway protection. While EPs recognize these indications well and expertly obtain definitive airways, postintubation management of mechanical ventilation often receives less emphasis. EPs must first select appropriate ventilator settings after intubating a patient. The five key variables to adjust include mode, tidal volume, respiratory rate, F_{IO_2}, and PEEP. Adjustments to tidal volumes and respiratory rates affect ventilation, whereas adjustments to F_{IO_2} and PEEP affect oxygenation.

EPs may choose from multiple ventilator modes, including volume-assist control, pressure-assist control, and pressure-regulated volume control, among others. In volume-targeted modes, the EP sets the desired tidal volume for a given breath, and the inspiratory pressures delivered will vary depending on the patient's pulmonary mechanics. Conversely, in a pressure-targeted mode, the EP sets the maximum inspiratory pressure for a given breath, and the tidal volume delivered will vary depending on the patient's pulmonary mechanics. Assist-control modes deliver the targeted breath at a mandatory frequency set by the EP (absent patient effort, these are termed "control breaths"), though patients can breathe at a higher frequency by triggering breaths (termed "assisted breaths") with the same target characteristics as those for control breaths. Most patients tolerate volume-assist control well, and its commonality and ease of use commend it as the best initial mode for most patients. Having selected a mode, the choice of the remaining settings depends upon the patient's characteristics and their specific pathophysiology. Two general strategies for commonly encountered pathophysiologic paradigms in the ED can guide selection of the remaining variables for most patients: a lung-protective strategy or an obstructive strategy.

LPV focuses on reducing the risk of ventilator-induced lung injury. A lung-protective strategy emphasizes LPV and is appropriate for any patient in the ED aside from those with obstructive lung diseases, such as chronic obstructive pulmonary disease or asthma. LPV aims to limit volutrauma and barotrauma by using tidal volumes between 6 and 8 mL/kg of ideal body weight. Data from prospective, randomized clinical trials demonstrate that these volumes reduce mortality as compared to volumes between 10 and 12 mL/kg in patients with the ARDS. Subsequent clinical data suggest that these volumes may also prevent the development of ARDS in all patients without it, including elective surgery/anesthesia. Given this information, EPs should avoid titrating tidal volumes to manage $Paco_2$. They should instead titrate the respiratory rate to meet ventilation goals. A rate of 16 to 18 bpm should achieve a normal $Paco_2$ for most patients, but rates exceeding 30 bpm may be necessary depending on disease severity. As for adjusting oxygenation, EPs often instinctively focus on Fio_2. However, this effect may be temporary, depending on the degree of shunt physiology present. Though many patients tolerate an initial PEEP of 5 cm H_2O, those requiring an Fio_2 exceeding 60% generally benefit from a PEEP between 10 and 12 cm H_2O. Prioritizing PEEP adjustment first can improve alveolar recruitment and, ultimately, oxygenation. For patients with ARDS, PEEP and Fio_2 titration tables are freely available online to guide adjustments to these variables.

An obstructive strategy primarily benefits patients with severe bronchospasm due to obstructive lung diseases. This strategy emphasizes longer exhalation times and the prevention of air trapping. Lower respiratory rates, generally between 8 and 10 bpm, achieve these goals. These rates often yield hypercapnia, which can be permitted depending on the degree of acidosis and associated hemodynamic derangements. EPs should adjust tidal volume, Fio_2, and PEEP settings in line with a lung-protective strategy, though higher PEEP support may negatively influence these patients' airway pressures.

EPs should frequently reevaluate the effectiveness of their chosen ventilatory strategy while the patient remains under their care, as conditions frequently change within the first several hours after intubation. An arterial or venous blood gas should be checked approximately 30 minutes after intubation to ensure the achievement of adequate ventilation. To avoid frequent blood gases, EPs can use $ETco_2$ to estimate $Paco_2$, as an elevated $ETco_2$ suggests an elevated $Paco_2$ and can spur adjustments to respiratory rate. However, they should avoid decreasing the respiratory rate based on a low $ETco_2$ alone, as multiple variables may confound a lower measured $ETco_2$. Similarly, pulse oximetry facilitates continuous measurement of oxygen saturation to guide titration of PEEP and Fio_2. Because skin pigmentation and melanin content affect the performance of pulse oximeters, EPs should consider initially correlating peripheral oxygen saturation measurements with an arterial oxygen saturation measurement using an arterial blood gas sample. Most patients tolerate goal oxygen saturations of 88% to 90%, depending on the underlying disease process.

EPs should also monitor plateau pressures with any PEEP or tidal volume adjustment. This pressure estimates alveolar pressures and serves as a safety threshold, with the optimal plateau pressure below 30 cm H_2O; above this, the risk for lung injury increases. In cases of elevated plateau pressures, consider first decreasing tidal volume in 1 mL/kg increments to a minimum of 4 mL/kg followed by decreasing PEEP when employing a lung-protective strategy. When employing an obstructive strategy, consider first decreasing the respiratory rate to prevent breath stacking. If these interventions fail to achieve acceptable plateau pressures, evaluate for other causes of reduced compliance such as mucous plugging, endotracheal tube displacement, pneumothorax, or inadequate sedation.

Appropriate analgesia and sedation facilitate synchronous mechanical ventilation. Inadequate analgesia and sedation can lead to ventilator dyssynchrony, increasing the risk for breath stacking, barotrauma, volutrauma, and other complications. Sedation should be titrated to promote synchrony and patient comfort at the lowest effective dose. Lastly, if analgesia and sedation are optimized but dyssynchrony persists, EPs can administer neuromuscular blocking agents to facilitate synchrony, though recent data did not find an associated mortality benefit.

PEARLS

- Employ one of the two major strategies when selecting initial mechanical ventilator settings: use a lung-protective strategy for most patients or an obstructive strategy in patients with severe bronchospasm.
- A LPV limits volutrauma and barotrauma through use of tidal volumes between 6 and 8 mL/kg of ideal body weight.
- An obstructive strategy limits air trapping by increasing expiratory time through use of respiratory rates between 8 and 10 bpm.
- Changes to tidal volume and respiratory rate affect ventilation, whereas changes to FIO_2 and PEEP affect oxygenation.
- Optimize a patient's analgesia and sedation to prevent ventilator dyssynchrony and its associated complications.

SUGGESTED READINGS

Mosier JM, Hypes C, Joshi R, et al. Ventilator strategies and rescue therapies for management of acute respiratory failure in the emergency department. *Ann Emerg Med*. 2015;66(5):529-541.

Weingart SD. Managing initial mechanical ventilation in the emergency department. *Ann Emerg Med*. 2016;68(5):614-617.

Wilcox SR, Richards JB, Fisher DF, et al. Initial mechanical ventilator settings and lung protective ventilation in the ed. *Am J Emerg Med*. 2016;34(8):1446-1451.

Wright BJ. Lung-protective ventilation strategies and adjunctive treatments for the emergency medicine patient with acute respiratory failure. *Emerg Med Clin N Am*. 2014;32(4):871-887.

SECTION XIX
TOXICOLOGY

231

ALCOHOL INTOXICATION AND WITHDRAWAL

KEVIN HANLEY AND KEVIN ROLNICK

ALCOHOL INTOXICATION

Alcohol intoxication and withdrawal are common ED presentations, yet their treatment can often be nuanced and complex. The first step to evaluate and treat patients for these entities is a careful social history to quantify the number of alcoholic beverages the patient consumes on average per day, week, or month as well as to determine the last time the patient consumed alcohol. If significant alcohol use is identified, the emergency physician must then consider the numerous metabolic and physiologic effects of alcohol.

Alcohol intoxication is associated with the "three Hs": hypoglycemia, hypothermia, and hypotension. While treatment of hypotension and hypothermia in alcohol intoxication is per usual interventions, treatment of hypoglycemia secondary to ethanol ingestion requires more specific interventions. Hypoglycemia is commonly seen in patients with a history of alcohol use disorder due to malnourishment and decreased gluconeogenesis. This should be identified quickly and treated by feeding the patient if their mental status allows or with IV dextrose if needed.

In addition, these patients are at high risk for vitamin deficiencies, most notably thiamine and magnesium. WE is an uncommon but not unheard of neurologic manifestation of thiamine deficiency and is missed in a large number of cases. Diagnosis is challenging, as symptoms resemble those of acute alcohol intoxication. Diagnosing WE is done on a clinical basis. The classic triad of ophthalmoplegia, ataxia, and confusion is rarely seen. Left untreated, WE may lead to Korsakoff syndrome, a form of dementia characterized by confabulation and amnesia and portends significant morbidity and mortality. Treatment of WE is high-dose parenteral thiamine, though the duration of therapy remains debated. Due to the high rates of thiamine deficiency, consider giving all patients with a history of alcohol use disorder thiamine prophylactically. The classic teaching that thiamine should be given before glucose to prevent the precipitation of WE is based on multiple case series and reports, and there is no clear evidence that this is true. If your patient requires treatment for hypoglycemia, it should be followed promptly by thiamine supplementation.

Clinicians should also be aware that patients with a history of alcohol abuse are at increased risk for occult trauma. In addition to a thorough physical examination, clinicians should maintain a low threshold for additional evaluation and imaging.

Alcohol Withdrawal

At the other end of the spectrum is alcohol withdrawal; remember, patients can have alcohol withdrawal even if their blood alcohol level is elevated. A large percentage of patients who use alcohol chronically and abruptly cease its use will develop acute AWS. AWS is a clinical spectrum that is characterized by autonomic hyperactivity after abrupt discontinuation or substantial reduction in use of alcohol in patients with a physical dependence.

The pathophysiology of AWS is complex. It is thought that chronic alcohol use induces CNS neurotransmitter remodeling. Abrupt cessation of alcohol results in an imbalance of neurotransmitter activity and CNS hyperexcitability.

It is important to determine the precipitating cause of AWS, as pathology like underlying infection or injury may have prompted alcohol cessation. Providers must maintain a high degree of clinical suspicion for alcohol withdrawal in patients who are critically ill or have a depressed level of consciousness. There are many well-validated tools for assessing the presence and severity of AWS, including CIWA, alcohol-withdrawal scale, and PAWSS.

Withdrawal symptoms typically begin 6 to 12 hours after the last drink. Patients may exhibit tremors, diaphoresis, nausea, vomiting, hypertension, and tachycardia. About 12 to 24 hours after the last drink, patients may develop visual and tactile hallucinations with an otherwise clear sensorium. Some patients with AWS will go on to develop seizures—typically generalized tonic-clonic seizures with little or no postictal period. DT represents the most severe manifestation of acute withdrawal and carries a very high mortality if untreated. It usually occurs 48 to 72 hours after the last drink, but can appear days later. Symptoms include disorientation, delirium, hyperthermia, seizures, and agitation and may last for 5 to 7 days even with treatment. Older patients, those with prior history of DTs, and those with a history of heavier drinking are at higher risk of developing DTs. AWS is a continuous spectrum of symptoms, but not all patients follow the same clinical course. It may start with mild symptoms and become progressively worse or start with DTs.

Early recognition and treatment of AWS is key. Not all patients require medical therapy or admission. Initial interventions should include decreasing stimulation, including providing reassurance and putting the patient in a dark, calm area. Benzodiazepines are the most common initially used drug class, though other therapies such as phenobarbital can be considered. The choice of benzodiazepine varies widely based on clinical practice. Longer acting benzodiazepines (eg, diazepam, chlordiazepoxide) or phenobarbital may be preferable as the protracted half-life acts as an effective auto-taper to reduce the risk of recurrent withdrawal. In older patients or those with advanced liver disease, the use of shorter acting agents may decrease the risk of oversedation. Patients with mild symptoms can be treated with oral formulations, whereas those with moderate-to-severe symptoms should be treated with IV medications. Symptom-triggered therapy is superior to fixed-dose therapy, and benzodiazepines should be titrated to the desired effect. Most benzodiazepines have a fast onset of action, and patients in severe withdrawal may need several rounds of medications to control symptoms. Patients should be frequently reassessed for response to therapy and need for additional medication. Escalation of therapy is warranted for those patients requiring very high doses of benzodiazepines and continuing to have worsening symptoms. This may include augmentation with phenobarbital and, in refractory cases, propofol and intubation.

PEARLS

- Perform a thorough physical examination and check a glucose level on "intoxicated patients" with altered mental status. Consider giving a dose of prophylactic parenteral thiamine.
- Determine why alcohol was abruptly discontinued.
- Alcohol-withdrawal symptoms do not always present in order—frequently reassess patients to determine need for escalated therapy.
- Many patients with alcohol withdrawal may require relatively high doses of benzodiazepines and/or phenobarbital to control withdrawal symptoms.

SUGGESTED READINGS

Allison M, McCurdy M. Alcoholic metabolic emergencies. *Emerg Med Clin North Am*. 2014;32(2):293-301.

Gold J, Nelson L. Ethanol withdrawal. In: Hoffman RS, Howland M, Lewin NA, Nelson LS, Goldfrank LR, et al., eds. *Goldfrank's Toxicologic Emergencies*. 10th ed. McGraw-Hill Professional Publishing; 2015.

Kosten TR, O'Connor PG. Management of drug and alcohol withdrawal. *N Engl J Med*. 2003;349(4):405-407.

Mirijello A, D'Angelo C, Ferrulli A, et al. Identification and management of alcohol withdrawal syndrome. *Drugs*. 2015;75(4):353-365.

Sachdeva A. Alcohol withdrawal syndrome: benzodiazepines and beyond. *J Clin Diagn Res*. 2015;9:VE01-VE07.

232

ACETAMINOPHEN TOXICITY: GETTING REACQUAINTED WITH MATTHEW AND RUMACK

PETER AIELLO AND VINCENT J. CALLEO

The most common cause of pharmacologic acute liver failure in the United States is APAP poisoning. Toxicity may result from intentional or unintentional ingestions, either acutely or chronically. It is important to remember that APAP is found in both prescription medications and multiple over-the-counter substances, including popular cough/cold remedies. Symptoms and signs of APAP toxicity are initially vague, including GI upset, but can progress to hepatotoxicity, multisystem organ failure, and death in severe cases.

Acute toxicity occurs with single acute ingestions of greater than 200mg/kg in the pediatric population or more than 10g in the adult population. Peak serum APAP concentrations normally occur quickly, often about 1 to 2 hours postingestion.

Ordinarily, APAP is metabolized mostly by conjugation with sulfate and glucuronide and is excreted in the urine. A small percentage is oxidized by the cytochrome P450 system to toxic NAPQI. This low level of NAPQI seen with nontoxic doses can then be conjugated with glutathione. Liver toxicity occurs when excessive NAPQI is produced and the body cannot detoxify it. The antidote for APAP poisoning is NAC. This works through many mechanisms, some of which include repleting glutathione and as well as directly detoxifying NAPQI.

When to Initiate Treatment

In an acute overdose, the Rumack-Matthew nomogram can be used to predict the risk of hepatotoxicity. This tool compares the time of ingestion to the APAP level; those above the treatment line should receive NAC therapy. However, it can only be used to risk stratify patients whose ingestion occurred within 4 to 24 hours of evaluation. Remember this nomogram is used for a single ingestion time with a known time of ingestion. Providers must obtain a meticulous history to ensure the nomogram is being correctly applied. If a patient presents before 4 hours postingestion, consider waiting until 4-hour postingestion time to obtain an APAP level.

Once the level returns, use the Rumack-Matthew nomogram to plot whether the level falls above the treatment line. At 4 hours postingestion, serum APAP concentrations above 150 mcg/mL require treatment. When applied to the correct patient population, APAP concentrations below the treatment line do not require antidotal therapy. The original treatment line was 200 mcg/mL at the 4-hour mark. The more conservative treatment line of 150 mcg/mL in the United States was plotted at 25% below the original line to add an additional safety buffer.

With sustained-release products or products that alter GI absorption, repeat levels should be considered. The absorption of these substances differs from immediate-release products. Situations may occur where these patients have nomogram "line crossing"; that is, patients not initially identified as needing NAC are found to require it based on a repeat level due to altered absorption.

If the ingestion time is unclear, use the earliest possible time of ingestion. This allows for the most conservative treatment approach so no patients who require NAC are missed. If the ingestion window is greater than 24 hours or cannot be determined, APAP and transaminase levels should be checked. If either level is elevated, NAC should be started; if the APAP is negative, the transaminase levels are normal, and the patient is doing well clinically, NAC is not indicated unless there is a concern the ingestion was within 4 hours in which case a 4-hour APAP level should be obtained.

Start NAC Empirically If APAP Level Will Result After 8 Hours

In patients who report a potentially toxic APAP ingestion but the APAP level will not result within 8 hours postingestion, NAC should be started while awaiting laboratory values. NAC is most effective when administered within 8 hours of ingestion; thus, empiric treatment is beneficial until therapy can be guided with objective data and the Rumack-Matthew nomogram.

Start NAC Empirically in Certain Patients with Liver Failure

Administration of NAC has been shown to decrease morbidity and mortality in APAP-induced liver failure, even once the APAP level is negative. It should be strongly considered in patients with APAP-induced hepatotoxicity.

Treat Chronic Ingestions Based on History and APAP/Transaminase Levels

Many patients are at risk for chronic APAP poisoning, including those with alcohol use disorder and malnourished patients.

If chronic toxicity is suspected (10 g or 200 mg/kg in 24 hours; or 6 g a day or 150 mg/kg/d in 48 hours), obtain both APAP and transaminase levels. An elevated APAP, AST, or ALT level should prompt administration of NAC. Providers must also consider other possible causes of liver failure.

Order an APAP Level in Patients With Any Suspected Ingestion

Studies have found universal APAP screenings beneficial in cases of intentional ingestion. One study demonstrated a treatable APAP level in 0.3% of all suspected ingestions that would have otherwise been missed based on history alone. Because APAP toxicity is common and the consequence of missing the diagnosis is potentially lethal, APAP levels should be strongly considered in any patient with altered mental status or intentional overdose.

Preparing Acetylcysteine for Administration

Providers should be familiar with NAC preparation and administration. NAC can be given IV or PO. When prepared IV, NAC should be prepared in suitable diluents, such as D5W or 0.45% sodium chloride. Providers must remember to carefully formulate NAC, particularly for small children. When using PO NAC, remember it has a pungent odor. Covering the top of the solution with a lid, having patients use a straw, and mixing it in a sweet drink may increase palatability. IV NAC is recommended for pregnant patients and those with signs of hepatotoxicity.

PEARLS

- APAP is found in a multitude of medications.
- Use the Rumack-Matthews nomogram to risk stratify who needs NAC.
- Start NAC empirically if APAP level will result after 8 hours.
- Treat chronic ingestions based on history and APAP/transaminase levels.
- Order an APAP level in patients with any suspected ingestion.

Suggested Readings

Burns MJ, Friedman SL, Larson AM. Acetaminophen (paracetamol) poisoning in adults: pathophysiology, presentation, and diagnosis. *UpToDate*. 2015.

Melanson P. Acetaminophen. *McGill Critical Care Medicine*. 2015. Accessed February 2, 2024. https://www.mcgill.ca/criticalcare/teaching/files/toxicology/acetaminophen

Nelson LS, Lewin NA, Howland MA, Hoffman RS, Goldfrank LR, Flomenbaum NE. Acetaminophen. In: *Goldfrank's Toxicologic Emergencies*. 9th ed. McGraw-Hill Education; 2011.

Rumack BH, Matthew H. Acetaminophen poisoning and toxicity. *Pediatrics*. 1975;55:871.

Sporer KA, Khayam-Bashi H. Acetaminophen and salicylate serum levels in patients with suicidal ingestion or altered mental status. *Am J Emerg Med*. 1996:14(5):446-447.

233

Toxic Alcohols

Sarah Mahonski

Methanol and ethylene glycol are toxic alcohols that, when ingested, cause significant morbidity and mortality. Acute ingestion of all alcohols causes inebriation, depending on the quantity ingested. The alcohols themselves are not acutely toxic, but their metabolites cause end-organ damage and are sometimes fatal. Toxic alcohol exposure should be considered in any patient presenting with an unexplained anion gap metabolic acidosis. Testing is not readily available at most hospitals in a clinically useful time frame, so clinicians must be adept at recognizing signs of toxic alcohol toxicity, using surrogate markers for diagnosis and initiating prompt treatment.

Alcohols are metabolized in the liver by ADH and ALDH to toxic metabolites. Ethanol binds ADH with a higher affinity than ethylene glycol or methanol; therefore, coingestion of a toxic alcohol with ethanol will initially prevent the production of toxic metabolites as ADH preferentially metabolizes the ethanol. Thus, it is uncommon, but not impossible, that an acidosis would be secondary to a toxic alcohol if the ethanol concentration is detectable. Alcoholic ketoacidosis should be considered in these situations and can be corroborated by ordering a beta-hydroxybutyrate concentration.

Methanol is found in windshield wiper fluid, model car fuel, solid catering cooking fuel, colognes, and perfumes. Toxicity occurs mainly from ingestion, but transdermal exposures resulting in toxicity are reported in small children or large exposures. Patients with methanol ingestion do not always experience inebriation. An elevated osmol gap is present initially, and development of an anion gap metabolic acidosis occurs over 12 to 24 hours. Methanol is metabolized to formic acid, which is toxic to the retina and the basal ganglia. If untreated, patients may experience irreversible vision loss and, occasionally, parkinsonism.

Ethylene glycol is used as antifreeze for car radiators as well as other commercial applications. Its sweet taste and fluorescent blue color due to an additive in antifreeze make it a target for unintentional ingestion by children. Ethylene glycol is metabolized to glycolic acid and later oxalic acid; patients initially present with an elevated osmol gap, with the production of an anion gap metabolic acidosis over 6 to 12 hours as metabolites develop. Oxalic acid precipitates in the renal tubules as calcium oxalate, leading to acute kidney injury and renal failure. This sometimes produces hypocalcemia and calcium oxalate crystals on urinalysis, but this is not always present. In addition, urine fluorescence secondary to the fluorescein additive in antifreeze is reported but is neither sensitive nor specific; therefore, this should not be used to rule in or rule out exposure.

Toxic alcohols should be considered if a patient has unexplained altered mental status, an increased osmol gap, or severe acidemia with an elevated anion gap. If suspected, serum ethylene glycol and methanol concentrations should be sent for confirmation but are not readily available with quick turnaround at most hospitals. An osmol gap is a surrogate marker of toxicity and is determined by calculating the serum osmolarity $[(2 \times Na) + (BUN/2.8) + (glucose/18) + (ethanol/4.6)]$ and comparing this to a measured osmolarity. For accuracy, the blood chemistry, ethanol, and measured osmolarity need to be collected from the same blood draw. A normal osmol gap varies in healthy humans from -14 to $+10$.

Therefore, a significantly elevated osmol gap greater than 50 is concerning for toxic alcohol exposure, but a low or normal osmol gap does not rule out a toxic alcohol. Glycolic acid is structurally similar to lactic acid; thus, on some analyzers, it is read as a false-positive elevated lactate. Thus, a lactate gap is seen with ethylene glycol toxicity when there is a discrepancy between a falsely elevated point-of-care lactate and a formal lactic acid measurement.

Treatment for methanol and ethylene glycol ingestions is ADH inhibition with fomepizole, to prevent the production of toxic metabolites. The dose of fomepizole is 15 mg/kg, followed by 10 mg/kg every 12 hours. If fomepizole is unavailable, ethanol is an alternative treatment, with maintenance of a serum concentration of 150 mg/dL. If an anion gap metabolic acidosis is already present, hemodialysis is used to remove the toxic metabolites, in addition to the parent compound. The decision to initiate hemodialysis should be made with consultation with a nephrologist, toxicologist, and poison control center. For methanol toxicity, adjunctive therapy with a sodium bicarbonate infusion is recommended to prevent retinal toxicity from formate via ion trapping. In addition, folic acid is given to assist with breakdown of formic acid to nontoxic byproducts. Similarly, with ethylene glycol toxicity, thiamine and pyridoxine are cofactors used to break down toxic metabolites and should be used adjunctively.

Toxicity from isopropyl alcohol is different than other toxic alcohols. Isopropyl alcohol is found in rubbing alcohol and many hand sanitizers. Given the higher molecular weight, isopropanol is more intoxicating than ethanol and is ingested for that reason. Large ingestions produce CNS depression, nausea, vomiting, and hemorrhagic gastritis. It is metabolized via ADH to acetone; therefore, it does not produce an acidosis but rather a ketosis. It is osmotically active and will produce an elevated osmol gap. Treatment is supportive with frequent reassessments and antacids as needed. Large ingestions in small children can be more severe, with vasodilatory shock. Isopropyl alcohol occasionally produces a falsely elevated creatinine.

PEARLS

- An unexplained anion gap metabolic acidosis should raise concern for toxic alcohols.
- All laboratory studies for an accurate osmol gap need to be obtained at the same time.
- A normal osmol gap does not rule out a toxic alcohol.
- Treatment includes prompt initiation of fomepizole and hemodialysis for severe or late cases.
- Isopropyl alcohol produces CNS depression, ketosis, without acidosis.

SUGGESTED READINGS

Hoffman RS, Smilkstein MJ, Howland MA, Goldfrank LR. Osmol gaps revisited: normal values and limitations. *J Toxicol Clin Toxicol*. 1993;31:81-93.

Howland MA. Fomepizole. In: Nelson LS, Howland M, Lewin NA, Smith SW, Goldfrank LR, Hoffman RS. eds. *Goldfrank's Toxicologic Emergencies*. 11th ed. McGraw-Hill Professional Publishing; 2019.

Roberts DM, Yates C, Megarbane G, et al. Recommendations for the role of extracorporeal treatments in the management of acute methanol poisoning: a systematic review and consensus statement. *Crit Care Med*. 2015;43(2):461-472.

Weiner S. Toxic alcohols. In: Nelson LS, Howland M, Lewin NA, Smith SW, Goldfrank LR, Hoffman RS. eds. *Goldfrank's Toxicologic Emergencies*. 11th ed. McGraw-Hill Professional Publishing; 2019.

234

Salicylate Poisoning: The Malicious Mimic

Robert W. Seabury

Salicylates are found in both prescription and nonprescription products, including tablets containing acetylsalicylic acid or bismuth subsalicylate and oils/liniments containing methyl salicylate.

Salicylate overdoses uncouple oxidative phosphorylation, causing metabolic acidosis. They also cause respiratory alkalosis by stimulating the medullary respiratory center, causing tachypnea and/or hyperpnea. Respiratory effects usually precede metabolic effects and may be accompanied by tinnitus and gastrointestinal complaints.

Salicylate poisonings are common overdoses and most often ingestions. They have high morbidity and mortality without early identification and treatment. This chapter highlights key points toward identifying and managing salicylate poisonings.

Some Salicylate Poisonings May Not Have Overdose History

Salicylate poisonings are divided into acute and chronic exposures. Acute exposures often have overdose history, as they are usually large, intentional ingestions in a suicide attempt. Chronic exposures may not have overdose history, as they are often nonintentional and due to therapeutic errors, such as accidently using multiple salicylate-containing compounds. Overdose history may be useful if positive, but negative or absent history may not exclude salicylate poisoning.

Consider Salicylate Poisoning If Mixed Respiratory Alkalosis With Metabolic Acidosis

Many salicylate poisonings are characterized by mixed respiratory alkalosis with metabolic acidosis. Additional symptoms can mirror more common diseases, such as AMS, fever, and respiratory distress. Many salicylate poisonings are misdiagnosed, thus delaying treatment and increasing mortality. Salicylate poisoning should be considered in adults with mixed respiratory alkalosis and metabolic acidosis. Pediatric patients may not have respiratory alkalosis, and salicylate poisoning should be considered with metabolic acidosis alone. Remember to consider salicylate toxicity in an older patient with an unexplained mixed picture acidosis as it often goes undiscovered early in the patient's hospital course.

Serum Salicylate Concentrations Must Be Repeated Until Down Trending

Suspected salicylate poisonings should have a serum salicylate concentration obtained. Delayed absorption can occur, and peak concentration may take more than 24 hours. Positive salicylate concentrations should be repeated every 2 hours until down trending and then every 4 hours until less than 30 mg/dL, and the patient is clinically improving and tolerating PO feeds. It may be reasonable in certain cases to repeat negative salicylate concentrations, as absorption can be delayed and toxicity can occur despite initially negative results.

Salicylate Concentrations Must Be Clinically Correlated Before Making Treatment Decisions

Chronic salicylate exposures have baseline tissue burden, and significant poisoning can occur at lower salicylate concentrations. Salicylates are intracellular poisons, and decreasing serum concentrations could mean increasing intracellular penetrance. A blood gas and serum electrolytes must be ordered with each salicylate concentration to evaluate clinical status. Decreasing and even near therapeutic salicylate concentrations may require aggressive treatment with worsening acidosis or clinical instability.

Give Intravenous Dextrose to Salicylate-Poisoned Patients With AMS and Blood Glucose Less Than 300 mg/dL

CNS glycolysis increases with worsening salicylate poisoning, depleting CNS glucose and causing CNS hypoglycemia and AMS despite normal blood glucose levels. Dextrose boluses can improve salicylate-induced AMS and may be reasonable in salicylate poisonings with AMS and blood glucose less than 300 mg/dL.

Endotracheal Intubation and Mechanical Ventilation Should Be Cautiously Utilized With Salicylate Poisoning

Though intubation and mechanical ventilation should be avoided, if possible, some salicylate poisonings may require it to prevent acidosis due to respiratory fatigue. Not maintaining preintubation minute ventilation and tidal volume can be dangerous, as it decreases serum pH and increases salicylate penetration. Respiratory acidosis is often a preterminal event and may be mitigated by maintaining preintubation minute ventilation and tidal volume, followed by aggressive titration to maintain a pH of 7.45 to 7.55.

AC Can be Considered in Any Salicylate Poisoning With a Protected Airway

AC drastically decreases salicylate absorption, and a single 1 g/kg dose can be considered in salicylate poisonings, as there are often absorptive delays. Repeat charcoal doses can be considered with increasing salicylate concentrations. AC should not be considered without a protected airway, as aspiration can lead to serious side effects, such as pneumonitis.

Serum and Urinary Alkalinization Are the Cornerstone Management for Salicylate Poisonings

Serum and urinary alkalinization decrease tissue penetration and increase salicylate elimination and are indicated with symptomatic salicylate poisoning or suspected salicylate poisoning with concentrations greater than 30 mg/dL. Sodium bicarbonate is given as a 1 mEq/kg bolus followed by a continuous infusion with 150 mEq in 1,000 mL D_5W at 1.5 to 2 times maintenance. The infusion rate is titrated to maintain serum and urinary pH of 7.45 to 7.55 and 7.5 to 8, respectively, and should be continued until the patient is clinically improving and salicylate concentrations are less than 30 mg/dL.

Hemodialysis Should Be Utilized for Severe Salicylate Poisonings

Hemodialysis is the definitive treatment for severe salicylate poisonings and should be considered in many cases, including patients with AMS, new hypoxia requiring supplemental oxygen, pH 7.20 or less, salicylate concentrations greater than 90 or greater than 80 mg/dL with impaired kidney function, and when standard therapy fails. Chronic salicylate poisonings may require hemodialysis at lower salicylate concentrations. Early toxicology and nephrology consultations are essential, and institutions without hemodialysis should consider early transfer in patients approaching severe salicylate poisoning.

PEARLS

- Some salicylate poisonings may not have overdose history, and salicylate poisoning should be considered in adults with mixed respiratory alkalosis with metabolic acidosis and pediatrics with metabolic acidosis.
- Salicylate overdoses can have delayed absorption, and salicylate concentrations should be repeated until down trending.
- Each salicylate concentration must be clinically correlated with a blood gas and serum electrolytes before making treatment decisions.
- Serum and urinary alkalinization are the cornerstone treatment for salicylate poisoning.
- Hemodialysis should be considered for severe salicylate poisoning, and early toxicology and nephrology consultation should be considered with worsening clinical status.

Suggested Readings

Juurlink DN, Gosselin S, Kielstein JT, et al. Extracorporeal treatment for salicylate poisoning: systematic review and recommendations from the EXTRIP workgroup. *Ann Emerg Med.* 2015;66(2):165-181.

Nelson LS, Howland MA, Lewin NA, Smith SW, Goldfrank LR, Hoffman RS, eds. *Goldfrank's Toxicologic Emergencies*. 11th ed. McGraw Hill; 2019.

Sheliza H, Wu PE. Salicylate toxicity from chronic bismuth subsalicylate use. *BMJ Case Reports*. 2020;13(11):e236929.

Truong D, Jaliawala HA, Nimri J, Wu H. Chronic salicylate toxicity presenting as stroke. A43. Critical Care Case Reports: Toxicology and Poisonings. American Thoracic Society International Conference Abstracts; 2020:A1668.

235

Managing the Hot and Bothered: Sympathomimetic Overdoses

Arun Nair

One of the most challenging groups of patients in emergency medicine are those who present with severe agitation. This difficult encounter is only made more complicated when the source of the agitation is pharmacologic. Many drugs (eg, cocaine and methamphetamine) and substances (eg, bupropion) can cause a hyperadrenergic state and lead to a sympathomimetic toxidrome. Getting a good history on these patients is frequently a Herculean feat as they are normally severely agitated and unable or unwilling to provide accurate information. Couple that with abnormal vital signs, difficulty obtaining IV access due to patient compliance, and concern for staff and patient safety, and you end up with an exigent experience. Remembering the following can help improve the overall encounter and ultimate patient outcome.

Treat the Patient First and Then Numbers

Remember the signs and symptoms of the sympathomimetic toxidrome, including agitation, hyperthermia, tachycardia, hypertension, and diaphoresis, to name a few; the next question becomes what to treat first. These patients are normally in a hyperadrenergic state, and the exact etiology is often unknown. Rather than focusing on the causative agent, first focus on treating the patient's symptoms. The main goal is symptom control and patient safety. Once agitated patients are adequately sedated, the vital sign and physical examination derangements frequently improve, often markedly. When an agitated patient needs sedation, what do you reach for?

Benzos, Benzos, and More Benzos...

Benzodiazepines are normally the first-line agents for sympathomimetic patients; depending on the degree of agitation, higher dose of benzodiazepines may be needed than in the average patient. Though some clinicians have strong preferences on first-line benzodiazepines, sometimes, the safest thing for the patient and staff is to use the medication with which the team has the most familiarity. That said, the use of rapidly acting, rapidly titratable benzodiazepines is highly desirable. Given their pharmacologic profile, IV midazolam and IV diazepam are some of the most commonly recommended agents used to sedate a sympathomimetic patient. Both midazolam and diazepam have a time of onset of about 3 to 5 minutes when given IV. This allows providers to redose the medication if needed and decreases the likelihood of dose stacking. Some patients may require large doses of benzodiazepines to safely control their agitation, and dose escalation is often needed; the dosing strategy should be tailored for each individual patient. IV dosing of benzodiazepines is strongly preferred whenever possible. However, in patients without IV access, agents such as midazolam or lorazepam are preferred for intramuscular administration. Benzodiazepines can potentially lower the respiratory drive, though this is less likely to occur with an appropriate dosing strategy in an agitated patient. However, patients should have their airways monitored after adequate sedation is obtained.

Historically, many other agents have been used for acutely agitated patients in the ED. Some of the most commonly used agents include substances like ketamine, various antipsychotics, and other sedatives such as dexmedetomidine. When approaching a sympathomimetic patient, the recommended initial approach is adequate benzodiazepine dosing to achieve adequate sedation. Mixing other pharmacologic agents can often make treating the patient more complex.

On some occasions, despite heroic efforts by the providers, patients are unable to be adequately sedated and require intubation for their safety as well as that of the staff. If intubation is needed, depolarizing agents such as succinylcholine should be avoided. There are a multitude of reasons for this, including altering the metabolism of certain drugs (eg, cocaine) and potentially worsening hyperkalemia. Once sedated, providers should continue to closely monitor the patient's physical examination (including muscle tone) and vital signs (including core temperature).

Patient Management

Patients with sympathomimetic toxicity often experience tachycardia and hypertension. These findings normally improve once the patient's agitation is controlled. However, in the event benzodiazepines are not controlling the hyperadrenergic state and the patient still has worrisome hypertension, other agents, such as phentolamine and nitroprusside, can be considered. It remains standard practice to avoid the use of beta-blockers due to the concern of unopposed alpha stimulation.

Any focal neurologic symptoms including severe headache necessitate a head CT, and chest pain begets a repeat ECG as well as a troponin. Cocaine can produce a number of clinical effects, including sodium channel blockade with resultant QRS widening. If QRS widening occurs, boluses of sodium bicarbonate should be considered until it narrows. Hyperthermia is one of the most concerning findings in patients with sympathomimetic toxicity. Patients who have unrecognized and untreated hyperthermia are at much higher risk for poor outcomes and death. Providers should frequently check for increased muscle tone and should also be monitoring core temperatures. In sympathomimetic patients whose temperature is greater than 38.8 °C (102 °F), active cooling should be considered. Frequently, patients may require aggressive measures, such as ice water immersion to rapidly lower their body temperature.

Often, these patients are part of a vulnerable population at higher risk for concomitant injuries. Providers should assess for other traumatic (ie, barotrauma from smoking) and medical etiologies when assessing patients who have sympathomimetic toxidromes. In addition, providers should consider checking screening labs, including acetaminophen, salicylate, and ethanol, along with a basic metabolic panel, blood gas, lactate, and creatine kinase. A screening ECG should also be performed. Labs and ECGs may need to be trended. Optimizing supportive measures should be pursued, and other medical causes for symptomatology should be explored.

PEARLS

- Prioritize treating agitation in patients with a sympathomimetic toxidrome.
- Benzodiazepines are the drug of choice and should be administered in a methodical manner.
- Hyperthermia may be life-threatening, and some patients may require aggressive cooling.
- Avoid beta-blockers in sympathomimetic patients.
- Monitor muscle tone in agitated patients, and consider rhabdomyolysis in severe agitation.
- Remember to expand your workup, and consider other causes for a patient's presentation.

Suggested Readings

DeSilva DA, Wong MC, Lee MP, et al. Amphetamine-associated ischemic stroke: clinical presentation and proposed pathogenesis. *J Stroke Cerebrovasc Dis*. 2007;16:185.

Nelson LS, Howland M, Lewin NA, Smith SW, Goldfrank LR, Hoffman RS. eds. *Goldfrank's Toxicologic Emergencies*, 11e. McGraw-Hill Education; 2019.

Richards JR, Albertson TE, Derlet RW, et al. Treatment of toxicity from amphetamines, related derivatives, and analogues: a systematic clinical review. *Drug Alcohol Depend.* 2015;1:150.

Riddell J, Tran A, Bengiamin R, Hendey GW, Armenian P. Ketamine as a first-line treatment for severely agitated emergency department patients. *Am J Emerg Med.* 2017;35(7):1000-1004.

236

EMERGING SUBSTANCES OF USE: WHAT'S OLD IS NEW AGAIN

CONOR YOUNG AND KAYLA DUELAND-KUHN

The landscape of substances and drugs of use is ever changing. New substances constantly emerge, and their novelty can make diagnosis and treatment challenging. This chapter focuses on some drug trends seen in recent years.

Fentanyl, Xylazine, and Other Adulterants

Opioids have been common recreational drugs for centuries. Their use has contributed substantially to overdose-related deaths in recent years. Fentanyl, though approved for medical use for decades, has become a common adulterant in many recreational substances, including heroin. Recent efforts by the US Centers for Disease Control and Prevention have led to expansion of awareness and availability of the emergency opioid-reversal agent naloxone. Providers should consider prescribing naloxone to anyone who is concomitantly prescribed opioids and/or is deemed high risk for overdose.

Fentanyl and other synthetic opioids have a very high affinity for mu-opioid receptors and can cause CNS depression and apnea, even at very low doses. This is the primary risk factor for overdose, especially when the user is not aware of its presence. Carfentanyl and fentanyl may be adulterants in heroin, methamphetamine, cocaine, and other illicit substances. Adulterated substances may also be introduced through pill-pressing techniques, meaning that individuals purchasing unregulated pharmaceuticals are also at risk for exposure.

Xylazine is a central alpha-2 agonist with sedative and analgesic properties, which has historically been used by the veterinary industry. Recently, it has been found to be an adulterant in heroin, fentanyl, cocaine, and pressed pills. When injected, xylazine can potentially cause significant tissue necrosis in addition to its other anticipated effects. Because it has different pharmacologic properties compared to opioids and yet produces a similar toxidrome, prehospital and ED staff may encounter patients who do not respond to opioid-reversal agents at the usual doses. When this happens in the context of a recreational drug overdose, clinicians should consider xylazine exposure and call the local poison control center or toxicology service for further guidance.

Novel Forms of THC

THC is the active ingredient in cannabis plants. Dried leaves, commonly referred to as marijuana, have been used recreationally for decades around the world. Many contemporary forms of THC, including THC for vape devices, are extremely concentrated. Edible THC products marketed as pharmaceuticals will typically have known concentrations, but products acquired through other means may have confusing labeling. Adults and children are often unaware of the amount of THC being ingested in noncommercial products. Some packaging of candy-like products containing THC may even look like the packaging of commercial products. This compounds the risk for unintentional ingestion and/or overdose. See Chapter 240 on THC for further information about presentation and management of this intoxicant.

DBZD

There are often many new DBZD derivatives produced illicitly, and their effect profiles are frequently unstudied. Benzodiazepines are GAB_{AA} agonists, which cause CNS depression in overdose. When combined with other CNS depressants such as alcohol, there is a much higher risk of respiratory depression. However, many DBZDs have been formulated to have much higher affinity for GAB_{AA} receptors, which may lead to a risk for significant toxicity after exposures occur.

The treatment for overdose is generally supportive, especially in the absence of respiratory depression. While there is the reversal agent available, flumazenil, caution should be exercised in its administration. Patients who chronically use benzodiazepines have likely developed tolerance to these substances, and reversal with flumazenil carries the risk for precipitated withdrawal. This can lead to significant, and even life-threatening sequelae, including seizures. Therefore, the risk of using flumazenil often outweighs the potential benefits, and the decision for its use should be carefully considered.

PHENIBUT

Phenibut (beta-phenyl-gamma-aminobutyric acid) is a GABA analog, which has been available since the 1960s. Current trends show that the compound has become more accessible after being marketed as an unregulated pharmaceutical. Many individuals have used this substance to try and decrease withdrawal symptoms when attempting to decrease chronic alcohol use. In the overdose setting, clinical effects include CNS depression, hypotension, hypothermia, and respiratory depression. Concomitant use of alcohol, benzodiazepines, barbiturates, and CNS depressants increases the risk for severe toxicity, especially respiratory depression. Providers should consider phenibut withdrawal when they encounter a patient with signs and symptoms of ethanol or benzodiazepine withdrawal but deny using the aforementioned substances. Dependence and subsequent withdrawal from phenibut can be particularly difficult to treat.

KRATOM

Kratom, much like many of the other emerging toxins discussed previously, is an old pharmaceutical, which has once again become prevalent in the unregulated market, particularly in patients who are trying to self-treat their opioid use disorder. The compound is derived from the leaves of the *Mitragyna speciosa* trees native to Southeast Asia. Large overdoses can produce findings consistent with an opioid toxidrome, and withdrawal is typically consistent with opioid withdrawal.

PEARLS

- Providers must be aware of new emerging substances of use when approaching an undifferentiated patient and should start by optimizing supportive care.

- Fentanyl is a common adulterant in both heroin and other nonopiate recreational drugs.
- Xylazine should be considered in patients with clinical features of an opioid overdose that do not respond to standard doses of naloxone.
- Phenibut is a $GABA_B$ agonist and can present with a sedative-hypnotic toxidrome.
- Large kratom ingestions can result in findings similar to opioid overdoses.

Suggested Readings

Brunetti P, Giorgetti R, Tagliabracci A, Huestis MA, Busardò FP. Designer benzodiazepines: a review of toxicology and public health risks. *Pharmaceuticals (Basel)*. 2021;14(6):560. PMID: 34208284.

National Institute of Drug Abuse. *Kratom*. Accessed January 21, 2023. https://nida.nih.gov/research-topics/kratom

United States Department of Health and Human Services. *Naloxone: the drug that saves lives*. https://www.hhs.gov/opioids/treatment/overdoseresponse/index.html.

United States Department of Justice Drug Enforcement Administration. *The growing threat of xylazine and it's mixture with illicit drugs: DEA joint intelligence report*. 2022. https://www.dea.gov/documents/2022/2022-12/2022-12-21/growing-threat-xylazine-and-its-mixture-illicit-drugs

237

Don't Forget Carbon Monoxide Toxicity in the Differential of HA

Joan Chou and Marvin Heyboer III

Workup and management of headache in the ED is frequently an arduous task due to its broad differential. Unfortunately, CO toxicity is often underdiagnosed because of its vague presentation. The long-term and often DNS can have significant impacts on quality of life. Bedside providers must have a high index of suspicion for CO as the cause of headache.

CO Incidence/Causes

Every year, more than 100,000 ED visits are related to CO exposure. This number may be an underestimation of CO frequency as it is likely underdiagnosed, given its vague symptoms. CO is produced from incomplete combustion of carbon-containing materials, such as kerosene, gasoline, wood, and charcoal. Vulnerable populations in regions across the country, especially those with harsh winters, have increased risk of CO exposure if they have suboptimal home heating systems. Whole households often present with vague symptoms, including headache and general malaise or fatigue. House fires are another common cause of CO exposure, and one must also consider concomitant cyanide poisoning in initial evaluation and resuscitation. A substantial proportion is also related to suicide attempts.

PATHOPHYSIOLOGY

CO binds to hemoglobin with greater than a 200 times affinity than oxygen, producing COHb. Its high affinity shifts the oxyhemoglobin dissociation curve to the left, resulting in global hypoxia. In addition, the unbound CO in the bloodstream is absorbed into tissue and binds to other cellular metabolism proteins, such as myoglobin and cytochromes; this prevents appropriate oxidative phosphorylation and ATP production. Furthermore, it causes intravascular neutrophil-mediated lipid peroxidation in tissues from superoxide generation along with oxidative stress, resulting in neuronal cell death. These more complex mechanisms by which CO causes tissue damage are still under investigation. They are thought to be the predominant reason the nervous and cardiac systems are most vulnerable to injury and contribute most to long-term morbidity and mortality.

PRESENTATION AND INITIAL ED MANAGEMENT

CO exposure can be either acute or chronic, has a wide range of nonspecific symptoms on initial presentation, and is why CO poisoning is often misdiagnosed as a viral illness. Common symptoms include headache, nausea, vomiting, dizziness, fatigue, lethargy, chest pain, and dyspnea. In addition, patients may present with neurologic symptoms, including loss of consciousness, transient confusion, slowed thinking and response, cerebellar dysfunction, visual changes, coma, and even death.

As with any toxic exposure, the mainstay of ED management is emergent stabilization and optimizing supportive care. Due to the varying causes and presentation of CO poisoning, the ED workup should evaluate for other coingestions and disease processes. Noninvasive pulse co-oximetry may be used to screen for CO exposure but should not take the place of serum COHb levels for diagnosis (pulse co-oximetry levels vary significantly in accuracy). In nonsmoking patients, normal CO level should be below 3%, while in smoking patients, their baseline CO level can be up to 10%. Diagnosing CO toxicity is done by looking at a myriad of factors, including patient history, the presence and severity of symptoms, and COHb levels. An ECG and troponin level should also be obtained as CO poisoning can cause acute myocardial injury, portending a worse outcome.

When CO exposure is suspected, patient should be immediately placed on a nonrebreather with 100% normobaric oxygen. In ambient air, the half-life of CO is approximately 5 to 6 hours, whereas administration of 100% oxygen decreases its half-life to 1.5 hours. In patients with COHb level greater than 25%, loss of consciousness, end-organ ischemia, and pregnant women with an elevated COHb level, HBO treatment should be considered. Fetal hemoglobin has even higher affinity to CO than adult hemoglobin, and CO can diffuse through the placenta. Also consider lowering the threshold for HBO treatment in the older patients as they are overall more vulnerable to systemic illness. Ideally, HBO should be initiated within 6 hours of CO exposure (although some experts in the field believe there may even be some benefit for treatment up to 24 hours after exposure). This may limit the benefit of transferring certain CO-poisoned patients to a hospital with 24/7 HBO services.

ROLE OF HBO IN CO POISONING

DNS resulting from neurologic injury is one of the most feared complications of CO poisoning, which includes, but is not limited to, cognitive sequelae. While DNS is most likely to occur in severe CO poisoning, it unfortunately has also been seen to occur in only mild or chronic CO exposure. Some studies suggest that there may be a genetic component to the risk of DNS development, but unfortunately, there currently is no emergent method of testing for these factors.

HBO therapy further decreases the half-life of CO to approximately 30 minutes. In addition, HBO has been hypothesized to provide additional benefit on the molecular level. It has been shown to inhibit intravascular neutrophil adherence to the endothelial wall by inhibiting the beta-2 integrin receptor on the neutrophil, which, in cerebral vasculature, prevents lipid peroxidation and neuronal cell death. HBO treatment for CO remains controversial, predominantly due to inconsistencies in methodologies as well as biases that may have influenced interpretation of the results. Nevertheless, several studies provide strong evidence supporting HBO therapy for severe CO poisoning to decrease the risk of DNS. For example, Weaver et al demonstrated that individuals treated with three HBO sessions in the first 24 hours were associated with 21% absolute reduction of neurologic sequelae 6 weeks post CO toxicity. Ultimately, additional research regarding the benefits and mechanisms with which HBO improves outcomes in CO toxicity would be beneficial.

PEARLS

- Have high index of suspicion for CO poisoning when patients present with vague viral-like illness, including headache and neurologic symptoms.
- Pulse co-oximetry can be helpful to screen for CO exposure; however, COHb blood level remains key in confirming diagnosis.
- Obtain a cardiac workup, as myocardial injury may predict worse outcome.
- Consider HBO treatment if patient is presenting within 6 and up to 24 hours of CO with symptoms of moderate-to-severe poisoning.

Suggested Readings

American College of Emergency Physicians Clinical Policies Subcommittee (Writing Committee) on Carbon Monoxide Poisoning; Wolf SJ, Maloney GE, Shih RD, Shy BD, Brown MD. Clinical policy: critical issues in the evaluation and management of adult patients presenting to the emergency department with acute carbon monoxide poisoning. *Ann Emerg Med.* 2017;69(1):98-107.e6.

Buckley NA, Juurlink DN, Isbister G, Bennett MH, Lavonas EJ. Hyperbaric oxygen for carbon monoxide poisoning. *Cochrane Database Syst Rev.* 2011;2011(4):CD002041.

Weaver LK. Clinical practice. Carbon monoxide poisoning. *N Engl J Med.* 2009;360(12):1217-1225.

Weaver LK. Carbon monoxide poisoning. *Undersea Hyperb Med.* 2020;47(1):151-169.

Weaver LK, Valentine KJ, Hopkins RO. Carbon monoxide poisoning: risk factors for cognitive sequelae and the role of hyperbaric oxygen. *Am J Respir Crit Care Med.* 2007;176(5):491-497.

238

DON'T FORGET SEROTONIN TOXICITY IN YOUR PATIENT WITH AGITATION

AHMED ALSAKHA AND CHRISTINE M. STORK

Treating patients with agitation is common in the ED. The differential diagnosis of patients exhibiting signs of agitation and alteration is vast and includes SS. This condition results from excess serotonin in the central nervous system. Although SS is the commonly used term for serotonergic excess, ST more aptly describes this phenomenon as the condition has a wide range of severity. The degree of toxicity ranges from mild to severe and is characterized by mental status changes, neuromuscular excitation, and autonomic instability.

ST most commonly results from the interaction of two or more xenobiotics with serotonergic properties and occasionally after overdose or high therapeutic doses of a single serotonergic xenobiotic. Many xenobiotics belonging to different therapeutic classes have been implicated in the development of ST (**Table 238.1**). SSRIs and other

TABLE 238.1 EXAMPLES OF XENOBIOTICS WITH A POTENTIAL OF CAUSING ST

SSRIs
Fluoxetine, paroxetine, sertraline, fluvoxamine, citalopram, escitalopram

SNRIs
Venlafaxine, desvenlafaxine, duloxetine

Atypical antidepressants
Trazodone, nefazodone, bupropion

Monoamine oxidase inhibitors
Moclobemide, clorgiline, tranylcypromine, isocarboxazid

Tricyclic antidepressants
Amitriptyline, amoxapine, desipramine, doxepin, imipramine, nortriptyline

Opioids
Fentanyl, tramadol, meperidine

Over-the-counter antitussives
Dextromethorphan

Antibiotics
Linezolid, ritonavir

Mood stabilizers
Lithium

Drugs of abuse
MDMA, LSD, ayahuasca preparations

Others
Methylene blue, St. John wort, ginseng, L-tryptophan

SNRIs, serotonin/norepinephrine reuptake inhibitors; SSRIs, selective serotonin reuptake inhibitors; ST, serotonin toxicity.

antidepressants are commonly prescribed, and their interactions with other serotonergic medications, including herbal supplements and over-the-counter medications, should be considered when evaluating a patient with agitation. A careful medication history with any recent additions or dosage changes is crucial to uncovering the diagnosis of ST. In addition to the serotonergic considerations, providers must remember that many agents possess unique properties. Some include seizures or QTc prolongation, and it is important to review the specific toxicities of each substance to which a patient may have been exposed.

The clinical diagnosis of ST is based on the presence of characteristic findings of mental status changes (agitation, confusion, anxiety, hypomania), neuromuscular excitation (clonus/myoclonus, hyperreflexia, rigidity/hypertonia, tremors/shivering), and autonomic instability (hyperthermia, tachycardia, diaphoresis, mydriasis, flushing) after exposure to serotonergic agents. One of the most widely used and validated tools to aid in the diagnosis of ST is the Hunter criteria. Hunter criteria stipulate that the diagnosis of ST is made based upon exposure to serotonergic drugs in the clinical setting of spontaneous clonus, inducible clonus AND agitation or diaphoresis, ocular clonus AND agitation or diaphoresis, tremor AND hyperreflexia, or hypertonia AND temperature above 100.4 °F (38 °C) AND ocular or inducible clonus. Certain findings such as clonus and hyperreflexia are rarely seen in other conditions. The clinical diagnosis of ST is often challenging in the clinical setting, and it is often confused with other conditions, such as NMS. One way to differentiate ST and NMS is through chronology; after medication changes are made, ST normally has its onset over hours to days, whereas NMS typically occurs over the course of weeks.

The treatment of ST is often accomplished by optimizing supportive measures, and the degree of intervention required depends on the severity of ST. First and foremost, any life-threatening vital signs derangements must be immediately addressed. Severe hyperthermia secondary to agitation and increased muscle rigidity often represents the most immediate life threat. This should be addressed by rapidly and aggressively cooling the patient to avoid catastrophic sequelae. This can be accomplished through a variety of manners, though one of the most effective forms of cooling for life-threatening hyperthermia is ice water immersion. Other therapies to treat agitation and increased muscle tone include the administration of benzodiazepines; two benzodiazepines that are often used for this purpose include midazolam and diazepam as they are both rapidly acting when given through the intravenous route, and therefore, patients can be frequently reassessed to ensure the desired effects are being achieved. Some cases of severe hyperthermia secondary to increased muscle tone may even require neuromuscular blockade and subsequent intubation. If this is needed, nondepolarizing agents such as rocuronium or vecuronium should be considered.

Another option in the management of ST is the administration of serotonin antagonists, such as cyproheptadine. This medication acts through 5-HT$_{2A}$ antagonism, the receptor believed to be responsible for the adverse effects of ST. Although this is frequently taught as the "antidote" for ST, its use is limited as it is only available orally and it also has anticholinergic properties that may worsen the clinical status of a patient with polypharmacy toxicity. Consultation with poison control centers or a toxicologist is recommended before the initiation of cyproheptadine.

Throughout the course of the patient's resuscitation, clinicians must pay close attention to the patient's core temperature and muscle tone to ensure proper response to treatment. Most cases require admission to the hospital with the majority improving within 24 to 72 hours after the discontinuation of the offending xenobiotics.

PEARLS

- Consider ST in your differential diagnosis of any patient with agitation in the ED.
- Discontinue any offending xenobiotics as soon as ST is suspected.
- Agitation, rigidity, and hyperthermia may lead to significant morbidity or mortality, and they should be treated aggressively.
- Close monitoring of vital signs, including a core temperature, should be performed.
- Use benzodiazepines as a first-line modality to control sedation and rigidity, and consider cyproheptadine in consultation with a toxicologist.
- Rapid cooling measures, including ice water immersion, should be implemented for life-threatening hyperthermia.

SUGGESTED READINGS

Boyer EW, Shannon M. The serotonin syndrome. *N Engl J Med*. 2005;352:1112-1120.
Buckley NA, Dawson AH, Isbister GK. Serotonin syndrome. *BMJ*. 2014;348:g1626.
Isbister GK, Buckley NA, Whyte IM. Serotonin toxicity: a practical approach to diagnosis and treatment. *Med J Aust*. 2007;187(6):361-365.
Stork CM. Serotonin reuptake inhibitors and atypical antidepressants. In: Nelson LS, Howland M, Lewin NA, Smith SW, Goldfrank LR, Hoffman RS, eds. *Goldfrank's Toxicologic Emergencies*, 11th ed. *McGraw Hill*; 2019.

239

BE SURE TO ASK ABOUT HERBAL REMEDIES

DANIELLA GIARDINA AND JEANNA M. MARRAFFA

Use of dietary and herbal supplements is common in the United States. In fact, it is estimated that nearly 60% of adults have used a dietary supplement at some point, with this percentage increasing with advancing age. Nearly 20% of patients use supplements on a regular basis. More than 20,000 ED visits in the United States annually are attributed to adverse events from dietary supplements. Herbal and dietary supplements are touted to be effective for a variety of health benefits, and many patients use these to prevent or treat underlying medical problems.

Supplements can cause adverse events and drug-drug interactions, which may go unrecognized if patients do not report use. When patients present to the ED, it is imperative for practitioners to explicitly ask questions regarding the use of herbal and dietary supplements as part of medication reconciliation. It is impossible to discuss every supplement or adverse event. This review is intended to provide an overview of the general approach to patients with the use of these agents as well as discuss scenarios where specific antidotal therapy is necessary in emergency stabilization.

Herbal supplements have a variety of uses and can be easily purchased in stores and on the internet. Despite not being well studied, they are often touted to prevent and treat illness. Some of the more common conditions that they are used for include depression, fatigue, pain, weight loss, sexual wellness, and overall immune support. The most common herbal supplements used in the United States include cranberry, turmeric, garlic, ginger, and gingko. Certain supplements are deemed as unsafe by the FDA but are neither regulated nor officially banned. One notable example of a banned substance is ephedra; sales of this substance were prohibited by the FDA in 2004. Kratom is a common substance that is not officially prohibited, although the FDA and DEA have considered regulations. The leaves of this tree may be used as a stimulant or for pain relief; many people also use this as an alternative to treat opioid use disorder.

Dietary supplements can be inherently toxic for a variety of reasons. As they are unregulated by the FDA, products may contain higher quantities of compounds than listed on the label. They also can be contaminated or adulterated with pharmaceutical products or even contain heavy metals. In addition, drug-drug interactions resulting in toxicity or the active ingredient may be toxic, even at low doses. Allergic reactions are likely underreported but can also occur. The information about product content, dose, and toxicities is often difficult to obtain, resulting in challenges and delays in accurate identification of the offending agent.

Herbal supplements may seem benign, but the spectrum of toxicity is similar to that of pharmaceuticals. Rapid stabilization and supportive care are paramount in managing these patients, similar to any toxic exposure. Basic diagnostic studies should be performed, including electrolytes and liver function tests, to help determine the course of treatment. In the case of an undifferentiated ingestion, laboratory results may also provide insight into the toxin. It is important to recognize the scenarios when targeted therapy is necessary. Benzodiazepines should be given to patients with sympathomimetic symptoms or seizure activity. Physostigmine may be considered in some patients with anticholinergic delirium; providers should talk with a toxicologist or poison center before giving physostigmine. Some supplements contain cardioactive steroids that cause toxicity similar to acute digoxin poisoning. In this scenario, treatment with digoxin Fab is warranted. Many herbal supplements have anticoagulant properties. Some may potentiate the activity of warfarin. Treatment may include prothrombin complex concentrate. Numerous dietary and herbal supplements are well-known hepatotoxins. In some scenarios, treatment with *N*-acetylcysteine may be considered. LiverTox is a free resource through the National Library of Medicine that has a list of medications and supplements that cause liver injury.

Herbal remedies continue to gain popularity, yet, in most cases, they are not adequately regulated nor studied. A patient may be using an herbal preparation for a specific effect, but they may be unaware of potential adverse reactions and interactions. It is important that practitioners have a general knowledge of the organ toxicities of common supplements and obtain a complete medication history, including the use of dietary or herbal supplements. Adverse events, drug interactions, and effects from contaminates can occur from these products. Clinical features may provide insight. Initial stabilization of these patients with general supportive care is the mainstay of therapy, although, in some situations, antidotal therapy is needed. Health care providers should include herbal and dietary supplements on the differential diagnosis.

TABLE 239.1 COMMON HERBAL REMEDIES

Agent	Common/Purported Use	Toxicity/Organ System	Specific Treatment
Aconitum (Aconite)	Inotropy, fever, restlessness	CV collapse, GI upset	Antiarrhythmic therapy
Ashwagandha	Immune support, stress relief	CNS depression (may potentiate effects of sedatives), GI upset	
Comfrey	Skin—burns, bruises, sprains	Hepatic disease	
Cranberry	UTI	Bleeding	
Elder	Laxative	GI upset	
Ephedra	Stimulant	Sympathomimetic—HTN, CVA, seizure, tachycardia	
Evening primrose	Used in the treatment of autoimmune diseases, cancer	May lower seizure threshold	
Garlic	Infection, HTN	Antiplatelet, may interact with anticoagulation	
Ginger	Antiemetic, stimulant	Increased risk of bleeding, may interact with anticoagulation	
Gingko	Antioxidant, digestion aid	Bleeding, may interact with anticoagulation, dermatitis, GI upset	
Ginseng	Many—stress relief, URIs, impotence	Stimulant effects, may reduce efficacy of warfarin	
Goldenseal	Abdominal and menstrual pain	GI upset, neuro effects/paralysis	
Green tea extract	Antioxidant, weight loss	Hepatotoxicity	
Kava	Stress relief	CNS depression, weakness, hepatotoxicity	
Kratom	Stimulant, pain relief	GI upset, withdrawal, psychosis, hepatic toxicity	Naloxone for respiratory depression; Buprenorphine for withdrawal
Licorice root	GI upset	Weakness; hyperaldosteronism (HTN, arrhythmia, hypokalemia)	
Melatonin	Insomnia		
St. John wort	Depression, anxiety	CYP3A4 inducer	
Valerian	Anxiety	CNS depression	
Yohimbe	Stimulant, sex drive, muscle development	HTN, weakness	

CNS, central nervous system; CV, cardiovascular; CVA, cardiovascular accident; GI, gastrointestinal; HTN, hypertension; UTI, urinary tract infection.

PEARLS

- Specifically ask about herbal remedies when taking a patient history. Patients may not consider them medications and may not mention them unless specifically prompted. Don't forget that pediatric patients may take herbal supplements as well.
- It is important to have a complete, reconciled medication list. The patient may be at risk for (or even experiencing) herbal-drug interaction. Anticoagulants (especially warfarin) and psychiatric medications are often implicated.
- Toxicity often comes from misuse or contamination, not an inherent property of the plant itself. The knowledge of many herbal preparations comes from indigenous medicine; however, modern consumers may be using these products differently than originally intended.
- Herbal supplements are generally not regulated by the FDA. Be wary that potentially dangerous products are easily attainable by patients.
- General treatment is withdrawal of the herbal remedy and supportive care (**Table 239.1**). However, there are cases in which targeted therapy is warranted. It is important to know which supplements require a specific antidote.

SUGGESTED READINGS

Ekor M. The growing use of herbal medicines: issues relating to adverse reactions and challenges in monitoring safety. *Front Pharmacol.* 2014;4:177. PMID: 24454289.

LiverTox. *Clinical and research information on drug-induced liver injury* [Internet]. National Institute of Diabetes and Digestive and Kidney Diseases; 2012. https://www.ncbi.nlm.nih.gov/books/NBK547852/

240

DUDE, DON'T MAKE THESE MARIJUANA MISTAKES

RAIZADA VAID AND MICHAEL HODGMAN

Marijuana is the common name for dried leaves, stems, and flowers of *Cannabis sativa*, the most used illicit substance in the world. Recreational use is legal in more than 20 US states, and as of 2023, many allow retail sales of cannabis and cannabis-derived products.

The principal active chemical component in marijuana is delta-9-THC. The THC content of cannabis has increased dramatically, from an average concentration of 4% to 6% several decades ago, to engineered strains now yielding concentrations exceeding 15% to 20%. Extracts, such as butane hash oil, may have THC concentrations exceeding 90% to 95%.

The past several years have also featured a surge in the popularity of THC-containing edibles. An unintended consequence has been an increase in unintentional exposure and intoxication of young children. As such, cannabis should be on the differential for any altered or intoxicated child.

The nonpsychoactive cannabinoid CBD, isolated from hemp, has been used to synthesize psychoactive delta-9 THC isomers and derivatives. These synthetic analogs include delta-8 THC and THC acetate ester. The past decade has also seen a proliferation of potent SCRAs. These bear little structural similarity to THC but can result in profound intoxication.

PHARMACOKINETICS/PHARMACODYNAMICS

Cannabinoid receptors are found both centrally and peripherally. The psychoactive effects of delta-9-THC and its analogs and isomers are modulated primarily through CB_1 receptors in the brain. The CB_2 receptor, found predominantly in peripheral tissues, is thought to have immunomodulatory effects. Many SCRAs have greater potency at CB_1 receptors, resulting in more profound intoxication.

The primary routes of exposure to cannabis are inhalation or ingestion. After inhalation, peak serum concentrations and symptom onset are seen within minutes, generally with a duration of maximal effect no more than 1 hour. In contrast, postingestion peak serum concentrations are delayed and unpredictable. Clinical effects may be delayed for up to an hour with a relatively more prolonged duration of intoxication.

THC is metabolized to an active metabolite, 11-hydroxy-THC, and then to inactive 11-carboxy-THC. As a lipid-soluble compound, THC can accumulate in lipid-rich tissues, particularly with chronic use. Once metabolized, THC metabolites are eliminated in both the urine and stool.

ACUTE TOXICITY

Common effects of marijuana use include perceptual alteration, relaxation, euphoria, and increased appetite. Clinical findings may include tachycardia, postural hypotension, and conjunctival injection. With more profound intoxication, ataxia, cognitive impairment, slurred speech, confusion, and sedation may be seen. Bradycardia rather than tachycardia sometimes occurs. Rarely, arrhythmias including life-threatening ventricular tachycardia have been reported. Other adverse clinical effects include dysphoria, anxiety, paranoia, agitation, and, rarely, acute psychosis.

Toddlers with exposure to cannabis may simply appear altered but can manifest more severe effects, including obtundation, agitation, irritability, respiratory depression, and coma. Other less common symptoms include apnea, seizures, bradycardia, and heart block.

After exposure to an SCRA, more severe manifestations may be seen, including severe agitation or deep sedation, profound bradycardia, and seizures.

DIAGNOSTIC TESTING AND MANAGEMENT

For patients with minor symptoms, a nonthreatening quiet environment and supportive care are effective. For any patient who is altered or intoxicated, perform routine rapid assessment. A careful physical examination should be done to evaluate for alternate diagnoses, complications, or injuries. Don't forget a core temperature and finger-stick glucose. Lastly, consider possible coexposure to other drugs.

Appropriate laboratory evaluation includes serum electrolytes in any patient who is altered, hepatic and pancreatic enzymes in patients with GI symptoms, and imaging studies as indicated by examination. Obtain a serum CK in patients who are agitated or hyperthermic or if there has been prolonged downtime. If there is any concern for suicidality, obtain acetaminophen and salicylate concentrations. The value of urine toxicology testing for THC in the altered adolescent or adult is extremely limited; however, in a presumably THC-naïve toddler, a urine positive for THC supports the diagnosis of cannabis intoxication.

Benzodiazepines are reasonable for patients who are agitated and not responding to nonpharmacologic measures. Psychotic symptoms related to cannabis intoxication may be brief and self-resolving. Antipsychotics should be considered in cases of prolonged symptomatology (remember to check for QT prolongation). Other management should be based on clinical findings.

Cannabinoid Hyperemesis Syndrome

CHS is associated with chronic, heavy marijuana use and should be considered in anyone presenting with recurrent or treatment-refractory vomiting and abdominal discomfort. A history of improvement with hot shower or baths is a clue to this diagnosis. This is a diagnosis of exclusion.

Treatment options include dopamine antagonists (such as droperidol or haloperidol), benzodiazepines, and/or topical capsaicin. Counsel patients that topical capsaicin may cause an unpleasant burning sensation. Although analgesics are sometime necessary, opioids should be avoided. Long term, the most important treatment is cessation of marijuana use.

Urine Drug Screening

Routine screening tests for THC are typically qualitative urine immunoassays directed toward delta-9-carboxy-THC. These antibodies cross-react with other THCs and THC metabolites to some degree. THC may be detectable in the urine for up to a week after single use and much longer in chronic users. For this reason, a positive urine test for THC in an adolescent or adult should not be assumed to represent acute intoxication. CBD will not cause a positive urine THC screen unless the product is contaminated with THC. The SCRAs will not be detected by urine THC tests and require specific testing.

Definitive testing for THC involves the use of more sensitive and specific testing, such as gas chromatography tandem mass spectrometry. For most routine encounters, this is rarely indicated, except for select cases with medico-legal implications.

PEARLS

- Most cannabis exposures can be managed with routine supportive care.
- The onset and duration of intoxication after ingestion are delayed and prolonged compared to that of inhalation.
- Edible cannabis exposure should be considered in any acutely altered child.
- Haloperidol or droperidol may alleviate symptoms of CHS.
- A positive urine immunoassay for THC does *not* equate to acute cannabis intoxication in adolescents or adults, while, in a naïve altered toddler, it supports the diagnosis.

Suggested Readings

Banister SD, Arnold JC, Connor M, Glass M, McGregor IS. Dark classics in chemical neuroscience: Δ9-tetrahydrocannabinol. *ACS Chem Neurosci*. 2019;10(5):2160-2175. PMID: 30689342.

Cao D, Srisuma S, Bronstein AC, Hoyte CO. Characterization of edible marijuana product exposures reported to United States poison centers. *Clin Toxicol (Phila)*. 2016;54(9):840-846. PMID: 27418198.

Crocker CE, Carter AJE, Emsley JG, Magee K, Atkinson P, Tibbo PG. When cannabis use goes wrong: mental health side effects of cannabis use that present to emergency services. *Front Psychiatry*. 2021;12:640222. PMID: 33658953.

Wang GS. Pediatric concerns due to expanded cannabis use: unintended consequences of legalization. *J Med Toxicol*. 2017;13(1):99-105. PMID: 27139708.

Wong KU, Baum CR. Acute cannabis toxicity. *Pediatr Emerg Care*. 2019;35(11):799-804. PMID: 31688799.

241

KNOW THE DIFFERENCES BETWEEN CALCIUM CHANNEL AND BETA-BLOCKER OVERDOSES

CURTIS GEIER AND KATHY LESAINT

The hallmark presenting symptoms of toxicity from both calcium channel blockers and beta-blockers are bradycardia and hypotension. Patients may present with vague complaints or remain asymptomatic early following ingestion and subsequently experience clinical deterioration. Early symptoms after overdose include fatigue, dizziness, and lightheadedness. Vital sign abnormalities result from decreased SA node function, causing sinus bradycardia, sinus pauses or sinus arrest, and impaired AV nodal conduction. In the case of large ingestions, shock resulting from impaired cardiac function and/or peripheral vasodilation will be present. The degree of impaired cardiac contractility relative to vasodilation may differ between classes and specific agents. Altered mental status, ranging from delirium to coma, and other organ dysfunction can result from impaired perfusion. Classic ECG findings from both classes may include a variety of AV nodal blocks or a junctional rhythm with a normal QRS duration, though exceptions do exist.

Among calcium channel blockers, dihydropyridine agents (amlodipine, nifedipine, etc) traditionally impair the vascular system more than chronotropy and inotropy, causing a predominant peripheral vasodilation that induces a reflex tachycardia. However, this distinction may be lost in massive ingestions. The nondihydropyridine agents, diltiazem and verapamil, affect both cardiac function and vascular tone. Calcium channel blocker toxicity also generally presents with hyperglycemia related to impaired pancreatic insulin secretion. This finding may be important in distinguishing between calcium channel and beta-blocker toxicity.

Beta-blocker toxicity may present with normoglycemia or even hypoglycemia. Susceptible patients may present with bronchospasm due to loss of beta-adrenergic–mediated bronchodilation. Propranolol, which possesses the most membrane-stabilizing activity of this class, readily crosses the blood-brain barrier, and toxicity can present with confusion, coma, or seizures in addition to a widened QRS interval. Sotalol uniquely inhibits delayed rectifying potassium channels, resulting in QT prolongation that may result in torsade de pointes in addition to its beta-blocking effects.

Initial management of toxicity from either calcium channel blockers or beta-blockers involves nonspecific emergency management of presenting symptoms. Contact your local poison center for specific recommendations. Patients with suspected calcium channel blocker or beta-blocker poisoning should be considered at risk for cardiovascular collapse and evaluated with an ECG, followed by cardiac and hemodynamic monitoring. Initiation of early GI decontamination and pharmacologic therapies before patients manifest severe poisoning is key. Activated charcoal given orally at a dose of either 50 g for adults or 1 g/kg in pediatric patients can decrease gastric absorption. For patients with ingestions of delayed or extended-release preparations, delayed administration of activated charcoal can be considered. Charcoal administration should be avoided in patients with altered mental status with a risk of aspiration. For sustained-release products, or large ingestions, whole bowel irrigation should be considered if the patient can safely tolerate; see Chapter 246.

Patients with altered mental status may require assisted ventilation or endotracheal intubation. Seizures resulting from lipophilic beta-blockers should be treated with benzodiazepines. Magnesium should be administered in the setting of prolonged QT interval. IV epinephrine or norepinephrine infusions are the initial vasopressor choices to treat both bradycardia and hypotension. There is limited role for hemodialysis in calcium channel blocker toxicity. Some beta-blockers, including nadolol, atenolol, sotalol, and acebutolol, can be cleared by hemodialysis.

Specific antidotes have varying efficacy based on the agent and degree of toxicity being managed. Often, multiple agents may be necessary to stabilize a patient experiencing significant toxicity. Glucagon is used in beta-blocker toxicity because of its ability to bypass the beta-receptor and ultimately increases myocardial contractility. For adults, the typical starting dose of glucagon is 5 mg IV administered as a bolus. There is limited evidence supporting patient outcomes with this therapy. Nausea is the most frequently encountered adverse effect of glucagon, while less common reactions include hypersensitivity/anaphylaxis and rebound hypoglycemia. IV calcium, either calcium chloride or calcium gluconate, should be considered as it may increase cardiac contractility; however, it may have limited effects on peripheral vasodilation or AV nodal blockade. Calcium chloride is ideally given via central venous access, if possible. High-dose insulin euglycemia therapy should be considered early if initial therapies are ineffective with beta-blocker or calcium channel blocker toxicity. See Chapter 245 for additional details.

IFE may be an effective therapy for patients in extremis despite optimizing therapeutic options. IFE may particularly be valuable in the case of severe verapamil or propranolol poisoning, as both are highly lipid soluble. The optimal dose and formulation of IFE are unknown; however, an initial bolus of 1.5 mL/kg of 20% lipid emulsion followed by an infusion of 0.25 mL/kg/min is a suggested protocol. IFE is normally reserved for patients who are in a peri-code setting or are hemodynamically unstable.

Other adjunctive pharmacotherapies and hemodynamic support have been studied, but there are limited data and should only be considered when aforementioned treatments have failed. Methylene blue, at an initial dose of 1 mg/kg IV bolus, has been utilized in dihydropyridine calcium channel blocker toxicity, specifically with amlodipine, resulting in lower vasopressor requirements. Transthoracic or IV cardiac pacing may induce capture and improve heart rate. Intra-aortic balloon counterpulsation is another invasive option to be considered in patients refractory to pharmacologic therapy. For refractory shock, ECMO or other mechanical cardiac assist devices should be considered if available, to support perfusion while the offending agent is metabolized or cleared.

PEARLS

- Patients presenting with toxicity from beta-blockers or calcium channel blockers may have hemodynamic instability due to impaired cardiac function and/or vasodilation.
- Calcium channel blocker toxicity frequently presents with hyperglycemia, while beta-blocker toxicity may present with normoglycemia or hypoglycemia.
- Initial management involves emergency stabilization, including seizure management or endotracheal intubation, if appropriate, followed by vasopressor initiation.
- High-dose insulin euglycemia therapy is effective and should be considered early.
- Call your local poison center in any suspected case of calcium channel or beta-blocker toxicity.

SUGGESTED READINGS

Engebretsen KM, Kaczmarek KM, Morgan J, Holger JS. High-dose insulin therapy in beta-blocker and calcium channel-blocker poisoning. *Clin Toxicol (Phila)*. 2011;49(4): 277-283.

DeWitt CR, Waksman JC. Pharmacology, pathophysiology and management of calcium channel blocker and β-blocker toxicity. *Toxicol Rev*. 2004;23:223-238.

242

DON'T STUMBLE ON THE DIALYZABLE TOXINS

DANIEL TIRADO AND VINCENT J. CALLEO

Managing a poisoned patient can be a complex and daunting task. Understanding the toxin is essential to determining the best way to deal with its effects. While many substances are amendable to pharmacologic treatment, others require additional measures to optimize care. One potentially lifesaving modality is dialysis.

WHAT MAKES A TOXIN DIALYZABLE?

Dialysis uses a closed circuit with a semipermeable membrane to separate molecules from the blood. Several factors must be considered trying to determine if dialysis will be effective for a particular toxin. The first factor is the size of the molecule; small molecules are more likely to be removed by dialysis than very large molecules. Another factor that affects a substance's amenability to dialysis is protein binding. As protein binding increases, the ability to successfully remove the substance via dialysis decreases. The V_d also influences whether dialysis will be effective; if a toxin has a high V_d, it will be less available in the serum and thus dialysis will be unlikely to remove it. Various forms of dialysis exist, including intermittent high-flux hemodialysis and continuous renal replacement therapy. For most poisonings, hemodialysis is the preferred modality of extracorporeal removal, though different techniques may be required based on individual patient characteristics.

SOME COMMON DIALYZABLE TOXINS

Although some toxins are not inherently dialyzable in and of themselves, dialysis is needed to manage their sequelae. However, there are many dialyzable toxins. We briefly discuss some of these more commonly ingested dialyzable toxins that an emergency physician is likely to encounter. As with the approach to any critically ill patient, remember to first address your primary and secondary survey and optimize supportive measures.

Salicylates (ASA) can be found in several products, including aspirin, oil of wintergreen, and bismuth subsalicylate. It also commonly exists in various combination medications. Salicylates are readily dialyzable, and a timely and appropriate initiation of dialysis can be lifesaving. Hemodialysis is strongly recommended if the salicylate level is greater than 100 mg/dL or if the level is greater than 90 mg/dL with renal impairment. Additional recommendations for hemodialysis include new hypoxemia and altered mental status that does not improve with dextrose administration. Acidosis (pH <7.20) should prompt the astute clinician to strongly consider hemodialysis. Severe salicylate toxicity poses major life-threatening effects, and nephrology should be consulted for dialysis if the patient appears to worsen clinically or if the salicylate levels are quickly rising (even if the level is below the aforementioned values). Providers must recall that chronic salicylism may require hemodialysis at lower levels than mentioned earlier.

Lithium is a metal that is most used in the treatment of not only bipolar disorder but also major depression. Although its mechanism of action is not well understood, its toxic effects are well established. Lithium is available in both immediate- and sustained-release formulations. It is primarily renally excreted, and any insult that affects kidney function may result in the accumulation of lithium to toxic levels. Lithium toxicity can be acute, acute on chronic, or chronic, and this should be considered when evaluating a lithium toxic patient. Symptoms of lithium toxicity are many and can include vomiting, tremor, ataxia, and altered mental status. Initial management of lithium toxicity normally includes fluid resuscitation with normal saline. Lithium does not bind to activated charcoal, but certain cases (ie, large ingestions of extended-release lithium) may benefit from whole bowel irrigation. Lithium is dialyzable, and hemodialysis should be considered in several conditions, including an isolated level greater than 5.0 mEq/L, levels greater than 4.0 mEq/L with renal impairment, altered mental status, or seizures.

Metformin is a commonly prescribed antidiabetic medication that can cause a profound lactic acidosis in either acute ingestions or as a result of drug accumulation due to other ongoing illnesses, including dehydration or sepsis. The mechanisms of metformin toxicity are complex but ultimately result in hyperlactatemia. Patients may present with a wide range of symptoms depending on the degree of toxicity and include nausea, vomiting, delirium, and alterations in mental status. Activated charcoal may be beneficial for those who have a suspected history of acute ingestion before presentation if it can be safely tolerated. Initial treatments largely center around optimizing supportive measures. Although metformin itself is not extremely dialyzable, dialysis is frequently needed for severe poisonings due to the markedly elevated lactate and profound acidosis. Although experts have differing opinions on when to initiate dialysis, most agree that dialysis is indicated for a lactate greater than 20 mmol/L or pH less than 7.0. It should also be strongly considered if patients are unresponsive to supportive therapy. Providers should have a lower threshold to consider dialysis for severe metformin poisonings if the patient has a rising lactate greater than 10 mmol/L as well as other comorbidities, including impaired renal or hepatic function.

The aforementioned toxins are but a few dialyzable substances. Additional information on some commonly encountered dialyzable toxins can be found in the guidelines from the Extracorporeal Treatments in Poisoning Workgroup. Given the complexities of dialysis, providers should remember to confer with their nephrology and toxicology colleagues to determine if a patient may benefit from this potentially lifesaving intervention.

PEARLS

- Optimizing supportive measures is key before determining if a patient is a candidate for dialysis.
- A toxin's size, volume of distribution, and protein-binding determine if it is dialyzable.
- High-flux hemodialysis is normally the preferred modality of extracorporeal removal for poisoned patients.
- Early consideration and involvement of nephrology is essential as it takes times to initiate dialysis.

Suggested Readings

EXTRIP. Blood purification in toxicology: reviewing the evidence and providing recommendations. February 2023. https://www.extrip-workgroup.org

Goldfrank LR, Flomenbaum NE, Lewin NA, Weisman RS, Howland MA, Hoffman RS. *Goldfrank's Toxicologic Emergencies.* Appleton & Lange; 1994.

Klaassen CD. In: Klaassen CD, ed. *Casarett & Doull's Toxicology: The Basic Science of Poisons*, 9th ed. McGraw Hill; 2018.

243

TCA Toxicities Still Happen

Rachel Gorodetsky

TCA toxicity is among the most classic poisonings. While still heavily emphasized in didactic education and board exams, they are far less frequently encountered in the modern era than in the past. Their place in therapy for the treatment of depression has grown smaller as many newer, safer antidepressants entered the market. TCAs are now much more likely to be prescribed at a low dose for sleep than for depression. It would be a mistake, however, to believe that TCA overdoses no longer occur. One of the reasons they remain so prevalent in toxicology instruction is because, despite their rarity, treating a patient affected by TCA poisoning can be a very challenging and humbling experience.

TCAs include amitriptyline, amoxapine, nortriptyline, imipramine, desipramine, and doxepin. Commonly referred to as "dirty drugs," these medications work through several mechanisms, have a narrow therapeutic index, and are often considered on the "deadly in small doses" list, meaning the ingestion of a single pill in a child weighing 10 kg or less could be potentially fatal.

The hallmark of TCA toxicity is the rapid onset of symptoms; delayed toxicity is extremely atypical. If severe poisoning is going to develop, it does so within the first few hours. Patients with a history of overdose who present asymptomatic can be cleared if they remain asymptomatic after a 6-hour observation with no other coingestants.

The four main features of TCA poisoning are as follows:

- Prolongation of the QRS interval due to cardiac sodium channel blockade
- Seizures from GABA antagonism
- Hypotension from blockade of alpha-1 adrenergic receptors
- Anticholinergic symptoms

Check Your ECG and Check It Often

The QRS interval on a 12-lead ECG is the most reliable metric for the severity of poisoning in a patient with a TCA overdose. In asymptomatic patients, an ECG at least every 2 hours is recommended to monitor for the development of toxicity. In symptomatic patients, ECGs are obtained as needed, as often as every 15 minutes, to determine progression of toxicity and response to treatment. About one in three patients with a QRS greater than 100 msec will develop seizures, and about one in two patients with a QRS greater than 160 msec will develop dysrhythmias. QRS intervals greater than 200 msec have been reported in severe toxicity. Finally, slowed conduction also causes an R wave on lead aVR, and the amplitude of the R wave is also associated with the severity of toxicity; an amplitude greater than 3 mm is associated with increased incidence of seizures and dysrhythmias.

Other than the ECG, standard monitoring of vital signs; basic labs including acetaminophen, aspirin, and ethanol levels; and mental status is also required. There are no specific drug levels to monitor for TCAs that are readily available to assist with clinical decision-making.

GI Decontamination

TCA overdoses are one of the few times where orogastric lavage may be clinically indicated. A patient who presents within an hour of ingestion should be considered a candidate for lavage. Intubation should be performed first to protect the airway, as aspiration is a major risk of gastric lavage. Activated charcoal should also be given if the patient presents early after ingestion and can safely tolerate it; this should be done either after lavage is completed or by itself if lavage is not performed. More information can be found in Chapter 246.

Managing Seizures

Seizures, usually brief and self-limited, are a common feature of TCA overdose. Seizures can be especially problematic by causing metabolic acidosis, which can exacerbate the cardiac toxicity. GABAergic agents are the preferred treatment for TCA-induced seizures. Benzodiazepines are first-line agents, followed by phenobarbital or propofol if needed.

BICARBONATE THERAPY IS OFTEN INDICATED

Beyond aggressive supportive care, which includes fluids, vasopressors, and benzodiazepines, IV sodium bicarbonate is a cornerstone of treatment for TCA toxicity. Sodium bicarbonate combats TCA toxicity from two different angles. First, bolus doses of 1 to 2 mEq/kg IV push work to increase the concentration gradient of sodium across the myocardial membrane, thus improving conduction and shortening the QRS interval. Second, an infusion of sodium bicarbonate, made by mixing 150 mEq of sodium bicarbonate in 1 L of D_5W, typically run at a rate of 100 to 200 mL/h in adults, can be used for serum alkalinization. Alkalinization drives the weakly basic TCAs into the unionized state, which decreases binding to sodium channels. A target serum pH of 7.45 to 7.55 is recommended.

The threshold QRS interval that is used as an indication to administer sodium bicarbonate varies by clinician, but greater than 100 msec is reasonable.

HOLD THE PHYSOSTIGMINE

Although the contraindication of physostigmine in the setting of TCA overdose represents typical medical education dogma with a less-than-impressive evidentiary basis, its use in patients affected by TCA poisoning is *not* recommended. Although patients may be displaying anticholinergic toxidrome, physostigmine is not recommended due to concerns for serious adverse outcomes, including asystole and seizures. The anticholinergic toxidrome is by far the least concerning feature of TCA overdose, and treatment should focus on the cardiac toxicity and seizures.

PEARLS

- Toxicity from TCA overdose develops early and evolves quickly.
- Clinical features include QRS prolongation, seizures, hypotension, and anticholinergic symptoms.
- Gastric lavage and activated charcoal are acceptable GI decontamination techniques for intubated patients who present within an hour of ingestion.
- Sodium bicarbonate is a mainstay of treatment for TCA toxicity.
- Physostigmine is contraindicated in TCA overdose.

SUGGESTED READINGS

Boehnert MT, Lovejoy FH Jr. Value of the QRS duration versus the serum drug level in predicting seizures and ventricular arrhythmias after an acute overdose of tricyclic antidepressants. *N Engl J Med*. 1985;313(8):474-479.

Bruccoleri RE, Burns MM. A literature review of the use of sodium bicarbonate for the treatment of QRS widening. *J Med Toxicol*. 2016;12(1):121-129.

Pai K, Buckley NA, Isoardi KZ, et al. Optimising alkalinisation and its effect on QRS narrowing in tricyclic antidepressant poisoning. *Br J Clin Pharmacol*. 2022;88(2):723-733.

Pentel P, Peterson CD. Asystole complicating physostigmine treatment of tricyclic antidepressant overdose. *Ann Emerg Med*. 1980;9(11):588-590.

244

Deadly in Small Doses

Timothy J. Bright and Vincent J. Calleo

Although many medications and substances are relatively benign in small amounts, a select subset are highly toxic at low doses. Some agents, collectively referred to as *xenobiotics*, are prescription medications, while others are substances commonly available in the home. Although not all encompassing, this chapter highlights many substances that are dangerous in small doses; a more detailed discussion of several substances can be found in the other chapters dedicated to these agents.

Two classes of medications that are extremely concerning in the overdose setting are CCBs and BBs. Both CCBs and BBs can precipitate profound hypotension, bradycardia, and even cardiovascular collapse. Nondihydropyridine CCBs, including verapamil and diltiazem, can be especially harmful as they antagonize both central and peripheral calcium channels, causing bradycardia, decreased cardiac contractility, and vasodilation. Amlodipine, nicardipine, and other dihydropyridine CCBs act primarily through peripheral vasodilation; this may cause hypotension and reflex tachycardia, though, in large overdoses, bradycardia is also seen. BBs have negative inotropic and chronotropic effects on the heart through blockade of the beta-receptors in the myocardium. Propranolol has the additional effect of sodium channel blockade, leading to QRS prolongation and can also lead to seizures. Sotalol, in contrast, additionally antagonizes the potassium channel, leading to QTc prolongation and torsades de pointes. As little as one to two pills of certain CCBs or BBs in pediatric patients or even double doses of certain CCBs or BBs in tolerant adults may cause life-threatening toxicity. Refer to Chapter 241 for specific management for these overdoses.

Antidysrhythmics, including flecainide, propafenone, ibutilide, and dofetilide, can also be dangerous, even at double the treatment dose in adults; pediatric patients who inadvertently ingest as little as one to two pills of certain antidysrhythmics are at risk for significant toxicity. Clinical findings vary on the individual agent but may include bradycardia, QRS and QTc prolongation, dysrhythmias, seizures, and cardiovascular collapse. Treatment is centered around optimizing supportive care and may include specific interventions such as sodium bicarbonate for QRS prolongation in the right clinical setting.

TCAs are well known for their significant toxicity. Significant toxicity can occur with as little as 10 to 20 mg/kg, meaning a small child weighing 10 kg can become significantly ill with just a single 100 mg amitriptyline pill. Though many TCAs have recognizable names, such as amitriptyline, amoxapine, imipramine, and nortriptyline, providers must also recognize other TCAs, such as doxepin, as delayed recognition may cause a delay in therapy initiation. In the overdose setting, findings can include an anticholinergic toxidrome, hypotension, QRS prolongation, and seizures. The treatment of TCA toxicity varies on presentation but frequently includes aggressive supportive care along with sodium bicarbonate for QRS prolongation, benzodiazepines for seizures, and vasopressors for hypotension.

Opioids can be highly dangerous, largely due to their potentially profound respiratory and CNS suppression in overdose. Significant toxicity can occur in many patients, particularly pediatrics, with as little as one to two pills ingested. Providers should determine which substance and formulation were ingested as it may affect monitoring parameters and treatment. Some immediate-release formulations need a minimum 6-hour observation period or until the child is at baseline (whichever occurs later), whereas many extended-release substances as well as methadone require a minimum 24-hour observation or back to baseline (whichever occurs later). Other substances such as buprenorphine also require prolonged observation in patients less than 2 years of age; providers should contact their local poison center or toxicology service for recommendations regarding specific agents. During monitoring, patients should be on a cardiac monitor with a pulse oximeter as well as end-tidal capnography, if possible. Treatment of opioid ingestions is supportive, and naloxone can be considered.

Antidiabetic medications are potentially lethal in small doses. Sulfonylureas, including glimepiride, glipizide, and glyburide, stimulate endogenous insulin release. Even a single pill in a toddler can cause profound, sometimes delayed, hypoglycemia. As such, ingestion of even one pill in a pediatric patient will typically require a 24-hour observation period with frequent glucose checks to allow early intervention for the treatment of hypoglycemia as needed. Treatment consists of enteral and parenteral glucose replacement as needed. In patients with refractory hypoglycemia, octreotide should be considered, which will decrease endogenous insulin release.

Benzonatate, commonly prescribed for cough, can be very dangerous at low doses. There have been multiple case reports of adults developing severe toxicity, including seizures, CNS and respiratory depression, conduction abnormalities, and cardiac arrest, from taking a few extra capsules. Pediatric patients are also at high risk for toxicity, and even a single dose of this medication in a small child can potentially be life-threatening. Management involves aggressive supportive care including benzodiazepines for seizure control, management of cardiac dysrhythmias as they arise, and airway control for CNS and respiratory depression. Lipid emulsion therapy can be considered in the peri-code setting.

Life-threatening salicylate toxicity is a feared sequelae after the ingestion of oil of wintergreen. Depending on the concentration, several grams of salicylate may be contained in one sip of oil of wintergreen; as such, catastrophic toxicity can occur, even with small volume ingestions. Refer to Chapter 234 for additional information on the clinical course and treatment of salicylate poisoning.

Many household chemicals are highly toxic in small amounts. One such chemical is HF acid, often found in wheel cleaning solutions and rust remover. Dermal exposure can cause severe pain and possible systemic/life-threatening toxicity, and even a single sip of HF acid can be life-threatening. HF acid can cause caustic injury, but it also depletes the body's supply of electrolytes, including calcium and magnesium. Exposures can lead to pain, hypocalcemia, hypomagnesemia, QTc prolongation, and fatal cardiac dysrhythmias. Frequent ECGs are often needed if patients have systemic toxicity. Treatment includes optimizing supportive care as well as calcium and magnesium supplementation. A toxicologist or poison center should be contacted for any HF acid exposure to assist with management.

Although not comprehensive, this discussion of xenobiotics should help providers recognize substances that are highly dangerous at small doses.

PEARLS

- Many xenobiotics are highly toxic in small doses.
- The list of substances that are highly toxic in small doses is long, so providers must remember to have a high index of suspicion with approaching ingestions.

- Pediatric patients are often much more susceptible to higher toxicity at lower amounts of drug due to their lower body weights.
- Aggressive supportive care is a mainstay of managing toxicologic emergencies, although some xenobiotics have specific antidotes.

Suggested Readings

Osterhoudt KC. The toxic toddler: drugs that can kill in small doses. *Contemp Pediatr.* 2000;3:73-90.

Ranniger C, Roche C. Are one or two dangerous? Calcium channel blocker exposure in toddlers. *J Emerg Med.* 2007;33(2):145-154.

245

Know the Indications for High-Dose Insulin Therapy

Kayla Bourgeois and William Eggleston

HDI, also called HIET, is an effective treatment for CCB or BB toxicity. Both BB and nondihydropyridine CCB (ie, diltiazem, verapamil) toxicity cause hypotension and bradycardia, while dihydropyridine CCB (ie, nifedipine, nicardipine) toxicity causes hypotension and reflex tachycardia. Because of the variable effects of these medications on inotropy, chronotropy, cardiac conduction, and peripheral vascular resistance, patients with moderate-to-severe BB or CCB toxicity typically require multiple therapies, including HIET. In addition, hypotension and decreased gastrointestinal motility can result in delayed and prolonged effects in patients with CCB or BB toxicity. Patients with severe toxicity often require admission to an intensive care unit and may progress to vasodilatory shock, cardiovascular shock, metabolic derangements, dysrhythmias, and death.

A stepwise approach for managing patients with CCB/BB toxicity begins with supportive care, including intravenous fluids and atropine to address hypotension and bradycardia. In patients who don't respond to supportive care, intravenous calcium and/or glucagon can be used to improve inotropy, chronotropy, and MAP. If the patient's vital signs remain unstable, both HIET and a direct-acting vasopressor (ie, norepinephrine) should be initiated and titrated to effect. HIET has shown benefit in animal models and observational human studies, with recent evidence suggesting that the combination of HIET and vasopressors improved cerebral perfusion pressure better than either agent alone. In addition, the onset of insulin's inotropic effects can take up to 40 minutes, and early initiation of vasopressors can serve as a bridge to manage hemodynamic instability. Patients with refractory hemodynamic instability despite HIET and multiple vasopressors may benefit from methylene blue or hydroxocobalamin for vasodilatory shock, ECMO, or intravenous lipid emulsion in the setting of cardiac arrest.

HIET exerts its inotropic effects by increasing carbohydrate uptake in cardiac myocytes. Under normal conditions, the heart relies primarily on free fatty acids for energy; however, in stressed states, the cardiac myocytes rely more heavily on carbohydrates as an energy source. A combination of factors, including decreased insulin release and increased insulin resistance, results in hyperglycemia, acidemia, and decreased cardiac output. HIET optimizes carbohydrate transport to support the metabolic demands of the cardiac myocytes and improve cardiac contractility. HIET also increases intracellular calcium stores, further increasing cardiac contractility. These effects may be more profound in patients with CCB toxicity because CCBs also inhibit endogenous insulin release from pancreatic beta-islet cells, but benefit has been shown in both CCB and BB toxicity.

HIET dosing protocols can vary by institutions, but HIET is typically initiated with a 1 unit/kg bolus of regular insulin, followed by 1 unit/kg/h continuous infusion. The infusion is titrated to achieve sufficient cardiac output, which can be assessed using bedside ultrasound, MAP, lactate clearance, or other markers of perfusion (typical doses range from 5 to 10 units/kg/h, but higher doses up to 20 units/kg/h are reported). In addition to the regular insulin bolus, patients with a blood glucose less than 300 mg/dL should receive a 0.5 g/kg intravenous dextrose bolus. Frequent finger-stick glucose measurements are needed to monitor for hypoglycemia, particularly when therapy is initiated or after dose adjustments are made. It is reasonable to assess a finger-stick glucose every 15 minutes for HIET initiation and dose changes, and to increase the time increments to 30 to 60 minutes once a patient has several stable readings.

Common adverse effects associated with HIET include volume overload, hypoglycemia, and hypokalemia. Volume overload typically occurs due to a combination of cardiogenic shock, renal hypoperfusion or acute kidney injury, and excess intravenous fluids from multiple medications. Standard insulin infusions are prepared as 1 unit/mL and can cause or exacerbate volume overload. It is reasonable to concentrate the HIET infusion (10-20 units/mL) to reduce the volume of the infusion as the dose is increased. However, it is important that obvious labels and infusion protocols are in place to prevent medication errors or adverse events from HIET. A continuous dextrose infusion should be used to maintain a serum glucose greater than 150 mg/dL. As with HIET, concentrated dextrose formulations can and should be used when possible. Oral or intravenous potassium supplementation should be used to maintain a serum potassium 3.5 to 4.5 mEq/L. HIET causes hypokalemia by transient intracellular shift of potassium, so careful monitoring and cautious repletion of potassium should be considered to avoid rebound hyperkalemia when the HIET is stopped. Consultation with a pharmacist is helpful to ensure that the HIET is appropriately concentrated and that other intravenous medications can be evaluated to reduce the patient's overall fluid load. Consider contacting your local poison center or toxicology group for additional guidance if HIET is being considered.

PEARLS

- Consider HIET in combination with vasopressors for patients with CCB or BB toxicity that is unresponsive to fluids, atropine, calcium, and glucagon.
- Initiate direct-acting vasopressors simultaneously with HIET.
- A bedside ultrasound, serum lactate, MAP, or other markers of perfusion can assist with patient monitoring during treatment with HIET.

- Hypervolemia, hypokalemia, and hypoglycemia are common adverse events that occur with HIET.
- Talk with your local poison center or toxicology group for additional guidance if HIET is being considered.

Suggested Readings

Cole JB, Arens AM, Laes JR, Klein LR, Bangh SA, Olives TD. High dose insulin for beta-blocker and calcium channel-blocker poisoning. *Am J Emerg Med*. 2018;36(10):1817-1824.

Katzung KG, Leroy JM, Boley SP, Stellpflug SJ, Holger JS, Engebretsen KM. A randomized controlled study comparing high-dose insulin to vasopressors or combination therapy in a porcine model of refractory propranolol-induced cardiogenic shock. *Clin Toxicol*. 2019;57(11):1073-1079.

Page CB, Ryan NM, Isbister GK. The safety of high-dose insulin euglycemia therapy in toxin-induced cardiac toxicity. *Clin Toxicol*. 2018;56(6):389-396.

St-Onge M, Anseeuw K, Cantrell FL, et al. Experts consensus recommendations for the management of calcium channel blocker poisoning in adults. *Crit Care Med*. 2017; 45(3):e306-e315.

246

What's the Latest on Decontamination?

Michael Keenan

Proper decontamination can be a potentially lifesaving intervention. The goal of decontamination is to minimize toxin exposure. Emergency medicine providers must remember to consider decontamination and weigh its risks against its benefits to determine the best method.

GI Decontamination

GI decontamination is a cornerstone of toxicologic management. Providers must critically think about whether GI decontamination is appropriate, and, if so, which method is best. GI decontamination methods are activated charcoal, whole bowel irrigation, and orogastric lavage. Induction of emesis is not recommended. Each form of GI decontamination has its benefits and indications, and a myriad of factors must be considered for each case.

First, providers must determine if the ingested substance is toxic. If it is not, then GI decontamination is unnecessary. If it is, it must be determined if a particular GI decontamination method would work for the substance ingested. The time of ingestion must also be considered. Contrary to traditional teaching, it is impossible to set a specific time beyond which GI decontamination will be ineffective—each case is unique and requires careful consideration. Instead, clinicians must think critically. Some drugs will delay gastric motility (eg, anticholinergics, opioids). Others are specially formulated to have delayed-release kinetics (eg, extended-release, sustained-release products). Finally, in large overdoses, many drugs form concretions that delay absorption. These instances provide a larger window for GI decontamination.

ACTIVATED CHARCOAL

Activated charcoal is produced from superheated carbonaceous materials. Its large surface area utilizes abundant intermolecular forces and adsorbs xenobiotics. Typical dosing is 1 g/kg in pediatrics and usually 50 g for adults. When considering activated charcoal for a toxicologic exposure, several key questions must be asked: (1) Is the ingestion toxic? (2) Does the xenobiotic adsorb to charcoal? (3) Does the provider think that there is still xenobiotic in the gut that could be bound? and (4) Does the provider feel the patient can safely tolerate charcoal? If the answer to all of these questions is yes, then activated charcoal should be considered. It is important to remember that many substances, including metals (eg, iron, lithium) and various liquids, do not adsorb well to charcoal, and it is not indicated for these exposures. If the ingested substance is caustic, and an endoscopy is being considered, activated charcoal should not be administered, as it will interfere with the ability to visualize the GI mucosa. It is important to remember there is an aspiration risk with activated charcoal. Therefore, it should only be given if the patient can protect their airway, or if the airway is already protected with an endotracheal tube in which case it can be administered through a nasogastric or orogastric tube.

MULTIDOSE ACTIVATED CHARCOAL

Some ingestions may benefit from repeat doses of activated charcoal. For example, ingestions of sustained-or extended-release products might benefit from a second dose of activated charcoal a few hours after the initial dose. Large ingestions of certain substances that potentially form bezoars (eg, aspirin) may be amenable to repeat doses of activated charcoal. Finally, some xenobiotics exhibit enterohepatic or enteroenteric recirculation. These properties are specific to certain drugs and provide an additional opportunity for them to adhere to charcoal. For these unique xenobiotics, a standard dose of charcoal is given, followed by half-standard doses every 4 to 6 hours. Patients must be able to safely tolerate the charcoal, and bowel sounds must be confirmed before giving repeat doses activated charcoal.

WHOLE BOWEL IRRIGATION

Whole bowel irrigation involves providing an electrolyte neutral solution in sufficient quantities to flush the GI tract. It is used for selected substance ingestions that may be life-threatening and is considered especially for sustained- or extended-release preparations, or for ingestions that do not adsorb to charcoal (eg, lead). It is also used in body packers to facilitate the evacuation of drug packets. There is an aspiration risk; therefore, it should only be done if patients can protect their own airway or if the airway is already protected with an endotracheal tube.

To perform whole bowel irrigation, a nasogastric or orogastric tube is placed, and the electrolyte neutral solution is titrated to a goal rate. For adults, the goal rate is 1.5 to 2 L/h. For smaller pediatric patients, the goal rate might be closer to 500 mL/h, depending on the size of the child. It is important to assess bowel sounds frequently as whole bowel irrigation cannot be run safely if GI motility is impaired. The irrigation is run until the rectal effluent is clear.

Gastric Lavage

Gastric lavage is rarely performed. Its use is limited to ingestions that are thought to be life-threatening and have limited therapeutic treatment options (eg, colchicine). To perform gastric lavage, a 36F to 40F orogastric tube must be placed and then placed to suction. A 250-mL bolus of saline is then instilled, and the tube is placed back to suction. This is repeated until the effluent is clear. There is an aspiration risk with this procedure, and patients must be able to protect their airway or, ideally, the airway should be protected with an endotracheal tube. The risks of inserting a large orogastric tube include iatrogenic injury during placement or inadvertent tracheal placement. Some institutions do not have an orogastric tube of the appropriate size. There are also inherent limitations in the size of the orogastric tube in pediatrics, and smaller tubes will not perform adequately, thus limiting its use in this population.

Dermal/Ocular Decontamination

A patient with a dermal exposure to a toxic substance should be decontaminated. The most important step in dermal decontamination is removal of clothing. In fact, removing clothing may remove up to 80% to 90% of contamination. Clothing should be placed in plastic bags and stored outside the ED. Once clothing is removed, powders or other solids remaining on the skin or hair should be wiped away. Copious irrigation with water plus a mild soap is adequate for most dermal exposures. Care should be taken to protect the mucus membranes (eyes, mouth, etc) and any open wounds to prevent contamination of these areas. Gas exposures do not normally require decontamination. However, if the exact nature of the exposure is in question, err on the side of performing decontamination.

Ocular decontamination is important to preserve vision. The eye should be irrigated with water or normal saline. Anesthetic drops can help facilitate patient cooperation. A Morgan lens may help in allowing for large volume irrigation. The pH of the eye should be monitored periodically with pH paper, and the irrigation should be continued until the pH is normal. Ophthalmology consultation should be considered.

PEARLS

- Decontamination should always be considered in toxicologic exposures.
- There is no hard time cutoff beyond which decontamination is ineffective—each case must be considered individually.
- The best method of decontamination will depend on the patient and the exposure.
- For dermal exposures, removing the clothing is the most important step in decontamination.
- Poison control can be contacted to assist in decontamination decisions: 1-800-222-1222.

Suggested Readings

Nelson LS, Howland MA, Lewin NA, Smith SW, Goldfrank LR, Hoffman RS. *Goldfrank's Toxicology Emergencies*. 11th ed. McGraw Hill; 2019.

Walter FG, Schauben JL, Thomas R, et al. *Advanced Hazmat Life Support*. 5th ed. University of Arizona; 2017.

SECTION XX

TRAUMA

247

MANAGING PENETRATING NECK INJURIES: HARD OR SOFT, SUPERFICIAL OR DEEP?

MELISSA JOSEPH AND RYAN F. COUGHLIN

Neck wounds can range from minor and superficial to life-threatening injuries fraught with significant morbidity and mortality. Since the degree of injury is not always obvious upon superficial inspection, an algorithmic approach is important to guide evaluation and determine which patients require imaging and surgical exploration.

Historically, the division of the neck "zones" was important for identifying underlying structures at risk for injury. Today a no-zone approach is recommended, which involves primary survey, prioritization of patient stabilization, evaluation for hard or soft signs of injury, examination of the wound, and advanced imaging and surgical consultation where indicated (**Table 247.1**).

TABLE 247.1 ZONES OF THE NECK AND CONTAINED VITAL STRUCTURES

NECK ZONE	ANATOMIC BORDER	STRUCTURES INVOLVED
Zone 1 (Highest mortality)	Superior: Cricoid cartilage Inferior: Clavicles and sternal notch	Common carotid arteries Vertebral and subclavian arteries Subclavian, innominate, and jugular veins Recurrent laryngeal and vagus nerves Trachea Esophagus Thoracic duct
Zone 2 (Most frequent)	Superior: Angle of mandible Inferior: Cricoid cartilage	Carotid arteries Jugular and vertebral veins Pharynx and larynx Recurrent laryngeal and vagal nerves Spinal cord Trachea
Zone 3	Superior: Skull base Inferior: Angle of mandible	Carotid and vertebral arteries Jugular veins Spinal cord Cranial nerves IX-XII Sympathetic trunk

Initiate Immediate Management in the Patient Who Is Unstable or When Hard Signs of Injury Are Present

Vigilantly monitor the patient for airway compromise and intervene emergently if there is evidence of tracheal injury, expanding hematoma, unstable vital signs, or decline in mental status. Patients with hard signs of injury (**Table 247.2**) warrant surgical exploration and definitive management. Life-threatening injuries most commonly involve damage to the aerodigestive tract and vascular structures.

Determine if the Wound Is Superficial or Deep

In the patient with neck wounds and no hard signs of injury, the initial step in evaluation is to determine whether the injury violates the platysma muscle, which is a superficial muscle that is situated between the superficial and deep cervical fascia. A penetrating injury that violates the platysma muscle is considered a PNI, and injury to deeper anatomic structures should be suspected. Thus, the platysma is an important structure to help distinguish superficial injuries that can be readily managed from PNI. Where it is unclear on initial bedside assessment whether or not the platysma is violated, maintain a low threshold to treat as PNI, obtain a CT scan, and involve surgical colleagues or transfer for higher level of care where feasible for exploration of wounds or removal of impaled objects. In settings where a surgeon and/or transfer is not available, a CT scan should be performed to determine if the wound is superficial or deep. Wounds that do not violate the platysma are unlikely to cause significant injury and do not always require further workup.

Obtain a CTA in Patients with PNI Who Are Stable With No Hard Signs of Vascular, Airway, Aerodigestive, or Neurologic Compromise

CTA of the neck is the modality of choice for evaluation of stable PNI. Patients with soft signs of neck injury (**Table 247.2**) despite a normal CTA, or those with nondiagnostic CTA, should undergo further evaluation. Additional tests may include MRI, duplex ultrasound, esophagography or esophagoscopy, and laryngoscopy depending on suspected injury. Management in pediatric patients similarly includes detailed physical examination and CTA for patients who are stable, with surgical exploration as warranted.

TABLE 247.2   HARD AND SOFT SIGNS OF NECK INJURY

HARD SIGNS	SOFT SIGNS
Airway compromise	Nonexpanding hematoma
Massive subcutaneous emphysema	Mild bleeding
Air bubbling through wound	Transient, fluid-responsive hypotension
Expanding or pulsatile hematoma	Small hemoptysis/hematemesis
Significant active bleeding	Voice change
Shock	Chest tube air leak
Neurologic deficit	Dyspnea
Massive hematemesis	
Pulse deficit	
Bruit/thrill	

The Patient Who Is Asymptomatic With Normal CTA and Reassuring Exam May Be Discharged

CTA has a high sensitivity (100%) and specificity (93.5%) for detecting significant injury. Discharge may be considered in patients with negative imaging and no hard or soft signs of injury. Those with a concerning trajectory of penetration should be observed with serial examinations or evaluated with additional imaging.

PEARLS

- PNI is defined as full-thickness violation of the platysma. When uncertain, err on the side of caution. Maintain a low threshold for treating as PNI when physical examination is equivocal.
- Patients with PNI and no hard signs of injury need to be imaged to determine risk. Based on imaging, those who are at high risk for decompensation should be urgently transferred to the nearest trauma center. After initial stabilizing interventions, transfer to a trauma center will allow for emergent surgical intervention and/or further diagnostic workup.
- Patients with hard signs of neck injury should be stabilized and managed operatively.
- Be prepared for a difficult airway. Distortion of anatomy, secretions, blood, and mechanical obstructions may complicate rapid sequence intubation. Intubation with ketamine sedation alone may be considered when there is concern that paralysis may further distort anatomy. Initiate a difficult airway algorithm, and be prepared for intervention with a surgical airway.
- Cervical spine immobilization is not necessary in patients with PNI who have a normal neurologic examination and mental status. Cervical collars limit full examination of the wound, spinal immobilization may inhibit airway protection, and unstable cervical spinal column injuries are rare in PNI.

Suggested Readings

Bell RB, Osborn T, Dierks EJ, Potter BE, Long WB. Management of penetrating neck injuries: a new paradigm for civilian trauma. *J Oral Maxillofac Surg*. 2007;65(4):691-705. PMID: 17368366.

Expert Panels on Neurologic and Vascular Imaging; Schroeder JW, Ptak T, et al. ACR Appropriateness Criteria® penetrating neck injury. *J Am Coll Radiol*. 2017;14(11S):S500-S505. PMID: 29101988.

Inaba K, Branco BC, Menaker J, et al. Evaluation of multidetector computed tomography for penetrating neck injury: a prospective multicenter study. *J Trauma Acute Care Surg*. 2012;72(3):576-583; discussion 583-584; quiz 803-804. PMID: 22491539.

Lustenberger T, Talving P, Lam L, et al. Unstable cervical spine fracture after penetrating neck injury: a rare entity in an analysis of 1,069 patients. *J Trauma*. 2011;70(4):870-872. PMID: 20805776.

McConnell DB, Trunkey DD. Management of penetrating trauma to the neck. *Adv Surg*. 1994;27:97-127. PMID: 8140981.

Prichayudh S, Choadrachata-anun J, Sriussadaporn S, et al. Selective management of penetrating neck injuries using "no zone" approach. *Injury*. 2015;46(9):1720-1725. PMID: 26117413.

Sperry JL, Moore EE, Coimbra R, et al. Western Trauma Association critical decisions in trauma: penetrating neck trauma. *J Trauma Acute Care Surg*. 2013;75(6):936-940. PMID: 24256663.

Tessler RA, Nguyen H, Newton C, Betts J. Pediatric penetrating neck trauma: hard signs of injury and selective neck exploration. *J Trauma Acute Care Surg*. 2017;82(6):989-994. PMID: 28521330.

Tisherman SA, Bokhari F, Collier B, et al. Clinical practice guideline: penetrating zone II neck trauma. *J Trauma*. 2008;64(5):1392-1405. PMID: 18469667.

248

SAVE A LIMB! VASCULAR INJURY IN PENETRATING EXTREMITY TRAUMA

TAYLOR MCCORMICK AND KELLY STEWART

Extremity injuries may initially be overlooked during the resuscitation of the patient with polytrauma with serious injuries. Vascular injuries can be occlusive, partially occlusive, or occult and include complete and partial transection, acute or delayed thrombosis, reversible arterial spasm, arteriovenous fistula formation, pseudoaneurysm formation, and intimal flaps with subsequent thrombus formation. The path of injury is typically predictable in stab wounds, and structures at risk can be anticipated depending on weapon trajectory. In contrast, damage from gunshot wounds is less predictable due to high-velocity concussive forces and bony ricochets. Life- and limb-threatening vascular injuries should be recognized, hemostasis achieved, and subtle arterial injuries identified to prevent delayed thromboembolic complications. Recognition and management priorities in penetrating extremity trauma are highlighted later.

PRIORITIZE HEMORRHAGE CONTROL

Hemostasis is paramount and is best achieved by direct pressure. Some wounds are not amenable to pressure dressing or tourniquets alone, and packing the wound cavity may aid in creating direct pressure on bleeding vessels. There are multiple hemostatic agents that can be used to assist with bleeding control for injuries that require packing. These products establish hemostasis by concentrating coagulation factors, adhering to tissues, and delivering procoagulant factors to the hemorrhaging site. Tourniquet application may be used when direct pressure fails or in a resource-limited setting. Ideally, tourniquets should be applied at least 2 to 3 inches above the site of the injury. Complication rates are low when tourniquets are applied correctly and provide essential hemostasis in transit to the hospital or while awaiting definitive operative repair.

HARD SIGNS OF VASCULAR INJURY REQUIRE SURGICAL EXPLORATION

An unstable patient with a "hard sign" of vascular injury should proceed immediately to the operating room without additional imaging. Surgical exploration within less than 6 hours from injury maximizes limb salvage in patients with "hard signs" of vascular injury (see **Table 248.1**). Over 90% of patients with hard signs will have a significant arterial injury requiring repair. Intraoperative angiography or preoperative CTA may be reasonable in a stable patient with hard signs for operative planning for complex injuries (eg, shotgun/multilevel gunshot wounds or mangled limb).

TABLE 248.1 HARD AND SOFT SIGNS OF VASCULAR INJURY	
HARD SIGNS	**SOFT SIGNS**
■ Absent distal pulses	■ Distal nerve deficit
■ Active pulsatile hemorrhage	■ Diminished pulses
■ Large expanding hematoma	■ Nonexpanding hematoma
■ Bruit or thrill	■ History of pulsatile or significant hemorrhage at time of injury

Evaluate a Patient for Soft Signs of Vascular Injury

Patients with penetrating extremity trauma without hard signs of vascular injury should be examined for "soft signs" (see **Table 248.1**), and an ABI, or API, should be measured. Up to 4% of patients with a normal physical exam will have a delayed presentation of an undetected vascular injury. This stresses the importance of ABI/APIs as an adjunct for the physical exam. Approximately 25% of patients with soft signs or abnormal ABI/APIs will have vascular injuries requiring surgical intervention. Patients without hard or soft signs of vascular injury and an ABI/API greater than 0.9 may be discharged.

Obtain a CTA in Patients With Soft Signs of Vascular Injury or Abnormal ABI/API.

Patients with soft signs of vascular injury or ABI/APIs less than 0.9 require further evaluation with advanced imaging. CTA has become the imaging modality of choice, as sensitivity and specificity are comparable to conventional angiography with less patient risk. CTA does not require an arterial puncture or on-site interventional radiologist, is quick and readily available, uses less contrast, and provides detailed anatomy of adjacent structures. Duplex Doppler ultrasound is less sensitive but may provide information when CTA is not available or if the patient has a contrast allergy.

Controversy Regarding Proximity Wounds

Both the definition and evaluation of proximity wounds are controversial. Variably defined as 1 to 5 cm from a major neurovascular bundle, some argue that proximity alone constitutes a soft sign. Others suggest special consideration for wounds in the thigh, as injury to the deep femoral artery may not manifest soft signs due to its location. The best available evidence suggests that in patients with a proximity injury without hard or soft signs and with a normal ABI/API, CTA is only indicated for shotgun wounds, which are known to have unpredictable fragment number, scatter, and velocity. Proximity to a major vascular structure in the absence of other findings is not an indication for additional workup.

PEARLS

- Penetrating extremity trauma has great potential for morbidity and mortality. Examine each patient thoroughly for hard and soft signs of injury and perform an ABI/API.
- Hemorrhage control with direct pressure or wound packing is a priority. Tourniquets are an effective adjunctive therapy when direct pressure is not possible or inadequate.

- CTA should be performed for patients with soft signs or abnormal ABI/APIs.
- Hard signs warrant emergent surgical exploration.
- Patients with a normal physical exam and ABI/APIs greater than 0.9 can be discharged home.

Suggested Readings

Fox N, Rajani RR, Bokhari F, et al. Evaluation and management of penetrating lower extremity arterial trauma: an Eastern Association for the Surgery of Trauma practice management guideline. *J Trauma Acute Care Surg*. 2012;73(5 Suppl 4):S315-S320.

Frykberg ER, Dennis JW, Bishop K, Laneve L, Alexander RH. The reliability of physical examination in the evaluation of penetrating extremity trauma: results at one year. *J Trauma*. 1991;31:502-511.

Inaba K, Branco BC, Reddy S, et al. Prospective evaluation of multidetector computed tomography for extremity vascular trauma. *J Trauma*. 2011;70(4):808-815.

Inaba K, Siboni S, Resnick S, et al. Tourniquet use for civilian extremity trauma. *J Trauma Acute Care Surg*. 2015;79(2):232-237.

Khoshmohabat H, Paydar S, Kazemi HM, Dalfardi B. Overview of agents used for emergency hemostasis. *Trauma Mon*. 2016;21(1):e26023. PMID: 27218055.

Manthey DE, Nicks BA. Penetrating trauma to the extremity. *J Emerg Med*. 2008;34(2):187-193.

Newton EJ, Love J. Acute complications of extremity trauma. *Emerg Med Clin North Am*. 2007;25(3):751-761.

249

Judicious Abdominal Imaging in Trauma

Caroline W. Burmon and Erick A. Eiting

Evaluation and management of patients with trauma has evolved with the advancement of technologies, such as CT and bedside ultrasound. Negative advanced imaging is reassuring and enables us to discharge patients earlier from the ED. Previously, many of these same patients required prolonged observation or were taken to the operating room for exploration.

The indications for CT imaging should be weighed against its availability, and bedside ultrasound should be used as a screening tool for the vast majority of patients with trauma. Two potential pitfalls to be avoided are the potential for overutilization and excessive radiation exposure and the urge to obtain imaging studies in critically ill patients that may lead to delays in operative management and definitive care. The indications and risks versus benefits of imaging must be carefully weighed to avoid these two potential pitfalls.

Imaging Indications Based on Mechanism of Injury

Injury patterns vary based on the mechanism of injury. The FAST examination can quickly provide information that guides management in both blunt and penetrating trauma with hemodynamic instability. The sensitivity of FAST in abdominal trauma ranges from 80% to 100% for volumes of free fluid greater than 200 to 400 mL. It has about 99% specificity with an experienced user with a positive predictive value of 94% and a negative predictive value of 95%. Unfortunately, FAST continues to have a lower sensitivity among stable patients, likely due to lower amounts of detectable free fluid (**Figure 249.1**).

Blunt Trauma

The physical examination can be used to screen for injury in awake, alert patients who have sustained blunt abdominal trauma and who do not have neurologic injury or impairment. Indications for CT include significant abdominal tenderness, evidence of peritonitis, referred pain, a positive FAST examination, gross hematuria, and an abdominal "seat-belt" sign; tenderness in the lower rib cage; or significant extremity injury or pain. Serial abdominal examinations can help identify patients with bleeding or viscous injury causing the slow development of peritonitis.

Penetrating Trauma

Mechanism of injury and patient stability dictate indications for imaging in penetrating trauma. Gunshot wounds are created at high velocity and cause significant injury to deep tissues. Abdominal CT can be informative but should be reserved for stable patients. Those with unstable vital signs will require laparotomy; imaging studies should not delay definitive operative management. Abdominal CT should be performed when there is suspicion of violation of the peritoneum and will better characterize injuries in hemodynamically stable patients with a positive FAST.

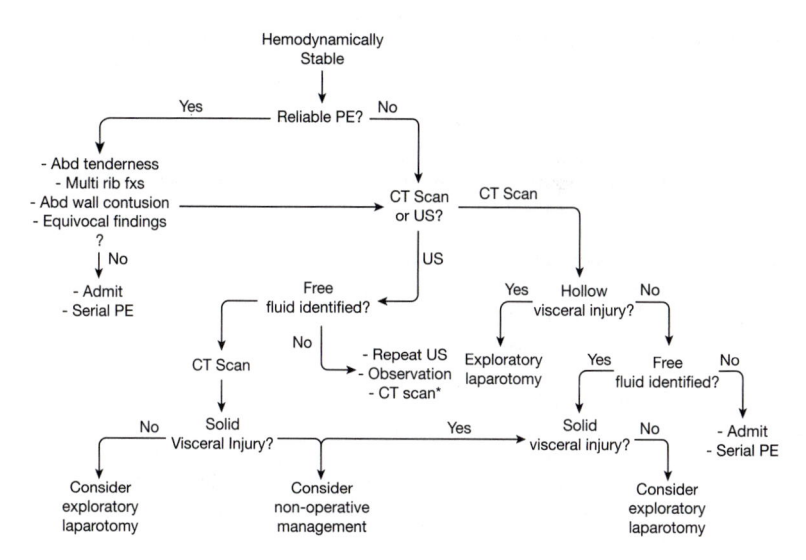

FIGURE 249.1 Suggested algorithm for imaging in blunt abdominal trauma as recommended by The Eastern Association for the Surgery of Trauma guidelines; PE, physical exam. (From Hoff WS, Holevar M, Nagy KK, Patterson L, et al. Practice management guidelines for the evaluation of blunt abdominal trauma: the EAST practice management guidelines work group. *J Trauma*. 2002 Sep;53(3):602-15. Figure 2.)

Imaging in Special Populations After Abdominal Trauma

Pediatrics

Most pediatric abdominal trauma is blunt, and the majority of injuries are managed nonoperatively. Children are most at risk for the consequences of radiation exposure, so CT must be ordered judiciously. Indications for CT in children are similar to those detailed earlier. FAST in the pediatric population has higher rates of false-negative and false-positive findings and as such should be interpreted carefully. The clinical scenario and abdominal examination should guide the decision for CT rather than ultrasound.

Pregnant Women

The FAST examination remains useful in pregnant women who sustain abdominal injury in trauma. Radiologist performed and interpreted pelvic ultrasound, and fetal monitoring can additionally diagnose traumatic obstetric emergencies, such as abruptio placentae, uterine rupture, or fetal injury. However, pregnancy should not preclude appropriate evaluation with CT for potential life-threatening visceral injuries. Discussion of the risks and benefits of imaging with pregnant patients is essential when possible. A CT scan of the abdomen and pelvis provides 25-mGy ionizing radiation, which can increase the risk of childhood cancer by about 1%. While the risk is small, this increase underscores the need to be thoughtful about imaging decisions.

Geriatric Patients

In contrast to children, there should be a lower threshold to image older patients. Patients over 65 years of age are 2 to 3 times more likely to die from trauma than their younger counterparts. They may initially look well but are at higher risk for complications secondary to their pathophysiology, including higher rates of bleeding from vascular injuries and comorbid conditions that require systemic anticoagulation and antiplatelet therapies. Decreased abdominal muscular tone can make patients less likely to develop peritonitis and make symptoms more difficult to interpret. Patients on nodal-blocking agents will exhibit a relative bradycardia, even when having significant bleeding, and older patients will be less able to compensate for acidosis and other manifestations of traumatic injury. Poor nutrition and diuretic medications often leave them dehydrated before trauma, which increases the challenge of resuscitative efforts.

In addition to imaging, careful consideration should be given to extended observation or inpatient admission for the older patient after trauma, ensuring appropriate social support systems and a safe discharge environment before discharging geriatric patients from the ED.

PEARLS

- Stable patients with normal mental status, benign abdominal and thoracic examination, absence of gross hematuria, and without a seat-belt sign do not require an abdominal CT after blunt abdominal trauma and can be evaluated with serial abdominal examinations.
- Avoid abdominal CT in patients who are unstable and have positive FAST or other indications for operative management.
- Keep a lower threshold to obtain additional imaging in geriatric patients due to higher rates of complication, including bleeding, and less reliable examination findings due to decreased abdominal muscular tone.

Suggested Readings

Chen MM, Coakley FV, Kaimal A, et al. Guidelines for computed tomography and magnetic resonance imaging use during pregnancy and lactation. *Obstet Gynecol.* 2008;112(2): 333-340.

Hoff W, Holevar M, Nagy KK, et al. Practice management guidelines for the evaluation of blunt abdominal trauma: the EAST practice management guidelines work group. *J Trauma.* 2002; 53:602-615.

Schwaub CW, Kauder DR. Trauma in the geriatric patient. *Arch Surg.* 1992;127(6):701-806.

Valentino M, Serra C, Pavlica P, et al. Blunt abdominal trauma: diagnostic performance of contrast-enhanced US in children—initial experience. *Radiology.* 2008;246(8):903-909.

250

When to Suspect Blunt Cerebrovascular Injury

Steven Straube and Ronald B. Tesoriero

Both adult and pediatric patients are at risk for BCVI. Although the carotid and vertebral arteries are the most commonly injured vessels, the subclavian artery and jugular veins are also at risk. Up to one-third of patients with BCVIs have multivessel injuries, any of which may result in cerebral ischemic events. Historically, BCVI in the patient with trauma was diagnosed after the development of neurologic deficits or decreased level of consciousness in the setting of a negative noncontrast CT of the head, with an incidence as low as 0.1%. However, only a minority of patients with BCVI will present with acute neurologic symptoms, and more recent series have demonstrated an incidence of nearly 3% in patients with polytrauma who undergo screening with CTA. Untreated BCVI confers a high morbidity (up to 58%) and mortality (up to 33%), with mortality most commonly due to stroke. The most common patterns of injury with BCVI are dissection, pseudoaneurysm, thrombosis, and distal embolization, while frank vascular disruption and exsanguination are rare. For those that develop stroke after BCVI 30-40% will be present on admission. In those that do not have symptoms on admission the largest number of strokes occur between 13 and 24 hours after injury. However, strokes may occur several days after injury with the median time to stroke being 48 hours. This latent phase allows for the diagnosis and treatment of BCVI, thereby giving the opportunity to decrease morbidity and mortality.

The most common mechanism of injury is via hyperextension with stretching of the internal carotid vessel over the lateral masses of the C1 and C2 vertebra, although injuries from direct blows or laceration from bony fragments of cervical fractures are also possible. Vertebral artery dissections can occur with even "minor" trauma such as with chiropractic manipulation or yoga, though they are most frequently associated with cervical spine fractures that involve the foramen transversarium in the C1 to C3 vertebra.

The expanded Denver Screening Criteria are a collective set of signs, symptoms, and risk factors developed to identify patients at the highest risk for BCVI. These are outlined in **Table 250.1**. A patient with a high-force injury and any of the listed signs or injuries should undergo diagnostic imaging to rule out vascular injury. Unfortunately,

TABLE 250.1	EXPANDED DENVER SCREENING CRITERIA

SIGNS AND SYMPTOMS OF BCVI

Arterial hemorrhage from neck/nose/mouth
Cervical bruit in patients <50 yr old
Expanding cervical hematoma
Focal neurologic deficit
Neurologic deficits not explained by imaging
Ischemic stroke on head CT or MRI

HIGH-RISK INJURY PATTERNS ASSOCIATED WITH BCVI

High energy transfer mechanism
Displaced midface fracture (Le Fort II-III)
Mandibular fracture
Complex skull fracture/basilar skull fracture/occipital condyle fracture
Severe TBI with GCS <6
Cervical spine fracture, subluxation, or ligamentous injury at any level
Near-hanging with anoxic brain injury
Clothesline-type injury or seat-belt abrasion with significant pain, swelling, or altered mental status
TBI with thoracic injuries
Scalp degloving
Thoracic vascular injuries
Upper rib fractures

BCVI, blunt cerebrovascular injury; CT, computed tomography; GCS, Glasgow Coma Scale; MRI, magnetic resonance imaging; TBI, traumatic brain injury.

even the liberal use of the expanded Denver Screening Criteria may miss patients with BCVI. Institutions that have adopted liberal cervical CTA screening of patients with blunt polytrauma have repeatedly demonstrated that up to 20% of patients with BCVI do not meet any screening criteria, with more than 50% having higher grade injuries.

CTA is the imaging modality of choice due to its availability, speed, cost-effectiveness, and ability to evaluate other cervical structures and injuries. Sensitivities as high as 97% to 100% and specificities of as high as 94% to 100% for vascular injury have been reported. Some limitations to CTA include streak artifacts from metallic foreign bodies and difficulty visualizing vessels coursing through bones. In patients at high risk for BCVI where CTA evaluation is limited by these factors, alternative diagnostic screening tests, such as DSA or MRA, may be necessary.

PEARLS

- Most patients with BCVI do not present with neurologic signs and symptoms.
- Patients meeting any of the expanded Denver Screening Criteria should undergo CTA, the diagnostic screening modality of choice.
- Untreated BCVI leads to significant stroke-related morbidity and mortality, and most patients develop stroke between 13 and 24 hours after injury.

SUGGESTED READINGS

Black JA, Abraham PJ, Abraham MN, et al. Universal screening for blunt cerebrovascular injury. *J Trauma Acute Care Surg*. 2021;90(2):224-231. PMID: 33502144.

Bruns BR, Tesoriero R, Kufera J, et al. Blunt cerebrovascular injury screening guidelines: what are we willing to miss? *J Trauma Acute Care Surg*. 2014;76(3):691-695. PMID: 24553535.

Cothren CC, Moore EE, Ray CE, et al. Cervical spine fracture patterns mandating screening to rule out blunt cerebrovascular injury. *Surgery*. 2007;141:76-82.

Geddes AE, Burlew CC, Wagenaar AE, et al. Expanded screening criteria for blunt cerebrovascular injury: a bigger impact than anticipated. *Am J Surg*. 2016;212(6):1167-1174. PMID: 27751528.

Harper PR, Jacobson LE, Sheff Z, Williams JM, Rodgers RB. Routine CTA screening identifies blunt cerebrovascular injuries missed by clinical risk factors. *Trauma Surg Acute Care Open*. 2022;7(1):e000924. PMID: 36101794.

Kim, DY, Biffl W, Bokhari F, et al. Evaluation and management of blunt cerebrovascular injury: a practice management guideline from the Eastern Association for the Surgery of Trauma. *J Trauma Acute Care Surg*. 2020;88(6):875-887.

O'Brien PJ, Cox MW. A modern approach to cervical vascular trauma. *Perspect Vasc Surg Endo-vasc Ther*. 2011;23(2):90-97.

251

CLOSING THE BOOK: USING A BEDSHEET TO STABILIZE PELVIC FRACTURES

MICHAEL GOTTLIEB AND STUART SWADRON

The most common causes of pelvic fractures are motor vehicle collisions and falls from substantial height. Pelvic fractures are associated with a significant risk of morbidity and mortality. There are three main patterns: lateral compression (most common), anteroposterior compression, and vertical shear. All of these may result in significant and life-threatening pelvic hemorrhage. Most bleeding in pelvic trauma is due to venous injury, but arterial injury may be identified in up to 15% of patients. Retroperitoneal bleeding from pelvic trauma can be severe; up to 4 L of blood can enter this potential space.

Once a pelvic fracture is identified, the pelvis should be stabilized to reduce further bleeding. The ideal treatment is external or internal fixation, which may be combined with angiographic embolization in the case of arterial bleeding. Studies have suggested that it is preferable to perform angiography before external fixation in unstable patients with pelvic fractures. However, in the initial resuscitation, other clinical priorities (eg, airway, breathing) may overshadow the identification and treatment of a potential pelvic fracture. In patients with risk of pelvic injury, the pelvis should be preliminarily stabilized while the patient is being evaluated and treated for concomitant injuries. This is primarily to prevent further shear injury to pelvic vessels rather than to tamponade any active bleeding as previously thought.

Multiple commercial devices exist to stabilize the pelvis while awaiting definitive care. However, if any of these devices are not immediately available, a bedsheet may also be utilized for this purpose. The bedsheet should be folded lengthwise and then wrapped around the patient's hips with the force directed inward on the greater trochanters. A common pitfall with this technique is wrapping the bedsheet over the iliac crests, which may actually worsen pelvic bleeding. Once the bedsheet is wrapped around the patient's pelvis, it should be pulled crosswise until it is snug (but not so tight as to pull the sides of the pelvis closer together). This may be augmented by taping the lower extremities in internal rotation. Towel clips or hemostats may also be used to hold the bedsheet in position during resuscitation.

While most patients with suspected pelvic fracture will receive an x-ray or computed tomography, point-of-care ultrasound could be utilized at the bedside to rapidly assess for this after completion of a FAST examination. This can be performed by sliding the ultrasound transducer inferiorly from the suprapubic view in the transverse orientation. Directly inferior to the bladder, the sonographer should see two hyperechoic, "L-shaped" structures in close proximity, which corresponds to the pubic symphysis (**Figure 251.1**). If these structures are widened or misaligned, a pelvic fracture should be suspected. However, a normal appearance is insufficient to exclude a pelvic fracture being present, as fractures can occur in other locations.

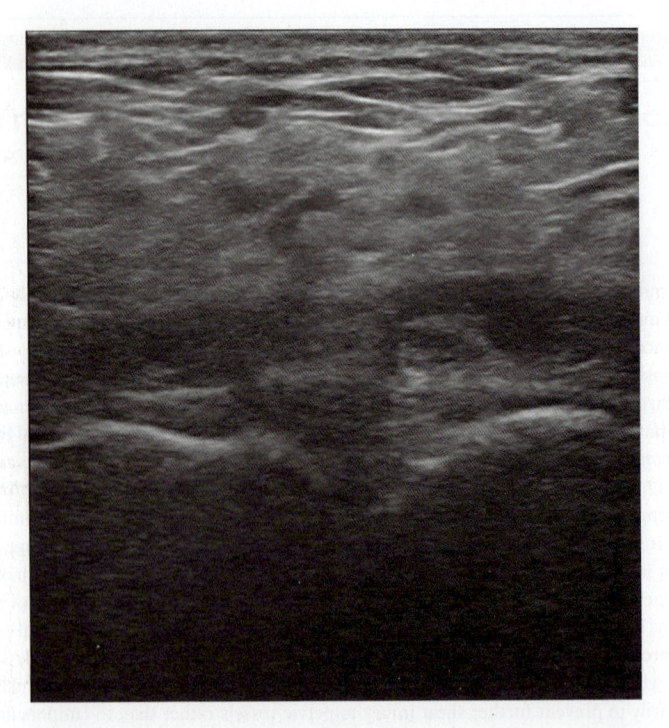

FIGURE 251.1 Pubic symphysis visualized with point-of-care ultrasound.

One particularly high-risk event during the resuscitation of a patient with polytrauma with a pelvic fracture is RSI. Clinicians may underestimate the degree of associated hemorrhagic shock, resulting in a profound and exaggerated drop in blood pressure after the administration of an induction agent. Furthermore, the muscle relaxation associated with the paralytic drug component of RSI may cause an acceleration of hemorrhage due to a loss of muscular tone across an unstable fracture site. When a pelvic fracture is suspected on primary survey, stabilize the pelvis before the administration of the RSI agents. A drop in blood pressure should be anticipated and mitigated by administration of blood products, fluids, and vasoactive agents as appropriate. Once other major injuries have been addressed, the patient should be admitted or transferred for definitive care.

PEARLS

- All major classes of pelvic fracture (with the exception of avulsion injuries) can cause life-threatening hemorrhage.
- In patients with polytrauma with suspected pelvic fracture, stabilize the pelvis before RSI.
- Pelvic binders are fastened snuggly over the greater trochanters, not across the iliac crests.
- A bedsheet secured with towel clips or hemostats can be used in the place of a commercially applied device.

Suggested Readings

Gardner MJ, Parada S, Chip Routt ML Jr. Internal rotation and taping of the lower extremities for closed pelvic reduction. *J Orthop Trauma*. 2009;23(5):361-364.

Giannoudis PV, Grotz MR, Tzioupis C, et al. Prevalence of pelvic fractures, associated injuries, and mortality: the United Kingdom perspective. *J Trauma*. 2007;63(4):875-883.

Ianniello S, Conte P, Di Serafino M, et al. Diagnostic accuracy of pubic symphysis ultrasound in the detection of unstable pelvis in polytrauma patients during e-FAST: the value of FAST-PLUS protocol. A preliminary experience. *J Ultrasound*. 2021;24(4):423-428.

Knops SP, Schep NW, Spoor CW, et al. Comparison of three different pelvic circumferential compression devices: a biomechanical cadaver study. *J Bone Joint Surg Am*. 2011;93(3):230-240.

Miller PR, Moore PS, Mansell E, et al. External fixation or arteriogram in bleeding pelvic fracture: initial therapy guided by markers of arterial hemorrhage. *J Trauma*. 2003;54(3):437-443.

Routt ML Jr, Falicov A, Woodhouse E, et al. Circumferential pelvic antishock sheeting: a temporary resuscitation aid. *J Orthop Trauma*. 2002;16(1):45-48.

252

SPINAL IMMOBILIZATION OR SPINAL MOTION RESTRICTION: WHICH IS BETTER?

JOSEPH PALTER

Spinal injuries remain a significant source of morbidity and health care costs for patients across the United States. The incidence of trauma-related spinal column injuries is estimated at 30,000 per year, with roughly one-third also representing acute spinal cord injuries. These data notwithstanding, 1 to 5 million patients per year are transported via EMS with cervical collar and backboard, suggesting overzealous use of spinal immobilization.

Spinal immobilization, defined as the use of rigid long backboard with straps and cervical collars for all patients with injury mechanisms that posed a potential for spinal injury, has been a hallmark of prehospital care for injured patients since the 1970s. Early research suggested that spinal immobilization decreased the likelihood of patients arriving with complete spinal lesions, though this likely ignored confounding factors such as improved EMS infrastructure and vehicle safety features. Spinal immobilization is not benign and the potential for hazard exists. Ironically, those patients whom spinal immobilization attempts to protect from further injury may actually be those most at risk for iatrogenic morbidity. It has been shown to negatively impact patients' respiratory status, intracranial pressure, skin/tissue pressure injuries, and comfort. Over the decades, no rigorous studies have demonstrated that spinal immobilization reduces further injury or improves short- or long-term neurologic outcomes.

In the early 2010s, a paradigm shift took place away from the term "spinal immobilization" to instead "spinal motion restriction." The goal of spinal motion restriction is to use adjunctive devices to maintain anatomic alignment of the spine and limit unwarranted movements, acknowledging that spine immobilization was not achieved by prior practices. In addition, a 2018 joint position statement from the ACS-COT, ACEP, and the NAEMSP provided consensus recommendations that spinal motion restriction should be applied to blunt trauma who additionally meet any of the following criteria: altered level of consciousness, midline neck or back pain, focal neurologic symptoms, anatomic deformity of spine, or any distracting injury or circumstance that impairs a reliable patient examination.

Special considerations for pediatric patients include the fact that age and communication ability alone should not necessitate spinal motion restriction without other appropriate clinical indicators. In addition, special attention should be paid to pediatric populations with regard to head-to-body ratio, in that additional padding may be required below the shoulders to avoid excessive cervical flexion.

Multiple studies have demonstrated that spinal motion restriction is unnecessary in the patient with penetrating trauma, even in the setting of suspected spinal column involvement. Haut et al reviewed over 45,000 cases and concluded that to potentially contribute to one patient's death, only 66 need to be immobilized, compared to over 1,000 patients that would need to be immobilized to see any benefit. In 2018, the EAST conducted a systematic review and meta-analysis of 24 studies and concluded that there was no mortality or neurologic outcome benefit from routine spinal immobilization of the patient with penetrating trauma, even in cases of direct neck trauma. The joint position statement from ACS-COT, ACEP, and NAEMSP also adopted the recommendation to avoid spinal motion restriction in patients with penetrating trauma.

Spinal motion restriction without spinal immobilization has not led to increased spinal cord injury, morbidity, or mortality, even with widespread adoption. In addition, overall treatment with either method seems to be decreasing. A study by McDonald et al retrospectively reviewed changes in practice patterns across their transition from spinal immobilization to a spinal motion restriction protocol, finding a significantly decreased rate of treatment with either method compared to prior levels of spinal immobilization, despite an increase in higher acuity patients across the study period. They also found increased utilization of cervical collar only treatment, which was preferentially applied to lower acuity patients. Castro-Marin et al reviewed over 100,000 cases comparing prespinal motion restriction protocols to postspinal motion restriction protocols and found no difference in their incidence of spinal cord injury, suggesting that their implementation of spinal motion restriction and decreased longboard use did not lead to greater morbidity.

Patients at risk for potential spinal column and spinal cord injury continue to require stabilization during transport, but the mass application of spinal immobilization has been replaced by a more targeted and nuanced practice of spinal motion restriction. Data to date suggest that spinal motion restriction does not contribute to greater morbidity during transport and should be adopted as the transport method of choice for patients with suspected spinal injuries.

PEARLS

- Spinal immobilization carries significant morbidity and may contribute to life-threatening complications such as airway compromise and increased intracranial pressure.
- Spinal motion restriction has replaced spinal immobilization, with an emphasis on reduction of routine and nonindicated use.
- Spinal motion restriction is not indicated for penetrating trauma.
- Pediatric patients should not have spinal motion restriction based on age and communication ability alone.

Suggested Readings

Castro-Marin F, Gaither JB, Rice AD, et al. Prehospital protocols reducing long spinal board use are not associated with a change in incidence of spinal cord injury. *Prehosp Emerg Care*. 2020;24(3):401-410.

Fischer PE, Perina DG, Delbridge TR, et al. Spinal motion restriction in the trauma patient—a joint position statement. *Prehosp Emerg Care*. 2018;22(6):659-661.

Haut ER, Kalish BT, Efron DT, et al. Spine immobilization in penetrating trauma: more harm than good? *J Trauma*. 2010;68(1):115-121.

McDonald N, Kriellaars D, Pryce RT. Patterns of change in prehospital spinal motion restriction: a retrospective database review. *Acad Emerg Med*. 2023;30:698-708.

Velopulos CG, Shihab HM, Lottenberg L, et al. Prehospital spine immobilization/spinal motion restriction in penetrating trauma: a practice management guideline from the Eastern Association for the Surgery of Trauma (EAST). *J Trauma Acute Care Surg*. 2018;84(5):736-744.

253

THE ABCs OF MAJOR BURNS

MARY CHEFFERS, RUBEN GUZMAN, AND STUART SWADRON

Major burns can be defined as those burns that meet burn center referral criteria as published by the American Burn Association. These criteria can be reviewed in **Table 253.1** and **Figure 253.1**. The majority of patients with major burn will be brought to the nearest ED by EMS professionals for stabilization. For emergency physicians, management of major burns should be focused on the essentials: securing the airway, appropriate fluid resuscitation, identifying concomitant injuries, stopping any continuing burns, treating pain, and obtaining definitive care.

AIRWAY

Prompt intubation for airway protection should be considered in anyone with suspected inhalation injury by mechanism or by physical findings. These include burns suffered in enclosed spaces, long exposure time, singed nose hairs, and soot in the nasopharynx or oropharynx. Airways of major burn patients can rapidly become edematous in the setting of fluid resuscitation as systemic tissue injury causes a capillary leak phenomenon. Intubation should be seriously considered in patient with burns exceeding 50% TBSA, as they often require large fluid volumes, experience severe SIRS reactions, and require large doses of opioid analgesia. In addition, intubation should be considered when a burn victim needs to be transported a long distance. Once intubated, a lung protective ventilation strategy with attention to avoiding both barotrauma and atelectrauma such as the National Institutes of Health ARDSNet protocol will help mitigate further complications of ventilator-induced lung injury.

TABLE 253.1 GUIDELINES FOR BURN PATIENT IMMEDIATE CONSULTATION WITH CONSIDERATION FOR TRANSFER

Thermal burns	■ Full thickness burns ■ Partial thickness ≥10% TBSA ■ Any deep, partial, or full thickness burns involving the face, hands, genitalia, feet, perineum, or over any joints ■ Patients with burns and other comorbidities ■ Patients with concomitant traumatic injuries ■ Poorly controlled pain
Inhalation injury	■ All patients with suspected inhalation injuries
Pediatrics (≤14 yr, or <30 kg)	■ All pediatric burns may benefit from a burn center referral due to pain, dressing change needs, rehabilitation, patient/caregiver needs, or nonaccidental trauma.
Chemical injuries	■ All chemical injuries
Electrical injuries	■ All high-voltage (≥1,000 V) electrical injuries ■ Lightning injury

Derived from the American Burn Association. Guidelines for burn patient referral. https://ameriburn.org/resources/burnreferral/

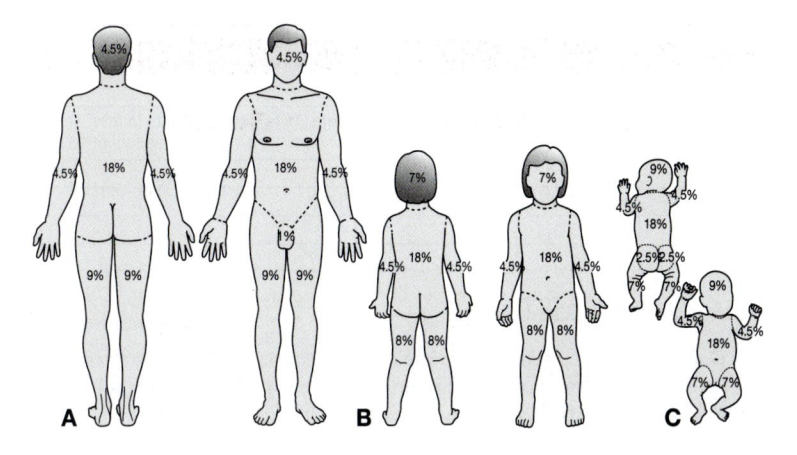

FIGURE 253.1 Rule of Nines: **(A)** adult, **(B)** child, and **(C)** infant.

Fluid Resuscitation

Fluid resuscitation in the ED will affect mortality associated with major burns. The goal is to maintain organ perfusion with the least amount of balanced crystalloid necessary. Both under- and over-resuscitation are associated with poor patient outcomes.

Over-resuscitation leads to complications, including prolonged ventilator time and associated morbidity; congestive heart failure; compartment syndrome of the abdomen, globe, and extremities; and extension of the zone of coagulation. Under-resuscitation may result in worsening shock and organ failure. This is thought to happen through the extension of the zone of coagulation and can contribute to hypovolemic and distributive shock. Hourly urine output can be used as an indicator of adequate resuscitation. Output goals are as follows: for adults, 0.3 to 0.5 mL/kg/h; for children weighing less than 30 kg, 1 mL/kg/h; and for children weighing more than 30 kg, 0.5 mL/kg/h.

Appropriate fluid resuscitation can be performed through accurate estimation of %TBSA of burn using accepted clinical tools such as the Wallace Rule of Nines, the Lund-Browder chart, or the Rule of Palms, and the Parkland or modified Brooke formulas, to estimate initial resuscitation volumes. Most reviews performed by burn centers suggest that the most common error lies in the *estimation of %TBSA* and not in the calculation of the subsequent fluid requirement.

Pearls in Applying %TBSA Estimation Tools

- Only partial-thickness burns and deeper burns should be counted, and *the zone of stasis or hyperemia surrounding the zone of injury should not be included in the calculation.* The area should be cleaned before the definitive calculation to distinguish between soiled areas bordering a wound and burn eschar.
- When noncontiguous burns are present, using the palm as a 1% estimate may be more accurate.
- The pediatric Lund-Browder chart is the most accurate tool to estimate %TBSA in children.

Parkland Formula: 4mL × Weight (kg) × % TBSA = Total Volume (mL) to be given over 24 hours
• ½ of volume is delivered over the first 8 hrs, the remainder in the last 16 hrs
• Timeclock starts at injury, not at ED arrival. Adjust rate as necessary

Weight (kg)	% TBSA	Total Volume (ml)	Rate (ml/hr) first 8 hours	Rate (ml/hr) subsequent 16 hrs
70	20	5600	350	175
70	50	14,000	875	430
80	20	6400	400	200
80	50	16,000	1000	500

FIGURE 253.2 Parkland example.

Once the %TBSA burned is calculated and the patient's weight is estimated, determining the initial 24-hour fluid resuscitation needs through a formula (such as Parkland) is fairly straightforward. Important considerations include the following:

- Fluid resuscitation formulas should be calculated only for burns with greater than 10% TBSA.
- All validated formulas calculate the volume delivered over a set time, starting the clock at the moment of injury, rather than the time of arrival at the ED.
- Lactated Ringer solution is the fluid of choice.
- Fluid resuscitation formulas provide half of the needed volume in the first 8 hours, with the reduction in the rate subsequent to that 8-hour mark.
- Children weighing less than 30 kg should receive dextrose-containing maintenance fluids in the form of D5 1/2 NS as well as lactated Ringer solution.

Example: (see **Figure 253.2**) Using the Parkland formula for an 80-kg patient, 20% TBSA burn means 6.4 L in the first 24 hours. In the first 8 hours, 3.2 L should be given, or 400 mL/h. If the patient arrives 2 hours after the injury, those 3.2 L need to be given in 6 hours, at a rate of close to 500 mL/h. In the example above, 3.2 L should be given over the remaining 16 hours, which means that fluids should be reduced to 200 mL/h after the 8-hour mark postinjury.

TRANSFER

Major burn patients should be transferred to burn centers. The American Burn Association referral criteria can be reviewed in **Figure 253.1** or easily found online. The threshold should be low for the transfer of these patients as care for burns involves multidisciplinary attention. Delaying transfer can cause serious harm to these patients, and when in doubt, the local burn center can be called for consultation. Any concomitant injury, including trauma, CO poisoning, cyanide poisoning, or electrical injury, should be addressed before transfer to allow for safe transfer.

Major burns are rare, but a clear management approach in the ED with a focus on protecting the airway, making accurate estimations of %TBSA of the burn, applying fluid resuscitation formulas precisely, and promptly transferring patients to burn centers will maximize their chance for success.

PEARLS

- Airway and breathing are always the first considerations in a patient with major burns. Prompt intervention with advanced airway management can be lifesaving.

- Both over- and under-resuscitation with fluids continues to be problematic. The greatest source of error is an inaccurate initial estimation of %TBSA.
- Early transfer to a burn center is important for patients who meet the criteria.

SUGGESTED READINGS

American Burn Association. *Guidelines for Burn Patient Referral*. https://ameriburn.org/resources/burnreferral/. American Burn Association; 2022.

Friedstat J, Endorf FW, Gibran NS. Burns. In: Brunicardi F, Andersen DK, Billiar TR, et al, eds. *Schwartz's Principles of Surgery*. 10th ed. McGraw-Hill; 2014.

Giretzlehner M, Dirnberger J, Owen R, Haller HL, Lumenta DM, Kamolz L-P. The determination of total burn surface area: how much difference? *Burns*. 2013;39(6):1107-1113.

Lang TC, Zhao R, Kim A, et al. A critical update of the assessment and acute management of patients with severe burns. *Adv Wound Care (New Rochelle)*. 2019;8(12):607-633. PMID: 31827977. https://www.researchgate.net/figure/Paediatric-Lund-and-Browder-Chart_fig1_319994658

Lee JO, Herndon DN. Burns and radiation. In: Mattox KL, Moore EE, Feliciano DV, eds. *Trauma*. 7th ed. McGraw-Hill; 2013.

Malbrain MLNG, Langer T, Annane D, et al. Intravenous fluid therapy in the perioperative and critical care setting: executive summary of the International Fluid Academy (IFA). *Ann Intensive Care*. 2020;10(1):64. PMID: 32449.

Swords DS, Hadley ED, Swett KR, Pranikoff T. Total body surface area overestimation at referring institutions in children transferred to a burn center. *Am Surg*. 2015;81(1):56-63.

254

OR VERSUS IR, WHERE SHOULD YOUR TRAUMA PATIENT GO?

MATTHEW CRAVENS AND COLMAN HATTON

IR strategies have a rapidly expanding role in the management of traumatically injured patients. This chapter discusses current, generally accepted indications for IR in trauma. Indications for IR involvement are likely to continue to expand as further research is done in this area and techniques evolve and will also depend heavily on your local IR availability and expertise. The Society of Interventional Radiology strongly recommends the development of institution-specific treatment algorithms for common traumatic scenarios for both adults and children.

Minimally invasive interventions such as angioembolization and covered stents have become preferred over operative interventions for certain injury patterns, in part due to their excellent safety profile. Common complications include those related to arterial access including retroperitoneal hematoma, pseudoaneurysm, arteriovenous fistula, dissection, distal embolization, as well as contrast-induced nephropathy and necrosis of the embolized organ.

The indications for IR in trauma are detailed by the organ system in the following section. A common theme across the indications for these injuries is that your patient must be "stable" at presentation or after initial resuscitation. Of course, the subjective definition of stability will be up to the clinicians at the bedside. In this chapter, we consider patients to be "stable" if they lack signs of hemorrhagic shock on presentation or have resolution of signs of shock after initial resuscitation in the trauma bay. The unstable trauma patient should generally proceed immediately to the OR—with the notable exception of isolated pelvic trauma.

INDICATIONS FOR IR IN TRAUMA BY ORGAN SYSTEM

Pelvis

Of all patients with traumatic pelvic bleeding, most are venous in origin and thus not amenable to angioembolization. However, in the hemodynamically unstable patient, arterial injury becomes more likely. The hemodynamically unstable patient with a presumed pelvic source of blood loss (ie, pelvic fracture on x-ray and no discernible intrathoracic or intra-abdominal bleeding on x-ray or FAST examination) should proceed directly to IR for bilateral internal iliac artery embolization.

If a patient is stable for contrasted CT imaging, extravasation may be seen in the pelvis. In general, if contrast extravasation is present, the patient should proceed to angiography. Note that your consultants may not take every patient immediately to IR as there is currently a lack of consensus for stable patients with "clinically insignificant" amounts of pelvic extravasation as CT technology is improved. Patients older than 60 years with major pelvic fractures are at particularly high risk for life-threatening bleeding and should be considered for angiography, regardless of hemodynamic status.

Spleen

The spleen is the most commonly injured solid organ in trauma and also highly amenable to IR embolization. This therapy is indicated for hemodynamically stable blunt splenic injuries with AAST grades IV to V, contrast extravasation, or clinical evidence of ongoing splenic bleeding. Studies have shown that a major advantage of angioembolization over operative splenectomy is preservation of immune function. Unstable patients should undergo splenectomy.

Liver

IR has become the treatment of choice for hemodynamically stable patients with blunt liver injury and ongoing evidence of bleeding or imaging evidence of an arterial source. Unstable patients and those with high-grade injuries (AAST grades IV-V) should be evaluated for operative intervention; however, high-grade injury is not an absolute contraindication to a trial of nonoperative management as operative intervention is associated with large-volume blood loss, coagulopathy, and bile leaks.

Kidney

Embolization is recommended for blunt renal grades III to IV injuries in the hemodynamically stable patient when surgical intervention is not warranted for other injuries. Embolization has the benefit of preservation of renal function compared to nephrectomy.

Aorta

In patients with grade III or IV blunt thoracic aortic injuries (pseudoaneurysm or rupture), endovascular repair is strongly recommended despite low-quality existing evidence.

Vascular

Covered stents may be deployed for traumatic injuries of large vessels, including the femoral veins, subclavian veins and arteries, and intercostal arteries.

Extremities

Endovascular therapy of the extremities is often limited by the need for osseous fixation. Embolization can be considered for extremity hemorrhage when the artery in question is expendable.

Pancreas

There is a paucity of evidence regarding IR for pancreatic injuries. Embolization may be considered if the patient is hemodynamically stable with active extravasation.

Penetrating abdominal injuries

IR for penetrating abdominal injury is an area to watch and occasionally considered for adjunct to operative management, but more studies are needed to guide recommendations.

Pediatric injuries

There is very limited guidance on the use of IR in patients with pediatric trauma, and clinicians should seek local guidelines and expertise. Current studies suggest a role in hemodynamically stable pediatric patients with AAST grades III to V renal injuries.

PEARLS

- IR can provide lifesaving intervention to the patients with traumatic injuries often with less risk than traditional OR management.
- The appropriate patient for IR is stable on presentation or after resuscitation; instability is an indication to proceed to the OR. Isolated pelvic trauma is the notable exception to this.
- IR can benefit patients with trauma to the pelvis, liver, spleen, kidney, aorta, or extremities.
- Institution-specific algorithms for common traumatic scenarios should be developed with input from emergency physicians, interventional radiologists, and trauma surgeons.

SUGGESTED READINGS

Cullinane DC, Schiller HJ, Zielinski MD, et al. Eastern Association for the Surgery of Trauma practice management guidelines for hemorrhage in pelvic fracture—update and systematic review. *J Trauma*. 2011;71(6):1850-1868.

Padia SA, Ingraham CR, Moriarty JM, et al. Society of Interventional Radiology position statement on endovascular intervention for trauma. *J Vasc Interv Radiol*. 2020;31(3): 363-369.e2.

Salcedo ES, Brown IE, Corwin MT, Galante JM. Angioembolization for solid organ injury: a brief review. *Int J Surg*. 2016;33(Pt B):225-230.

Stassen NA, Bhullar I, Cheng JD, et al. Nonoperative management of blunt hepatic injury: an Eastern Association for the Surgery of Trauma practice management guideline. *J Trauma Acute Care Surg*. 2012;73(5 suppl 4):S288-S293.

Stassen NA, Bhullar I, Cheng JD, et al. Selective nonoperative management of blunt splenic injury: an Eastern Association for the Surgery of Trauma practice management guideline. *J Trauma Acute Care Surg*. 2012;73(5 suppl 4):S294-S300.

255

GETTING IT RIGHT IN GLOBE RUPTURE

AMANDA CORREIA

Globe rupture is a can't miss sight-threatening emergency. The leading cause of trauma associated blindness, globe rupture is the colloquial term that refers to any ocular injury that results in an open globe including laceration, perforation and rupture. An open globe injury should be considered in anyone presenting to the ED with trauma and eye pain, or when traumatic facial injuries are present such as periorbital ecchymosis, eyelid laceration, and facial fractures in patients unable to provide symptoms or history.

Traumatic globe rupture can be the result of both blunt and penetrating trauma. Blunt trauma to the orbit or orbital rim leads to an increase in intraocular pressure such that the globe ruptures at its weakest points. In patients without a history of eye surgery, this most commonly occurs posterior to the insertion of the extraocular muscles on the sclera and the limbus, where the cornea meets the sclera. In patients with previous eye surgery, the rupture most commonly occurs at the location of the prior incision site. In penetrating trauma, a foreign object acts as a projectile causing direct injury to the globe.

THE EXAM

Visual inspection provides helpful clues to the presence of an open globe injury. The affected side may have significant periorbital swelling, large subconjunctival hemorrhage, and hyphema. In the case of significant periorbital swelling, gentle retraction of the eyelids should occur to visualize the orbit; however, one must take care not to evert the eyelids as this could lead to increasing pressure on an open globe. Large penetrating intraorbital foreign bodies may be visualized and should not be removed by the emergency physician.

The pupil may appear irregularly shaped or demonstrate a pathognomonic teardrop pupil. The affected eye may have traumatic mydriasis, damage to the iris sphincter, or a third nerve palsy. In addition, an afferent pupillary defect may be appreciated on examination indicating severe damage to the optic nerve and retina.

When globe rupture is obvious or there is a strong suspicion for rupture, intraocular pressure should not be measured as this may worsen the injury and result in extrusion of intraocular contents. In addition, in this scenario fluorescein staining is contraindicated; however, if there is diagnostic uncertainty, applying fluorescein dye and obtaining a positive Seidel sign (extravasation of aqueous humor) is diagnostic of an open globe injury.

Globe rupture may or may not be associated with vision loss; however, obtaining an accurate initial visual acuity is important as worsening of vision can indicate progression to endophthalmitis.

In addition to performing visual inspection and slit lamp exam, a CT of the orbits may be obtained to evaluate for the presence of globe rupture. The sensitivity of CT is up to 68% for detecting an open globe injury and additionally is helpful in identifying intraocular foreign bodies. Ocular ultrasound should be avoided when there is concern for globe rupture as pressure on the globe from the probe may worsen the injury. Patients with high concern for globe rupture should undergo prompt ophthalmologic consultation regardless of imaging findings due to poor sensitivity.

ED Role

It is up to the emergency medicine physician to promptly recognize globe rupture and start treatment. Once suspected, there should be no further manipulation of the globe as it may worsen the condition and ophthalmology should be emergently consulted. In anticipation of surgery, patients with open globe injuries should be made NPO. A hard eye shield should be placed over the affected side, and the head of the bed should be elevated if spinal precautions allow. Antiemetics and pain medication should be administered to prevent further elevation in intraocular pressure.

Antibiotic coverage against both gram-positive and -negative organisms (such as IV vancomycin and ceftazidime or other third-generation cephalosporin) should be administered to prevent progression to endophthalmitis. Tetanus prophylaxis should be provided for those patients without an up-to-date vaccine or unknown vaccination status in the setting of penetrating injury.

For patients with traumatic globe rupture that require intubation, the physician should utilize induction agents that will most likely contribute to first-pass success. Since the 1970s, ketamine has been implicated in raising intraocular pressure; however, there is limited data to support this. Most recently, meta-analyses in 2014 and 2015 found no significant change in ICP after the administration of ketamine both in populations of otherwise healthy individuals and those with traumatic brain injuries.

PEARLS

- Globe rupture should be suspected in any patient presenting to the ED with eye pain and trauma.
- Measuring intraocular pressure in a suspected globe rupture is absolutely contraindicated.
- The affected eye should be patched, and broad-spectrum antibiotics, antiemetics, and pain medication should be administered to avoid elevations in intraocular pressures.
- Ophthalmology should be consulted in all patients felt to be at high risk for globe rupture regardless of the presence of rupture on CT.

Suggested Readings

Guilherme S, Iyeke LO, Vazquez TL, Rai RS, Richman M. Globe rupture—a case report and review of emergency department diagnosis and management. *Cureus*. 2022;14(10):e30007. PMID: 36381828.

Loflin R, Koyfman A. When used for sedation, does ketamine increase intracranial pressure more than fentanyl or sufentanil? *Ann Emerg Med*. 2015;65(1):55-56.

Pelletier J, Koyfman A, Long B. High risk and low prevalence diseases: open globe injury. *Am J Emerg Med*. 2023;64:113-120.

Wang D, Deobhakta A. Open Globe Injury: Assessment and Preoperative Managment. *Am Acad Opthalmol*. Accessed January 31, 2021. https://www.aao.org/eyenet/article/open-globe-injury.

Zeiler FA, Teitelbaum J, West M, et al. The ketamine effect on ICP in traumatic brain injury. *Neurocrit Care*. 2014;21:163-173.

256

TRAUMATIC CARDIAC ARREST

MATTHEW E. ANTON AND MATTHEW A. ROGINSKI

Traumatic cardiac arrest (TCA) is defined as the loss of spontaneous cardiac output after traumatic injury. Management of TCA differs from advanced cardiac life support algorithms described by the American Heart Association. A medical cause of arrest should always be considered, as the pathophysiology of TCA differs from medical causes of cardiac arrest. TCA outcomes are influenced by the amount of time the patient is pulseless prehospital, whether there are signs of life, and the mechanism of trauma. Penetrating trauma has a lower mortality rate than blunt trauma, and the best outcomes occur in penetrating cardiac injuries with brief duration of arrest. In this chapter, we will review outcomes related to traumatic arrest and ED-focused interventions.

SIGNS OF LIFE

Signs of life are defined as cardiac electrical activity, detection of a blood pressure, respiratory effort, and pupillary reactivity. They stratify which patients without a detectable pulse may benefit from invasive interventions. Patients with traumatic injuries may be profoundly hypovolemic in a low-flow state without a palpable pulse. Assessing for additional signs of life aids in determining which patients should have ongoing resuscitation. Point-of-care echocardiography is a useful tool to assess for cardiac activity.

REVERSIBLE CAUSES OF TCA

The acronym "HOTT"—hypovolemia, oxygenation, tamponade, and tension pneumothorax—is helpful in remembering the reversible causes of TCA. Ideally, these etiologies of TCA should be addressed simultaneously when multiple providers are performing different roles. When only one clinician is present, HOTT is a guide for the immediate resuscitation tasks. While a thoracotomy may address multiple etiologies, we recommend less invasive treatments be attempted first based on the patient presentation such as pelvic binding, additional IV access and blood product resuscitation, and oxygenation through a patent airway.

Hypovolemia

The overwhelming majority of patients experiencing trauma without a pulse have hemorrhagic shock. Obtaining rapid large-bore intravenous access is a resuscitation priority. Peripheral access may be challenging in the patients with hypotension due to hypovolemia, in which case intraosseous or central venous access should be obtained. Warmed blood product transfusion should be initiated in a balanced manner. Crystalloid fluid infusion should be avoided when possible. Depending on the site of blood loss, stopping the hemorrhage with direct compression, a tourniquet, pelvic binder, or thoracotomy is critical.

Oxygenation

Hypoxemia is a potentially reversible cause of arrest as well as a cause of significant morbidity related to traumatic arrest. Ideally, the patient may be endotracheally intubated while simultaneously undergoing other procedures. If this is not possible, the patient may be bag-mask ventilated through a patent airway or supraglottic device while other

Table 256.1	Checklist for Traumatic Arrest

Consider likelihood of medical arrest.
Obtain large-bore intravenous access and rapidly infuse blood products.
Oxygenate
Decompress bilateral hemithoraces.
Assess for cardiac tamponade.
Bind unstable pelvis and stop obvious hemorrhage.
Assess indication for thoracotomy.

reversible causes of cardiac arrest are addressed. Endotracheal intubation should not occur before addressing other reversible causes of cardiac arrest.

Tamponade and Tension Pneumothorax

Both penetrating and high-energy blunt trauma can cause a pneumothorax that contributes to arrest. Bilateral chest decompression with thoracostomies is recommended over needle decompression. A point-of-care echocardiogram can assess for a pericardial effusion and evidence of cardiac tamponade. These pathologies can also be treated during a thoracotomy (see **Table 256.1**).

THE ED THORACOTOMY

The primary intervention studied in the patient experiencing trauma without a pulse is the EDT or resuscitative thoracotomy. Ideally, a thoracotomy can quickly address cardiac tamponade, cardiac injuries, air emboli, pulmonary bleeding, and allow for aortic cross-clamping. It also allows for cardiac massage, defibrillation, and decompression of the hemithorax.

Results have varied across the literature, and the main trauma societies have made recommendations based on factors such as time since arrest, mechanism of injury, and signs of life. Penetrating thoracic trauma has the best outcomes after EDT. Even without signs of life, the survival rate after EDT was found to be 8.3% with EDT versus 0.2% survival rate without EDT.

TCA from blunt trauma is associated with worse outcomes. Patients with blunt trauma who arrive in refractory shock have a 2% survival rate after EDT and less than 1% survival rate without vital signs. Trauma societies recommend performing EDT in patients without a detectable pulse with signs of life for both penetrating and blunt trauma. Patients should be declared dead if they have received cardiac compressions for more than 10 minutes in blunt trauma, more than 15 minutes in penetrating trauma, and more than 5 minutes in extremity trauma without return of circulation. The ED clinician should consider the surrounding resources such as equipment, ED and hospital staffing, and their own experience when considering which patient receives a thoracotomy. Without surgical resources for definitive management, thoracotomy may only provide temporary improvement. Either the immediate availability of a surgeon or the availability of rapid transfer to a facility with surgical capability is paramount to possible patient survival (see **Table 256.2**).

REBOA and Emerging Technologies

REBOA is a less invasive procedure to stop subdiaphragmatic bleeding by occluding the aorta with a balloon device inserted through the femoral artery. REBOA is appealing

TABLE 256.2	PATHOLOGIES TO ADDRESS IN AN ED THORACOTOMY

Pericardial tamponade release and cardiac hemorrhage control
Cardiac massage and direct defibrillation
Thoracic aortic cross-clamping
Bronchovenous air embolism evacuation
Pneumothorax
Pulmonary hemorrhage control

because it can be used with less technical skill and less morbidity than an EDT; however, there is insufficient evidence to recommend its application in the patient experiencing trauma without a pulse. Institutional protocols should be developed in conjunction with vascular surgery and should only be performed if an acute care surgeon is immediately available.

PEARLS

- Evaluate the patient for signs of life: cardiac electrical activity, detectable blood pressure, respiratory effort, and pupillary reactivity.
- Immediately treat reversible causes of traumatic arrest: hypovolemia, hypoxemia, cardiac tamponade, tension pneumothorax.
- Considerations for the ED thoracotomy include time since arrest, local expertise, and system capabilities.

SUGGESTED READINGS

Evans CC, Petersen A, Meier EN, et al. Prehospital traumatic cardiac arrest: management and outcomes from the resuscitation outcomes consortium epistry-trauma and PROPHET registries. *J Trauma Acute Care Surg*. 2016;81(2):285-293.

Lockey DJ, Lyon RM, Davies GE. Development of a simple algorithm to guide the effective management of traumatic cardiac arrest. *Resuscitation*. 2013;84(6):738-742.

Moore EE, Burlew CC. Emergency department thoracotomy. In: Moore EE, Feliciano DV, Mattox KL, eds. *Trauma*. 8th ed. McGraw Hill Education; 2017:244-245.

Ohlén D, Hedberg M, Martinsson P, et al. Characteristics and outcome of traumatic cardiac arrest at a level 1 trauma centre over 10 years in Sweden. *Scand J Trauma Resusc Emerg Med*. 2022;30:54.

Seamon MJ, Haut ER, Van Arendonk K, et al. An evidence-based approach to patient selection for emergency department thoracotomy: a practice management guideline from the Eastern Association for the Surgery of Trauma. *J Trauma Acute Care Surg*. 2015;79(1):159-173.

Western Trauma Association. *Resuscitative Thoracotomy*. Western Trauma Association. Published October 12, 2020. Accessed March 29, 2023. https://www.westerntrauma.org/western-trauma-association-algorithms/resuscitative-thoracotomy/introduction/

257

Know When to Drain a Pericardial Effusion in Trauma

Calixto Romero

The Patient
Patients with trauma who experience chest wall injuries are at risk of developing hemopericardium. Most commonly, the development of traumatic hemopericardium is secondary to penetrating causes, but blunt injury can also lead to the condition. Early identification of traumatic hemopericardium offers the best chance for survival. The presentation of someone with a life-threatening hemopericardium is the same as any other cause of cardiac tamponade. While classically described as "Beck's Triad" of symptoms, including hypotension, neck vein distention, and muffled heart sounds, patients with hemopericardium who are developing tamponade will only present with these descriptive diagnostic physical exam findings a minority of the time (12% for muffled heart sounds, and 37% for the hypotension and JVD). Identification of neck vein distention has inherent interrater reliability issues, and muffled heart sounds are difficult to determine in the trauma bay. For those reasons, exposure of the chest and historical details of the trauma are of utmost importance.

Diagnostic Consideration
Bedside ultrasound should be used to rapidly diagnose pericardial effusion and tamponade in a patient who is sick and with crashing trauma. On bedside echocardiography, the diagnosis of pericardial effusion can be made with a single cardiac window but should be evaluated in multiple views to identify the extent of the effusion. Identification of a pericardial effusion in the parasternal long-axis view allows for the clinician to quickly identify the pericardial sac as it sits between the heart and the descending thoracic aorta. If black/anechoic fluid sits deeper than the descending thoracic aorta, it is likely not a pericardial effusion but rather a pleural effusion. RV diastolic collapse can be identified by putting the machine into M-mode while in the parasternal long axis and placing the marker over the septal leaflet of the mitral valve and the free wall of the RV. Cardiac tamponade is evident if the RV-free wall is dipping down at the same moment that the mitral leaflet is at its peak opening. Other findings suggestive of cardiac tamponade include pulsus paradoxus, right atrial systolic collapse, and a large plethoric IVC.

To Drain or Not to Drain?
Patients with trauma with pericardial effusion undergoing tamponade physiology will require treatment, often based on the resources available—if a trauma surgeon is available, they should be involved in the care and decision-making. Blunt and penetrating trauma causing hemopericardium and tamponade physiology can often be temporized with pericardiocentesis but ultimately may require emergent surgical intervention for treatment. Specific indications for emergent pericardiocentesis are hemodynamic instability, impending deterioration, or cardiac arrest. Relative contraindications should be considered, including uncorrected coagulopathy, INR greater than 1.5, platelets less than 50,000 cells/mcL, and a posterior or loculated effusion.

Pericardiocentesis should never delay definitive management of traumatic hemopericardium. However, if definitive care is not going to be delayed and the procedure is to temporize them until they can receive definitive management, the procedure is indicated and should strongly be considered. Optimization with oxygen and blood product resuscitation should be performed before any attempts at positive pressure ventilation, as cardiac tamponade will drastically reduce preload and can precipitate cardiac arrest upon induction.

THE PROCEDURE

Before the advent of ultrasound, a landmark-guided approach was used. Using either a pericardiocentesis kit (Seldinger kit with a drain catheter) or a triple lumen central line kit, the clinician palpates the xiphoid process and inserts a needle at a 45° angle directed toward the left shoulder. If using a central line kit, be aware that the end-hole catheter may become occluded more easily when up against the myocardium and may require repositioning. This should be performed with ultrasound guidance due to its shorter length. Negative pressure is applied and the needle is advanced until the operator begins to aspirate back fluid (in the setting of hemopericardium, blood), at which point the angiocatheter can be advanced into the space.

Ultrasound can be used to obtain imaging to guide the procedure in apical four chamber, parasternal, or subcostal views, enhancing your chance of first-pass success and decreasing the risk for iatrogenic injury. Place the catheter into the pericardial space using standard Seldinger technique, and aspirate fluid until the patient's hemodynamics improve. The catheter needs to be left in place as this space likely is to continue to fill with blood. The provider should suture the catheter in place, place appropriate dressings, and then continue to monitor the patient's hemodynamics while coordinating definitive care.

PEARLS

- In a patient with pericardial effusion that is exhibiting tamponade physiology for which the effusion can be explained by blunt or penetrating chest trauma, pericardiocentesis can be used to temporize the patient until they can receive definitive care for the condition.
- From a physiologic standpoint, trying to avoid positive pressure ventilation is best. Patients with pericardial effusion and tamponade physiology will have reductions in preload and will require additional volume to optimize their hemodynamics for positive pressure ventilation.

SUGGESTED READINGS

Alerhand S, Adrian RJ, Long B, Avila J. Pericardial tamponade: a comprehensive emergency medicine and echocardiography review. *Am J Emerg Med*. 2022;58:159-174.

Huang YK, Lu MS, Liu KS, et al. Traumatic pericardial effusion: impact of diagnostic and surgical approaches. *Resuscitation*. 2010;81(12):1682-1686.

Lee, TH, Ouellet JF, Cook M, Schreiber MA, Kortbeek JB. Pericardiocentesis in trauma: a systematic review. *J Trauma Acute Care Surg*. 2013;75(4):543-549.

Omoto K, Tanaka C, Fukuda R, Tagami T, Unemoto K. Comparison of the effectiveness of pericardiocentesis and surgical pericardiotomy in the prognosis of patients with blunt traumatic cardiac tamponade: a multicenter study using the Japan Trauma Data Bank. *Acute Med Surg*. 2022;9(1):e768.

258

ANTICOAGULANT AND ANTIPLATELET REVERSAL IN TRAUMA

ELIZABETH MALIK AND SAMANTHA HUNT

WHO NEEDS REVERSAL?

From therapeutically anticoagulated patients in the outpatient setting to trauma patients with developing coagulopathy, there are many situations where anticoagulation reversal should be considered. Most often, reversal is indicated when a patient with potentially life-threatening bleeding is known to be taking a PO anticoagulant in the outpatient setting. One glance at a patient's medication list or problem list should trigger clinicians to consider anticoagulation reversal.

Less common reasons for coagulopathy reversal in trauma patients include TIC, advanced liver disease, disseminated intravascular coagulation, certain malignancies, and autoimmune conditions. TIC was initially thought to be caused by largely extrinsic factors, including clotting factor depletion, hypothermia, and crystalloid fluid administration; however, more recently, it is thought to occur secondary to largely intrinsic processes, which overall leads to an imbalance of procoagulant and anticoagulant factors, platelet depletion and dysfunction, dysfunctional endothelium, and excessive fibrinolysis. These patients will require reversal of their coagulopathy in instances of severe or life-threatening bleeding. In the discussion that follows, "severe bleeding" includes hemorrhage causing hypotension, tachycardia, altered mental status, or life-threatening bleeding, including intracranial hemorrhage or retroperitoneal hemorrhage.

VITAMIN K ANTAGONISTS (WARFARIN, COUMADIN)

The two main components of warfarin reversal therapy include vitamin K and either PCC containing factors II, IX, and X (as well as factor VII in four-factor PCC, also known as KCENTRA) or FFP, which contains all clotting factors and von Willebrand factor.

In severe acute bleeding, do not wait for an INR result to begin reversal. Give 10 mg IV vitamin K over 30 minutes and either PCC or FFP. PCC and FFP are only effective for about 8 hours, and vitamin K does not begin working for 6 to 12 hours; thus, the combination of the two is needed for both acute and subacute stabilization of patients with severe hemorrhage. IV vitamin K administration is optimal, as it has the fastest onset working within 6 to 12 hours. Avoid subcutaneous, intramuscular, or PO administration as it results in much slower time to steady state. PCC is preferred to FFP due to greater overall concentration of clotting factors, less volume to infuse resulting in decreased risks of fluid overload, faster infusion time and shorter preparation time since no thawing is needed, and no need for blood-type matching.

In patients on warfarin without serious bleeding but with supratherapeutic INR, recommendations are less clear overall. In general, management depends on INR, with options including withholding warfarin and monitoring INR and withholding warfarin and giving PO vitamin K. PO administration of vitamin K results in reduction of the INR over a period of about 24 to 48 hours rather than the rapid reduction in 6 to 12 hours seen with IV administration.

Clinical Setting	INR	Intervention
Serious or life-threatening bleeding	Any	PCC or FFP vitamin K 10 mg IV Hold warfarin
Minimal bleeding	>5	Vitamin K 1-2.5 mg IV or PO Hold warfarin
Without bleeding	≥10	Vitamin K 5 mg PO Hold warfarin
Without bleeding	5.1-9.9	Vitamin K 1-2.5 mg PO Hold warfarin
Without bleeding	≤5	Hold warfarin

FFP, fresh-frozen plasma; INR, international normalized ratio; IV, intravenous; PCC, prothrombin complex concentrates; PO, by mouth.

Direct Thrombin Inhibitors (Bivalirudin, Argatroban, and Dabigatran)

Dabigatran (Pradaxa) is the only direct thrombin inhibitor with a specific reversal agent. In the setting of severe bleeding, use idarucizumab 5 g IV, which directly binds dabigatran and inactivates it. A normal thrombin time reliably rules out dabigatran effect, while a normal PTT argues against clinically significant dabigatran effects without ruling it out. Dabigatran can also be removed via hemodialysis in severe cases. For reversal of bivalirudin or argatroban, we can attempt reversal with PCC; however, this is not a direct reversal agent. Hemodialysis is less effective in the removal of bivalirudin or argatroban.

Factor Xa Inhibitors (Rivaroxaban, Apixaban, Edoxaban, Fondaparinux)

The reversal agent of choice for these agents is four-factor PCC. Use the INR to roughly correspond to a significant drug level; however, a normal INR does not exclude clinically significant anticoagulation, especially in the setting of trauma. Consider giving vitamin K 10 mg IV if the INR is elevated. Andexanet alfa is a new specific reversal agent for Xa inhibitors; however, this medication has limited data to support its use, so it is not yet routinely used.

Antiplatelet Agents

There are limited data to guide the management of aspirin-, NSAID-, clopidogrel-, and ticagrelor-induced prolonged bleeding time in acute traumatic hemorrhage. While platelet transfusion can be considered, it has not been shown to be effective at improving outcomes in traumatically injured patients on aspirin. We recommend using standard accepted transfusion ratios for bleeding trauma patients.

TXA and TEG

The administration of TXA within 3 hours of a trauma has shown mortality benefit in bleeding patients, even those not taking anticoagulants or antiplatelet agents. Give TXA 1 g IV loading dose followed by an additional 1 g over the next 8 hours. If available, TEG can guide specific transfusion agents, including FFP, cryoprecipitate, platelets, and TXA in treating TIC.

PEARLS

- In the actively bleeding anticoagulated patient, ongoing monitoring of coagulation labs (PT/INR, PTT, thrombin time, fibrinogen, platelet counts, etc) is essential to monitor ongoing reversal needs.
- Warfarin reversal requires both vitamin K and PCC.
- Direct thrombin inhibitors are reversed with PCC. Consider idarucizumab if the patient is on dabigatran.
- Xa inhibitors are reversed by PCC plus vitamin K if INR is elevated.

SUGGESTED READINGS

Briggs A, Gates JD, Kaufman RM, Calahan C, Gormley WB, Havens JM. Platelet dysfunction and platelet transfusion in traumatic brain injury. *J Surg Res*. 2015;193(2):802-806.

Fischer K, Bodalbhai F, Awudi E, Surani S. Reversing bleeding associated with antiplatelet use: the role of tranexamic acid. *Cureus*. 2020;12(9):e10290.

Özgönenel B, Rajpurkar M, Lusher JM. How do you treat bleeding disorders with desmopressin? *Postgrad Med J*. 2007;83(977):159-163.

Pandya U, Malik A, Messina M, Albeiruti AR, Spalding C. Reversal of antiplatelet therapy in traumatic intracranial hemorrhage: Does timing matter? *J Clin Neurosci*. 2018;50:88-92.

Peck KA, Ley EJ, Brown CV, et al. Early anticoagulant reversal after trauma: a Western Trauma Association critical decisions algorithm. *J Trauma Acute Care Surg*. 2021;90(2):331.

Roberts I, Shakur H, Coats T, et al.. The CRASH-2 trial: a randomised controlled trial and economic evaluation of the effects of tranexamic acid on death, vascular occlusive events and transfusion requirement in bleeding trauma patients. *Health Technol Assess*. 2013;17(10):1-79.

Tran HA, Chunilal SD, Harper PL, et al. An update of consensus guidelines for warfarin reversal. *Med J Aust*. 2013;198(4):198-199.

259

Fluids, PRBCs, or Whole Blood for Trauma?

ALISON MARSHALL AND KALLE J. FJELD

What do you reach for in volume resuscitation of the patient experiencing traumatic hemorrhage? Fluids, PRBCs, or whole blood? The pendulum has swung over the years from blood to crystalloid and back again. Ultimately, the goal is to decrease mortality and morbidity in these critically ill patients. Emerging data suggest that whole blood with dynamic monitoring of coagulopathies may be the answer.

PRBCs AND "BALANCED TRANSFUSION"

PRBC transfusion has become the cornerstone of trauma resuscitation. However, transfusion ratio protocols for PRBC:plasma:platelets continue to vary widely. Several trials have illustrated decreased death from hemorrhage at 3 and 6 hours in severe trauma when utilizing a 1:1:1 transfusion ratio that mimics whole blood. A balanced protocolized hemostatic resuscitation approach of 1:1:1 PRBC is recommended for trauma patients presenting acutely to the ED. It is important to note that despite this early survival benefit, no difference in mortality at 24 hours and 30 days has been shown. This may be due to the high risk of nonhemorrhagic causes of death in this patient population during their subsequent recovery course.

Whole Blood

Combat data illustrate improved 24-hour and 30-day survival when using WFWB in severe trauma. However, there are no clinical trials comparing WFWB to a 1:1:1 transfusion ratio. While further investigation is warranted, whole blood should be considered if available in patients with potential need for massive transfusion.

Crystalloids

Crystalloids should not be a significant component of trauma resuscitation. They have been associated with increased complications and in-hospital mortality in the patient experiencing traumatic hemorrhage. Aggressive crystalloid resuscitation causes myriad detrimental effects. Complications range from the obvious such as pulmonary edema, ARDS, and renal failure to the less obvious and more insidious coagulopathy, disruption of cellular membrane potentials, and increased inflammatory mediators. When possible, avoid crystalloids in this patient population in favor of resuscitation with available blood products.

Trauma-Induced Coagulopathy

Trauma patients rapidly become coagulopathic. Both hemodilution and hypothermia are recognized mechanisms. More recently, a third distinct entity is emerging in the literature—TIC. TIC results in failure of functional clotting culminating in diffuse, difficult to control bleeding. Although the pathogenesis of TIC remains incompletely understood, activated protein C, endothelial disruption, platelet dysfunction, and fibrinogen/fibrin dysregulation are thought to be major drivers. Targeted resuscitation utilizing point-of-care TEG, which has been shown to decrease blood product use and improve patient outcomes, can define a variety of patterns of TIC in real time, thus introducing a novel approach to targeted resuscitation.

Special Populations

There is limited evidence to inform pediatric volume resuscitation in trauma. In contrast to adults, initial crystalloid resuscitation has not been associated with increased mortality. However, data may be limited by the logistical challenge of implementing weight-based, balanced transfusion ratios in patients with small total blood volumes when products require time to thaw. Therefore, a balanced ratio of PRBC:plasma:platelets may be beneficial in pediatric patients in hemorrhagic shock and should be considered. When available, implementation of TEG to facilitate goal-directed resuscitation may also benefit pediatric patients at high risk for coagulopathy. Increased risk of coagulopathy should additionally be considered in patients who are pregnant or have cirrhosis. In this population, consideration of early cryoprecipitate can be lifesaving.

Additional Considerations

Close attention to the basic tenets of trauma resuscitation still hold: (1) Hypothermia worsens coagulopathies and should be avoided; (2) give calcium early and regularly in massive transfusion to avoid severe hypocalcemia (an independent predictor of mortality), we recommend 1 to 2 g calcium chloride or 3 to 6 g calcium gluconate with every 6 units of PRBC; and (3) if given within the first 3 hours, TXA reduces the risk of death in patients with bleeding trauma.

PEARLS

- A balanced transfusion ratio of 1:1:1 PRBC:plasma:platelets should be protocolized in severe trauma.
- Whole blood may have a mortality benefit over PRBCs as illustrated in combat data.
- Minimize crystalloid resuscitation in traumatic hemorrhage.
- Where available, utilize TEG for dynamic evaluation and treatment of TIC.
- Avoid hypothermia, give calcium, give TXA when appropriate, and consider early cryoprecipitate in trauma patients who are pregnant or have cirrhosis.

Suggested Readings

Chang R, Cardenas JC, Wade CE, Holcomb JB. Advances in the understanding of trauma-induced coagulopathy. *Blood*. 2016;128(8):1043-1049.

Drucker NA, Wang SK, Newton C. Pediatric trauma-related coagulopathy: balanced resuscitation, goal-directed therapy and viscoelastic assays. *Semin Pediatr Surg*. 2019;28(1):61-66.

Holcomb JB, del Junco DJ, Fox EE, et al. The prospective, observational, multicenter, major trauma transfusion (PROMMTT) study: comparative effectiveness of a time-varying treatment with competing risks. *JAMA Surg*. 2013;148(2):127-136. PMID: 23560283.

Holcomb JB, Tilley BC, Baraniuk S, et al. Transfusion of plasma, platelets, and red blood cells in a 1:1:1 vs a 1:1:2 ratio and mortality in patients with severe trauma: the PROPPR randomized clinical trial. *JAMA*. 2015;313(5):471-482.

Roberts I, Shakur H, Coats T, et al. The CRASH-2 trial: a randomised controlled trial and economic evaluation of the effects of tranexamic acid on death, vascular occlusive events and transfusion requirement in bleeding trauma patients. *Health Technol Assess*. 2013;17(10):1-79. PMID: 23477634.

Spinella PC, Perkins JG, Grathwohl KW, Beekley AC, Holcomb JB. Warm fresh whole blood is independently associated with improved survival for patients with combat-related traumatic injuries. *J Trauma*. 2009;66(4 Suppl):S69-S76. PMID: 19359973.

SECTION XXI
ORTHOPEDICS

260

ADMIT DISPLACED SUPRACONDYLAR FRACTURES FOR NEUROVASCULAR CHECKS

DANIELLE SUTTON

Supracondylar fractures are some of the most commonly encountered fracture patterns in young children and account for over half of all pediatric elbow fractures. In 70% of patients, these result from an injury caused by a FOOSH in which force is transmitted through the olecranon to a weak supracondylar area resulting in a fracture. These fractures occur most commonly in children between the ages of 3 and 10 years, with peak incidence between 5 and 7 years of age.

There are two primary types of supracondylar fractures, those that occur during extension or hyperextension and those that occur during flexion. More than 95% of these fractures are the extension type, those caused by a FOOSH. In the flexion type, the mechanism is usually a fall from height onto a flexed elbow. Key findings on physical examination include swelling, deformity, and decreased range of motion of the elbow joint. Be sure to evaluate for ipsilateral forearm fractures ("floating elbow") and bruising/puckering of the skin in the antecubital fossa, which may indicate underlying injury to the brachial artery and median nerve. Neurovascular injuries occur in approximately 12% of all supracondylar fractures, and this rate increases with the degree of displacement. In extension-type fractures, the median nerve is injured most commonly, specifically the AIN. The integrity of the AIN can be tested using the strength of the patient while holding the "OK" sign using the thumb and index fingers. The median, radial, and ulnar nerves can be evaluated by asking the patient to show you "rock, paper, scissors" accordingly. In flexion-type injuries, the ulnar nerve may be injured. Motor impairment at the time of injury is almost always caused by neuropraxia and usually improves within 3 months. Further workup is not needed unless the deficit persists beyond this period. Any injury with an absent radial pulse requires an immediate orthopedic consult. Management of a pulseless extremity may differ based on whether the hand has evidence of perfusion (color, temperature, capillary refill) but regardless should be treated as a true orthopedic emergency.

Anterior-posterior and lateral radiographs of the elbow are required to make the diagnosis. Radiographic evaluation should focus on the AHL, the presence or absence of fat pads, and the different ossification centers of the elbow. A posterior fat pad that is

TABLE 260.1	CRITOE Mnemonic for Elbow Ossification Centers in Children	
Ossification Center	Age Ossification Becomes Visible (yr)	Age Ossification Fuses (yr)
Capitellum	1	12
Radial head	3	15
Internal (medial) epicondyle	5	17
Trochlea	7	12
Olecranon	9	15
External (lateral) epicondyle	11	12

displaced by hemorrhage (referred to as a "sail sign") is always abnormal and indicative of a fracture. CRITOE is a well-known mnemonic used to help predict when ossification centers appear and subsequently fuse (**Table 260.1**). A common error is to confuse a medial epicondyle growth center for a fracture, as it is the last to fuse in a pediatric elbow. If there is doubt, comparing radiographs with the opposite uninjured elbow may be helpful.

In a normal radiograph, the AHL should pass through the middle third of the capitellum. If the capitellum is anterior to the AHL, this is diagnostic for a flexion-type supracondylar fracture. A capitellum that is seen posterior to the AHL is diagnostic of an extension-type supracondylar fracture. Extension-type supracondylar fractures are separated into the classifications based on their treatment (**Table 260.2**).

Regardless of the type of fracture, the elbow should initially be splinted in a position of comfort at approximately 20° to 30° flexion and elevated above the level of the heart. Avoid splinting the limb in full extension as this could damage the neurovascular bundle, especially in displaced or unstable fractures. In addition, splinting at greater than 90° flexion increases the forearm compartment pressures, putting the patient at risk for compartment syndrome.

TABLE 260.2	Classification of Extension-Type Supracondylar Fractures	
	Characteristics	ED Treatment
Type I	Minimally or nondisplaced fracture (fat pad abnormality)	Splint with a posterior long arm in slight flexion and discharge home with close follow-up within 24 h
Type II	Displaced fractures or those with an AHL that passes anterior to the capitellum on the lateral radiograph, with intact posterior cortex	Pediatric orthopedist evaluation with choice of closed reduction vs percutaneous pinning. Hospital admission for neurovascular checks
Type III	Significant displacement of the distal humerus with disruption of the posterior cortex	Pediatric orthopedist evaluation with closed or open reduction, percutaneous pin placement, and hospitalization for neurovascular checks

AHL, anterior humeral line.

Compartment syndrome should be suspected in any patient with increasing narcotic pain medication requirements or if paresthesias develop. Severely displaced fractures, floating elbows, and those with vascular injuries are at increased risk for compartment syndrome. Management for compartment syndrome involves emergent transfer to the OR for fasciotomy. The feared complication of compartment syndrome is the development of Volkmann ischemic contracture. Volkmann contracture results from an untreated compartment syndrome of the forearm and is characterized by fixed flexion at the wrist and elbow, with the forearm in pronation and the metacarpophalangeal joints in extension. If there is any concern for compartment syndrome or if the patient is at high risk for the development for compartment syndrome, an orthopedic consult and admission for serial examinations is reasonable. Most type II and III supracondylar fractures will be splinted and admitted in preparation for surgical repair.

PEARLS

- Supracondylar fractures with significant displacement are at high risk for neurovascular complications and poor outcomes. Admission and observation for significantly displaced fractures is indicated.
- Evaluate for ipsilateral forearm fractures and the presence of a radial pulse.
- Increasing pain and paresthesias should raise suspicion for compartment syndrome.

Acknowledgments

We gratefully acknowledge the contributions of previous edition authors, Allison S. Luu and Eric Wei, as portions of their chapter have been retained in this revision.

Suggested Readings

Abzug JM, Herman MJ. Management of supracondylar humerus fractures in children: current concepts. *J Am Acad Orthop Surg*. 2012;20(2):69-77.

Armstrong DG, MacNeille R, Lehman EB, Hennrikus WL. Compartment syndrome in children with a supracondylar fracture. Not everyone has risk factors. *J Orthop Trauma*. 2020;35(8):e298-e303.

Brubacher JW, Dodds SD. Pediatric supracondylar fractures of the distal humerus. *Curr Rev Musculoskelet Med*. 2008;1(3/4):190-196.

Carson S, Woolridge DP, Colletti J, Kilgore K. Pediatric upper extremity injuries. *Pediatr Clin North Am*. 2006;53(1):41-67.

Cheng JC, Wing-Man K, Shen WY, et al. A new look at the sequential development of elbow-ossification centers in children. *J Pediatr Orthop*. 1998;18(2):161-167.

Duffy S, Flannery O, Gelfer Y, Monsell F. Overview of the contemporary management of supracondylar humeral fractures in children. *Eur J Orthop Surg Traumatol*. 2021;31(5): 871-881.

261

KNOW THE DIFFERENCE BETWEEN JONES AND PSEUDO-JONES FRACTURES

KAITLYN MCBRIDE AND ANDREW B. MOORE

The proximal fifth metatarsal is the most common site of midfoot fractures in children over 10 years old and adults and accounts for approximately 45% to 70% of all metatarsal fractures. The best-known injury pattern is the Jones fracture, which was first described in 1902 by Sir Robert Jones after he injured his foot dancing. Throughout the years, others have further classified fractures of the fifth metatarsal based on three main anatomic and radiographic zones. The prognosis and management of the various fracture types varies based on the zone of the fracture location, which comes down to millimeters and highlights the importance of correctly identifying the fracture type (see **Figure 261.1**). The oblique x-ray is the most helpful for determining fracture location.

ZONE 1 TUBEROSITY AVULSION FRACTURES: PSEUDO-JONES

Tuberosity avulsion fractures of the fifth metatarsal are often referred to as pseudo-Jones fractures and represent the majority of fractures at the base of the fifth metatarsal. Standard AP, lateral, and oblique foot radiographs are usually sufficient to make the diagnosis. If there is malleolar tenderness in addition to tenderness at the base of the fifth metatarsal, ankle films are also indicated according to the Ottawa Ankle Rule. The fracture itself can have a transverse or oblique appearance and occurs proximal to the intermetatarsal joint between the fourth and fifth metatarsals, sometimes also including the tarsometatarsal articulation.

The typical mechanism of injury is inversion of the foot and ankle while in plantar flexion (eg, a basketball player landing awkwardly after a jump or runner inverting the ankle on an uneven surface) causing tension in the peroneus brevis tendon and lateral cord of the plantar aponeurosis to avulse the tuberosity. Patients often present complaining of a "sprained ankle" due to the mechanism and relatively mild symptoms.

Treatment of nondisplaced fracture is symptomatic and includes compression dressing with primary care follow-up in 1 week. Fractures with less than 3 mm of

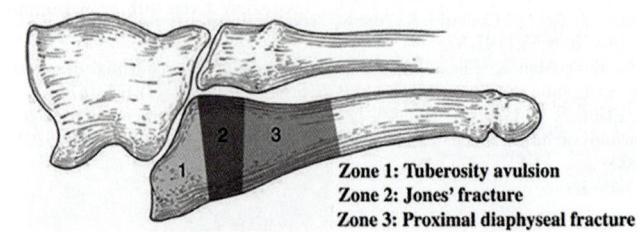

FIGURE 261.1 Fifth metatarsal fractures. (Modified from Lawrence SJ, Botte MJ. Jones' fractures and related fractures of the proximal fifth metatarsal. *Foot Ankle*. 1993;14(6):358-365, Figure 3.)

Zone 1: Tuberosity avulsion
Zone 2: Jones' fracture
Zone 3: Proximal diaphyseal fracture

displacement can generally be treated with 2 weeks of a short leg walking boot (± compression dressing) with a goal of preventing significant plantar flexion. Evidence supports improved outcomes with early weight bearing. Orthopedic referral is indicated if there is greater than 3 mm of displacement, 10° of plantar angulation, a step-off of more than 1 to 2 mm on the articular surface of the cuboid, or symptomatic nonunion. All of these may ultimately require operative intervention.

Multiple metaphyseal blood vessels and branches of the nutrient artery supply the tuberosity of the fifth metatarsal. Prognosis for these fractures is excellent and radiographic union is typically seen at 4 to 8 weeks. Complications are unusual but include nonunion or prolonged discomfort. These are more common if there is a step-off on the articular surface and in older patients.

ZONE 2 METAPHYSIS/DIAPHYSIS—JONES FRACTURE

The Jones fracture is an acute fracture of the junction of the diaphysis and metaphysis of the fifth metatarsal—this is where the widened part of the bone begins to thin out as it becomes the shaft of the bone (typically within 1.5 cm of the metatarsal tuberosity) and extends toward the intermetatarsal joint (typically between the fourth and fifth metatarsals). Jones fractures are frequently accompanied by phalanx fractures. Blood supply to the metaphysis-diaphysis falls in a watershed area from the nutrient artery and can lead to healing complications.

The mechanism of a Jones fracture is typically a sudden change in direction with the heel off of the ground. This creates either a vertical or lateral force on the forefoot. It is often reported in contact sports with quick acceleration and directional changes. A patient will typically present with pain and tenderness in the lateral foot. Jones fractures are thought to be more common in people with a high-arched foot shape, resulting in increased loading on the lateral foot.

Zones 2 and 3 of the metatarsal can further be divided into three Torg classifications, which help to determine management in delayed presentations. Torg I represents acute fractures, Torg II represents delayed union with a widened fracture line and sclerosis, and Torg III represents nonunion with a history of recurrent symptoms or trauma.

Initial treatment includes ice, elevation, and immobilization in a posterior short leg splint with strict non–weight-bearing status and orthopedic follow-up within 3 to 5 days. Definitive treatment is typically a short leg, non–weight-bearing cast for 6 to 8 weeks in the nonathlete population and early intramedullary screw fixation in the athlete population or those with greater than 2 mm of displacement. Athletes generally can return to play in 8.5 weeks.

Prognosis is guarded because of a high incidence of delayed healing and nonunion due to the watershed area of blood supply to this region. Even with proper immobilization, up to 60% later require surgery due to nonunion or refracture and bone grafting might be necessary.

ZONE 3 PROXIMAL DIAPHYSIS—STRESS FRACTURES

Diaphyseal stress fractures are seen distal to the ligamentous attachments of the bone (1.5 cm into the diaphysis). These fractures are typically symptomatic for several days before presentation and are typically from chronic overloading of the bone leading to a stress fracture. Obesity is a risk factor for zone 3 fractures.

The treatment is similar to the Jones fracture with immobilization and non–weight bearing for 6 to 10 weeks, but the prognosis for nonunion is even worse than with Jones fractures. Early surgery is recommended for the acute fracture and for Torg II and III fractures.

> **PEARLS**
>
> - A pseudo-Jones fracture occurs when an inversion injury causes an avulsion fracture whereas a Jones fracture occurs when a lateral force encounters the foot while the heel is off of the ground.
> - An avulsion fracture of the fifth metatarsal occurs proximal to the intermetatarsal joint between the fourth and fifth metatarsals.
> - While an avulsion fracture can be treated with a short leg walking boot and early weight bearing, both Jones fractures and fifth metatarsal stress fractures require prolonged immobilization and strict non–weight-bearing status with possible surgical intervention, particularly in the athlete population.

SUGGESTED READINGS

Bica D, Sprouse RA, Armen J. Diagnosis and management of common foot fractures. *Am Fam Physician*. 2016;93(3):183-191.

Bowes J, Buckley R. Fifth metatarsal fractures and current treatment. *World J Orthop*. 2016;7(12):793-800.

Cheung CK, Lui TH. Proximal fifth metatarsal fractures: anatomy, classification, treatment and complications. *Arch Trauma Res*. 2016;5(4):e33298.

Chloros GD, Kakos CD, Tastsidis IK, et al. Fifth metatarsal fractures: an update on management, complications, and outcomes. *EFORT Open Rev*. 2022;7(1):13-25.

Stiell IG, Greenberg GH, McKnight RD, et al. Decision rules for the use of radiography in acute ankle injuries. Refinement and prospective validation. *JAMA*. 1993;269(9):1127-1132.

262

ALWAYS SEARCH FOR OTHER INJURIES IN PATIENTS WITH SCAPULA FRACTURE

JOHN W. MARTEL AND JOSEPH M. MINICHIELLO

Scapula fracture is an uncommon injury, with annual incidence of 10 to 12 per 100,000 in the United States. Although uncommon, it is typically associated with high-energy blunt force traumatic mechanisms, including motor vehicle collisions and falls from height, and often occurs in conjunction with other serious injuries. Comprising less than 1% of all fractures, it is associated with a 10% to 15% mortality rate, and over 90% of patients have concomitant injuries whose diagnoses may be delayed or overlooked entirely if not carefully considered. In particular, there is risk of coexisting multisystem thoracic, orthopedic, intracranial, intra-abdominal, and neurovascular injuries. Specifically, there is a very high reported incidence (75%-98%) of associated injuries to the ipsilateral lung, chest wall, and shoulder girdle; the prevalence of concurrent acute aortic injury has been reported to be similar in blunt trauma patients, irrespective of scapula fracture presence, and any association may have been overestimated in the past. Scapula fracture is also uncommon in children, with the vast majority resulting from high-energy traumatic mechanisms. Pediatric scapula fracture may result from nonaccidental trauma, with one study suggesting that scapula fracture is the second most common injury from nonaccidental trauma after rib fractures.

During physical examination, fully conscious patients commonly maintain the affected shoulder in a position of adduction with the extremity itself held close to the chest wall. In the appropriate clinical context, a variety of shoulder findings, including ipsilateral ecchymosis, hematoma, focal tenderness, or crepitus, should raise suspicion for scapula fracture as well as a wide variety of potentially serious associated injuries. Scapula fracture occurs primarily in the body, followed by the neck, glenoid, and acromion in descending order. Three-view shoulder radiograph (AP, trans-scapular lateral, and axillary lateral views) aids in rapid diagnosis via evaluation of both the glenohumeral structures and the scapular body. Occasionally, scapula fracture may also be seen on chest radiograph; however, it may not be initially appreciated clinically on portable chest radiograph in the critically injured patient. CT more effectively delineates the fracture extent and is also useful in comprehensive evaluation of associated serious multisystem injuries in the hemodynamically stable patient. Therefore, if there is clinical suspicion for scapula fracture, then CT should be obtained without need to obtain x-ray first.

With regard to injury patterns, rib fractures and acute intrathoracic pathology (including pneumothorax, hemothorax, and lung contusions) are considered to be the most common co-occurring injuries associated with scapula fracture, seen in up to two-thirds of cases in some combination. In addition, skull fracture and intracranial injuries, including intracranial hemorrhage and cerebral contusion, occur in up to 40% of patients. Furthermore, up to 10% of cases are associated with injury to regional vasculature, including the brachial, subclavian, and axillary arteries. It is also prudent to conduct thorough surveillance for multifocal orthopedic injuries, with special focus on the axial skeleton, pelvis, and extremities. Not surprisingly, a 10-year retrospective review of blunt trauma admissions at two large, urban level 1 trauma centers reported that patients with scapular fracture tended to have higher injury severity scores and underlying thoracic injuries. Similarly, a retrospective review of the National Trauma Database reported that concomitant injuries to the thorax, upper extremities, and pelvis were associated with greater frequency in patients with scapula fracture.

Fortunately, isolated scapula fracture is generally not associated with permanent disability. The vast majority are managed nonoperatively per sling placement and early range of motion, with the exception being unstable fracture that requires operative intervention. Given the high-energy mechanisms that typically result in scapula fractures and the frequency of patients presenting with concomitant injuries, careful consideration of traumatic mechanism, injury pattern, and thorough trauma evaluation is required in order to avoid missing potentially life-threatening comorbidities.

PEARLS

- Scapula fractures are typically associated with high-energy mechanisms.
- Over 90% of patients have concomitant injuries, including very high incidence of injuries to ipsilateral lung, chest wall, and shoulder girdle.
- When scapula fracture is identified, carefully consider the mechanism and evaluate closely for potentially life-threatening concomitant injuries.

Suggested Readings

Baldwin KD, Ohman-Strickland P, Mehta S, Hume E. Scapula fractures: a marker for concomitant injury? A retrospective review of data in the national trauma database. *J Trauma*. 2008;65:430-435.

Brown CV, Velmahos G, Wang D, Kennedy S, Demetriaes D, Rhee P. Association of scapular fractures and blunt thoracic aortic injury: fact or fiction? *Am Surg*. 2005;71:54-57.

Cole PA, Freeman G, Dubin JR. Scapula fractures. *Curr Rev Musculoskelet Med*. 2013; 6(1):79-87.

Veysi VT, Mittal R, Agarwal S, Dosani A, Giannoudis PV. Multiple trauma and scapula fractures: so what? *J Trauma*. 2003;55:1145-1147.

263

Don't Miss the Proximal Fibula Fracture in Patients With Ankle Fracture

Danielle Sutton

One of the most common musculoskeletal injuries evaluated in the ED is the twisted ankle. Significant research has been conducted on the evaluation of the injured ankle in the ED, with the creation of rules to help aid in the differentiation between a sprain and a fracture via history and physical examination alone. However, not all ankle injuries are isolated to the distal extremity. Specifically, one rare but significant injury pattern of the ankle injury can throw the clinician off track because it also causes a fracture near the knee. It is known as the Maisonneuve fracture.

The Maisonneuve fracture is a spiral fracture of the proximal third of the fibula that is significant because it implies disruption of the distal tibiofibular syndesmosis and associated injury. This fracture pattern is caused when an external rotation force is applied to the fixed foot. The force of the injury runs from the distal tibia, up through the interosseous membrane and ends at the proximal third of the fibula. This force creates an injury pattern that first causes an injury in the deltoid ligament and/or fracture of the medial malleolus. Next, there is a rupture of the distal tibiofibular syndesmosis with occasional fracture of the posterior malleolus. Finally, the force causes a rotational and valgus stress on the proximal fibula causing a proximal fibular fracture. The characteristic feature of the Maisonneuve fracture is a spiral or oblique fracture at the fibular neck or immediately proximal to the neck.

The mechanism of injury of the Maisonneuve fracture is most often sports related, followed by injuries caused by slipping on ice, walking or running, and finally by motor vehicle accidents and falls from height. Patients may complain of only ankle pain and resultant inability to ambulate and not complain of proximal fibular pain. This may be due to the minimal weight-bearing demands of the proximal fibula. On examination, there is typically tenderness over the deltoid ligament (on the medial side) and the tibiofibular syndesmosis without lateral ligamentous or distal fibular tenderness. While there will likely not be any obvious deformity or swelling over the proximal fibula, there is usually tenderness to palpation. Moreover, the patient may complain of decreased sensation in the dorsum of the foot. This is a result of an injury to the peroneal nerve as it crosses over the head of the fibula.

The lack of a historical complaint of proximal fibular pain is precisely why we need to conduct a thorough radiographic examination, extending to at least the proximal fibula of any patient with a complaint of an ankle injury. An x-ray of the ankle often demonstrates a widening of the distal tibiofibular joint as well as a fracture of the medial malleolus and/or posterior malleolus. However, in some cases, the proximal fibular fracture can occur with only soft tissue damage at the level of the ankle (see **Figure 263.1**). Only films of the tibia-fibula or knee, if ordered, will demonstrate the proximal fibula fracture. Furthermore, ankle films may not demonstrate any obvious pathology, leaving little to suspect on the basis of ankle films alone that a high fibular fracture may be present. Thus, without recognition of the injury pattern and examination of the proximal fibula, many patients with Maisonneuve fracture patterns (and therefore syndesmotic injuries) are missed. Tibial and fibular radiographs should not necessarily be obtained routinely but should be obtained if there is bony tenderness over the proximal fibula in the setting of an ankle injury or if an ankle fracture is appreciated on x-ray. Obtaining a CT of the ankle may be helpful if there is suspicion for associated injuries and to determine whether the distal fibula is sitting correctly in the fibular notch.

Treatment of a Maisonneuve injury is commonly surgical due to syndesmotic disruption but depends on the nature of injury to the ankle mortise. Failed diagnosis can lead to long-term pain and arthritis. With proper diagnosis and management,

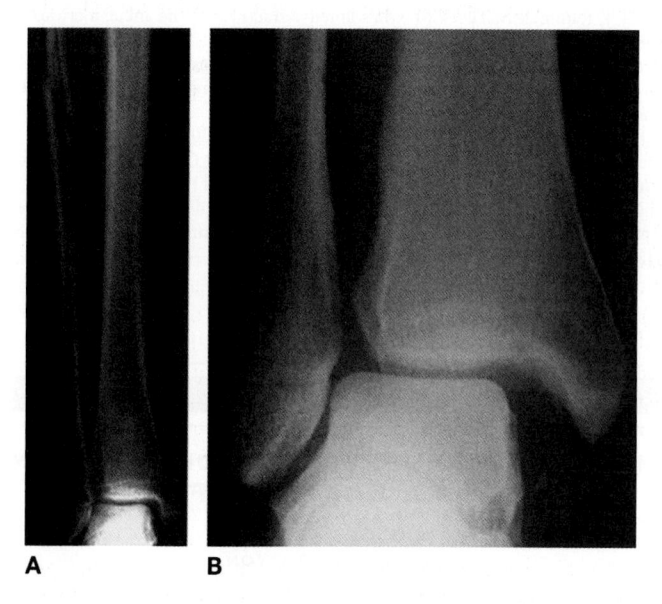

FIGURE 263.1 A Maisonneuve fracture with a proximal fibula fracture (**A**) and lateral displacement of the talus and widening of the syndesmosis (**B**). (From Tornetta P, Ricci W, Court-Brown CM, McQueen MM, McKee M, eds. *Rockwood and Green's Fractures in Adults*. 9th ed. Wolters Kluwer; 2020. Figure 64.12.)

nevertheless, the long-term functional outcome is typically good. As an emergency physician, it is important to properly immobilize the leg. In isolated proximal fibula fractures, a cam boot or short leg splint, with or without a knee immobilizer, is sufficient for discharge with outpatient orthopedic referral. If there are associated posterior malleolar fractures (which can occur in as many as 77%-83% of Maisonneuve fractures) or evidence of ankle mortise widening, orthopedic surgery should be consulted to discuss advanced imaging, need for reduction, and plans for surgery.

PEARLS

- The Maisonneuve fracture is a spiral fracture of the proximal third of the fibula with associated disruption of the ankle. It presents most commonly as a sprained ankle.
- Management is often surgical to fix the syndesmosis, and delays in diagnosis may result in complications.
- Diagnostic delays can occur because of a failure to examine and, if necessary, image the proximal fibula in ankle injuries.
- The absence of an actual ankle fracture in some cases (only soft tissue injury) may lead the clinician to underestimate the severity of this injury.

Suggested Readings

Bartoníček J, Rammelt S, Tuček M. Maisonneuve fractures of the ankle: a critical analysis review. *JBJS Rev*. 2022;10(2):e21.00160.

Duchesneau S, Fallat LM. The Maisonneuve fracture. *J Foot Ankle Surg*. 1995;34(5):422-428.

Kalyani BS, Roberts CS, Giannoudis PV. The Maisonneuve injury: a comprehensive review. *Orthopedics*. 2010;33(3):196-197.

Millen JC, Lindberg D. Maisonneuve fracture. *J Emerg Med*. 2011;41(1):77-78.

Stufkens SA, van den Bekerom MP, Doornberg JN, van Dijk CN, Kloen P. Evidence-based treatment of maisonneuve fractures. *J Foot Ankle Surg*. 2011;50(1):62-67.

Taweel NR, Raikin SM, Karanjia HN, Ahmad J. The proximal fibula should be examined in all patients with ankle injury: a case series of missed maisonneuve fractures. *J Emerg Med*. 2013;44(2):e251-e255.

264

Check for Snuffbox Tenderness and Don't Miss a Scaphoid Fracture

Danielle Sutton

Wrist pain is a very common chief complaint in the ED, and emergency physicians must be aware of the high rate of scaphoid fractures among patients with acute wrist pain. The scaphoid bone is the most commonly fractured carpal bone, and injury most frequently occurs from a FOOSH with force transmitted via axial loading of the wrist. Classically, scaphoid fractures have a male predominance and often occur in the third decade of life, though they may also be seen in younger individuals who play contact sports.

The scaphoid is a crescent-shaped bone in the wrist and the largest of the proximal carpal bones. Its anatomy can be remembered by dividing it into thirds: the proximal pole, the middle third (waist), and the distal pole. The scaphoid receives its vascular supply from the palmar carpal branch of the radial artery. This branch enters the scaphoid at the distal end and then travels retrograde toward the proximal pole. The waist and proximal pole of the scaphoid are, therefore, dependent on an intact *distal* blood supply, which will frequently become compromised after fracture. Due to its tenuous blood supply, missed fractures are at particular risk for nonunion and avascular necrosis and patients are at risk for developing SNAC arthritis.

When a history suspicious for scaphoid fracture exists, clinical examination of the wrist will often help solidify the diagnosis. Examination will classically reveal tenderness and/or swelling over the anatomical snuffbox (best tested with the wrist in slight volar flexion and ulnar deviation). Tenderness will also be elicited with palpation over the scaphoid tubercle on the volar aspect of the hand and with axial loading of the thumb metacarpal. All three of these quick bedside maneuvers are sensitive for detecting scaphoid fractures.

Wrist x-rays should include posterior/anterior and lateral views, a pronated oblique view, and an additional dedicated scaphoid view (involves placing the patient's hand in full pronation with as much ulnar deviation of the wrist as tolerated). This is the best view to visualize the waist, which is the most frequently fractured portion of the scaphoid. A clear fracture line is obviously indicative of fracture; however, up to 20% of scaphoid fractures will have negative x-rays. Some helpful subtle findings, such as obliteration or displacement of the scaphoid fat pad, may indicate the presence of a fracture as well. Traditionally, empiric immobilization with repeat radiographs within 1 to 3 weeks has been recommended when there is a high clinical suspicion for a scaphoid fracture despite negative radiographs. This allows more time for any fracture to present itself, while keeping the patient immobilized in the interim. Obtaining advanced imaging such as MR or CT, in the acute setting, has been generally reserved for athletes needing prompt diagnosis for return to play, but recent literature advocates for advanced imaging acutely in the ED or in the outpatient setting as it is thought to help decrease the morbidity associated with prolonged immobilization and help guide definitive management. Both MR and CT have excellent sensitivity and specificity for identifying scaphoid fractures with MR having the ability to detect occult fractures even within a few hours of injury. There is also emerging data for using ultrasound in the diagnosis of scaphoid fractures with one study citing its diagnostic accuracy around 98%; however, this was a relatively small study and this method is still being validated. The Herbert classification is the most commonly used classification system in orthopedic literature to define a fracture as stable versus unstable and is helpful in guiding management (**Table 264.1**).

Splinting or casting after a scaphoid fracture focuses on immobilization of the scaphoid and usually requires placement of a thumb spica cast or splint, and is the appropriate immediate management in the ED regardless of the fracture type. In patients with stable fractures (distal pole and non-displaced waist), it is reasonable to cast with follow-up in a few weeks with orthopedic surgery. Most distal pole fractures will heal within 6 to 8 weeks of casting and most non-displaced waist fractures can often also

TABLE 264.1	HERBERT CLASSIFICATION OF SCAPHOID FRACTURES
CLASSIFICATION	**DESCRIPTION**
Type A	Stable fracture in the acute phase (non-displaced waist fracture and fracture of the tubercle)
Type B	Unstable fracture in the acute phase (comminuted fracture, fracture dislocation, distal oblique fracture, proximal pole fracture, displaced waist fracture)
Type C	Old fracture with evidence of delayed union
Type D	Old fracture with nonunion

be managed conservatively. Unstable fractures as outlined by the Herbert classification system require urgent orthopedic referral in the outpatient setting and include:

- Fractures of the proximal pole, displaced waist fractures, and any unstable fracture (Often CT/MR needed to diagnose)
- Greater than 1 mm displacement of fracture segments (CT/MR may be necessary)
- Delayed presentation (delayed presentation over 4 weeks after the initial scaphoid injury carries a nonunion rate as high as 40% as opposed to 3% when diagnosed and addressed in under 4 weeks)

PEARLS

- The scaphoid is the most commonly fractured carpal bone. The most common mechanism of injury is a fall onto an outstretched hand.
- Snuffbox tenderness, tenderness upon palpation of scaphoid tubercle, and pain with axial loading of the thumb metacarpal are physical exam findings that should increase suspicion for scaphoid fracture.
- Immobilize the wrist in a thumb spica splint/cast in patients whom you clinically suspect occult scaphoid fractures or have a proven fracture of any type with appropriately timed orthopedic follow-up.
- Consider advanced imaging (CT or MRI) to aid in decision-making.

SUGGESTED READINGS

Bond CD, Shin AY, McBride MT, Dao KD. Percutaneous screw fixation or cast immobilization for nondisplaced scaphoid fractures. *J Bone Joint Surg Am*. 2001;83(4):483-488.

Carpenter CR, Pines JM, Schuur JD, Muir M, Calfee RP, Raja AS. Adult scaphoid fracture. *Acad Emerg Med*. 2014;21:102.

Fowler JR, Hughes TB. Scaphoid fractures. *Clin Sports Med*. 2015;34(1):37-50.

Herbert TJ, Fisher WE. Management of the fractured scaphoid using a new bone screw. *J Bone Joint Surg Br*. 1984;66(1):144-123.

Langhoff O, Andersen JL. Consequences of late immobilization of scaphoid fractures. *J Hand Surg Br*. 1988;13(1):77-79.

265

Calcaneal Fracture? Don't Miss a Spinal Injury!

Michael Abraham

Calcaneus fractures are a source of debilitating disease and are important to quickly identify. The incidence of calcaneal fracture is 11.5 per 100,000, with a male-to-female predominance of 2.4:1. These fractures have high rates of acute and long-term complications. They are often the result of high-impact trauma, most often occurring after an axial load injury on the foot after a fall (or jump!) from 6 feet or more. In one study, 72% of calcaneus fractures occurred after a fall.

Plain films are the initial study of choice for confirming the presence of a calcaneal fracture. Lateral and axial (Harris) views of calcaneus as well as an AP view of the foot are indicated. Additional views or CT may be required to further define the extent of the fracture or for surgical planning. Open fractures, any neurovascular injury, fractures with dislocation, and acute compartment syndrome are potential findings that require emergent orthopedic surgical consultation. Some complications are present and some will develop over time, that is, compartment syndrome. It is important to be cognizant of late complications such as of skin necrosis, which can commonly occur when there is posterior displacement of the calcaneus, and adjust your disposition based on possibility of developing a late complication.

Initial management of calcaneus fracture includes elevation of the limb about the level of the heart, as well as icing of the injury. A bulky compression dressing (also referred to as a bulky Jones splint) should be applied. Of course, analgesia is indicated. Frequent skin exams are required to assess for skin necrosis and compartment syndrome. Surgical repair may be indicated for displaced and comminuted fracture patterns involving the articular spaces of the foot.

It has been shown that up to 50% of patients with calcaneal fractures have other associated injuries. The most commonly seen concomitant injuries are to the lower limbs (13.2%) and thoracolumbar spine (12%). In addition, about 5% of patients have bilateral calcaneal fractures. It is therefore important to do a careful head-to-toe examination of the axial and appendicular skeleton and a neurologic exam that includes motor function, sensation, reflexes, and proprioception. Patients with calcaneal and spinal injuries often have less neurologic deficits present, likely due to force dispersion, and may present with an incomplete spinal injury. In patients with a high-force mechanism or signs of injury on examination, imaging of the axial skeleton (eg, x-ray or CT of the thoracolumbar spine) is appropriate. CT has a higher sensitivity for detecting spinal fractures.

PEARLS

- Calcaneus fracture results from high-impact trauma such as a fall from significant heights and is often associated with other injuries.
- Carefully examine the other calcaneus, thoracolumbar spine, and lower limbs for concomitant injuries.

- Adequate initial radiographic views to assess for calcaneal fracture include lateral and axial (Harris) views of the calcaneus, as well as an AP view of the foot.
- Clinicians should be aware of possible compartment syndrome and skin necrosis of the foot as a result of calcaneus fracture. Emergent orthopedic consultation is indicated if either appears imminent.

SUGGESTED READINGS

Antevil JL, Sise MJ, Sack DI, et al. Spinal computed tomography for the initial evaluation of spine trauma: a new standard of care? *J Trauma*. 2006;61(2):382-387.

Boruah T, Sareen A, Sreenivasan R, et al. Concomitant spine and calcaneum fractures: a possible indication of less extensive injury. *Spinal Cord Ser Cases*. 2022;8(1):1.

Mitchell MJ, McKinley JC, Robinson CM. The epidemiology of calcaneal fractures. *Foot (Edinb)*. 2009;19(4):197-200.

Walters JL, Gangopadhyay P, Malay DS. Association of calcaneal and spinal fractures. *J Foot Ankle Surg*. 2014;53(3):279-281.

266

BEWARE OF BENIGN-APPEARING HIGH-PRESSURE INJECTION INJURIES

ANDREW B. MOORE AND EMILY SCHAEFFER

High-pressure injection injuries may appear benign on examination but have an exceptionally high risk of negative outcomes including amputation. Initial presentation may be limited to a small puncture wound or a vague neurologic deficit. Thus, physicians must be diligent in investigating the mechanism of injury and the specific tools associated with the injury. Common causes of high-pressure injection injury are paint guns, grease guns, and other occupational tools. These injuries most commonly affect young men. Common injury patterns include injuries to the nondominant index finger due to attempts to explore a clogged nozzle (**Figure 266.1**).

Delay in presentation is common, as the injected material may not cause discomfort for several hours. The injected agent disturbs the surrounding tissues, inflammatory processes take effect, leading to swelling, pain, and paresthesia. Compression of blood vessels and nerves results in an edematous, tense, pale finger with limited range of motion on examination. The injection site may appear only as a small punctate lesion. The emergency physician should remain suspicious of systemic injuries proximal to the area of insult as foreign material from high-pressure injuries have been noted to travel substantial distances proximally along tendon sheaths and neurovascular bundles.

Determination of the material injected may impact initial management. Organic solvents, such as paint, paint thinner, fuels, and oil, tend to be more caustic and have a

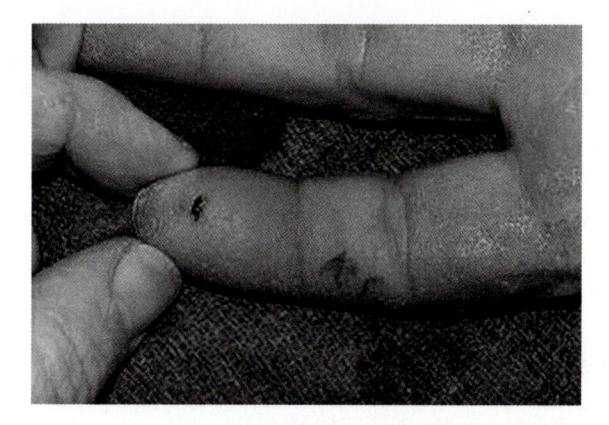

FIGURE 266.1 Common injury patterns include injuries to the nondominant index finger due to attempts to explore a clogged nozzle.

higher rate of amputation. High-pressure water and air injections tend to result in less inflammation.

Radiography with plain film may assist the clinician in making the diagnosis as findings may include radiopaque substances in the case of a paint injection or increased radiolucency due to tissue disruption from air or water. Administration of a third-generation cephalosporin to provide coverage for both gram-positive and gram-negative bacteria is indicated. In addition, tetanus prophylaxis is indicated in patients with inadequate coverage. The use of steroids is controversial and should likely be made in consultation with a surgical specialist. Surgical debridement is the definitive management and should not be delayed.

Avoid the use of compression, icing, or digital blocks as these may exacerbate ischemia.

Ultimately, time to surgical debridement is of the utmost importance, as amputation rates can be as high as 50%. Surgical debridement within 6 hours of injury may decrease amputation rates. Surgical exploration is needed to not only eradicate the offending chemical and irrigate the necrotic tissue but also decompress surrounding nerves and vessels. There is limited published data regarding the overall functional outcome of these patients.

The astute emergency clinician should focus their efforts on recognizing high-pressure injection injuries early, identifying the total area of insult, and reducing time to surgical intervention to improve patient outcomes.

PEARLS

- High-pressure injection injuries often have a benign appearance on examination.
- Injection injuries are associated with significant soft tissue destruction.
- Plain radiographs of the affected extremity may help reveal the true extent of the underlying injury.
- Third-generation cephalosporins and tetanus prophylaxis are indicated in this injury.

- Minimizing time to surgical exploration and debridement is the most important factor in preventing a devastating outcome and minimizing the chance of amputation.

Acknowledgments

We gratefully acknowledge the contributions of previous edition author, Jennifer Farah, as portions of their chapter have been retained in this revision.

Suggested Readings

Amsdell SL, Hammert WC. High-pressure injection injuries in the hand: current treatment concepts. *Plast Reconstr Surg*. 2013;132(4):586e-591e.

Hogan CJ, Ruland RT. High-pressure injection injuries to the upper extremity: a review of the literature. *J Orthop Trauma*. 2006;20(7):503-511.

Kennedy J, Harrington P. Pneumomediastinum following high pressure air injection to the hand. *Ir Med J*. 2010;103(4):118-119.

Rosenwasser MP, Wei DH. High-pressure injection injuries to the hand. *J Am Acad Orthop Surg*. 2014;22(1):38-45.

267

Lisfranc Injury: Danger in the Midfoot

Brian L. Fuquay

The Lisfranc joint is a TMT joint complex that is prone to injury. It constitutes roughly 0.2% of all fractures and is considered one of the causes of significant disability from injuries to the mid- and forefoot. It can occur from both low- and high-energy mechanisms where an axial load is applied to the plantar flexed foot. Low-energy mechanisms include ground-level falls and athletic injuries. High-energy mechanisms include falls from height, crush injuries of the foot, and motor vehicle collisions. While history and physical examination with careful attention to plain radiographs are important, plain radiographs are not always diagnostic due to bony overlap, especially on the lateral view. Delayed or missed diagnosis of a Lisfranc injury leads to chronic instability, deformity, and pain. Up to 20% of these injuries may not be accurately diagnosed on initial plain radiographs, making them a high-risk injury for emergency physicians to miss.

A brief review of foot anatomy helps in understanding Lisfranc injuries. The forefoot is composed of five metatarsal bones and their associated phalanges. The midfoot also consists of five bones: three cuneiforms (medial, middle, and lateral), the cuboid, and the navicular. The Lisfranc or TMT joint consists of the articulations between the metatarsals and the three cuneiforms and cuboid, all very critical to the stability of the foot. The Lisfranc joint is composed of three longitudinal components, the medial column (medial cuneiform and first metatarsal), middle column (middle and lateral cuneiforms with the second and third metatarsals), and the lateral column (the cuboid and the fourth and fifth metatarsals). The Lisfranc ligament runs from the plantar medial cuneiform to the base of the second metatarsal, while the second through fifth metatarsals are interconnected through a series of intermetatarsal ligaments, thus connecting the medial column to the lateral four metatarsals and serving as the primary soft tissue support of the TMT articulation.

A Lisfranc injury can result from both direct and indirect trauma; most commonly, direct trauma includes crush injuries associated with significant soft tissue injury, vascular insufficiency, and compartment syndrome of the foot. About one-third of all Lisfranc injuries come from low-energy mechanism, with the remainder usually coming from high-impact forces. Most common indirect injury patterns are due to forced external rotation, axial loading of a foot in plantar flexion, or twisting of an axially loaded foot in a fixed equinus position where forced abduction of the forefoot causes dislocation of the second metatarsal and lateral metatarsal displacement. For example, when first described by French war surgeon Jacques Lisfranc de St. Martin, a soldier who fell off his horse with his foot still in the stirrups might have sustained this type of injury.

In general, patients with Lisfranc injuries tend to present with midfoot tenderness, forefoot and midfoot edema, and an inability to bear weight. If the examination of the foot reveals midfoot edema and plantar arch ecchymosis, this is essentially pathognomonic for Lisfranc injury. Other physical examination findings suggestive of TMT joint injury include the "piano key test," where one can induce pain or subluxation by dorsiflexion and plantar flexion (or abduction and adduction) of the first and second metatarsals.

AP, oblique, and lateral x-ray views are utilized for initial assessment of Lisfranc injury. The AP is used to assess the alignment of the first and second TMT joints by determining whether the medial border of the second metatarsal lines up with that of the middle cuneiform. The oblique is used to assess the other TMT joints, by determining whether the medial border of the fourth metatarsal lines up with the cuboid. Lateral radiograph may show dorsal dislocation or subluxation between the first and second metatarsals. In addition, avulsion fractures of the second metatarsal or medial cuneiform, also known as the "fleck sign," or greater than 2 mm of diastasis between the first and second metatarsals, suggest TMT joint injury (see **Figure 267.1**).

Many Lisfranc injuries present with non–weight-bearing radiographs in the ED, making this a commonly missed diagnosis. If a Lisfranc injury is clinically suspected despite normal imaging, either weight-bearing or stress views of the foot should be obtained, including oblique, lateral, and AP views. Stress or weight-bearing imaging allows increased diastasis of the Lisfranc joint in patients with subtle Lisfranc injuries, increasing diagnostic accuracy. On normal AP x-ray of the foot, the medial border of the second metatarsal should line up with the medial border of the cuneiform. Any displacement greater than 2 mm between the first and second metatarsals is diagnostic of ligamentous Lisfranc injury. Comparison x-ray views of the unaffected foot can also aid in the diagnosis. Given the pain and discomfort of obtaining these views, the patient should receive analgesia before obtaining films and receive clarification on why additional images are needed.

Management of Lisfranc injuries depends on the degree of displacement. Even minimally displaced (2 mm of displacement) are unstable and require orthopedic consultation from the ED, with specific attention placed on monitoring for compartment syndrome. These injuries will usually require transarticular fixation or arthrodesis depending on a number of factors determined by the treating orthopedic surgeon.

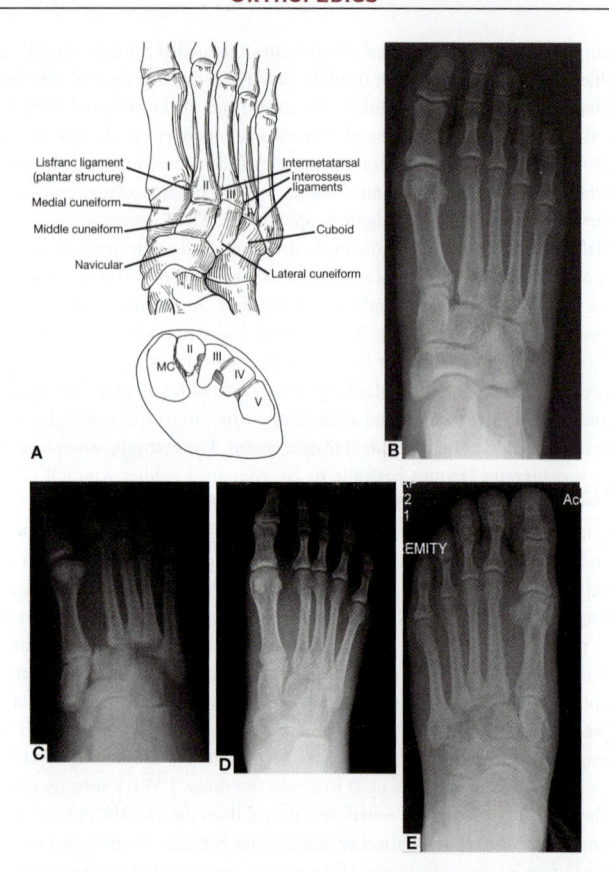

FIGURE 267.1 Lisfranc injuries. A: Drawing shows dorsal and coronal views of bone, joint, ligament anatomy of Lisfranc complex. B: Isolated disruption of second TMT joint. C: Severe disruption of Lisfranc complex including medial cuneiform. D: A more subtle Lisfranc injury with intercuneiform instability. E: Subtle Lisfranc injury with medial cuneiform subluxation and fracture. Note first and second TMT joints are at about the same level. (From Early JS, Kitaoka HB, Campbell JT. Tarsometatarsal (Lisfranc) Reduction and Fixation. In: Kitaoka HB, ed. *Master Techniques in Orthopaedic Surgery: The Foot and Ankle*. 3rd ed. Wolters Kluwer; 2014:229–248. Figure 17.1.)

PEARLS

- Lisfranc injury occurs from injury to the TMT joint and, if not diagnosed and properly managed, can lead to significant disability to the patient. Midfoot tenderness and edema, plantar ecchymosis, and inability to bear weight on examination should raise suspicion for Lisfranc injury.
- When a Lisfranc injury is suspected, foot radiographs can reveal malalignment of the TMT joints and/or the fleck sign. Weight-bearing or stress views, or

- Patients with a Lisfranc injury or suspected injury should be splinted with instructions to remain non–weight bearing. Minimally displaced injuries can be urgently referred to orthopedics as outpatient, while displaced injuries with significant soft tissue edema should be monitored for compartment syndrome and evaluated by an orthopedic surgeon in the ED.

SUGGESTED READINGS

Aronow MS. Treatment of the missed Lisfranc injury. *Foot Ankle Clin.* 2006;11(1):127-142.
Mantas JP, Burks RT. Lisfranc injuries in the athlete. *Clin Sports Med.* 1994;13(4):719-730.
Peicha G, Labovitz J, Seibert FJ, et al. The anatomy of the joint as a risk factor for Lisfranc dislocation and fracture dislocation. An anatomical and radiological case control study. *J Bone Joint Surg Br.* 2002;84(7):981-985.
Schenck RC Jr, Heckman JD. Fractures and dislocations of the forefoot: operative and nonoperative treatment. *J Am Acad Orthop Surg.* 1995;3(2):70-78.
Trevino SG, Kodros S. Controversies in tarsometatarsal injuries. *Orthop Clin North Am.* 1995;26(2):229-238.
Watson TS, Shurnas PS, Denker J. Treatment of Lisfranc joint injury: current concepts. *J Am Acad Orthop Surg.* 2010;18(12):718-728.

268

TIBIAL PLATEAU FRACTURES CAN BE SUBTLE

LAUREN E.R. BRADY AND ERIC R. FRIEDMAN

The tibia serves as the major weight-bearing bone of the lower leg. It can be divided into the proximal tibia, tibial shaft, and distal tibia. The proximal tibia consists of the tibial plateau, which forms the inferior portion of the knee joint (the remainder of the knee joint is formed by the femur). The medial and lateral condyles, separated by the intercondylar eminence, comprise the tibial plateau. The intercondylar eminence is an important landmark, as it is where the ACL, PCL, and menisci all attach. The tibial shaft connects the proximal and distal portions of the bone. The distal tibia makes up the medial malleolus and comprises the superior articular surface of the ankle joint (the remainder of the ankle joint is formed by the fibula and talus).

Proximal tibia fractures in adults are more common than those in other regions of the tibia, while they are much less common than tibial shaft or distal tibial fractures in pediatric patients. Proximal fractures generally occur from high-energy trauma, such as a dashboard to knee injury in a motor vehicle crash, or direct trauma to a hyperextended knee (ie, during contact sports). However, in older adults, they can also occur from lower impact injuries, such as simple falls or twisting movements, so it is crucial to have a higher suspicion of injury when evaluating knee/leg pain in the older population. Proximal tibia fractures are generally categorized as those involving the tibial plateau or the intercondylar notch. Another subtype is an avulsion fracture of the tibial tubercle, which occurs primarily in children. Tibial plateau fractures make up roughly 1% of all fractures, and they more commonly involve the lateral condyle, as it is thinner and weaker than the medial side.

Plain films, including AP, lateral, and oblique views, are the initial diagnostic imaging of choice for suspected tibial plateau fractures (see **Figures 268.1** and **268.2**). They can provide information on fracture location/type, displacement, and angulation. The lateral view (either standing or cross-table) is important, as it can show a fat-fluid level, which can indicate an intra-articular injury. However, tibial plateau fractures can be difficult to see on plain radiographs, especially if there is no depression of the tibial plateau. Some studies estimate the sensitivity of plain films for tibial plateau fractures to be only around 85%. When a two-view x-ray is the sole imaging, the sensitivity can drop below 80%. Therefore, if radiographs are equivocal and clinical suspicion is high,

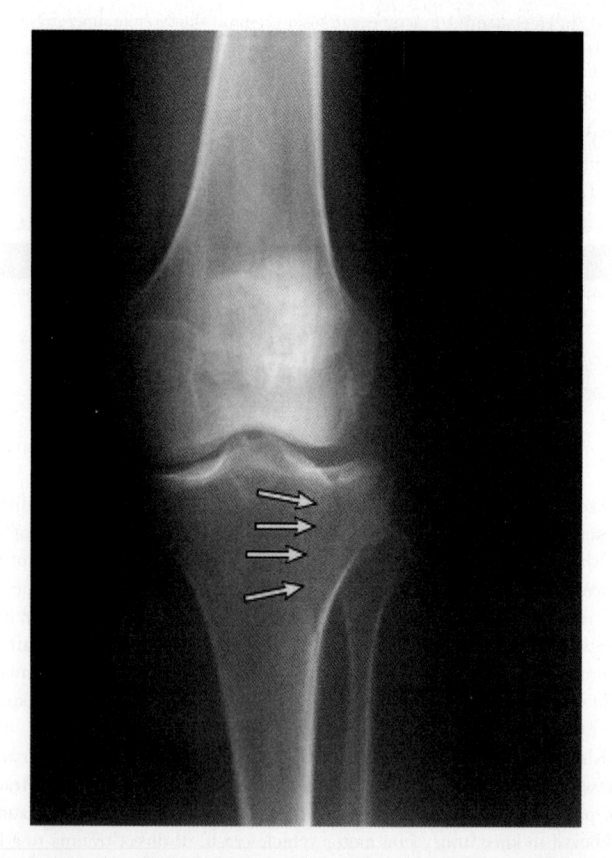

FIGURE 268.1 An anteroposterior radiograph with arrows revealing a nondisplaced lateral tibial plateau fracture. (Courtesy of Scott Koehler, MD.)

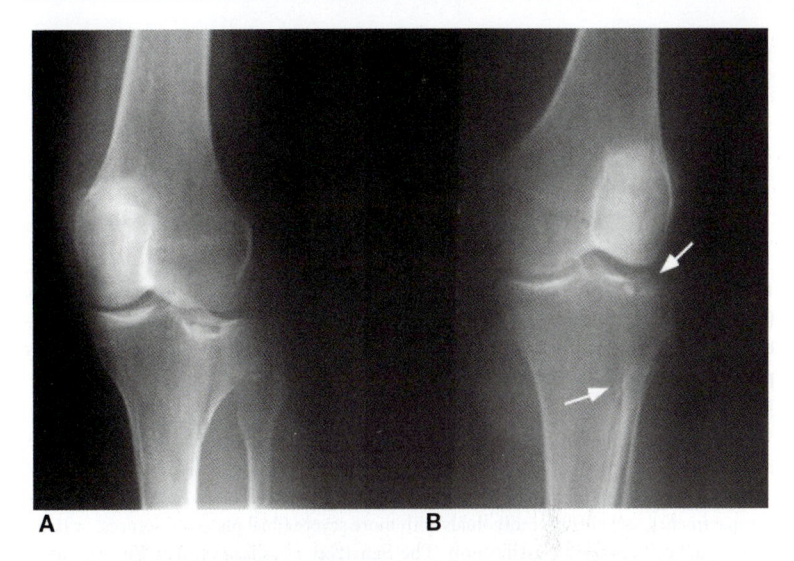

FIGURE 268.2 Two oblique radiographs of the same knew demonstrate the usefulness of these views in cases of suspected fracture. The fracture of the lateral tibial plateau appears as a curvilinear area of radiolucency in one oblique view (**A**), while the same fracture is less easily appreciated in the other view (**B**). The arrows indicate the beginning and end of the lateral tibial plateau fracture. (Courtesy of Scott Koehler, MD.)

CT and/or MRI should be attained to better classify a suspected tibial plateau injury, as well as associated injuries. While CT is generally quicker, and more readily available in most EDs, certain fractures have a higher likelihood of concurrent ligament/meniscal tears (which all attach to the intercondylar eminence), including Segond fractures (avulsion fractures of the lateral condyle) and those of the tibial spine and posteromedial tibial plateau. In these instances, MRI can be considered depending on the available resources and consultant preferences. Damage to the fibula should also be assessed when diagnosing tibial plateau injuries, as fibular head fractures are found in roughly 30% of cases. Similarly, the common peroneal nerve, given its close proximity, is the most likely nerve to be damaged with tibial plateau fractures.

The initial treatment for most tibial plateau fractures diagnosed in the ED includes knee splinting in complete extension (or 5°-10° of flexion for intercondylar fractures) and strict non–weight bearing with crutches, along with general supportive care measures used with most musculoskeletal injuries (ice, compression, elevation, and analgesics) until outpatient orthopedic evaluation can be achieved. Elevation is especially important with tibial plateau fractures as the compartments in the lower leg are small, and even a small amount of edema can lead to compartment syndrome. Emergent orthopedic consult in the ED is necessary for any open fractures, or those compromising vascular structures or causing compartment syndrome. Fractures involving any degree of depression or displacement, or those with suspected or known ligament/meniscus injury, should have urgent orthopedic follow-up within 48 hours.

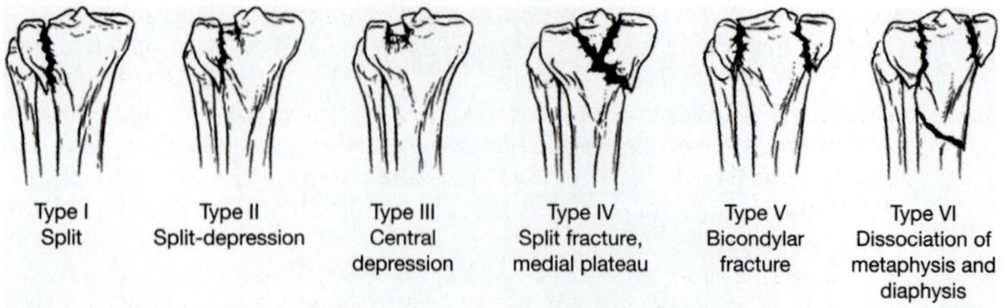

Type I	Type II	Type III	Type IV	Type V	Type VI
Split	Split-depression	Central depression	Split fracture, medial plateau	Bicondylar fracture	Dissociation of metaphysis and diaphysis

FIGURE 268.3 The Schatzker classification system of tibial plateau fractures. (Reprinted and published with permission from Berkson EM, Virkus WW. High-energy tibial plateau fractures. *J Am Acad Orthop Surg*. 2006;14:20-31. © 2006 by American Academy of Orthopaedic Surgeons.)

The most common significant short-term complication of tibial fractures is ACS because three of the four compartments of the lower leg border the tibia. The risk of ACS is increased in individuals on anticoagulants, as they can bleed excessively into the compartments, as well as in individuals with more severe tibial plateau fractures, or those with a higher Schatzker classification. The Schatzker classification (see **Figure 268.3**) grades tibial plateau fractures into six types and is used by many orthopedic surgeons to help with surgical planning. When diagnosed quickly and managed appropriately, most uncomplicated tibial plateau fractures have good outcomes, and patients can eventually return to their daily activities. More complicated fractures have an increased likelihood of developing chronic gait abnormalities, osteoarthritis of the knee joint, and/or requiring a total knee replacement down the road.

PEARLS

- Make sure you get at least a three-view radiograph when evaluating for tibial plateau fractures.
- If a patient cannot bear weight and clinical concern is high, consider getting a CT/MRI in the ED.
- When evaluating tibial plateau injuries, it is important to evaluate for other commonly associated injuries, such as ACL/PCL, menisci, fibular head, and common peroneal nerve.
- If a tibial plateau fracture is diagnosed, we recommend the patient be non–weight bearing and placed in a knee immobilizer.
- Educate patients on the symptoms of ACS upon discharge.

SUGGESTED READINGS

Berkson EM, Virkus WW. High-energy tibial plateau fractures. *J Am Acad Orthop Surg*. 2006;14(1):20-31.

Chapman J, Cohen J. Proximal tibial fractures in children. *UpToDate*. https://www.uptodate.com/contents/proximal-tibial-fractures-in-children?sectionName=Physeal%20fractures&topicRef=6551&anchor=H14&source=see_link#

Fields KB. Proximal tibial fractures in adults. *UpToDate*. https://www.uptodate.com/contents/proximal-tibial-fractures-in-adults?source=mostViewed_widget#references

Markhardt BK, Gross JM, Monu JU. Schatzker classification of tibial plateau fractures: use of CT and MR imaging improves assessment. *Radiographics*. 2009;29(2):585-597. PMID: 19325067.

Modarresi S, Jude CM. Radiologic evaluation of the acutely painful knee in adults. *UpToDate*. https://www.uptodate.com/contents/radiologic-evaluation-of-the-acutely-painful-knee-in-adults?search=Radiologic%20evaluation%20of%20the%20acutely%20painful%20knee%20in%20adults&source=search_result&selectedTitle=1~150&usage_type=default&display_rank=1

Mustonen A. *Imaging of Knee Injuries With Special Focus on Tibial Plateau Fractures*. Doctoral Dissertation. University of Helsinki; 2009. https://core.ac.uk/download/pdf/14918491.pdf

Wennergren D, Bergdahl C, Ekelund J, Juto H, Sundfeldt M, Möller M. Epidemiology and incidence of tibia fractures in the Swedish Fracture Register. *Injury*. 2018;49(11): 2068-2074. PMID: 30220634.

Zheng ZL, Yu YY, Chang HR, Liu H, Zhou HL, Zhang YZ. Establishment of classification of tibial plateau fracture associated with proximal fibular fracture. *Orthop Surg*. 2019;11(1):97-101. PMID: 30734492.

269

CAN I REDUCE THE SHOULDER DISLOCATION WITH A FRACTURE?

JUSTIN LACKEY AND IAN J. DEMPSEY

The shoulder is the most commonly dislocated large joint due to its relatively small articular surface with large bearing surface, allowing for unrestricted range of motion. Longer delay from initial injury increases the risk for unsuccessful reduction. Prompt restoration of glenohumeral alignment is critical to avoid chronic complications. Initial evaluation of patients with dislocation and determination of appropriate candidates for ED reduction are both essential and time sensitive. Traditional teaching has urged against attempted reduction of shoulder dislocations with associated fractures, but the exact scope of this recommendation has not always been clear. Regardless of the presence of associated fracture, emergent indications and contraindications to reduction are unchanged. Injuries associated with vascular compromise should be promptly reduced in the ED in consultation with orthopedic surgery. Chronic dislocations, conservatively defined as those occurring more than 72 hours since the time of injury, should not undergo ED manipulation due to the increased risk for iatrogenic fracture and axillary artery injury.

GLENOLABRAL PATHOLOGY

The bony Bankart lesion and the Hill-Sachs defect occur due to impaction of the posterolateral humeral head against the anteroinferior glenoid rim. The Hill-Sachs defect is a cortical depression of the posterolateral head of the humerus that is seen in up to 90% of traumatic anterior dislocations. The bony Bankart lesion is a fracture of the anteroinferior glenoid rim. The reverse Hill-Sachs lesion is an analogous cortical lesion of the anterosuperomedial humeral head, which is seen in the majority of posterior glenohumeral dislocations. Historically, identifying the Hill-Sachs defect and the bony Bankart lesion on plain radiographs required dedicated projections such as the West Point and Stryker notch views, but CT and MR imaging are now preferred, and, given the proliferation of these modalities, the emergency physician should be prepared to appropriately incorporate these findings in their clinical decision making.

PROXIMAL HUMERUS FRACTURES

Nearly 20% of shoulder dislocations are complicated by proximal humerus fractures. Traditionally, these fractures have been classified according to the Neer classification scheme (**Figure 269.1**), which categorizes fractures based on the degree of displacement of the four "parts" of the humerus: the humeral head, humeral shaft, the greater tuberosity, and the lesser tuberosity.

Traditional teaching has discouraged closed manipulation of any shoulder dislocation with associated fracture, citing the risk for conversion to a three-part or four-part

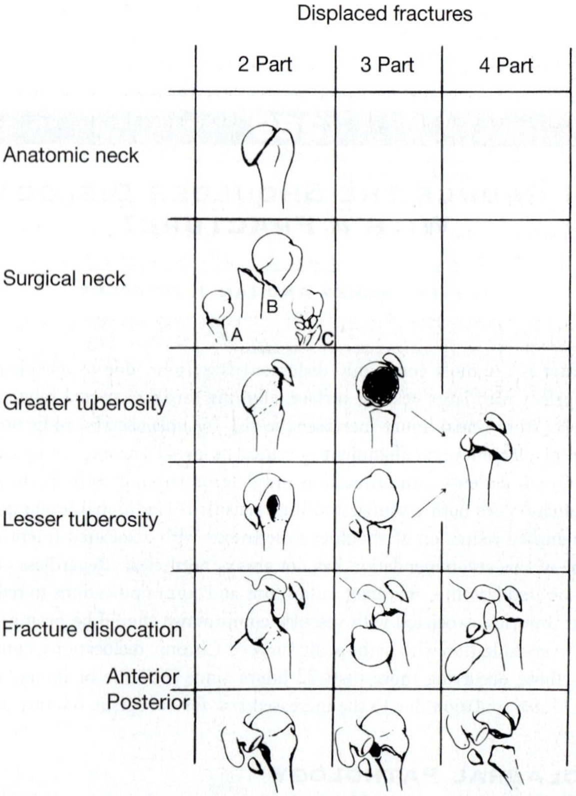

FIGURE 269.1 Neer classification of proximal humerus fractures. (From Neer CS II. Displaced proximal humeral fractures. Part I. Classification and evaluation. *J Bone Joint Surg Am.* 1970;52:1077-1089, used with permission. Copyright © 1970 by *The Journal of Bone and Joint Surgery*, Incorporated.)

fracture during attempted closed reduction, which is associated with increased risk for avascular necrosis of the humeral head and subsequent poor clinical outcomes. However, there have been multiple studies that have demonstrated the safety of ED reduction of some fracture-dislocation morphologies. There are no consensus recommendations for which fracture patterns are appropriate for manipulation, and individual consideration of the risks and benefits for every patient is essential.

Fractures of the greater tuberosity are the most common proximal humerus fracture associated with anterior glenohumeral dislocation, and the incidence increases with age, likely due to a change in the underlying mechanism of injury in older patients. Attempted closed reduction of patients with isolated fractures of greater tuberosity is often appropriate, and the risk for iatrogenic fracture is low (**Figure 269.2**). Older patients, postmenopausal females, those with osteoporosis, and large fractures (>40% of humeral head) warrant discussion with an orthopedic surgeon due to the possibility of increased risk for iatrogenic fracture, but multiple studies have shown safe closed manipulation of this population. If manipulation is attempted, procedural sedation is encouraged to increase relaxation, and manipulation should be limited to two attempts as additional attempts are unlikely to be successful. Finally, the Hippocratic reduction technique should be avoided altogether, as its use was prevalent in many cases of iatrogenic fracture. While several methods may be appropriate based on patient-specific factors, the Stimson technique can be very effective for patients who tolerate prone positioning. All patients with associated greater tuberosity fractures require close orthopedic surgery follow-up due to the risk for fragment migration.

Patients with fractures of the humeral neck should receive emergent orthopedic evaluation before attempted manipulation. Nondisplaced neck fractures are at high risk for displacement during attempted reduction, which can worsen functional outcomes.

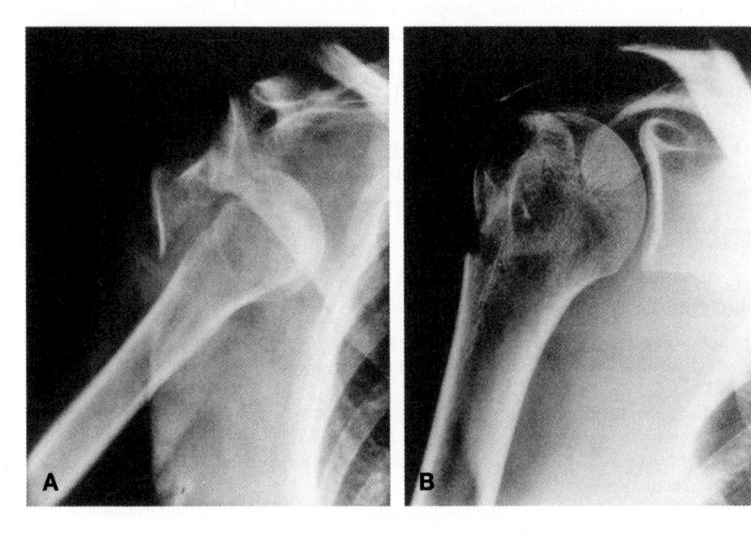

FIGURE 269.2 "Pre- and postreduction." Anterior dislocation with two-part greater tuberosity fracture (**A**) on initial presentation and (**B**) following closed reduction. (From Iannotti JP, Williams GR. *Disorders of the Shoulder: Diagnosis and Management*. Lippincott Williams & Wilkins; 2007.)

Displaced fractures are unlikely to demonstrate worsening alignment, but are infrequently reduced into a satisfactory position and should only be manipulated in direct consultation with orthopedic surgery. If necessary, these patients should undergo transfer for closed reduction under general anesthesia.

SPECIAL POPULATIONS

Both inferior glenohumeral dislocations (luxation erecta) and posterior glenohumeral dislocations have a significant risk of associated proximal humerus fracture. Posterior dislocations commonly co-occur with lesser tuberosity fractures. A similar approach to that proposed for the management of isolated greater tuberosity fracture with limited attempts under maximal relaxation is reasonable. Due to the relatively low incidence of these injuries relative to anterior dislocations, there is no objective data to guide the management of these fracture-dislocation injuries and they should be managed on a case-by-case basis in close consultation with orthopedic surgery.

Finally, all pediatric patients presenting with proximal humerus fracture dislocations should be taken to the operating room for attempted reduction under general anesthesia.

PEARLS

- Anterior glenohumeral dislocation is common, and the emergency physician is capable of prompt and effective reduction.
- Bony Bankart and Hill-Sachs lesions are common in anterior shoulder dislocations and are not contraindications to reduction in the ED.
- An isolated fracture of the greater or lesser tuberosity in association with dislocation is not a strict contraindication to reduction. Manipulation should be limited to two attempts; procedural sedation should be used if possible; and methods of high mechanical stress, such as the Hippocratic method, should be avoided.
- Humeral neck fractures should not be manipulated in the ED without direct discussion with orthopedic surgery.
- Patients with posterior and inferior fracture dislocations and all pediatric patients with fracture dislocations should be considered on a case-by-case basis and managed in close consultation with orthopedic surgery.

SUGGESTED READINGS

Green A, Choi P, Lubitz M, Aaron DL, Swart E. Proximal humeral fracture-dislocations: which patterns can be reduced in the emergency department? *J Shoulder Elbow Surg.* 2022;31(4):792-798.

Hasebroock AW, Brinkman J, Foster L, Bowens JP. Management of primary anterior shoulder dislocations: a narrative review. *Sports Med Open.* 2019;5(1):31.

Murthi AM, Ramirez MA. Shoulder dislocation in the older patient. *J Am Acad Orthop Surg.* 2012;20(10):615-622.

Neer CS. Displaced proximal humeral fractures: part I. Classification and evaluation. 1970. *Clin Orthop Relat Res.* 2006;442:77-82.

Popkin CA, Levine WN, Ahmad CS. Evaluation and management of pediatric proximal humerus fractures. *J Am Acad Orthop Surg.* 2015;23(2):77-86.

270

LEAVING IT ALL UP TO CHANCE

TORI SHANK AND ERIC R. FRIEDMAN

Chance fracture is a flexion-distraction injury to the vertebra caused by sudden deceleration and flexion causing strain on the vertebra and associated ligaments. This fracture is often seen as a result of motor vehicle accidents that occurred when vehicles were only equipped with lap belts, and it became known as the "seat belt fracture." With the passenger only strapped in at the waist, a rapid deceleration of the vehicle causes the torso to flex quickly forward over the pressure point of the lap belt. Chance fracture, however, tends to occur after falls and other flexion-distraction injuries, as more recent car manufacturing has developed the shoulder harness. It still occurs in association with seat belts, and this is why it is heavily associated with the "seat belt sign." Chance fracture is sometimes subtle and can be hard to identify, and may be mistaken as compression or burst fracture on initial imaging. Identification of this unstable spinal fracture is paramount in the ED as it can stave off permanent disability and neurologic impairment.

Chance fracture has the highest incidence among children and young men and is defined as injury through the anterior and posterior aspects of the vertebra. This fracture most often occurs in the thoracolumbar region. However, in the pediatric population, there can often be injury to the mid-lumbar region. The fracture itself extends through the anterior, middle, and posterior columns of the vertebra and therefore can have associated ligamentous injury. The extent of ligamentous involvement may dictate management especially if the posterior ligamentous complex is involved, as this makes the spinal column unstable. Another important factor associated with chance fracture is the high correlation with intra-abdominal injury, particularly perforation and mesenteric injury. These associated injuries occur at a rate of about 50% but have been reported to be as high as 90%. Therefore, appropriate imaging is important not only for fracture management, but identification and management of life-threatening abdominal injuries.

Plain films may be appropriate first-line imaging, if hemodynamically stable and if there is not high clinical suspicion for intra-abdominal injury. CT, however, is the most appropriate form of imaging to determine the extent of injury. CT abdomen-pelvis is appropriate, but sagittal spinal reconstructions are needed for fracture identification. In the spine, there will be evidence of a horizontal fracture through the vertebral body and spinous process, and increased length of the intervertebral segment. MRI may be used as an adjunctive imaging study when management is unclear, as this will give a better idea of the extent of ligamentous injury and mechanical instability of the injury. However, MRI is probably more appropriate for presurgical planning, not ED management.

Most patients can be managed conservatively with TSLO bracing or hyperextension cast and follow-up. Bracing is indicated for up to 8 to 12 weeks for appropriate healing. Compliance with the brace may be an issue as it should be worn for an extended period. Surgical instead of conservative management may be a consideration in the obese patient population, regardless of neurologic findings or kyphosis, due to improper orthosis from TSLO bracing and subsequent poor healing. Conservative management does have a high rate of success, with most patients recovering without any disability. Surgical management is warranted in the presence of neurologic symptoms or in the setting of mechanical instability, defined as associated kyphosis if the curve is greater than 15°. It should be noted that neurologic symptoms are only present in a small subset of patients. Regardless of symptoms, these patients warrant a neurosurgical or orthopedic consult as chance fracture is an unstable fracture. Inappropriate management of these patients can result in permanent disability from worsening kyphosis as well as neurologic sequelae.

PEARLS

- Chance fracture is a flexion-distraction injury to the vertebra.
- "Seat belt sign" or history of lap belt use should raise clinical suspicion for chance fracture and intra-abdominal injury.
- CT of the abdomen/pelvis is the most appropriate imaging for identification of fracture and associated intra-abdominal injury.
- Neurologic symptoms or associated kyphosis greater than 15° warrant surgical management.

Suggested Readings

Durel R, Rudman E, Milburn J. Clinical images—a quarterly column: chance fracture of the lumbar spine. *Ochsner J*. 2014;14(1):9-11. PMID: 24688326.

Koay J, Davis DD, Hogg JP. Chance fractures. [Updated 2022 Aug 22]. In: *StatPearls* [Internet]. StatPearls Publishing; 2023. https://www.ncbi.nlm.nih.gov/books/NBK536926/

Savitsky E, Votey S. Emergency department approach to acute thoracolumbar spine injury. *J Emerg Med*. 1997;15(1):49-60. PMID: 9017488.

Tyroch AH, Mcguire EL, Mclean SF, et al. The association between chance fractures and intra-abdominal injuries revisited: a multicenter review. *Am Surg*. 2005;71(5):434-438.

SECTION XXII

PROCEDURES/SKILLS

271

SEDATION PEARLS AND PITFALLS: PROCEDURAL SEDATION IN THE EMERGENCY DEPARTMENT

BENJAMIN CORNWELL AND J. DAVID GATZ

Procedural sedation is a common and essential technique in the ED. While overall safe when performed by a well-trained clinician, it is important to anticipate common errors and complications that may occur and tailor each sedation to the needs of an individual patient. This chapter reviews key aspects of the patient assessment, setup, and pharmacologic selection so as to maximize safety.

PATIENT ASSESSMENT

A thorough history and physical examination are important before any procedural sedation. Most fundamental is to review/assess the following:

- Vital signs
- Mental status
- Airway patency
- Cardiopulmonary status
- Pregnancy
- Neck/pharyngeal/facial anatomy
  - Macroglossia or micrognathia
  - Short neck
  - History of cervical fusion
  - Facial hair
- Comorbidities
  - History of obstructive sleep apnea
  - Obesity
  - Congestive heart failure
  - History of difficult intubations

If a patient has undergone procedural sedation in the past, knowing if they have an allergy or adverse reaction to an agent is crucial in selecting the appropriate medication. Preprocedural fasting has been studied in both general anesthesia and procedural sedation, and while the American Association of Anesthesiologists has guidelines including 2 hours of fasting for clear liquids and 6 hours after solid foods, shortened fasting has not shown increased rates of serious adverse events during procedural sedation. Currently, there is no evidence to support a specific fasting period before ED procedural sedation. The American College of Emergency Physicians provides a Level B recommendation to not delay procedural sedation in adults or pediatrics based on fasting time. Lastly, consent must be obtained from the patient for both the sedation and any associated procedures. For pediatric sedations, consent must be obtained from a parent or guardian, but involving the patient in discussion of the procedures (depending on age) may help a younger patient tolerate the procedure.

PROCEDURE SETUP

All appropriate resources should be brought into the patient's room and established before beginning any procedural sedation. With regard to the patient, they should have reliable IV access—ideally at more than one site. Make sure the IV will be accessible throughout the planned procedure. The patient should be monitored with regular blood pressure measurements (ideally on the arm opposite of medication administration), continuous cardiac monitoring, continuous pulse oximetry, and continuous capnography. Empiric administration of oxygen in the absence of capnography may inhibit early recognition of respiratory depression as patients can temporarily maintain a normal oxygen saturation despite apnea. Concurrent oxygen administration and capnography allow brief episodes of respiratory depression to be supported while also being recognized on capnography.

Airway equipment should be readily available. Typically, a bag-valve mask and suction system should be set up in the room. The readiness of more advanced equipment (eg, airway adjuncts and intubation equipment) will depend on the performing clinician's preference. All team members should perform a "time-out" before beginning the procedure that identifies all parties, reviews plan for sedation (including anticipated dosages), and reviews plan for the concomitant procedure.

PHARMACOLOGIC SELECTION

There are numerous choices in medications to accomplish a safe and successful procedural sedation (**Table 271.1**). An emergency clinician must consider the level of sedation required as well as the desired duration of effect when selecting the appropriate medication. Particular attention should be given to the level of sedation (ranging from anxiolysis to deep) as an increase in complications may occur at increased sedation. Levels of sedation are as follows:

- Minimal sedation: near-normal level of alertness, but minimally impaired coordination and cognitive function. Patient does not require ventilatory or cardiovascular support.
- Moderate sedation: depressed level of consciousness, responds purposefully to verbal commands. Patients maintain their airways, breathe spontaneously, and cardiovascular function is typically at baseline.
- Deep sedation: depressed level of consciousness where patients cannot be easily aroused, but respond to painful or repeated stimuli. May require assistance in maintaining a patent airway and/or ventilation.
- General anesthesia: unresponsive to all stimuli and no protective airway reflexes. Invasive positive-pressure ventilation is usually required, and cardiovascular function may be depressed.

TABLE 271.1 MOST COMMON SEDATIVE OPTIONS

MEDICATION	DOSE	ANALGESIC PROPERTIES	AMNESTIC PROPERTIES	ANXIOLYTIC PROPERTIES	PEARLS	PITFALLS
Fentanyl	1 mcg/kg IV	X			Rapid onset/offset Minimal CV effects	Chest wall rigidity Respiratory depression at higher doses
Midazolam	0.05-0.1 mg/kg IV		X	X	Rapid onset	Paradoxical agitation in pediatrics
Propofol	0.5-1 mg/kg IV		X	X	Short duration Rapid onset	Hypotension Respiratory depression
Ketamine	1-1.5 mg/kg IV 3-4 mg/kg IM 6-9 mg/kg IN	X	X		Provides analgesia and sedation Maintains airway reflexes	Emergence phenomena Emesis Hypertension and tachycardia
Etomidate	0.15 mg/kg IV		X		Rapid onset/recovery	Myoclonus Respiratory depression
Ketamine-propofol	1:1 mixture: 0.5 mg/kg ketamine IV and 0.5 mg/kg propofol IV	X	X	X	Hemodynamic stability Analgesia and sedation	
Nitrous oxide	30%-70% concentration		X		Rapid onset	Availability Emesis

CV, cardiovascular; IM, intramuscular; IN, intranasal; IV, intravenous.

There are a variety of options for medications that can be used for procedural sedation, each with complications that a clinician must consider before use. Propofol has become a more commonly used agent. It is an isolated sedative that does not provide any analgesia, so it should be paired with an opioid or other analgesic for more painful procedures. It has a very rapid onset and offset, while also providing anxiolysis and amnesia. Propofol can, however, induce hypotension, especially in patients who are already volume depleted. Fentanyl is an opioid that has a favorable profile for its use as an analgesic during procedural sedation. It has a rapid onset of action, a duration of 30 to 40 minutes, and can be easily reversed. Complications include chest wall rigidity and glottic spasms, both of which are typically seen at higher doses.

Benzodiazepines may also be considered for procedural sedation, as they provide both amnestic and anxiolytic properties. Midazolam is typically used, as it has a rapid onset of action with longer durations up to 2 hours when administered IV. In the pediatric population, benzodiazepines can cause paradoxical agitation, a reaction that has not been shown in the adult population. In addition, midazolam carries a higher risk for apnea, bradycardia, and hypotension.

Ketamine is a commonly used agent, especially in the pediatric population. Importantly, it does not have a dose-dependent response, and once the dissociative dose is reached additional medication will not yield further decreased consciousness. Ketamine has analgesic and amnestic properties and has a favorable hemodynamic profile with decreased rates of hypotension and bradycardia. Vomiting is a common side effect but can typically be treated with antiemetics such as ondansetron. An emergence phenomenon is relatively common but is typically not clinically significant.

Ketamine has also been used with propofol, termed "ketofol," as an additional option. "Ketofol" is commonly dosed in a 1:1 mixture as a single dose, with 0.5 mg/kg of ketamine and 0.5 mg/kg of propofol. This combination minimizes each agent's disadvantages. Ketamine induces dissociation and analgesia while maintaining hemodynamic stability, while propofol causes sedation with rapid onset. When used in combination, lower doses of each are typically used when compared to using each agent individually. These benefits, however, are only seen in the adult population, and ketamine alone remains a recommended choice for pediatric sedation.

Etomidate is another sedative agent used more frequently for short procedures such as cardioversion. It has a very quick onset of action in 30 to 60 seconds with recovery in about 5 to 10 minutes. Side effects can include myoclonus, and although there is a risk of adrenal suppression, there have not been any studies showing a clinically significant effect.

PEARLS

- Unique patient characteristics such as comorbidities, allergies, anatomy, and type of procedure being performed must all be considered when selecting the appropriate sedation strategy.
- Patients undergoing sedation must be closely monitored using telemetry, blood pressure readings, pulse oximetry, and ideally continuous capnometry. Clinical observation is also paramount.
- Plan for adverse events and have rescue equipment readily available.

- Available resources as well as predicted risk of sedation must be considered. Certain sedations are more safely performed in a controlled operating room under the care of an anesthesiologist.
- Children can more commonly pass to a deeper level of sedation unintentionally.

SUGGESTED READINGS

Bhatt M, Kennedy RM, Osmond MH, et al. Consensus-based recommendations for standardizing terminology and reporting adverse events for emergency department procedural sedation and analgesia in children. *Ann Emerg Med*. 2009;53(4):426-435.

Coté CJ, Wilson S. Guidelines for monitoring and management of pediatric patients before, during, and after sedation for diagnostic and therapeutic procedures. *Pediatrics*. 2019;143(6):e20191000.

Miller KA, Andolfatto G, Miner JR, et al. Clinical practice guideline for emergency department procedural sedation with propofol: 2018 update. *Ann Emerg Med*. 2019;73(5):470-480.

272

ARTHROCENTESIS TIPS

BENJAMIN CORNWELL AND J. DAVID GATZ

Arthrocentesis, the aspiration of synovial fluid from a joint space, is a valuable diagnostic and therapeutic tool. Emergency clinicians must know the appropriate indications to perform this vital procedure, understand how to troubleshoot a challenging arthrocentesis, and be familiar with potential complications.

INDICATIONS AND CONTRAINDICATIONS

The most common indication for arthrocentesis is to aid in the diagnosis of an acutely swollen atraumatic joint, which carries a broad differential, the most serious of which is septic arthritis. Other diagnoses or indications to consider include crystal arthropathies, tense hemarthroses, evaluating for a communicating laceration, or occasionally administering medicine. Certain patient populations are at higher risk of septic arthritis including older adults, as well as those with a history of immunosuppression, diabetes, alcoholism, intravenous drug use, prosthetic joints, or chronic arthritis. Acute flares of chronic inflammatory joint conditions, including the crystal arthropathies, can present like septic arthritis and may even present concomitantly with septic arthritis. Arthrocentesis is a relatively benign procedure with rare absolute contraindications (overlying abscess) and few relative contraindications (overlying cellulitis, bacteremia, and severe coagulopathies). Use of anticoagulants is not a contraindication to joint aspiration.

TECHNIQUE

Arthrocentesis can be accomplished using one of three approaches: the landmark approach, the indirect ultrasound-guided approach, and the direct ultrasound-guided approach. The landmark approach relies on a thorough understanding of joint anatomy and may be difficult in those with an obese body habitus or distortion of classic anatomic landmarks. This approach may also miss other important diagnoses, such as abscesses and hematomas. The indirect ultrasound-guided approach relies on locating the target effusion using ultrasound visualization, approximating the depth to the target, and marking the skin for needle entry. Once the target has been acquired and depth approximated, the ultrasound is no longer used for procedural guidance. Conversely, the direct ultrasound-guided approach relies on dynamic and continuous visualization of needle entry into the target space. This last approach is preferred, as it results in greater accuracy and a decreased complication rate.

When performing the direct ultrasound-guided approach, the patient should be placed in a supine position, except during shoulder arthrocentesis when the patient should remain upright. A high-frequency linear transducer should be used for the elbow, wrist, knee, ankle, and foot. A low-frequency transducer, such as the curvilinear probe, should be used for the shoulder and hip. A 20-gauge needle (3.5 inches in length) is recommended for both the shoulder and knee joints, while a 22-gauge (3.5 inches or 1.5 inches) can be used for smaller joints. The clinician should hold the needle in the dominant hand and maintain control of the probe with the nondominant hand. Once the area of interest is centered on the screen, the needle is inserted into the skin at equidistance away from the probe and tracked along its trajectory to the joint space. The needle should ideally be visualized with an in-plane approach and the entire length of the needle identifiable throughout the procedure.

Ultrasound-guided arthrocentesis should especially be considered in the pediatric population. Pediatric patients have smaller joints, smaller effusions, and may be less able to tolerate a more uncomfortable landmark-based approach. Ultrasound is equally useful in the pediatric population as in adults in identifying and draining an effusion. Consider using local anesthetic with epinephrine for any patients (adult or pediatric) who are at an increased risk of bleeding.

Synovial Fluid Interpretation

Arthrocentesis allows for synovial fluid analysis including joint WBC count, Gram stain, and culture. Though most sources designate a "positive" result for septic arthritis if the WBC is greater than 50,000 cells/mL, a significant proportion of patients can have a WBC below that value. Furthermore, joint aspirate culture only identifies the causative organism in 65% of patients.

Complications and Pitfalls

Potential complications of arthrocentesis include iatrogenic infection and injury to neurovascular structures. Ultrasound reduces these risks by allowing direct visualization of the joint effusion and additionally decreases the time required and the number of attempts to perform.

Note that the gold standard of diagnosis for a septic joint remains the clinical suspicion of an experienced physician. A negative Gram stain and culture do not fully exclude the possibility of septic arthritis. Patients who are believed to have septic arthritis must be promptly treated with antibiotics and discussed with orthopedic surgery about possible surgical washout.

Special consideration should be given to patients with a history of a total knee or hip replacement. Aspiration of hip fluid following a replacement is not routinely performed by emergency medicine clinicians, and prompt consultation with an orthopedic specialist is recommended. A knee replacement is not an absolute contraindication for joint aspiration; however, consultation with an orthopedic surgeon should similarly be considered. Workup in the ED is similar; however, it includes lab values such as erythrocyte sedimentation rate and c-reactive peptide. An acute infection is more suspected when CRP levels are greater than 100 mg/L and synovial WBC count greater than 10,000 WBC/mcL with at least 90% polymorphonuclear cells.

PEARLS

- Emergency clinicians must consider septic arthritis in patients presenting with an atraumatic, acutely swollen joint.
- Chronic inflammatory joint diseases increase a patient's risk of developing septic arthritis.
- Ancillary lab tests should be considered within the context of the clinical scenario and should not be used alone to rule out septic arthritis.
- Ultrasound-guided arthrocentesis is preferred over the traditional landmark-based approach, with the direct ultrasound approach with in-plane needle visualization to be utilized whenever possible.

SUGGESTED READINGS

Carpenter CR, Schuur JD, Everett WW, et al. Evidence based diagnostics: adult septic arthritis. *Acad Emerg Med*. 2011;18(8):781-796.
Long B, Koyfman A, Gottlieb M. Evaluation and management of septic arthritis and its mimics in the emergency department. *West J Emerg Med*. 2019;20(2):331-341.
Okano T, Mamoto K, Di Carlo M, et al. Clinical utility and potential of ultrasound in osteoarthritis. *Radiol Med*. 2019;124(11):1101-1111.

273

LUMBAR PUNCTURE AND THE CHAMPAGNE TAP

KEVIN HANLEY

Without proper setup and planning, perform an LP can quickly escalate into a frustrating and time-consuming experience. This procedure follows the mantra that 90% of success is preparation. This chapter discusses high-yield tips and current evidence to perform a successful LP and attain that "champagne tap."

CONSENT AND CONTRAINDICATIONS

Determine if an LP is the correct course of action and obtain consent. Relative contraindications include suspected elevated ICP, systemic anticoagulation or thrombocytopenia (platelets less than 50,000/mcL), or the presence of obstruction caused by previous spinal surgery. Infection in the tissues near the puncture site is an absolute contraindication.

Administer Antibiotics ASAP
Time is of the essence if evaluating for meningitis. Empiric antibiotics should be given without delay. If the LP is performed within 2 hours of antibiotic administration, culture yield from the CSF sampling should not be affected. Consider a simultaneous dose of intravenous steroids, which has been shown to decrease mortality and the risk of poor neurologic outcome in bacterial meningitis.

CT if Concerned About ICP
Intracranial imaging prior to LP, usually via CT, may be necessary to rule out increased ICP as this could risk brainstem herniation. Several criteria, if all negative, represent a 97% negative predictive value of the patient experiencing increased ICP and may obviate the need for head CT: age above 60 years, immunocompromised status, history of central nervous system disease, seizure within 1 week of presentation, presence of papilledema, or current neurologic symptoms consistent with altered mental status or cerebral ischemia.

Stay Sterile
Maximize efficiency and reduce patient anxiety by avoiding the need to break sterility during the procedure. Make sure that all equipment is available within arm's reach including one to two extra spinal needles. Consider marking the spinous processes above and below the target site prior to getting sterile, so the course of the spine can be more easily visualized during the procedure. If the processes are difficult to palpate, ultrasound can be used to locate them and to see their depth. Ensure the spinal needle is long enough to traverse the distance from the skin to the canal.

Midazolam a Must?
Patients may be understandably anxious. Treating such anxiety may improve patient compliance and increase the chance of a successful tap. Unless otherwise contradicted, a small dose of midazolam or other benzodiazepine can be a helpful anxiolytic. Midazolam has a faster onset and shorter duration of action compared to other benzodiazepines.

Position, Position, Position
Patient positioning is the single most important factor for success. A recent study showed the lateral decubitus position and upright position yield equal success rates, but lateral decubitus is required for an opening pressure. The patient's shoulders and hips must be aligned, and the back should be arched as much as possible to increase the gap between the spinous processes. The patient's sterile drape should cover their hips, so these can be palpated while maintaining sterility. The posterior, superior iliac crests align with the L4 spinous process, and the needle can be safely inserted one space above or below L4 in the L3 to L4 or L4 to L5 interspace. Anesthetize both potential tracts by first creating a wheal and then injecting deeper along a perpendicular tract. The wheal should be small—larger wheals may make palpation of the spinous processes difficult.

Once the site is identified and the patient is in the correct plane, the needle should be inserted, aimed toward the umbilicus. The bevel of the needle should be inserted longitudinally with the dural fibers (bevel up if in lateral decubitus and bevel to either side if sitting upright). The stylet should be removed periodically as the needle is advanced to check for fluid. There may be a tactile "pop" when the needle enters the spinal canal. If the patient reports a shooting pain down one of their legs, the needle should be redirected away from that leg. If the needle hits bone, the best practice is to withdraw and redirect it toward the head, matching the angle of the spinous processes. If there is difficulty obtaining fluid in one space, the needle should be removed and LP attempted in the other space with a new needle (as the prior needle may be occluded by a small blood clot in the tip).

PREVENT POST-LP PAIN

As many as one-third of all patients who receive LPs will complain of a postprocedural headache beginning 1 to 2 days after the procedure is performed. Many prevention methods have been studied including lying supine over a pillow immediately after the procedure, preprocedural IV fluid bolus, and early ambulation. None of these have shown significant benefit. Instead, use of atraumatic (or noncutting) needles instead of cutting needles, insertion of the needle parallel to dural fibers, and replacement of the stylet before withdrawing the spinal needle all have a role in preventing a post-LP headache. If a patient presents to the ED for post-LP headache, treatment includes IV or PO caffeine (though these have a high recurrence rate) or a blood patch, which is insertion of 10 to 30 mL of the patient's blood into the epidural space.

PEARLS

- Determine if an LP is the correct course of action, obtain consent, and ensure you are prepared prior to sterilization.
- Do not delay antibiotics to perform LP.
- A small dose of midazolam can be a helpful anxiolytic.
- Patient positioning is key—the more time you spend ensuring correct positioning, the higher the likelihood of a successful procedure.

SUGGESTED READINGS

Boon JM, Abrahams PH, Meiring JH, Welch T. Lumbar puncture: anatomical review of a clinical skill. *Clin Anat*. 2004;17(7):544-553.

Cognat E, Koehl B, Lilamand M, et al. Preventing post-lumbar puncture headache. *Ann Emerg Med*. 2021;78(3):443-450.

Joffe AR. Lumbar puncture and brain herniation in acute bacterial meningitis: a review. *J Intensive Care Med*. 2007;22(4):194-207.

Mason Jess. *Lumbar Puncture Tutorial*. Video. EMRAP; 2016. https://www.emrap.org/episode/lumbarpuncture/lumbarpuncture

Thundiyil JG, O'Brien JF, Tymkowicz AE, Papa L. Is lateral decubitus or upright positioning optimal for lumbar puncture success in a teaching hospital? *J Emerg Med*. 2023;64(1):14-21.

274

Tapping the Belly: Paracentesis in the Emergency Department

Ryan Bierle and Brian Parker

Indications

Patients with ascites commonly require diagnostic and therapeutic paracentesis. The etiology of ascites can be diverse, but the majority of patients presenting to the ED will have underlying liver pathology. A recent study showed that performing early paracentesis within 12 hours of admission resulted in multiple improved patient-oriented outcomes including decreased incidence of hepatic encephalopathy, hepatorenal syndrome, infection, length of stay, and in-hospital mortality.

It is important to understand the indications for ED paracentesis. This procedure can be therapeutic, diagnostic, or both. A frequent indication for diagnostic paracentesis is a suspicion of SBP. The clinical presentation of SBP can be subtle, even asymptomatic, and has been estimated to be present in 10% of hospitalized patients with ascites. However, it is most frequently seen in large-volume ascites, and classic symptoms include fever, diffuse abdominal pain or tenderness, and worsening encephalopathy. In addition, paracentesis is also indicated for first-time ascites, respiratory compromise, and tense ascites causing abdominal compartment syndrome. Therapeutic paracentesis may also lower esophageal variceal pressures during upper gastrointestinal bleeding.

Contraindications

The absolute contraindications to a paracentesis are disseminated intravascular coagulation and an acute abdomen requiring surgical evaluation. Other considerations include issues that may increase the risk of collateral damage (distended urinary bladder or bowel, pregnancy, abdominal adhesions) and signs of abdominal wall cellulitis at planned insertion sites. Although most textbooks recommend correction of elevated INR or thrombocytopenia, the American Gastroenterological Association no longer recommends routine correction of these factors prior to paracentesis.

Technique

Proper technique for a paracentesis begins with an understanding of the landmarks. The most common puncture sites are below the umbilicus and lateral to the rectus muscles. The area should be inspected with ultrasound to identify any underlying vascular structures and to locate a large fluid pocket that does not have any bowel near it. Consider rolling the patient toward the puncture to increase fluid volume at the site.

The two sensate structures in the needle path are the skin and peritoneum. Once the optimum site has been located, a 25-gauge or smaller needle is used to anesthetize the superficial skin and deep peritoneum. The aspiration needle is then inserted at a 45° angle and advanced while aspirating until ascitic fluid is obtained. Peritoneal fluid should be sent for analysis in cases of first-time ascites and if there is concern for infection.

Emergency clinicians can confidently remove small volumes of ascites (<100 mL) without concern for fluid shifting that would affect the patient's perfusion status (post-paracentesis circulatory dysfunction). As the aspirated volume increases, attention to hemodynamic stability becomes critical. Fluid should be removed slowly to minimize the possibility of hypotension, tachycardia, electrolyte imbalances, and renal impairment. Albumin administration can also help reduce the frequency of reactions. The dose of albumin is 6 to 8 g/L of ascitic fluid removed and should be infused if more than 5 L of fluid is removed.

COMPLICATIONS

Paracentesis is a safe procedure when performed correctly with a reported complication rate of less than 1%. Complications can be divided into hemorrhagic and nonhemorrhagic categories.

Hemorrhagic complications are rare but pose the most serious risk, and can present as overt shock to complaints (eg, abdominal pain). Unrecognized or delayed bleeding can lead to life-threatening hemodynamic instability. Examples include abdominal wall hematomas, inferior epigastric artery injuries, and hemoperitoneum. Patients who develop a significant rectus sheath hematoma should be investigated for an inferior epigastric artery injury and pseudoaneurysm with contrast-enhanced CT. Hemoperitoneum may be an acute or delayed complication. It occurs due to the drop in intraperitoneal pressure from the paracentesis, which can lead to mesenteric variceal rupture. A diagnostic paracentesis that demonstrates bloody fluid may assist in the diagnosis, and further imaging in the form of CT, ultrasound, or angiography may direct therapy.

Nonhemorrhagic complications are generally more benign. Paracentesis poses a risk of small bowel perforation and iatrogenic bacterial seeding, both of which can lead to secondary infection and abscess formation. Patients showing new signs of peritonitis, fever, rigors, or unexplained symptoms of shock following paracentesis should be evaluated with imaging, surgical consultation, and repeat paracentesis.

Perhaps the most frustrating complication for an emergency clinician is the persistent leakage of peritoneal fluid from the puncture site. To minimize this complication, consider using a small needle gauge or the Z-track technique. The Z-track technique entails putting downward traction on the skin at the puncture site prior to advancing the needle. Once fluid is aspirated, the skin is released to form a seal around the needle tract. A figure-8 suture may be used at the insertion site for persistent leakage.

Mechanical complications of paracentesis can be reduced and first puncture success improved with ultrasound guidance. Ultrasound can detect the location of the largest pocket of fluid and identify structures to avoid (eg, liver, spleen, bowel, bladder). Noting the distance to the center of the pocket of fluid to drain allows for accurate determination of how far the needle can safely be advanced. Furthermore, if the fluid pocket is relatively small, ultrasound can be used (with a sterile probe cover) for dynamic guidance to track the needle tip continuously and reduce the likelihood of iatrogenic injury.

PEARLS

- Paracentesis is typically performed below the umbilicus in the left lower quadrant where dullness to percussion is greatest.
- Place the patient in a recumbent position and roll them toward the desired puncture site.
- The Z-track technique and smaller needle gauge help reduce the risk of persistent peritoneal fluid leaks.
- The epigastric arteries are usually found along the lateral third of the rectus; avoiding these areas will help reduce potentially lethal complications of paracentesis.

- Use of ultrasound will help identify what structures to avoid and where to place the needle for highest first pass success.

SUGGESTED READINGS

Alvaro D, Caporaso N, Giannini EG, et al. Procedure-related bleeding risk in patients with cirrhosis and severe thrombocytopenia. *Eur J Clin Invest*. 2021;51(6):e13508.

De Gottardi A, Thévenot T, Spahr L, et al. Risk of complications after abdominal paracentesis in cirrhotic patients: a prospective study. *Clin Gastroenterol Hepatol*. 2009;7(8):906-909.

Katz MJ, Peters MN, Wysocki JD, Chakraborti C. Diagnosis and management of delayed hemoperitoneum following therapeutic paracentesis. *Proc (Bayl Univ Med Cent)*. 2013;26(2): 185-186.

O'Leary JG, Greenberg CS, Patton HM, Caldwell SH. AGA clinical practice update: coagulation in cirrhosis. *Gastroenterology*. 2019;157(1):34-43.e1.

Sharzehi K, Jain V, Naveed A, Schreibman I. Hemorrhagic complications of paracentesis: a systematic review of the literature. *Gastroenterol Res Pract*. 2014;2014:985141.

275

WHAT NERVE! ULTRASOUND-GUIDED REGIONAL NERVE BLOCKS

CASEY LEE WILSON AND JON HALLING

Emergency clinicians are skilled acute pain specialists. Managing complex injuries and painful conditions is a core aspect of training and clinical practice. Pain is best controlled when it is considered on a continuum and approached from a multimodal standpoint. Clinicians should start with less invasive methods, such as oral analgesics, and escalate to parenteral opioids or procedural sedation guided by patient condition. In the emergency setting, regional anesthesia in the form of peripheral nerve blockade provides a safe and effective adjunct for many acutely painful conditions. Blocks significantly reduce pain levels and the quantity of required opioid analgesics, particularly if initiated early in patient care.

POTENTIAL BENEFITS

Historically, nerve blocks have been performed using anatomic landmarks. But up to 30% of nerve blocks fail when a landmark technique is utilized. With bedside ultrasound almost universally available, UGRA has become an expanding adjunct in emergency pain management. Ultrasound provides real-time needle localization to minimize the effects of anatomic variability and avoid iatrogenic injury. It also allows the operator to directly visualize deposition of local anesthetic around the nerve. In 2020, the American College of Surgeons endorsed ultrasound-guided nerve blocks as best practice for opioid-sparing analgesia. The ACEP similarly released a 2021 policy statement advocating for UGRA as a core skill that should be supported by hospital credentialing.

Peripheral nerve blockade performed with sonographic guidance has been proven to result in lower volumes of anesthetic administered, faster onset, more effective analgesia, and fewer complications. Nerve blocks such as the interscalene brachial plexus block can be utilized for anterior shoulder dislocation reductions that would otherwise require a resource-intensive and potentially risky procedural sedation. Blocks, therefore, hold particular promise in low-resource and critical access facilities, and may save time, space, and risk.

COMMON NERVE BLOCKS

Femoral Nerve/Fascia Iliaca Compartment Blocks. Painful hip fractures in the older adults are a great example of why UGRA can be so helpful. Geriatric patients, who constitute over 80% of hip fractures in the United States, are at greater risk of opioid-induced adverse events (eg, delirium, hypotension, aspiration). Femoral nerve/fascia iliaca compartment blocks can avoid these complications. A recent systematic review and meta-analysis found that ultrasound-guided nerve blocks were superior to parenteral opioids in reducing pain and the need for rescue analgesia in hip fractures.

Lower Extremity Blocks. Successful analgesia requires knowledge of the anatomy of the peripheral nervous system. Sometimes more than one peripheral nerve must be blocked to achieve appropriate analgesia. Popliteal sciatic blocks are wonderful adjuncts for lower limb injuries such as ankle fractures and dislocations. Posterior tibial nerve blocks are an excellent analgesic option for isolated injuries to the plantar surface of the foot, including lacerations, foreign bodies, and calcaneal fractures.

Upper Extremity Blocks. Forearm nerve blocks provide adequate analgesia to the hand but less so for more proximal injuries such as distal forearm fractures which can be managed with the aid of brachial plexus blocks. One of the most useful blocks for the upper extremity is the supraclavicular brachial plexus block, sometimes referred to as the "spinal of the arm." Its applications are broad in the ED, providing adequate analgesia to assist in distal radius and ulnar fracture reductions.

TECHNIQUE

The choice of local anesthetic and ultrasound-guided in-plane technique is relatively universal regardless of the block. Patient should be awake and alert, able to communicate throughout the procedure, and connected to a cardiac monitor. The patient's cardiac rhythm, blood pressure, and oxygen saturation must be monitored during the block period. A thorough assessment and documentation of a neurovascular exam should be performed prior to any nerve block. Best practice involves constant needle tip visualization on ultrasound and aspirating frequently when advancing the needle. One should withdraw the needle several millimeters if significant resistance is encountered or if the patient feels painful paresthesias, as this may represent intraneural injection.

In choosing which local anesthetic to administer, one must consider the indication for the nerve block, the onset of clinical effects, desired duration of analgesia, and institutional preference. Lidocaine is a wonderful short-acting choice for procedures such as laceration repair, but the addition of epinephrine to lidocaine assists with the length of analgesia and can alert clinicians of intravascular injection due to immediate tachycardia. Bupivacaine is an attractive choice for indications such as pain control in hip fractures, but it is considerably more cardiotoxic at doses that exceed the 2.5 mg/kg limit. If available, ropivacaine (the levoisomer of bupivacaine) provides long-acting analgesia with less cardiotoxic potential. Care must be taken to avoid exceeding recommended weight-based local anesthetic dosing, especially in pediatric patients. A double-person verification of the toxic threshold should be verbalized and documented in the medical record.

RISKS AND COMPLICATIONS

Regional nerve blocks are not without risk. Fortunately, the most common complications (eg, bleeding, risk of infection) are easily managed. Clinicians should be familiar with unique complications associated with individual blocks. For example, while the interscalene brachial plexus block is incredibly effective during shoulder reductions, it may cause a phrenic nerve palsy leading to a transient sensation of breathlessness. Similarly, the interscalene block may lead to a temporary Horner syndrome and hoarseness.

There is a risk of inadvertent vascular injection resulting in systemic effects. This is rare, especially under ultrasound guidance, but clinicians must know the signs and symptoms of LAST. Subtle symptoms, such as tinnitus or a "funny taste in the mouth," can occur immediately if intravascular injection has occurred. In the case of large volume blocks deposited in a highly perfused space, absorption can lead to symptoms of LAST within 5 minutes of supratherapeutic injection. LAST will typically first manifest with signs of central nervous system excitation, such as perioral numbness and agitation. These may progress to refractory seizures, coma, and even cardiovascular collapse. Anyone performing a nerve block should know the unique treatment for LAST—intralipid therapy and supportive care.

PEARLS

- Consider a femoral nerve/facia iliaca compartment block for older patients with femur fractures.
- Use ultrasound-guided peripheral nerve blockade as an adjunct to systemic therapy for the management of acute pain.
- A thorough assessment and documentation of a neurovascular exam should be performed prior to any nerve block.
- An understanding of the various indications, complications, anatomy, and pitfalls of each nerve block is essential to procedural safety and success.

SUGGESTED READINGS

Beaudoin FL, Nagdev A, Merchant RC, et al. Ultrasound-guided femoral nerve blocks in elderly patients with hip fractures. *Am J Emerg Med*. 2010;28(1):76-81.

Bhoi S, Sinha TP, Rodha M, et al. Feasibility and safety of ultrasound-guided nerve block for management of limb injuries by emergency care physicians. *J Emerg Trauma Shock*. 2012;5(1):28-32.

Brown JR, Goldsmith AJ, Lapietra A, et al. Ultrasound-guided nerve blocks: suggested procedural guidelines for emergency physicians. *POCUS J*. 2022;7(2):253-261.

Liebmann O, Price D, Mills C, et al. Feasibility of forearm ultrasonography-guided nerve blocks of the radial, ulnar, and median nerves for hand procedures in the emergency department. *Ann Emerg Med*. 2006;48(5):558-562.

Zaki HA, Iftikhar H, Shallik N, et al. An integrative comparative study between ultrasound-guided regional anesthesia versus parenteral opioids alone for analgesia in emergency department patients with hip fractures: a systematic review and meta-analysis. *Heliyon*. 2022;8(12):e12413.

276

A Needling Issue: Decompressing Tension Pneumothorax

Arun Nair

Recognize Who Needs Needle Decompression

When your patient in respiratory distress is becoming increasingly tachycardic and now has distended neck veins—think tension pneumothorax! Those at risk classically include history of COPD with blebs, tall thin men, substance use with a bong or pipe, and anyone with chest trauma. But not all pneumothoraxes require decompression; often those less than 10% to 15% in size can be managed noninvasively. The only specific subset that requires *the needle* is unstable patients and those with impending respiratory or hemodynamic compromise.

Recognize that an existing needle in the chest does not guarantee the pneumothorax is decompressed. Many prehospital needle decompression attempts never reach the pleural space. Even if successful, subsequent kinking may allow the pneumothorax to reaccumulate. Listen to the patient, assess the vitals, and decide if another needle attempt is indicated. A tension pneumothorax should never be diagnosed by radiograph!

Landmarks

The debate of where, anatomically, to perform needle decompression is complex and one location does not appear to be universally superior to the other. Classically, the literature has supported an anterior approach, in which the emergency clinician inserts an 18-gauge needle into the second ICS at the midclavicular line. But clinicians may confuse the mammillary for the midclavicular line or misidentify the second ICS. These mistakes increase the risk of iatrogenic injury. The following technique is recommended:

- Find the sternal notch and slide your finger down until you feel a bony ridge—this is the angle of Louis and where the second rib attaches.
- Track your fingers laterally on the second rib until halfway between the sternal notch and AC joint.
- The ICS just below marks the spot for needle entry. Depending on habitus and sex, this site can be anywhere in relation to the nipple.

In the morbidly obese or extensively muscled patient, consider placement at the midaxillary line of the fifth ICS (the same location for a chest tube) as the chest wall tends to be thinner with less overlying muscle and no major blood vessels. To locate the correct spot:

- Position your open palm facing the patient's affected side with fingertips touching the bed and thumb extended.
- Next tuck your hand into their axilla until your thumb overlies the deltopectoral groove.
- Then push up/cephalad as far as you can go without allowing the shoulder to raise. The breadth of your palm at the fifth MCP should approximate the fifth ICS at the midaxillary line.

In large patients, the chest wall may still be too thick and you should consider using a longer needle (spinal needle) or even a quick cut down to the rib before needle placement. Keep in mind that the more overlying tissue there is, the greater the risk for the catheter to kink and for the pneumothorax to reaccumulate.

Finger Thoracostomy

If your patient is crashing and there are signs of significant trauma to the thorax, forget the needle—*give 'em the finger*! Follow the same steps to identify the fifth ICS, although now your target is the sixth rib. Using a scalpel, make a 4-cm incision parallel to the rib and down to the level of the bone. Use a curved Kelly clamp to enter the pleural space, remembering the neurovascular bundle runs just below each rib (the reason why you only cut/enter the chest immediately above a rib). More specifically, palm the Kelly clamp with the finger loops resting on your palm and curved tip pointing away from you, then grasp the clamp with your thumb and third to fifth digits. This frees your pointer finger to rest along the top clamp so that just a few centimeters of the instrument are visible pointing down past your fingertip. Place the tip of the Kelly on the sixth rib and in a controlled motion, drive it cephalad and into the pleural cavity—your pointer finger automatically acts as a stop to prevent the Kelly from plunging too deep. From here, spread open the Kelly parallel to the rib and prepare for the rush of air and blood.

What About the Bougie?

One potential trick when delivering the chest tube, rather than using a finger to maintain the tract, is to instead use a bougie as the "wire" for a modified Seldinger technique. After entrance into the chest cavity with the Kelly and quick confirmation of the pleural space with a full finger sweep, advance a bougie cephalad just far enough to ensure that it will not fall out. This frees up both hands while maintaining the tract (similar to a central line). It may also prevent accidental injury on a sharp fragment of broken while trying to guide a thoracostomy tube. Keep in mind this will only work for larger diameter tubes.

Don't Forget the Ultrasound Machine!

Ultrasound can rapidly differentiate air versus fluid in the chest, evaluate the heart, and even find an impalpable ICS while someone is grabbing a needle. Don't forget that ultrasound is useful after decompression too, as it can assess reaccumulation of a pneumothorax or see if the needle is still in the pleural space.

PEARLS

- Tension pneumothorax is a clinical diagnosis, NOT a radiologic finding.
- Clinically silent pneumothoraxes may not require invasive procedures or can await sterile chest tube placement.
- Needle placement does not guarantee decompression. Know your landmarks for both the second and fifth ICSs as body habitus significantly affects success.
- A finger thoracostomy should only take seconds but still requires technique and care.

Suggested Readings

Azizi N, Ter Avest E, Hoek AE, et al. Optimal anatomical location for needle chest decompression for tension pneumothorax: a multicenter prospective cohort study. *Injury*. 2021;52(2):213-218.

Nelson M, Chavda Y, Stankard B, McCann-Pineo M, Nello A, Jersey A. Using ultrasound to determine optimal location for needle decompression of tension pneumothorax: a pilot study. *J Emerg Med*. 2022;63(4):528-532.

Osterman J, Kay AB, Morris DS, Evertson S, Brunt T, Majercik S. Prehospital decompression of tension pneumothorax: have we moved the needle? *Am J Surg*. 2022;224(6):1460-1463.

Shah K, Tran J, Schmidt L. Traumatic pneumothorax: updates in diagnosis and management in the emergency department. *Emerg Med Pract*. 2022;25(5 suppl 1):1-28.

277

Is Ultrasound Sufficient for Line Confirmation?

Samantha A. King and Brian Euerle

Time is precious when treating critically ill patients in the ED. Emergency clinicians understandably embrace techniques or protocols that expedite decisions concerning therapies and patient dispositions. One such technique is the use of point-of-care ultrasound to confirm CVC position—a necessary step before use. Ultrasound confirmation, if reliable, would allow more rapid treatment of critically ill patients compared to the traditional use of a confirmatory CXR.

Malposition of the CVC is a significant complication that confirmation is intended to detect. In general, the tip of the catheter should be located in a large central vein, such as the SVC or IVC. If the tip is located in a smaller vein, thrombosis is more likely. Catheters may also inadvertently perforate a vein, resulting in an extravascular location of the tip in the pericardial, pleural, or peritoneal cavities with subsequent hemorrhage. Unrecognized intra-arterial placement of the catheter can be the cause of significant morbidity. For these reasons, confirmation of CVC location is essential.

Ultrasound-Guided Line Placement

Intravascular access for peripheral and central veins is a fundamental skill set for clinicians working in the ED. Traditionally, central venous access was obtained using a landmark-based technique. The U.S. Agency for Healthcare Research and Quality has strongly recommended the use of ultrasound guidance for the placement of central venous catheters since 2001. Ultrasound guidance offers several advantages, the most important being fewer complications and greater safety for patients.

Preassessment is an important first step in ultrasound guidance and proper CVC placement. Potential sites should be evaluated for ease of access, evidence of thrombosis and venous patency, and proximity to arterial structures. After preassessment, ultrasound should be used for direct visualization and placement of the catheter by visualizing the needle insertion into the vessel and confirmation of the wire location in the vein prior to dilation.

POSTPLACEMENT CONFIRMATION WITH ULTRASOUND

Historically, CXR has been the gold standard for confirmation of IJ and subclavian vein central lines to evaluate the location of the catheter tip. The time required to obtain a CXR before the line is used may significantly delay patient care. There are also limitations to the accuracy of CXR as a means of confirmation, and misidentification of the catheter tip is possible. Consequently, additional methods have been developed for bedside ultrasonographic evaluation of CVC placement.

Confirmation of venous access begins with the previously described preprocedural ultrasound guidance and subsequently includes postprocedural ultrasound of the catheter itself. The catheter should be visualized within the vein without piercing into artery or soft tissue. It is important to make sure the catheter has not gone through the back wall of the vein. A backwalled catheter can be seen by observing the catheter traversing through the posterior wall of the vein, and if saline is flushed, it would result in fluid collection outside the vein.

Unfortunately, ultrasound cannot directly visualize the entire length of the catheter to evaluate the tip location. The ideal position is typically thought to be within the entrance of the RA or the SVC-RA junction. If the tip can be visualized, this is considered confirmation, but these locations are typically not amenable to direct visualization by transthoracic ultrasound. Ultrasound line confirmation has, therefore, typically been through visualization of secondary signs.

The most common and widely published method of confirmation is the visualization of agitated saline, which can be produced simply by rapidly pushing 5 mL of a saline flush, within the RA on transthoracic echo (apical four-chamber or subxiphoid view). Pooled meta-analysis of saline-flush studies with visualization of the central line within the vessel and not in alternative vessels (subclavian vein, IJ vein, etc) and visualization of the flush within 2 seconds have shown sensitivities of 0.64 to 0.89 and specificities consistently greater than 0.90 for detection of misplacement. These studies require the ability to visualize the RA, which may prove difficult in patients who are obese or distended and is thus a potential limitation. However, more recent literature suggests that this time delay should be shorter; delays as little as 0.5 seconds have been proposed. The optimal time delay will depend in part on what is considered the ideal tip location. Delays of less than 2 seconds likely indicate location within the SVC; even shorter delays may indicate a location closer to the junction. However, the literature offers no consensus on this point. Published protocols such as ECHOTIP use a delay of less than 1 second. For patients unable to meet these criteria, an alternative line placement confirmation is required prior to use. These methods have not been well studied in the pediatric population and caution should be used in extrapolating.

EVALUATION OF POSTPROCEDURAL COMPLICATIONS

A radiograph obtained to evaluate the location of the tip of the catheter also may be used to assess for pneumothorax, a significant potential complication of central line placement. Multiple studies have shown the reliability of ultrasound in detecting a pneumothorax in less time than is required for detection by CXR. Additional complications, such as arterial or soft tissue placement of catheters, may also be observed by postprocedural vascular ultrasound.

PEARLS

- Malposition of a CVC can result in significant patient morbidity.
- Ultrasound can help confirm the location of a central venous catheter with high specificity in less time than the traditional method of confirmation using CXR.
- Ultrasound has reasonable sensitivity (0.70-0.80) to detect CVC malposition and excellent sensitivity and specificity to detect pneumothorax.
- In patients with uncomplicated ultrasound-guided CVC insertion, visualization of the catheter within the correct vessel, not visualizing the CVC in an incorrect vessel, and rapid visualization of saline flush (<1 second) likely confirm the correct placement of a CVC.

Suggested Readings

Greca A, Iacobone E, Elisei D, et al. ECHOTIP: a structured protocol for ultrasound-based tip navigation and tip location during placement of central venous access devices in adult patients. *J Vasc Access*. 2023;24(4):535-544.

Montrief T, Auerbach J, Cabera J, Long B. Use of point-of-care ultrasound to confirm central venous catheter placement and evaluate for postprocedural complications. *J Emerg Med*. 2021;60(5):637-640.

Saugel B, Scheeren TWL, Teboul JL. Ultrasound-guided central venous catheter placement: a structured review and recommendations for clinical practice. *Crit Care*. 2017;21(1):225.

Smit JM, Haaksma ME, Lim EHT, et al. Ultrasound to detect central venous catheter placement associated complications: a multicenter diagnostic accuracy study. *Anesthesiology*. 2020;132(4):781-794.

Smit JM, Raadsen R, Blans MJ, et al. Bedside ultrasound to detect central venous catheter misplacement and associated iatrogenic complications: a systematic review and meta-analysis. *Crit Care*. 2018;22(1):65.

278

Nasopharyngoscopy in the ED

Michael Billet

Nasopharyngoscopy, as the name suggests, is a method of visualizing the pharynx via the nasal route using a flexible endoscope. As opposed to oral visualization, nasopharyngoscopy can provide a more complete inspection of the pharynx without activation of the pharyngeal gag reflex. This is of great use to the emergency medicine clinician for both diagnostic and interventional purposes. Nasopharyngoscopes have traditionally been fiberoptic devices that may include a video assist feature. Modern devices more commonly consist of digital cameras on the end of a flexible wand but are similar in function. Physical and mental preparation of the patient is essential for a successful procedure.

Indications and Patient Assessment

Common diagnostic uses of nasopharyngoscopy include assessment for foreign bodies, burns, vocal cord dysfunction, and swelling from allergic reactions or angioedema. Nasopharyngoscopy is a useful adjunct if nasotracheal intubation is required. As with any procedure involving the airway, the patient should be assessed for neck mobility, mouth opening, Mallampati score, and a history of adverse reactions to local or general anesthetics if these are to be used. The nares should also be inspected for any injury, septal deviation, inflammation, or other conditions that could impede passage of the nasopharyngoscope. Coagulopathy is a relative contraindication; the risks and benefits of the procedure should be weighed closely in patients with a bleeding diathesis, and care should be taken not to injure the sensitive mucosa. Suspected injury to the cribriform plate or bony midface is a contraindication, as is suspicion for epiglottitis or croup in children.

Patient Preparation

The patient should be seated upright with the head against an unmoving seatback if possible. Maintaining a neutral to slightly extended neck position will facilitate passage of the scope from the nasopharynx into the oropharynx. Benzocaine or lidocaine achieves rapid and potent local anesthesia when atomized into the nostril, though clinicians should be mindful of the increased dose of medication present if using higher concentration formulations to avoid systemic toxicity. Lidocaine jelly or ointment is useful to anesthetize the posterior tongue. Finally, gargled 1% lidocaine will aid in anesthetizing the supraglottic area.

Purely diagnostic nasopharyngoscopy being performed in a stable patient (eg, sensation of foreign body in a patient with a patent airway) may not require any additional preparation aside from topical anesthetic and a thorough briefing of the patient. A topical vasoconstricting agent such as oxymetazoline can be useful if inflammation is present. Anxiolytics can be provided if needed in an otherwise cooperative patient. A respiration-preserving sedative such as ketamine can be administered if the patient is not able to cooperate with the procedure.

Procedural Considerations

A water-soluble lubricant should be applied near the tip of the scope, taking care to avoid covering the lens or camera. True fiberoptic devices may benefit from applying antifog solution or the patient's saliva to the glass lens; fogging is less of an issue with fully digital devices with their plastic lenses and heat-producing electronics. With the patient seated upright, the scope is held parallel to the floor and inserted into the more patent nostril toward the back of the head. If done correctly, the scope will smoothly pass between the inferior turbinate and the floor of the nasal cavity as one would insert a nasogastric tube. Insertion at an angle can cause discomfort or injury to the sensitive mucosa. It may be tempting to use the camera at this point, but doing so will merely delay passage into the posterior nasopharynx. Once the turbinates have been passed, the camera can be used to inspect the nasopharynx before manipulating the scope inferiorly into the posterior oropharynx. From this position, the posterior tongue and vallecula can be inspected, followed by the vocal cords and surrounding structures.

If nasotracheal intubation is being considered, the physician should load an endotracheal tube onto the nasopharyngoscope before performing nasopharyngoscopy to avoid repeated removal and insertion of the scope. Once the scope has been advanced into the hypopharynx, the lubricated tube is advanced and held in position above the vocal cords, using the scope as a stylet. When both are in position, a respiration-preserving sedative can be administered if not already given. The scope is passed through the vocal cords during exhalation followed immediately by the tube.

Compared to the orotracheal route, nasotracheal intubation entails a longer path to the vocal cords. Endotracheal tubes used for orotracheal intubation have lengths proportional to their outside diameter. Consequently, small diameter tubes may not have necessary length, but larger tubes may not pass through the nasal cavity. Ideally, a specific nasotracheal tube should be used, but this may not be available in an emergent situation. A simple way of determining the largest (and therefore longest) possible tube is to first pass a nasopharyngeal airway device into the nostril, as both are sized by their outside diameter.

CONSIDER THE AVAILABLE RESOURCES

If there is a question of airway stability, consider intubation in an operative setting by anesthesiology. In the ED, nasotracheal intubation is by its very nature only performed in patients without a clear oral route, so standard supraglottic airways may not be useful. In a failed airway situation, a front-of-neck airway may be the only option.

PEARLS

- Adequate analgesia and mental preparation of the patient are of prime importance to successfully performing nasopharyngoscopy.
- Patients with reduced neck mobility, suspected airway obstruction, or who cannot actively participate in the procedure are at higher risk for failure or complication.
- The nasopharyngoscope should be inserted horizontally in a seated patient and smoothly pass the turbinates to avoid injury and pain.
- If stability of the airway is in question, consider intubation in an operative setting with surgical backup.

SUGGESTED READINGS

Folino TB, Mckean G, Parks LJ. Nasotracheal intubation. In: *StatPearls [Internet]*. StatPearls Publishing; 2022.
Tonna JE, DeBlieux PM. Awake laryngoscopy in the emergency department. *J Emerg Med*. 2017;52(3):324-331.

279

FOLEY CATHETER FOLLIES

ARTHUR J. POPE AND CHINEZIMUZO IHENATU

Foley catheter insertion is a simple yet essential procedure, providing both diagnostic information and therapeutic relief. It is important to recognize when Foley catheterization is indicated and how to perform this fundamental skill to reduce injury and other nosocomial and iatrogenic complications.

Foley Catheterization Indications

Acute urinary retention is one of the most common reasons for Foley catheter placement in the ED. Other therapeutic indications include neurogenic bladder, patients experiencing incontinence with severe sacral or groin wounds (to assist the healing process), continuous bladder irrigation, and administration of intravesical medication. Urinary catheters are also used in a diagnostic capacity. For example, they may be placed in the setting of shock to accurately measure urine output. Other diagnostic indications include measurement of postvoid residual volumes, obtaining sterile urine samples, and performing imaging procedures such as retrograde urethrography. Foley catheter placement is contraindicated in patients who are suspected to or found to have a urethral injury (eg, bloody urethral meatus or high-riding prostate). Recent urethral or bladder surgery and urethral strictures are relative contraindications.

Insertion

A standard Foley kit should come with all necessary equipment. Placement of the catheter will vary slightly between patients with male or female anatomy. To prevent patient discomfort, the best catheter choice for a patient is usually the softest and narrowest functional catheter. The Foley catheter size for an average female urethra is 14F to 16F, while 16F to 18F is appropriate for most average adult males. Choose catheter sizes below the average size in patients with known strictures or scarring that leads to narrow urethras. Larger sizes may be appropriate for patients at risk of catheter obstruction, such as those experiencing hematuria with clots.

Tips on Insertion

- Sterility is key to avoiding CAUTIs. Keep one hand sterile at all times.
- Female patients should be placed in lithotomy or frog-leg position.
- Male patients should have the penis held perpendicular to the body.
- If there is resistance with insertion, ask the patient to take a deep breath and relax as this may be due to external sphincter tightening. Do NOT force the catheter when met with resistance.
- When inflating the balloon, make sure to inject the full 10 mL of sterile water. Injecting less may lead to dislodged catheters into the urethra and cause trauma. Avoid using saline, as it may lead to crystallization and valve malfunction. Avoid using air, which may allow the balloon to float in the bladder and lead to possible kinks in the catheter.

Risks of Catheterization

Foley catheterization is not an entirely benign procedure. Chief among the risks are CAUTIs. Colonization can occur within 48 hours of insertion. The best way to avoid CAUTIs is to avoid catheterization when possible. Urethral trauma is a risk associated with insertion and improper removal. Trauma can range from minimal discomfort and hematuria to vena cava air embolism and false passage creation necessitating surgical intervention. Trauma can lead to strictures and scarring as well.

Difficult Uterine Catheterization/ Troubleshooting

Anxiety and stress about the procedure can make Foley catheter placement difficult. Prior to placing the catheter, reassure patients and address any questions or concerns they may have. Anticipate difficult catheterizations in patients with previous genitourinary procedures and pelvic organ anatomic variants. Catheterization can be difficult for patients who have experienced childbirth, patients with prostatic hyperplasia, and patients who are morbidly obese. In patients who are morbidly obese, use an assistant to maintain traction and consider Trendelenburg positioning to improve visualization and ensure sterility. If the penis is buried, apply pressure to the base of the penile shaft to expose the glans and have an assistant insert the catheter. However, in this patient population, a guidewire may be necessary. In female patients, a prolapsed vagina or atrophic vaginitis can lead to difficult insertion. In the latter case, the urethra retracts and lies in a more anterior anatomic position. To troubleshoot both cases, insert the nonsterile index finger in the vaginal orifice and apply pressure superiorly. If unable to visualize the urethra, this technique will straighten the urethra and allow the finger to guide the Foley through the urethral opening. It is important to obtain the consent of the patient prior to using this technique.

In patients with prostatic hyperplasia, the proceduralist may notice resistance in advancement at 16- to 20-cm mark. In these circumstances, the use of a coudé catheter may prove beneficial, as the firm curved tip will help maneuver around the narrow prostatic urethra. In addition, using a larger size (eg, 24F) may also help, as smaller sizes are less firm and are prone to kinking at the bladder neck.

Free flow of urine indicates proper insertion. If there is no urine flow, this could be due to wrong site insertion (most likely with female anatomy), obstructed catheter, or an empty bladder. Test the Foley by flushing the catheter with saline. One can also gently massage the bladder in an attempt to provoke urinary flow. Consider consulting urology for catheter placement if the patient has had recent urologic surgery, phimosis, meatal stenosis, or known urethral strictures.

PEARLS

- Assess appropriateness of catheter placement to prevent CAUTIs and avoid other risks.
- Anticipate difficult placements by contextualizing abnormal anatomy and assessing past medical and surgical history.
- Never use force to advance a catheter. It's okay to call urology for help.

SUGGESTED READINGS

Meddings J, Saint S, Fowler KE, et al. The Ann Arbor criteria for appropriate urinary catheter use in hospitalized medical patients: results obtained by using the RAND/UCLA appropriateness method. *Ann Intern Med*. 2015;162(9 suppl):S1-S34.

Ortega R, Ng L, Sekhar P, et al. Female urethral catheterization. *N Engl J Med*. 2008;358(14):e15.

Thomsen TW, Setnik GS. Male urethral catheterization. *N Engl J Med*. 2006;354(21):e22.

280

MIND THE PRESSURE! BALLOON TAMPONADE FOR UGIB

AARON ALINDOGAN AND BRIAN PARKER

The nauseated and pale-appearing patient who presents with bloody emesis will humble even the most seasoned emergency clinician. While the ABCs of the medical resuscitation do not change, this critically ill patient requires contemporaneous initiation of all modems of resuscitation. Two large-bore peripheral IVs are crucial in this patient, and in the case of hemorrhagic shock, blood product transfusion should already be underway. The airway should be secured with respect to the patient's shock index. Assuming the patient has not aspirated an entire lung's volume of blood, judicious management of the ventilator should also be observed. Furthermore, pharmacologic agents ought to be implemented: antibiotics (eg, ceftriaxone) to reduce mortality and rebleeding in cases of variceal bleeding, high-dose proton-pump inhibitor infusion to reduce rebleeding and need for blood transfusion in cases of bleeding ulcers, and somatostatin analogs (eg, octreotide) to selectively vasoconstrict the splanchnic system and decrease flow to the portal system. Some of the most dire cases, however, will further benefit from a BTD.

INDICATIONS

Unstable UGIB demands prompt recognition and decisive action, which can stave off portending hemorrhagic shock or respiratory failure and subsequent hypoxic arrest. A BTD is indicated in cases of refractory bleeding in an unstable and intubated patient with suspected variceal hemorrhage.

CONTRAINDICATIONS

BTD is contraindicated in the stable patient and in those lacking a definitive airway. Relative contraindications include recent gastroesophageal surgery and a history of esophageal stricture.

TUBE TYPES AND TECHNIQUE

There are three common BTDs. The main differences between these tubes are the number of balloons and the total amount of air that can be utilized. Most hospitals only carry one of the following types: the LNT, the SBT, and the Minnesota tube. It is imperative every emergency clinician familiarize themselves with whichever type is present within their own clinical site(s).

The Minnesota tube has both a gastric (inflated to 500 mL) and esophageal balloon (30-45 mL) and four ports for independent gastric and esophageal inflating and suctioning. SBT also has two balloons (250 and 30-45 mL, respectively) but has three ports, lacking an esophageal suction port. The LNT is simplest, with one gastric balloon (inflated to 600 mL) and its respective gastric inflation and suction ports (**Figure 280.1**).

The procedure requires the most readily available BTD, a large volume (≥60 mL) syringe, bulb inflater, manometer, three-way stop cocks, "Christmas tree" Luer-lock converters, 1 L of crystalloid, Kerlix gauze, McGill forceps, and padded hemostats. The following steps are advised:

1) Make sure x-ray technician is readily available.

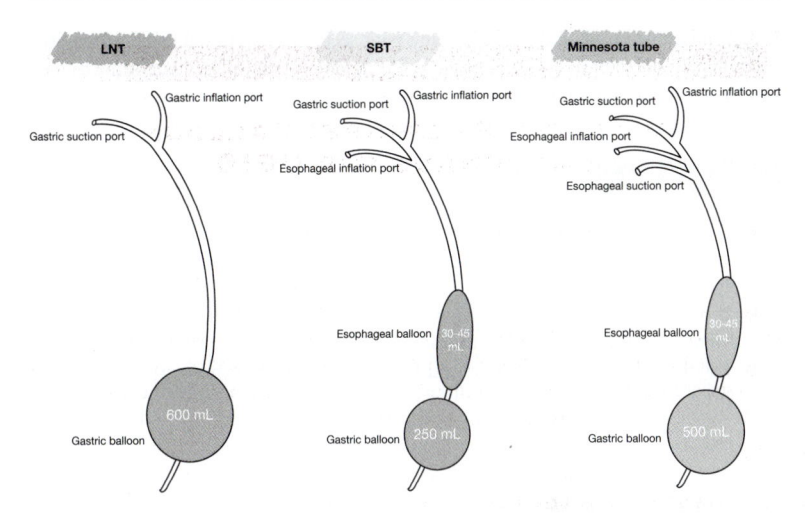

FIGURE 280.1 Three common balloon tamponade devices. LNT, Linton-Nachlas tube; SBT, Sengstaken-Blakemore tube and the Minnesota tube. Illustrated by Dr Alindogan.

2) Gather all equipment and test integrity of each balloon submerged in water. Place three-way stop cocks in each inflation port. Place Christmas tree Luer-locks in each suction port. There are case reports of submerging the tube in ice water to increase the stiffness of the tube, but this has not been definitively shown to improve insertion.
3) Lubricate and insert the deflated BTD about 50 cm. Consider using laryngoscopy and McGill forceps. A "super stiff" or "extra-stiff" guidewire; an Eschmann stylet, commonly called a "bougie"; or pediatric-sized "bougie" can be used to help assist in insertion. Insert the straight end into the most proximal port to prevent folding of the distal ports when removing the stylet after confirmed placement in the stomach.
4) While auscultating over the stomach, inflate the gastric balloon about 50 mL.
5) Obtain chest x-ray or KUB to confirm placement in the stomach.
6) Inflate gastric balloon to indicated volume as earlier (Minnesota to 500 mL, SBT to 250 mL, LNT to 600 mL) in 50-mL increments. Do not exceed 15 mm Hg on manometry. Clamp just distal to inflation port with padded hemostats.
7) Apply traction using Kerlix and 1-L crystalloid bag suspended over an IV pole in order to apply 1 kg of traction. Be sure to mark the depth of the tube at the mouth to monitor for displacement.
8) Perform gastric suction and lavage.
9) For continued bleeding with a Minnesota and SBT, inflate the esophageal tube while measuring with a manometer to 30 and up to 45 mm Hg. Then clamp just distal to its port with padded hemostats.

COMPLICATIONS

The feared risk of BTD is esophageal or gastric ulceration and perforation, which is why these devices are only temporizing and bridging measures. Patients ultimately need endoscopy or an emergent TIPS. Most clinicians will be inexperienced with this rare procedure, which may account for increased rates of complications. Failure to check for compromised balloons, underinflation, and poor securement with too much or too little traction may all result in device migration. Overinflation or misplacement of the balloon can lead to airway compromise, aspiration resulting in respiratory failure, or large vessel occlusion.

PEARLS

- The early recognition of the patient with hemorrhagic GI bleeding is important, and early placement of a BTD may help stabilize the patient until definitive treatment can be arranged.
- If a bougie or Eschmann stylet is utilized, they are radiopaque and can help identify correct placement of the tamponade device in the stomach.
- Esophageal balloon pressures need to be checked with manometry to prevent pressure necrosis.

SUGGESTED READINGS

Bari V, Subramanian RM. Practical strategies related to the application of balloon tamponade therapy in acute variceal bleeding. *Crit Care Explor*. 2022;4(8):1-5.

Bridwell R, Long B, Ramzy M, Gottlieb M. Balloon tamponade for the management of gastrointestinal bleeding. *J Emerg Med*. 2022;62(4):545-558.

Powell M, Journey JD. Sengstaken-Blakemore tube. In: *StatPearls* [Internet]. NLM NCBI. Accessed June 5, 2022. https://www.ncbi.nlm.nih.gov/books/NBK558924/.

281

PEARLS FOR PROPER SPLINT PLACEMENTS

TIANYU TANG AND STEVEN STRAUBE

Splinting helps immobilize musculoskeletal injuries to promote healing. Although the most common indications are for fractures, splint immobilization is also used for certain tendon and ligament injuries. The goal is to immobilize the injury to avoid further malalignment or deformity. Splinting also provides compression to the area, helping to decrease edema and pain. Splinting is appropriate for adult and pediatric populations although, if available, casting material can be applied to pediatrics immediately. Splinting is beneficial because it is non–circumferential, allowing room for edema. See **Table 281.1** for a brief summary of splint options and their indications.

GENERAL PROCEDURE

Ensure easy access to all aspects of the extremity. For upper extremities, consider hanging the fingers from an IV pole using finger traps. For distal upper extremity splints, have the patient or an assistant hold the hand up in the air. For lower extremities, either hang the toes from an IV pole using finger traps or have the patient lay prone and flex 90° at the knee.

For patient comfort, apply a stockinette or a couple of circumferential layers of cotton padding directly to the extremity. Avoid wrinkles to prevent pressure sores. Splints can be applied in the following eight steps:

1) Measure and lay out six layers of cotton padding at appropriate length, specific to each splint type and patient.
    a) If using fiberglass that comes with padding, stretch to extend the cotton padding beyond the fiberglass to cover up the splintered fiberglass edges. You can also use extra cotton padding or trim the fiberglass edges.
2) Lay out 10 layers of plaster (or the fiberglass) of sufficient length. Keep in mind that the plaster will shrink a bit with water.
3) Activate the splint material.
    a) Plaster: Soak thoroughly with hot water. It is easiest to do this with a tub of water on the ground to have access to the entire length of the plaster.
    b) Fiberglass: Rinse fiberglass quickly with room temperature water; fiberglass hardens more quickly with warmer water.
4) Dry splint material.
    a) Plaster: Prime the layers together and wring out extra water by running the layers together through two fingers.
    b) Fiberglass: Use a towel to wring out the excess water.
5) Place one more layer of cotton padding on top of the wet plaster or fiberglass with the six layers of cotton padding at the bottom.
    a) If using fiberglass that comes with padding, can skip this step.
6) Apply the side with multiple layers of cotton padding to the patient's skin.
    a) If using fiberglass that comes with padding, it does not matter which side is applied to the patient.
7) Wrap the splinted extremity circumferentially with Bias wrap, or elastic wrap if Bias is unavailable. Overlap 50% with each round. Be sure not to wrap too tightly.
8) Tape the edge to secure.

Special Considerations

Always perform a neurovascular examination before and after splint application. Injured extremities will swell. With a rigid, immobile splint, there is risk of neurovascular compression causing compartment syndrome, nerve palsies, or pressure wounds. It is vital that patients elevate the extremity above the level of the heart to reduce swelling.

Do not set the extremity down on a hard surface until after the plaster or fiberglass has completely solidified to avoid compression injuries. When molding, use the palms of your hands.

Patients with fractures requiring splints often have overlying skin lacerations and abrasions. As long as these wounds are not in connection with the fracture (ie, it is not an open fracture), clean out the wound and place a petroleum-coated gauze on the wound and proceed with splinting.

TABLE 281.1 SPLINT TYPE AND INDICATIONS

SPLINT	FRACTURE/INJURY	POSITIONING	PLASTER/FIBERGLASS LENGTH	NOTES
Hand and wrist				
Thumb spica	Scaphoid, trapezium, lunate, first metacarpal, thumb (metacarpophalangeal joint) MCP dislocation, first phalanx, ulnar collateral ligament injuries	Wrist extended 20°, thumb holding soda can	Radial mid-forearm to thumb (distal interphalangeal joint) DIP	If using plaster, can cut the thumb length into thirds for ease of wrapping the thumb circumferentially
Ulnar gutter	Fourth or fifth metacarpal/ proximal or middle phalanx	Wrist extended 20°, fourth and fifth fingers mostly straight and flexed 70° at MCP	Ulnar mid-forearm to most distal DIP	Place a thin layer of cotton padding between fingers
Radial gutter	Second or third metacarpal/ proximal or middle phalanx	Wrist extended 20°, second and third fingers mostly straight and flexed 70° at MCP	Radial mid-forearm to most distal DIP, leaving thumb free	Cut hole in splint before application to keep thumb free. Cotton padding between fingers
Volar	Triquetrum, pisiform, trapezoid, capitate, hamate, wrist drop, carpal tunnel syndrome	Wrist extended 20°	Volar mid-forearm to distal palmar crease	
Sugar tong	Distal radius and/or ulna	Wrist extended 20°	Dorsal MCP around elbow to proximal palmar crease	
Aluminum U-shaped splint	Distal phalanx	DIP in extension for distal phalanx fracture and mallet finger, DIP slightly flexed for Jersey finger	Just distal to (proximal interphalangeal joint) PIP	
Buddy tape	Middle and proximal phalanx fractures	Fingers straight	One tape at the proximal phalanx and another at the middle phalanx	Tape partners: second and third, fourth and fifth. Cotton pad between fingers

Forearm and humerus

Posterior long arm	Supracondylar, proximal or midshaft radius and/or ulna, olecranon/coronoid	Elbow flexed at 90° and palms facing torso	Ulnar surface from mid-humerus to the distal palmar crease volarly and MCP joints dorsally
Double sugar tong	Supracondylar, proximal or midshaft radius and/or ulna	Elbow flexed at 90° and palms facing torso	Regular sugar tong and another sugar tong from distal deltoid insertion around elbow to similar length on medial side
Coaptation	Humerus shaft	Elbow flexed at 90°	Acromioclavicular joint around elbow to axilla
Cuff and collar	Proximal humerus	Elbow flexed with hand in direction of opposite shoulder and palms facing torso	Can use wrist restraint and straps from regular sling

Lower extremities

Posterior short leg	All stable distal lower extremity injuries including foot injuries, Achilles tendon rupture	Ankle at 90° (except for Achilles tendon rupture plantar flexed)	Two inches distal to fibular head to great toe
Stirrup	Ankle sprain	Ankle at 90°	Lateral mid-calf around the heel to medial mid-calf
Short leg	All unstable distal lower extremity injuries (distal tibia/fibula fractures)	Ankle at 90°	Posterior short leg with stirrup splint
Knee/posterior long leg	Distal femur fractures, knee injuries, and proximal tibia and fibula fractures	Knee in extension	Posterior proximal leg to 3 inches above the malleoli. Extend to include short leg splint if indicated

	For calcaneus fractures, provide significantly extra padding to calcaneus (bulky Jones)
	Use three separate layers of plaster to cover lateral, dorsal, and medial sides
	Commercial velcro knee immobilizers are superior to these splints

PEARLS

- Hang the extremity using finger/toe traps to have easy access to all sides of the extremity.
- Prepare all materials at appropriate length before starting the procedure.
- Perform a complete and thorough neurovascular examination before and after splinting.
- Elevate the extremity to reduce swelling, pain, and risk of neurovascular compression.
- Assess for open fracture before splinting.

SUGGESTED READINGS

Boyd A, Benjamin H, Asplund C. Splints and casts: indications and methods. *Am Fam Physician*. 2009;80(5):491-499.

Denq W, Delasobera EM. SplintER series: splint principles 101. *AliEM*. September 19, 2017. https://www.aliem.com/splinter-series-splint-principles-101/

Denq W, Hockstein M. SplintER series: common ED splint techniques 104. *AliEM*. July 4, 2018. https://www.aliem.com/splinter-series-104/

Hockstein M, Denq W. SplintER series: splint application principles 102. *AliEM*. November 20, 2017. https://www.aliem.com/splinter-series-splint-application-principles-102/

Ross RI. *Splinting techniques*. Emergency Medicine Residents' Association. Accessed December 29, 2022. https://www.emra.org/globalassets/emra/publications/reference-cards/emra_sportsmedicine_splint_guide.pdf

282

CHEST TUBE PLACEMENT IN THE PATIENTS WHO ARE OBESE

NEIL A. RAY AND ANTHONY J. NASTASI

Chest tube placement is most commonly used for patients with a large pneumothorax, pleural effusion, or hemothorax, as a way to relieve the pressure on the cardiopulmonary system. While potentially lifesaving, it is one of the most invasive and painful procedures performed in the ED. For that reason, it is essential to be familiar with both the procedures and how to troubleshoot in patients who may have a higher risk of complications—such as the patients who are obese.

Nearly a third of ED patients are obese, and while that proportion varies by region, at least some of these patients will require a chest tube. The general procedure and approach are largely the same compared to patients who are lean, but performing the procedure on patients who are obese carries a higher complication rate and requires extra attention to preparation and setup.

CONTRAINDICATIONS AND COMPLICATIONS

There are no absolute contraindications, but relative contraindications include bleeding conditions (such as coagulopathy or anticoagulation), pleural abnormalities (such as pleurodesis, prior pulmonary surgery, or multiple pleural adhesions), and skin infection overlying the insertion site. Correction of coagulopathy should strongly be considered when possible.

Complications of chest tube placement include tube malposition, as well as bleeding, reexpansion pulmonary edema (most often with removal of >1.5 L of fluid), iatrogenic injury (eg, to the lung, heart, esophagus, mediastinum, diaphragm, and intra-abdominal organs), and downstream infection.

SETUP

Chest tube insertion in any patient begins with careful preparation and setup but is especially important for patients who are obese. This begins with careful identification of chest tube needs, typically based on the patient's clinical picture and radiography. Chest radiographs may have poor penetration in patients who are obese, making them harder to meaningfully interpret.

Patient positioning is important for patients who are obese as redundant soft tissue and increased adipose and subcutaneous tissue can impede easy intrathoracic access. The patient should be supine and up to 60° semi-upright to allow the diaphragm to lower with gravity. This reduces both risk of injury and aspiration risk if using sedation, which is higher in patients who are obese. Secure the ipsilateral arm above the patient's head. Place padding like a rolled blanket or towel underneath the patient's shoulder for elevation to minimize the redundant soft tissue to drape into the intended access site. A helper can manipulate soft tissue or use tape to secure the tissue out of the way of your incision site.

Adequate analgesia is essential. Patients should receive both systemic analgesia, such as intravenous opioids or NSAIDs, and liberal local anesthetic at the planned incision site and tube trajectory. The maximum dose of subcutaneous lidocaine is 5 mg/kg ideal body weight, and 7 mg/kg for lidocaine with epinephrine. Procedural sedation is another great adjunct in conscious patients, keeping in mind the increased risk of sedation-related complications in patients who are obese including apnea, desaturation, and obstruction.

TECHNIQUE

Traditional chest tubes are preferred over pigtail catheters, as pigtails have been associated with drainage failure in this population. For insertion site selection, the British Thoracic Society has outlined a "triangle of safety" delineated by the anterior border of the latissimus dorsi, lateral border of the pectoralis major, and an imagined horizontal line at the nipple (can use inframammary fold in those with breasts). The most common incision misplacement is too far caudally. These specific landmarks can be difficult to identify in patients who are obese, as well as those with darker skin tones, so excellent lighting and a thorough physical exam identifying these landmarks in advance are helpful.

The first step is to prepare the entire ipsilateral chest, leaving the axilla, midline chest, and costal margin visible after draping. Make an adequate incision of at least 2 cm, possibly larger in more patients who are obese. Larger incisions are usually required to accommodate digital guidance of the tube through the subcutaneous tissue. Dissect the fat and subcutaneous tissue with a curved Kelly clamp. To avoid the neurovascular bundle, go immediately above the rib, traditionally between the fourth and fifth intercostal space. Visual inspection alone is likely not possible in patients who are obese, so rely on tactile confirmation and guidance throughout the procedure. It is key to use your nondominant hand to guide and provide the tactile feedback of the clamp tapping the rib. Once you meet the parietal pleura resistance, close the clamp and apply axial pressure to puncture through. Open the clamp before removing it to widen the pleural hole, replacing the clamp with your finger. Removing the finger prematurely can cause loss of the subcutaneous tract. Insert the chest tube superoposteriorly, twisting the tube as you insert to prevent tube kinking.

The ideal depth is when the sentinel hole is inside the pleural space. Measurements on the tube begin at the sentinel hole. Most adults require about 10 cm, but patients who are obese may need deeper insertion. Inserting too far risks nearby organ injury. Chest tube size is the same as in patients who are lean. Attach the tube to a chest drainage system, and secure the tube with a number 1 or 0 silk/nylon suture. Cover tube with gauze and tape. Obtain a chest x-ray for confirmation of appropriate tube positioning.

PEARLS

- Patients who are obese make up a large portion of ED patients and insertion of chest tubes in these patients is often technically more challenging with higher complication rates.
- Chest tube insertion in patients who are obese is largely the same as in patients who are lean but requires additional attention to preparation and setup.
- Additional measures to consider include excellent lighting, semi-upright positioning, soft tissue manipulation and positioning, elevating the patient to avoid redundant tissue impeding access, and heavy utilization of tactile feedback throughout the procedure from site selection to tube insertion.
- Remember the limitations of chest radiographs in patients who are obese and the additional risks of procedural sedation.
- Tubes may need to be inserted further in patients who are obese compared to patients who are lean, but avoid over-insertion and its associated risks.

Suggested Readings

Dev SP, Nascimiento B Jr, Simone C, Chien V. Videos in clinical medicine. Chest-tube insertion. *N Engl J Med*. 2007;357(15):e15.

Kirsch T, Sax J. Tube thoracostomy. In: *Roberts and Hedges' Clinical Procedures in Emergency Medicine*. 6th ed. Saunders; 2013:189-211.

Laws D, Neville E, Duffy J; Pleural Diseases Group, Standards of Care Committee, British Thoracic Society. BTS guidelines for the insertion of a chest drain. *Thorax*. 2003;58(2 suppl 2):ii53-ii59.

283

Pitfalls in US-Guided IV Placement

Kevin J. Flanagan and Sarah Sommerkamp

PIV placement is among the most common invasive procedures in the ED. Traditional landmark-based PIV placement depends on visible or palpable veins and may be complicated by many factors (eg, body habitus and chronic comorbidities). Difficulty with PIV access can cause significant delays in patient care. When required, alternatives to failed PIV placement include consultation with a vascular access service, insertion of a CVC, or USGPIV placement. USGPIVs have improved safety and minimized complication profiles when compared to CVCs. Thorough consideration of the target vein, procedural preparation, and mechanics will offer emergency clinicians the best chance of procedural success.

Pitfalls in Selecting a Target Vein

It is important to choose an appropriate vein. Some factors to consider include vein depth, available IV catheter length, vessel diameter, tortuosity, and proximity to nearby neurovascular structures. In general, deeper veins are more difficult and require a longer catheter. Catheters with insufficient residual length within the vessel are at greater risk of dislodgement. Ideal vessels have a larger diameter (preferably >0.4 cm) and shallower depth (<2.5 cm). Vessel segments with observed tortuosity, proximal bifurcations, internal valves, or surrounding neurovascular structures should be avoided, if possible.

While the antecubital veins are commonly visible on ultrasound, this location is suboptimal because of the patient's arm movement and "kinking" of the catheter. Forearm veins, though smaller, are a favorite location for ultrasonographers as they are frequently superficial and straight. The basilic and brachial veins are also common targets. The basilic vein is preferred as it does not run adjacent to the artery. The ideal vessel is patient-specific and requires surveying of the individual's arm.

Please note that USGPIVs are not always the best or most efficient line. Less commonly accessed veins like EJ or those of the lower extremity, when visible, have similar success rates to USGPIV placement and do not require the setup time associated with ultrasound. When vessels are visible, the landmark approach is the preferred method to obtain PIV access.

Pitfalls in Procedural Preparation

Inadequate preparation before attempting USGPIV can result in multiple procedural interruptions and poor outcomes. Preparation includes ultrasound machine and patient positioning, skin sterilization, and infection prevention measures. The ultrasound must be positioned, so the ultrasonographer has enough space to access and view the arm for probe and ultrasound manipulation. The probe must be oriented, so the probe marker aligns with the corresponding direction on screen to avoid misdirection while advancing the needle. Special care to avoid contamination of the insertion site should always be taken. This includes wiping the linear probe with a towel followed by the appropriate cleaner, using a barrier like a transparent film dressing over the probe, and utilizing single-use sterile ultrasound gel packets. Preparation also includes ensuring appropriate IV catheters are available for USGPIV placement. A minimum of 1.88-inch catheter is suggested to reduce the risk of decannulation.

PITFALLS IN PROCEDURAL MECHANICS

Even after all the above preparations are completed, the ultrasonographer should be ready to encounter several common pitfalls during USGPIV placement. While both short-axis (ie, cross-sectional) and long-axis (ie, longitudinal) approaches can be used, higher success rates have been observed by those using a short-axis orientation. One common challenge is venous collapse. Clinicians should maintain only light pressure from the probe to prevent accidental vein compression. A proximal tourniquet is helpful to decrease collapsibility. A blood pressure cuff inflated to 150 mm Hg has been identified as superior to the tourniquet but is larger and occupies the area frequently used for cannulation of the basilic and brachial veins.

Failure to center the needle or anticipate the correct needle trajectory are additional common pitfalls. Centering the needle may be accomplished by placing the probe over the needle without piercing the skin and seeing a ring-down artifact. Correct trajectory can be estimated by visualizing a 45° right triangle to approximate the point of insertion that will reach the target vessel at the desired location and with the correct angle for penetration and catheterization (**Figure 283.1**). The probe and needle should then be set up at this location for insertion.

Simultaneous movement of both the needle and probe increases the risk an operator will lose visualization of the needle tip. Once the needle is inserted into the skin, immediately appreciate the bright hyperechoic dot that represents the needle tip and stop advancing the needle. Then advance the probe alone until the needle is no

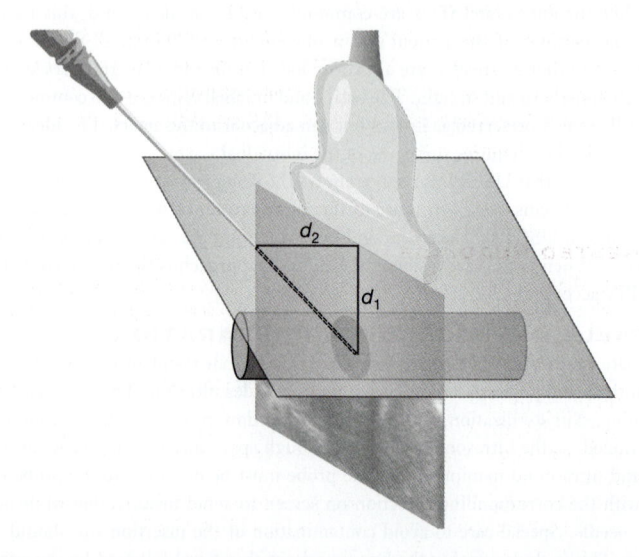

FIGURE 283.1 Approximating point of insertion. Depth of target vessel (d_1); distance from probe of needle insertion (d_2). d_1-d_2.

longer seen. Once the needle disappears stop moving the probe and begin moving the needle again until just the tip is visualized. Only one hand should be moving at a time. Continue this approach with small adjustments as needed to direct the needle into the vessel. The ultimate goal is to visualize the needle in the vessel, forming a target sign. Consider advancing the needle further into the vessel, which will ensure it is not just tenting the anterior wall.

PITFALLS IN CONFIRMATION OF PROCEDURAL SUCCESS

Clinicians should not depend on the flash to predict correct placement of the PIV. A hematoma from initial vessel puncture may cause a falsely reassuring and premature flash. The flash may initially be falsely absent as it can take a long time to reach the visible area of the long needle, causing clinicians to overshoot the vessel. The catheter should not meet significant resistance to advancement in an appropriately placed PIV. Blood draws and saline flushes should both be easy in a properly placed line.

Ultrasound can be used to confirm placement. Using the same probe, place the window immediately proximal to the anticipated end of the catheter and, using an agitated flush, inject the sterile saline into the vessel. A moment of hyperechoic flash should highlight the proximal vein confirming correct placement. Hypoechoic enlargement around the vessel would instead represent a failed attempt and access will need to be reattempted at a more proximal site. Securing the IV is crucial as the ultrasound gel must be removed to adequately attach the transparent film dressing.

PEARLS

- Choose a vessel that is large in diameter, not too deep, straight, and ideally separated from any artery or nerve.
- Ensure catheter is at least 1.88 inches in length to minimize risk of decannulation.
- Check that the probe marker corresponds to the correct direction on the screen.
- Use a gradual step-wise method wherein only one hand moves at a time.
- Look for the "target sign" as the indication of successful placement, and confirm with agitated saline and ultrasound if needed.

SUGGESTED READINGS

Mahler SA, Wang H, Lester C, Skinner J, Arnold TC, Conrad SA. Short- vs long-axis approach to ultrasound-guided peripheral intravenous access: a prospective randomized study. *Am J Emerg Med*. 2011;29(9):1194-1197.

McCarthy ML, Shokoohi H, Boniface KS, et al. Ultrasonography versus landmark for peripheral intravenous cannulation: a randomized controlled trial. *Ann Emerg Med*.2016;68(1):10-18.

Rose JS, Sylvester PJ, Abo AM. Vascular access. In: Ma O, Mateer JR, Reardon RF, Byars DV, Knapp BJ, Laudenbach AP, eds. *Ma and Mateer's Emergency Ultrasound*. 4th ed. McGraw Hill; 2021.

Shokoohi H, Armstrong P, Tansek R. Emergency department ultrasound probe infection control: challenges and solutions. *Open Access Emerg Med*. 2015;7:1-9.

284

LIFESAVING PROCEDURES IN AN AUSTERE ENVIRONMENT

ANNE WALKER AND LISA TENORIO

Although we hope to never have to perform lifesaving interventions in remote and unfamiliar terrain, it is important to be equipped and able to handle life-threatening medical emergencies in austere environments. We focus on three topics that can change the course of a wilderness resuscitation: airway management, FT, and hemorrhage control.

AIRWAY MANAGEMENT

In a backcountry environment, the most common cause of airway compromise is trauma. If safe, the conscious patient should be allowed to sit up to better protect their own airway. For an unconscious patient breathing spontaneously, preferentially perform a jaw thrust. Deciding to move forward with intubation is a major commitment. Once intubated, the patient will likely require 24-hour ventilatory support until reaching definitive care. A supraglottic device such as an LMA may also be used. While an LMA is simpler to place and does not require airway visualization, it does not reliably protect against the aspiration of gastric contents. Many newer LMAs allow for a bougie to pass through the tube, making later exchange of the LMA for an endotracheal tube possible. If equipment is malfunctioning or not available, digital intubation can be performed by using a finger to palpate the glottic fold.

Cricothyrotomy is usually performed as a last resort or after failed endotracheal intubation. There can be, however, indications to proceed directly with cricothyrotomy (eg, airway obstruction, significant facial trauma, unclearable vomiting/hemorrhage, edema, trismus).

If there is time, clean the neck and subcutaneously inject lidocaine with epinephrine in the anterior neck to mitigate bleeding upon incision. Palpate landmarks using the "tracheal handshake," with the nondominant thumb and middle finger, grab the trachea and palpate the cricothyroid membrane with the index finger. Identify the thyroid cartilage superiorly and the cricoid cartilage inferiorly by either starting at the manubrium and walking the index finger upward or by starting at the laryngeal prominence, representing the thyroid cartilage, and walking downward. Make a vertical midline incision with a scalpel (or pocket knife), followed by a horizontal stab incision through the anterior membrane. Insert a bougie, stylet, or tube into the airway. Pass a 6-0 or 6-5 ET tube over the bougie until the balloon is just out of sight, then inflate the balloon. If using improvised tubing, secure with tape and mark the tube at the appropriate skin location to monitor for dislodgement.

FINGER THORACOSTOMY

Any serious blunt or penetrating thoracic trauma may cause a TPX, in which a continuous leakage of air into the potential space between the visceral and parietal pleura progressively collapses the lung and mediastinum. If not treated within minutes, cardiac arrest may ensue. Once a TPX is identified (unequal chest rise, unilateral lung sounds with unstable vitals, tracheal deviation), plan for pleural decompression—either by NT or FT. Although NT is faster to perform, FT is not limited by needle length or bore size and allows for visual and tactile confirmation of the parietal pleura. Additionally, there is no chance of catheter "kinking" or traveling along the subcutaneous tissue.

Identifying landmarks is essential in FT. If too low, you risk entering the peritoneal cavity. If too high, you could cause damage to the brachial plexus or axillary vasculature. The ideal location is the fourth or fifth ICS at the mid or anterior axillary line. After identifying your preferred ICS, confirm visually and by palpation that it is above the level of the xiphoid process to ensure you are indeed in the thoracic cavity. If time allows, prep the skin with betadine or chlorhexidine. Palpate the landmark previously identified, just superior to the rib. It is critical to avoid the neurovascular bundle traveling along the inferior aspect of each rib. Using a scalpel or blade, make a generous incision spanning the ICS. Using a closed Kelly clamp, hemostat, needle driver, or your finger, slide over the superior aspect of the inferior rib and puncture the pleura. Open the instrument to stretch the pleural tissue. Using a single finger, palpate the inner border of the rib and assess for lung expansion.

Ideally, a chest tube would be placed following this procedure as the hole may seal off during prolonged transit. If no chest tube is placed, a commercial chest seal or a dressing occluded on three sides can be the next best option. Contraindications to FT can be localized trauma (rib fractures), which could increase the risk of injury to the rescuer by sharp bone fragments.

Hemorrhage Control

In an austere environment, it is important to address major bleeds early. Control of massive hemorrhage with tourniquets, hemostatic dressings, and pelvic binding can prevent adverse outcomes. The first step to control bleeding is to apply direct manual pressure to the area for 3 to 5 minutes. A pressure dressing, a tightly wrapped, small, folded piece of gauze directly over the bleeding site, is also an option. Hemostatic products should be used in noncompressible sites but can also be used in extremity wounds. These products come in various forms, such as gauze, granules, or wafer, for different wound types/shapes. Having at least two different forms of hemostatic products in a wilderness first aid kit is ideal.

A tourniquet should be used if direct pressure is unsuccessful or if there is massive extremity hemorrhage. Place the tourniquet 2 to 3 inches above the site of bleeding, avoiding a joint. Tighten by turning the windlass until distal pulse is absent and secure. Use multiple tourniquets if needed. An improvised tourniquet can be created with any piece of clothing or material. Wider material is safer and more effective. Most importantly, create a windlass. A pen, pencil, stick, pole, or other stiff object is placed through the knot, cranked down, and secured. Controlled bleeding can be checked by slowly releasing the tourniquet if it has been present for less than 2 hours. If more than 2 hours, it should not be removed until in a hospital setting due to theoretical risk of releasing metabolic acidosis and hyperkalemia.

Internal bleeding from a pelvic fracture should be suspected with any fall from height or if the patient is endorsing pain near the pelvic area. In wilderness settings, the physical exam can be unreliable, and rocking the pelvis can worsen bleeding. Thus, if there is any suspicion of pelvic fracture, apply a pelvic binder. This can help approximate the bony fragments, allowing for better hemostasis and preventing vessel rupture by sharp bony fragments—primarily to the sacral venous plexus. If a commercial pelvic binder is unavailable, a sheet, piece of clothing, poncho, or sleeping bag can be used along with a windlass to tighten and secure. It should be centered over the greater trochanters.

PEARLS

- Cricothyrotomy should be considered more readily in an austere environment.
- FT requires minimal equipment and is more reliable than NT.
- Hemostasis by direct pressure, hemostatic dressings, tourniquet placement, or fracture reduction are vital techniques to prevent a patient who has experienced trauma from going into shock.
- Maintain a low threshold to suspect pelvic fracture. Pelvic binders may be lifesaving.
- Anticipate what can be used as an improvised tourniquet or pelvic binder, but remember that the windlass is the most important aspect.

SUGGESTED READINGS

Bennett BL, Christensen R. TCCC chest trauma guideline update: tension pneumothorax. *Wilderness Medicine Magazine*. 2022;39(1). https://wms.org/magazine/magazine/1336/TCCC-chest-trauma-guideline-update/default.aspx

Littlejohn LF. Treatment of thoracic trauma: lessons from the battlefield adapted to all austere environments. *Wilderness Environ Med*. 2017;28(2S):S69-S73.

285

SHUNT TAP: TRICKS OF THE TRADE

RICCARDO SERRO AND WAN-TSU W. CHANG

HC is typically defined as an imbalance between CSF production and reabsorption, leading to either an increase in ICP or CSF accumulation. While congenital HC is less common than iNPH, the treatments available vary little between the pediatric and adult populations. Diversion of CSF to other body cavities was first suggested in 1908 using rubber conduits to "shunt" fluid from the lateral ventricles to the superior sagittal sinus and peritoneum, respectively. Lumbo-peritoneal, ventriculo-pleural, and ventriculo-ureteral shunts were popularized in the 1920s, while the first ventriculoatrial CSF diversion was performed in 1952.

SHUNT SYSTEM

All shunt systems are comprised of three essential parts:

1) *Proximal shunt catheter*. This is made of silicone, either non-, silver- or antibiotic-impregnated, and drains CSF from a cerebral ventricle or subarachnoid cistern. Of note, recent variations use Teflon-derived polymers to decrease the rates of obstruction and film formation. Common designs include 32 side holes.
2) *Pressure or flow-sensitive shunt valve*. Since 1956, when the first mechanical Holter-Spitz slit valve was implanted in children with obstructive HC, several fixed and adjustable

valves have been developed and introduced into clinical practice. Programmable valves, such as Strata (Medtronic) and Certas (Integra Codman), are among the most popular shunt valves currently in use. Fixed-pressure valves are nonetheless still common, especially in systems implanted before the advent of programmable shunts and in resource-limited settings. All valves have a reservoir chamber.

3) *Distal tubing*. This is usually composed of non-impregnated or antibiotic-impregnated silicone and tunneled from the shunt valve to the target cavity (peritoneum, pleura, or atrium) and ends with a millimeter-wide hole at the catheter tip.

A functional shunt, therefore, drains CSF from the cerebral ventricles or subarachnoid space to another body cavity, allowing for variable flow that is constantly influenced by several factors. Among them, rate of CSF production, absorption capacity of the target body cavity, valve setting, as well as body position and habitus, have a prominent role in the ability of these systems to effectively relieve ICPs.

Causes of Shunt Failure

Despite several advancements in valve/catheter design and operative care, these systems still experience frequent malfunction and failure, with a rate of approximately 40% at the 5-year mark. Congenital and obstructive HC are the most common factors that predispose shunt failure, with the age of the first surgery being inversely related to the risk of shunt replacement. Infections are also a significant cause of shunt replacement, with *Staphylococcus epidermidis*, *Staphylococcus aureus*, and gram-negative rods being the most commonly detected organisms.

The clinical presentation of shunt failure varies. It can range from obvious HC (with changes in mental status, nausea/vomiting, etc) to more subtle signs such as changes in bowel/urinary habits, lethargy, or irritability. Fever may occur in cases of shunt infections. This variation makes the diagnosis of malfunctioning shunt systems particularly challenging. It requires a systematic approach that incorporates imaging, clinical assessment, laboratory tests, and neurologic evaluation.

Workup of Shunt Failure

Workup of shunt failure begins with a thorough history, including symptoms, confirmation of valve type, setting, previous complications/revisions, and the proximal and distal location. Physical examination should include fundoscopic evaluation to assess for papilledema as a sign of increased cerebral pressure before shunt tapping. Laboratory analyses include screening labs and inflammatory indexes. Imaging workup revolves around ventricular size, shape, intraventricular/parenchymal blood, shunt and valve position. This can be acquired via head CT without contrast or, in pediatric patients, with brain MRI. Before and after MRI, it is vital to check and reset programmable valves to their intended level. Radiographs of the head, neck, chest, and abdomen will also provide important information about the system's integrity, valve model, and setting (radiograph examples of common valves are available online). Abdominal CT can sometimes help in distal failures to investigate the presence of a pseudocyst. After imaging workup, the shunt can be pumped to assess for early refilling of the valve chamber.

To avoid iatrogenic shunt obstruction, tapping should only be performed after imaging evaluation of ventricular size and catheter position in relation to the ependymal layer and brain tissue. Tapping is safe to perform if the ventricles are not slit-like and the catheter's tip is not lying in the proximity of the ependyma/brain matter. Of note, in communicating HC a lumbar puncture should be attempted to preserve shunt sterility and obtain a CSF sample.

Finally, it is important to be aware that while "positive" results (ie, no CSF obtained from the tap) have a high positive predictive value, a "negative" tap does not reliably exclude the possibility of shunt failure.

Shunt Tap—Considerations and Steps

- **Supplies**
    - Chlorhexidine wash
    - Isopropyl alcohol
    - Iodine (Duraprep, 3M)
    - 25G butterfly needle
    - 4×4 gauzes
    - OR towels
    - Gloves
    - Three-way stopcock
    - 5-mL syringe
    - 5-mL tube
    - Extension tube
    - Manometer
- **Technique**
    - Shave the scalp overlying the valve reservoir and disinfect the overlying skin widely.
    - Topical anesthetics such as lidocaine cream or 1% lidocaine can be applied to the skin.
    - Drape the valve reservoir with blue towel, leaving only the access point uncovered.
    - Connect the 25G butterfly needle via a plastic extension to a three-way stopcock and manometer open to the patient. A 5-mL syringe can also be attached to the stopcock.
    - Tap the valve reservoir using the 25G butterfly needle. Gentle backpressure can be applied to the syringe. If CSF return is spontaneous or under 1 cm^3 of negative pressure, the tap is considered to have good flow. On the other hand, if the tap necessitates lower pressure (up to 2-3 cm^3 of negative pressure) or if no CSF is obtained, the tap is considered to have poor flow.

Opening pressure can be measured by leveling the base of the manometer at the tragus in the supine position. It is important that the patient is not in pain, uncomfortable, or performing a Valsalva maneuver during this measurement. Distal shunt flow can be assessed by finding the proximal catheter and compressing it to prevent backflow into the ventricles. This lets CSF flow distally toward the absorption site (peritoneum, atrium, etc) and allows to measure a distal opening pressure. Finally, CSF can be sampled for lab analysis and tested for xanthochromia, cell count, protein and glucose concentration, Gram stain, culture, and other parameters based on clinical evaluation.

Complications are possible while performing a shunt tap. CSF over drainage, ventricular collapse, and catheter/valve occlusion by choroid/ependyma aspiration are rare events. The most feared complication of a shunt tap is certainly CSF infection. To prevent this occurrence, careful antisepsis must be performed before the procedure, and sterility must be maintained throughout the tap.

> **PEARLS**
>
> - Obstruction, disconnection, and infection are the most common etiologies of shunt failure.
> - Exhaustive clinical, laboratory, and radiographic evaluation must be carried out before pumping the valve reservoir and considering a shunt tap.
> - Neurosurgery should be involved to facilitate the shunt workup and perform the tap. Emergent tapping can be carried out using a 25G needle, assuming a valve or distal catheter failure and a patent proximal catheter.
> - Manometry and CSF collection play a pivotal role in shunt failure workup. Consider performing a lumbar tap in communicating HC if concerned for CSF infection.

Suggested Readings

Iskandar BJ, McLaughlin C, Mapstone TB, Grabb PA, Oakes WJ. Pitfalls in the diagnosis of ventricular shunt dysfunction: radiology reports and ventricular size. *Pediatrics*. 1998;101:1031-1036.

Mihalj M, Dolić K, Kolić K, Ledenko V. CSF tap test—obsolete or appropriate test for predicting shunt responsiveness? A systemic review. *J Neurol Sci*. 2016;362:78-84.

Paff M, Alexandru-Abrams D, Muhonen M, Loudon W. Ventriculoperitoneal shunt complications: a review. *Interdisc Neurosurg*. 2018;13:66-70.

286

Tips and Tricks for the Bedside Hip Reduction in the Emergency Room

Nikita Paripati and Mei Ling Liu

Hip dislocations are common and time-sensitive orthopedic injuries. Young patients typically present after high-energy trauma, while older patients and those with prosthetic hips may experience dislocation after low-energy trauma. Approximately 90% of dislocations are posterior. Timely bedside reduction reduces the risk of sciatic nerve injury and avascular necrosis. However, bedside reduction is challenging and typically requires procedural sedation. Other complications include femoral head osteonecrosis, posttraumatic arthritis, and recurrent dislocations. Familiarity with techniques and pitfalls is crucial for performing a bedside hip reduction.

Physical Examination

When assessing patients with a suspected hip dislocation, a thorough physical examination is essential to determine the extent of injury. In posterior dislocations, the leg is shortened, adducted, and internally rotated. In anterior dislocation, the leg is extended (superior) or flexed (inferior), abducted, and externally rotated. Perform a thorough skin and neurovascular examination checking pulses, strength, sensation, and skin integrity. Evaluate for signs of compartment syndrome and specifically assess for sciatic nerve damage, such as sensory deficits on the lateral leg and foot or weakness with ankle dorsiflexion. An open dislocation, indicated by a skin break, requires urgent antibiotic administration to reduce risk of infection.

DIAGNOSTIC TESTS

To evaluate for posterior versus anterior dislocation, obtain AP and lateral view hip radiographs. Also, obtain radiographic imaging of the knee to assess for injury below the joint. In a posterior dislocation, the femoral head will appear smaller than the contralateral femoral head, whereas in an anterior dislocation, it will appear larger. On an AP view for posterior dislocations, the femoral head is posterior and superior to the acetabulum, while for anterior dislocations, it is medial or inferior to the acetabulum. If there is evidence of a femoral head, neck, or acetabular fracture, consult orthopedic surgery for open reduction. Obtain a postreduction CT scan of the hip to evaluate for acetabular fractures and retained bony fragments that may be difficult to detect on plain films. Up to 70% of patients may have an associated acetabular fracture, and 33% may have loose intra-articular bodies post-injury.

PROCEDURAL SEDATION

There are various approaches to procedural sedation, but the key components are ensuring adequate sedation, pain control, and muscle relaxation. Consider concomitant use of an analgesic agent. Fentanyl is often ideal due to its rapid onset and short duration of action. Common sedative options include benzodiazepines, etomidate, propofol, or ketamine. Literature has shown success with propofol alone due to muscle relaxation or the combination of ketamine + propofol ("ketofol"). Etomidate can theoretically cause myoclonus which would be less preferred during an orthopedic reduction. Intra-articular and hematoma blocks can be used as local analgesia but may be inadequate for achieving muscle relaxation. Moderate sedation is generally sufficient to safely reduce a hip; however, consider deep sedation or general anesthesia in the subset of patients whose hip has been dislocated for greater than 6 hours. Consider OR reduction for pregnant and geriatric patients.

REDUCTION TECHNIQUE

When deciding on the appropriate reduction technique for a posterior hip dislocation, consider the number of assistants available, clinician comfort, extent of the patient's injury, and optimal patient positioning. No single technique has been demonstrated to have superior efficacy compared to others (**Table 286.1**). Excessive strain on the lower leg during these maneuvers can potentially cause ligamentous injury to the knee or fibular fractures.

The Allis technique is a well-established reduction maneuver for posterior hip dislocations. Position the patient supine with both the hip and knee flexed to 90°. This technique often requires an assistant who applies downward pressure on the pelvis. The clinician should then apply traction toward the ceiling while gently internally and externally rotating the leg. The disadvantages of this technique include difficult positioning for the clinician if they are standing on the bed, which increases the risk of lower back injury and/or falling.

TABLE 286.1 PATIENT POSITIONING AND TECHNIQUE

NAME	PATIENT POSITIONING	TECHNIQUE	NUMBER OF PEOPLE NEEDED	ADVANTAGES	DISADVANTAGES
Allis	Supine	Assistant stabilizes pelvis against the bed. Clinician grasps affected proximal tibia and pulls upward applying traction toward the ceiling.	1–2		Risk of fall, injury to lower back
Captain Morgan	Supine on a backboard	Clinician places their knee underneath patient's affected knee. They then plantar flex/lift knee while simultaneously pushing patient's ankle downward.	1	Requires only one clinician	Difficult in patients with long legs
Whistler	Supine w/both knees flexed	Clinician places arm under patient's affected knee with palm extending onto unaffected knee. This arm acts as a lever while the provider's arm applies downward pressure on the ankle.	1	Requires only one clinician	Possible injury to clinician's forearm
East Baltimore Lift	Supine	Two clinicians place their arms underneath the patient's knees with their hands on each other's shoulders. Clinicians slowly stand up while a third clinician holds countertraction to patient's ankles.	2	Controlled, steady reduction	Multiple clinicians needed
Lefkowitz	Supine	Clinician uses their knee as a fulcrum under the affected leg and applies downward force on the patient's lower leg.	1	Requires only one clinician; controlled, steady reduction	Can cause injury to patient's knee

After successful reduction, place a pillow between the patient's legs to maintain abduction position. Subsequently, place the patient in either a knee immobilizer or hip abduction brace if available. Generally, the patient may be discharged home after appropriate reduction if there are no other associated injuries. Ensure the patient has a clear understanding of dislocation precautions. Patients should follow toe touch weight bearing on the injured leg, avoid bending the hip past 90°, crossing midline, and internal rotation.

When to involve orthopedics:

1) If there is evidence of a femoral head, neck, or acetabular fracture
2) If unable to reduce hip despite two attempts
3) If there is a neurovascular deficit upon presentation and postreduction
4) If a patient presents more than 6 hours after dislocation
5) Prosthetic hip joint (especially if recent surgery)

PEARLS

- Perform reduction *within 6 hours* to prevent avascular necrosis in native hip dislocations.
- Obtain a postreduction CT for *all* native hip dislocations to identify common concomitant injuries (eg, acetabular fractures).
- For prosthetic hips, the femoral head is no longer present and the urgency of reduction is based primarily on pain control and extent of other injuries.
- Choose a reduction technique based on the patient's injuries and number of available assistants. More than one technique may be attempted.

Suggested Readings

Dela Cruz JE, Sullivan DN, Varboncouer E, et al. Comparison of procedural sedation for the reduction of dislocated total hip arthroplasty. *West J Emerg Med*. 2014;15(1):76-80.

Frymann SJ, Cumberbatch GLA, Stearman ASL. Reduction of dislocated hip prosthesis in the emergency department using conscious sedation: a prospective study. *Emerg Med J*. 2005;22(11):807-809.

Gottlieb M. Hip dislocations in the emergency department: a review of reduction techniques. *J Emerg Med*. 2018;54(3):339-347.

SECTION XXIII
PEDIATRICS

287

RECOGNIZE CHILD ABUSE EARLY

CAROL C. CHEN

Child abuse and neglect remains a significant problem in the United States, with an estimated 618,000 children suffering from child maltreatment in 2020 and an increase in the number of related deaths by 1.2% from 2016 to 2020. Children under the age of 1 year experienced a disproportionately high victimization rate at 25.1 per 1,000.

ED visits represent missed opportunities to recognize abused children who eventually return with more serious injuries and sometimes even death. A comparison of the rates of missed abusive head trauma showed that there was no change between 1999 and 2016. This demonstrates the importance of emergency medicine physicians being able to recognize child abuse early.

Sentinel injuries are critically important to understand because they have been recognized as much more common in children who have been abused than those who have not. Sheets et al found that of 200 confirmed abused infants, 27.5% of them had had a previous sentinel injury compared to only 8% of 100 infants with an intermediate concern for abuse, and none of 101 confirmed nonabused infants. Unfortunately, there is no international consensus on a list of specific sentinel injuries; however, there are several overlapping injuries noted across different guidelines. For example, the above mentioned study found the following types of sentinel injuries in the confirmed abused cohort that is discussed in further detail later: bruising (80%), intraoral injury (11%), and fractures (7%).

When providers fail to recognize sentinel injuries during ED visits, these abused children can return as victims of escalating violence with even more severe injuries.

However, before discussing the details of sentinel injuries and how to recognize them, it is important to first point out that recognition begins with routine screening of all children who come into the ED, especially those whose chief complaint includes injury. This is in contrast to the current system of screening, which relies upon gestalt and intuition and can be riddled with subjective judgments and unconscious biases.

Clinical decision rules exist, which can help guide routine screening and identify sentinel injuries. TEN-4-FACESp is a validated bruising clinical decision rule for use in children to indicate a potential risk for abuse and those children that warrant further evaluation. It has been shown to be 96% sensitive and 87% specific for distinguishing abusive bruising from nonabusive bruising.

TEN refers to bruising in the following areas: torso (chest, abdomen, back, buttocks, genitourinary area), ears, and neck. 4 refers to the age of the child that this rule can be used for—up to 4 years for bruising in concerning locations or ANY bruising in a child younger than 4 months. Infants who have not yet begun cruising (≤4 months) are at the highest risk for abuse. FACES refers to bruising in the following areas:

- Frenulum
- Angle of the jaw
- Cheeks (fleshy part)
- Eyelids
- Subconjunctivae

p refers to patterned bruising, such as bruising that may look like fingerprints.

Additional sentinel injuries to evaluate for include intraoral injuries, such as a frenulum tear or a contusion of the tongue, fractures of the ribs, scapula, vertebrae, and sternum, as well as classic metaphyseal corner fractures of long bones. Any fracture in a nonambulatory infant and infants or toddlers with midshaft humerus or femur fractures, especially without a clear history of significant trauma or inborn risk factor, should raise the suspicion for abuse. In addition, any child who presents with multiple fractures warrants closer inspection.

Lastly, a provider should be suspicious of any injury in an infant or child that is not consistent with the patient's age or developmental stage, or that cannot be adequately explained by the caregiver.

Once a child with concerns for abuse has been identified, next steps include further evaluation, specialty referrals, and, finally, disposition from the ED. The US-specific guidance on the detailed workup of suspected abuse can be found in the AAP 2015 report "The Evaluation of Suspected Child Physical Abuse." A report to CPS is mandated of all providers who care for such a child; this requirement is not absolved by the transfer of the child to another institution to make a report. If available, consults to social work and pediatric or child abuse specialists should be made. CPS can often assist with deciding if a child is safe to be discharged from the ED and with which family or community member. However, if there is any doubt or further concerns about a child's safety, they can be admitted to a pediatric ward for further evaluation and disposition.

PEARLS

- ED visits represent critical, often-missed opportunities to recognize child abuse earlier and avoid escalating violence and even death.
- The use of a standard screening protocol rather than clinical gestalt or other subjective judgments to identify infants and children at highest risk for abuse will result in less missed cases and avoid biases.
- Sentinel injuries are common among abused infants and children (vs nonabused children) and include certain types of bruising, intraoral injuries, and specific fracture patterns.
- The TEN-4-FACESp bruising clinical decision rule has very good sensitivity and specificity for identifying which children should undergo additional evaluation for potential abuse.
- Any concerns or evaluation for potential child abuse should be reported and additional resources activated.

SUGGESTED READINGS

Berger RP, Lindberg DM. Early recognition of physical abuse: bridging the gap between knowledge and practice. *J Pediatr*. 2019;204:16-23.

Christian CW, Committee on Child Abuse and Neglect, American Academy of Pediatrics. The evaluation of suspected child physical abuse. *Pediatrics*. 2015;135:e1337-e1354.

Pierce MC, Kaczor K, Lorenz DJ, Bertocci G, Fingarson AK, Makoroff K. Validation of a clinical decision rule to predict abuse in young children based on bruising characteristics. *JAMA Netw Open*. 2021;4(4):e215832.

Sheets LK, Leach ME, Koszewski IJ, Lessmeier AM, Nugent M, Simpson P. Sentinel injuries in infants evaluated for child physical abuse. *Pediatrics*. 2013;131:701-707.

US Department of Health and Human Services, Administration for Children and Families, Administration on Children, Youth and Families, Children's Bureau. Child maltreatment; 2020. Accessed December 14, 2022. https://www.acf.hhs.gov/cb/report/child-maltreatment-2020

288

KEEP THE BABY WARM! AND OTHER STEPS IN NEONATAL RESUSCITATION

CAROLINE BURKE AND HEIDI WERNER

The delivery of a newborn in the ED is usually unplanned and can be wrought with chaos. Current neonatal resuscitation guidelines target situations in a labor and delivery unit with reliable equipment, specially trained staff, and a controlled environment. Deliveries in the ED, in contrast, often occur without specialized clinical teams or equipment available. This presents a unique set of challenges when resuscitating the newly born in the ED, and emergency providers need to be trained to handle these situations.

BASIC RESUSCITATION

Approximately 10% of newborns will require basic resuscitation after birth, and providers should be prepared when a delivery occurs. Designate team members focused on neonatal resuscitation. Gather basic supplies including warm blankets, a radiant warmer, a bulb suction, a neonatal-sized bag-valve mask, and an oxygen source. Consider calling the hospital's delivery or NICU team if available.

Once the infant is born, ask three questions: *Is the baby term gestation? Is the baby breathing or crying? Do they have good tone?* If the answer to all these questions is "yes," then the baby can stay with mom, placed skin-to-skin, and dried and warmed on the mother's chest. Consider delayed cord clamping, which can have significant benefits, particularly for preterm infants including improved transitional circulation, better establishment of red blood cell volume, decreased need for blood transfusion, and lower incidence of necrotizing enterocolitis and intraventricular hemorrhage. If the answer to any of the earlier questions is "no," the baby should be brought to the warmer for further evaluation. If the gestational age is unclear, a general rule is that term infants will have wrinkles across the entire plantar surface of the foot, scrotal rugae, or touching labia majora.

Initial resuscitation consists of warming, drying, and stimulating the baby using warm blankets, to encourage the infant to cry. If the baby is still not crying, bulb suction should be used to remove secretions from the oropharynx and the nares. Reposition the airway into a "sniffing" position. HR can be checked by listening with a stethoscope, palpating the umbilical cord at the stump, or with a three-lead ECG. A normal HR is more than 100 beats/min. These initial steps should take no longer than 60 seconds. By 1 minute of life, if the baby is gasping or not crying, or if the HR is less than 100 beats/min, then PPV should be initiated after suctioning.

Once PPV has been initiated, apply an O_2 monitor to the pre-ductal (right) hand. Do not be surprised by a low oxygen saturation! Normal initial pulse oximetry on room air is 70% and gradually increases to 90% after 10 minutes of life. Breaths should be delivered at 40 to 60 breaths per minute with an inflation pressure of 20 to 25 cm H_2O. The initial delivered O_2 concentration should be room air (21%) for newborns 35 weeks gestation or more, and 21% to 30% for less than 35 weeks. 100% oxygen can be toxic for newborns and is reserved for difficult resuscitations. If there is no chest movement and increase in heart rate within 15 seconds of PPV, corrective steps including airway repositioning, mask adjustment, pressure increase, and advanced airway placement may be needed. Provide PPV until the baby is initiating breaths and the HR is more than 100 beats/min.

These steps will often result in clinical improvement, evidenced by an improved HR, tone, and respiratory effort. If not, the baby will require more advanced resuscitation.

WARMING THE BABY

Warming a baby after delivery is one of the most important steps in resuscitation, but it can be difficult given the rapid nature of ED deliveries. Delivery rooms are typically 26 °C (78 °F), much warmer than the typical ED! Cold neonates can be more difficult to resuscitate, and initial measures may not be successful in the setting of hypothermia (<36.5 °C). Fortunately, there are many practical ways to warm infants in limited resource settings.

Every ED should have a radiant warmer available, which should be turned on in preparation as soon as you expect a delivery. Warm blankets should be available immediately after delivery and used to dry the infant. Placing the child skin-to-skin with the mother for the resuscitation is another technique often used in resource-limited settings.

Premature infants can be even more difficult to keep warm due to their immature body systems and increased heat losses. Infants less than 32 weeks, or weighing less than 1,500 g (~3.5 lb), should receive additional means of warmth by immediately being placed in a plastic wrapping. If special plastic bags for infants are not readily available, biohazard bags, large resealable plastic bags, and food-grade plastic wrapping can be used instead. The baby should be wrapped immediately after birth and covered from the neck down; additional resuscitation can be performed with this in place.

ADVANCED RESUSCITATION

Around 1% of births will require advanced resuscitation. If effective PPV with supplemental oxygen based on gestation has been provided for more than 30 seconds and the HR is less than 60, start chest compressions. Chest compressions should be delivered with a ratio of 3:1 coordinated with breaths, with a target of 90 chest compressions and 30 breaths per minute (120 events per minute). If giving chest compressions, 100% FIO_2 and intubation should be considered. If the infant's HR remains less than 60 beats/min after adequate PPV and chest compressions, epinephrine and volume expansion may be indicated. Peripheral venous access can be difficult in neonates; therefore, umbilical venous catheters or intraosseous access may be required. Advanced resuscitation is a rare event in the ED, and as such, providers with less exposure to these clinical situations should periodically review the skills needed.

PEARLS

- At birth, ask three key questions: Is the baby term? Is the baby breathing or crying? Do they have good tone?
- If the answer to any is "no," begin basic neonatal resuscitation with warming, drying, and stimulating the infant to cry.
- Keep the baby warm with warm blankets, radiant warmers, mother's chest, or plastic wrapping for very small or premature infants.
- Term infants should be initially resuscitated with oxygen concentration of 21% (room air).
- Although rare, be familiar with advanced resuscitation techniques.

SUGGESTED READINGS

Aziz K, Lee HC, Escobedo MB, et al. Part 5: Neonatal resuscitation: 2020 American Heart Association Guidelines for cardiopulmonary resuscitation and emergency cardiovascular care. *Circulation*. 2020;142:S524-S550.

Gupta AG, Adler MD. Management of an unexpected delivery in the emergency department. *Clin Pediatr Emerg Med*. 2016;17(2):89-98.

Weiner GM, Zaichkin J, eds. Positive-pressure ventilation. In: *Textbook of Neonatal Resuscitation*. 8th ed. American Academy of Pediatrics; 2021:65-116.

289

THE PEDIATRIC AIRWAY: LEARN IT, LIVE IT, CONTROL IT!

ALEXANDRA BARBOSA AND GARRETT S. PACHECO

While infrequent, pediatric emergency airway management requires heightened attentiveness to prevent deterioration in the critically ill child. Prominent differences exist between the pediatric and adult airway including the location of the airway, size and shape of the epiglottis, low oxygen reserve, and risk for rapid oxygen desaturation. Hemodynamic instability and hypoxemia are factors associated with increased risk of peri-intubation cardiac arrest. It is imperative to optimize resuscitation before intubation and ensure provider familiarity with anatomic and physiologic differences when caring for these critically ill patients.

Younger children, particularly infants, have anatomic differences that require consideration before intubation. Glottic visualization is more difficult due to a large occiput with a more cephalad larynx that creates a sharp angle with the floppy, omega-shaped epiglottis. The pediatric arytenoids and vocal cords incline anteriorly, producing an angle that can cause the ETT to catch on the anterior commissure during insertion. These anatomic features are important when positioning the patient for intubation. Proper patient positioning may decrease the time for intubation and subsequent risk of hypoxemia. Patients may be positioned with 20° torso elevation and placed in "flextension" position. Flexion of the neck at the upper cervicothoracic joint and extension of the head at the atlanto-occipital joint improve the laryngeal view by aligning the external auditory meatus with the sternal notch. This position may be achieved by placing a small, rolled towel under the shoulders in infants or by elevating the head in older children and adults.

The pediatric airway is also a physiologically difficult airway due to lower FRC, increased closing volume, and more rapid oxygen desaturation. Diseased states lead to decreased oxygen reserve and increased metabolic demand, making these differences more pronounced. The consequences of prolonged hypoxemia may lead to seizure, bradycardia, and hemodynamic compromise, causing cardiac arrest. Sedatives and neuromuscular blockade further decrease FRC, particularly in infants.

Cuffed tracheal tubes are appropriate for full-term infants and older children, with decreased need for reintubation and decreased air leak, which subsequently improve ventilation. Appropriate ETT size is important to facilitate tube delivery past the narrowest point of the airway, and pressure from cuff inflation must be carefully monitored to prevent tracheal injury.

Recent evidence supports improved first-pass success and reduced esophageal intubations with VL compared to DL in pediatric patients. Devices used in VL include standard geometry blades (curved and straight) as well as hyperangulated blades. These VL devices perform similarly in children, but standard blades perform better in very small infants.

Anesthesia literature has demonstrated increased "safe apnea time" with the application of HFNO. HFNO decreases dead space, potentially provides PEEP during apnea, and provides heated and humidified oxygen at flow rates that exceed the patient's inspiratory flow rate.

NIPPV may also be used to improve recruitment and oxygenation before intubation. During the apnea period, the airway operator can transition to the combined use of HFNO with gentle face mask ventilation. mRSI, that is face mask ventilation during the apnea period, is a safe and effective option. When using a BVM in pediatric patients, a pop-off valve can be used to prevent barotrauma and overdistension.

The physiologically difficult airway is associated with an increased risk of adverse events, including cardiac arrest. Children are particularly vulnerable to experiencing cardiac arrest with the peri-intubation presence of hypoxemia and hemodynamic instability. Improved oxygenation strategies and optimization of hemodynamics before intubation may help mitigate some risks associated with the physiologically difficult airway.

Intubation and mechanical ventilation further alter hemodynamics by increasing intrathoracic pressure, leading to an increase in right atrial pressure and subsequent decrease in preload. Decreased preload may exacerbate pre-intubation hypotension or precipitate cardiac depression leading to hypotension. Patients who are not volume responsive may need vasoactive medications to improve inotropy and systemic vascular resistance. "Bolus-dose pressors" include epinephrine (1 mcg/kg, 1/10th of the code dose) have demonstrated safety and effectiveness for pediatric patients with acute hypotensive episodes or experiencing a prearrest condition. To avoid dilution errors, an epinephrine or norepinephrine (0.1 mcg/kg/min) infusion can be initiated.

Risks and benefits must be evaluated for induction agent selection in pediatric patients. Propofol and midazolam have known effects of myocardial depression and sympatholysis leading to hypotension and thus should be avoided in patients at risk. Ketamine has sympathomimetic activity leading to increased heart rate and blood pressure and has additional benefits, including bronchodilation. However, patients with catecholamine depletion may experience myocardial depression with ketamine. Etomidate is considered to be "hemodynamically neutral" relative to other induction agents. There is ongoing concern that etomidate may cause adrenal suppression, worsening shock in septic pediatric patients.

PEARLS

- Pediatric patients have anatomic and physiologic differences that must be addressed by positioning and optimization of oxygenation.
- VL should be the first-line option to increase first-pass success without adverse events in pediatric emergency airway management.
- For patients with hypoxemia requiring intubation, preoxygenation, apneic oxygenation, and face mask ventilation during the apnea period may increase the oxygen reservoir and prevent worsening hypoxemia and potential peri-intubation arrest.
- Hemodynamics should be optimized with appropriate resuscitation, and vasoactive medications can be used if needed.
- Careful induction selection is necessary for physiologically compromised children.

Suggested Readings

Long E, Barrett MJ, Peters C, Sabato S, Lockie F. Emergency intubation of children outside of the operating room. *Paediatr Anaesth*. 2020;30(3):319-330.

Pacheco GS, Patanwala AE, Mendelson JS, Sakles JC. Clinical experience with the C-MAC and GlideScope in a pediatric emergency department over a 10-year period. *Pediatr Emerg Care*. 2021;37(12):e1098-e1103.

Pokrajac N, Sbiroli E, Hollenbach KA, Kohn MA, Contreras E, Murray M. Risk factors for peri-intubation cardiac arrest in a pediatric emergency department. *Pediatr Emerg Care*. 2022;38(1):e126-e131.

Reiter PD, Roth J, Wathen B, LaVelle J, Ridall LA. Low-dose epinephrine boluses for acute hypotension in the PICU. *Pediatr Crit Care Med*. 2018;19(4):281-286.

Soneru CN, Hurt HF, Petersen TR, Davis DD, Braude DA, Falcon RJ. Apneic nasal oxygenation and safe apnea time during pediatric intubations by learners. *Pediatr Anesthesia*. 2019;29(6):628-634.

290

ALL THAT BARKS IS NOT CROUP

STEVEN S. BIN

Croup (laryngotracheitis) is a URI in infants and young children that presents with stridor and a characteristic barky cough. While the presence of stridor with croup represents a common upper respiratory diagnosis in children, it is important for the ED physician to maintain a high index of suspicion to differentiate croup from other chronic or life-threatening causes of stridor.

Stridor is the high-pitched respiratory sound produced by turbulent airflow passing through a narrowed upper airway when breathing and is often the most prominent sign of an evolving upper airway obstruction. Due to the smaller size of the upper airway in younger children relative to adolescents and adults, a small amount of edema or secretions results in an exponential increase in airway resistance and reduction in airflow. This predisposes younger children to develop stridor and increased work of breathing due to the inflammation from routine respiratory illnesses.

For all patients in the ED with stridor, the first priority is to assess for airway patency and the need for any urgent or emergent airway interventions. A thorough history and physical exam will guide the tempo of the evaluation. The history should include any previous intubation and birth history, onset of stridor being sudden, chronic, or recurrent, fever, relationship to feeding or positioning, history of choking or trauma, and any episodes of cyanosis or apnea. An initial examination should focus on the work of breathing, retractions—intercostal/subcostal/suprasternal retractions, nasal flaring, the ability to protect the airway, drooling, level of consciousness, air entry, and oxygen saturation. Hypoxia and fatigue in the setting of an isolated upper airway obstruction are signs of an impending complete airway obstruction. Every effort should be made to minimize noxious stimuli before definitive interventions and therapies are initiated, as this will often exacerbate a child's agitation and worsen their stridor and symptoms.

In croup, viral inflammation results in swelling of extrathoracic airway structures, and this manifests as the classic croupy "seal-like" or "barky" cough. If the swelling progresses, *inspiratory* stridor is heard and children often present to the ED in varying degrees of respiratory distress. Croup typically starts as a respiratory infection and is often associated with rhinorrhoea and fever. It is most prevalent in the fall to early winter months with the uptick in respiratory viruses, including Parainfluenza viruses types 1 to 3, RSV, adenovirus, and SARS-CoV-2 variants. It occurs in children between 6 and 36 months of age and is less frequently diagnosed beyond 6 years of age. It is more commonly seen in males (ratio 1.4:1), and patients often present in the late evening or early morning.

Most cases of croup are mild (minimal to no stridor, minimal to no increased work of breathing, normal activity) and self-limited with symptoms lasting a few days. The mainstay of treatment includes dexamethasone (PO/IM). In contrast, children with moderate (audible stridor at rest, increased work of breathing with retractions, fussy) and severe (significant stridor and retractions, decreased air entry, cyanosis, lethargy) symptoms are treated with dexamethasone (PO/IM) and racemic epinephrine nebulization to reduce inflammation and obstruction. Both modalities/therapies have resulted in a dramatic reduction in bounce-back ED revisits, the need for hospital admissions, and length of inpatient days in patients with croup. Patients are typically observed for 2 to 4 hours after racemic epinephrine to assess the need for additional treatments before discharge or admission after 2 to 3 doses of racemic epinephrine.

While croup represents the most common cause of stridor in the febrile child, other infectious causes should be considered, including bacterial tracheitis, epiglottitis, and retropharyngeal abscess. Bacterial tracheitis should be suspected in a child who presents with high fever and toxic appearance or develops marked worsening of symptoms after having mild croup symptoms. Dysphagia and drooling are common. Epiglottitis would present as an ill-appearing child with a muffled voice and tripod positioning (ie, neck extended and mouth open to maximize airway caliber). A retropharyngeal abscess may not present with stridor, but rather will have fever, limited neck extension, and neck fullness.

In a child without fever, the sudden development of stridor without URI symptoms should prompt all ED providers to consider a FBA or ingestion. Discerning if there was an abrupt choking episode or sudden onset of cough is often all that is required to suspect a FB. Do not attempt to relieve a partial obstruction in the ED as this could dislodge the FB and worsen the degree of obstruction. Children with partial obstruction caused by FBA should be definitively managed in the operating arena. Manage these patients "expectantly," contact subspecialists early in the evaluation, and be prepared in case the child progresses to a complete airway obstruction where immediate intervention is required.

Stridors due to congenital pathologies include laryngomalacia, laryngeal cysts and webs, vascular rings, and other airway abnormalities such as Down syndrome with subglottic stenosis. In a child with a history of hemangiomas, development of stridor should raise concern for an expanding vascular abnormality. These may cause symptoms soon after birth or may develop over weeks or months.

The diagnosis of croup is made clinically, and routine laboratory testing or radiographs are not required unless standard treatments are refractory, there is an atypical course, recurrent episodes, or other diagnoses are being considered. Plain films of the neck and chest may identify radiopaque FBs, and a steeple sign is pathognomonic for subglottic swelling from the croup versus epiglottitis. Subspeciality consultation with otolaryngology or pulmonary for direct visualization of the airway with flexible airway bronchoscopy may be required for complete evaluation of chronic stridor.

PEARLS

- Patients with stridor and barky cough often have croup, yet stridor represents a partial airway obstruction, and other life-threatening causes should be considered.
- In the setting of an unwitnessed choking episode or sudden cough in a child without fever or URI symptoms, a FBA should be high on the differential diagnosis.
- Any interventions that exacerbate a child's agitation may worsen their stridor and symptoms, precipitating the progression of an airway obstruction.
- Recurrent episodes of stridor, progressive symptoms, cyanosis, apnea, or respiratory distress all require further evaluation and referral to otolaryngology for airway bronchoscopy.

SUGGESTED READINGS

Baiu I, Melendez E. Croup. *JAMA*. 2019;321(16):1642.
Eskander A, De Almeida JR, Irish JC. Acute upper airway obstruction. *N Engl J Med*. 2019; 381(20):1940-1949.
Pfleger A, Eber E. Assessment and causes of stridor. *Paediatr Respir Rev*. 2016;18:64-72.

291

PEDIATRIC PROCEDURAL SEDATION IN THE ED: DEALER'S CHOICE

JORDAN A. JUSTICE

Bedside procedures necessitating the use of procedural sedation are frequent in EDs. Procedural sedation has proven to be a safe and inexpensive way to facilitate many procedures that may be impeded due to pain and lack of patient cooperation. If age-appropriate distraction techniques will not suffice for a particular procedure, procedural sedation may be the preferred option.

Before beginning sedation, evaluate the patient's airway and cardiovascular status. There are no absolute contraindications; however, relative contraindications include craniofacial/airway abnormalities, difficult airway, or ASA classification III or higher. In these circumstances, the patient may benefit from sedation in the operating room by a pediatric anesthesiologist. While a period of fasting is ideal, the ACEP has issued a Level B recommendation to not delay necessary procedural sedation in adult or pediatric patients based on fasting time, as duration of fasting has not reduced the risk of emesis or aspiration.

Preparation should include proper monitoring and ensuring all necessary equipment is easily accessible. Monitoring should include cardiac rhythm, respirations, noninvasive blood pressure, pulse oximetry, and capnography. Capnography is especially useful as an increasing end-tidal CO_2 or drop-off in respirations will be the first indicator of respiratory depression. Emergency airway equipment should be immediately available in the event of decompensation.

Consider using supplemental oxygen for several minutes before and during sedation to maximize Pa_{O_2} and safe apnea/hypoventilation time. Devices such as nasal cannula may be anxiety provoking for young children and can be applied after sedation has begun.

When circumstances permit, sedation should be administered and managed by a physician not involved in performing the procedure. Thus, one can concentrate on patient monitoring and managing potential complications. Familiarity with the procedure being performed is required in order to anticipate the duration of sedation and the need for additional analgesia during or after the procedure.

Numerous sedative-hypnotics and analgesic agents are available for procedures requiring brief sedation. The choice of agent is largely based on the physician's comfort and institutional availability. Commonly used agents in the ED are shown in **Table 291.1**.

Table 291.1 Commonly Used Agents in the ED

Medication	Dosing	Notes on Side Effects and Potential Complications
Ketamine ■ Short-acting NMDA antagonist ■ Dissociative "trance-like" state ■ Preserves airway reflexes and respiratory drive ■ Amnestic and analgesic properties	IV: 1-1.5 mg/kg with repeat dosing of 0.5-1 mg/kg PRN IM: 4-5 mg/kg with repeat dosing of 2-4 mg/kg PRN IN: Variable	■ Nausea and vomiting (consider premedicating with antiemetic) ■ Emergence phenomenon (brief, resolves spontaneously) ■ Watch for increased airway secretions (consider alternate agent for ENT/airway procedures) ■ Laryngospasm (rare—administer slowly to reduce risk)
Midazolam ■ Short-acting benzodiazepine ■ Anxiolytic and amnestic properties; lacks analgesic properties (may need to add opioid for painful procedures)	PO: 0.25-0.5 mg/kg IV: 0.05-0.1 mg/kg IN: 0.2-0.5 mg/kg	■ Respiratory depression (increased risk if combined with opioid) ■ Paradoxical reaction in 1%-3% of children (hyperactivity, aggression, inconsolability; self-limited) ■ Flumazenil can reverse effects (avoid in patients with seizure disorder or on chronic benzodiazepines)
Propofol ■ Short-acting general anesthetic ■ Anesthetic and amnestic properties (may need to add opioid for painful procedures) ■ Rapid onset and short recovery time ■ Commonly combined with a second agent (ketamine, fentanyl)	IV: 1-2 mg/kg with repeat dosing of 0.5 mg/kg PRN ■ If combined with ketamine or fentanyl, consider lower initial bolus (0.5 mg/kg)	■ Administer slowly and watch for respiratory depression and hypotension ■ Avoid as long-term infusion due to the risk of propofol infusion syndrome
N2O ■ Inhaled anesthetic gas ■ Anesthetic, amnestic, anxiolytic, and analgesic properties ■ Rapid onset and short recovery time	Administered through demand-valve mask or continuous flow system ■ Either fixed 50/50 concentration of N_2O and oxygen or titratable concentration of N_2O up to 70%, depending on the system	■ Contraindicated in pregnancy ■ Nausea and vomiting can occur (consider premedicating with antiemetic) ■ Generally excellent safety profile

ENT, ear, nose, and throat; IM, intramuscular; IN, intranasal; IV, intravenous;
NMDA, *N*-nitrosodimethylamine; N_2O, nitrous oxide; PO, by mouth; PRN, pro re nata (as needed).

Other sedatives such as dexmedetomidine and etomidate can also be used for procedural sedation. It is vitally important to be familiar with the safety profile, duration of action, contraindications, and adverse effects of the agent you're using. Consider the effect of multiple agents being used in conjunction—for instance, the use of opiates may reduce the amount of sedative needed to achieve adequate sedation.

Observe the patient in the ED per institutional policy after the sedation until the patient has returned to a baseline mental status and can tolerate PO liquids. Remember to provide additional pain control after discharge PRN.

PEARLS

- Preparation—Always have emergency airway equipment, backup airway equipment, medications, and suction at bedside. Anticipate and prepare for potential complications.
- Become very familiar with the agent being used—contraindications, adverse effects, onset of action, and recovery time. Consider the additive effects of multiple agents.
- Ensure the patient has recovered from sedation and that pain is well controlled before discharge.

Suggested Readings

Babl FE, Oakley E, Seaman C, et al. High-concentration nitrous oxide for procedural sedation in children: adverse events and depth of sedation. *Pediatrics*. 2008;121:e528.

Godwin SA, Burton JH, Gerardo CJ, et al. Clinical policy: procedural sedation and analgesia in the emergency department. *Ann Emerg Med*. 2014;63:247-258.

Green SM, Roback MG, Krauss BS, et al. Unscheduled procedural sedation: a multidisciplinary consensus practice guideline. *Ann Emerg Med*. 2019;73:E51-E65.

Kennedy RM, Luhmann JD. Pharmacological management of pain and anxiety during emergency procedures in children. *Paediatr Drugs*. 2001;3:337.

Zempsky WT, Cravero JP; American Academy of Pediatrics Committee on Pediatric Emergency Medicine and Section on Anesthesiology and Pain Medicine. Relief of pain and anxiety in pediatric patients in emergency medical systems. *Pediatrics*. 2004;114:1348.

292

Urinary Tract Infection in Young Children

Cornelia Latronica

UTI is one of the most common bacterial infections in children. Approximately 7% of children less than 2 years presenting to the ED with fever have a UTI. UTI should be considered in young infants presenting with vague symptoms. Risk factors for UTI include female gender, circumcision status, history of UTI, congenital anomalies, vesicoureteral reflux, nephrolithiasis, bladder dysfunction, and constipation. Periurethral microflora may also impact the risk for development of UTI.

Up to 90% of UTIs are caused by *Escherichia coli*. Other organisms include *Enterococcus* and *Enterobacter* spp., *Proteus, Klebsiella*, and *Staphylococcus saprophyticus* in sexually active adolescents. Less common organisms are seen in patients with recent surgery, instrumentation, urinary tract anomalies, or immunocompromise.

In 2018, Shaikh et al developed a calculator, updated in 2022 (https://uticalc.pitt.edu/), to estimate the pretest probability of UTI in otherwise healthy children aged 2 months to 2 years. The revised calculator uses the clinical risk factors of age, temperature, history of UTI, sex, circumcision status, presence of an alternate source for fever, and duration of fever. The threshold to detect 95% of UTIs is a calculated risk of 2% or higher. The calculator subsequently incorporates UA results to calculate a posttest probability of UTI and aid in the decision to treat. Use of the calculator was found to reduce testing when compared with the AAP algorithm, decrease the number of missed UTIs, and reduce treatment delays.

UA with microscopy and urine culture, obtained by urethral catheterization or SPA, remains the gold standard for diagnosis of UTI in non-toilet-trained children. SPA may be reserved as modality for boys with phimosis and girls with labial adhesion for whom catheterization is not possible and empiric treatment is not acceptable. Urine obtained by bag collection has contamination rates exceeding 80% and false positive rates of 95% to 99%. A study by Lavelle et al found that bag urine samples may be effectively utilized to exclude UTI when initiated in triage, with reduction of urethral catheterization by approximately 50% and without increased length of stay. Additional studies have evaluated the utility of other noninvasive methods of urine collection in children. Two such techniques include the Quick-Wee method by Kaufman et al (suprapubic stimulation with cold saline-soaked gauze) and a bladder stimulation technique by Herreros et al (manual suprapubic tapping alternating with lumbar massage). In a single small prospective study, success rates for obtaining urine by the bladder stimulation technique were 38% to 53%. The technique was found to have comparable contamination rates with catheterization and increased parental satisfaction.

The AAP defines UTI by the presence of more than 50,000 CFU/mL of pathogenic bacteria from a specimen obtained by catheterization (>100,000 CFU/mL on clean catch specimens), along with a UA positive for LE or WBCs on microscopy. While this is the currently accepted definition of UTI, it remains debated and is likely to continue to evolve. Challenges to the definition include the determination of the number of CFU/mL on urine culture, the threshold of the WBC count on microscopy, and the inadequate specificities of single markers (eg, LE, nitrite) on UA. Several studies argue that some children with fewer than 50,000 CFU/mL may have true UTI. Conversely, others may have asymptomatic bacteriuria, which is the colonization of the bladder in the absence of an inflammatory reaction, such that urine culture is positive by the above definition but UA is negative. Species including *Enterococcus* and *Klebsiella* may cause symptomatic infection in the absence of pyuria. Sterile pyuria is the presence of a UA positive for WBC and LE with a negative culture and may be seen in conditions such as nephritis, cystitis, or urethritis related to noninfectious disease processes (eg, Kawasaki disease). LE, released by the lysis of neutrophils and macrophages, is sensitive but not specific for UTI. The presence of nitrite on UA is specific but not sensitive. *Enterobacteriaceae* species elaborate nitrate reductase, which converts urinary nitrate to nitrite. The accumulation of urinary nitrite requires urinary stasis, which is limited in infants without voluntary bladder control who void frequently.

Distinguishing cystitis from pyelonephritis is important in determining the length of antibiotic therapy. The recommended first-line treatment for cystitis is 3 to 5 days of a first-generation cephalosporin (eg, cephalexin) or nitrofurantoin. First-line outpatient antibiotic therapy for pyelonephritis is a 7- to 10-day course of cephalosporin, amoxicillin-clavulanate, or trimethoprim/sulfamethoxazole and may be considered in patients as young as 2 months old who are well-appearing and can tolerate oral medication. Amoxicillin is not preferred due to high rates of antibiotic resistance. Following the initiation of treatment, up to 68% of patients improve within 24 hours and 92% by 72 hours. Urine cultures should be followed to ensure appropriate therapy. Rates of reoccurrence of UTI after an initial episode range from 12% to 30%. Renal ultrasounds should be obtained in children younger than 24 months after the first UTIs and for older children with recurrent UTI to evaluate for anatomic anomalies.

PEARLS

- A UTI calculator may be a clinically useful tool in children aged 2 months to 2 years without known urogenital anomalies.
- Positive indicators of UA with microscopy and culture are both needed to establish the diagnosis of UTI.
- Multiple markers of UA must be interpreted in the clinical context for diagnosis.
- Urine obtained by bag collection has high contamination rates and should not be used to diagnose UTI but may be used to exclude it.
- First-generation cephalosporin is appropriate therapy for most young children with UTI.

Suggested Readings

Lavelle JM, Blackstone MM, Funari MK, et al. Two-step process for ED UTI screening in febrile young children: reducing catheterization rates. *Pediatrics*. 2016;138(1):e20153023. PMID: 27255151.

Ravichandran Y, Parker S, Farooqi A, DeLaroche A. Bladder stimulation for clean catch urine collection: improved parent and provider satisfaction. *Pediatr Emerg Care*. 2022;38(1):e29-e33. PMID: 34475366.

Shaikh N, Hoberman A, Hum SW, et al. Development and validation of a calculator for estimating the probability of urinary tract infection in young febrile children. *JAMA Pediatr*. 2018;172(6):550-556. PMID: 29710324.

Subcommittee on Urinary Tract Infection, Steering Committee on Quality Improvement and Management; Roberts KB. Urinary tract infection: clinical practice guideline for the diagnosis and management of the initial UTI in febrile infants and children 2 to 24 months. *Pediatrics*. 2011;128(3):595-610. PMID: 21873693.

293

BEWARE PEDIATRIC APPENDICITIS

CHRISTYN MAGILL

Appendicitis in the pediatric population can be a diagnostic challenge as it presents variably in different age groups. Presenting symptoms of nausea, vomiting, fevers, and anorexia often overlap with other common pediatric illnesses that cause abdominal pain including viral GI illnesses or urinary tract infections. Historical features and scoring systems may help identify children more likely to require evaluation for appendicitis.

HISTORY

Historical features can help differentiate acute appendicitis from other childhood illnesses. The duration of symptoms is important. Acute appendicitis evolves over hours to days, not weeks. Are symptoms getting better, worse, or staying stable? Is the pain colicky? Has there been any diarrhea, especially bloody diarrhea? Is there burning or pain with urination, or hematuria? Is there a history of gynecologic disorders or any gynecologic or abdominal surgeries? Have they had menses yet? Are there any sick contacts with similar symptoms? What other systemic symptoms do they have, such as rash, headache, sore throat, or myalgias? Have they traveled anywhere recently, especially out of the country?

SCORING SYSTEMS

Several scoring systems have been developed to classify and quantify pediatric appendicitis risk (**Table 293.1**). The oldest and best-studied scoring systems are the Alvarado score and the PAS, which have high sensitivity but low specificity, and have insufficient positive predictive value to be used alone to determine the need for surgery. Newer scoring tools include the pARC, the AIR, and the PALabS. These weighted scoring systems were validated in different age groups, thus applicability to your specific patient may be limited. Common variables across all the scoring systems include right lower quadrant pain, WBC count, and ANC as part of the scores, as these are the most sensitive markers to predict appendicitis. The calculated scores correlate with suggestions that may guide further workup and management and may be found at www.MDcalc.com.

WORKUP—IMAGING

"Why not just CT the abdomen/pelvis?" Multiple studies address the concern that children are at a significantly higher lifetime risk for development of solid organ tumors following the ionizing radiation associated with CT scans of the abdomen/pelvis. Thus, ultrasound is the preferred initial imaging choice.

"What if I can't obtain a diagnostic ultrasound?" Some surgeons may consider operative management for patients with scores in the high-risk category without imaging. If the patient's score is intermediate or equivocal and ultrasound is not an option, the surgeon may request a CT scan or may admit for serial abdominal exams. If you do not have a surgeon, or if the patient's score is in the intermediate range, then consider transferring the patient to a center where pediatric subspecialty care, ultrasounds, or serial abdominal exams are available.

WORKUP—LABS

The initial workup in the ED for a child with suspected appendicitis often includes a CBC with differential, C-reactive protein, comprehensive metabolic panel (if there is

TABLE 293.1 COMMON PEDIATRIC APPENDICITIS SCORING SYSTEMS

	ALVARADO SCORE	PEDIATRIC APPENDICITIS SCORE (PAS)	PEDIATRIC APPENDICITIS RISK CALCULATOR (PARC)
Year developed	1986	2002	2018
Applicable age (yr)	4–80	3-18	5-18
Exclusions		Children with known gastrointestinal disease, pregnancy, or previous abdominal surgeries. Pain should be less than 4 d duration.	Children under 5 yr old, pregnancy, previous abdominal surgery, inflammatory bowel disease, chronic pancreatitis, sickle cell anemia, cystic fibrosis, any medical condition affecting the ability to obtain an accurate history, history of abdominal trauma within the previous 7 d
Right lower quadrant/right iliac fossa pain	✓	✓	✓
Temperature	≥99.1 °F (37.3 °C)	≥100.4 °F (38 °C)	
Rebound tenderness	✓		
Migration of pain to right lower quadrant	✓	✓	✓
Anorexia	✓	✓	
Nausea/vomiting	✓	✓	
White blood cell (WBC) count	>10,000	>10,000	✓
Polymorphonuclear leukocytes (PMN)	>75%	>75%	✓
Practice setting (community vs pediatric ED)			✓
Sex			✓
Duration of pain			✓
Pain with walking		✓	✓
Abdominal guarding			✓
Additional tip	Tends to be more accurate at the extremes.	Useful when abdominal pain is less than 4 d in duration.	Performed better than PAS in a validation study.

concern for alternative pathology or electrolyte changes from GI losses), urinalysis, and pregnancy test for females of childbearing age. Labs can be helpful to risk-stratify patients with indeterminate ultrasound studies. If a positive imaging study results before the labs are drawn, it may not be necessary to obtain labs, although that should be a joint decision made after discussion with the pediatric surgeon.

TREATMENT

Adequate analgesia is paramount. Opioid administration for severe pain will not obscure crucial examination findings and may be appropriate and necessary for adequate pain control. A 20 mL/kg crystalloid fluid bolus may be beneficial for patients with vomiting and concern for dehydration. Acute appendicitis is strongly suggested by either a high appendicitis score or diagnostic imaging with evidence of an enlarged noncompressible tubular structure with or without peri-appendiceal fat stranding or an appendicolith. Patients may be managed with IV fluids, IV antibiotics (eg, ceftriaxone plus metronidazole, ampicillin/sulbactam, or piperacillin/tazobactam), analgesics (opioids or NSAIDs), antiemetics (eg, ondansetron), and a surgical consult. Although more recent trends and literature suggest treatment of uncomplicated acute appendicitis with antibiotics alone, the current standard of treatment is still surgical appendectomy.

Stable patients who fall into the intermediate "gray zone" due to either nondiagnostic imaging or inability to image with persistent pain or tenderness may be treated with IV fluids, antiemetics, and analgesics. These patients may be transferred to a tertiary pediatric center or may be admitted for observation and serial abdominal exams without antibiotics.

Patients with vital sign abnormalities, evidence of shock, or patients with ruptured appendicitis should be adequately resuscitated and given broad-spectrum antibiotics.

COMPLICATIONS

Perforated appendicitis that develops into an abscess or phlegmon may be treated with IV antibiotics alone, antibiotics plus percutaneous drainage, or laparoscopic surgical drainage and removal. Complications include post-appendectomy wound infection, intra-abdominal abscess formation, and ileus.

PEARLS

- Scoring tools can be useful when diagnosing acute appendicitis in the pediatric population.
- Treating pain with opioid or nonsteroidal medications does not mask or delay the diagnosis of appendicitis.
- First-line diagnostic imaging is an abdominal ultrasound.
- You don't need to have a definitive diagnosis to transfer a patient to a tertiary pediatric center.
- You can safely wait to give antibiotics until after surgical consult unless the patient is unstable/septic.

SUGGESTED READINGS

Cotton DM, Vinson DR, Vazquez-Benitez G, et al. Validation of the pediatric appendicitis risk calculator (pARC) in a community emergency department setting. *Ann Emerg Med.* 2019;74(4):471-480.

Di Saverio S, Podda M, De Simone B, et al. Diagnosis and treatment of acute appendicitis: 2020 update of the WSES Jerusalem guidelines. *World J Emerg Surg*. 2020;15(1):27.

Fawkner-Corbett D, Hayward G, Alkhmees M, Van Den Bruel A, Ordóñez-Mena JM, Holtman GA. Diagnostic accuracy of blood tests of inflammation in paediatric appendicitis: a systematic review and meta-analysis. *BMJ Open*. 2022;12(11):e056854.

Huang L, Yin Y, Yang L, Wang C, Li Y, Zhou Z. Comparison of antibiotic therapy and appendectomy for acute uncomplicated appendicitis in children: a meta-analysis. *JAMA Pediatr*. 2017;171(5):426-434.

Schneider C, Kharbanda A, Bachur R. Evaluating appendicitis scoring systems using a prospective pediatric cohort. *Ann Emerg Med*. 2007;49(6):778-784, 784.e1.

Snyder MJ, Guthrie M, Cagle S. Acute appendicitis: efficient diagnosis and management. *Am Fam Physician*. 2018;98(1):25-33.

294

DIAGNOSES NOT TO MISS IN THE ACUTELY LIMPING CHILD

GREGORY HAND AND GUYON J. HILL

Limp is a common pediatric chief complaint whose myriad causes may range from benign and self-limited conditions to life-threatening diagnoses. A high index of suspicion must be maintained for causes such as osteomyelitis or NAT that can be easily missed yet have severe consequences for the health of the child.

INFECTION

Rapid recognition of septic arthritis is essential to preserve the joint and prevent long-term disability. Usually affecting the knee or hip, other joints may also be involved. Children generally appear ill, are febrile, and are reluctant to bear weight or permit range of motion. Pain with axial load, an effusion, and a warm and tender joint may be present on physical examination. A CBC, ESR, CRP, and blood cultures can be useful in any limping child where infection is a concern. One study showed the probability of septic arthritis was 74% with the presence of both an inability to bear weight and CRP higher than 2.0 mg/dL. Children with neither had less than a 1% chance. Another study showed 100% sensitivity and 87% specificity for an elevated CRP and a temperature greater than 101 °F. The diagnosis is confirmed via synovial fluid analysis following aspiration. When considering osteomyelitis, radiographs may show findings of bone destruction or periosteal inflammation; however, a normal radiograph does not rule out the diagnosis. Elevated inflammatory markers indicate the need for imaging such as MRI or bone scan. Risk factors include patients who are immunocompromised, puncture wounds, and ulcers. A history of trauma is not elicited in the majority of cases. Abscesses in various locations, discitis, cellulitis, Lyme disease, or myositis should also be in the differential for limping children.

INJURY

The toddler's fracture is a non-displaced spiral fracture of the tibia usually from an insignificant mechanism. Most are in the distal tibia, found in ambulating children under

6 years of age, and are typically not associated with abuse unlike other spiral fractures of long bones. AP and lateral radiographs may be normal and obtaining an internal oblique view increases the sensitivity of visualizing the fracture line. Obtaining a history can be difficult in nonverbal children, unwitnessed events, or victims of NAT. High suspicion of NAT should be given to injuries that do not match the mechanism or child's developmental stage. It is important to recognize concerning radiographic findings that may be suggestive of NAT such as fractures in various stages of healing, vertebral fractures, metaphyseal-epiphyseal injuries (ie, corner fractures), bilateral long bone fractures, or transverse fractures.

Inflammation

The most common cause of nontraumatic limp in a child is TS. This benign inflammatory process predominantly affects the hip and will self-resolve with supportive care. Septic arthritis must be ruled out first, as TS is a diagnosis of exclusion. A typical presentation is several days of limping in a well appearing, afebrile child following a recent viral illness. The leg is typically abducted and in external rotation, but unlike septic arthritis can usually be fully ranged. It can be helpful to treat a possible patient with TS with an NSAID while the evaluation is ongoing as symptomatic improvement can aid disposition.

Neoplastic

Malignancies such as leukemias, lymphomas, or various tumors may cause a child to limp. The most common malignant tumors are osteosarcoma and Ewing sarcoma that are found in the distal femur or proximal tibia. The symptoms may be subtle and are often attributed to other injuries. Suspicion should be increased with history of "B symptoms," pain at rest or at night, or lack of trauma. Numerous benign tumors such as osteoid osteomas, osteochondromas, and bone cysts can cause similar symptoms. Radiographs in malignancy show no clear margins while benign tumors grow slower and typically manifest sclerotic changes.

Structural

SCFE usually affects children in their early adolescence. The diagnosis is typically made with pelvic AP and bilateral frog-leg lateral radiographs that show the classic appearance of ice cream slipping off a cone at the femoral epiphysis. LCP disease is idiopathic avascular necrosis of the femoral head. Plain radiographs in the early stages are frequently normal and MRI is the best modality if suspicion is high. The presentation can be similar to TS but with a different time course. TS is self-limited and lasts 1 to 2 weeks whereas LCP can last 18 to 24 months. ED management of this disorder consists of making the patient non-weightbearing and ensuring orthopedic follow-up.

It is also important to consider causes of limp not localized to the lower extremities. Examples of these include intra-abdominal or retroperitoneal pathologies, such as appendicitis, rheumatologic causes, and spinal abnormalities.

PEARLS

- Elevated CRP is the most useful laboratory study in the diagnosis of septic arthritis, especially when combined with an inability to bear weight.
- Ensure you look at all views of radiographs as subtle findings in pediatric injuries can be very easy to miss. Many fractures will initially have normal radiographs.

- Consider NAT as a possible cause when the injury doesn't match the mechanism or the developmental age of the child or is well known to occur with abuse.
- Serious diagnoses such as septic arthritis and osteomyelitis can still have normal laboratory values.

SUGGESTED READINGS

Herman MJ, Martinek M. The limping child. *Pediatr Rev*. 2015;36(5):184-195.

Kocher MS, Mandiga R, Zurakowski D, Barnewolt C, Kasser JR. Validation of a clinical prediction rule for the differentiation between septic arthritis and transient synovitis of the hip in children. *J Bone Joint Surg Am*. 2004;86(8):1629-1635.

McQueen A, Place AE. Oncologic emergencies. In: Fleisher GR, Ludwig S, eds. *Textbook of Pediatric Emergency Medicine*. 8th ed. Lippincott Williams and Wilkins; 2021:918-919.

Payares-Lizano M. The limping child. *Pediatr Clin North Am*. 2020;67(1):119-138.

Singhal R, Perry DC, Khan FN, et al. The use of CRP within a clinical prediction algorithm for the differentiation of septic arthritis and transient synovitis of the hip in children. *J Bone Joint Surg Br*. 2011;93(11):1556-1561.

295

BACK PAIN IN KIDS IS NEVER NORMAL

RACHEL E. TSOLINAS AND EMILY C. Z. ROBEN

Back pain in children is highly unusual and warrants concern by emergency physicians. Although often benign, the symptom may reflect abnormalities in the spinal column and viscera. Lumbago, involving the lower aspect of the 12th ribs to the gluteal folds, may be indicative of a serious illness that, if missed, can lead to permanent neurologic dysfunction or death. Younger children with back pain raise suspicion for etiologies such as discitis, vertebral osteomyelitis, and malignancy. The differential is broader for children older than 10 years and includes nonspecific etiologies, spondylolysis, spondylolisthesis, kyphosis, lumbar disk herniation, benign tumors, and rheumatologic causes. Adolescent rates of back pain approach that of adults.

HISTORY AND PHYSICAL EXAM

Clinicians should inquire about "red-flag" features of low back pain including constitutional symptoms (eg, fatigue, weight loss, night sweats), neurologic symptoms (eg, bladder or bowel impairment, weakness, numbness), and nonmechanical pain (eg, pain at rest).

The physical examination should be completed with the patient fully undressed and in a gown. A complete spine examination should be conducted, with particular attention to stance, gait, symmetry, motion, and tenderness. In addition, providers should be mindful of skin abnormalities (hair patches, unusual macules, hemangiomas) and complete a thorough neurologic examination of all muscle groups, deep tendon reflexes, and sensations.

Workup

Many children presenting to the ED with low back pain will require some laboratory and radiographic workup. If the cause of low back pain is quite clear, the child may not require any workup at all (eg, carrying a heavy load, engaging in new vigorous physical activity, no tenderness or other abnormalities on physical exam). Patients with no discernible etiology or with "red-flag" symptoms or signs should undergo a more comprehensive workup. Laboratory studies should include complete blood count, erythrocyte sedimentation rate, C-reactive protein, and blood cultures; depending on the symptoms, exam, and family history, it may also be useful to add RF, ACCP, ANP, and HLA-B27. Initially, posteroanterior and lateral radiographs of the entire spine should be obtained. For patients who have an abnormal neurologic exam, prominent neurologic symptoms, constitutional symptoms, and prolonged persistent pain should undergo MRI. The MRI should include contrast if infection, inflammation, or tumor is suspected. CT and bone scans have limited clinical indications due to high radiation exposure but are an option if MRI is not feasible.

Can't Miss Diagnoses

Spinal infection presents insidiously in children via absence of classic findings such as fever and elevated inflammation markers. For those younger than 5 years, discitis is more common and may present with refusal to sit upright, increased fussiness, and tenderness over affected areas with trunk flexion pain. Vertebral osteomyelitis rates are higher in the adolescent population and may be secondary to bacteremia, Pott disease (tuberculosis infection of the vertebra), or sickle cell disease with vasoocclusive crises of the spine. Fever, spinal pain, and neurologic deficits raise concern for an epidural abscess. MRI is the study of choice to diagnose all types of spine infections. Early neurosurgical consultation is imperative.

Infections located outside of the spine may also present with back pain. Providers should also search for localized infections (eg, pyelonephritis), systemic infections (eg, influenza), skin infections (eg, cellulitis, varicella/shingles), and infections with referred pain (eg, pneumonia, pelvic inflammatory disease, pancreatitis).

Both benign and malignant neoplasms may present with low back pain. The most common tumor in children with lumbago is vertebral osteoid osteoma; however, primary bone malignancies (eg, Ewing sarcoma, osteoblastoma, osteosarcoma) should remain on the differential. Other non-bone tumors (eg, neuroblastoma, Wilms tumor) and hematologic malignancies can also present with back pain. An emergent neurosurgical consultation is indicated for tumors compressing the spinal cord.

CES is a rare spinal emergency and can be permanently disabling syndrome if not rapidly recognized. The compression of lumbar and sacral nerve fibers below the conus medullaris may present simply as lower back pain. The classic presentation of CES includes bladder or rectal dysfunction, paresthesias in the lower extremities, saddle anesthesia, motor deficits, and decreased reflexes. Be aware that these red-flag symptoms are not always present in children. The most common etiologies for CES are spinal infection and malignancy.

Spinal trauma is also a common cause of low back pain in children. Direct trauma to the back can cause vertebral fracture or spinal epidural hematoma, both of which would present with back pain. Acute back pain in a child with known cancer should raise suspicion for a pathologic spinal fracture. Repetitive microtrauma may lead to spondylolysis (stress fracture vertebral pars interarticularis), spondylolisthesis (cephalic vertebrae slippage relative to caudal vertebrae), or intervertebral disk herniation.

Rheumatologic diseases and inflammatory arthritides should also be considered in pediatric patients, particularly when back pain is worsened with activity. Inflammatory markers such as RF, ACCP, ANA, and HLA-B27 are often outside the ED scope of practice; however, these studies can assist outpatient provider workup in identifying ankylosing spondylitis, inflammatory bowel disease-associated arthritis, reactive sacroiliitis, and psoriatic arthritis. And always remember, psychogenic back pain is a diagnosis of exclusion!

PEARLS

- Low back pain is less common in children than adults; the rate of back pain in adolescents approaches that of adults.
- Consider low back pain a "red flag" for children younger than 4 years.
- Benign causes of low back pain in children include overuse, minor musculoskeletal injuries, and mild systemic infections. Ominous causes of low back pain in children include infections, malignancy, trauma, and rheumatologic conditions.
- All children with low back pain should undergo workup with labs and imaging unless there is a clear, identifiable, benign cause for the pain. Start with radiographs, followed by MRI as needed.

Suggested Readings

Bachur RG, Shaw KN, Chamberlain J, Lavelle J, Nagler J, Shook J. *Fleisher & Ludwig's Textbook of Pediatric Emergency Medicine*. Lippincott Williams & Wilkins; 2020.

Biagiarelli FS, Piga S, Reale A, et al. Management of children presenting with low back pain to emergency department. *Am J Emerg Med*. 2019;37(4):672-679.

Devlin VJ. Pediatric back pain. In: Devlin VJ, ed. *Spine Secrets E-Book*. Elsevier Health Sciences; 2020:342.

Hartvigsen J, Hancock MJ, Kongsted A, et al. What low back pain is and why we need to pay attention. *Lancet*. 2018;391(10137):2356-2367.

Hébert JJ, Beynon AM, Jones BL, et al. Spinal pain in childhood: prevalence, trajectories, and diagnoses in children 6 to 17 years of age. *Eur J Pediatr*. 2022;181(4):1727-1736.

296

Kid ECGs Are Not Just Little Adult ECGs

Krista Young and Ian H. Law

Cardiac physiology changes with age during childhood, and the respective changes can be reflected on ECG. Some of these expected ECG patterns are only seen in pediatric tracings, and so it is important to differentiate normal from pathologic. This section will review common findings seen specifically in normal pediatric ECGs.

During fetal circulation, the right ventricle (RV) is the dominant chamber. It pumps against a relatively high-resistance pulmonary circulation in utero. As a result, the RV is larger and thicker than the left ventricle, and at birth, a neonate's ECG appears similar to an adult with RV hypertrophy. Specifically, the axis will be rightward; a dominant R wave in V1; Q waves in the inferior (II, III, aVF) and left precordial leads (V5, V6); and inverted T waves in V1 through V3 after the first week of life.

Examine the axis by reviewing leads I and aVF. Normally, the QRS complex will be positive (upward deflection) in both leads. However, in neonates, lead I may be overall negative leading to a more rightward axis. After birth, intrathoracic pressures dramatically decrease with initial breaths, with subsequent decreased pulmonary vascular resistance and increased systemic vascular resistance. After a few days, the ductus arteriosus normally closes, and systemic output becomes left ventricle dependent. By early childhood or 3 to 4 years of age, the heart takes on the more adult-appearing normal axis with a larger and thicker left ventricle.

Remembering that V1 through V3 are right-sided precordial leads, a positive dominant R wave is also normally seen in childhood. Many children also display an rsr′ pattern (two peaks/"bunny ears"), often interpreted as a partial right bundle branch block or right ventricular conduction delay using adult criteria, but the QRS duration is near normal. In children, if the second peak (r′) is not 10 mm greater than the first peak, this is a normal variant that usually disappears by age 5 (**Figure 296.1**).

Likewise, small and narrow isolated Q waves that point downward or are negative can be normally seen in the inferior and left precordial leads in asymptomatic, otherwise healthy patients. However, use caution as deep Q waves can be a sign of an underlying pathologic process including myocardial ischemia/infarction, ventricular hypertrophy, and hypertrophic cardiomyopathy. Patients with new chest pain may be worrisome if several adjacent leads show similar changes and/or if new Q waves are seen that were not on a previous ECG. In general, pathologic Q waves are one small box (40 msecond) or greater in width.

During ventricular repolarization, in children, the T-wave pattern is negative or inverted in V1 through V3 representing a juvenile T-wave pattern after the first week of life until around puberty. If the juvenile T-wave pattern is still seen into adolescence, this may be a normal variant called persistent juvenile T waves. Inverted T waves beyond V2 after puberty suggest a possible RV cardiomyopathy and require further evaluation. Inverted T waves in the lateral precordial leads (V5, V6) suggest a left ventricular cardiomyopathy and warrant cardiology follow-up.

Due to the smaller size necessitating faster rates to maintain cardiac output, rates will appear tachycardic by adult standards and are routinely above 100 until 4 years of age. Conduction intervals like PR and QRS will also be decreased because less time is needed for the electrical impulse to move through the heart.

Two other special findings that are commonly mistaken for abnormal by those less familiar with pediatric ECGs are sinus arrhythmia and benign early repolarization (BER). When a patient is in sinus rhythm, the ECG shows consistent P-wave morphology in the expected axis for age followed by a QRS. In healthy children, the P-P interval can sometimes vary with respirations and is called sinus arrhythmia. This finding is physiologically normal and is due to transient decreases in vagal tone on inspiration causing an increase in heart rate which is restored and reversed on expiration. With age, baroreceptor sensitivity and the ability for the carotids to stretch most likely decrease, and the incidence of sinus arrhythmia decreases. Comparatively, in older adults, a pronounced

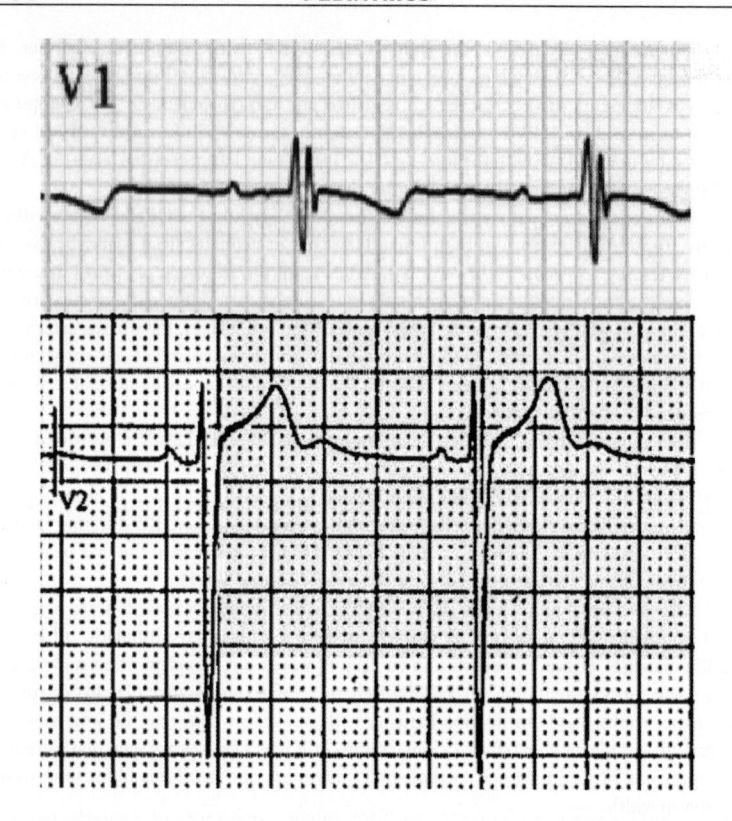

FIGURE 296.1 Examples of normal ECG variants in healthy children. Top: Tracing demonstrates an rsr' pattern (two peaks/"bunny ears") with normal QRS duration and r' peak less than 10 mm than the r peak in lead V1. Bottom: Tracing demonstrates an upsloping ST-segment in lead V2, an example of benign early repolarization.

sinus arrhythmia is often pathologic due to heart disease or digoxin toxicity and not related to respirations.

The J-point is the junction of the QRS complex and the ST segment. During J-point elevation, there is an upsloping ST-segment elevation in the mid-precordial leads, most commonly V2 and V3 (**Figure 296.1**). In adults, if the ST-segment elevation is flat it could represent pericarditis or an acute MI. In healthy children, the upsloping ST-segment elevation represents BER. The physiologic basis is not known, but this finding can be seen until the age of 50.

During childhood, specific normal findings are seen on the ECG that represent the healthy, growing pediatric heart. Knowing normal from abnormal can be difficult in this population as some normal findings mimic concerning findings in the adult population. Remembering normal ECG findings can reassure practitioners, patients, and families alike.

PEARLS

- Due to fetal circulation, in the early stage of childhood, the RV is larger and thicker, and shows right axis deviation on ECGs at birth.
- Additional right-sided findings include juvenile T-wave inversion, R waves in the right precordial leads, or a normal variant of rsr' in V1.
- Isolated inferior and left precordial Q waves can be normal when short and narrow in otherwise healthy children.
- Pediatric ECGs have faster heart rates (>100 beats/min) and shorter conduction intervals.
- Sinus arrhythmia and BERs are normal but commonly mistaken during childhood.

SUGGESTED READINGS

Dickinson D. The normal ECG in childhood and adolescence. *Heart*. 2005;91(12):1626-1630.
Goodacre S. ABC of clinical electrocardiography: paediatric electrocardiography. *BMJ*. 2002;324(7350):1382-1385.
O'Connor M, McDaniel N, Brady W. The pediatric electrocardiogram. *Am J Emerg Med*. 2008;26(2):221-228.
Park M, Guntheroth W. *How to Read Pediatric ECGs*. 4th ed. Mosby/Elsevier; 2006:35-61, 86-88, 107-108.
Tipple M. Interpretation of electrocardiograms in infants and children. *Images Paediatr Cardiol*. 1999;1(1):3-13.

297

WHAT'S NEW IN MANAGING PEDIATRIC DIABETIC KETOACIDOSIS

HILARY ONG AND MIMI LU

DKA is a common reason for children with IDDM to present to EDs. The three laboratory criteria for DKA include hyperglycemia (>200 mg/dL or >11 mmol/L), ketosis (ketonuria or serum beta-OH butyrate >3 mmol/L), and anion gap metabolic acidosis (venous pH < 7.3 or HCO_3 <15 mmol/L). DKA is the leading cause of death in children with diabetes, most commonly due to cerebral edema. Children with either type 1 or type 2 insulin-dependent diabetes can develop DKA. Clinically apparent cerebral edema occurs in approximately 0.5% of episodes of DKA in children and is fatal in nearly 25% of affected children. Even those who survive are at high risk for long-term neurologic consequences.

Management of DKA is focused on reversing the catabolic state by administering insulin and replacing fluids and electrolytes. It was previously believed that rapid administration of initial fluids may lead to shifts in serum osmolality, resulting in worsening cerebral edema. However, a recent PECARN randomized clinical trial showed no difference in rapid administration (20 mL/kg vs 10 mL/kg bolus) nor type (0.45% NS vs 0.9% NS) of fluids in neurologic decompensation. The International Society for Pediatric and Adolescent Diabetes guidelines from 2014 recommend NS rather than LR based on expert opinion. LR administration may lead to electrolyte imbalances and an increased risk of cerebral edema. However, more recent studies report a potential decrease in cases of cerebral edema in pediatric patients with DKA who received LR fluid.

It is critical to administer a continuous infusion of insulin (regular insulin 0.05-0.1 units/kg/h) to reverse the catabolic state and metabolic acidosis. The infusion is continued until laboratory values normalize (pH > 7.3, HCO_3 >15, beta-hydroxybutyrate <1 mmol/L, and resolved anion gap). Administration of intravenous bicarbonate will not reverse the catabolic state and is associated with an increased risk of cerebral edema. A common error is to stop the insulin infusion when serum glucose starts to decrease, but insulin must be continued until ketosis and acidosis are resolved. A two-bag fluid system can be used to allow for the addition of dextrose to avoid hypoglycemia when the blood glucose falls below 300 mg/dL. One liter bag should contain NS with 20 mEq/L of potassium chloride and 20 mEq/L of potassium acetate. The second bag has the same fluid and electrolyte content with D10W added. The two bags of fluids are titrated according to the patient's blood glucose level at a rate 1.5 times the maintenance fluid rate for pediatric patients.

Cerebral edema is life-threatening and constitutes a clinical diagnosis with subtle initial presenting symptoms. The etiology in DKA is likely multifactorial due to vasogenic, osmotic, and cytotoxic insults. Patients may present with headache and vomiting, altered mental status, focal neurologic deficits, bradycardia, and decreased oxygen saturation. Established risk factors for pediatric DKA associated with increased risk of developing cerebral injury/edema are age younger than 3 years, new-onset diagnosis of IDDM, severely abnormal laboratory values (eg, pH < 7.1, low serum bicarbonate, high BUN, low Pco_2, failure of serum sodium to rise with treatment), and treatment with IV bicarbonate. Cerebral edema typically occurs 4 to 12 hours following initiation of treatment for DKA. However, this complication can manifest as late as 48 hours following the initiation of treatment for DKA (despite the resolution of ketoacidosis) and has been described in 5% to 10% of affected children on initial presentation before initiation of treatment.

When cerebral edema is suspected, treatment must be initiated immediately and should not be delayed for advanced brain imaging. The head of bed should be elevated to 30° and medications administered to address increased ICP. Hyperosmolar therapy reduces blood viscosity and draws water out of brain tissue, resulting in transient reductions in ICP. Options include intravenous mannitol at a dose of 1 g/kg given over 10 minutes or intravenous hypertonic (3%) saline at a dose of 5 to 10 mL/kg over 10 minutes. Although less acutely life-threatening than cerebral edema, thrombotic events are more common in children than adults with DKA and include CVT and DVT.

Children in DKA are often acutely ill and may decompensate precipitously, even before treatment is initiated. Rapid recognition of the severe complications of pediatric DKA and directed therapy are essential.

PEARLS

- Cerebral edema is a rare but life-threatening condition in children with DKA and is a clinical diagnosis. Monitor the patient closely for neurologic decompensation and treat early with hyperosmolar therapy if concerned.
- Risk factors associated with cerebral edema in pediatric patients with DKA include age younger than 3 years, severe acidosis, decreasing sodium levels, low P_{CO_2}, low serum bicarbonate, and high BUN. Avoid using intravenous bicarbonate.
- Fluid repletion is essential in management of DKA. The two-bag IV fluid system is used to rehydrate and to avoid hypoglycemia as ketosis improves. Fluid type, bolus, or infusion rate are likely not associated with the development of cerebral edema.

SUGGESTED READINGS

Bergmann KR, Abuzzahab MJ, Nowak J, et al. Resuscitation with Ringer's lactate compared with normal saline for pediatric diabetic ketoacidosis. *Pediatr Emerg Care*. 2021;37(5): e236-e242.

Bialo S, Agrawal S, Boney C, et al. Rare complications of pediatric diabetic ketoacidosis. *World J Diabetes*. 2015;6(1):167.

Glaser N, Ghetti S, Casper C, et al.; PECARN. Childhood diabetic ketoacidosis, fluid therapy and cerebral injury: the design of a factorial randomized controlled trial. *Pediatr Diabetes*. 2013;14:435-446.

Kuppermann N, Ghetti S, Schunk JE, et al. Clinical trial of fluid infusion rates for pediatric diabetic ketoacidosis. *N Engl J Med*. 2018;378(24):2275-2287.

Lavoie M. Management of a patient with diabetic ketoacidosis in the emergency department. *Pediatr Emerg Care*. 2015;31(5):376-380.

Long B, Koyfman A. Emergency medicine myths: cerebral edema in pediatric diabetic ketoacidosis and intravenous fluids. *J Emerg Med*. 2017;53(2):212-221.

298

MAKE PALS YOUR PAL

RASHEED ALHADI AND EFRAT ROSENTHAL

Pediatric critical care resuscitations are stressful, highly emotional, and fortunately rare. Similar to any emergent situation, preparation and structure are essential for success. The American Heart Association developed the PALS program as a standardized approach to the critically ill pediatric patients including cardiac arrest, post-arrest management, shock, cardiac arrhythmias, and respiratory failure.

PALS serves as an internationally recognized tool to help adult and pediatric emergency providers with these daunting scenarios. PALS highlights important differences in the resuscitation of critically ill pediatric patients compared to adult patients.

Systematic Approach

PALS requires rapid identification of the child's age and weight. This informs vital sign ranges, weight-based medication dosing, and equipment sizes. Involving team members and other resources in dose calculations can allow the team leader to focus on other elements of the resuscitation.

PALS supports the use of the Broselow tape that estimates medication dosing based on the patient's height. Locate the Broselow tape, familiarize yourself with its use, and lay it out before the patient arrives when possible. There are also great apps and pocket cards available. It is important to be comfortable with whatever resource you decide to use.

The initial resuscitation steps remain the same for children and adults: IV, O_2, monitoring. Beware that IV placement can agitate and worsen a tenuous patient at high risk for airway or respiratory compromise. If access is emergently needed, consider a proximal tibial or humeral IO if two IV attempts have been made without success.

Pediatric Assessment

PALS utilizes the PAT as a quick observational tool to categorize patients as sick or not sick (**Figure 298.1**). The PAT has three components: appearance, breathing, and circulation. Abnormalities in any of the three can give insight into the underlying disease process. The assessment of appearance can be remembered by the mnemonic TICLS (tone, irritability, consolability, look [gaze], and speech [cry]). The breathing assessment involves looking for tripoding, nasal flaring, head-bobbing, retractions, and accessory muscle use. Circulation assessment involves examining the skin for pallor, mottling, and cyanosis that could signal poor peripheral perfusion and oxygenation. The PAT should be immediately followed by the primary survey and followed by a SAMPLE history (signs and symptoms, allergies, medications, past medical history, last meal, and events).

PALS Algorithms

When the PAT indicates that a child is critically ill, PALS can help! Key similarities and differences between PALS and ACLS as well as important 2020 updates are listed in **Table 298.1**.

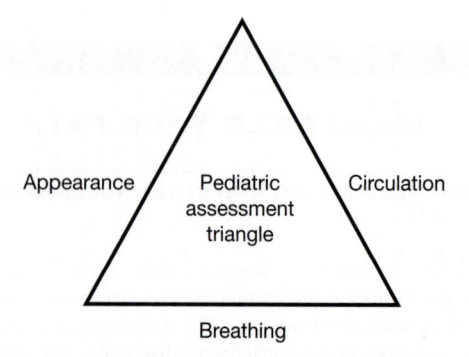

FIGURE 298.1 Pediatric assessment triangle.

TABLE 298.1 SUMMARY OF PALS VERSUS ACLS SIMILARITIES AND DIFFERENCES AND PALS 2020 UPDATES

Algorithm	Similarities	Differences	Updates
Cardiac arrest	■ High quality CPR with minimal interruptions at a rate of 100-120 beats/min ■ Early defibrillation for shockable rhythms ■ Epinephrine every 3-5 min regardless or rhythm ■ Sodium bicarbonate and calcium are not routinely recommended.	■ Etiology of cardiac arrest in children is likely respiratory vs primary cardiac in adults ■ Most reliable pulse for infants (brachial) vs children and adults (carotid, femoral) or apply three lead ECG ■ Method (infants: two-thumb encircling chest for two-rescuers and two-finger technique for one rescuer; children: one or two hand technique). Adequate depth: 1/3 AP chest diameter ■ Medications AND defibrillation are weight based in PALS. ■ Compression-ventilation CPR ratio 15:2 (two rescuers) or 30:2 (one rescuer)	■ Early epinephrine within 5 min improved outcomes ■ Cricoid pressure is no longer routinely used. ■ Cuffed ETT recommended for all ages. ■ Breath delivery rate of 1 breath every 2-3 sec (20-30/min). Previously 1 breath every 6 sec (10/min)
Post-arrest management	■ Reverse the underlying etiology of arrest. ■ Maintain hemodynamics goals to optimize neurologic recovery. ■ Follow targeted temperature management.	N/A	■ Identify post-arrest nonconvulsive seizures with routine EEG if encephalopathic. ■ Evaluate and address psychological, physical, and social impact post-arrest.
Shock	■ IV, O₂, monitor and primary survey ■ Fluid resuscitation, vasopressor choice, and targeted treatments depending on etiology	■ Recognize shock early. Children decompensate rapidly. ■ Use physical exam to identify and categorize shock. Repeat to monitor response to treatment. ■ For neonates and young infants consider ductal-dependent congenital heart defects. Start a prostaglandin E1 infusion. Beware of apnea.	■ Septic: • 10-20 mL/kg crystalloid, up to 40-60 mL/kg, avoid fluid overload. • Vasopressor: epi (cold) vs norepi (warm shock) first line; dopamine second line in fluid-refractory septic shock ■ Hemorrhagic: • 1:1:1: matched blood products similar to adults

AP, anterior-posterior; CPR, cardiopulmonary resuscitation; ECG, electrocardiogram; EEG, electroencephalogram; ETT, endotracheal tube; IV, intravenous; PALS, pediatric advanced life support.

PEARLS

- **Remember that for children:**
  1. Respiratory failure is the leading cause of cardiac arrest.
  2. Normotensive shock is common and kids decompensate quickly. Act early!
- **Utilize the PAT.** Repeat it.
- **Double check your medication dosing and equipment sizing.** The adult dose is the max dose. Dedicate a reliable team member to read out or calculate doses.
- **Involve parents and guardians** in the resuscitation as they can provide history, comfort the patient, and better process the resuscitation.
- **Make PALS your PAL.** Find comfort that there are many similarities between PALS and ACLS. Respect the key differences. Review PALS early and often.

SUGGESTED READINGS

American Academy of Pediatrics, and American Heart Association. *Pediatric Advanced Life Support: Provider Manual*. American Heart Association; 2020.

Andersen LW, Berg KM, Saindon BZ, et al. Time to epinephrine and survival after pediatric in-hospital cardiac arrest. *JAMA*. 2015;314:802-810.

Dieckmann RA, Brownstein D, Gausche-Hill M. The pediatric assessment triangle: a novel approach for the rapid evaluation of children. *Pediatr Emerg Care*. 2010;26(4):312-315.

Herman ST, Abend NS, Bleck TP, et al. Consensus statement on continuous EEG in critically ill adults and children, part I: indications. *J Clin Neurophysiol*. 2015;32:87-95.

Topjian AA, Raymond TT, Atkins D, et al. Part 4: Pediatric basic and advanced life support: 2020 American Heart Association guidelines for cardiopulmonary resuscitation and emergency cardiovascular care. *Circulation*. 2020;142(16_suppl_2):S469-S523.

299

IS PROCALCITONIN HELPFUL IN YOUNG INFANTS?

MONICA CHARPENTIER AND SIMA PATEL

Identifying the young infant (<90 days old) with a SBI such as meningitis, bacteremia, or urinary tract infection in the ED is a unique challenge. Clinical signs and symptoms are not reliable predictors of serious illness in this age group and infants are at higher risk of morbidity and mortality due to immune system immaturity, minimal vaccine-induced immunity, and lower physiologic reserve. Fever may be the only indicator of SBI in well-appearing infants. As the consequences of a missed bacterial illness may be severe, these infants often receive a substantial diagnostic workup, parenteral antibiotics, and hospital admission. Biomarkers are an evolving tool to distinguish the febrile young infant with an SBI from one with a self-limiting viral illness and to reduce unnecessary hospital admissions and antibiotic use.

HISTORICAL GUIDELINES

Biomarkers used to assess risk of bacterial illness in young infants have included WBC, ANC, ABC, CRP, ESR, UA, and CSF. CRP and ANC have demonstrated higher accuracy than WBC alone. Combined clinical and laboratory analysis algorithms such as the Boston, Philadelphia, and Rochester criteria have a high negative predictive value, missing less than 10% of serious bacterial illnesses but with lower positive predictive values and higher false-positive rates.

PCT: THE NEW BIOMARKER ON THE BLOCK

PCT is a newer laboratory biomarker used to identify young infants with SBI. PCT is a peptide that under normal physiologic circumstances is found at very low levels. PCT production is thought to be increased by the inflammatory pathways associated with bacterial infections, while PCT levels are actually reduced by the alternative inflammatory pathway in response to viral illnesses. PCT is released within a few hours of bacterial illness, leading to high concentrations detectable earlier in the illness course than other biomarkers such as CRP. Current data indicate that PCT is a more accurate test than WBC, ANC, and CRP alone.

Many small studies have shown improvement in accuracy and specificity when combining PCT with other laboratory biomarkers compared to single markers alone. A 2019 PECARN study derived a clinical prediction rule using only the UA, ANC, and PCT levels. Unlike the prior clinical practice guidelines, this tool did not use a priori thresholds for laboratory values, does not require a lumbar puncture to be performed, and is more generalizable, including infants even with clear respiratory symptoms.

2021 AAP GUIDELINES

The AAP provided their first guidelines for management of febrile infants in 2021. Their guidelines apply exclusively to well-appearing infants born at term and stratify by age: 8 to 21 days, 22 to 28 days, and 29 to 60 days of age. The guidelines recommend the use of PCT for all three groups, if available, using a cutoff of greater than 0.5 ng/mL.

PCT AND AGE: HOW LOW CAN YOU GO?

There are a few important caveats to using PCT as a biomarker in premature infants and infants within the first week of life. There is a physiologic increase in the levels of PCT during the first few days of life before falling and peaking later in premature infants than in term infants. Age-specific nomograms for both preterm and term infants have not yet been definitively established in large cohorts. The NeoPIns trial found that use of PCT-guided decision-making was superior to standard care in reducing antibiotic administration for suspected early-onset neonatal sepsis. Small studies suggest that PCT appears to be a more sensitive indicator of both early-onset and late-onset neonatal sepsis compared to CRP.

PRACTICAL CONSIDERATIONS AND CONFOUNDERS

PCT offers several practical benefits in evaluating a young infant in the ED: It requires a very small blood sample (200 mcL), can provide risk stratification without more invasive and time-consuming procedures such as a urinary catheterization or lumbar puncture, and can have a short turn-around time.

While PCT levels rise earlier than CRP, they may still be normal in the immediate hours after illness or fever onset, and thus should not be the exclusive criterion used for risk stratification. If an infant is ill-appearing, clinical judgment should supersede biomarkers, and laboratory evaluation should not delay antibiotic administration. Obtaining a PCT in the ED may be useful in deciding the duration of antibiotics, as PCT can be trended over time and there is strong data supporting the use of PCT trends to reduce antibiotic administration in the intensive care unit.

While PCT appears to be among the most specific inflammatory markers for bacterial infection, several other conditions may lead to an increase in PCT, such as burns, ischemia, maternal preeclampsia, perinatal asphyxia, and intracranial hemorrhage, although these are not well-studied. For children and young infants presenting to the ED with fever and any of these other confounders, we do not recommend basing antibiotic administration on PCT levels alone.

PEARLS

- Young infants are at higher risk for a serious bacterial illness and may present with nonspecific clinical signs and symptoms.
- PCT may have the best sensitivity and specificity for identification of significant bacterial infections in young infants.
- Special consideration must be given to neonates in the first week of life and preterm infants as nomograms for PCT are not clearly defined.
- Guidelines incorporating PCT for diagnostic workup and management of the febrile young infant from the AAP and PECARN are best established and widely used.
- PCT has limitations and should be used in conjunction with validated guidelines and clinical judgment.

Suggested Readings

Eschborn S, Weitkamp JH. Procalcitonin versus C-reactive protein: review of kinetics and performance for diagnosis of neonatal sepsis. *J Perinatol*. 2019;39(7):893-903. PMID: 30926891.

Hui C, Neto G, Tsertsvadze A, et al. Diagnosis and management of febrile infants (0-3 months). *Evid Rep Technol Assess (Full Rep)*. 2012;(205):1-297. PMID: 24422856.

Olaciregui I, Hernández U, Muñoz JA, Emparanza JI, Landa JJ. Markers that predict serious bacterial infection in infants under 3 months of age presenting with fever of unknown origin. *Arch Dis Child*. 2009;94(7):501-505. PMID: 19158133.

Pantell R, Roberts K, Adams W, et al. Evaluation and management of well-appearing febrile infants 8 to 60 days old. *Pediatrics*. 2021;148(2):e2021052228.

Stocker M, van Herk W, El Helou S, et al. Procalcitonin-guided decision making for duration of antibiotic therapy in neonates with suspected early-onset sepsis: a multicentre, randomised controlled trial (NeoPIns). *Lancet*. 2017;390(10097):871-881. PMID: 28711318.

300

The Hard Truth of Constipation—Don't Miss the Potentially Serious Causes of Constipation

Jennifer Guyther and Carmen Avendano

Between 5% and 30% of the pediatric population experience constipation. Patients present with fewer than three bowel movements per week, acute abdominal pain, stool retention, and crying. Constipation can be divided into two main types: organic (5%) versus functional (95%). For reference, normal stooling patterns are as follows. Newborns transition from meconium to a green/brown stool and then a yellow/brown milk stool by 4 or 5 days of life. After 3 weeks of life, babies may go up to 2 weeks without passing stool. Older children stool between several times per day to once every several days. The NASPGHAN defines constipation as a delay or difficulty in defecation for more than 2 weeks that causes significant distress to the patient. Other definitions that are well known include Rome IV criteria: two or fewer defecations in the toilet per week, at least one episode of fecal incontinence per week, history of retentive posturing or excessive volitional stool retention, history of painful or hard bowel movements, presence of a large fecal mass in the rectum, or history of a large diameter stool. Key historical questions include frequency and consistency of stools, pain or bleeding with defecation, abdominal pain, vomiting, toilet training history, soiling, appetite change, diet, prior surgeries, family history, suspected foreign body ingestion, and medications.

Worrisome signs suggesting a secondary cause of constipation or other serious conditions include onset during the neonatal period, failure to pass meconium, weight loss or poor weight gain, bilious vomiting, family history of Hirschsprung disease, delayed motor milestones, fever, bloody stools, distended abdomen, prior abdominal surgery, abnormal bowel sounds, suspected foreign body ingestion, and ribbon-like stool. The differential diagnosis for abdominal pain is broad, and thus we will only touch on differential diagnosis for organic causes of constipation, which includes Hirschsprung disease, hypothyroidism, milk protein allergy, celiac disease, imperforate/stenotic anus, intestinal obstruction, cystic fibrosis, spinal cord dysfunction, and botulism. Special attention should be paid to the abdominal, perineal, and neurologic exam. Concerning findings include abdominal distention, sacral dimpling, midline pigment abnormalities or hair tufts, an abnormal anus or an empty rectal vault despite palpable stool on abdominal exam. A digital rectal exam is only needed if the history or exam is abnormal.

Current evidence does not support routine abdominal radiographs or blood work for evaluation of fecal impaction unless worrisome signs are present. Multiple scoring systems for assessing stool burden have been proposed, but they do not have high inter-reader reliability. The Choosing Wisely campaign has encouraged a decrease in the ordering of abdominal radiographs for abdominal pain given the lack of correlation between the clinical history of constipation and the fecal load seen on imaging.

An elimination diet may be beneficial for milk protein allergy but often not for 2 to 4 weeks. Most children with cow's milk allergy also react to goat and sheep's milk and some to soy milk, so hydrolyzed formulas such as Nutramigen and Alimentum may

TABLE 300.1	ORAL MEDICATIONS USED TO TREAT CONSTIPATION	
MEDICATION	**MECHANISM**	**DOSE**
Polyethylene glycol	Opposes absorption of water by the large bowel; not absorbed or metabolized	Disimpaction: 1-1.5 g/kg/d for 3-6 d Maintenance: 0.4 g/kg/d (max, 100 g/d)
Lactulose	Draws fluid into large bowels, increasing peristalsis (safe at all ages)	1-2 g/kg/d
Milk of magnesia	Promotes osmotic retention of fluid (can lead to toxicity in infants)	2-5 yr: 0.4-1.2 g/d 6-11 yr: 1.2-2.4 g/d 12-18 yr: 2.4-4.8 g/d
Mineral oil	Makes the stool slippery; slows colonic absorption of water	1-3 mL/kg/d (max 90 mL)
Bisacodyl	Acts on intestinal mucosa, altering water and electrolyte secretion	3-10 yr: 5 mg/d >10 yr: 5-10 mg/d
Senna	Acts on intestinal mucosa, altering water and electrolyte secretion	2-6 yr: 2.5-5 mg/d 6-12 yr: 2.5-12 mg/d >12 yr: 15-20 mg/d
Sodium picosulfate	Acts on intestinal mucosa, altering water and electrolyte secretion	1 mo-4 yr: 2.5-10 mg/d 4-18 yr: 2.5-20 mg/d

be preferable in these cases. Adding fiber or water to the diet does not relieve constipation unless they are deficient. Medication options to treat constipation are listed in **Table 300.1**.

Future considerations for constipation diagnosed in the ED could include sending patients home with a constipation action plan in discharge paperwork to include information on disimpaction (if enema not used) and maintenance therapy for successful treatment.

PEARLS

- Constipation is a delay or difficulty in defecation for more than 2 weeks that causes significant distress to the patient.
- Rectal examination, blood work, and radiographs are needed only if the patient's history or the physical exam raises concern.
- Always consider secondary causes of constipation such as Hirschsprung disease and botulism and look for clues in the history and physical exam findings.
- For fecal disimpaction, consider PEG at 1 to 1.5 g/kg/day for 3 to 6 days or enemas. Once disimpaction has been achieved, continue maintenance therapy with PEG, 0.4 g/kg/day. Lactulose is also the first-line treatment and is considered safe for all ages.

SUGGESTED READINGS

Gfroerer S, Rolle U. Pediatric intestinal motility disorders. *World J Gastroenterol*. 2015;21:9683-9687.

Kearney R, Edwards T, Bradford M, Klein E. Emergency provider use of plain radiographs in the evaluation of pediatric constipation. *Pediatr Emerg Care*. 2019;35(9):624-629.

Khan L. Constipation management in pediatric primary care. *Pediatr Ann*. 2018;47:e180-e184.

Madani S, Tsang L, Kamat D. Constipation in children: a practical review. *Pediatr Ann*. 2016;45:e189-e196.

Tabbers MM, DiLorenzo C, Berger MY, et al. Evaluation and treatment of functional constipation in infants and children: evidence-based recommendations from ESPGHAN and NASPGHAN. *J Pediatr Gastroenterol Nutr*. 2014;58:258-274.

Trapani S, Montemaggi A, Indolfi G. Choosing wisely in pediatric healthcare: a narrative review. *Front Pediatr*. 2023;10:1071088.

301

Mishaps in Pediatric Myocarditis

Madeline Grade and Margaret Lin-Martore

The gravest mishap of pediatric myocarditis is to miss the diagnosis altogether. Albeit rare (annual estimated incidence varies between 1 and 2 cases per 100,000), this diagnosis is critical to consider, as it can cause considerable morbidity or mortality in an otherwise healthy child.

Myocarditis, defined as inflammation of the myocardium, can lead to necrosis of cardiac myocytes and subsequent cardiac dysfunction. Complications include heart block, ventricular aneurysm, dilated cardiomyopathy, and congestive heart failure. In developed countries, viral infection is the most common cause (eg, parvovirus B-19, human herpesvirus-6, and enteroviruses including coxsackie). Worldwide, common etiologies include protozoal (eg, Chagas disease) and rheumatic carditis. Considering the recent coronavirus disease (COVID) pandemic, it is important to note that both the COVID-19 vaccine and post-COVID multisystem inflammatory syndrome in children can trigger myocarditis, though both varieties appear to have better clinical outcomes than traditional viral myocarditis. Many other infections, toxins, and autoimmune disorders can trigger myocarditis. In the majority of cases, no specific cause is identified.

Patient Assessment

Classically, children present with dyspnea, fever, chest pain, tachycardia, and signs of volume overload after a viral prodrome. However, not all cases are so straightforward, especially given the potential variations in time course, trigger, and severity. Since half of cases can be missed on the initial visit, repeat visits for persistent viral symptoms should prompt the consideration of additional workup. Unfortunately, there is no definitive noninvasive diagnostic test (the traditional gold standard is endometrial biopsy). In practice, myocarditis is a clinical diagnosis surmised from a constellation of symptoms, exam findings, and test results. Thus emergency clinicians must maintain a high degree of clinical suspicion.

In more subtle presentations, the first exam clue may be persistent unexplained tachycardia. While tachycardia in a febrile pediatric patient is most often benign, one should reconsider if it fails to improve with antipyretics. Other exam findings may include tachypnea, abnormal auscultation (eg, rales, murmur, gallop), hepatomegaly, and edema (rare in children). In more severe cases, children may appear sick, cyanotic, hypotensive, and in respiratory distress.

Diagnostic Studies

Point-of-care ultrasound is an invaluable adjunct to the physical exam. A bedside assessment of cardiac function and volume status are particularly useful for distinguishing between distributive and cardiogenic shock in a patient with undifferentiated hypotension. This important step can prevent the potentially devastating error of giving a large fluid bolus to a child with left ventricular dysfunction. Ultrasound findings in myocarditis may include reduced systolic function, regional wall motion abnormalities, pericardial effusion, B-lines, plethoric inferior vena cava, and pleural effusions.

The presence or absence of lab or imaging findings can be highly variable in myocarditis. The classic finding on chest radiography is cardiomegaly (40% of cases), and overall, only 60% are abnormal. Electrocardiogram is abnormal in over 93% of patients, though sensitivity is low, and specificity is unknown. The most common finding is sinus tachycardia. Other potential findings include low voltage, widened QRS, prolonged QT interval, conduction block, ventricular or atrial arrhythmias, and signs of ischemia. Laboratory evaluation, especially warranted if the patient appears unwell and the differential includes infection or metabolic derangements, may reveal an elevated leukocyte count, inflammatory markers, B-type natriuretic peptide, or troponin (none of which are sensitive or specific). In recent years, cardiac magnetic resonance imaging has demonstrated promising diagnostic utility, but it is impractical in the emergency setting.

Management

Once a high degree of clinical suspicion exists, management of myocarditis must proceed swiftly, as these patients are at risk of rapid decompensation and cardiac dysrhythmias. Patients require continuous cardiac monitoring and often admission to pediatric intensive care units. Treatment is generally supportive and focuses on providing circulatory support, optimizing volume status, and preventing respiratory decompensation.

Low cardiac output in myocarditis should be managed with inotropic support, often milrinone in the intensive care setting. In cases of concurrent cardiogenic shock, epinephrine or dobutamine can offer vasopressor support in addition to inotropy; however, they may also confer higher arrhythmogenic risk. Alternatively, recent literature suggests concurrent arginine vasopressin and calcium chloride infusion as a safer alternative for improving perfusion pressure. Arrhythmias should be managed promptly, with care taken to avoid antiarrhythmic agents with significant negative inotropic effects (eg, beta-blockers) as they may exacerbate acute heart failure. In severe cases, patients should be transferred to a center capable of early mechanical circulatory support (eg, ventricular assist device, extracorporeal membrane oxygenation), as this may be lifesaving.

A variety of systematic reviews have investigated the utility of steroids or intravenous immune globulin in acute myocarditis, neither of which has demonstrated significant benefit. Furthermore, immunosuppressive therapy in the acute phase of illness may in fact exacerbate viral replication and worsen the disease course.

Careful fluid optimization is essential. Avoid negligent fluid administration and utilize diuretics as needed to reduce cardiac strain from volume overload. If a definitive airway must be obtained, it is critical to anticipate possible peri-intubation hypotension and cardiac arrest. Temporize with noninvasive positive pressure ventilation, and if intubation is necessary, have push-dose pressors on hand.

Racial disparities impact outcomes, and unfortunately children of racial and ethnic minorities have higher rates of in-hospital mortality. With early recognition and treatment, many patients with pediatric myocarditis can survive and achieve full restoration of cardiac function. However, even in mild cases, complete recovery may take months to years, and more severe cases may eventually require heart transplant. Thoughtful communication with parents or guardians about the potential for prolonged recovery should not be overlooked.

PEARLS

- The greatest risk in myocarditis is to miss the diagnosis. Maintain a high clinical suspicion, particularly in pediatric patients experiencing persistent unexplained tachycardia.
- Check volume status with ultrasound before administration of fluids in undifferentiated shock, as this can cause acute respiratory decompensation in myocarditis.
- Supportive treatment includes supplemental oxygen, inotropic support, maintenance of adequate perfusion pressure, and careful fluid optimization.
- Consider early mechanical circulatory support in severe cases.

SUGGESTED READINGS

Karki KB, Towbin JA, Harrell C, et al. Concurrent use of calcium chloride and arginine vasopressin infusions in pediatric patients with acute cardiocirculatory failure. *Pediatr Cardiol.* 2019;40(5):1046-1056.

Law YM, Lal AK, Chen S, et al. Diagnosis and management of myocarditis in children: a scientific statement from the American Heart Association. *Circulation.* 2021;144:e123-135.

Olsen J, Tjoeng YL, Friedland-Little J, Chan T. Racial disparities in hospital mortality among pediatric cardiomyopathy and myocarditis patients. *Pediatr Cardiol.* 2021;42(1):59-71.

Patel T, Kelleman M, West Z, et al. Comparison of multisystem inflammatory syndrome in children-related myocarditis, classic viral myocarditis, and COVID-19 vaccine-related myocarditis in children. *J Am Heart Assoc.* 2022;11(9):e024393.

Pomiato E, Perrone MA, Palmieri R, Gagliardi MG. Pediatric myocarditis: what have we learnt so far? *J Cardiovasc Dev Dis.* 2022;9(5):143.

302

THE KITCHEN SINK—PEDIATRIC STATUS ASTHMATICUS

MAHNOOSH NIK-AHD

Asthma is a relatively common childhood diagnosis and during respiratory season, severe asthma exacerbations resulting in status asthmaticus are not uncommon. Status asthmaticus is defined by a severe asthma exacerbation that does not respond to typical treatments, sometimes complicated by acute respiratory failure.

Signs of a severe exacerbation include signs of bronchoconstriction including inspiratory and expiratory wheezing, or diminished wheezing due to poor air flow into the lungs. A lack of wheezing occurs when bronchoconstriction is so severe that this impedes air movement. Therefore, a lack of wheezing with increased work of breathing should signal alarm, rather than reassurance. Other signs include agitation as a result of hypoxemia or lethargy due to hypoxemia/hypercarbia, severe tachypnea or inability to speak in short sentences, accessory muscle use, grunting, head bobbing, cyanosis, and decreased oxygen saturation (SpO_2 <92%).

The mainstay of treatment is bronchodilation and anti-inflammatory therapies. Start with continuous albuterol 20 mg/h for at least 1 hour and ipratropium 250 mcg if less than 20 kg and 500 mcg if at least 20 kg. Due to a national shortage of continuous albuterol in the United States, you may also consider albuterol 2.5 mg/3 mL mixed with ipratropium in the dose described via three back-to-back nebulized treatments over the course of 1 hour. We recommend early peripheral IV access both for the risk of decompensation and to administer magnesium 50 mg/kg IV (maximum 2 g IV) for further bronchodilation. Due to the risk of hypotension with magnesium, consider a concurrent IV bolus of isotonic fluid. Give dexamethasone 0.6 mg/kg IV with a maximum of 16 mg or methylprednisolone 2 mg/kg; max 60 mg IV.

If the child is having a severe exacerbation and you are concerned about impending respiratory failure, remember that epinephrine 0.01 mg/kg IM (1 mg/mL concentration; max 0.5 mg IM) is a potent bronchodilator and can be used in respiratory distress in severe asthma exacerbation as well as for anaphylaxis. Epinephrine IM can be repeated every 5 to 15 minutes. This can serve as a bridge to treatment with inhaled beta-agonists. If you give epinephrine IM, you should avoid other bronchodilators such as terbutaline via the IM or subcutaneous routes.

If you choose to start terbutaline, you may give a bolus of 10 mcg/kg IV (max 300 mcg) over 10 minutes and then start a continuous infusion at 0.1 to 0.4 mcg/kg/min. Terbutaline can also be given IM at a dose of 0.01 mg/kg IM (1 mg/mL solution; max 0.4 mg). Terbutaline IM, like epinephrine IM, can be repeated; specifically, terbutaline IM can be repeated every 20 minutes for three total doses. Remember to not give both terbutaline IM and epinephrine IM—choose one. However, giving epinephrine IM does not prevent use of terbutaline IV, though use of both may lead to worse adverse effects. With terbutaline, watch for hypokalemia and obtain a baseline ECG. Because terbutaline infusions cause systemic beta-agonist effect compared to nebulized beta-agonist therapy, the hypokalemia seen with terbutaline is often more pronounced, though it rarely requires repletion. Terbutaline has not been shown to decrease the rate of pediatric floor or PICU admissions, but is worth considering as we try to throw the kitchen sink at a patient in our best attempts to stave off intubation.

Arterial blood gases are rarely helpful in the management of pediatric asthma. Instead, follow end-tidal CO_2. VBGs can also be helpful to monitor the degree of hypercarbia. Intubation should be avoided as much as possible because there is high risk for barotrauma and cardiovascular collapse in asthma. In addition, mechanical ventilation rarely provides better respiratory support than the patient's own breathing pattern. If you must intubate, preoxygenate and use ketamine for RSI induction at 1 to 1.5 mg/kg IV. We recommend permissive hypercapnia with tidal volumes (often 6-8 mL/kg) that allow you to keep inspiratory pressures to less than 40 cm H_2O and a plateau pressure of less than 30 cm H$_2$O, with a lower respiratory rate (6-12 breaths/min), an inspiratory time between 1 and 1.5 seconds, and expiratory time between 6 and 12 seconds. While younger patients may require higher respiratory rates, the I:E ratio should be set low. The goal is to minimize breath stacking and worsening hyperinflation, which could increase intrathoracic pressure and decrease cardiac output.

In cases not requiring immediate intubation, consider heliox as an adjunctive therapy. Heliox has been shown to help stave off invasive mechanical ventilation, improve laminar airflow, which will also improve deposition of nebulized treatments. Noninvasive mechanical ventilation such as HFNC or BiPAP can also help you avoid intubation in the appropriate clinical setting. Nebulized treatments such as albuterol can also be used in conjunction with these noninvasive modalities by discussing with your respiratory therapist how to add them in line with HFNC or BiPAP.

PEARLS

- Lack of wheezing suggests lack of air flow and a more severe presentation.
- Epinephrine IM is not just for anaphylaxis—use it for its bronchodilatory effect. It can serve as a bridge toward inhaled beta-agonist therapy.
- Treat severe exacerbations aggressively and early with continuous albuterol, ipratropium, magnesium IV, and steroids IV.
- Avoid intubation, consider noninvasive ventilation such as HFNC or BiPAP.
- Talk to your respiratory therapist about the in-line use of albuterol with HFNC or BiPAP.

Suggested Readings

Adair E, Dibaba D, Fowke JH, Snider M. The impact of terbutaline as adjuvant therapy in the treatment of severe asthma in the pediatric emergency department. *Pediatr Emerg Care.* 2022;38(1):e292-e294. PMID: 33136831.

Doymaz S, Schneider J. Safety of terbutaline for treatment of acute severe pediatric asthma. *Pediatr Emerg Care.* 2018;34(5):299-302. PMID: 26959519.

Doymaz S, Schneider J, Sagy M. Early administration of terbutaline in severe pediatric asthma may reduce incidence of acute respiratory failure. *Ann Allergy Asthma Immunol.* 2014;112(3):207-210. PMID: 24468309.

Kneyber MCJ, de Luca D, Calderini E, et al. Recommendations for mechanical ventilation of critically ill children from the Paediatric Mechanical Ventilation Consensus Conference (PEMVECC). *Intensive Care Med.* 2017;43(12):1764-1780. PMID: 28936698.

Scarfone R. Acute asthma exacerbations in children younger than 12 years: emergency department management. UpToDate, November 16, 2022.

Shein SL, Speicher RH, Filho JO, Gaston B, Rotta AT. Contemporary treatment of children with critical and near-fatal asthma. *Rev Bras Ter Intensiva.* 2016;28(2):167-178. PMID: 27305039.

303

OVERSCANNING THE PEDIATRIC PATIENT WITH TRAUMA

JENNIFER GUYTHER AND MIMI LU

Resuscitation of the traumatically injured pediatric patient differs from that of the adult based on both underlying pathophysiology and injury patterns, especially in the setting of blunt trauma. When caring for the injured pediatric patient, physicians must balance the risk of radiation and resource utilization against the diagnosis of a clinically significant injury. Studies have shown that following evidence-based algorithms and clinical decision rules can safely reduce the number of CT scans obtained while not missing critical diagnoses.

PECARN derived a clinical prediction rule that has been extensively validated and is able to accurately identify children with minor head injuries at very low risk of clinically significant brain injury and do not require a CT (**Table 303.1**). Studies also note that observation is more appropriate than CT scan for patients presenting with the isolated symptom of vomiting after head injury. Despite awareness of this rule, children with minor head injuries still receive CT scans 10% to 40% of the time. Rapid MRI protocols are increasingly available and represent a reasonable radiation-free alternative for stable patients at higher risk for clinically significant brain injury.

While cervical spine injuries are less common than in adults, children have a higher risk of permanent neurologic damage and mortality. There is a wide variation in clinical protocols for cervical spine clearance and no prospectively validated clinical guideline has been published. Cervical spine injuries should be considered in the setting of a high-risk mechanism of injury, unresponsiveness, torticollis, rigidity of the neck muscles, significant neck pain, or neurologic symptoms. While cervical spine XRs are less sensitive than CT scan, it is the preferred initial study to decrease radiation exposure if the indications for a CT scan are not met (**Table 303.1**), and the patient is unable to range the neck or has a high-risk mechanism of injury (axial load, fall >1 m, high-speed MVC/rollover, ejection, bike or motorized recreational vehicle).

A CXR can help identify conditions such as hemothorax or pneumothorax. Although CXR is less sensitive (41%-60%) for detecting injuries found on CT scan, thoracic CT scan rarely changes management and does not impact morbidity and mortality, yet exposes the child to 25 to 150× as much radiation. Thoracic CT imaging should be obtained only after careful consideration and discussion with the trauma team, if available.

In blunt abdominal trauma, several clinical predication rules have been studied to determine the necessity of CT scans including PECARN, Streck, and BaTiC. The PECARN study is most frequently used (**Table 303.1**). The role of FAST in the hemodynamically stable child after blunt abdominal trauma is evolving. Test characteristics of FAST have variable reliability and accuracy in children; when combined with the physical exam, it has better test characteristics than the physical exam alone. Whereas the RUQ view is the most sensitive in adults, the pelvic view is the most sensitive in children, with fluid most commonly collecting in the rectovesicular or rectouterine pouch. The FAST may appear initially negative with a free fluid volume under 100 mL. Trace pelvic free fluid may be physiologic in children, thus limiting specificity. Pediatric injury patterns

TABLE 303.1 CLINICAL DECISION RULES FOR OBTAINING CT IMAGING IN BLUNT PEDIATRIC TRAUMA

	CRITERIA	INTERPRETATION	CAVEATS
Head			
PECARN <2 yr	(i) GCS ≤14, palpable skull fracture or signs of AMS (ii) Occipital, parietal, or temporal scalp hematoma; history of LOC ≥5 sec; not acting normally per parent or severe mechanism of injury	If yes to (i): CT If no to (i) and yes to (ii): Observation recommended over CT If no to both: CT not recommended	Severe mechanism: MVC with patient ejection, death of another passenger, rollover; pedestrian or bicyclist w/o helmet struck by motorized vehicle; fall from >0.9 m; head struck by high-impact object
PECARN 2 yr and older	(i) GCS ≤14 or signs of basilar skull fracture or signs of AMS (ii) History of LOC or history of vomiting or severe headache or severe mechanism of injury	Same as children <2 yr	Severe mechanism: same as for children <2 except height of the fall is >1.5 m
C-Spine			
NEXUS	Alert Developmentally normal neurologic exam No posterior midline cervical tenderness No distracting injuries No hypotension No intoxication	If all criteria are met, no imaging is required.	Children >3 yr
NICE	GCS <13 Intubated Focal neurologic signs Paresthesia Strong clinical suspicion of injury despite negative XR Inability to obtain adequate XRs Bony injury detected on XR	If any criteria are present, CT is recommended.	
Abdomen			
PECARN	Evidence of abdominal wall trauma or seat belt sign GCS score of <14 Abdominal tenderness Evidence of thoracic wall trauma Complaints of abdominal pain Decreased breath sounds Vomiting	0/7 = low risk, no CT indicated	

AMS, altered mental status; CT, computed tomography; GCS, Glasgow coma scale; LOC, loss of consciousness; MVC, motor vehicle crash; XR, x-ray.

commonly result in solid organ lacerations without hemoperitoneum, making the FAST a less sensitive means for detecting important intra-abdominal injury.

Liberal use of CT scanning in the pediatric patient with blunt injuries increases both radiation exposure and resource utilization without significant changes to morbidity and mortality. Clinical decision rules, such as those put forth by PECARN, should be incorporated into the management of the pediatric patient with trauma.

PEARLS

- Use clinical decision rules to determine if a CT scan is warranted in the pediatric patient with blunt trauma.
- A CXR is a reasonable screening tool for intrathoracic trauma and a thoracic CT scan is unlikely to change patient management.
- Remember to apply your age-appropriate neurologic exam and vital signs when using the clinical decision rules.
- Cervical spine XRs are a reasonable screening tool if the patient has a high-risk mechanism of injury with limitation of neck mobility when a CT scan is not indicated.
- The PECARN clinical decision rule for CT in blunt abdominal trauma does not require blood work.

Suggested Readings

Copley PC, Tilliridou V, Kirby A, Jones J, Kandasamy J. Management of cervical spine trauma in children. *Eur J Trauma Emerg Surg*. 2019;45(5):777-789.

Kuppermann N, Holmes JF, Dayan PS, et al. Identification of children at very low risk of clinically-important brain injuries after head trauma: a prospective cohort study [published correction appears in *Lancet*. 2014;383(9914):308]. *Lancet*. 2009;374(9696):1160-1170.

Liang T, Roseman, E, Gao M, Sinert R. The utility of the focused assessment with sonography in trauma examination in pediatric blunt abdominal trauma: a systematic review and meta-analysis. *Pediatr Emerg Care*. 2021;37(2):108-118.

Lynch P, Samoilov L, Brahm G. Thoracic imaging in pediatric trauma: are CTs necessary? *Pediatr Emerg Care*. 2023;39(2):98-101.

Ozcan A, Ahn T, Akay B, Menoch M. Imaging for pediatric blunt abdominal trauma with different prediction rules. *Pediatr Emerg Care*. 2022;38(2):e654-e658.

304

Pediatric Status Epilepticus: Pearls and Pitfalls of Emergency Management

Lane Epps and Shruti Kant

Status epilepticus is the most common neurologic emergency in childhood. The estimated incidence is 17 to 23 per 100,000 children per year, and 30-day mortality is 2% to 6%. Early treatment is critical because prolonged seizure activity can cause neuronal injury, hypoxemia, and death. Status epilepticus is defined as continuous seizure activity or multiple seizures without return to baseline, lasting greater than 5 minutes. It can be further characterized as early (5-30 minutes), established (>30 minutes), and refractory, defined as ongoing seizure activity despite administration of two appropriately dosed ASMs. A three-step approach can be used to manage status epilepticus.

INITIAL MANAGEMENT AND FIRST-LINE THERAPY

Step 1 (0-10 minutes): Initial management includes assessing airway, breathing, and circulation while administering a benzodiazepine. Place the patient on cardiac monitoring and pulse oximetry, administer oxygen via nonrebreather to avoid hypoxia, and establish IV access. A BVM and airway adjuncts should be accessible. After the primary survey, administer a benzodiazepine (**Table 304.1**). Collect preliminary diagnostics, including complete vital signs with a rectal temperature, finger-stick glucose, venous blood gas, complete blood count, basic metabolic panel, magnesium, calcium, and ASM levels in patients with a known seizure disorder. Serum lactate is often elevated, but a normal lactate does not rule out seizure activity. Treat reversible causes of seizure, such as hypoglycemia, hypocalcemia, and hyponatremia; for example $D_{10}W$ for hypoglycemia or 3% hypertonic saline for hyponatremia. A second dose of benzodiazepine can be given after 3 to 5 minutes for ongoing seizure activity. More than two doses of benzodiazepine increase the risk of respiratory depression with limited clinical utility.

SECOND-LINE THERAPY

Step 2 (10-30 minutes): If two doses of benzodiazepine and treating immediately reversible causes of seizure are inadequate, give a loading dose of a second-line ASM

TABLE 304.1 ASMs FOR STATUS EPILEPTICUS

TIME AFTER ED ARRIVAL	DRUG	ROUTE	DOSE	NOTES
0-10 min (first line)	Lorazepam	IV/IO	0.1 mg/kg (max 4 mg)	IV/IO doses can be repeated once after 3-5 min. If IV/IO access is not established within 3-5 min, use an alternative route.
	Diazepam	IV/IO PR	0.2 mg/kg (max 10 mg) 0.5 mg/kg (max 20 mg)	
	Midazolam	IN/IM BUC	0.2 mg/kg (max 10 mg) 0.3-0.5 mg/kg (max 10 mg)	
10-30 min (second line)	Fosphenytoin	IV/IO	20 mg/kg (max 1,500 mg)	All have similar efficacy, but consider previous response, clinical context (eg, levetiracetam in trauma), and potential adverse events.
	Levetiracetam	IV/IO	60 mg/kg (max 4,500 mg)	
	Valproate	IV/IO	40 mg/kg (max 3,000 mg)	
>30 min (third line)	Midazolam	IV/IO	0.2 mg/kg bolus, then 0.05-0.1mg/kg/h gtt (max 2 mg/kg/h)	Requires RSI when starting infusion. Iatrogenic hypotension may occur and require treatment with fluids and vasopressors.
	Pentobarbital	IV/IO	5-15 mg/kg bolus, then 0.5 mg/kg/h gtt (max 5 mg/kg/h)	

ASMs, anti-seizure medications; BUC, buccal; ED, emergency department; gtt, continuous infusion; IN, intranasal; IO, intraosseous; IV, intravenous; PR, per rectum; RSI, rapid sequence intubation.

(Table 304.1). Levetiracetam, fosphenytoin, and valproate were found to be equally effective and have similar adverse event rates in the ESETT. Continue to monitor respiratory status closely and prepare for RSI, but support respiration with a BVM if feasible to allow ongoing neurologic assessment. Reassess 10 to 15 minutes after giving a second-line ASM, and give an alternate ASM if needed. Consult pediatric neurology early on site or through the nearest children's hospital.

MANAGEMENT OF REFRACTORY STATUS AND ADDITIONAL DIAGNOSTIC WORKUP

Step 3 (>30 minutes): After two second-line ASMs have been given, perform RSI and prepare a continuous infusion of a third-line ASM. Midazolam is often preferred to pentobarbital because it causes less hypotension and respiratory depression, but this can occur at higher doses. Fluid resuscitation and vasopressors may be needed to treat iatrogenic hypotension. If there is concern for trauma (accidental, nonaccidental) or increased intracranial pressure (hemorrhage, meningitis), obtain a noncontrast CT of the head. A head CT is also recommended for patients with first-time seizures with ongoing status or persistent altered mental status. Consider lumbar puncture if there is concern for intracranial infection. In these patients, broad-spectrum antibiotics should be given empirically even if a lumbar puncture cannot be performed. Many patients become more responsive within 30 minutes of termination, but some patients have a prolonged postictal state. Common reasons for a prolonged postictal period are prolonged seizure activity, sedation, and ongoing nonconvulsive or subclinical status epilepticus. Patients who do not return to their neurologic baseline within a few hours after termination of generalized convulsions should be admitted for further evaluation and continuous EEG monitoring.

SPECIAL CONSIDERATIONS

Propofol and etomidate have antiepileptic properties, so they are often used for RSI induction if additional sedation is needed. Ketamine is also a reasonable induction agent due to growing evidence that it can terminate refractory status. Neuromuscular blockade with a paralytic such as rocuronium is recommended to maximize first-pass intubation success. Succinylcholine can be considered if there are no contraindications, but is often avoided due to the risk of hyperkalemia in the setting of undiagnosed neuromuscular disease.

There is limited evidence supporting specific treatment in the neonatal period (0–28 days), but phenobarbital is often used as a first-line agent. Fosphenytoin, levetiracetam, and lidocaine are reasonable second-line agents for seizures refractory to phenobarbital.

PEARLS

- **Remember the ABCs**—Open the airway, suction secretions, and start oxygen via nonrebreather. Be prepared for RSI, but it is often possible to avoid intubation.
- **Treatment before diagnosis**—Administer a benzodiazepine within the first 3 to 5 minutes. Repeat the dose once after 3 to 5 minutes if the initial dose was inadequate and not given in the prehospital setting. Load a second-line ASM (Table 305.1) if the patient is still seizing 3 to 5 minutes after the second dose of benzodiazepine.

- **Identify and address underlying causes**—Measure core temperature and finger-stick glucose, obtain basic labs, look for signs of trauma or infection, and consider possible ingestions.
- **Anticipate next steps**—If you are considering using a third-line ASM, prepare for RSI and a continuous infusion simultaneously. Consult pediatric neurology early.

SUGGESTED READINGS

Abend NS, Bearden D, Helbig I, et al. Status epilepticus and refractory status epilepticus management. *Semin Pediatr Neurol*. 2014;21(4):263-274.

Brophy GM, Bell R, Claassen J, et al. Guidelines for the evaluation and management of status epilepticus. *Neurocrit Care*. 2012;17(1):3-23.

Chin RF, Neville BG, Peckham C, et al. Incidence, cause, and short-term outcome of convulsive status epilepticus in childhood: prospective population-based study. *Lancet*. 2006;368(9531):222-229.

Jafarpour S, Stredny CM, Piantino J, Chapman KE. Baseline and outcome assessment in pediatric status epilepticus. *Seizure*. 2019;68:52-61.

Kapur J, Elm J, Chamberlain JM, et al. Randomized trial of three anticonvulsant medications for status epilepticus. *N Engl J Med*. 2019;381(22):2103-2113.

305

EASY DOES IT: BE CAUTIOUS WITH THE PEDIATRIC PATIENT WITH CYANOSIS WHO HAS UNDERGONE CARDIAC SURGERY

Christyn Magill

Children with complex CHD are living longer and healthier lives as a result of improved management. Community ED physicians, however, are unlikely to be familiar with children with single ventricle physiology (approximately every 1 per 10,000 births) and endorse feeling "uncomfortable" with managing these patients. Lack of comfort in caring for these children is understandable, as they are at high risk of interstage morbidity and mortality. Children with CHD seek medical attention at a higher rate than children without CHD, so it is likely that you will care for a child with CHD during your career. An understanding of the basics of the physiology is critical to avoid mismanagement and catastrophic complications that happen secondary to failure to recognize key aspects of care.

Children with single ventricle physiology, such as those with hypoplastic left heart syndrome among other lesions, undergo three surgical stages to allow their one functional ventricle to provide systemic circulation. Pulmonary circulation occurs as a result of *passive* blood flow driven by systemic venous return. The first surgery is done before the newborn leaving the hospital, often referred to as a Norwood or BT shunt.

This creates an arterial shunt to provide pulmonary blood flow (see **Figure 305.1A**). These children will have baseline oxygen saturations of about 75% to 85%. This is the most tenuous stage of palliation—overall 1-year survival sans transplant is 69%. Once the child makes it to the second stage of palliation, at about 4 to 6 months of age (called a Glenn or hemi-Fontan), survival is often more than 90%. The arterial shunt is removed and replaced with a venous shunt, connecting the SVC to the pulmonary arteries to give passive blood flow to the lungs (see **Figure 305.1B and C**). Since the IVC is not altered and continues to contribute deoxygenated blood to the mixture that becomes systemic blood, the child remains cyanotic. The third stage of palliation, called a Fontan, occurs between 18 months and 3 years of age. This completes the routing of venous return to the lungs where the SVC and IVC are anastomosed to the pulmonary arteries. After the third surgery, the child will have normal or near-normal oxygen levels and is not as fragile as the child between the first and second stages of palliation.

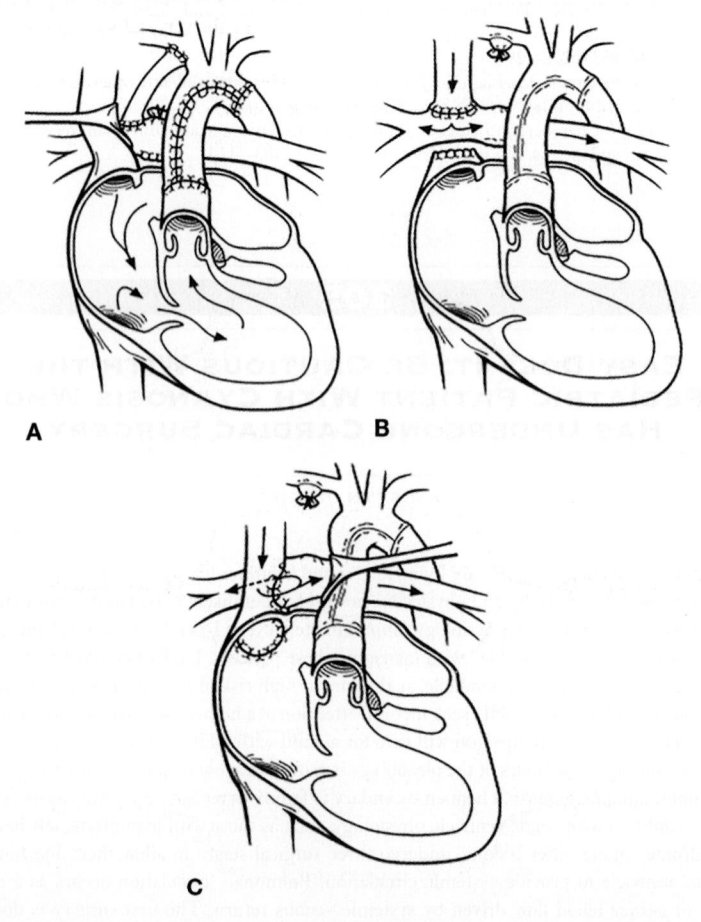

FIGURE 305.1 (A) BT shunt. (B) Bidirectional Glenn. (C) Hemi-Fontan.

The remainder of this chapter focuses on the child between the first and second stages of palliation, as they are the most medically fragile. The parents should be able to tell you two key pieces of information—how many surgeries the child has had (stage of palliation) as well as the baseline oxygen saturation. This information helps you correctly manage these complicated children.

After the first stage of palliation, the circulatory system is in a parallel circuit; blood must balance its flow between the lungs and the systemic circulation through the shunt (see **Figure 305.2**). If the pulmonary vascular resistance is high or preload is too low, then the lungs are undercirculated (see **Figure 305.2**). Conversely, when blood floods the lungs, the child can be overcirculated (see **Figure 305.2**).

Overcirculation of the lungs is less common—unless we cause it iatrogenically. Overcirculation is indicated by an oxygen saturation of more than 85% and means too much blood is getting to the lungs. This can be caused if the shunt is too large or if there are collaterals, but these rarely cause an acute ED presentation. More common is exogenous oxygen causing pulmonary vasodilation. This is usually our fault; a child comes in with an oxygen saturation of 80% (normal for them!), and someone slaps a nonrebreather on the child to "fix" the hypoxia. The result is pulmonary vasodilation, overcirculation to the lungs, and steal of systemic blood flow. If not fixed quickly, this can lead to rapid deterioration and cardiac arrest. Respiratory complaints are a common reason for ED presentation, so remind staff that these babies are not expected to have normal oxygen saturations.

Parallel Circuit
Q_T (flow) $= Q_P + Q_S$

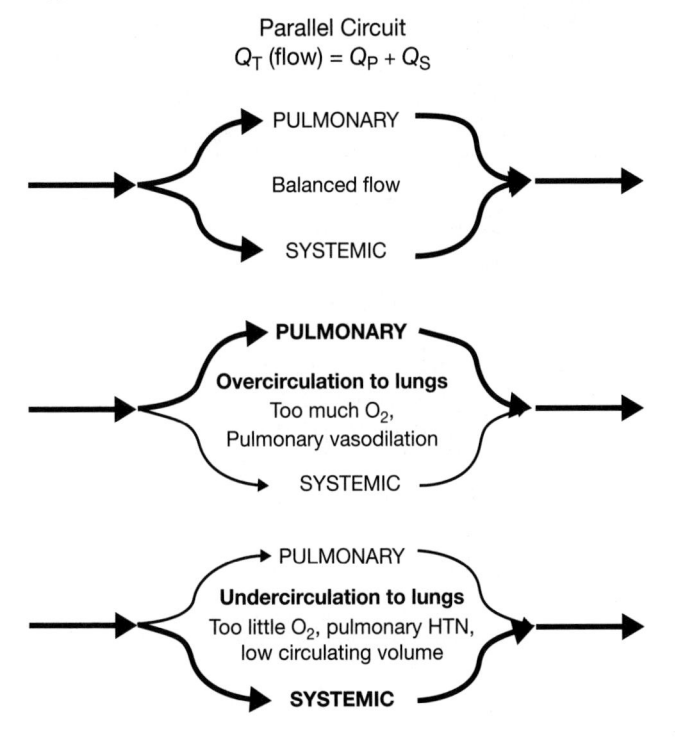

FIGURE 305.2 Parallel circulation after first-stage palliation. HTN, hypertension.

More commonly you will see undercirculation to the lungs. Recall that the child with single ventricle is dependent on *passive* venous return to perfuse the lungs. They are susceptible to dehydration and prone to cardiovascular collapse with seemingly benign illnesses. Undercirculation is represented by a pulse oxygenation of less than 70%. Usually, this is from dehydration from a GI or a respiratory illness, and less commonly by shunt obstruction, a shunt that is too small, or increased pulmonary vascular resistance like pulmonary hypertension. Your careful management can save a life. Gently correct any relative hypoxia—aim for 75% to 85%, but don't overshoot or you will get in trouble as noted previously. Most importantly in the ED, don't be afraid to give gentle fluid boluses to correct dehydration. If these children dependent on preload are dehydrated, they can't get enough blood to the lungs. Give 5 to 10 mL/kg of crystalloid fluid (or blood for increased oxygen-carrying capacity) and reassess frequently—you will be surprised how quickly it helps. Call the pediatric cardiologist *early* to help you make decisions on management and disposition. Most often a first-stage palliation child will be watched overnight in the hospital to maintain preload.

In short, with single ventricle physiology children, what you do *not* do matters as much as what you do. Give enough oxygen, but not too much. Give enough fluid, but not too much. Use the oxygen saturations to guide your management decisions. Most importantly, don't be afraid of these interesting and complicated children, and you will make a difference in their lives.

PEARLS

- The parents are your best friends—ask them what is normal and abnormal for their child.
- Know the stage of surgery—be cautious if there has only been one!
- Use the pulse oxygen to guide your management. Keep sats between 75% and 85%.
- Small changes in oxygen and fluids make big differences.
- Early cardiology consultation and consideration of transfer is important—always phone a friend.

Suggested Readings

Cashen K, Gupta P, Lieh-Lai M, Mastropietro C. Infants with single ventricle physiology in the emergency department: are physicians prepared? *J Pediatr.* 2011;159:273-277.e1.

Chauhan M, Mastropietro CW. Hypoplastic left heart syndrome in the emergency department: an update. *J Emerg Med.* 2014;46:e51-e54.

Friedman KG, Salvin JW, Wypij D, et al. Risk factors for failed staged palliation after bidirectional Glenn in infants who have undergone stage one palliation. *Eur J Cardiothorac Surg.* 2011;40(4):1000–1006.

Islam S, Kaul P, Tran DT, Mackie AS. Health care resource utilization among children with congenital heart disease: a population-based study. *Can J Cardiol.* 2018;34(10):1289-1297.

Prentice E, Morey N, Richards K, et al. Emergency department use after stage II palliation for children with single ventricle lesions. *Pediatr Emerg Care.* 2015;31:343-347.

SECTION XXIV
GERIATRICS

306

DO NOT UNDERESTIMATE THE POTENTIAL MORBIDITY OF ABDOMINAL PAIN IN OLDER ADULTS

CHRISTINA L. SHENVI

Abdominal pain is the most common non-injury-related chief complaint in the ED. Older adults with abdominal pain are more likely than younger adults to have a dangerous or deadly underlying cause that could require surgery. The risk of serious causes increases with advancing age.

HIGH INDEX OF SUSPICION FOR DANGEROUS ETIOLOGIES

About 50% of older adults who present with abdominal pain require admission, and they are admitted for longer periods than younger adults. Patients who are admitted have a 5% to 10% mortality rate, and 20% to 30% require surgery or an intervention. The two most common indications for surgery in older adults are biliary disease and bowel obstructions. In younger adults, no specific cause of pain is found during their ED visit 36% of the time, whereas in older adults, only 22% have no identifiable cause.

There are many different dangerous causes of abdominal pain in older adults. These causes should be considered high in the differential diagnosis, and a focused history and physical examination should be used to decide what further workup is indicated. In each older adult with abdominal pain, consider the following in the differential: aortic dissection, aortic aneurysm rupture, mesenteric ischemia, bowel perforation, cholecystitis, diverticulitis, appendicitis, and bowel obstruction.

DO NOT BE FALSELY REASSURED BY VITAL SIGNS, EXAM, AND LABS

Older adults may have deceptively reassuring exams. For example, older adults with peritonitis are less likely than younger patients to exhibit the classic signs of peritoneal rigidity, fever, and leukocytosis. In fact, 30% of older adults with peritonitis lack a fever and leukocytosis. They may be taking medications that prevent the expected response of tachycardia attributed to pain, infection, or fever. In addition, severe pain out of proportion to an otherwise benign exam may suggest mesenteric ischemia, a challenging diagnosis associated with considerable morbidity. Because of the limitations of physical exams, diagnoses are more often ambiguous or delayed.

Older adults are more likely than younger patients to have a positive urinalysis without a clinically significant urinary tract infection and as such, an abdominal pain workup should not anchor on a urinary tract infection with mild pyuria. Older adults, particularly those who are incontinent, immobile, or in a long-term care environment, often have chronic incidental pyuria and bacteriuria. If the patient has abdominal pain, it should not be attributed to mild abnormalities on a urinalysis without at least considering and exploring other possibilities. In fact, sterile pyuria is often seen in abdominal infections unrelated to the urinary system.

Use Appropriate Imaging

Bedside ultrasound can help rapidly identify certain high-risk causes of abdominal pain, such as aortic aneurysms, aortic dissection, cholecystitis, cholelithiasis, free fluid, and bowel obstructions. If the ultrasound is positive, it can help facilitate rapid disposition and appropriate surgical consultation. However, in many cases, a CT or formal ultrasound will also be needed. In older adults, the risk:benefit ratio for CT scanning generally favors imaging. Older adults are less likely to have negative downstream effects of radiation exposure and are more likely to suffer the negative consequences of delayed diagnosis of acute intra-abdominal pathology.

Think Outside the Abdomen

Abdominal symptoms can also occur from problems originating outside the abdomen. For example, patients with a myocardial infarction may have upper abdominal pain or nausea and vomiting. A patient with left upper quadrant or right upper quadrant pain could actually have a lower lobe pneumonia or pulmonary embolism. Patients with vomiting but a nontender abdomen may have an intracranial hemorrhage. Patients with DKA may present with abdominal pain and vomiting but have no intra-abdominal pathology. Remember to consider causes outside the abdomen that could cause pain or nausea.

Avoid Anchoring

Patients often try to explain away their pain or symptoms and relate it to something they have experienced. For example, they may attribute their paint to indigestion, or a "stomach bug" that other family members have also had. Be cautious when anchoring to what they tell you. They may be correct, but you should still consider the highly morbid conditions that could be present and perform the necessary exam or tests to rule them out.

PEARLS

- Keep the more serious causes of pain higher on the differential diagnosis, such as aortic dissection or rupture, mesenteric ischemia, bowel perforation, cholecystitis, diverticulitis, appendicitis, and bowel obstruction.
- Be aware that older adults with abdominal infections may lack fever and leukocytosis.
- Do not shorten the workup after finding a mildly abnormal urinalysis, as many older adults have incidental pyuria and bacteriuria.
- Have a low threshold for obtaining advanced imaging for older adults with abdominal pain.
- Think of causes outside of the abdomen.
- Do not anchor to what the patient tells you.

Suggested Readings

Hendrickson M, Naparst TR. Abdominal surgical emergencies in the elderly. *Emerg Med Clin North Am*. 2006;21:937-969.

Laurell H, Hansson LE, Gunnarsson U. Acute abdominal pain among elderly patients. *Gerontology*. 2006;52:339-344.

Lewis LM, Banet GA, Blanda M, Hustey FM, Meldon SW, Gerson LW. Etiology and clinical course of abdominal pain in senior patients: a prospective, multicenter study. *J Gerontol A Biol Sci Med Sci*. 2005;60(8):1071-1076.

Magidson PD, Martinez JP. Abdominal pain in the geriatric patient. *Emerg Med Clin North Am*. 2016;34(3):559-574.

Martinez JP, Mattu A. Abdominal pain in the elderly. *Emerg Med Clin North Am*. 2006;24:371-388.

Ragsdale L, Southerland L. Acute abdominal pain in the older adult. *Emerg Med Clin North Am*. 2011;29:429-448.

Sangiorgio G, Biondi A, Basile F, Vacante M. Acute abdominal pain in older adults: a clinical and diagnostic challenge. *Minerva Chir*. 2020;75(3):169-172.

307

Rib, Hip, and Vertebral Compression Fractures

Sean Heavey and Katren Tyler

A fragility fracture is a fracture resulting from a low-energy event such as a fall from a standing height. The most common sites for fragility fractures are hip, pubic rami, spine, proximal humerus, and distal radius; VCF are the most common fragility fracture. A fragility fracture is diagnostic for osteoporosis and is common in older adults, especially women. Most fragility fractures are associated with GLF. This chapter focuses on the diagnosis and specific management of low-energy fragility fractures. For older adults with pain following a GLF, with nondiagnostic plain films, consider advanced imaging to exclude occult fractures. In general, topical pain relief, such as lidocaine patches or NSAID gels, will be ineffective for fractures. Systemic NSAIDs should be used with caution in older adults.

Hip Fractures

Hip fractures are a common injury in older patients and are associated with short- and long-term mortality. Women account for about 75% of hip fractures in the United States. Although the incidence of hip fractures in men is much lower, the 12-month mortality for hip fractures in men approaches 40%. Even for patients with limited mobility at baseline, operative fixation provides significant analgesia and should be offered to most patients.

Pain in the affected hip ranges from minor to severe, and occasionally, patients have been weight-bearing on a hip fracture for days to weeks. Many patients with hip fractures are relatively pain-free at rest. For this reason, it is critical to move the leg as part of the physical examination, ideally with a rotational component.

Most hip fractures are identified on plain films of the hip and pelvis. If these films are negative or nondiagnostic and the patient still experiences pain with weight-bearing, advanced imaging is recommended. MRI is the most sensitive for detecting occult hip fractures but is often less accessible, time consuming, and may require sedation. Selective MRI after a CT scan is a possible solution for identifying occult hip fractures if the CT scan is negative.

Many health systems and EDs have care coordination pathways for hip fractures. Hip fracture pathways include multimodal analgesia with acetaminophen, careful use of opioid analgesics, and regional anesthesia of the femoral nerve. Preoperative regional anesthesia of the femoral nerve has been recommended by orthopedic societies as integral to the care of patients with hip fractures. There are multiple approaches to providing regional anesthesia of the femoral nerve; the FICB is one of the simplest and safest methods and can be performed with or without ultrasound guidance.

In the hospital, operative fixation within 48 hours is associated with improved outcomes. Pathways to minimize delirium include comanagement with geriatric expertise, early mobilization, and medication reconciliation (**Figure 307.1**).

VCF

VCF are the most common fragility fracture and range from relatively painless to extremely painful. VCF can be spontaneous and progressive or occur following a low-velocity trauma such as a fall. Management is determined by the degree of compression, pain, and general patient mobility. Spinal cord compression or other neurologic impairments are uncommon.

Acute fractures associated with less than 50% loss of vertebral height may be operatively managed with kyphoplasty or vertebroplasty. Subacute fractures are usually managed with pain control. Pain control includes acetaminophen, topical lidocaine, judicious use of opioids, and intranasal calcitonin. Thoracolumbar bracing may help with pain but should not be used long term because of atrophy of core musculature. In addition, braces are not universally well tolerated.

Rib Fractures

Pain limits both mobility and deep inspiration, increasing the risk of atelectasis and pneumonia; pneumonia is the most common complication of rib fractures. Management should include analgesia sufficient to allow respiration and mobility. Analgesic requirements may range from acetaminophen to regional anesthesia, including serratus anterior blocks. Incentive spirometry of less than 1 L is associated with worse outcomes following blunt chest trauma. Evidence for improved outcomes with the use of incentive spirometry following with an isolated rib fracture is lacking. For patients with significant comorbidities or multiple rib fractures, consideration should be given to multimodal analgesia and admission for monitoring. Critical care monitoring is usually unnecessary for isolated rib fractures in older adults.

Pelvic Fragility Fractures

The pelvis is another location vulnerable to osteoporosis, and nondisplaced acetabular and pubic rami fractures are commonly seen in older patients following a GLF. Pubic rami fractures are often identified when a patient is being evaluated for hip or groin pain following a fall. Management is usually conservative, unless ongoing pain requirements necessitate operative intervention.

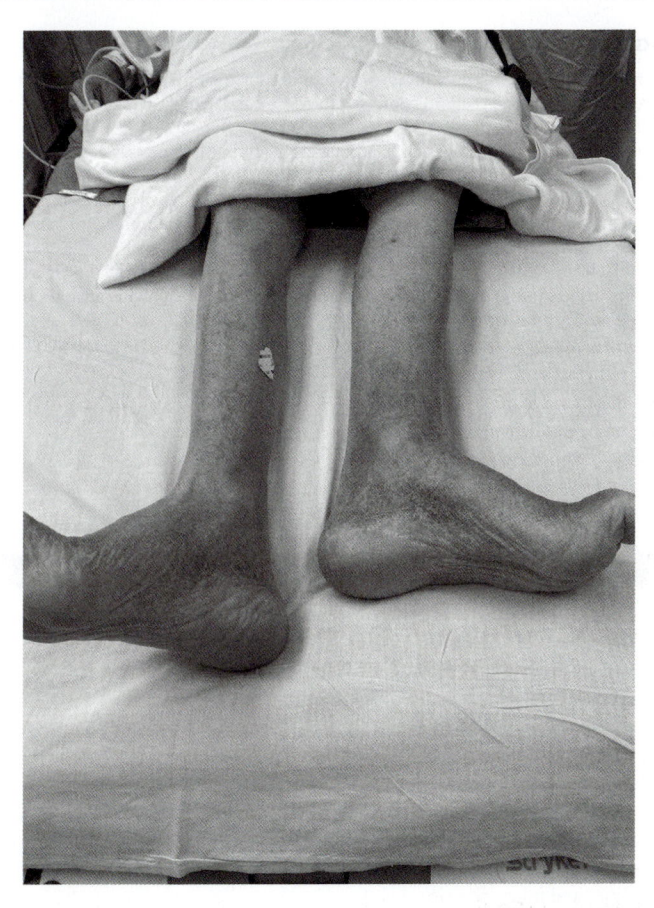

FIGURE 307.1 Left hip fracture with a shortened and externally rotated left leg.

PEARLS

- Fragility fractures are diagnostic for osteoporosis and can result from low-energy trauma, mostly GLF.
- Maintain a high index of suspicion for fragility fractures in patients who have fallen and still have pain.
- Osteoporosis reduces the sensitivity of plain films to detect fractures; advanced imaging may be required to detect occult fractures. CT scans are usually sufficient.
- Attention to pain requirements is critical for older patients as both untreated pain and excessive opioids can contribute to the development of delirium.

SUGGESTED READINGS

Boucher E, Rosgen B, Lang E. Efficacy of calcitonin for treating acute pain associated with osteoporotic vertebral compression fracture: an updated systematic review. *CJEM*. 2020;22(3):359-367.

Davidson A, Silver N, Cohen D, et al. Justifying CT prior to MRI in cases of suspected occult hip fracture. A proposed diagnostic protocol. *Injury*. 2021;52(6):1429-1433.

Kolodychuk N, Krebs JC, Stenberg R, Talmage L, Meehan A, DiNicola N. Fascia iliaca blocks performed in the emergency department decrease opioid consumption and length of stay in patients with hip fracture. *J Orthop Trauma*. 2022;36(3):142-146.

Naar L, El Hechi MW, van Erp IA, et al. Isolated rib cage fractures in the elderly: do all patients belong to the intensive care unit? A retrospective nationwide analysis. *J Trauma Acute Care Surg*. 2020;89(6):1039-1045.

Patel D, Liu J, Ebraheim NA. Managements of osteoporotic vertebral compression fractures: a narrative review. *World J Orthop*. 2022;13(6):564-573.

Switzer JA, O'Connor MI. AAOS management of hip fractures in older adults evidence-based clinical practice guideline. *J Am Acad Orthop Surgeons*. 2022;30(20): e1297-e1301.

308

THE GERIATRIC PATIENT WITH TRAUMA IS SICKER THAN YOU REALIZE

SARAH BETH SPIEGEL AND SURRIYA AHMAD

Trauma is the fifth leading cause of death in older adults who account for 30% of all trauma-related deaths. Studies have demonstrated that age is an independent predictor for morbidity and mortality in traumatic injuries, even when accounting for medical comorbidities and injury severity.

Numerous factors contribute to the high morbidity and mortality rate of geriatric patients with trauma. Impairments in hearing and vision, deconditioning, and polypharmacy make the older adults more susceptible to falls and other traumatic injuries. Older adults are more likely to be on multiple medications such as anticoagulants, beta-blockers, and calcium channel blockers that alter physiologic responses to trauma. It is vital to obtain a medication list early in their presentation. In addition, one should scrutinize the events leading to the injury, especially falls, to determine if the injury mechanism was from environmental causes (often referred to as "mechanical") or the result of an acute medical condition. Assess capacity and the overall reliability of your historian when obtaining a history. Older adults, especially those with dementia, may underreport their pain or the circumstances leading to a fall. Addressing goals of care and identifying a health care proxy are important to do early, even if a patient appears stable. The Clinical Frailty Scale is a screening tool for frailty in patients with trauma, which has been shown to highlight those at risk of increased length of stay and mortality.

The undertriage of geriatric patients with trauma likely further accounts for increased mortality rates in this group. Traditional trauma triage criteria based on injury mechanism and vital signs were largely studied in young healthy men and frequently lead to undertriage of geriatric patients with trauma. Regardless of indication for definitive surgical care, trauma centers improve functional outcomes through multidisciplinary teams of geriatricians, physical therapists, and occupational therapists. Current ATLS guidelines recommend trauma center evaluation for all patients over 55 years of age who present for traumatic injury despite injury mechanism, severity of injuries, and vital signs with unique considerations for older adults.

With respect to airway management, degenerative skeletal conditions like osteoarthritis can limit cervical mobility and mouth opening making direct laryngoscopy intubation challenging. Application of a cervical collar can further complicate airway management. For these reasons, video-assisted intubation with a hyperangulated laryngoscope is recommended. During rapid sequence intubation, consider low-dose sedation (reduce dose by 20%-40%) to protect against post-intubation hypotension.

Aging decreases chest wall compliance, respiratory muscle strength, and capacity for oxygen exchange. These physiologic changes lead to limited respiratory reserve and ability to compensate for chest wall injuries. The reflexive tachycardia in response to hypoxia seen in younger patients may be blunted. Geriatric patients with trauma may not appear to be in respiratory distress despite impending respiratory failure. Thresholds to provide supplemental oxygen to geriatric patients with trauma even with perceived minor injuries should be low.

Apparently "normal" vital signs in geriatric patients may be falsely reassuring due to underlying chronic conditions such as baseline hypertension or use of certain medications. Research suggests using a SBP of 110 as a cutoff for hypotension in patients over 65 years old.

No combination of physical exam and history has been shown to reliably predict the presence of traumatic brain injury in older adults. Dementia, delirium, or depression can make it more difficult to identify changes in mental status in older adults. Age-related brain atrophy can contribute to delayed neurologic symptoms as there is more space for blood to accumulate before symptoms develop. Geriatric patients have a higher rate of cord stenosis and kyphosis leading to a higher incidence of cervical spine injuries, even without radiographic abnormality. Patients with a focal neurologic deficit and normal CT should be evaluated with MRI to evaluate for ligamentous or more subtle spinal cord injury.

Impaired thermoregulation increases these patients' susceptibility to hypothermia. Once exposed and evaluated for injuries, place warm blankets on patients to prevent hypothermia. Consider getting a core temperature (eg, rectal) on all geriatric patients with trauma.

Blunt trauma, including falls and motor vehicle collisions, is the predominant mechanism of injury in older adults. Falls are the leading cause of injury-related death in patients over 65. Age-related changes in gait, stability, balance, strength, and reaction time contribute to the increased rate of falls.

Burns are the fourth leading cause of unintentional injury mortality in adults over 65 years of age. The high rate of burn-related trauma in this patient population may be secondary to decreased reaction time, sensory impairment, dementia, and difficulty evacuating fires. All geriatric burn victims should be evaluated and treated at designated burn centers.

In older adults, many deaths associated with firearm-related injuries are secondary to intentional self-harm. Notably, men over 85 years old have the highest rate of successful suicide across age groups.

The care of geriatric patients with trauma requires a multidisciplinary approach, with careful attention to the unique needs and vulnerabilities of this patient population.

PEARLS

- Assess capacity early and the overall reliability of your historian. Clarify goals of care early including identifying advanced directives and designated health care proxies.
- Avoid under triage of geriatric patients with trauma. Have a low threshold to obtain cross-sectional imaging in older patients even with seemingly minor mechanisms of injury.
- Mechanical falls are often not just mechanical—consider the underlying cause in older adults who present after a fall.
- Obtain a medication list in the geriatric patient with trauma with special attention to anticoagulants, beta-blockers, and calcium channel blockers.

SUGGESTED READINGS

American College of Surgeons. Geriatric trauma. In: Merrick C, ed. *Advanced Trauma Life Support Student Course Manual*. 10th ed. 2018:214-224.

Centers for Disease Control and Prevention. *Fatal Injury Reports, National and Regional, 1999–2014*. 2014.

Hashmi A, Ibrahim-Zada I, Rhee P, et al. Predictors of mortality in geriatric trauma patients: a systematic review and meta-analysis. *J Trauma Acute Care Surg*. 2014;76(3):894-901.

Lachs DK, Stern ME, Elman A, et al. Geriatric burn injuries presenting to the emergency department of a major burn center: clinical characteristics and outcomes. *J Emerg Med*. 2022;63(2):143-158.

Thompson A, Gida S, Nassif Y, et al. The impact of frailty on trauma outcomes using the Clinical Frailty Scale. *Eur J Trauma Emerg Surg*. 2022;48(2):1271-1276.

Tintinalli J, ed. Trauma in the elderly. In: *Tintinalli's Emergency Medicine: A Comprehensive Study Guide*. 8th ed. McGraw Hill; 2016:1688-1692.

309

RESPECTING THY ELDERS: DEFINING, DETECTING, AND REPORTING OF GERIATRIC ABUSE

ALEXANDER ZIRULNIK AND SHAN W. LIU

It is estimated that around 10% of older adults (>60 years) face some form of abuse annually. However, this is likely underestimated, given factors such as victims' fear of retaliation, fear of forced removal from home settings, loss of financial security, perceived shame, or cognitive impairment. Geriatric abuse is defined by the CDC as "an intentional act or failure to act that causes or creates a risk of harm to an older adult." This term encompasses several forms of abuse, including physical, sexual, emotional, psychological, and financial abuse. These are often not mutually exclusive, and many victims suffer from multiple forms of abuse. Often, geriatric abuse is committed by someone with the perception of trust and commonly involves family members or friends. While geriatric abuse has been reported in institutions, it is more commonly seen in home or community-based settings. Victims suffer from increased mortality, nursing home placement, and increasing levels of anxiety and depression. Self-neglect is another important form of geriatric abuse, commonly seen in emergency settings, that often requires further investigation, safety screening, and capacity assessment.

As the number of older adults has increased in the United States, so have the prevalence of ED visits among this age group. Between 2014 and 2017, the CDC reported 20% of all ED visits were made by older adults. Victims of geriatric abuse are twice as likely to visit the ED than nonvictims. EM providers remain an important vanguard in the detection, reporting, and treatment of victims of geriatric abuse. However, the rate of detection and reporting remains staggeringly low. In the United States, as few as 1 in 24 cases of geriatric abuse is reported to appropriate authorities. In one study, the diagnosis of geriatric abuse was made in 0.01% to 0.02% of national ED visits, greater than two orders of magnitude lower than the estimated national prevalence. Health care professionals have reported several barriers to identifying and caring for victims, including a lack of adequate training. Other barriers likely include uncertain decision-making capacity of victims, lack of knowledge regarding reporting to legal agencies, skepticism of the legal system, perceived inadequate time to complete a thorough evaluation, difficulty distinguishing between accidental trauma or abuse, or even denial by the victim themselves. Often, victims of geriatric abuse suffer from a form of cognitive impairment, a spectrum of disorders affecting roughly 12% of adults aged 65 years or above in the United States. Nearly half of individuals with dementia has suffered from some form of geriatric abuse.

Other difficult factors in identifying geriatric abuse include a lack of awareness of previous functional status, common accidents such as falls, and normal physiology of aging. Several studies have looked at and identified common physical examination findings associated with neglect or physical abuse (**Table 309.1**). Documentation of these physical examination findings is important and may be better supplemented with photographs. While there are no gold standard screening tools to aid in the detection of geriatric abuse, the National Center for Elder Abuse has a list screening tools on their website. The BASE, ED Senior AID tool, and EASI are commonly used screening tools that take only minutes to complete in the ED.

TABLE 309.1 PHYSICAL EXAMINATION FINDINGS ASSOCIATED WITH GERIATRIC ABUSE OR NEGLECT

- Weight loss/cachexia/signs of malnutrition or dehydration
- Poor hygiene
- Isolated facial or neck injuries combined with no upper and lower extremity injuries
- Injuries to the left face/neck (assailants are often right handed)
- Ear injuries
- Bite marks
- Burns
- Open wounds, cuts, punctures, untreated injuries in various stages of healing
- Evidence of physical restraint (wrist or ankle abrasions or scars)

When identified, decision-making capacity of victims is important to determine if they have capacity to decline care or intervention. It is important that if care is declined, that a safety plan is established, and a list of resources is given. Social work consultation remains an important asset in geriatric abuse cases in the ED. In most states, health care professionals, including EM providers, must report geriatric abuse to law enforcement agencies or adult protective services. Improved recognition of geriatric abuse and knowledge surrounding reporting should increase reporting.

EM providers can utilize screening tools such as the EASI or BASE and recognition of distinctive physical examination findings to improve their detection and reporting of geriatric abuse in the ever-growing population of older adults in the United States.

PEARLS

- Only 1 in 24 cases of geriatric abuse are reported to appropriate authorities or agencies.
- Victims of geriatric abuse commonly present to the ED but are missed due to underrecognition and poor screening.
- There are several screening tools available to aid EM providers, such as the BASE, ED Senior AID tool, and EASI.
- Geriatric abuse should be reported to law enforcement or adult protective services and is mandatory in most jurisdictions.
- ED social work or services are vital resources for older patients.

SUGGESTED READINGS

Ashman JJ, Schappert SM, Santo L. Emergency department visits among adults aged 60 and over: United States, 2014-2017. *NCHS Data Brief*. 2020;(367):1-8.

Centers for Disease Control and Prevention. Subjective cognitive decline—a public health issue. Centers for Disease Control and Prevention; 2019. Accessed January 14, 2023. https://www.cdc.gov/aging/data/subjective-cognitive-decline-brief

Dong X, Simon MA. Association between elder abuse and use of ED: findings from the Chicago Health and Aging Project. *Am J Emerg Med*. 2013;31(4):693-698.

Evans CS, Hunold KM, Rosen T, Platts-Mills TF. Diagnosis of elder abuse in U.S. Emergency Departments. *J Am Geriatr Soc*. 2017;65(1):91-97.

Mercier É, Nadeau A, Brousseau AA, et al. Elder abuse in the out-of-hospital and emergency department settings: a scoping review. *Ann Emerg Med*. 2020;75(2):181-191.

Mosqueda L, Burnight K, Gironda MW, Moore AA, Robinson J, Olsen B. The abuse intervention model: a pragmatic approach to intervention for elder mistreatment. *J Am Geriatr Soc*. 2016;64(9):1879-1883.

Rosen T, Stern ME, Elman A, Mulcare MR. Identifying and initiating intervention for elder abuse and neglect in the emergency department. *Clin Geriatr Med*. 2018;34(3):435-451.

Rosen T, LoFaso VM, Bloemen EM, et al. Identifying injury patterns associated with physical elder abuse: analysis of legally adjudicated cases. *Ann Emerg Med*. 2020;76(3):266-276.

310

Pain Medications and Procedural Sedation in Older Adults

Jessica Kuxhause and Lauren Cameron-Comasco

While acute pain is a frequent presenting complaint for patients of all ages, older adults are less likely to have this pain adequately treated compared to their younger counterparts. It is known that older adults are more susceptible to adverse risks associated with analgesia and sedation, due to higher rates of nutritional deficiencies, polypharmacy, frailty, cognitive impairment, and comorbidities. Less appreciated is that untreated pain can also precipitate delirium and lead to poorer outcomes. A patient-tailored multimodal approach can improve pain levels, patient satisfaction, and quality of life as well as reduce length of stay and readmission rates among older ED patients.

The golden rule for dosing medications in older adults is "start low and go slow," meaning a small initial dose followed by stepwise, repeat dosing, if necessary. This strategy requires frequent reassessments and potentially retreatments to achieve pain control while minimizing adverse effects. The goal is early assessment in the initial evaluation, subsequently after each intervention, and before disposition.

Accurately assessing pain level can be difficult in nonverbal or cognitively impaired individuals. In this population, pay close attention to facial expressions, behaviors (such as pain avoidance), agitation, and physical examination findings. Caregivers and family can also provide critical insight into a patient's condition.

More so than in younger patients, selecting a pain control intervention in the older adult is a fine balance between adverse effects and pain relief. When choosing a therapy, consider patient factors such as comorbidities, medications, and patient preferences. Nonpharmacologic, alternative, and nonsystemic interventions are first line and may be used either alone or in conjunction with pharmacologic modalities. Consider warm or cold compresses, compression, elevation, massage, and physical/occupational therapy. Topical analgesics such as topical NSAIDs, capsaicin, and lidocaine patches (5%) can be effective for MSK and neuropathic pain syndromes with less risk of toxicity. In addition, consider nonanalgesic therapies targeting the underlying etiology, such as for GI-related pain, trial antiemetics, antacids, and proton-pump inhibitors. Use caution with muscle relaxants, which can cause dizziness and sedation. Steroids, though considered beneficial in many conditions, can have serious toxicity and adverse effects, especially in patients on anticoagulation. This limits their utility in older adults.

Indications for systemic analgesics parallel those in younger adults, with some dosing adjustments. Acetaminophen remains the first-line choice for mild (0-3/10) level acute pain as well as for mild persistent pain due to its low-risk profile. Dosing recommendations range from 325 to 500 mg every 4 hours to 500 to 1,000 mg every 6 hours. Maximal daily dose is 4 g. Note maximum in hepatic impairment or alcohol abuse is 2 to 3 g daily.

NSAIDs are on the Beers criteria of inappropriate medications for older adults due to their high-risk profile, particularly in those with cardiovascular disease, GI bleeding, impaired renal function, and concomitant medications (eg, anticoagulation, ACE inhibitors, and diuretics). As toxicities are dose and time dependent, use lowest dose possible for the shortest possible duration. Dosing recommendations are 200 mg up to 3 times per day; counsel patients on warning signs and symptoms.

Opioids remain the standard of care for moderate-to-severe pain in older adults, if no contraindications; however, dose adjustments must be made to account for physiologic changes in metabolism and clearance. Dose adjustments for opioids should be 25% to 50% lower than standard dosing. Oral agents are preferred for moderate pain (4-6/10), with typical options from the ED being oxycodone or hydrocodone dosed at 2.5 to 5 mg every 4 to 6 hours. For severe pain (7-10/10), IV options, such as morphine or hydromorphone, are recommended. Use morphine with caution and at lower dosing in patients with renal insufficiency, and hydromorphone with caution in hepatic dysfunction. Hydromorphone 0.5 to 2 mg every 3 to 4 hours can be used and is a good adjunct for breakthrough pain. Opioids to avoid include codeine, which has increased CNS side effects, and meperidine, which has neurotoxic metabolites. Counsel patients on side effects, including CNS depression, nausea, vomiting, and constipation. Consider pretreatment with antiemetics, and always include a bowel regimen with your opioid prescriptions.

Regional anesthesia is effective in MSK complaints, such as fractures and dislocations, by providing the benefit of anesthesia without systemic side effects or prolonged required hemodynamic monitoring. For hip fractures, the FNB and FICB target the femoral nerve and/or nerves under the fascia iliaca. While both are similarly effective for analgesia, the FICB is technically easier to perform. Rib fractures are painful and can result in serious sequelae, and while opioids provide analgesia, they can also cause counterproductive effects, such as respiratory depression and sedation. Use the SAPB for lateral rib fractures, which targets the cutaneous intercostal nerve branches by injecting a large volume dilute anesthetic into the fascial plane between the serratus anterior and latissimus dorsi muscles.

Other procedures for the ED practitioner's toolkit include hematoma blocks for distal radius and fractures, intra-articular posterior shoulder injections for shoulder reductions, and SPGBs for intractable headaches or migraines.

In regional anesthesia, anesthetic choice is determined by the ED's formulary as well as desired effects: Lidocaine is slightly faster onset (10-20 minutes) but shorter duration (3-8 hours), while ropivacaine and bupivacaine are slower onset (15-30 minutes) with longer duration (ropivacaine 5-12 hours, bupivacaine 6-30 hours). Using ultrasound for blocks improves efficacy and reduces risks such as nerve and vascular injury. In case of anesthetic toxicity, ensure monitoring and resuscitative equipment is ready and intralipid available in case of anesthetic toxicity; to best prevent, always aspirate before injection. As always, perform using sterile technique to minimize infection risk.

Procedural sedation of older adults can be challenging, with increased risk of complications. As always, choose the medication after careful consideration of patient factors. In general, use a lower starting dose given at a slower administration rate, with less frequent dosing intervals. Anticipate challenges with supplemental oxygen and bedside resuscitative equipment. Short-acting medications (propofol, etomidate) are preferred, given their short onset/offset times and ease of titratability. For longer procedures, ketamine is a reasonable choice that preserves airway protective reflexes and blood pressure. Avoid benzodiazepines, which are an independent risk factor for delirium, particularly if the patient is also receiving opioids. In combination, these medications carry higher risk of adverse events, including death.

> **PEARLS**
>
> - Controlling pain is as important as identifying its etiology.
> - "Start low and go slow."
> - Treat pain with multimodal approach.
> - Consider alternative treatments, such as topical therapies and regional anesthesia.
> - Appropriately choose and dose medications after consideration of patient factors.

Suggested Readings

Hwang U. The quality of emergency department pain care for older adult patients. *J Am Geriatr Soc*. 2010;58(11):2122-2128.

Hwang U, Platts-Mills TF. Acute pain management in older adults in the emergency department. *Clin Geriatr Med*. 2013;29(1):151-164.

Lin C, Darling C, Tsui BCH. Practical regional anesthesia guide for elderly patients. *Drugs Aging*. 2019;36:213-234.

Weaver CS, Terrell KM, Bassett R, et al. ED procedural sedation of elderly patients: is it safe? *Am J Emerg Med*. 2011;29(5):541-544.

311

Overdiagnosing and Overtreating UTIs in the Older Person

Robert Anderson

The fascination with urine dates back thousands of years. Hippocrates was one of the earliest physicians to study urine and felt that no other organ system provided more clues to health than the urinary system. Some 1,000 years later, Theophilus Protospatharius's treatise on urine, *De Urinis*, became a staple for medical students for nearly 600 years.

In current clinical practice, the captivation with UA in the specific context of the older adult continues. The UA is often part of an older person's testing, regardless of the presenting issue; it is frequently ordered in patients with slight confusion or if there is malodorous or cloudy urine. However, in isolation, none of those attributes are indications to order a UA.

Remarkably, there is no universal definition of symptomatic UTI in older adults. The interpretation of the standard UA can be fraught with error. For example, there is an array of different evaluations depending on the dipstick used, white cells can be reported in variable measurements, and the sediment can be challenging to interpret.

Who to Test

The reality is that a significant portion of older adults are harboring bacteria and/ or WBCs in their urine without clinical symptoms or acute disease. Up to 50% of older women living in facilities have asymptomatic bacteriuria/pyuria. Up to 15% of community-dwelling men have asymptomatic bacteriuria/pyuria. Screening for and treating asymptomatic older adults is not recommended.

While unnecessary use of antibiotics has downstream consequences, the real-time issues are premature closure and confirmation bias. Falsely attributing an older person's presentation to a UTI could be disastrous if, for example, a subdural hematoma is the ultimate cause for the confusion. A UTI causing delirium should be a diagnosis of exclusion.

To be clear, a UA should absolutely be obtained on all older adults presenting with sepsis or septic shock. Outside of septic older adults, the UA should only be requested if there are signs or symptoms attributable to the urinary tract. Without signs or symptoms consistent with a UTI, a UA is of no value.

Symptoms and Signs of a UTI

Guidelines differ on the number of signs and symptoms needed to support a diagnosis of UTI. For an older adult with cognitive issues, examining for signs may be more important than eliciting symptoms.

In older adults without cognitive impairment, symptoms such as dysuria, frequency, urgency, and new or worsening incontinence are typical and not age related. Importantly, signs of a UTI, including fever, costovertebral angle tenderness, or suprapubic tenderness, should be present in most older adults, regardless of cognitive status. Most people with advanced dementia syndrome or other neurologic deficits should still respond to painful stimuli. Keep in mind that fever has been defined as a 2° increase from baseline.

Interpreting the Results

In nonseptic older adults, a UA should only be ordered if there is a significant pretest probability for a UTI. If the LE, nitrite, or blood are positive on the urine dipstick, most labs reflex to the sediment exam. The sediment exam, or microscopy, is performed manually by counting WBCs, RBCs, and bacteria. This is usually reported as cells per HPF. However, WBCs can also be counted visually in a device called a hemocytometer with units reported as WBCs per microliter. The proper attention to units is paramount to the proper interpretation of results.

Because of the high degree of variability in reporting, it is unclear how to interpret positive LE or nitrites on the dipstick. If they are both negative, a UTI is ruled out. It is unclear how to interpret bacteria, glitter cells, or clumping WBCs on the sediment exam. The significance of bacteria in the sediment is unknown at the time of initial reporting and until culture results are available.

In contrast, a more consistent definition of pyuria exists in older adults defined as 10 or more WBCs per HPF. This value is supportive of an inflammatory process in the urinary tract of older adults.

Putting It All Together

In the nonseptic older adult with symptoms and/or signs attributable to the urinary tract, a UA should be ordered. If that UA shows 10 or more WBCs per HPF, a presumptive diagnosis of UTI can be made. The urine culture will confirm the diagnosis. However, a positive urine culture in the absence of symptoms and/or signs is of low utility, defines asymptomatic bacteriuria, and should not be treated with antibiotics.

PEARLS

- Older adults who present with sepsis or septic shock should have a UA ordered.
- Up to 50% of older adults harbor bacteria and/or WBCs.
- In patients with dementia, utilize objective findings to support your decision to order a UA, such as fever, CVA tenderness, and suprapubic tenderness.
- The number of WBCs or bacteria in the urine from a nonseptic older adult is meaningless without the accompanying clinical suspicion of a UTI. People with positive urine cultures without symptoms do not have a UTI and should not be treated with antibiotics.
- Pyuria in an older adult is defined as 10 or more WBCs per HPF.

SUGGESTED READINGS

Chu CM, Lowder JL. Diagnosis and treatment of urinary tract infections across age groups. *Am J Obstet Gynecol*. 2018;219:40-51.

Detweiler K, Mayers D, Fletcher SG. Bacteriuria and urinary tract infections in the elderly. *Urol Clin North Am*. 2015;42:561-586.

Juthani-Mehta M, Datunashvili A, Tinetti M. Tests for urinary tract infection in nursing home residents. *JAMA*. 2014;312(16):1687-1688.

Mody L, Juthani-Mehta M. Urinary tract infections in older women, a clinical review. *JAMA*. 2014;311(8):844-854.

Pallin DJ, Ronan C, Montazeri K, et al. Urinalysis in acute care of adults: pitfalls in testing and interpreting results. *Open Forum Infect Dis*. 2014;1(1):ofu019.

Pescatore R, Niforatos JD, Rezaie S, et al. Evidence-informed practice: diagnostic questions in urinary tract infections in the elderly. *West J Emerg Med*. 2019;20(4):573-577.

Rowe TA, Juthani-Mehta M. Urinary tract infection in older adults. *Aging Health*. 2013;9(5):1-15.

Rowe TA, Juthani-Mehta M. Diagnosis and management of urinary tract infections in older adults. *Infect Dis Clin North Am*. 2014;28:75-89.

312

BE ATTENTIVE TO INATTENTION: DELIRIUM MANAGEMENT PEARLS IN THE ED

BRIANNA KLUCHER AND DANYA KHOUJAH

Delirium is a common neuropsychiatric condition characterized by waxing and waning disturbance in attention, awareness, and cognition, not attributable to a preexisting neurocognitive disorder and developing secondary to one or more medical triggers such as infection or medication side effects. Although prevalent among older adults in the ED, it is commonly missed. Delirium is associated with prolonged hospitalization, increased mortality, and long-term declines in independence and cognitive function. Identification is paramount and relies on screening those at risk, early recognition of those affected, timely intervention to treat underlying causes, and avoidance of possible precipitants for those at risk.

Delirium occurs in 8% to 10% of older adults in the ED and can be multifactorial. It usually develops in vulnerable older adults with underlying risk factors, such as dementia, advanced age, or visual or hearing impairment. When these predisposed individuals are exposed to a precipitating insult, delirium ensues. Common triggers include infection, metabolic disorders, and dehydration. Iatrogenic insults include medications, ED boarding, procedures, and untreated pain.

Early recognition is a critical factor in improving outcomes in geriatric delirium. All older adults, or at least those who are high risk, should be screened for delirium. Clinical gestalt is the most commonly reported approach to delirium identification; however, misses 50% to 85% of patients, making it insufficient to rely on. A validated highly sensitive screening tool should be used, such as the DTS and the 4AT, which take less than 30 seconds to administer. Those who screen positive should have the diagnosis confirmed with a more specific tool such as the bCAM, which is validated in ED settings and takes 2 minutes to administer.

Uncover the Underlying Cause Using a Systematic Approach

A thorough history and physical examination of patients with delirium are of paramount importance. Obtaining a comprehensive medication list (including over-the-counter medications and herbal supplements) with special attention to drugs with anticholinergic properties and CNS effects is essential. Vital signs may be normal even in critical illness, as older adults may not mount fever or tachycardia. Patients should be fully undressed to look for signs of infection, medication patches, indwelling catheters, or evidence of trauma or abuse.

The workup should include a complete blood cell count, basic metabolic panel, blood glucose, and an electrocardiogram to uncover common delirium precipitants. When clinical symptoms of an infection are present, urinalysis and chest x-ray are frequently obtained to address common sources of infection. Head CTs are unlikely to uncover a clinically significant acute abnormality in patients without a focal neurologic deficit, decreased level of consciousness, suspected trauma, or anticoagulant use. Additional workup including lumbar puncture should be considered on an individual basis. Delirium is often multifactorial and one should not be misled by asymptomatic bacteriuria or other vague findings without completing a thorough assessment.

Nonpharmacologic Intervention Is First Line

The mainstay of delirium treatment lies in addressing the underlying cause and prioritizing nonpharmacologic intervention. Reorientation, reassurance, and decreasing unfamiliar stimuli are first line for treatment of delirium. The presence of caregivers, or utilizing sitters if available, is a priority for care. If medications are required, low-dose oral antipsychotics are preferred, as they preserve patient autonomy and have lower side effects than parenteral preparations. Benzodiazepines are reserved for those with alcohol withdrawal or with suspected seizures. Physical restraints should be a last resort for patients who are hyperactive and putting themselves or others at risk of harm until medications take effect.

Most patients benefit from admission for treatment of underlying conditions and for monitoring safety while altered. Admission has been shown to reduce ED returns and future hospitalizations. However, discharge can be considered in select patients if the underlying cause is identified and there is appropriate supervision at home with a clear follow-up plan. If a patient wishes to leave against medical advice, capacity should be thoroughly assessed and documented, and family members/next-of-kin should be involved. Remember that capacity may fluctuate in delirium.

The best approach to delirium is prevention by promptly treating underlying causes and avoiding precipitating iatrogenic insults for all at-risk individuals. A family or staff member should be available for frequent reorientation and to engage the patient with cognitively stimulating activities. Lights should be kept bright during daytime hours and darkened in the evening to avoid circadian rhythm disruption. The use of home glasses and hearing aids improves sensory deficits. Excess stimuli such as noise and alarms should be minimized. Adequately treating pain is a key intervention: use nonsedating medications if feasible. Careful attention should be paid to hydration, toileting, and safe mobility. Patients' home medications including those with CNS effects should be continued to avoid withdrawal unless the medication is the presumed trigger. Pharmacologic measures are not helpful for prevention. Prophylactic antipsychotic administration typically worsens and prolongs delirium rather than prevents it and is best avoided.

PEARLS

- Use the DTS tool for all at-risk patients, and then the bCAM scoring for early recognition of delirium.
- Prevention and treatment of delirium relies on early interventions targeting pain, dehydration, disorientation, and sensory deficits.
- Pharmacologic intervention with antipsychotics should be reserved for hyperactive delirium with acute risk to personal or others' safety.
- All patients should receive a workup of complete blood cell count, basic metabolic panel, blood glucose, chest radiograph, and electrocardiogram. Additional workup should be performed on an individual basis, including urinalysis when symptoms of UTI or altered mental status are present.
- Most patients benefit from admission for treatment of underlying conditions and for monitoring safety while altered. Discharge may be considered if the underlying cause is identified and improving and there is appropriate supervision at home.

SUGGESTED READINGS

Carpenter CR, Hammouda N, Linton EA, et al. Delirium prevention, detection, and treatment in emergency medicine settings: a geriatric emergency care applied research (GEAR) network scoping review and consensus statement. *Acad Emerg Med*. 2021;28(1):19-35.

Eagles D, Khoujah D. Rapid fire: acute brain failure in older emergency department patients. *Emerg Med Clin North Am*. 2021;39(2):287-305.

Lee S, Chen H, Hibino S, et al. Can we improve delirium prevention and treatment in the emergency department? A systematic review. *J Am Geriatr Soc*. 2022;70(6):1838-1849.

Oliveira JE Silva L, Berning MJ, Stanich JA, et al. Risk factors for delirium in older adults in the emergency department: a systematic review and meta-analysis. *Ann Emerg Med*. 2021;78(4):549-565. PMID: 34127307.

313

Evaluating the Asymptomatic Patient with Dementia

Surriya Ahmad and Richard Sinert

Dementia describes a deterioration of intellectual faculties, which include memory, attention, learning, and judgment. AD is the most common cause of dementia.

The global annual incidence of dementia is 4.6 million; the National Institutes of Health reports that in the United States, at least 5 million older adults have AD. The Centers for Disease Control and Prevention estimates doubling the senior population over the next 25 years, resulting in 19.6 million more senior adult ED visits. It is estimated that 22% of older adults seen in the ED have a form of cognitive impairment.

Dementia is often complicated by emotional disturbance and personality changes. The most common tools to detect dementia in the ED are the Mini-Cog and SPMSQ, which identify a continuum from mild to severe cognitive impairment. However, a recent meta-analysis found that the AMT-4 was the most specific, and the BAS was the most sensitive. After a positive dementia screen, we recommend communicating with providers and having specialty consultations, including social work, case management, and outpatient geriatric referral.

A 78-year-old female with PMHx HTN, type II diabetes mellitus BIBEMS from a nursing home for a report of hitting staff. No family or caregivers are present in the ED.

A typical presentation of an asymptomatic patient with dementia coming from home or a long-term care facility is for agitation or other behavioral issues. Other catalysts for ED visits could be caregiver burden, related social and medical concerns, or simple unfamiliarity with the patient's baseline mental status by a new staff member.

The evaluation before discharge often encompasses medical and psychiatric conditions. Is this dementia of organic origin or depression? Older people with depression are at an increased risk of dementia. Likewise, depression can mimic dementia and can exacerbate and predispose patients to dementia. Due to the complex association between depression and dementia, older adults should also be evaluated for depression during their visit.

In evaluating a clinically stable patient with cognitive impairment, first establish the patient's baseline through discussion with a representative at the long-term care facility, a physician, a nurse, a family member, or a friend. Consider caregiver burden as a cause for ED presentation. Older adult abuse must also be considered in cases of trauma. Engaging the social work team to help obtain this vital collateral information may be helpful.

Obtaining a good history and performing a thorough physical exam is paramount in determining the cause of the ED presentation. Information about recent critical events like illness, falls, or trauma and comparing behaviors over time may be helpful. Although the patient may seem asymptomatic at the ED evaluation, recent events could elucidate the actual cause of the visit. Concurrent findings may be uncovered in an older adult, requiring a more in-depth assessment.

A medical evaluation should be undertaken if the patient is not at baseline. At a minimum, review a patient's medication list, address new medications added, and assess whether a patient adheres to currently prescribed medications. Although there is no unified expert consensus, clinical context may dictate a workup that includes a complete blood count, basic metabolic panel, hepatic panel, thyroid stimulating hormone, urinalysis, urine toxicology screen, medication levels, ECG, chest x-ray, and a head CT. Initiate an appropriate trauma evaluation if the history is deemed necessary. A more expanded workup for reversible causes of dementia, including vitamin B_{12}, folic acid, RPR, and HIV, can be considered.

Special considerations for patients with dementia include agitation, addressing pain levels and environmental triggers, and communication barriers in the emergency department setting. Utilize tools when possible to aid in communication that aim to improve comfort and experience among older adults in the ED, such as eyeglasses, hearing amplifiers, and other physician-specific strategies, such as allowing extra time, sitting face to face, and maintaining eye contact.

Once free of infection, trauma, or other causes, patients may benefit from a psychiatry or geriatric psychiatry evaluation at the ED physician's discretion.

PEARLS

- Determine the patient's baseline mental status and whether the patient deviates from it.
- Lower the threshold to initiate concurrent infection and trauma workups if the history or physical suggests recent illness or frequent falls or trauma.
- Consider how much caregiver burden may be pertinent to the patient's visit.
- Be mindful of the unique needs of a patient with dementia, including special considerations regarding agitation and difficulties with communication, and utilize tips to improve communication with older adults in the ED.

Suggested Readings

Ahmad S. Communicating with older adults in the emergency department. *SAEM Pulse.* 2022;37(4):18-19.

Carpenter CR, Banerjee J, Keyes D, et al. Accuracy of dementia screening instruments in emergency medicine: a diagnostic meta-analysis. *Acad Emerg Med.* 2019;26(2):226-245.

Carpenter CR, Bassett ER, Fischer GM, Shirshekan J, Galvin JE, Morris JC. Four sensitive screening tools to detect cognitive dysfunction in geriatric emergency department patients: brief Alzheimer's Screen, Short Blessed Test, Ottawa 3DY, and the caregiver-completed AD8. *Acad Emerg Med.* 2011;18(4):374-384.

Centers for Disease Control and Prevention. *The State of Aging and Health in America.* U.S. Department of Health and Human Services; 2013.

Lichen IM, Berning MJ, Bower SM, et al. Non-pharmacologic interventions improve comfort and experience among older adults in the emergency department. *Am J Emerg Med.* 2021;39:15-20.

Mutter MK, Snustad D, Bond M. *Evaluating Dementia and Delirium in the Emergency Department.* Accessed September 6, 2015. https://www.reliasmedia.com/articles/136204-evaluating-dementia-and-delirium-in-the-emergency-department

Santangelo I, Ahmad S, Liu S, et al. Examination of geriatric care processes implemented in level 1 and 2 geriatric emergency departments. *J Geriatr Emerg Med.* 2022;3(4): 10.17294/2694-4715.1041.

Valkanova V, Ebmeier KP, Allen CL. Depression is linked to dementia in older adults. *Practitioner.* 2017;261(1800):11-15.

314

DEFINING GOALS OF CARE IN YOUR GERIATRIC ED PATIENT

JOSEPHINE LO BELLO AND BALAKRISHNA VEMULA

Emergency physicians are trained to save lives. In fact, most of our education and time in the clinical space is spent thinking about how to identify, treat, and often reverse time-sensitive diseases or injuries. However, life-extending interventions may not always be concordant with the wishes of our patients.

Seventy-five percent of older adults with a life-limiting illness will visit the ED in their last 6 months of life. The decisions we make, from those as dramatic as intubation to those that seem far more routine, such as the decision to admit someone to the hospital, represent crossroads in a patient's care, especially for those older adults who may have limitations in their care goals or priorities in their lives that would be disrupted by our interventions. Ideally, conversations outlining these goals of care will have been initiated in the outpatient setting, though patients often do not present with advanced directives or have had these discussions. The ED may become the default to navigate these challenging circumstances and initiate critical conversations.

How

There are numerous barriers to having these conversations in the ED—limited time and oftentimes limited context are two such barriers. Both of these can make the conversation challenging to have in the delicate manner to which such a discussion is entitled. There are ways to set oneself up for success despite these barriers and steps to follow within the conversation itself as a guide to navigating a difficult subject.

Set Yourself Up for Success

- Sit down
  - Studies demonstrate that sitting down in the exam room increases the perception of how long the clinician spent with a patient in addition to providing a more comforting environment for the patient.
- Allow for protected time
  - If you anticipate a longer conversation, inform the team, just as you might prior to starting a time-consuming procedure.
- Anticipate clinical deterioration and begin these conversations early
- Invite family, friends, and/or care partners
  - In-person discussions are often preferred, but if not possible, telephone or videoconferencing with family, friends, or care partners during such discussions may be considered. Engagement of loved ones can provide support and strength to an overwhelmed patient and valuable context for the clinical team.

Have a Framework in Mind

It can be challenging to initiate such an intimate conversation with a patient with whom you have no long-term relationship. "REMAP," published in the *Journal of Oncology Practice*, provides a framework for goal-based care conversations and a helpful tool for navigating these conversations.

- R: Reframe the situation
  - When considering the patient's clinical condition, we create a mental model for that patient's illness severity and trajectory, which the patient may not understand. Ask the patient what their understanding is of their illness, particularly whatever underlying condition might be driving their chief complaint. With their permission, then, offer your perspective. Speak simply and use direct language (eg, *"I'm worried that you are getting sicker"; "I'm worried that your breathing is getting worse"*).
- E: Expect emotion, empathize
  - Telling a patient they are sick, even if they already know it in their gut, is hard to say and harder to hear. Take a beat, pause, and try to validate whatever reaction the patient or their family may have (eg, *"I know that's not what you wanted to hear, I'm so sorry"; "I can see you're scared, and that's completely understandable"*).
- M: Map what is most important; A: Align with what the patient values
  - These next two steps go hand in hand—ask the patient what is important to them and then reiterate your understanding of what they are telling you (eg, *"As I listen to you, it sounds like the most important things to you are"*).
- P: Plan medical treatments that match patient values
  - This may translate into admission and intubation should their condition decline, intravenous antibiotics with an accompanying do-not-resuscitate order, or even discharging the patient with the appropriate resources (eg, *"Here are the ways we could help your breathing while letting you stay awake and talk to your family"*).

Have Reasonable Expectations

The ED is an overwhelming place, and difficult conversations can be overwhelming for patients and providers alike. Due to the combination of time pressure from the clinical team and the high likelihood that this may be the first time a patient has been asked about their goals, an initial conversation may not result in an answer or a clear plan. However, initiating this conversation and giving patients and their families the tools to advocate for themselves has significant value and opens the door to future discussions to address dynamic clinical conditions.

PEARLS

- Set yourself up for success: Sit down and notify your team.
- Anticipate potential clinical deterioration and have this conversation early.
- Involve family when appropriate.
- REMAP provides a valuable framework.
- Remember that your conversation may not result in an immediate clear decision, but initiating the discussion in the first place has value in and of itself.

Suggested Readings

Childers JW, Back AL, Tulsky JA, Arnold RM. REMAP: a framework for goals of care conversations. *J Oncol Pract.* 2017;13(10):e844-e850. PMID: 28445100.

Ouchi K, George N, Schuur JD, et al. Goals-of-care conversations for older adults with serious illness in the emergency department: challenges and opportunities. *Ann Emerg Med.* 2019;74(2):276-284.

Smith AK, McCarthy E, Weber E, et al. Half of older Americans seen in emergency department in last month of life; most admitted to hospital, and many die there. *Health Aff (Millwood).* 2012;31:1277-1285.

315

Know How to Cognitively Screen Your Geriatric Patient

Rachel M. Skains, Jin H. Han, and Richard E. Kennedy

Annual ED visits among adults aged 65 or older are rapidly increasing, creating a paradigm shift in the emergency care model to address unique geriatric syndromes. Nearly a third of older patients presenting to the ED have CI, which is subdivided into acute (delirium) and chronic (dementia) forms. Delirium is the most common form of acute CI, defined as acute loss of cognition that is often medically reversible. Because of its poor prognosis and unique considerations, a dedicated chapter on delirium is provided (see Chapter 312). Dementia is the most common form of chronic CI and is a slowly progressive loss of cognition. PLWD are more likely to receive diagnostic testing in the ED, be admitted, and have ED revisits. More than two-thirds of patients in the ED with CI lack documentation or a history of dementia, making prompt recognition and management of CI in the ED critically important. Thus, knowing how to cognitively screen your geriatric patient is essential for every emergency provider to deliver high-quality care.

Impact of Missing CI

Despite its high prevalence, CI is a neurocognitive disorder frequently undetected by emergency providers, often due to a lack of routine screening. This has serious implications for ED care practices, such as involving family and caregivers in medical decision-making, obtaining comprehensive geriatric assessments (eg, functional status for fall prevention), identifying behavioral or psychological disturbances, and modifying pain management. Older patients in the ED with CI may be unable to provide accurate histories, which can lead to inadequate diagnostic workups, underdiagnoses, missed interventions, and inadvertent discharges home. If discharged from the ED, these patients may not be able to comprehend discharge instructions, potentially leading to noncompliance.

Routine CI Screening Recommendations

The "Geriatric ED Guidelines" advise emergency providers to perform routine cognitive screening of all geriatric patients with documentation at the initial ED encounter. In 2022, the Geriatric Emergency care Applied Research (GEAR) 2.0 network published a scoping review focused on identifying the most accurate and pragmatic approach for detecting CI in the ED. Over 27 global cognitive assessments have been evaluated in the ED to detect CI and dementia. Of these screening instruments, the Ottawa 3DY (O3DY), 4 A's Test (4AT), and SIS have the highest sensitivity and negative predictive value for clinical use in the ED setting. The SIS, which consists of three-item temporal orientation (year, month, day of week) questions followed by three-item object recall (naming three objects), was the fastest to administer, taking less than 1 minute. Several of these instruments can be found in online medical calculators, such as MDCalc, including the 4AT and AMT-4 for easy implementation into routine ED practice. The "Geriatric ED Guidelines" recommend the Short Blessed Test (SBT), which consists of six items assessing orientation, attention, and short-term recall with high sensitivity but takes nearly 5 minutes to perform with complicated scoring. Any of these ED-valid screens can be

OPTIMAL ED CARE PRACTICE FOR PERSONS WITH CI

Regardless of the cognitive assessment used, recognizing CI is critical for providing optimal ED care. If CI is detected, collateral history from family and caregivers should be obtained to determine baseline mental status and confirm the reason for ED visit. For CI that is not previously documented, potentially reversible causes should be considered for ED diagnostic workup, including depression, drugs/toxins, hypothyroidism, normal pressure hydrocephalus, space-occupying brain lesions, and vitamin deficiencies (eg, B12, folate). However, less than 1% of PLWD have resolution of CI due to reversible etiologies.

For patients with CI who are admitted, the degree of CI should be communicated with the admitting team as dementia is a powerful risk factor for developing delirium during hospitalization. Early implementation of multicomponent delirium prevention interventions, including reorientation, mobility, sleep hygiene, sensory aids, hydration, and nutrition, and minimizing ED length of stay, is essential to improving patient safety and care transitions. If patients with CI are discharged from the ED, every effort should be undertaken to ensure that discharge instructions are understood and carried out, such as using the Teach-Back method and involving family, caregivers, case managers, and/or social workers. It is important to note that a positive CI screen is not a formal diagnosis of dementia; however, in those without a history of dementia, primary care providers should be notified as referrals for cognitive evaluation and management after the ED visit is important to improve patient outcomes.

PEARLS

- CI is prevalent in over a third of older patients in the ED.
- Emergency providers often fail to recognize CI in the ED due to lack of routine screening.
- CI has significant implications and considerations for ED care practice.
- Several ED-valid screening instruments exist to detect CI and routine CI screening is recommended for all geriatric patients in adult EDs.
- If CI is detected, it is important to (1) obtain an accurate history, (2) communicate with the admitting or primary care team, and (3) refer for additional cognitive evaluation.

SUGGESTED READINGS

Carpenter CR, Banerjee J, Keyes D, et al. Accuracy of dementia screening instruments in emergency medicine: a diagnostic meta-analysis. *Acad Emerg Med*. 2019;26(2):226-245.

Dresden SM, Taylor Z, Serina P, et al. Optimal emergency department care practices for persons living with dementia: a scoping review. *J Am Med Dir Assoc*. 2022;23(8):1314.e1-1314.e29.

Han JH, Suyama J. Delirium and dementia. *Clin Geriatr Med*. 2018;34(3):327-354.

Hustey FM, Meldon SW. The prevalence and documentation of impaired mental status in elderly emergency department patients. *Ann Emerg Med*. 2002;39(3):248-253.

Nowroozpoor A, Dussetschleger J, Perry W, et al. Detecting cognitive impairment and dementia in the emergency department: a scoping review. *J Am Med Dir Assoc*. 2022;23(8):1314-1315.e55.

316

SAFELY DISCHARGING YOUR OLDER PATIENT TO HOME

KYLE BURTON AND CAMERON J. GETTEL

Transitioning care from the ED to the outpatient and ambulatory care setting is a central responsibility of emergency clinicians, with particular attention required in the older adult population. Given higher rates of frailty, cognitive impairment, and sensory deficits, older adults and their family members face challenges accurately executing discharge instructions in a busy ED environment. Furthermore, barriers to family support, a lack of aged-care facilities, and problems with accessing primary care services have been proposed as reasons that older adults are at increased risk of ED revisits and mortality during the care transition period.

HIGH RISK IDENTIFICATION

Several tools can be used to recognize older patients who warrant focused attention on discharge coordination. Identifying age-related vulnerabilities is essential to recognizing those with increased risk for adverse post-discharge outcomes. One such tool is the ISAR survey, which is used to predict negative outcomes in older ED patients. This self-reporting screening tool asks simple "yes/no" questions related to functional dependence, recent hospitalization, impaired memory and vision, and polypharmacy. Developed and validated in Canadian EDs, the ISAR is one of the most used tools in geriatric EDs. While this survey attempts to rapidly identify those at risk for negative outcomes, more comprehensive and focused evaluation will be required to support optimal patient service.

CLINICAL APPROACH

The Institute for Healthcare Improvement 4-Ms model helps clinicians develop a safe discharge plan by understanding Medications, Mentation, Mobility, and what Matters most to the patient. Addressing these core issues is paramount for ED clinicians to ensure successful care transitions after emergency care among older adults.

MEDICATIONS

ED clinicians should avoid prescribing PIMs. Beers Criteria provides a list of medications to avoid in older patients including the rationale for such recommendations. The STOPP/START criteria is also validated to help reduce PIMs among older patients and has demonstrated success in doing so. It is important to take patient preferences, life expectancy, and comorbidities into consideration while discussing medication regimens. Upon discharge, ED clinicians should confirm that the patient, their caregiver(s), and the patient's primary provider(s) are updated with the new prescription plan.

MENTATION

A brief assessment to identify cognitive impairment can be used if clinical suspicion of cognitive impairment (eg, delirium, dementia) arises, as this would allow referral for neuro-psycho-social testing and appropriate resource provision to caretakers. This is critical as the presence of delirium in the ED has been found to be associated with a significantly higher 6-month mortality. The DTS or bCAM can be used to reliably identify delirium which may be important in determining if a patient requires admission for further workup to identify underlying etiologies or may be discharged safely.

MOBILITY

Older adults in the ED are at high risk of functional decline in the days, weeks, and months following an ED visit. A sizable portion of the population may warrant evaluation by a physical therapist, allocation of ambulatory assistive devices, and education for patients and their caretakers regarding home safety best practices, particularly after fall-related ED visits. ED clinicians should consider standardized testing such as The TUG test, when evaluating older adults' mobility in the context of discharge considerations.

WHAT MATTERS

ED clinicians should ensure that older patient care management, disposition, and the ultimate follow-up care plan are patient-centered and aligned with desired outcomes. Multidisciplinary expert stakeholders developed a conversation guide that explores patients' 1) concerns about healthcare in the ED and 2) outcome most desired from the ED visit. According to recent qualitative work, researchers identified the feasibility of incorporating these two "What Matters" questions in the ED and the short time (mean of 3 minutes) needed to identify older adults' priorities. Eliciting older adults' concerns and desired outcomes from the outset of the clinical encounter has real merit in aligning the workup and disposition with that desired by the patient.

ANCILLARY SERVICES

Ancillary services, such as physical therapy, social work, care management, and pharmacists, can support the safe discharge of older patients and be especially helpful in navigating care transitions to independent living in the community. When compared to controls, ED-based transitional care nurse contact was associated with lower risk of inpatient admission during both index ED visits and 30 days following the visit. Another important group that is often overlooked is the informal caregivers (eg, family and friends) of the older adult. ED clinicians must anticipate discharge needs in collaboration with the caregivers, and when possible, assess caregiver burden and their capacity to carry out instructions.

PEARLS

- Older patients discharged from the ED have a higher rate of ED return and adverse health outcomes during the post-discharge course than other patient populations.
- A holistic approach to ED discharge requires addressing Medications, Mentation, Mobility, and what Matters most to the patient.
- Dedicated care transition staff can help facilitate a safe handoff from ED care to the older patient's outpatient care team.

SUGGESTED READINGS

Conneely M, Leahy S, Dore L, et al. The effectiveness of interventions to reduce adverse outcomes among older adults following Emergency Department discharge: umbrella review. *BMC Geriatr*. 2022;22(1):462.

Jacobsohn GC, Jones CMC, Green RK, et al. Effectiveness of a care transitions intervention for older adults discharged home from the emergency department: a randomized controlled trial. *Acad Emerg Med*. 2022;29(1):51-63.

Southerland LT, Pearson S, Hullick C, Carpenter CR, Arendts G. Safe to send home? Discharge risk assessment in the emergency department. *Emerg Med Australas*. 2019; 31(2):266-270.

317

PERFORM MOBILITY TESTING IN YOUR OLDER PATIENT WITH A GROUND LEVEL FALL

FREDERICK R. MURPHY JR AND PHILLIP D. MAGIDSON

Every year, 35% of adults 65 years of age and older fall, accounting for over 2.8 million ED visits. Although many GLFs do not lead to an ED visit or are otherwise not reported to PCPs, falls are a leading cause of traumatic injuries with an increased fall-related death rate by 30% from 2007 to 2017. GLFs often have a multisystem impact and are associated with a 30% increased risk of future falls, increased functional decline, and depression within the next 6 months. As such, it is important for EMPs to be able to evaluate and identify those patients who may be at increased risk for future falls.

MOBILITY ASSESSMENT

GLFs are often multifactorial and may be the result of polypharmacy, frailty, unsafe living conditions, age-related sensory impairment (such as hearing and visual impairment), and underlying acute medical pathology. In the ED, EMPs often focus on acute medical consequences of falls while many times failing to consider the etiology of the fall or evaluating the mobility. Use of evidenced-based, functional mobility tests can help provide an objective evaluation of an individual's fall risk. These tests, however, can be time consuming and are often unfamiliar to ED staff, which further limit adoption. Although no mobility test has perfect prognostic risk value for future falls, use of these tests may help the provider identify the most appropriate disposition including identifying patients who may safely be discharged home thus avoiding unnecessary health-care resource utilization.

Although formal consultation with PT or OT for all older adult GLF patients is ideal, pragmatically, such consultation is not possible. EMPs should be familiar with how to mobilize older adult patients using functional mobility measures that require minimal staff, time to complete, and space to administer. **Table 317.1** reviews some of these measures. In addition to the completion of these tests and associated timing, it is important for the EMP to observe the quality of the patient's movement. Quality of movement includes ensuring patient's feet are clearing the floor, each foot passes the other, and continuous movement forward.

Sarcopenia, age-related loss of skeletal muscle mass and strength, as well as frailty, may impact the aforementioned mobility assessments in older adults. Frailty, a geriatric syndrome of physiologic decline, closely related to mobility impairment, decreased walking speed, and physical activity intolerance, is important for EMPs to recognize as frail older adults seen in the ED are known to be at increased risk of in-hospital and post-procedural mortality. Numerous frailty screening tools exist and should be something EMPs become familiar with and use in tandem with mobility assessment tools, as they continue to care for an increasing number of older adults.

POST-ASSESSMENT INTERVENTIONS

Older adults with concern for mobility challenges or gait instability as evidenced by a visit for a GLF and abnormalities on functional mobility assessment testing should be counseled on future fall prevention and referred to more specialized care.

TABLE 317.1 FUNCTIONAL MOBILITY ASSESSMENT TOOLS

TEST	EQUIPMENT REQUIRED	PATIENT INSTRUCTIONS	INTERPRETATION
Timed Get Up and Go	Chair with arms; 10 feet of level, unobstructed space; use of usual assistive device is acceptable.	Rise from the chair, walk 10 feet, turn around, and then return to sitting position. This should be timed.	A time of ≥13.5 sec is abnormal and associated with increased risks of falls.
Five Times Sit to Stand Test	Chair with arms	Rise to standing, then return to seated position. Should be completed total of 5 times. Should not use chair arms.	A time of >15 sec suggests a high recurrence of falls in community-dwelling older adults.
One-Leg Balance	None	Stand on one leg (of their choice), flex the opposite knee, and raise foot off the floor for 5 sec.	Failure to complete was predictive of injurious falls in community-living older adults.

ED-specific care processes, a key component for geriatric ED accreditation and encouraged by the 2014 Geriatric Emergency Department Guidelines, aimed at fall interventions might include a PT or OT referral pathway, dedicated mobility aids in the ED or printed material for families, caregivers, and patients. The Centers for Disease Control and Prevention offers a comprehensive website with patient-specific educational material related to falls in older adults. Furthermore, the "Stay Independent" of STEADI program provides a simple questionnaire aimed at identifying those at increased risk of falls. This questionnaire can be provided to patients and their caregivers to complete during or after an ED visit and discussed with a PCP or other outpatient provider.

PEARLS

- Remember to consider the reason for a fall while evaluating for acute injuries including the role frailty or sarcopenia may play.
- Use a functional mobility assessment tool for older adults who present after a noninjurious GLF.
- Develop a care process or referral pathway to physical or OT for older adults suspected to be a higher risk for repeat falls.
- Train providers and nursing staff in implementation of functional mobility measures.

SUGGESTED READINGS

American College of Emergency Physicians, American Geriatrics Society, Emergency Nurses Association, Society for Academic Emergency Medicine, Geriatric Emergency Department Guideline Task Force. Geriatric emergency department guidelines. *Ann Emerg Med.* 2014;63(5):e7-e25.

Burns E, Kakara R. Deaths from falls among persons aged ≥65 years—United States, 2007–2016. *MMWR Morb Mortal Wkly Rep.* 2018;67:509-514.

Centers for Disease Control and Prevention. *Deaths From Older Adult Falls.* 2020. https://www.cdc.gov/falls/data/fall-deaths.html

Centers for Disease Control and Prevention. *Older Adult Fall Prevention.* 2022. https://www.cdc.gov/falls/index.html

Centers for Disease Control and Prevention, National Center for Injury Prevention and Control. *Web-Based Injury Statistics Query and Reporting System (WISQARS).* 2024. https://www.cdc.gov/injury/wisqars/

Covino M, Salini S, Russo A, et al. Frailty assessment in the emergency department for patients ≥80 years undergoing urgent major surgical procedurals. *J Am Med Dir Assoc.* 2022;23(4):581-588.

Sturnieks DL, Sherrington C. Gait impairment and falls. In: Busby-Whitehead J, Durso SC, Arenson C, Elon R, Palmer MH, Reichel W, eds. *Reichel's Care of the Elderly: Clinical Aspects of Aging.* Cambridge University Press; 2016:107-115.

318

TOO MUCH OF A GOOD THING: POLYPHARMACY IN OLDER ADULTS

FINNELLA MORGAN AND JONATHAN HANSEN

Fatigue, weakness, dizziness, falls, abdominal pain, and confusion are common, nonspecific complaints for which older adult patients present to the ED for evaluation. Although the potential causes for these symptoms are many, one culprit that is often overlooked is the role medications may play in patients seeking care in the ED.

Medication administration both during an ED visit and at the time of discharge may need to be tailored to the specific needs of older adults including dosing considerations, review of outpatient medications, and communication with ambulatory providers to ensure decreased risk of adverse drug events and interactions.

PHARMACOKINETICS

Advancing age comes with significant changes in pharmacokinetics. In simple terms, pharmacokinetics is how the body interacts with a drug in four key areas: absorption, distribution, metabolism, and excretion. Medication absorption is affected by increased gastric pH and delayed gastric emptying. The medication volume of distribution is affected by increased body fat, decreased total body water, and decreased albumin production. Warfarin, for example, is highly protein bound. In older adults with decreased albumin, the concentration of free warfarin and its anticoagulation effects are increased. Thus, conservative warfarin dosing is preferred in this population.

In the older patient population, it is especially important to consider metabolism and excretion. The major site for drug metabolism is the liver; however, in older adults, decreased hepatic mass, blood flow, and cytochrome p450 production lead to significant changes in drug metabolism. Medications that undergo first-pass metabolism such as morphine are most affected by these changes. Aging also negatively impacts GFR which declines even in older adults without kidney disease. As such, medications that are metabolized or excreted by the kidneys may need dosing adjustments. Such medications include common antibiotics such as piperacillin-tazobactam and vancomycin as well as pain medications such as morphine and gabapentin.

It is important that clinicians appreciate creatinine clearance and not just serum creatinine when renally dosing medications, as age-related reductions in muscle mass may show a normal serum creatinine despite a decreased GFR. Failure to make this distinction may result in inappropriately high dosing of certain medications.

Tramadol, a common pain medication known to lower the seizure threshold, exemplifies the impact of these pharmacokinetic issues at play. Tramadol depends on cytochrome 2D6 to be metabolized to its active metabolite and its excretion is dependent on the kidneys. The significant changes in metabolism and excretion in older adults can lead to increased drug half-life which perpetuates its adverse effects. Tramadol is often thought to be safer in older adults given its weaker opioid receptor activation properties; however, it offers a similar adverse effect profile to other opioid medications with less desirable pharmacokinetics making it a poor choice for geriatric patients.

POLYPHARMACY

Advancing age also comes with increasing chronic medical conditions and often accompanying daily medication regimens. A National Canadian Survey found that more than half of adults over the age of 65 reported taking four or more medications which increases the risk of medication interactions and dosing errors. Furthermore, socio-economic factors, cognitive impairment, age-related sensory decline such as macular degeneration and vision loss also impact safe adherence to complex regimens. In many instances, multiple providers may be writing similar or conflicting prescriptions for patients who are often left with little support in reconciling proper medication regimens.

PRESCRIBING BEST PRACTICES FOR GERIATRIC PATIENTS

A team-based approach has been shown to benefit geriatric patients in the management of their acute and chronic conditions. Ideally, this occurs for all patients, but it is particularly important for patients who take five or more medications, use high-risk medications, or who are at increased risk for adverse drug events. The goal of the multidisciplinary team approach is to recognize drug-drug interactions, minimize polypharmacy, and decrease high-risk medication use when appropriate.

The astute emergency provider should look for opportunities to take this team-based approach, such as consulting with their ED pharmacist or a patient's primary care provider when feasible. Unfortunately, this is not always possible and so one must look for other ways to remain vigilant.

One resource that may be beneficial to the ED provider is the STOPP and START Tool. This is an evidence-based medication review system designed to identify PIMs in the older adults. It can help identify potential adverse medication side effects as well as potential alternative treatment options.

The American Geriatric Society publishes the Beers Criteria for Potentially Inappropriate Medication Use in Older Adults. This comprehensive guideline highlights medications and their potential harm in the geriatric population. The medications included in this list are not absolute contraindications but should be avoided unless clinically necessary.

PEARLS

- In older adults, pharmacokinetic changes may significantly alter drug absorption, distribution, metabolism, and excretion.
- Patients on five or more medications should be considered high risk for drug-drug interactions and adverse medication reactions.
- Adverse drug interactions and medication reactions in older adults may contribute to vague complaints and presentations to the ED.
- Consider consulting a clinical pharmacist, primary care doctor, or geriatric specialist when determining the appropriate medications to start or stop in the ED.
- Utilize drug information resources such as the Beers Criteria to assess appropriateness of medications and their potential risk for harm in the geriatric population.

Suggested Readings

Geriatric Emergency Department Guidelines Task Force, American College of Emergency Physicians, American Geriatrics Society, Emergency Nurses Association. Geriatric emergency department guidelines. *Ann Emerg Med*. 2014;63(5):e7-e25.

Swedko PJ, Clark HD, Paramsothy K, Akbari A. Serum creatinine is an inadequate screening test for renal failure in elderly patients. *Arch Intern Med*. 2003;163(3):356-360.

SECTION XXV
WOUND CARE

319

SUTURES: WHAT, WHEN, WHY, AND WHY NOT?

BOBBI-JO LOWIE

Lacerations are incredibly common and account for 8.2% of all ED visits. When repairing a laceration, the goal of management includes obtaining a functional closure with optimal strength, maintaining low risk for infection, and minimizing scar formation. Multiple factors affect the clinician's approach to wound management including the location, length, depth, the type and tension across the tissue involved, wound contamination, and the time elapsed since the injury occurred. Ideal wound closure includes achieving apposition of the wound edges while minimizing tension and avoiding inversion or dead space.

A full history of the mechanism and timing of injury, as well as comorbidities and tetanus status, should be obtained to ensure proper wound care and repair. Before repair, wounds should be anesthetized and examined through full range of motion to evaluate for foreign bodies, and neurovascular and/or tendon injuries. Proper anesthesia and pain control can allow for better examination of patient injuries. Nerve blocks can also be considered to help in areas (fingers, toes, and lips) where tissue infiltration with anesthetic may lead to tissue distortion. X-ray, ultrasound, and/or CT imaging can be employed to evaluate for foreign bodies as well as important underlying injuries.

Any wound presenting to the ED should be considered contaminated and irrigated with copious amounts of water before repair. Potable tap water is sufficient for irrigation and sterile water or saline is not required. The volume and pressure of irrigation required are debated, but more volume is likely better and enough pressure to irrigate the wound without causing tissue damage is ideal. This is, unfortunately, difficult to quantify clinically. Current literature also suggests that sterile gloves are not required when repairing lacerations in the ED.

Two techniques commonly employed for primary closure in the emergency setting are percutaneous (skin) and dermal (deep) sutures and can be placed in interrupted or continuous manner. Percutaneous sutures pass through both the epidermal and dermal layers of the skin; dermal sutures pass through the dermis without ever penetrating the epidermis. Sutures should not be placed within adipose tissue, as this layer provides no support for wound closure.

Dermal sutures can be used alone or together with percutaneous sutures for wound closure. Dermal sutures, alone, are indicated for closure that will later be covered by a cast, or in patients who develop keloids, have poor follow-up for removal, and in whom suture removal will be challenging or traumatic. Dermal sutures are often the only technique available to close lacerations involving macerated or avulsed tissue, where percutaneous closure is impossible. While percutaneous sutures alone can close wounds under low or medium tension, dermal sutures are a useful adjunct for gaping wounds or wounds under high tension. Excessive tension across a wound interrupts capillary blood flow to the wound edge and can delay healing and cause local ischemia and cellular necrosis. Placing an interrupted dermal suture in each quadrant of the wound will allow the wound edge to be brought together in apposition while removing the tension across the epidermal surface. This type of dermal placement will also reinforce the tissue enough to allow for early suture removal, which can improve the final cosmetic outcome.

When choosing materials for repair, the wound, patient, and characteristics of the materials used should be considered. Sutures provide the most strength, but different suture types have varying characteristics. Nonabsorbable sutures, nylon and Prolene, have minimal tissue reactivity but require eventual follow-up for removal. Absorbable sutures, chromic gut and Vicryl, have moderate to high tissue reactivity but absorb without removal in 2 to 4 weeks. These can be helpful in patients with poor follow-up. Staples are quickly placed but result in more scarring and require removal. Tissue adhesive is quick to place and dissolves, which negates the need for follow-up, but cannot be used on high-tension wounds.

Although all sutures have the potential to increase the risk of infection, dermal sutures are associated with higher rates of infection than percutaneous sutures and are even more pronounced with a continuous dermal closure. Conversely, dermal sutures have little to no effect on infection rates in clean or noncontaminated lacerations. While there are clear indications and benefits to using dermal sutures, in contaminated wounds, this has to be balanced against the increased risk of infection. Current literature supports using dermal sutures to close dead space only in noncontaminated or minimally contaminated wounds using as few sutures as possible. Ideally, wounds should be repaired as soon as possible, though patients may present late in the course of injury. Wounds that are highly contaminated, infected, or at high risk of infection may be left to heal by secondary intention. This will result in scarring and clear patient counseling should take place.

PEARLS

- The goal of wound repair is a functional closure with low risk for infection and minimal scar formation.
- Wounds should be irrigated with copious amounts of water and probed for foreign bodies and deeper injury before repair.
- Indications for dermal sutures include wounds covered by a cast, wounds in patients who develop keloids, or patients in whom suture removal will be difficult.
- Sutures provide the best tensile strength of all wound closure options.
- Dermal sutures are associated with higher rates of infection and should be avoided in contaminated wounds.

Acknowledgments

We gratefully acknowledge the contributions of previous edition authors, Hollynn Larrabee and R. Alissa Mussell, as portions of their chapter have been retained in this revision.

Suggested Readings

Berk WA, Welch RD, Bock BF. Controversial issues in clinical management of the simple wound. *Ann Emerg Med.* 1992;21(1):72-80.

Lloyd JD, Marque MJ, Kacprowicz RF. Closure techniques. *Emerg Med Clin N Am.* 2007;25:73-81.

Nicks BA, Ayello EA, Woo K, Nitzki-George D, Sibbald RG. Acute wound management: revisiting the approach to assessment, irrigation, and closure considerations. *Int J Emerg Med.* 2010;3(4):399-407.

Otterness K, Singer AJ. Updates in emergency department laceration management. *Clin Exp Emerg Med.* 2019;6(2):97-105.

Weiss EA, Oldham G, Lin M, et al. Water is a safe and effective alternative to sterile normal saline for wound irrigation prior to suturing: a prospective, double-blind, randomised, controlled clinical trial. *BMJ Open.* 2013;3(1):e001504.

320

Pitfalls in Emergency Department Abscess Incision and Drainage

Annie Rominger

ED management of cutaneous abscesses has changed significantly over the past 10 years. The recent literature guiding these changes recommends ultrasound during initial evaluation, debunks packing, and favors LD over classic I&D. There is a movement toward less invasive techniques and a more conservative approach to the use of wound cultures and antibiotics.

When considering an abscess for drainage, one pitfall is not using ultrasonography to evaluate the area. Multiple studies have shown a significant decrease in cutaneous abscess treatment failure rate with POCUS plus I&D compared to blind I&D. In clinically unclear cases, correctly identifying an abscess by physical examination had a sensitivity of 44% compared to 92% with POCUS. In addition, POCUS guides the procedure by visualizing the depth, size, and margins of the abscess cavity and identifies other structures, like blood vessels or nerves, that may result in complications. Ultrasonography also identifies associated cellulitis which can aid in the decision to treat with antibiotics following drainage. The current medical research supports POCUS as a standard clinical practice when evaluating abscesses in the ED.

Another pitfall to avoid is not consulting a surgeon when indicated. It is important to consider patient risk factors, comorbid conditions, and abscess location. The following conditions are associated with higher rates of complications: perirectal abscesses, anterior or lateral neck masses (from congenital cysts), hand abscesses (excluding paronychias or felons), an abscess adjacent to vital nerves or vessels, abscesses located in the central facial triangle, and breast abscesses. If any of these are present, a surgeon should be consulted, or prompt follow-up for wound evaluation and definitive care be sought within 48 hours.

Wound packing used to be the common practice following the I&D of a cutaneous abscess in the ED. Recent studies show similar outcomes in patients with abscesses less than 5 cm who had an I&D with packing compared to those who did not have packing. In addition, packing is associated with a higher cost and postoperative pain with no added benefit. Therefore, it is reasonable to forego wound packing in small cutaneous abscess less than 5 cm, with consideration for LD instead.

The current literature favors LD of cutaneous abscesses in the ED over traditional I&D. LD is associated with either a similar failure rate or a lower failure rate than conventional I&D. LD is a less painful procedure, has a better cosmetic outcome, has fewer return visits and lower health care costs than I&D. This is particularly true in the pediatric population where LD has repeatedly shown to have lower failure rates and better overall outcomes.

Another pitfall, particularly in children, is not having adequate analgesia or sedation for an abscess drainage. Abscess drainage is a very painful procedure and despite local injection, it can still be very uncomfortable. Failure rates are higher if the abscess is inadequately drained and if patient pain or anxiety limits the practitioner's ability to adequately perform the procedure, other medications may be needed. It is important to provide an oral analgesic or consider a nerve block of the area in addition to local infiltration. In young children, providing an oral anxiolytic (midazolam) in addition to an analgesic is often recommended. Depending on the age of the patient and location of the abscess, sedation is occasionally needed to guarantee an adequate drainage with appropriate pain control.

Wound cultures are typically not required for an uncomplicated abscess in a healthy patient. *Staphylococcus aureus* has been isolated in 60% to 75% of uncomplicated abscesses with MRSA accounting for 50% to 70% of those isolates. Therefore, it should be assumed that the uncomplicated abscess is caused by a *S. aureus* infection, specifically MRSA. There are certain cases, however, when a wound culture is indicated. These include a severe, rapidly spreading local infection, systemic signs, failure of initial treatment, extremes of age, immunocompromised state, or recent travel to a developing country.

The use of antibiotics in the treatment of cutaneous abscesses is still debated and is situation dependent. The provider needs to consider the risks and benefits to the patient, type and location of the infection, local resistance patterns, patient follow-up and preference when deciding to initiate antibiotics. A recent meta-analysis showed an increased risk of treatment failure in patients not treated with antibiotics following drainage of a cutaneous abscess. The same study showed similar cure rates using TMP-SMX and clindamycin which were both superior to cephalosporins. A newer medication, dalbavancin, has emerged and was approved for use in the United States in 2014 for the treatment of adults with acute bacterial skin and soft tissue infections. The treatment is a single IV infusion of 1,500 mg which should be considered in patients without follow-up or who are unable to access oral antibiotics due to their social situation. It is a low cost, generally well-tolerated option. However, not all patients with an abscess require antibiotic therapy. In healthy individuals with an initial, single, uncomplicated abscess without surrounding cellulitis and the ability to follow up in the outpatient setting, systemic antibiotics are not indicated.

PEARLS

- Consider patient risk factors, comorbidities, and high-risk locations before draining a cutaneous abscess in the ED.
- Use point-of-care ultrasound when evaluating a suspected cutaneous abscess in the ED.
- In the ED, use LD instead of I&D for patients with an uncomplicated cutaneous abscess.
- Ensure adequate pain control and consider anxiolysis or even sedation in young children before draining a cutaneous abscess in the ED.
- The use of antibiotics following ED drainage of a cutaneous abscess should be a case-to-case decision and consider a one-time dose of dalbavancin in adults with lack of follow-up and/or limited access to antibiotics.

SUGGESTED READINGS

Gottlieb M, Avila J, Chottiner M, et al. Point-of-care ultrasonography for the diagnosis of skin and soft tissue abscesses: a systematic review and meta-analysis. *Ann Emerg Med*. 2020;76:67-77.

Goulding M, Haran J, Sanseverina A, Zeoli T, Gaspari R. Clinical failure in abscess treatment: the role of ultrasound and incision and drainage. *Clin J Emerg Med*. 2022;24(1):39-43.

Long B, April MD. Is loop drainage technique more effective for treatment of soft tissue abscess compared with conventional incision and drainage? *Ann Emerg Med*. 2019;73(1):19-21.

Schechter-Perkins EM, Dwyer KH, Amin A, et al. Loop drainage is noninferior to traditional incision and drainage of cutaneous abscesses in the Emergency Department. *Acad Emerg Med*. 2020:27(11):1150-1157.

Schmitz G, Gottlieb M. Managing a cutaneous abscess in the Emergency Department. *Ann Emerg Med*. 2021;78(1):44-47.

Stevens DL, Bisno AL, Chambers HF, et al. Practice guidelines for the diagnosis and management of skin and soft tissue infections: 2014 update by the Infectious Diseases Society of America. *Clin Infect Dis*. 2014;59(2):e10-e52.

Vermandere M, Aertgeerts B, Agoritsas T, et al. Antibiotics after incision and drainage for uncomplicated skin abscesses: a clinical practice guideline. *BMJ*. 2018;360:k243.

321

PLANTAR PUNCTURE WOUND PEARLS AND PITFALLS

R. GENTRY WILKERSON

Puncture wounds to the plantar surface of the foot are a common presentation to the ED with increased incidence during summer months. There is limited data driving evidence-based management of plantar puncture wounds. Much of the data is from retrospective reviews of patients who already have complications of wounds. Immediately following the injury, the wounds often have a benign appearance causing many to not seek medical care. Most of these wounds heal without need for medical intervention; however, in some cases, these wounds can have devastating long-term outcomes even with appropriate medical care.

Evaluation should begin with a thorough medical history in addition to obtaining details of the incident including timing of injury, type of penetrating object, type of footwear worn at time of injury, and care rendered by the patient. It is also important to ask if the penetrating object was intact if removed by the patient. Risk factors for serious infection include older age, history of diabetes, and contamination of the wound. An immunization history will determine the need for tetanus prophylaxis with tetanus toxoid. Patients without prior or incomplete tetanus immunization require administration of tetanus immune globulin.

The physical examination should determine the location of the puncture wound and assess the integrity of the surrounding soft tissue. The neurologic and vascular function both proximal and distal to the wound should be evaluated. Patzakis classified plantar puncture wounds based on location dividing the foot into three zones: zone 1 extends from the metatarsal necks to the toes, zone 2 extends from the distal calcaneus to the proximal metatarsal neck, and zone 3 is over the calcaneus. The external surface of the foot should be washed. If the wound defect is large enough, the wound can be gently irrigated. High-pressure irrigation should be avoided due to risk of causing injury to tissue and potential for pushing retained foreign bodies or bacteria deeper into the wound. Simple probing of the wound may falsely reassure the provider that a foreign body is absent and may result in pushing the foreign body deeper into the wound. For simple puncture wounds presenting acutely but at risk for contamination or retained fragments, some recommend that providers extend the length of simple puncture wounds and gently explore and irrigate the area. A regional nerve block will facilitate wound exploration by providing superior pain control.

Any concern for retained foreign body mandates further evaluation. The clinician should consider that the retained object might be part of the footwear and not the penetrating object itself. Plain radiographs will detect most metallic objects. Glass fragments larger than 2 mm should be visualized regardless of the lead content of the glass. Ultrasound may have increased sensitivity for detection of wood and other radiolucent objects as well as abscesses. False positives may occur as a result of trapped air within the wound, presence of sesamoid bones, and calcifications. Other imaging modalities to consider are CT and MRI.

Patients who present shortly after the injury do not require laboratory studies. Patients who seek delayed medical care typically do so because of persistent or increasing pain and development of signs of infection. In cases of suspected infection, laboratory tests to consider are complete blood cell count, blood cultures, erythrocyte sedimentation rate, and c-reactive protein although no laboratory test can rule out infection. In cases of osteomyelitis, a bone biopsy with culture will help direct antibiotic therapy.

Most plantar puncture wounds are allowed to heal by secondary intention without suturing closed. For patients who seek medical care for plantar puncture wounds, the overall risk of infection is 2% to 10%. The risk of infection increases with increasing depth of wound, wound located in zone 1, presence of devitalized tissue, presence of retained foreign bodies, and delay in presentation more than 48 hours. The goal of antibiotic prophylaxis is to prevent infectious complications such as cellulitis, abscess, osteochondritis, osteomyelitis, and pyogenic arthritis. The organisms commonly associated with these infections are *Staphylococcus aureus*, beta-hemolytic streptococci, and *Pseudomonas aeruginosa*. Pseudomonal infection is associated with puncture wounds through rubber-soled athletic shoes. There are no prospective, randomized trials assessing the efficacy of prophylactic antibiotics. In one retrospective study of 96 adult patients who developed infectious complications, half the patients received prophylactic antibiotics and half did not. This suggests no benefit to prophylactic antibiotics to an undifferentiated patient population. Infections that occur in patients with diabetes have a much worse clinical course than patients without diabetes. In one study, patients with diabetes were found to have a 46-fold increased risk of lower extremity amputation. Despite the lack of prospective data, patients with diabetes may be the population who benefit from prophylaxis. If the provider opts to place the patient on prophylactic antibiotics, then coverage for *Pseudomonas* and methicillin-resistant *S. aureus* should be considered.

Patients with simple, acute presentations of plantar puncture wounds can be discharged from the ED. They should be provided with detailed wound care instructions and signs of infection should be reviewed. They should be given follow-up in 2 to 3 days for wound reevaluation. Some patients may benefit from being given crutches and placed on non-weight-bearing status until at least the first reevaluation.

PEARLS

- The care provider should perform a very detailed history regarding the wound.
- Extension of the wound may be required to allow for appropriate irrigation and wound exploration.
- Plain radiographs may locate metallic objects and most glass pieces over 2 mm in size, but ultrasound is superior for detection of other radiolucent objects.
- Uncomplicated, plantar puncture wounds that present early in healthy patients likely do not benefit from antibiotic prophylaxis.
- Patients with diabetes have a greatly increased risk of requiring amputation if an infection develops.

Suggested Readings

American College of Emergency Physicians: Clinical policy for the initial approach to patients presenting with penetrating extremity trauma. *Ann Emerg Med*. 1999;33(5):612-636.

Chachad S, Kamat D. Management of plantar puncture wounds in children. *Clin Pediatr (Phila)*. 2004;43(3):213-216.

Eidelman M, Bialik V, Miller Y, Kassis I. Plantar puncture wounds in children: analysis of 80 hospitalized patients and late sequelae. *Isr Med Assoc J*. 2003;5(4):268-271.

Fisher MC, Goldsmith JF, Gilligan PH. Sneakers as a source of *Pseudomonas aeruginosa* in children with osteomyelitis following puncture wounds. *J Pediatr*. 1985;106(4):607-609.

Rubin G, Chezar A, Raz R, Rozen, N. Nail puncture wound through a rubber-soled shoe: a retrospective study of 96 adult patients. *J Foot Ankle Surg*. 2010;49(5):421-425.

322

DO NOT BELIEVE THE ADAGE THAT EPINEPHRINE CANNOT BE USED FOR DIGITAL BLOCKS

BENNETT A. MYERS AND MICHAEL C. BOND

Finger and toe injuries are commonly encountered in the ED. Due to the vascularity of the digits, these wounds are associated with an increased risk of bleeding. Vascular supply to each finger and toe is from arteries that run along the medial and lateral sides of each digit. In the hand, each finger is innervated by four nerves that arise from the median or ulnar nerves. The toes have similar innervations that arise from the tibial and peroneal nerves. Achieving hemostasis, while providing adequate analgesia, is essential when treating these injuries. Proper hemostasis not only allows for thorough exploration of the wound but improves visualization during repair. For most digit injuries (ie, lacerations, nail injuries, tendon repair), a digital nerve block can be performed to achieve analgesia. A digital block can also be useful in the management of a fracture, dislocation, ingrown nail, felon, paronychia, or subungual hematoma.

The digital nerve block is done by injecting anesthetic at the base of a finger or toe near the proximal nerve, allowing for effective regional anesthesia of the entire digit. This allows for minimal amount of anesthetic to be used to achieve adequate pain control. In addition, the digital block avoids injection of the anesthetic directly into the wound, which can distort the anatomy, be more painful for the patient, and make repair more difficult. Lidocaine, an amide, is the most commonly used anesthetic for digital blocks. Longer-acting anesthetics, such as bupivacaine, can also be used if prolonged duration of action is needed (4-8 hours for bupivacaine). For patients who are allergic to amide anesthetics, an ester anesthetic, such as procaine, can be used. Lidocaine or other anesthetics can be combined with epinephrine (lidocaine 1% or 2% with epinephrine 1:100,000 or 1:200,000) for anesthesia, The benefit of including epinephrine in the digital nerve block is a faster onset of anesthesia, prolonged analgesic effect, and decreased systemic absorption of the anesthetic which decreases risk of systemic toxicity. Since the digital arteries run in close proximity with the digital nerves, the epinephrine can induce vasoconstriction of the arteries, although this effect tends to wear off after 60 to 90 minutes. The traditional teaching for a digital block has been to use a local anesthetic without epinephrine with concern that epinephrine can decrease circulation to the distal finger or toe, leading to necrosis and possible loss of digits. Therefore, the common adage is to avoid using epinephrine when anesthetizing patients to treat digit injuries.

The original data regarding epinephrine in digital nerve blocks come from the late 19th to mid-20th century. There are multiple case reports of local anesthetic use that was associated with digital necrosis. The majority of the studies were not performed in the ED, nor were they designed to determine the safety of epinephrine. Half the cases of necrosis occurred when epinephrine was not even used. Upon further review of these cases, it is likely that digital necrosis occurred due to infections, postoperative burns, improper use of tourniquets, or older anesthetics such as cocaine and procaine. Prolonged storage of procaine can cause increased acidity (documented pH of 1) due to hydrolysis, increasing risk of tissue necrosis.

Over the last several decades, there have been many studies that show the safety of epinephrine in digital nerve blocks. Literature review in the fields of emergency medicine, plastic surgery, hand surgery, dermatology, and podiatry all concur that epinephrine is safe to include in digital blocks. One recent case series looked at poison center data from accidental discharges of epinephrine autoinjectors (used for treatment of anaphylaxis) into the hand and fingers over a 6-year period. All the patients had complete resolution of symptoms with no long-term complications. They reported that most patients with ischemic symptoms were simply observed until symptom resolution, although a few patients were treated with vasodilatory measures: phentolamine injection, topical nitroglycerin paste, and terbutaline treatments reported. The authors inferred that this study supported the safety of epinephrine in digital blocks, especially compelling given the dose of epinephrine delivered by the autoinjector is 100 times the dose used for digital blocks. Other prospective studies have looked at the effect of blood flow parameters with inclusion of epinephrine in the digital block. Fingertip blood capillary measurements (pH, CO_2, PCO_2, PO_2, HCO_3, SaO_2) did not show a significant difference between patients receiving digital blocks with and without epinephrine. In addition, color Doppler ultrasonography showed transient vasoconstriction related to epinephrine, but returned to normal flow within 90 minutes of the injection. Most authors caution use of epinephrine in patients with peripheral vascular disease or Raynaud phenomenon due to theoretically increased risk for ischemia, although there is no specific data to support this.

In conclusion, it is safe to use epinephrine in digital nerve blocks in the majority of patients. For patients with peripheral vascular disease, caution should be used before any digital block (with or without epinephrine).

PEARLS

- Epinephrine in digital blocks can result in a faster onset and prolonged duration of anesthesia.
- The data cited to avoid use of epinephrine in digital blocks were based on older case reports that had more plausible reasons for digital ischemia.
- Epinephrine can lead to a transient vasoconstriction of digital arteries that has no long-term complications.
- Use caution with epinephrine for digital blocks in patients with peripheral vascular disease or Raynaud syndrome.

SUGGESTED READINGS

Altinyazar HC, Ozdemir H, Koca R, et al. Epinephrine in digital block: color Doppler flow imaging. *Dermatol Surg.* 2004;30:508-511.

Arp AS, Multani JK, Yen RW, et al. The anesthetic effects of lidocaine with epinephrine in digital nerve blocks: a systematic review. *J Am Podiatr Med Assoc.* 2023;113:21-66.

Ilicki J. Safety of epinephrine in digital nerve blocks: a literature review. *J Emerg Med.* 2015;49(5):799-809.

Muck AE, Bebarta VS, Borys DJ, Morgan DL. Six years of epinephrine digital injections: absence of significant local or systemic effects. *Ann Emerg Med.* 2010;56:270-274.

Sönmez A, Yaman M, Ersoy B, et al. Digital blocks with and without adrenalin: a randomised-controlled study of capillary blood parameters. *J Hand Surg Eur.* 2008;33:515-518.

Thompson, CJ, Lalonde DH, Denkler KA, Feicht AJ. A critical look at the evidence for and against elective epinephrine use in the finger. *Plast Reconstr Surg.* 2007;119:260-266.

When Are Prophylactic Antibiotics Indicated for Wounds?

Annie Rominger

The foundation of good wound care includes irrigation, exploration, and selective closure. The decision to prescribe antibiotics is based on the likelihood that an infection will develop, the consequences of the infection, and the potential adverse effects of the antibiotics. It is important not to abandon basic wound care, particularly irrigation and debridement if antibiotics are initiated. A recent study looking at care for contaminated wounds showed infection rates of 17% in patients who had wound irrigation but no antibiotics, 40% in those who had no irrigation but received antibiotics, and 2.6% in those who had irrigation and received antibiotics.

There are three parts of the epidemiologic triangle that should be considered when assessing and treating wounds in the acute setting. The first part, the "host," considers specific characteristics of patients that put them at an increased risk of wound infection. Patients with comorbid conditions, including diabetes, vascular insufficiency, increased age, obesity, renal failure, and immunosuppression, should be treated with prophylactic antibiotics for high-risk wounds. The type and location of the wound is important to consider. Lacerations or wounds that are greater than 5 cm require extensive debridement; are grossly contaminated; result from a mammalian bite; have associated puncture wounds; have a prolonged time since injury; and/or are located on the lower extremities, hands, or intraorally are at increased risk of infection.

The next part of the epidemiologic triangle is the "agent," or potential microorganism of infection. Overall, the incidence of wound infection ranges from 4% to 6%, with the majority caused by skin flora, specifically *Staphylococcus aureus* and *Streptococcus pyogenes*. *Pasteurella multocida*, *Eikenella corrodens*, and anaerobic bacteria are associated with mammalian bites while *Vibrio* and *Aeromonas* can complicate wounds that occur in marine environments. Both *Vibrio* and *Aeromonas* are gram-negative organisms that can cause aggressive infection and may not be covered by antibiotics that target skin flora. Therefore, it is important to target the potentially contaminating organism when prescribing prophylactic antibiotics.

The final part of the triangle is the "environment." Environmental exposures pose unique infectious risks. As mentioned above, freshwater injuries can be contaminated with *Aeromonas*, whereas saltwater wounds are associated with *Vibrio vulnificus*. Wounds may also be contaminated with dirt, soil, feces, or saliva. These wounds are at risk of infection with *Clostridium perfringens* and *Clostridium tetani*, gram-positive anaerobes that cause gas gangrene and tetanus, respectively. Tetanus vaccination should be documented in patients with contaminated wounds and tetanus immunoglobulin and/or vaccine administered if indicated (**Table 323.1**).

Wounds involving deep structures (eg, joints) or associated with fractures are orthopedic emergencies and are at substantial time-dependent risk of infection; thus, antibiotic prophylaxis should not be delayed. Additional deep structure injuries that have a higher risk of infection and should receive prophylactic antibiotics include extensor tendon injuries or ear wounds with exposed cartilage.

TABLE 323.1 TETANUS TREATMENT RECOMMENDATIONS		
NUMBER OF TETANUS VACCINES	**TIME SINCE LAST VACCINATION**	**TREATMENT**
<3	Any	TIG, Td
>3	<5 yr	None
>3	>5 yr	Td

TIG, tetanus immune globulin; Td, tetanus and diphtheria.

Mammalian bite wounds are at increased risk of infection due to the mechanism of injury (puncture and crush), the wound location (commonly face and hands), and the inoculation of multiple organisms. It is important that these wounds are copiously irrigated. Current recommendations do not include prophylactic antibiotics for dog bites except in patients who are older than 50, have major puncture wounds, require extensive debridement, have wounds to the hands, have wounds that are sutured, or are immunocompromised. Cat bites result in puncture wounds and are at a high risk of infection so should be routinely treated with prophylactic antibiotics (**Table 323.2**). They are also indicated in human bite wounds.

Intraoral lacerations frequently become infected. Limited data suggest that antibiotic prophylaxis is beneficial for intraoral wounds that extend from the intraoral cavity to the external skin surface, are larger than 1 cm or gaping, or are full thickness (**Table 323.2**).

Puncture wounds can introduce organisms into deep subcutaneous tissues and should be considered for antibiotic prophylaxis based on the mechanism and depth of wound. If the wound is through a rubber-soled shoe, there is an increased risk of contamination with *Pseudomonas aeruginosa* and should be given appropriate prophylactic antibiotics (**Table 323.2**). Of note, puncture wounds from Crotalid envenomation do not require prophylactic antibiotics but should be evaluated for tetanus risk.

TABLE 323.2 ANTIBIOTIC PROPHYLAXIS RECOMMENDATIONS FOR VARIOUS TYPES OF WOUNDS	
TYPE/NATURE OF WOUND	**ANTIBIOTIC RECOMMENDATION**
Involve deep structures	Cephalexin, clindamycin
Intraoral wounds	Penicillin, clindamycin
Mammalian bite	Amoxicillin with clavulanic acid
	Pcn allergy: cefuroxime/doxycycline + clindamycin
	Children with pcn allergy: cefuroxime + clindamycin
Soil/feces/saliva contamination	Amoxicillin with clavulanic acid
	Pcn allergic: cephalosporin
Puncture through rubber-soled shoe	Ciprofloxacin
Water (salt/fresh)	Doxycycline and third generation cephalosporin or ciprofloxacin
	Children: aminoglycoside and TMP/SMX

Pcn, penicillin; TMP/SMX, trimethoprim-sulfamethoxazole.
[a]Prophylactic courses range from 3 to 5 days

In summary, healthy patients with clean, simple wounds do not benefit from prophylactic antibiotics. Consideration of the epidemiologic triangle, shared decision-making, follow-up plan, and meticulous documentation are important when treating these injuries.

PEARLS

- Antibiotic prophylaxis is no substitute for good wound care, particularly irrigation.
- Healthy patients with clean, simple wounds should not receive prophylactic antibiotics.
- Consider the epidemiologic triad, host, agent, and environment when determining the need for prophylactic antibiotics.
- Wounds associated with fractures, certain mammalian bites, puncture wounds, and larger intraoral injuries often benefit from antibiotic prophylaxis.
- Tetanus risk should be considered in contaminated wounds.

SUGGESTED READINGS

Byrkit BN, LaScala EC, MenkinSmith L, et al. Characterization of prophylactic antimicrobial therapy practices for patients with marine-associated injuries in the Emergency Department. *J Pharm Pract*. 2023;36(1):53-59. PMID: 34098786.

Gottlieb M, Peska GM. Prophylactic antibiotics are not routinely indicated for dog bites. *Ann Emerg Med*. 2020;76(1):86-87.

Hoff WS, Bonadies JA, Cachecho R, et al. East Practice Management Guidelines Work Group: update to practice management guidelines for prophylactic antibiotic use in open fractures. *J Trauma*. 2011;70(3):751-754.

Mark DG, Granquist EJ. Are prophylactic oral antibiotics indicated for the treatment of intraoral wounds? *Ann Emerg Med*. 2008;52(4):368-372.

Murray CK. Field wound care: prophylactic antibiotics. *Wilderness Environ Med*. 2017;28:S90-S102.

Raz R, Miron D. Oral ciprofloxacin for treatment of infection following nail puncture wounds of the foot. *Clin Infect Dis*. 1995;21(1):194-195.

324

EYELID LACERATIONS: WHEN TO REPAIR AND WHEN TO REFER

ANNIE ROMINGER

It is important for EP to recognize eyelid lacerations that are appropriate for them to repair and those that should be referred to a specialist. Inappropriately managed lid lacerations can lead to eyelid and tear duct dysfunction, which results in significant patient discomfort and/or poor cosmetic outcomes.

The eyelid is composed of several layers, including the skin, orbicularis muscle, and the orbicularis septum (**Figure 324.1**). The orbicularis septum separates superficial eyelid structures from deeper structures, including orbital fat and the levator palpebrae muscle. The levator muscle is important for eyelid function and inserts at the tarsal plate along the eyelid margin. The eyelid margin is the mucocutaneous junction of the eyelid with skin and the orbicularis muscle anteriorly and the deep tarsus and conjunctiva posteriorly. Puncta are located in the medial eyelid margins and connect via canaliculi to the lacrimal duct system (**Figure 324.1**).

Eyelid laceration repair should only be considered after the eye has been thoroughly evaluated for injury. In greater than 50% of patients with eyelid lacerations, there is a concurrent ocular injury. In addition, 25% of open globe injuries have associated eyelid or periorbital lacerations. If globe rupture is suspected, laceration repair should not be performed because increased pressure on the globe can worsen the injury.

The history and mechanism of injury are important when assessing eyelid lacerations, specifically the time of injury, previous ocular history, and possible foreign bodies. Plain radiographs, ultrasound, or computed tomography can be used to evaluate for retained foreign bodies since they can lead to infection and discomfort. A fluorescein

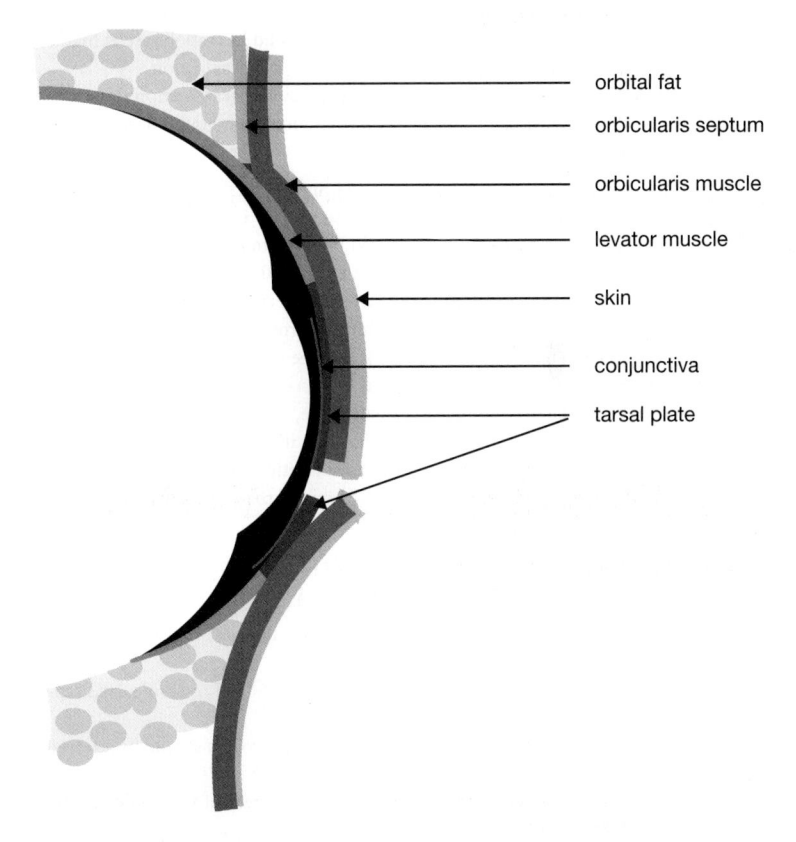

FIGURE 324.1 Eyelid anatomy.

examination should be performed to evaluate for corneal abrasions which are commonly seen with eyelid lacerations. In children, it may be difficult to get a reliable eye examination and may require ophthalmology consult for an examination under sedation. In addition, the eyelid is highly vascular, and laceration repair can be deferred up to 24 hours if there is no associated ocular injury and the patient requires specialist evaluation and repair.

It is important to determine whether the eyelid laceration is simple or complex by assessing the location, depth, and size.

1) Location. Any laceration that involves the lid margin or communicates with the lacrimal duct system is complex and should be referred to a specialist for repair. If the eyelid margin is not aligned perfectly, it can heal with eyelid notching. Injuries to the medial eyelids should be evaluated for lacrimal duct involvement. To evaluate the lacrimal duct system, place a drop of fluorescein into the eye and examine the laceration with a blue light. If any fluorescein is detected within the wound, there is lacrimal duct involvement.
2) Depth. The presence of fat within an eyelid laceration indicates that the orbicularis septum has been violated and deeper structures, like the levator muscle, may be injured and require specialist repair. Ptosis is another key exam finding to suggest that the levator muscle is compromised. Any full-thickness lid lacerations are at high risk of other ocular injuries and require urgent ophthalmologic evaluation.
3) Size. Avulsion injuries are considered complex lacerations because improper management can cause wound tension that affects lid function and should be repaired by a specialist.

The EP can repair simple eyelid lacerations. Small (<25% of lid width), superficial, horizontal lacerations can be left to heal by secondary intention. Tissue adhesive is an option for small lacerations, but care should be taken to prevent the adhesive from entering the eye. If the laceration needs repair, a small, 6-0 or 7-0 nylon suture, or 6-0 rapidly absorbing suture, may be used with a simple interrupted or running technique. Uncooperative patients or young children should have procedural sedation for the repair to avoid complications. The ends of the suture should be cut short to avoid irritating the eye. If the wound is near the lid margin, then the sutures most proximal to the margin should be buried or incorporated into the next suture tie, effectively tying them down and keeping them away from the eye. Puncturing the eye with the suture needle can occur. The provider can prevent this by using an ocular anesthetic and inserting a Morgan lens into the eye to shield the globe during repair. If nonabsorbable sutures are used, they should be removed in 5 to 7 days.

PEARLS

- Eyelid lacerations are associated with other ocular injuries, so a thorough eye examination must be performed.
- The presence of fat in the laceration indicates penetration of the orbicularis septum and injury to deeper structures.
- Any laceration that involves the lid margin or lacrimal system should be referred for repair.
- Avulsion injuries or lacerations through the full thickness of the eyelid require specialty referral.

- Small, simple, eyelid lacerations can be repaired by the EP with care to avoid injury to the eye (ie, Morgan lens) or irritation from the suture tails.

Suggested Readings

Ali SN, Budny PG. "Minding the ends": a simple technique for repair of lower eyelid lacerations. *Emerg Med J*. 2004;21:263.
Chang EL, Rubin PA. Management of complex eyelid lacerations. *Int Ophthalmol Clin*. 2002;42:187.
Hatton MP, Thakker MM, Ray S. Orbital and adnexal trauma associated with open globe injuries. *Ophthalmic Plast Reconstr Surg*. 2022;18:458-461.
Huang J, Rossen J, Rahmani B, Mets-Halgrimson R. Pediatric eyelid and canalicular lacerations: epidemiology and outcomes. *J Pediatr Ophthalmol Strabismus*. 2023;60(1):33-38.
Nelson CC. Management of eyelid trauma. *Aust N Z J Ophthalmol*. 1991;19:357-363.

325

Ear Injuries and Lacerations

Sarah B. Dubbs

Ear injuries generally occur as a result of blunt trauma or mammalian bites. Appropriate management of these injuries is critical to prevent serious complications, permanent physical deformity, and medicolegal risk. The irregular contour of the ear, blood supply, and underlying cartilaginous structures can make these injuries difficult to manage.

One of the first steps in evaluating an ear injury is to determine whether the underlying cartilage has been injured or exposed. When cartilage is involved, injuries should be classified as complete or incomplete avulsions. Plastic surgery or otolaryngology (ENT) should be consulted emergently for complete avulsion injuries. Avulsed tissue should be reattached as quickly as possible. Detached tissue can be cleaned in cold saline, but this is best done in consultation with the specialist. Consultation should also occur for partial avulsion injuries with very small pedicles of tissue.

The decision to repair external ear injuries in the ED is dependent on the extent of tissue loss, the time elapsed since the injury, and any associated injuries. Proper repair of ear injuries and lacerations requires appropriate anesthesia. Small lacerations can be anesthetized with local infiltration of lidocaine. It has been traditionally taught to avoid the use of epinephrine in this region. However, hemostasis is important for repair and prevention of an auricular hematoma, and there is evidence to support that epinephrine does not lead to complications when used for repair of ear injuries and other acral or distal areas. A regional auricular block may be required for large or complicated lacerations. Some patients, such as children or easily agitated patients, may require procedural sedation for proper repair.

The emergency clinician can consider primary closure if the injured portion of the ear is on a wide pedicle and demonstrates good distal capillary refill. The perichondrium and subcutaneous layers should be sutured closed with absorbable sutures. The skin should be approximated with 5-0 or 6-0 nonabsorbable sutures (ie, nylon or polypropylene). Rapid absorbing 5-0 or 6-0 sutures may be acceptable in children when there is concern for difficult removal. Use the contralateral ear for comparison to help guide the repair of the affected ear. Patients should receive specialist follow-up after primary closure, as the repair can be revised if the cosmetic outcome is not satisfactory.

Allowing ear wounds to heal by secondary intention may be appropriate in select patients, namely patients with diabetes, patients who are immunocompromised, or those with heavily contaminated wounds. Small wounds to the concave portions of the auricle (conchal bowl and antihelix) heal particularly well by secondary intention, provided the surrounding ear is intact to provide structural support. The wound requires copious irrigation even when primary closure is not performed. In addition, the wound should be covered with antibacterial ointment and any crusting removed. Exposed cartilage should be avoided, as the overlying skin provides its vascular supply. Patients who do not have their wounds closed in the ED should be referred for follow-up within 1 to 2 days with an ENT or plastic surgeon.

The primary complications of ear injuries are infection, auricular hematoma, and poor cosmetic appearance. Antibiotic prophylaxis should be prescribed if the patient sustained their injury from a human or animal bite. The clinician should also consider antibiotics for contaminated or macerated injuries. Auricular hematomas are usually the result of blunt trauma to the auricle. The skin adheres to the perichondrium, which supplies blood to the cartilage, and the unique anatomy of the ear does not allow for significant expansion of the subcutaneous tissue. Blood accumulates in the subperichondrial space and disrupts blood supply to the underlying cartilage. To prevent formation of an auricular hematoma, a pressure dressing should be placed after wound closure, and patients should be given strict instructions to return for any signs of swelling. Auricular hematomas should be drained as soon as possible to prevent the development of fibrocartilaginous overgrowth and deformity of the ear. Two approaches have been described in the literature to aid with the drainage of these hematomas. Generally, smaller hematomas can be drained with needle aspiration, whereas larger hematomas should be drained with incision and drainage. Following drainage, patients should be regularly followed for at least 1 week to ensure there is no recurrence. Hematomas more than 7 days old should be referred to a specialist.

PEARLS

- Consult ENT or plastic surgery emergently for complete avulsion injuries.
- Many small lacerations to the concave portions of the ear can be allowed to close by secondary intention provided the supporting peripheral structure of the ear is intact.
- Pressure dressings should be placed after repair to prevent auricular hematoma.
- All patients with ear lacerations closed in the ED should be referred to ENT or plastic surgery for follow-up.

Acknowledgments
We gratefully acknowledge the contributions of previous edition authors, Anas Sawas and Eric J. Morley, as portions of their chapter have been retained in this revision.

Suggested Readings
Flores S, Herring AA. Ultrasound-guided greater auricular nerve block for emergency department ear laceration and ear abscess drainage. *J Emerg Med*. 2016;50(4):651-655.

Häfner HM, Röcken M, Breuninger H. Epinephrine-supplemented local anesthetics for ear and nose surgery: clinical use without complications in more than 10,000 surgical procedures. *J Dtsch Dermatol Ges*. 2005;3(3):195-199.

Hyden A, Tennison M. Evaluation and management of sports-related lacerations of the head and neck. *Curr Sports Med Rep*. 2020;19(1):24-28.

326

Just Under the Surface: Tendon and Nerve Injuries

Sarah B. Dubbs

It is easy for clinicians to make errors in diagnosis and management of tendon and nerve injuries because they can be hidden just under the surface of a wound. This is especially challenging in very busy emergency and urgent care settings. These injuries require prompt and accurate assessment to prevent long-term complications and optimize outcomes for patients. Due to the intricate anatomy, wounds on the upper extremities should be approached with caution when it comes to tendon and nerve injuries—especially the extensor side of the hand and forearm. The following principles will prevent clinicians from the pitfalls of tendon and nerve injuries in wounds.

Know the Mechanisms of Injury
Understanding the mechanisms of tendon and nerve injuries helps in identifying high-risk scenarios. For example, lacerations, crush injuries, or penetrating trauma are more likely to result in significant tendon or nerve damage. Tendon and nerve injuries may coexist with other injuries, such as fractures or vascular damage. Identifying the specific mechanism prompts thorough evaluation and appropriate interventions of other concomitant injuries.

Copiously Irrigate the Wound
Copious irrigation of a wound involves the thorough cleansing of the affected area using a large volume of solution. This process is crucial for removing debris, foreign particles, and bacteria from the wound, thereby reducing the risk of infection and promoting optimal healing. Sterile solution is often used, but nonsterile potable water from a faucet is safe to utilize. A good rule of thumb is to use at least 100 mL/cm of wound. High volume plus pressure of the irrigation help to dislodge contaminants, preparing the wound bed for further evaluation and treatment.

Properly Examine the Wound
When assessing a wound, it is imperative to examine it through full range of motion, within a bloodless field. This approach allows for a comprehensive evaluation of the injury and base of the wound, ensuring that no underlying tendon, nerve damage, or foreign body is overlooked. By moving the affected limb or joint through its complete range of motion, clinicians can assess the integrity of surrounding structures, identify any limitations or abnormalities, and gauge the extent of functional impairment. Performing the examination in a bloodless field, achieved through techniques such as elevation or the use of a tourniquet, enhances visibility and reduces the risk of contamination, enabling a more accurate assessment of the wound and facilitating appropriate decision-making regarding management and treatment strategies.

Perform Functional Testing
Thorough functional testing must accompany appropriate visualization of the wound to identify tendon and nerve injuries. For example, the Elson test is the most reliable way to diagnose a central slip injury. For the Elson test, the patient is asked to bend the PIP joint over the edge of a table while extending the middle phalanx against resistance. Central slip injury will cause weak, but present PIP extension while the DIP joint is rigid or even hyperextended. A reassuring exam is where the DIP remains floppy because the extension force is now placed entirely on maintaining extension of the PIP.

Assess Neurovascular Status
Always assess neurovascular status before and after any intervention. Changes in sensation, motor function, or circulation should raise suspicion for complications such as compartment syndrome or vascular compromise. Prompt action is crucial if there are concerning findings.

Appropriately Splint and Immobilize
Splinting can facilitate healing by limiting movement and thus tension on partial tendon injuries. Improper splinting or immobilization can exacerbate complications. Always splint in a position of function. Ensure proper alignment and immobilization of the affected limb to prevent further damage and promote healing. Avoid excessive pressure or constriction that could compromise blood flow or exacerbate nerve compression.

Ensure Patient Education and Follow-Up
Inadequate patient education and follow-up can lead to poor compliance and outcomes. Take the time to explain the nature of the injury, treatment plan, expectant course, and potential complications such as permanent disability and/or deformity. Emphasize the importance of good wound care, follow-up appointments, and potential physical therapy for optimal recovery. Return precautions should include symptoms of infection and any change in functional status that could indicate neurovascular compromise.

Consultation and Referral
Don't hesitate to consult or refer to specialists when needed. Tendon and nerve injuries may require specialized interventions such as surgical repair. Often, this can be done in a delayed fashion; however, temporary tendon repair by the emergency clinician or consultant may need to be done more urgently. For high-risk wounds, such as lacerations over the extensor finger, referral to a hand surgeon for evaluation is still wise despite a reassuring exam. For example, the central slip lies millimeters under the surface of the skin and is easily injured with superficial laceration. Injury causes palmar migration of

the collateral and lateral bands, unopposed pulling of the lumbrical muscles, leading to a Boutonniere deformity.

DOCUMENTATION

If it wasn't documented, it didn't happen. Accurate documentation of the mechanism of injury, findings on examination, interventions performed, and instructions given to the patient is extremely important for patient care and medicolegal protection. Specifically, document efforts to copiously irrigate the wound and examine it in a bloodless field through full range of motion, as well as the neurovascular examinations done before and after intervention.

Avoiding common errors in wound-related tendon and nerve injuries requires a comprehensive approach that involves thorough assessment and intervention, good patient education and communication, and safe handoff to consulting clinicians when indicated. By being vigilant, understanding the complexities of these injuries, and seeking appropriate consultation when needed, emergency and urgent care clinicians can optimize the outcomes for patients presenting with these injuries.

PEARLS

- Obtain a thorough history of the mechanism of injury.
- Use extra caution with wounds on the extensor surfaces of the hand and forearm.
- Visualize the wound in a bloodless field through full range of motion.
- Understand the complex anatomy and how that translates to examining the findings indicative of injury.
- Document thoroughly; tendon and nerve injuries are high risk!

SUGGESTED READINGS

Davenport, M. Arm, forearm, and hand lacerations. In: Tintinalli JE, Ma OJ, Yealy DM, et al, eds. *Emergency Medicine: A Comprehensive Study Guide*. 9th ed. McGraw-Hill Education.
Klifto CS, Capo JT, Sapienza A, Yang SS, Paksima N. Flexor tendon injuries. *J Am Acad Orthop Surg*. 2018;26(2):e26-e35. PMID: 29303923.

327

WHAT DO I DO WITH ROAD RASH?

JOYCE WAHBA AND MANPREET SINGH

Road rash is defined as a skin abrasion from a fall, typically involving sliding on a rough surface. In the ED, road rash is often seen in patients involved in accidents with bicycles, motorcycles, or motor vehicles. There is a paucity of evidence for the management of road rash in the ED; however, some basic principles have been accepted.

Step 1: Assessment
As with any patient with trauma, the first few steps of ATLS are to assess the ABCs. Afterward, clothing is removed to assess disability and exposure which will reveal the road rash. It is important to remember that road rash can be a marker for deeper injuries and to assess these areas properly and order any necessary imaging studies. Road rash is a misnomer as it is not a rash but in fact a friction burn with possible thermal burn. Under this definition, burn principles can be applied to properly assess the severity of the road rash. These measures include TBSA and depth which can help guide fluid resuscitation and burn center criteria.

Step 2: Anesthesia
Multimodal pain management is the best approach. Depending on the severity of the patient's injuries, anesthesia may include nonopioid oral medications (acetaminophen, ibuprofen), topical agents (anesthetic creams, local injections), opioids (oxycodone, morphine), or in severe cases, procedural sedation. Anesthesia is imperative with these patients to be able to properly clean the wound. Some recommend using field blocks with lidocaine or applying 4% LET cream directly to the wound.

Step 3: The Scrub
It is recommended to start with cool running water. Sink water is easily accessible and offers continuous gentle running water. This will allow removal of most large debris with minimal effort or pain. This initial step also allows assessment of the patient's ability to tolerate further debridement and whether more anesthesia will be required. As with thermal burns, cool water is preferred over warm water because it offers additional numbing effects and helps to dissipate some of the thermal energy.

After the gentle cool running water, it is important to scrub the wounds to remove as much dirt, debris, and dead skin as possible. Debridement can be accomplished with available items including a clean toothbrush, a washcloth, or a surgical scrub sponge with antibacterial soap. Some suggest using more aggressive techniques, such as a scalpel, to scrape and dig out remaining dirt; however, most agree that gentle scrubbing with running water is the most effective method.

Step 4: Dressings
There is no consensus on the best dressing for road rash. Nonadherent dressings covered with an absorbent dressing tend to be the best choice, as they absorb weeping discharge without sticking to the wound. Ointments, such as petroleum jelly or Vaseline, are recommended to keep the wound moist and prevent scabbing. Newer literature suggests that bacitracin is not recommended as many may develop an allergic contact dermatitis. Silver sulfadiazine is associated with poorer wound healing and is not recommended. If the road rash involves a joint, splinting can be considered for pain control. Dressings should be changed on a regular basis until the wound stops weeping. Regular dressing changes will also allow for frequent reevaluation of the wound to assess for signs of infection. Some commercial dressings have proven benefits; however, they are more expensive and less accessible (eg, biosynthetic dressings, silver or silicon-containing dressings, or hydrogel dressings).

Step 5: Cosmetics
Removing embedded organic particulate matter is vital in preventing traumatic tattooing. This type of tattooing occurs via the reepithelialization process and can be prevented by removing as much debris as possible. The initial ED management will have the biggest

effects on cosmetic outcomes, as particulate matter will become harder to remove after the reepithelialization process has begun. Topical agents, such as Mederma and vitamin E, have not demonstrated evidence-based reduction in scarring.

It is important to note that patients with darker skin tones may have more visible burn scars. Sun protection for the next year is the best way to minimize scarring. This can be achieved with clothing and sunscreen, preferably containing zinc or titanium with SPF30+. Dermatologists have methods for removing traumatic tattooing via lasers, injections, and micro incisions; however, these methods can be very expensive and have their own limitations.

PEARLS

- Road rash should be treated as a friction burn and as a marker for possible deeper injuries.
- Multimodal pain control should be attempted before cleaning out the wounds.
- Wounds should be initially cleaned with gentle cool running water and then scrubbed out, removing as much organic particulate matter to prevent traumatic tattooing.
- Dressings should be nonadherent, and wounds should be kept moist with ointments to prevent scabbing and subsequent scarring.

SUGGESTED READINGS

Jacob SE, James WD. From road rash to top allergen in a flash: bacitracin. *Dermatol Surg*. 2004;30(4 Pt 1):521-524. PMID: 15056142.

Orman R, Swaminathan A. "Introduction—road rash." EM:RAP. November 2017. Accessed September 2023. https://www.emrap.org/episode/supersickdka/introduction

"Road rash! Part I & II." Laceration Repair. Accessed September, 2023. https://lacerationrepair.com/wound-blog/road-rash-part-i/

Wasiak J, Cleland H, Campbell F, Spinks A. Dressings for superficial and partial thickness burns. *Cochrane Database Syst Rev*. 2013; 2013(3):CD002106.

328

WHAT'S NEW IN THE CARE OF MINOR BURNS

ASLAM ABBASI AKHTAR

More than one million burn injuries occur annually in the United States. The majority of these are minor burns that can be discharged from the ED and do not require transfer to a burn center. This chapter discusses the classification, disposition, and management of minor burns.

Burn Classification by Depth

The nomenclature used to describe the severity of burns based on degree (first, second, and third) has transitioned to a more anatomic approach based on depth injury. Briefly, superficial burns involve the epidermis only and are painful, dry, blanch with pressure, and do not blister. They generally heal within 1 week. Partial-thickness burns involve the epidermis and portions of the dermis and are classified into superficial partial-thickness and deep partial-thickness. Superficial partial-thickness burns are painful, moist, red, blanch with pressure, and form blisters within 24 hours. They normally heal in 1 to 3 weeks. Deep partial-thickness burns that extend to the deeper dermis are less painful (may only be painful to pressure), blister, do not blanch, and can be wet or waxy dry in appearance. They may heal in 2 to 9 weeks but will scar. Distinguishing a deep partial-thickness burn from a full-thickness burn may be challenging. Full-thickness burns are dry; leathery; and may be white, gray, or black in appearance. They are insensitive to pain and do not blanch. Without surgery, these wounds heal with severe scarring and contracture.

Minor Burn Criteria

Burn centers across the country are staffed by burn specialists and receive transfers from local hospitals based on predetermined criteria. These criteria may be hospital-specific, and clinicians should be aware of their hospital's guidelines and transfer processes. In general, a burn may be treated as minor without need for emergent burn center referral if they meet the following criteria: superficial burns and partial-thickness burns with less than 10% of TBSA in patients 10 to 50 years of age. Superficial burns are not included in the calculation of TBSA. In addition, there should be no suspicion of inhalational injury; no high-voltage injury; no circumferential burns; and no involvement of the face, hands, genitalia, feet, or major joints. Importantly, patient comorbidities and social circumstances should also be taken into consideration as they may preclude the necessary wound care and warrant burn center evaluation. For outpatient burn care, the clinician must also consider the goals of outpatient burn management: rapid healing, infection prevention, patient comfort, compliance, cost, maintaining full function, and returning the patient to full productivity during the treatment period. Furthermore, the possibility of physical abuse should be considered. Scald burns with demarcated edges, circular burns the diameter of a cigarette, or burns in the perineal area of a child in a dipping pattern may suggest physical abuse.

Initial Management of Minor Burns

Burns can be distracting injuries, and it is imperative to evaluate the patient for other traumatic injuries. In a hemodynamically stable patient, clothing and jewelry around the burn should be promptly removed. In the immediate acute phase after a burn, cooling the burn should be done by applying cool tap water or saline for 5 minutes. Applying ice should be avoided due to the potential of increasing burn depth and soaking in water can cause maceration. Adequate pain control should be achieved using nonopiates (NSAIDs/acetaminophen) and opiates if necessary. It is imperative to reduce discomfort during wound care as a painful experience may reduce the patient's willingness to engage in the subsequent sessions. Tetanus immunization should be updated, and tetanus immunoglobulin should be given to patients who have not received a complete primary immunization. If a patient is being transferred, the burn can be covered with a clean bedsheet or nonadherent dressing. All dressings will be removed on arrival at the burn center.

Wound Care

The burn should be cleaned using mild soap and water. Betadine, alcohol, or hydrogen peroxide should be avoided as they can impair healing. Sloughed or necrotic skin should be gently removed. It is an acceptable practice to remove blisters that are in an area causing discomfort or that are likely to rupture during wound care. Blisters should not be aspirated using a needle alone as the overlying skin provides an enclosed space and a medium for potential microbial growth. Rather, the entire blister should be gently removed such that there is no loose skin remaining.

Superficial burns, involving epidermis only, for example, mild sunburn with no blistering, do not require dressings or any topical antibiotic. A nonscented moisturizing lotion can be applied. Some physicians may elect to use bacitracin for its emollient properties, although no antimicrobial treatment is required. For partial-thickness burns deemed minor, a topical antibiotic such as bacitracin can be used for its antimicrobial and emollient properties. While aloe vera does have antimicrobial properties, there is no evidence to suggest it provides improved outcomes and fresh aloe may result in seeding of soil-based microbes. SSD was previously the mainstay of burn treatment; however, data suggest that SSD is inferior to other comparative agents and seems to have a negative impact on some of the outcomes related to wound healing. Hence, SSD as an agent of choice in the management of burns should be discouraged. There is no role for topical steroids or toothpaste as they may irritate the burn, increase the risk of infection, and impair healing. Systemic antibiotics are not recommended for prophylaxis.

Partial-thickness burns can be dressed using gauze that is placed over a topical antibiotic and nonadherent dressing such as Xeroform. An elastic gauze roll such as Kerlix can be used as a gentle wrap to assist in keeping the deeper dressings in place. Dressings should be changed once a day unless otherwise specified by a burn specialist. During dressing changes, the burn can be gently cleaned using water and mild soap. If a dressing becomes adherent, briefly soaking in water can help loosen the dressing. Patients should take round-the-clock analgesia for pain control. Pruritus around the burn is common, and a systemic antihistamine (oral diphenhydramine or a less-sedating antihistamine such as cetirizine) is an effective adjunct. Patients discharged from the ED should have follow-up in 1 to 2 days for a wound check and to ensure satisfactory dressing changes are occurring at home.

PEARLS

- Clinicians should be aware of local burn center transfer criteria and transfer processes.
- In addition to objective burn characteristics (type of burn, TBSA, etc), consider patient's comorbidities when deciding if transfer/referral to burn center is warranted.
- Treat pain adequately with nonopiates and opiates if necessary. A patient's early experience with wound care is likely to impact adherence to their wound care regimen.
- Avoid SSD given its association with poorer healing outcomes. Systemic antibiotics are not recommended for prophylaxis.
- Urgent follow-up is imperative to assess wound healing and home wound care.

Suggested Readings

American Burn Association. Multiple educational resources and a listing of US burn centers. http://www.ameriburn.org

DeKoning EP. Thermal burns. In: Tintinalli JE, John Ma O, Yealy DM, et al, eds. *Tintinalli's Emergency Medicine: A Comprehensive Study Guide*. 9th ed. McGraw-Hill Education; 2020.

Schaefer TJ, Szymanski KD. Burn evaluation and management. [Updated 2023 Aug 8]. In: StatPearls. StatPearls Publishing; 2023.

Wasiak J, Cleland H, Campbell F, Spinks A. Dressings for superficial and partial thickness burns. *Cochrane Database Syst Rev*. 2013(3):Cd002106.

329

Do Not Miss a Foreign Body in a Wound

Tiffany Fan

Open wounds are frequently seen in the ED and must be evaluated for potential foreign bodies. A thorough history regarding the injury mechanism should be obtained to determine whether a foreign body is likely. Foreign bodies can be categorized based on composition: metallic, inorganic, or organic; this will guide your evaluation and choice of imaging.

All wounds should be copiously irrigated with normal saline or tap water to allow adequate visualization and exploration of the wound in a bloodless field. It is not recommended to use antiseptic solutions for cleaning as this may inhibit wound healing. Exam of the wound should include wound depth and margins, signs of neurovascular or tendon injury, signs of infection, and visualization or palpation of a foreign body. Imaging should be considered if the wound depth is not fully visualized, the patient reports severe pain, the patient perceives a foreign body, or if the object can shatter or fragment (eg, glass, thorns, and wood).

Radiographs are standard in the evaluation of radiopaque foreign bodies and can detect approximately 80% of foreign bodies that are 2 mm or larger. Sensitivity may be increased by obtaining multiple views, as bone or surrounding structures may obstruct an object in a single view.

For radiolucent foreign bodies, ultrasound is an easily accessible imaging modality. Pooled data suggest ultrasound is 72% sensitive and 92% specific for detecting foreign bodies in wounds. Using a high-frequency linear transducer, a foreign body will appear as a hyperechoic object often with an acoustic shadow, which helps to differentiate the foreign body from other anatomical structures. A water or saline bath may be beneficial to allow ultrasound evaluation of areas that are difficult to image, such as web spaces between fingers or toes. While ultrasound is highly sensitive for radiolucent foreign bodies, acoustic shadowing from calcifications, tendons, or bones may limit diagnostic accuracy by obscuring smaller objects. A negative ultrasound does not exclude the presence of a foreign body.

If there is a high suspicion for foreign body and the patient reports a foreign body sensation, advanced imaging such as CT (if radiopaque) and MRI (if radiolucent) may be considered. CT may also evaluate for associated complications, such as deep space infections or involvement of specific anatomic structures. MRI may be particularly useful to evaluate the involvement of nerves or blood vessels; however, it should be avoided if a metallic foreign body is suspected.

Once identified, foreign bodies should be evaluated for removal on a case-by-case basis. Not all foreign bodies require removal, particularly if the object is biologically inert, as there is a risk for iatrogenic injury. Organic foreign bodies, such as wood, must be removed as they often lead to inflammation and infection. Chemically reactive material, such as metal, may lead to allergic reactions and toxicity. Deeply embedded foreign bodies that involve other anatomic structures such as nerves, blood vessels, tendons, joints, or bone require removal. However, risks of ED-attempted removal should be weighed and, in some cases, evaluation by a specialist should be considered. Antibiotic prophylaxis is not recommended in simple nonbite wounds in immunocompetent patients; however, for contaminated wounds, risks and benefits of antibiotics should be considered. In addition, patients should be evaluated for tetanus immunization history and vaccinated if indicated.

PEARLS

- Foreign body wounds should be appropriately irrigated with copious amounts of saline or tap water before wound exploration in a bloodless field. Antiseptic solution should be avoided.
- Ultrasound is a readily accessible and useful tool for evaluation of radiolucent foreign bodies.
- Radiographs may miss a radiopaque foreign body; therefore, CT should be considered if there is high clinical suspicion.
- Not all foreign bodies require removal. Risks of attempted removal should be carefully considered.

SUGGESTED READINGS

Davis J, Czerniski B, Au A, Adhikari S, Farrell I, Fields JM. Diagnostic accuracy of ultrasonography in retained soft tissue foreign bodies: a systematic review and meta-analysis. *Acad. Emerg. Med.* 2015;22(7):777-787.

Richard L. Soft tissue foreign bodies. In: Tintinalli JE, Stapczynski J, Ma O, Yealy DM, Meckler GD, Cline DM, eds. *Tintinalli's Emergency Medicine: A Comprehensive Study Guide.* 8e. McGraw Hill; 2016.

Rupert J, Honeycutt JD, Odom MR. Foreign bodies in the skin: evaluation and management. *Am Fam Physician.* 2020;101(12):740-747.

330

FINGERNAIL FAUX PAS

SARAH ZYZANSKI

Digital injuries are a common presentation to the ED and are often complicated by concomitant damage to the fingernail. Nails contribute to the overall fine motor function and cosmetic appearance of the hand, and it is critical that repair of injuries in this location minimize infection, promote favorable cosmesis and function, and ensure healthy regrowth of the nail.

Before attempting to repair fingernail injuries, clinicians must understand the anatomy and growth process of the nail. The visible, utilitarian portion of the nail is referred to as the nail plate, which is attached to the underlying nail bed; the two only separate at the distal aspect of the digit. The nail plate is flanked on three sides by the lateral and proximal nail folds. Beneath the proximal nail fold is the germinal matrix where constant production of keratinized cells results in nail growth. Disruption of this matrix via injuries to the proximal nail fold, therefore, can threaten the regeneration of the nail. A visible portion of the germinal matrix is the lunula, the white crescent shape just distal to the proximal nail fold. The lunula then transitions into the sterile matrix, the portion of the nail bed extending from the lunula to the distal end of the finger where the nail plate then separates from the nail bed and extends from the digit. The sterile matrix serves as a secondary, albeit minor site of nail growth (**Figure 330.1**).

Digits and nails play a crucial role in many daily activities; therefore, injuries to this area are frequent and diverse. Injuries can present in the form of lacerations and avulsions

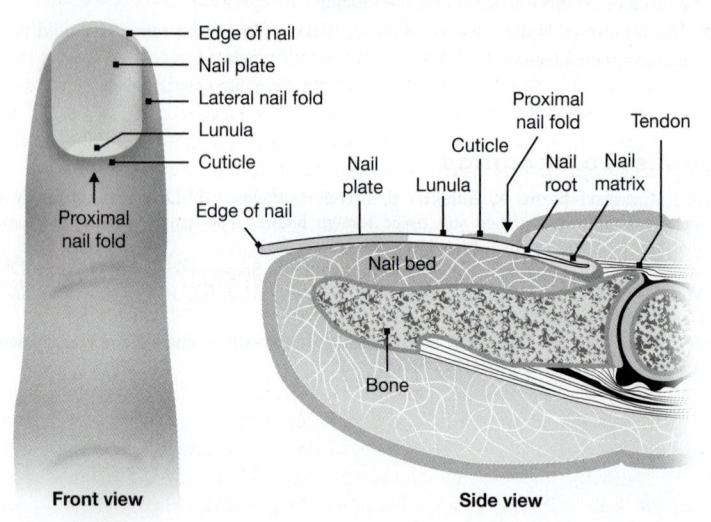

FIGURE 330.1 Fingernail anatomy.

to the nail plate only, the nail bed, or to the germinal matrix as well as crush injuries resulting in damage to the nail only or concurrent with fractures in the distal phalanx. A systematic approach to digital injuries and detailed examination should guide clinicians in management and result in avoidance of complications. Often an adequate examination requires a digital block and thorough cleaning of the affected area for adequate visualization of the extent of injuries, and specific tendon, bone, and nail damage. Clinicians must assess for tendon injury to the flexor digitorum profundus as well as extensor digitorum via range of motion and strength testing at the DIP via maintaining the PIP in extension. Crush injuries to the digit are frequently associated with underlying distal phalanx fractures; therefore, plain radiographs of the affected area are indicated. Clinicians may then evaluate and document the extent of damage to the fingernail and matrix with The Van Beek Criteria which are as follows:

SI: Small subungual hematoma (<25% nail bed surface)
SII: Sterile matrix laceration, large subungual hematoma (>50% nail bed surface)
SIII: Sterile matrix laceration with tuft fracture
SIV: Sterile matrix fragmentation
SV: Sterile matrix avulsion
GI: Small subungual hematoma proximal nail (<25% nail bed surface)
GII: Germinal matrix laceration, large subungual hematoma (>50% nail bed surface)
GIII: Germinal matrix laceration and fracture of distal phalanx
GIV: Germinal matrix fragmentation
GV: Germinal matrix avulsion

Management of fingernail and nail bed injuries depends on the injuries noted on examinations mentioned earlier. All injuries should be irrigated for infection prevention, and patients should receive tetanus vaccination as needed.

For lacerations and avulsions to the distal finger, fingernails should be removed if injuries involve the nail folds or if there is complex damage to the nail plate that will interfere with nail growth. A hemostat or other clamp should be used to first blunt dissect the nail plate off its underlying bed. Once the clamp can be inserted beneath the nail plate as proximally as possible, the nail may be removed with distal traction. Lacerations that extend through skin and nails should not be repaired until the nail is removed. The nail bed can be repaired with 6-0 absorbable sutures with transition to nonabsorbable outside of the nail bed. Once a nail is removed and any associated lacerations are repaired, clinicians should splint the proximal nail fold to retain patency of the germinal matrix and allow for new nail growth to occur. Clinicians may use the native nail if clean and predominantly intact, though more commonly should use the foil encasing the nonabsorbable sutures by cutting the foil into a shape that fits beneath the proximal nail fold and suturing the piece of foil in place. There is no role for prophylactic antibiotics unless there is an associated tuft fracture. In simple nail bed lacerations, infection prevention is adequate with extensive irrigation and dedicated wound care alone.

Crush injuries may result in subungual hematomas alone or may be complicated by lacerations/avulsions or underlying fractures. Distal phalanx "tuft" fractures can be managed with a finger splint for DIP immobilization. Complicated or displaced phalanx fractures, fingertip amputations, or extensive nail fold injuries will require a hand specialist as these may require complex or surgical repair. The presence of a subungual hematoma requires trephination if there is significant associated pain or if more than 50% of the nail is involved. Trephination can be achieved with electrocautery most often, though clinicians may use a large bore needle to drain the hematoma. Nails may need to be removed in scenarios where there is a subungual hematoma and nonintact nail folds or matrix for direct visualization of underlying structures.

Once repair of all injuries is complete, patients may be discharged home with a follow-up planned for wound check and removal of material that may have been used for stenting. More complex injuries should be dispositioned in conjunction with hand specialists.

PEARLS

- Fingernails are highly functional and cosmetic, and injuries to fingernails often present with concomitant injuries in deeper structures; therefore, an in-depth examination often involving digital blocks and radiographs is indicated before repair.
- Significantly damaged fingernails should be removed for adequate examination of underlying nail bed as well as promotion of nail regeneration.
- Damage to the germinal matrix requires stenting of the proximal nail fold to allow for regrowth of new nails.
- Subungual hematomas without obvious nail fold or matrix injuries can be managed with trephination alone and generally results in immediate and considerable pain reduction.

Suggested Readings

Hawken JB, Giladi AM. Primary management of nail bed and fingertip injuries in the Emergency Department. *Hand Clin*. 2021;37(1):1-10.

Patel L. Management of simple nail bed lacerations and subungual hematomas in the Emergency Department. *Pediatr Emerg Care*. 2014;30(10):742-745; quiz 746-748.

331

Scalp Wounds

Nicole Titze

Scalp wounds and lacerations account for a significant amount of ED visits each year. The scalp presents a unique challenge for repair due to its difference in anatomy and blood supply. The skin is stretched over bone making it prone to injury, and its extensive blood supply can lead to significant hemorrhage. There are five layers of the scalp, which can be remembered through the mnemonic SCALP: the *S*kin, *C*onnective tissue layer, *A*poneurosis (galea) and muscle, *L*oose areolar connective tissue, and the *P*ericranium. Knowing these layers can help manage laceration repair and hemorrhage control. Lacerations most commonly involve the loose areolar layer, leading to bleeding from the musculoaponeurotic layer which contains the temporal artery.

Injury to the scalp is most commonly due to blunt trauma and can be associated with more severe injuries. It is important to assess the mechanism of injury and determine if there is evidence of skull fractures or intracranial injuries. A thorough medical history should be obtained including tetanus vaccination status, any immunocompromised state, or conditions interfering with wound healing such as diabetes, cancer, medications, drug and alcohol use, and prior keloid formation. Initial management includes achieving hemostasis and assessing for foreign bodies, contamination, skull fractures, or traumatic brain injury. If the wound is actively bleeding, direct pressure for 15 minutes with or without infiltration of lidocaine with epinephrine can be helpful. If hemostasis cannot be achieved with these measures, the edges of the scalp wound should be everted using manual manipulation, hemostats, or skin hooks. The laceration should then be closed using sutures.

If there is concern for a skull fracture or an intracranial injury, imaging should not be delayed and the patient should be taken to the CT scanner before laceration repair. If there is penetration into the cranial vault or significant skin loss, the appropriate surgical team should be notified (eg, neurosurgery, plastic surgery). If there is concern for nonvisualized foreign body, an XR can be obtained to assess for radiopaque objects. Radiolucent foreign bodies can be visualized through ultrasound.

Generally, primary closure is preferred. In scalp lacerations, delayed closure should be considered if there are obvious signs of infection such as erythema, edema, warmth, or purulent drainage. If closure is delayed saline-soaked gauze packing can be provided to facilitate secondary healing. If the patient is high risk for infection, empiric antibiotics can be considered.

In children or apprehensive adults, the use of LET is helpful. This can be used as a single anesthetic agent or in conjunction with infiltration of local anesthetics. In young children, anxiety can be severe and a dose of intranasal versed or procedural sedation may be necessary.

Before closure, irrigation should be performed. For moderate lacerations between 2.5 and 5 cm in length, irrigation with 100 to 150 mL of tap water should be sufficient. Lacerations larger than 5 cm may benefit from 200 mL or more.

There are several different techniques for scalp laceration closure, including staples, hair apposition, and suturing. Staples are generally preferred as they are fast, cheap, and provide good cosmetic results. Hair apposition is an option for straight lacerations smaller than 10 cm with at least 1 cm of hair length present. This technique can be time consuming, though much less painful, and without the need for follow-up. Hair apposition is accomplished by taking a strand of hair from each side of the laceration and twisting them around each other. Tissue glue is then applied. If hair is short, surgical clamps may be used to twist hair. Patient instructions should include refraining from washing hair for 2 days.

Sutures are indicated if there is significant bleeding, if staples are not available, or if the patient is bald. Absorbable sutures should be used for galeal lacerations larger than 0.5 cm. The skin can be closed in any manner discussed, and pressure dressing should be applied for 24 hours.

Complications of scalp lacerations include wound infections, bleeding, and scarring. Wound infections are rare with scalp lacerations as there is good blood supply to the area. Most scalp lacerations do not require antibiotic prophylaxis, though they should be considered if significant contamination or retained foreign body is present, wound is inflicted by an animal or human bite, or in patients with immunocompromised status.

Due to the good blood supply, scalp lacerations tend to have profuse bleeding. Scarring is usually only a concern if there are chronic medical problems predisposing to poor wound healing or prior keloid formation.

Once repaired, patients should be instructed to leave the wound open to air (unless pressure dressing is necessary). If sutures or staples were placed, the wound can be cleansed with water and soap after 24 to 48 hours. Staples and nonabsorbable sutures should be removed 7 to 10 days after placement. Return precautions should include return if any signs or symptoms of infection.

PEARLS

- Ensure there is no traumatic brain injury before laceration repair.
- Scalp lacerations can cause a significant amount of bleeding. Control this by using direct pressure, everting laceration edges, and/or suture repair.
- Irrigate and explore the wound extensively to ensure no foreign body is present.
- Scalp lacerations can be repaired with staples, hair apposition, and sutures.

SUGGESTED READINGS

Almulhim AM, Madadin M. Scalp laceration. In: *StatPearls*. StatPearls Publishing; 2022.

Azmat CE, Council M. Wound closure techniques. In: *StatPearls*. StatPearls Publishing; 2022.

Hock MOE, Ooi SBS, Saw SM, Lim SH. A randomized controlled trial comparing the hair apposition technique with tissue glue to standard suturing in scalp lacerations (HAT study). *Ann Emerg Med*. 2002;40(1):19-26.

Karaduman S, Yürüktümen A, Güryay SM, Bengi F, Fowler JR. Modified hair apposition technique as the primary closure method for scalp lacerations. *Am J Emerg Med*. 2009;27(9):1050-1055.

SECTION XXVI
COVID-19

332

KNOW THE VARYING CLINICAL PRESENTATIONS OF COVID-19

RAWAN SAFA AND STEPHEN Y. LIANG

The clinical presentation of COVID-19 can range anywhere from asymptomatic infection to severe disease with respiratory failure requiring mechanical ventilation. Throughout the COVID-19 pandemic, EDs have played a vital role in the timely recognition and frontline management of this disease with many faces.

In general, COVID-19 can be divided into asymptomatic versus symptomatic disease, with the latter further stratified into nonsevere, severe, and critical diseases. Asymptomatic patients are infected but are not experiencing symptoms; however, they can transmit the virus to others. Many are identified on routine screening as part of hospital admission for another problem or in preparation for a surgical procedure. Clinically asymptomatic infections have historically accounted for almost a third of positive SARS-CoV-2 tests.

Approximately 98% of patients with symptomatic disease develop their symptoms within 12 days of exposure. Most have a nonsevere disease, marked by mild symptoms involving multiple systems. COVID-19 frequently manifests with respiratory symptoms, including congestion, rhinorrhea, and sore throat. Gastrointestinal symptoms may include abdominal pain, nausea, vomiting, and diarrhea. Neurologic symptoms can include headaches, confusion, altered mental status, and even seizures or strokes. Cardiac complications of infection, including acute coronary syndrome, dysrhythmia, and myocarditis, may present with the constellation of symptoms typically encountered with these conditions. Unusual and/or uncommon symptoms may include rash and conjunctivitis; loss of taste or smell was a distinctive symptom of COVID-19 but may be less common with emerging variants. The presence of fever is variable.

Unfortunately, no clinical features reliably distinguish COVID-19 from other viral infections with high specificity and testing is therefore necessary to establish the diagnosis. Atypical presentations of COVID-19 underscore the importance of testing and isolation when clinical suspicion for COVID-19 exists, even if symptoms are mild.

Severe disease occurs in over 15% of patients with COVID-19 presenting to the ED. The severity of the disease is most closely correlated to the patient's respiratory status. Severe disease is defined as hypoxia or greater than 50% lung involvement. Hypoxia is identified as an oxygen saturation greater than 90% or signs of severe respiratory distress (eg, accessory muscle use, inability to speak in full sentences).

Critical disease comprises approximately 5% of symptomatic disease and has been less commonly encountered with the emerging and more highly transmissible SARS-CoV-2 variants (eg, Omicron) than the original virus. Critical diseases can include ARDS, respiratory failure, multiorgan injury, sepsis, septic shock, and other conditions requiring life-sustaining therapies (eg, mechanical ventilation, vasopressors). Hematologic complications, including venous thromboembolic events, are common in critically ill patients with COVID-19.

Reported rates of ED presentation, hospitalization, need for life-sustaining therapies, and even mortality associated with COVID-19 vary significantly depending on several factors, including patient age and comorbidities, access to healthcare, and the availability of therapeutics. Early in the pandemic, patients were more likely to present with a critical illness, with higher mortality rates reported. As the pandemic has progressed, ICU survival rates for patients with COVID-19 have improved significantly.

Risk factors for progression to severe COVID-19 include age 65 years or above, overweight/obesity (BMI >25), pregnancy, diabetes mellitus, chronic kidney disease, cardiovascular disease, chronic lung disease, cancer, solid organ or hematopoietic stem cell transplantation, and HIV, to name a few. It is important to recognize that immunocompromised patients and the older individuals can have muted disease presentations despite their heightened risk for progression to severe disease. Poor prognostic factors include an initial oxygen saturation below 88% as well as laboratory abnormalities encountered in severe or critical disease (eg, lymphopenia, elevated C-reactive protein and ferritin, elevated serum levels of proinflammatory cytokines and chemokines, elevated lactate dehydrogenase level, elevated liver function enzymes).

Evaluation of COVID-19 in the ED should focus on establishing SARS-CoV-2 infection and assessing disease severity, including evidence of end-organ damage. Emergency physicians should remain vigilant of the wide range of clinical presentations possible with COVID-19 and incorporate an analysis of risk factors for disease progression into decision-making with respect to diagnostic evaluation, management, and patient disposition.

PEARLS

- COVID-19 can be broadly divided into asymptomatic versus symptomatic disease, with the latter further broken down into nonsevere, severe, or critical disease.
- Patients with medical comorbidities (eg, older and immunocompromised) may be at substantial risk of disease progression even if initially asymptomatic or mildly symptomatic.
- Poor prognostic factors may include hypoxia (SpO_2 <88%) on ED presentation, abnormal laboratory workup, and existing comorbid diseases.

Suggested Readings

Bellou V, Tzoulaki I, Evangelou E. Risk factors for adverse clinical outcomes in patients with COVID-19: a systematic review and meta-analysis. *medRxiv*. 2020. Published in *Eur Respir J*. 2022;59:2002964.

Long B, Carius BM, Chavez S, et al. Clinical update on COVID-19 for the emergency clinician: Presentation and evaluation. *Am J Emerg Med*. 2022;54:46-57. PMID: 35121478.

Payán-Pernía S, Gómez Pérez L, Remacha Sevilla ÁF, Sierra Gil J, Novelli Canales S. Absolute lymphocytes, ferritin, C-reactive protein, and lactate dehydrogenase predict early invasive ventilation in patients with COVID-19. *Lab Med*. 2021;52(2):141-145. PMID: 33336243.

333

Don't Miss MIS-C

M. Kaitlin Parks and Tara Copper

MIS-C is an inflammatory condition impacting cardiac, gastrointestinal, mucocutaneous, dermatologic, and neurologic systems in children associated with SARS-CoV-2. While overall rare, MIS-C can lead to life-threatening illness in previously healthy children. With similarities to Kawasaki disease and toxic shock syndrome, MIS-C demonstrates more predominant cardiac dysfunction and gastrointestinal symptoms. It occurs in less than 0.05% of previously infected children but is likely underreported/underdiagnosed particularly in milder cases. Definitions have slight differences across organizations but include a pediatric patient with recent SARS-CoV-2 infection or exposure presenting with fever, laboratory evidence of inflammation, and evidence of severe organ system involvement in two or more systems without an alternative plausible diagnosis.

Immune dysfunction is thought to drive the process with evidence of IgG mediated activation of monocytes and CD8+ T cells and T cell lymphopenias. Cardiac dysfunction may be related to direct injury from inflammation, myocarditis from viral infection, stress cardiomyopathy, or a combination. Further investigation to understand the pathophysiology of MIS-C remains ongoing.

MIS-C usually affects school-age children (median 8-11 years) but has been seen in children ages 1 to 20, and there is a rare adult correlate (MIS-A). There is not a significant difference based on sex. It affects children of all racial and ethnic backgrounds. Early in the COVID-19 pandemic, Black and Hispanic children seemed more affected, while later in the pandemic, rates remained high in Black children and increased in White children. Unlike severe acute COVID-19, which affects primarily children with underlying medical conditions, MIS-C is seen more commonly in healthy children. It can follow COVID-19 disease or asymptomatic SARS-CoV-2 infection. Peaks in MIS-C cases follow peaks of SARS-CoV-2 transmission by 2 to 6 weeks although there have been case reports of MIS-C occurring over 6 weeks from infection.

The most common presenting signs and symptoms include fever, abdominal pain, diarrhea, vomiting, and even shock. Other frequently seen symptoms include rash, conjunctivitis, and neurocognitive symptoms (**Table 333.1**). Length of fever is typically 5 days or more. Gastrointestinal symptoms can result from terminal ileitis/colitis, mimicking appendicitis. Cardiac dysfunction can cause shock and pulmonary edema with resulting tachypnea and increased difficulty breathing. Primary respiratory dysfunction is not typically seen. Neurocognitive symptoms are usually isolated to headache, irritability, and lethargy though rarely encephalopathy, seizures, demyelination, and stroke may occur.

Initial laboratory evaluation can be approached based on the severity of clinical presentation and institutional availability. CBC with differential, CMP, CRP, ESR, pro-BNP, troponin, ferritin, PT/PTT, and D-dimer should be considered. Advanced testing (fibrinogen, LDH, triglycerides, cytokine panel, SARS-CoV-2 serology) can be obtained where available. Laboratory testing should be initiated prior to targeted treatments, which may cause expected changes in test values. Children with MIS-C show elevated CRP, elevated ferritin, elevated troponin, and lymphopenia. Many also demonstrate elevated ESR, elevated BNP, and thrombocytopenia.

TABLE 333.1	COMMON PRESENTING SIGNS AND SYMPTOMS OF MIS-C
PRESENTING FEATURES	**PATIENTS (%)**
Fever	100
GI symptoms	60-100
Myocardial dysfunction	51-90
Rash	45-60
Shock	32-76
Conjunctivitis	30-81
Respiratory failure (NiPPV/intubation)	28-52
Mucus membrane involvement	27-76
Neurocognitive symptoms	29-58
Effusions (pleural, pericardial, ascites)	24-57

GI, gastrointestinal; MIS-C, multisystem inflammatory syndrome in children; NiPPV, noninvasive positive pressure ventilation.

Other important ED diagnostics include an ECG and a cardiac ultrasound. ECG may show nonspecific ST or T wave changes, and about 20% of hospitalized children with MIS-C have a first-degree AV block. Children with ECG changes warrant telemetry monitoring as some may progress to a higher degree of AV block. Cardiac ultrasound can be used to evaluate left ventricular size and systolic function, right ventricular size, and systolic function, as well as the presence of a pericardial effusion. Those more facile with ultrasound can evaluate valvular dysfunction and assess for coronary artery dilation or aneurysm as well as signs of pulmonary, intracardiac, or intra-arterial thrombus.

Timely diagnosis of MIS-C and identification of cardiac dysfunction can inform earlier supportive and therapeutic interventions. MIS-C can cause distributive shock due to systemic inflammation as well as cardiogenic shock. Managing shock in MIS-C is no different than in other conditions and should include hemodynamic monitoring, judicious fluid resuscitation, and the use of pressors when appropriate. Empiric antibiotics are recommended for those with systemic illness pending completion of an infectious workup. Antipyretics and other supportive care should be given as needed. Specific treatments are based on expert opinion as data on the treatment and outcomes of MIS-C remain limited. Early consultation with pediatric subspecialists (Critical Care, Rheumatology, Cardiology, Infectious Disease, Hematology) is encouraged, particularly with respect to specific therapeutics including steroids, IVIG, aspirin, immunomodulators (eg, anakinra), and anticoagulation. Antivirals are not recommended but should be considered in children with positive SARS-CoV-2 RT-PCR and respiratory failure. IVIG may be initiated in the ED if transfer to definitive pediatric care is prolonged.

PEARLS

- The most common presenting symptoms of MIS-C include fever, shock, and GI symptoms. Other typical features include rash, conjunctivitis, and neurocognitive symptoms.

- Unlike severe, acute COVID-19, MIS-C is seen more commonly in healthy children.
- Evaluation includes CBC, CMP, CRP, ESR, troponin, BNP, D-dimer, ferritin, PT/PTT, ECG, cardiac ultrasound, and SARS-CoV-2 RT-PCR. Advanced testing (fibrinogen, LDH, triglycerides, cytokine panel, SARS-CoV-2 serology) can be performed if available or upon transfer to a pediatric center.
- Treatment of MIS-C includes supportive management of myocardial dysfunction, IVIG, and, in more severe cases, steroids, immunomodulators, aspirin, and anticoagulation.
- Despite the potential for severe illness, most children experience full recovery.

Suggested Readings

Centers for Disease Control and Prevention. Information for healthcare providers about multisystem inflammatory syndrome in children (MIS-C). Centers for Disease Control and Prevention; 2023. Accessed January 11, 2023. https://www.cdc.gov/mis/mis-c/hcp_cstecdc/index.html

Home. Multisystem inflammatory syndrome in children (MIS-C) interim guidance. 2022. Retrieved January 11, 2023. https://www.aap.org/en/pages/2019-novel-coronavirus-covid-19-infections/clinical-guidance/multisystem-inflammatory-syndrome-in-children-mis-c-interim-guidance

Riphagen S, Gomez X, Gonzalez-Martinez C, Wilkinson N, Theocharis P. Hyperinflammatory shock in children during COVID-19 pandemic. *Lancet.* 2020;395(10237):1607-1608.

Som MB, Friedman K. COVID-19: multisystem inflammatory syndrome in children (MIS-C) clinical features, evaluation, and diagnosis. UpToDate; 2022. Accessed January 11, 2023. https://www.uptodate.com/contents/covid-19-multisystem-inflammatory-syndrome-in-children-mis-c-clinical-features-evaluation-and-diagnosis

334

In It for the Long Haul: Long COVID

Michael Kim and Stephen Y. Liang

While those infected with SARS-CoV-2 commonly develop symptoms 4 to 5 days after exposure, a subset of individuals can experience persistent or new symptoms long after the initial infection. First described as "post-COVID-19 syndrome," *long COVID* refers to the persistence or development of symptoms weeks or months after the initial infection. According to the World Health Organization, new symptoms generally occur 3 months from the onset of COVID-19 and last for at least 2 months. They can be continuous or relapsing and remitting in nature, with most individuals recovering from the initial microbiologic infection. Diagnosis of long COVID can be challenging due to the wide range of symptoms, the lack of testing to confirm preceding SARS-CoV-2 infection, and the onset of symptoms long after acute infection.

PREVALENCE

Due to these challenges in diagnosis, it is difficult to accurately estimate the prevalence of long COVID. In a cross-sectional study by Perlis et al conducted between February 2021 and July 2022 in the United States, 14.7% of those who reported a positive COVID-19 test result more than 2 months before participation continued to experience symptoms associated with acute infection. The Office for National Statistics in the United Kingdom found that an estimated 2.1 million people (3.3% of the population) reported having long COVID as of December 2022. Some evidence suggests that most patients hospitalized for COVID-19 continue to have symptoms of long COVID, while the prevalence of residual symptoms in patients treated on an outpatient basis is much lower.

PATHOPHYSIOLOGY

The complications from acute infection, such as end-organ damage, inflammation, and the sequelae of critical illness and hospitalization, can contribute to the development of long COVID (**Figure 334.1**). The virus invades many tissues due to the ubiquitous expression of the angiotensin-converting enzyme 2 (ACE2) receptor, and subsequent inflammation can lead to dysregulated immunologic response and virus-induced cytokine storm. Furthermore, vascular inflammation can lead to hematologic changes and eventual thromboembolic formations that could affect other organs, including the nervous, gastrointestinal, and renal systems. Central nervous system involvement may lead to neurodegeneration, disruption of the blood-brain barrier, and persistent neuropsychiatric symptoms. Social and financial impacts of COVID-19 can also contribute to long

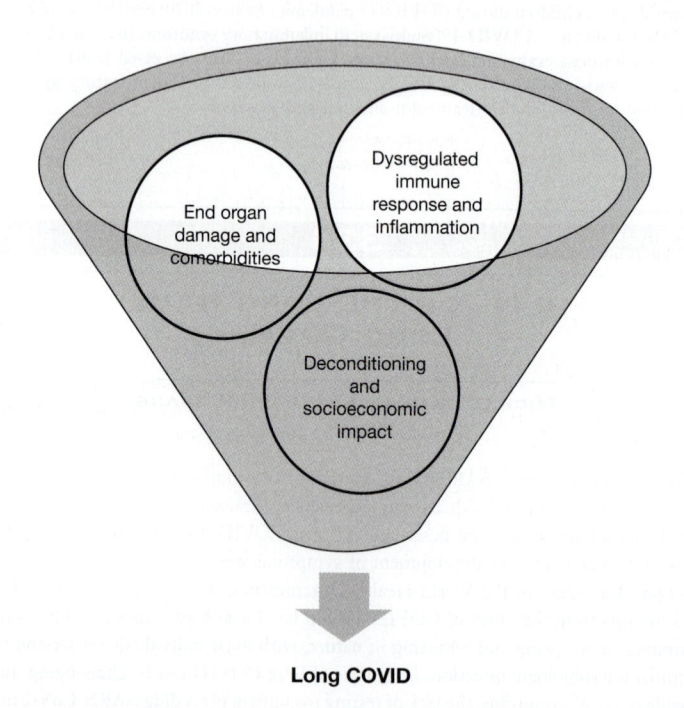

FIGURE 334.1 Long COVID: complications and sequelae.

COVID, affecting not only psychological issues but also the management of chronic medical conditions such as diabetes and cardiovascular disease.

Symptoms

A wide range of symptoms has been reported after an acute SARS-CoV-2 infection, which range from the persistence of old symptoms to new symptoms that arise after initial infection and viral recovery. Fatigue, breathlessness, cough, chest pain, palpitations, headache, joint pain, myalgia and weakness, insomnia, diarrhea, and neurocognitive issues, including memory and concentration problems, have been commonly reported.

Multiple studies highlight fatigue as one of the most common complaints, affecting more than half of patients who recover from initial infection. Respiratory symptoms include cough, shortness of breath, and chest tightness. Multiple studies have looked at the long-term effects on the respiratory system and have found abnormalities in pulmonary function tests, spirometry, and diffusion capacity. Other studies have also observed continuing effects involving the cardiovascular system, manifesting as persistent palpitations and chest pain. Myocardial infarction, vasculitis, heart failure, arrhythmias, coronary artery aneurysms, and aortic aneurysms can arise after recovery from acute illness. Cardiovascular manifestations are prominent in the hyperinflammatory state that typically occurs 2 to 6 weeks after viral infection, called MIS. In the pediatric population (MIS-C), cardiovascular effects, including circulatory failure and myocardial dysfunction, predominate; coronary artery dilation and aneurysm formation were more prevalent in those with MIS-C than those with Kawasaki disease, a similar inflammatory syndrome. Thromboembolic diseases, such as pulmonary embolism, have been observed in acute infections. However, no strong evidence exists to suggest that patients are at higher risk of thromboembolism post-SARS-CoV-2 infection.

Headache, vertigo, cognitive dysfunction known as "brain fog," and loss of taste and smell are frequently reported neurologic symptoms of long COVID. Mental health problems such as anxiety, depression, and post-traumatic stress disorder are also common and can persist for many months and possibly years. Other reported symptoms include musculoskeletal weakness and cutaneous manifestations such as urticaria, rash, and alopecia.

Management

The diagnosis of long COVID can be difficult and requires a detailed history and clinical examination. While demonstration of SARS-CoV-2 seropositivity can help confirm the diagnosis, antibody levels are known to wane over time, and therefore, a negative serology may not rule out past SARS-CoV-2 infection. Criteria such as Raveendran's criteria can help ascertain the likelihood of long COVID but should not hinder the management of symptoms described by patients, even if the diagnosis is doubtful. Management of long COVID should involve a personalized, holistic, and multidisciplinary approach due to the diverse spectrum of symptoms and burden. Close follow-up with a primary care physician can help manage different therapeutic modalities, including physiotherapy, psychological support, and medications. Patients are also at risk of worsening underlying comorbidities and may need further management of chronic medical conditions.

Future Studies

Due to the novelty of the disease, more long-term global studies are necessary to understand long COVID. Challenges include establishing clear diagnostic criteria, establishing long-term follow-up, and identifying risk factors that may predispose certain individuals to COVID. Race, ethnicity, and other socioeconomic differences may present barriers to accessing healthcare for long COVID. As some studies have demonstrated lower incidence of long COVID in those who completed the primary vaccine series before acute illness, the impact of vaccination on the risk for long COVID warrants further investigation.

PEARLS

- Long COVID refers to the persistence or development of symptoms weeks or months after initial SARS-CoV-2 infection.
- Due to challenges in diagnosis, it is difficult to accurately estimate the prevalence of long COVID, but it is thought likely to be underreported.
- The most common symptoms include fatigue, cardiopulmonary symptoms such as chest pain and shortness of breath, and neuropsychiatric symptoms including headaches, cognitive dysfunction, and post-traumatic stress disorder.
- The management of long COVID should involve a personalized, holistic, and multidisciplinary approach due to the wide range of symptoms and burden.
- Due to the novelty of the disease, long-term global studies are needed to better understand long COVID and identify potentially modifiable risk factors.

Suggested Readings

Akbarialiabad H, Taghrir MH, Abdollahi A, et al. Long COVID, a comprehensive systematic scoping review. *Infection*. 2021;49(6):1163-1186. PMID: 34319569.

Carfi A, Bernabei R, Landi F; Gemelli Against COVID-19 Post-Acute Care Study Group. Persistent symptoms in patients after acute COVID-19. *JAMA*. 2020;324(6):603-605.

Perlis RH, Santillana M, Ognyanova K, et al. Prevalence and correlates of long COVID symptoms among US adults. *JAMA Netw Open*. 2022;5(10):e2238804.

Raveendran AV, Jayadevan R, Sashidharan S. Long COVID: an overview [published correction appears in *Diabetes Metab Syndr*. 2022;16(5):102504] [published correction appears in *Diabetes Metab Syndr*. 2022;16(12):102660]. *Diabetes Metab Syndr*. 2021;15(3):869-875. PMID: 33892403.

Silva Andrade B, Siqueira S, de Assis Soares WR, et al. Long-COVID and post-COVID health complications: an up-to-date review on clinical conditions and their possible molecular mechanisms. *Viruses*. 2021;13(4):700. PMID: 33919537.

335

How Accurate Are the COVID-19 Tests

Addie Burtle

In the early months of the COVID-19 pandemic, molecular testing emerged as the backbone of SARS-CoV-2 diagnosis. Although physical examination and imaging findings may be suggestive, contributing to overall clinical gestalt, they are neither sensitive nor specific enough to be relied on alone. Furthermore, the emergence of new viral variants can lead to changes in the predominant manifestations of SARS-CoV-2 infection with regard to both physical examination and imaging. Molecular diagnostics have, thus far, proven robust against all of the wild-type variants. RT-PCR testing is consequently the most common diagnostic used to detect SARS-CoV-2 in US EDs. Although RT-PCR has favorable test characteristics compared to alternative options, a major shortcoming of the SARS-CoV-2 diagnostic landscape is the lack of a true testing reference standard.

One significant limitation inherent to RT-PCR is that it can only implicate the presence of viral RNA—it cannot, alone, answer the question of whether a patient is infected or simply was infected. In prior respiratory pandemics, multiple positive tests were required to meet the case definition. Alternatively, a composite standard, such as a positive test along with the presence of certain symptoms, was used to minimize false positives. Composite standards prove challenging for SARS-CoV-2; however, given that approximately 35% of infections are asymptomatic. Current practice is to rely upon a single positive RT-PCR test to diagnose SARS-CoV-2 infection. As a result, this creates a significant risk of both false positives and false negatives.

The amplification process of PCR not only has the potential for tremendous sensitivity but also creates a risk of magnifying leftover RNA fragments from a recent infection, or even minute amounts of contamination, into what might be perceived as a positive signal. Lateral flow immunochromatographic RAT, which lacks the exponential amplification seen in PCR, has somewhat lower sensitivity. But, in trade, it offers greater specificity for diagnosing active infections. The RT-PCR process iterates through up to 40 cycles of replication, with each successive cycle representing a shift toward sensitivity with a commensurate reduction in specificity. Furthermore, when lab reports omit cycle count, this risks creating a false impression that RT-PCR is a binary test. Positivity at a low cycle count typically represents an unequivocal infection. The highest high-cycle counts are seen with negative tests. There is a middle range, however, which represents a spectrum of uncertainty. Ultimately, each laboratory faces the challenging task of enacting a cycle threshold to serve as the cut point between positive and negative. The omission of cycle count from test reporting erases this complex gradient of probability. As a thought experiment, one can consider the added difficulty in diagnosing heart failure exacerbation if, for example, serum BNP was reported simply as positive or negative.

Sensitivity of RT-PCR

FDA Emergency Use Authorization requires a minimum of 95% sensitivity and 98% specificity for RT-PCR; however, it must be noted that this is a laboratory analytic threshold using reference samples, and real-world performance is another story. Clinical data from numerous studies show that the sensitivity of nasopharyngeal swabs for SARS-CoV-2 is typically around 70%-80%—meaning that perhaps one in four "true positives" is missed. Thus, if clinical suspicion is high enough in the setting of a negative test, retesting is a reasonable consideration. Particularly given the large body of literature that shows viral load does not always mirror the onset and degree of symptoms. The degree of viral load, as well as variations in the manner and thoroughness of swab collection, may explain the suboptimal performance of RT-PCR in clinical studies.

RT-PCR False Positives

False positives due to a variety of real-world examples have been documented, including sample contamination by infected staff, carry-forward contamination from lab equipment, and contamination of testing reagents. The latter case is perhaps most interesting, as studies of contaminated primers/probes have shown that low-level contamination will produce sporadic false positives, and these positives may appear only with a high cycle count (ie, they produce weak positives). This is much harder to detect than gross contamination, which would be expected to produce an implausibly high proportion of positives with low cycle values.

Even with excellent specificity, when testing is employed in a low-prevalence context, RT-PCR may produce an unacceptable operational false positive rate. This is illustrated in multiple analyses of real-world SARS-CoV-2 testing, in which high specificity (≥99%) is found, but the proportion of false positive tests ranges from 26% to 84%, depending on context. The clinical takeaway is that when the pretest probability is similar to the false positive rate, the predictive value of the test approaches that of a coin flip.

RT-PCR testing is a powerful and useful tool, but it must be applied thoughtfully and its limitations considered. Testing exists and evolves to support clinical reasoning. Reciprocally, clinical reasoning must adapt to the evolving nuances of diagnostic testing.

PEARLS

- Nasopharyngeal PCR is 70%-80% sensitive → 25% false negative rate.
  - If clinical suspicion remains high after a negative PCR, consider retesting.
- PCR testing cannot distinguish between an *active* and *recent* infection.
  - In select cases where this distinction is important, there may be a role for RAT.
- PPV and NPV are tied to disease prevalence.
  - Consider pretest probability both when ordering a test and interpreting the result.

Suggested Readings

Braunstein GD, Schwartz L, Hymel P, Fielding J. False positive results with SARS-CoV-2 RT-PCR tests and how to evaluate a RT-PCR-positive test for the possibility of a false positive result. *J Occup Environ Med*. 2021;63:e159.

Carpenter CR, Mudd PA, West CP, Wilber E, Wilber ST. Diagnosing COVID-19 in the emergency department: a scoping review of clinical examinations, laboratory tests, imaging accuracy, and biases. *Acad Emerg Med*. 2020;27:653-670.

Mayers C, Baker K. Impact of false-positives and false-negatives in the UK's COVID-19 RT-PCR testing programme. UK Government; 2020. https://www.gov.uk/government/publications/gos-impact-of-false-positives-and-negatives-3-june-2020/impact-of-false-positives-and-false-negatives-in-the-uks-covid-19-rt-pcr-testing-programme-3-june-2020

Woloshin S, Patel N, Kesselheim AS. False negative tests for SARS-CoV-2 infection – challenges and implications. *N Engl J Med*. 2020;383:e38.

336

What Pharmacologic Management Matters in COVID-19

Julianne Yeary and Stephen Y. Liang

As the ED serves as the gateway to healthcare for many, emergency clinicians play a critical role in the treatment of patients with COVID-19. Pharmacologic targets of SARS-CoV-2 include host-receptor attachment, penetration, biosynthesis of viral mRNA, and maturation of viral particles. An important protein that facilitates binding and fusion of SARS-CoV-2 with host cell membranes is the spike protein, which binds to ACE-II receptors found in the lungs and other organs. Infection with SARS-CoV-2 causes an array of host complications with the most common and devastating being lung injury. The immunologic response of the host to infection is responsible for continued organ damage and the progression of disease.

To date, pharmacologic management of COVID-19 has hinged on disease severity and progression. The NIH COVID-19 Treatment Guidelines dichotomize therapeutic approaches by nonhospitalized versus hospitalized patients. Patient risk factors for disease progression help further guide medical decisions surrounding therapeutics. Risk factors to consider include age greater than 65 years, BMI greater than 25, pregnancy, CKD, DM, immunosuppressive disease or treatment, cardiovascular disease or hypertension, chronic lung disease, sickle cell disease, neurodevelopmental disorders or other medical complexity conditions, or having a medical-related technologic dependence.

Remdesivir is approved by the FDA for the treatment of COVID-19 in nonhospitalized and hospitalized patients. Remdesivir binds to viral RNA-dependent RNA polymerase, thereby inhibiting viral replication. The greatest benefit from remdesivir is derived early in the course of COVID-19 and should be started as soon as possible in patients meeting high-risk criteria and requiring hospitalization. Patients who have progressed to respiratory failure requiring MV or ECMO are less likely to benefit from remdesivir. Remdesivir is generally well tolerated; however, side effects may include GI upset (eg, nausea), elevated transaminase levels, increased PT, and rarely, hypersensitivity reactions.

Nirmatrelvir/ritonavir (Paxlovid) is an antiviral that has been approved by the FDA for the treatment of nonhospitalized patients with COVID-19. Nirmatrelvir is a protease inhibitor that inhibits viral replication by cleaving two polyproteins. Ritonavir "boosts" nirmatrelvir levels through P450 3A4 inhibitor activity. A barrier to the use of this antiviral has been its many potential drug-drug interactions. Medications that should be avoided include several neurologic agents (carbamazepine, phenytoin, and clozapine), cardiovascular medications (antiarrhythmics, most statins, ticagrelor, and rivaroxaban), and immunosuppressants (tacrolimus). Dose reductions should be considered with apixaban, digoxin, cyclosporine, and most benzodiazepines. Rebound COVID-19 symptoms have been observed in patients receiving nirmatrelvir/ritonavir; however, this has not led to progression toward severe disease.

Other agents that have been studied in nonhospitalized patients include molnupiravir and mAbs to decrease hospitalization and death in high-risk patients. Molnupiravir has not been shown to be as effective as other agents and is associated with teratogenicity, which excludes its use in pregnant women; men and women of childbearing age prescribed with this medication must adhere to appropriate contraception to avoid pregnancy during and for 4 to 90 days after treatment. Molnupiravir is reserved for patients who have absolute contraindications to receiving nirmatrelvir/ritonavir or remdesivir and are at high risk of disease progression and/or death.

A number of mAbs (bamlanivimab/etesevimab, casirivimab/imdevimab, sotrovimab, bebtelovimab, tixagevimab/cilgavimab) were brought to market for treatment of COVID-19 and work by inhibiting viral entry into the cell by binding to the SARS-CoV-2 spike protein or targeting human ACE-II receptors, decreasing viral attachment. However, the NIH has concluded that mAbs should no longer be used, given their limited efficacy against emerging variants.

Corticosteroids dampen host immune response to COVID-19; their use is currently limited to those with disease progression (eg, requiring escalation of oxygen therapy) and requiring hospitalization. The NIH recommends dexamethasone (or an equivalent dose of another corticosteroid) for hospitalized patients requiring oxygen therapy; it is not recommended for nonhospitalized patients given the lack of efficacy and concern for additional harm.

Patients progressing to severe disease and those requiring invasive MV and critical care may be eligible to receive additional therapeutics, including JAK inhibitors (baricitinib or tofacitinib) or IL-6 inhibitors (tocilizumab or sarilumab). The NIH recommends oral baricitinib or IV tocilizumab in patients with rapidly progressing oxygen requirements or systemic inflammation.

Data on existing therapeutics are limited for patients less than 12 years of age; therefore, the NIH has extrapolated adult studies to pediatric patients. Supportive care is recommended for nonhospitalized patients less than 12 years of age. Hospitalized patients between the ages of 2 and 11 years should receive remdesivir and corticosteroids if escalation of care and oxygen supplementation are needed. Baricitinib and tocilizumab may be considered in pediatric patients with severe disease or requiring MV or ECMO.

As the COVID-19 pandemic continues to progress, emergency clinicians must recognize which patients are at greatest risk for disease progression, understand the mechanisms by which current and emerging therapeutics combat disease, and initiate therapeutics when clinically appropriate (**Table 336.1**).

PEARLS

- Nonhospitalized patients with COVID-19 meeting high-risk criteria for disease progression should receive either oral nirmatrelvir/ritonavir (Paxlovid) or intravenous remdesivir.
- Remdesivir is recommended for all patients who are hospitalized with COVID-19 early in their disease course.
- Corticosteroids should be reserved for patients who are hospitalized with COVID-19 requiring oxygen supplementation and are not recommended in nonhospitalized.
- Immunomodulating agents may be considered in hospitalized patients with progressing severe disease.

TABLE 336.1 COVID-19 THERAPEUTICS

NONHOSPITALIZED PATIENTS

MEDICATION (IN ORDER OF PREFERENCE)	SYMPTOM ONSET	ADULT (>12 YR, >40 KG)	PEDIATRICS (<12 YR)	EFFICACY (% REDUCTION IN DEATH AND HOSPITALIZATIONS)	NOTES
Nirmatrelvir/ritonavir [Paxlovid]	5 d	300/150 mg oral bid × 5 days	Not recommended	88%	Drug–drug interactions
Remdesivir	7 d	100 mg IV daily × 3 d	Not recommended	87%	Cost; feasibility
Molnupiravir *Last line option for severe risk*	5 d	800 mg oral bid × 5 d must be 18 yrs of age	Not recommended	30%	Teratogenic; avoid in pregnancy or lactating women; contraception required

Treatments NOT recommended given lack of efficacy and emerging resistant variants:
Monoclonal antibodies, chloroquine/hydroxychloroquine with or without azithromycin, lopinavir/ritonavir, metformin, colchicine, fluvoxamine, ivermectin, or inhaled corticosteroids.

HOSPITALIZED PATIENTS

SEVERITY OF ILLNESS	MEDICATION	ADULT (>12 YR)	PEDIATRICS (2-11 YR)	EFFICACY	NOTES
No oxygen therapy needed	Remdesivir	200 mg × 1 followed by 100 mg daily × 5 d or until discharge	Only if requiring oxygen therapy	↓ mortality	Limited efficacy progressing disease (MV or ECMO)
Require oxygen therapy	Dexamethasone *(or equivalent corticosteroid)*	6 mg daily × 10 d	0.15 mg/kg to max 6 mg daily × 10 days	↓ mortality and MV days	Monitor hyperglycemia, infection risk
Disease progression and systemic inflammation; MV; critical care	Immunomodulators *(JAK inhibitors or IL-6 inhibitors)*	Baricitinib oral or tocilizumab IV *(tofacitinib and sarilumab alternatives)*	Baricitinib or Tocilizumab Recommended: dosing per package insert. (Tofacitinib only if Baricitinib unavailable. Consult specialist)	↓ risk of respiratory failure and death	Cost; infection risk

ECMO, extracorporeal membrane oxygenation; IL-6, interleukin 6; IV, intravenous; JAK, Janus kinase; MV, mechanical ventilation.

Suggested Readings

Beigel JH, Tomashek KM, Dodd LE, et al. Remdesivir for the treatment of COVID-19 – final report; PINETREE trial. *NEJM*. 2020;383(19):1813-1826.

COVID-19 Treatment Guidelines Panel. Coronavirus disease 2019 (COVID-19) treatment guidelines. National Institutes of Health. Accessed December 28, 2022. https://www.covid19treatmentguidelines.nih.gov/

Hammond J, Leister-Tebbe H, Gardner A, et al. Oral nirmatrelvir for high-risk, nonhospitalized adults with COVID-19; EPIC-HR trial. *NEJM*. 2022;386:1397-1408.

NIH COVID-19 Treatment Guidelines. Drug-drug interactions between ritonavir-boosted Nirmatrelvir (Paxlovid) and concomitant medications. 2022. https://www.covid19treatmentguidelines.nih.gov/therapies/antivirals-including-antibody-products/ritonavir-boosted-nirmatrelvir--paxlovid-/paxlovid-drug-drug-interactions/

RECOVERY Collaborative Group. Dexamethasone in hospitalized patient with COVID-19. *NEJM*. 2021;384(9):693-704.

RECOVERY Collaborative Group. Baricitinib in patients admitted to hospital with COVID-19 (RECOVERY): a randomized, controlled, open-label, platform trial and updated meta-analysis. *Lancet*. 2022;400(10349):359-368.

WHO Solidarity Trial Consortium. Remdesivir and three other drugs for hospitalized patients with COVID-19: final results of the WHO Solidarity randomized trial and updated meta-analyses. *Lancet*. 2022;399(10339):1941-1953.

Yuki K, Fugiogi M, Koutsogiannaki S. COVID-19 pathophysiology: a review. *Clin Immunol*. 2020;215:108427.

337

Mechanical Ventilation in the Patient with COVID-19

Robert J. Stephens and Brian M. Fuller

Mechanical ventilation is necessary in about 375,000 ED patients annually. Patients who are ventilated in the ED carry a high morbidity and mortality burden, with as many as one in four dying while hospitalized. The COVID-19 pandemic strained the healthcare system, especially the ED, with an increase in the number of boarding patients, including those mechanically ventilated. Literature over the past decade demonstrates that this early period of critical illness is pivotal in determining clinical outcomes. Emergency physicians, therefore, play a key role in the care of critically ill patients with COVID-19 who require ventilation beyond initial airway management.

Overall, there is nothing unique with respect to ventilator management of patients with COVID-19 versus other etiologies of respiratory failure. We, therefore, recommend a systematic approach that can be applied to most patients requiring intubation and mechanical ventilation in the ED for acute hypoxic respiratory failure and may be at significant risk for acute lung injury. All patients with COVID-19 who require intubation should be considered to have early ARDS or "pre-ARDS" if they do not meet strict criteria and should be ventilated using lung protective ventilation to prevent ventilator-associated lung injury. In contrast, the approach to patients with expiratory flow limitation (ie, status asthmaticus, decompensated COPD) focuses on management with higher tidal volumes and lower respiratory rates to avoid intrinsic PEEP.

Target a Protective Tidal Volume

High tidal volume can cause excessive lung stretch (ie, volutrauma) and contribute to ventilator-associated lung injury. Use of higher tidal volume ventilation has been associated with worse outcomes in ARDS. Mechanical ventilation data from the ED have demonstrated a high prevalence of potentially injurious high tidal volume use. The first step is to target protective tidal volumes appropriate for each patient. Tidal volume should range between 6 and 8 mL/kg PBW, calculated from height and gender. As such we recommend measuring the height of each patient immediately after intubation to determine an initial tidal volume setting. Tables of recommended tidal volumes by PBW for common heights are freely available at www.ardsnet.org.

Minute ventilation can be adjusted to prevent severe hypercarbia and acidosis, but in ARDS the use of a permissive hypercapnia approach should be favored over the normalization of arterial blood gas values (suggested pH threshold of 7.15 is usually well tolerated).

Assess and Limit Distending Pressures

Elevated airway pressures can also reflect alveolar overdistension and risk for ventilator-associated lung injury. The two pressures easily obtained from all modern ventilators are the peak (determined by resistance and respiratory system compliance) and plateau (determined by respiratory system compliance) pressures. Soon after intubation, perform an inspiratory hold maneuver on the ventilator to measure plateau pressure. Plateau pressure (P_{plat}) should, in general, be limited to less than 30 cm H_2O. However, in patients with lower chest wall and abdominal compliance (eg, obesity, ascites), a higher plateau pressure can be tolerated. In patients with a P_{plat} greater than 30, driving pressure (P_{plat}—PEEP) can be used to further assess pulmonary mechanics. Driving pressure is essentially tidal volume indexed to the compliance of the respiratory system and a marker of global lung strain. A driving pressure of less than 15 cm H_2O is a commonly referenced limit but has not been studied prospectively. After PEEP setting and optimization of compliance, if driving pressure is elevated, tidal volume can be decreased by 1 mL/kg PBW and driving pressure reassessed after several minutes.

Adequate PEEP to Prevent Atelectrauma

Cyclic recruitment and de-recruitment of alveoli causes injury to the alveoli as they collapse and reopen. This can cause significantly more injury to lungs in the early phases of injury. All patients with hypoxic respiratory failure should be ventilated with at least 5 cm H_2O of PEEP. The optimal approach to PEEP titration remains controversial and should be individualized. In the ED, we recommend a simple approach that allows for recruitment with PEEP and avoidance of unnecessarily high FIO_2 and hyperoxia. PEEP and FIO_2 should be titrated in concert and ARDSNet has both high- and low-PEEP titration tables, also available freely at **www.ardsnet.org**. Evidence does not suggest clinical benefit of one strategy versus the other.

Oxygen is often overdosed in patients with respiratory failure in the ED. Oxygenation goals should be an arterial partial pressure of oxygen of 55 to 80 mm Hg or pulse oximetry of 88% to 95%. To avoid hyperoxia in the ED, which has been associated with worse outcomes, we recommend initiating mechanical ventilation with an FIO_2 of 30% to 40% immediately after intubation (not 100% FIO_2), and only uptitrating FIO_2 in combination with PEEP.

Prevent Aspiration

VAP is a major source of morbidity and mortality in critically ill patients who require mechanical ventilation. Few interventions have demonstrated benefit in preventing VAP other than minimizing number of days exposed to mechanical ventilation. However, aspiration prevention is a mainstay of VAP prevention. Simply elevating the head of bed to greater than 30° after intubation reduces microaspiration around the endotracheal tube and is an evidence-based, inexpensive, and easily performed intervention to substantially reduce the risk of VAP.

PEARLS

- Have a systematic approach to the management of the ventilator in patients who require intubation in the ED (**Figure 337.1**).
- Patients with COVID-19 infection who require mechanical ventilation are particularly at risk for developing acute lung injury and ARDS.
- High volumes, high pressures, atelectasis, hyperoxia, and aspiration all play a role in the pathogenesis of ventilatory-associated lung injury.
- Practice lung protective ventilation by targeting low tidal volumes (6-8 mL/kg PBW), avoiding injurious plateau and driving pressures.

Use protective volumes → Titrate settings for tidal volume of 6-8 mL/kg PBW

Assess distending pressures → Measure plateau pressure and decrease tidal volumes to maintain P_{plat} <30 cm H_2O

Avoid atelectasis and hyperoxia → Titrate FiO_2 and PEEP based on ARDSNet tables

Prevent aspiration → Raise head of bed to >30°

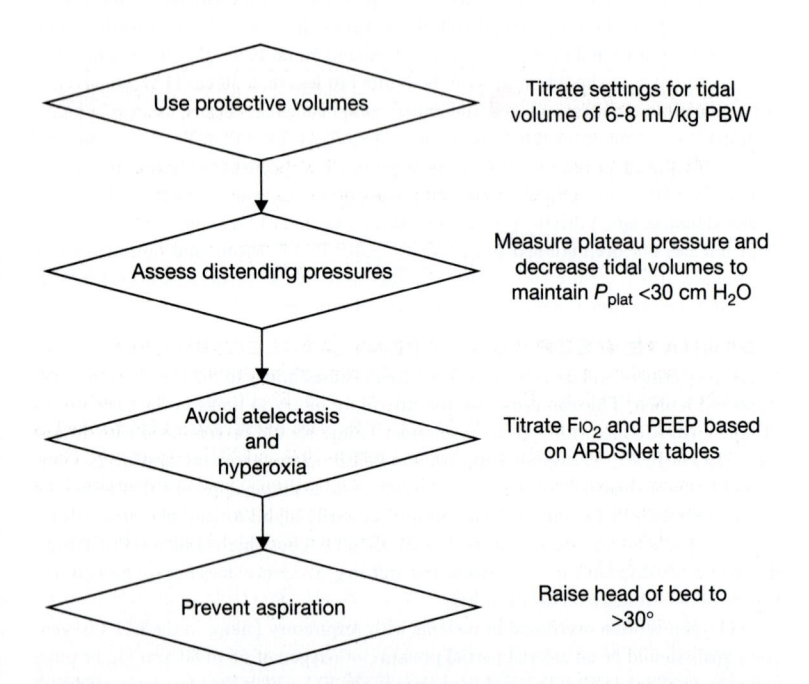

FIGURE 337.1 Algorithm for ventilator management for provision of lung protective ventilation. FiO_2, fraction of inspired oxygen; PBW, predictive body weight; PEEP, positive end expiratory pressure; P_{plat}, plateau pressure.

- Titrate PEEP and FIO_2 to prevent atelectasis and achieve adequate oxygenation without hyperoxia.
- Raise the head of bed to prevent aspiration.

SUGGESTED READINGS

Fuller BM, Ferguson IT, Mohr NM, et al. A quasi-experimental, before-after trial examining the impact of an emergency department mechanical ventilator protocol on clinical outcomes and lung-protective ventilation in acute respiratory distress syndrome. *Crit Care Med*. 2017;45(4):645-652.

Fuller BM, Page D, Stephens RJ, et al. Pulmonary mechanics and mortality in mechanically ventilated patients without acute respiratory distress syndrome: a cohort study. *Shock*. 2018;49(3):311-316.

Page D, Ablordeppey E, Wessman BT, et al. Emergency department hyperoxia is associated with increased mortality in mechanically ventilated patients: a cohort study. *Crit Care*. 2018;22(1):9.

Stephens RJ, Siegler JE, Fuller BM. Mechanical ventilation in the prehospital and emergency department environment. *Respir Care*. 2019;64(5):595-603.

The Acute Respiratory Distress Syndrome Network. Ventilation with lower tidal volumes as compared with traditional tidal volumes for acute lung injury and the acute respiratory distress syndrome. *N Engl J Med*. 2000;342:1301-1308.

338

BEATING THE BEAST: EVOLUTION OF COVID-19 VACCINES

NICHOLAS MAXWELL AND STEPHEN Y. LIANG

Vaccines have played a central part in combating COVID-19. Several platforms exist worldwide, including inactivated vaccines, viral vector vaccines, protein subunit vaccines, and mRNA vaccines (**Table 338.1**). In the United States, BNT162b2 (Pfizer-BioNTech) and mRNA-1273 (Moderna) COVID-19 mRNA vaccines were granted EUA by the US FDA in December 2020 and full approval for adults in 2021 and 2022, respectively. These vaccines contain mRNA encoding the SARS-CoV-2 spike protein used by the virus to bind to ACE-II receptors found in host epithelial cells present in the airway and other organs. In doing so, mRNA vaccines elicit protective host immunity against SARS-CoV-2. mRNA from the vaccine neither enters the host cell nucleus nor modifies host cell DNA. Ad26.COV2.S (Janssen/Johnson & Johnson) is a viral vector COVID-19 vaccine that received EUA in 2021 with use later limited to certain settings by the FDA in 2022. NVX-CoV2373 (Novavax) is a protein subunit vaccine that was granted EUA approval in 2022.

VE against COVID-19 varies widely depending on the type of vaccine received, completion of the primary series as well as subsequent boosters, time elapsed since the primary series and/or last booster, prevalent variants at the time of exposure, and comorbid conditions. mRNA vaccines have tended to perform better than other COVID-19 vaccine

TABLE 338.1	PRIMARY COVID-19 VACCINE SERIES AVAILABLE IN THE UNITED STATES		
	VACCINE TYPE	DOSES FOR PRIMARY SERIES	AVAILABLE TO AGES
BNT162b2 (Pfizer-BioNTech)	mRNA	2 doses 3-8 wk apart[a]	6 mo and older
mRNA-1273 (Moderna)	mRNA	2 doses 4-8 wk apart	6 mo and older
Ad26.COV2.S (Janssen/ Johnson & Johnson)	Viral vector	Single dose	18 yr and older
NVX-CoV2373 (Novavax)	Protein subunit	2 doses 3-8 wk apart	12 yr and older

[a]Those between 6 months and 4 years old are to get a bivalent vaccine for third dose 8 weeks after their second dose to complete their primary series.

platforms; in one case-control analysis, VE against hospitalization from COVID-19 was 93% for mRNA-1273 (Moderna), 88% for BNT162b2 (Pfizer-BioNTech), and 71% for Ad26.COV2.S (Janssen/Johnson & Johnson). Protection against infection and symptomatic disease wanes over time after vaccination, while protection from severe disease is fairly well sustained. Variability in protection has been seen with emerging SARS-CoV-2 variants. Those who are immunocompromised (eg, primary immunodeficiency, malignancy, solid organ transplant, or hematopoietic stem cell transplantation) may be more susceptible to severe disease despite vaccination.

VE against infection may decrease below 50% as early as 150 days postvaccination. The receipt of a booster can improve VE to as high as 70% or even 95% in certain settings. Likewise, a booster can improve the immune response even in groups previously suspected to have a limited response to vaccination, such as the immunocompromised. Those with prior COVID-19 infection who receive a booster will also mount a demonstrable increase in protective antibody levels. As SARS-CoV-2 variants with significant changes to the spike protein emerge and circulate, updated boosters incorporating these variants will likely be necessary to achieve optimal protection during the COVID-19 pandemic. As of early 2023, bivalent COVID-19 mRNA boosters have been developed by Pfizer-BioNTech and Moderna, incorporating mRNA from the original SARS-CoV-2 virus and two prevalent Omicron variants, BA.4 and BA.5. Early data suggest that these bivalent boosters significantly improve protection. Patients may receive the bivalent booster as early as 2 months after their primary series or once symptoms resolve and the isolation period is complete after having a COVID-19 infection. The selection of which mRNA booster to receive does not depend on which primary vaccine series the patient received. Updated COVID-19 vaccine and booster guidance can be found at https://www.cdc.gov/coronavirus/2019-ncov/vaccines/.

EDs can play a vital role in advancing public health through COVID-19 prevention, building upon successful models with influenza and tetanus immunization. COVID-19 vaccines and boosters can be administered concurrently with seasonal influenza and other vaccines when clinically appropriate. SARS-CoV-2 testing in the absence of symptoms is not necessary to receive either the primary series or booster. ED visits present unique opportunities to dispel myths and misconceptions surrounding COVID-19 vaccines and to initiate primary series or provide updated boosters, particularly when regional surges in cases are occurring or anticipated. This may be particularly important among patient populations with limited access to or interaction with the healthcare system or primary care.

PEARLS

- COVID-19 mRNA vaccines are highly efficacious and widely available in the United States.
- VE against infection and symptomatic disease varies depending on vaccine platform, prevalent variants, time since vaccination, and comorbid conditions.
- Vaccine-mediated protection against severe disease is better sustained over time than protection against general infection and nonsevere disease.
- Boosters are important to address emerging variants and waning immunity.
- EDs are well-positioned to serve the public through education about and the provision of COVID-19 primary vaccines and boosters.

Suggested Readings

Andrews N, Stowe J, Kirsebom F, et al. COVID-19 vaccine effectiveness against the Omicron (B.1.1.529) variant. *N Engl J Med*. 2022;386(16):1532-1546. PMID: 35249272.

Lee ARYB, Wong SY, Chai LYA, et al. Efficacy of COVID-19 vaccines in immunocompromised patients: systematic review and meta-analysis. *BMJ*. 2022;376:e068632. PMID: 35236664.

Self WH, Tenforde MW, Rhoads JP, et al. Comparative effectiveness of moderna, Pfizer-BioNTech, and Janssen (Johnson & Johnson) vaccines in preventing COVID-19 hospitalizations among adults without immunocompromising conditions—United States, March-August 2021. *MMWR Morb Mortal Wkly Rep*. 2021;70(38):1337-1343. PMID: 34555004.

Ssentongo P, Ssentongo AE, Voleti N, et al. SARS-CoV-2 vaccine effectiveness against infection, symptomatic and severe COVID-19: a systematic review and meta-analysis. *BMC Infect Dis*. 2022;22(1):439. PMID: 35525973.

Tenforde MW, Weber ZA, Natarajan K, et al. Early estimates of bivalent mRNA vaccine effectiveness in preventing COVID-19-associated emergency department or urgent care encounters and hospitalizations among immunocompetent adults—vision network, nine states, September-November 2022. *MMWR Morb Mortal Wkly Rep*. 2022;71(5152):1616-1624. PMID: 36580430.

339

Complications and Myths in COVID-19 Vaccinations

Olena Kostyuk

The global effort to develop safe and effective COVID-19 vaccines has made significant progress since the introduction of the first vaccine in December 2020. While authorized vaccines commonly have mild side effects (such as pain, redness, and swelling) and mild systemic effects (such as low-grade fever, fatigue, headache, muscle, or joint pain), there have been rare reports of serious adverse reactions during postmarketing surveillance.

These include anaphylaxis, vaccine-induced thrombotic thrombocytopenia, myopericarditis, Guillain-Barré syndrome, and so forth. However, it is important to note that despite these rare cases, the overall benefit-risk ratio strongly supports COVID-19 vaccination for people of all ages and genders. Addressing misinformation and vaccine hesitancy remains crucial in promoting vaccine safety and public health.

Currently, there are two main types of COVID-19 vaccines available for use in the United States: mRNA vaccines (Pfizer-BioNTech or Moderna) and the protein subunit vaccine (Novavax). As of April 2023, the bivalent mRNA vaccines have replaced the original monovalent mRNA vaccines. Additionally, the adenovirus vector vaccine Janssen (Johnson & Johnson) is no longer available or recommended by the CDC in the United States.

Anaphylaxis

Adverse events, including anaphylaxis, have been reported following COVID-19 vaccination, possibly due to the polyethylene glycol component in mRNA vaccines. However, continued safety monitoring of mRNA COVID-19 vaccines in the United States has confirmed that anaphylaxis following vaccination is rare, with rates of 4.7 cases per million for Pfizer-BioNTech and 2.5 cases per million for Moderna as of January 2021. These rates are comparable to those observed with other vaccines. Treatment protocols for anaphylaxis caused by COVID-19 vaccines are similar to those for other severe allergic reactions. If moderate or severe allergic reactions occur after the first vaccine dose, it is not recommended to administer the second dose. Alternatively, individuals who received an mRNA vaccine as their first dose may consider a non-mRNA vaccine as a substitute (eg, protein subunit vaccine).

VITT

VITT is a rare condition that can occur within 2 to 42 days following the COVID-19 vaccination. It is characterized by the development of arterial and/or venous thrombosis, along with thrombocytopenia, elevated D-dimer, and positive antibodies against PF4. The condition is caused by the formation of anti-PF4 antibodies, which cross-react with vaccine antigens, leading to platelet activation and consumption and subsequent arterial and venous thrombosis. Most cases of VITT have been reported after receiving mRNA vaccines.

Venous thrombosis in VITT can occur at multiple sites, including cerebral venous sinus, splanchnic veins, and extremities. Individuals who experience severe headaches, visual changes, abdominal pain, back pain, shortness of breath, leg pain or swelling, petechiae, easy bruising, or bleeding within 42 days after vaccination should be evaluated for VITT. Diagnostic tests such as CBC with platelet count, PF4 ELISA, D-dimer, fibrinogen, and imaging techniques can aid in timely diagnosis and management.

Treatment for VITT typically involves high-dose IVIG and, in refractory cases, plasma exchange. Therapeutic-dose anticoagulants, such as direct oral anticoagulants (dabigatran, apixaban, rivaroxaban, edoxaban, and fondaparinux) or parenteral direct thrombin inhibitors (bivalirudin and argatroban), should be administered to prevent further thrombotic complications.

Myocarditis and Pericarditis

Rare cases of myocarditis and pericarditis have been reported following the COVID-19 vaccination, particularly with mRNA vaccines. These cases primarily affect adolescent and young adult males, occurring within 7 days after the second dose, but can also happen after the first dose or a booster.

The exact underlying mechanisms behind myocarditis and pericarditis postvaccination are not fully understood, but potential factors include molecular mimicry between viral spike proteins and cardiac proteins, immune system activation, and a nonspecific innate inflammatory response.

Patients usually presented 2 to 3 days after the second dose of mRNA vaccination with chest pain, some preceded by fever and myalgia. Laboratory tests show elevated troponin and C-reactive protein levels indicative of myocardial inflammation, while an ECG may reveal ST-segment elevation. A transthoracic echocardiogram often shows mildly reduced to normal left ventricular ejection fraction and global hypokinesia.

Treatment approaches may involve NSAIDs, colchicine, or corticosteroids; in younger patients (≤18 years old), IVIG may be combined with corticosteroids. Notably, most reported cases have shown complete clinical recovery within 1 to 3 weeks after the onset of myocarditis or pericarditis.

GBS

According to a Vaccine Safety Datalink analysis, there is no increased risk of GBS associated with the Pfizer-BioNTech or Moderna COVID-19 vaccines. However, it was found that the risk of GBS within the initial 21 days following the Janssen (Johnson & Johnson) COVID-19 vaccination is 21 times higher compared with Pfizer-BioNTech or Moderna vaccines.

COMPLICATIONS OF COVID-19 VACCINES DURING PREGNANCY

Pregnancy is an independent risk factor for severe COVID-19, and vaccination is the best way to reduce the risk of infection and limit morbidity and mortality.

Vaccine side effects in pregnant women are similar to those in nonpregnant individuals, with mild to moderate symptoms; severe allergic reactions are rare.

Studies have shown no increased risk of adverse pregnancy outcomes or fetal anomalies after COVID-19 vaccination. The rates of preterm birth and NICU admission have not significantly increased.

COVID-19 VACCINATION IN CHILDREN

COVID-19 vaccination in children aged 5 to 11 years resulted in mostly mild-to-moderate reactions, with a higher occurrence after the second dose. According to the VAERS, 97% of reported adverse events were nonserious. Among the 194 serious VAERS reports, there were 15 confirmed cases of myocarditis, with eight cases occurring in boys after the second dose (2.2 per million doses). Furthermore, a Vaccine Safety Datalink analysis of 726,820 doses administered found no safety signals. These findings provide reassuring evidence regarding the safety of the COVID-19 vaccination in this age group.

PEARLS

- Universal vaccination is the most effective strategy to protect against COVID-19.
- Authorized COVID-19 vaccines (mRNA and protein subunit) have demonstrated a strong safety profile.
- Rare serious adverse reactions have been reported postvaccination, including anaphylaxis, VITT, myopericarditis, and GBS.
- The overall benefit-risk ratio strongly supports the COVID-19 vaccination for all ages and genders, including pregnant women and children.

Suggested Readings

Ahmed SH, Shaikh TG, Waseem S, Qadir NA, Yousaf Z, Ullah I. Vaccine-induced thrombotic thrombocytopenia following coronavirus vaccine: a narrative review. *Ann Med Surg.* 2022;73:102988.

Badell ML, Dude CM, Rasmussen SA, Jamieson DJ. COVID-19 vaccination in pregnancy. *BMJ* 2022;378:e069741.

Fatima M, Khan MHA, Ali MS, et al. Development of myocarditis and pericarditis after COVID-19 vaccination in children and adolescents: a systematic review. *Clin Cardiol.* 2023;46:243-259.

Fragkou PC, Dimopoulou D. Serious complications of COVID-19 vaccines: a mini-review. *Metabol Open.* 2021;12:100145.

Hanson KE, Goddard K, Lewis N, et al. Incidence of Guillain-Barré syndrome after COVID-19 vaccination in the vaccine safety datalink. *JAMA Netw Open.* 2022;5(4):e228879.

Hause AM, Shay DK, Klein NP, et al. Safety of COVID-19 vaccination in United States children ages 5 to 11 years. *Pediatrics.* 2022;150(2):e2022057313.

Shimabukuro TT, Cole M, Su JR. Reports of anaphylaxis after receipt of mRNA COVID-19 vaccines in the US—December 14, 2020-January 18, 2021. *JAMA.* 2021;325(11):1101-1102.

SECTION XXVII
CLINICAL PRACTICE

340

IMPROVING PATIENT TRUST: TIPS FOR PATIENT SATISFACTION

TODD D. MORRELL

Patient satisfaction is essential to patient care. In recent history, the subject of patient satisfaction has been a source of frustration for providers and administrators. We have developed a habit of reducing this complex subject to patient surveys with worn and unrevealing questions, often in an attempt to improve satisfaction scores in a superficial manner. However, stepping back from tired surveys, patient satisfaction is the patient's experience of our care, and that experience holds the care together. The degree of satisfaction is the measure of the degree to which we emergency physicians and providers have been able to understand and empathetically meet the needs and hopes of our patients. Our success determines if our patients will entrust their health and concerns to us.

While ED volumes dropped temporarily during the COVID-19 pandemic, they have soared since. Compounded by staffing and flow problems, the patient experience has only worsened as we emerge from the pandemic with long waits, crowded departments, limited privacy, and extended boarding. The situation is further complicated by a new distrust of medicine and physicians on the part of some patients. Now more than ever, it is vital that we can understand our patients and communicate our commitment to their best interests.

Patient experience is complex, and no single behavior or phrase will guarantee every patient's satisfaction, but there are essential principles that apply to most patients. In the ED communication, patient-centered care, empathy, and comfort each impact the patient experience.

Communication with patients is bidirectional. Listening not only to the details of the patient's history but also to their hopes for the visit and then reflecting those to the patient demonstrates that we understand why they are there. Many patients are seeking relief from pain some are looking for reassurance concerning a potentially serious diagnosis and some have come out of frustration with their inability to access care elsewhere. Regardless of the reason for the visit, reflecting it back to the patient in an understanding manner assures that we have understood their concerns, which in turn increases their trust in our care. Communicating test results promptly, following up with the patient to understand their response to treatments, and communicating delays are all important.

At the end of the visit, whether the patient is admitted or discharged, we should explain diagnoses, next steps in care, and precautions.

Communication need not end at discharge. Follow-up phone calls from emergency physicians are sadly uncommon, but there may be no easier way to become the best physician your patient has ever met. A timely phone call to a patient gives them the opportunity to ask additional questions and will occasionally reveal a worsening condition that may need to be returned to the ED. Most patients will find the phone call exceptional and will be respectful of the physician's time.

Patient-centered care is an often-recited phrase, which can deplete it of meaning. Nevertheless, it is an important concept, and there are opportunities in the ED to properly orient our care around the patient. Understanding the patient's values and priorities can help direct care. Some patients come with an agenda to be admitted, while others are adamant that they be discharged home. Not every request can be accommodated, but when possible, care and communication should be centered around these desires. Understanding the goals of care for the older individuals and the chronically ill can also afford opportunities to orient around patient desires. Respect for patient privacy during the physical exam or sensitive conversations are also opportunities to respect the patient.

The physical environment and patient comfort are important elements of patient satisfaction. Unfortunately, many aspects of the ED are not conducive to patient comfort. It is often bright and loud and affords little privacy. This makes it all the more important that the emergency physician attend to patient comfort where possible. The efforts need not be large ones: adjusting the patient's bed, getting a warm blanket, and, if there is no reason for the patient to be NPO, offering water, will all go a long way in improving patient comfort. Attention to the patient's family also communicates concern for their experience. Returning to the room with an extra glass of water is a very small action that can help patients see their care as exceptional.

Empathy is a difficult quality to teach or quantify, yet patients often cite it as an important attribute in physicians. Empathy and compassion are often inherent in the areas listed earlier: communication, patient-centeredness, and concern for comfort. Yet, there are still opportunities for simple "I understand" statements. When a patient has come to the end of their ED care and has no definitive diagnosis, an "I understand" statement such as "I understand that it is frustrating to not have a name for what is going on, but even without a name, we can still do these things to make you feel better." Statements such as these can still be meaningful.

Attending to the patient's experience is an essential element of providing care and should be an end in and of itself. However, multiple positive associations also demonstrate the benefits of maximizing patient satisfaction. Patients are more likely to be compliant with therapy when they trust the provider and are satisfied with their care. The risk of medical malpractice is reduced, even in the setting of unexpected outcomes. Patients who are highly satisfied with their care are likely to tell friends and relatives, improving institutional reputation and increasing institutional loyalty.

In a time of constant surveys and online reviews, patient satisfaction may seem like a belabored subject. However, at its heart, it is an essential part of being a compassionate provider. Even in the midst of a hectic ED, a bit of attention to being the kind of physician our mothers tell people we are will go a long way toward being an effective physician whom patients will tell their family about.

PEARLS

- Patient-centered care, empathy, and comfort each impact the patient's experience.
- Understanding patients' values and priorities helps direct care.
- High satisfaction should be an end in itself, but it is also associated with increased compliance, decreased lawsuits, and institutional loyalty.

SUGGESTED READING

Garmel G. 10 tips to improve patient satisfaction in the emergency department. Academic Life in Emergency Medicine; 2018. Accessed February 25, 2023. https://www.aliem.com/10-tips-improve-patient-satisfaction/

341

YOUR PATIENT HAS DIED: HOW TO DELIVER BAD NEWS TO FAMILY MEMBERS

HEIDI MARIA TEAGUE

While providers in the ED encounter innumerable challenges caring for patients, delivering bad news to family members is one of the most intimidating. Although the ED is not the ideal location for end-of-life care, it is unfortunately not an uncommon outcome of an ED encounter. Acknowledging that delivering bad news is a difficult and emotional task is a step toward providing supportive patient- and family-centered care. Communicating a bad outcome does not have to be the most stressful and unsettling challenge that we face. Tools and resources are available in the literature to help guide us when breaking bad news. Training and role-playing exercises can support the development of the skills and confidence needed to deliver bad news with compassion and sensitivity, leading to more positive emotional outcomes for family, loved ones, and ourselves.

Family members may be in a state of shock or disbelief when hearing that their loved one has died, but we can take steps to decrease their burden and allow for emotional healing to begin. In our hectic environment, we must pause and prepare prior to delivering bad news. Before meeting with the family, gather all relevant information, including the patient's medical history and events leading to their death. Identify a private and quiet setting for the conversation, even if that is simply a quiet corner. Have items such as tissue, water, and appropriate seating. Whenever available, include hospital chaplaincy, social workers, or other support services. Approach family members with sensitivity and compassion, using clear and simple language without medical jargon. Begin with introductions, providing names and roles of the ED team members, and obtaining family members' names and relations to the patient. Consider using the Ask-Tell-Ask approach to portray empathy and respect. Ask: Begin by asking what the family's knowledge of the incident is so far. Tell: Obtain permission to tell them what you know, providing a clear summary of the event without medical terms using culturally and educationally appropriate language. Conclude your summary with a direct and clear statement: "I'm sorry to tell you that your loved one has died." After delivering the bad news, pause and allow family members time to process the information and express their emotions. Ask: Give them the opportunity to ask questions, allowing them to feel heard. Understand they might express disbelief, anger, shock, or sadness. Provide honest and clear responses to any questions or concerns. If the cause of death is unknown, explain that further investigation will be needed. Acknowledge their feelings, providing empathy and support. For example, "I wish there was more we could have done; I'm very sorry for your loss." "We understand this is difficult news to hear, and we are here to support you. Is there anyone I can call for you?" "Please take your time and let us know if there is anything we can do to help." Be aware of and respect cultural, spiritual, and religious beliefs, involving an appropriate liaison to ensure family needs are being met if necessary.

Be prepared to provide practical information and resources. If possible, solicit assistance from social work and chaplaincy to provide information regarding funeral arrangements, support groups, or counseling services. When delivering bad news to family members after a death, also remember the emotional toll events have on ED providers. Consider instituting debriefing protocols for the ED team and options for closure, such as sending the family a sympathy card.

Many of us feel underprepared to communicate a patient's death effectively and empathetically to family members and loved ones. It is important to recognize that improving our patients' outcomes and providing lifesaving care are our goals. While ED providers often perceive a patient's death as a failure, it is often a natural outcome of a patient's medical illness that is out of our control. Rather than seeing death as failure, learning to communicate a patient's death to family members in a culturally sensitive and compassionate manner should be viewed as an opportunity for personal growth. Short education sessions involving simulation, role-playing, feedback, and debriefing can help prepare us for managing bad news. Having the SPIKES protocol and six steps developed by oncology providers, Setting, Perception, Invitation, Knowledge, Emotion, and Strategy, available to providers and incorporating the Ask-Tell-Ask approach to communication can enhance educational training and provide ED providers with both the skills and confidence they need.

Delivering bad news about a patient's death to family members is difficult. It requires compassion, sensitivity, and clear communication. Preparing for the conversation, using clear and simple language devoid of medical jargon, and providing emotional support and practical information can help ease the burden of grief and support loved ones. While never easy, delivering bad news is an essential part of providing compassionate and patient-centered care.

PEARLS

- View the patient's death not as a failure but as an opportunity to provide compassionate communication to support families and loved ones.
- Understand what the family and loved ones' knowledge of the situation is. Ask to share what you know.
- Use direct, empathetic communication using basic language.

- Include hospital chaplaincy, social workers, or other support services available in the conversation, if available.
- Provide training and role-play scenarios to improve physician/staff comfort with the delivery of bad news.

SUGGESTED READINGS

Elmer J, Mikati N, Arnold RM, Wallace DJ, Callaway CW. Death and end-of-life care in emergency departments in the US. *JAMA Netw Open*. 2022;5(11):e2240399.

Geller DE, Dowling Evans D. Death and dying in the emergency department. *Adv Emerg Nurs J*. 2020;42(2):81-89.

Harris D, Gilligan T. Delivering bad news. *Med Clin North Am*. 2022;106(4):641-651.

Meier DE. The human connection of Palliative Care: ten steps for what to say and do [Video]. YouTube; 2013. https://www.youtube.com/watch?v=7kQ3PUyhmPQ

Servotte J-C, Bragard I, Szyld D, et al. Efficacy of a short role-play training on breaking bad news in the emergency department. *West J Emerg Med*. 2019;20(6):893-902.

342

DISCHARGE DOCUMENTATION: KEEP IT CLEAR, CONCISE, YET COMPLETE

ALBERT FIORELLO

You are ready to send your patient home with a prescription and instructions for close follow-up. There are now only two things left to do: Prepare the discharge instructions and discharge the patient. In some cases, these last steps could be as important, if not more important, than what you have done thus far. Your thorough diagnostic evaluation and excellent treatment in the ED could be negated by the patient failing to follow your discharge and follow-up instructions. Compliance with recommended treatment after discharge from the ED has been shown to be related to patient satisfaction with the discharge instructions. In one study, an independent predictor of not filling prescriptions was dissatisfaction with discharge instructions, whether it be dissatisfaction with the explanation of the medical problem, instructions for treatment, or instructions for follow-up.

Lack of comprehension of discharge instructions is a significant barrier to receiving appropriate care following discharge. In one study, patients were interviewed immediately after discharge, and 78% demonstrated some deficiency in comprehension of their discharge instructions. Possibly more concerning, of those demonstrating a deficiency in comprehension, only 20% perceived difficulty with comprehension. Adding written instructions to verbal instructions helps reinforce the instructions and gives the patient something to refer to after discharge. A meta-analysis demonstrated that adding written instructions to verbal instructions increased recall from 47% to 58%. Unfortunately, some premade complaint or diagnosis-based instructions are written at a level that is difficult for some patients in ED with lower health literacy to understand. Patients with lower incomes and those who have not graduated from high school have been shown to be at higher risk of not understanding discharge instructions, particularly when there is a language barrier.

ED discharge instructions should contain:

- The diagnosis or clinical impression: If an exact diagnosis is not known at the conclusion of the ED visit, general complaint-based instructions can be provided. For example, instructions for "abdominal pain" may be more appropriate than instructions for "gastroenteritis" if the diagnosis is not certain. Aftercare instructions for the condition should be provided, such as splint care and wound care.
- The expected course for their condition: Patients should be informed what to expect after discharge and, maybe more importantly, what not to expect. If unexpected signs or symptoms arise, the patient needs to know that they should return to the ED for reevaluation.
- Information regarding medications provided in the ED as well as any prescriptions written: This should include precautions regarding any potentially sedating medications and appropriate restrictions. If you recommend changing any of the patient's current medications, this should be clearly stated in the instructions. If prescriptions were electronically sent to a pharmacy, the address and phone number of the pharmacy should be included.
- Follow-up instructions: These instructions should be *action-specific and time-specific* (eg, "follow up with your primary care Dr Jones in his office at 232 Main Street (999-999-9999) within 1 week," rather than simply "follow with your PCP"). Engaging the patient in selecting a time for follow-up and making actual follow-up appointments prior to leaving the ED may improve follow-up compliance and decrease no-show rates.
- Diagnostic studies performed: Any abnormal findings or incidental findings, such as a lung nodule requiring follow-up, should be highlighted and specific follow-up instructions included. Any diagnostic studies with pending results should be listed with a plan for follow-up on those results.
- Return to activity/work/school instructions: Specific notes with restrictions should be provided as needed.
- If the institution has an electronic patient portal, instructions on accessing the portal should be included so that the patient may access their records.

Many EMRs will suggest or prepopulate discharge instructions based on the complaint or entered diagnosis. These are a good starting point for developing a patient's discharge instructions, but the emergency physician should know what is included in these premade instructions and modify them as needed. For example, instructions for an ankle sprain may recommend the use of Tylenol for pain. But this would not be appropriate for a patient with advanced liver disease. So, it is important for the emergency physician to personalize the discharge instructions for each patient. When personalizing the instructions, avoid the use of abbreviations that may be unfamiliar to the patient (eg, f/u in AM with PCP or 1 tab q6h PRN).

Although written discharge instructions are important and helpful, they are not a substitute for verbal instructions and provide the patient with an opportunity to have questions answered. A "teach-back" method where patients repeat what they understand about their discharge instructions may improve knowledge retention and resource utilization.

Ideally, both written and verbal instructions should be provided in the patient's primary language. If it is not possible to provide written instructions in their language, at least a verbal review of the instructions should be provided through a translator.

The EMR can reduce the time required to prepare discharge instructions for patients, but sometimes the EMR can produce overly lengthy instructions that are actually counterproductive. It is important to highlight the important details when reviewing them with the patient. The goal is that take-home messages are clear, concise, and complete.

PEARLS

- Use premade complaint or diagnosis-based discharge instructions, but know the content of those instructions and personalize them as needed for each patient.
- Provide instructions in a way that can be understood by the patient.
- Ensure that the patient understands their instructions, including the next steps in their care.

SUGGESTED READINGS

Hesselink G, Sir O, Koster N, et al. Teach-back of discharge instructions in the emergency department: a pre-post pilot evaluation. *Emerg Med J*. 2022;39(2):139-146.

Hoek AE, Anker SCP, Van Beeck EF, Burdorf A, Rood PPM, Haagsma JA. Patient discharge instructions in the emergency department and their effects on comprehension and recall of discharge instructions: a systematic review and meta-analysis. *Ann Emerg Med*. 2020;75(3):435-444.

Sheikh H, Brezar A, Dzwonek A, Yau L, Calder LA. Patient understanding of discharge instructions in the emergency department: do different patients need different approaches? *Int J Emerg Med*. 2018;11(1):5.

Vinson DR, Patel PB. Facilitating follow-up after emergency care using an appointment assignment system. *J Healthc Qual*. 2009;31(6):18-24.

343

ADVANCED PRACTICE PROVIDER SUPERVISION IN THE EMERGENCY SETTING

MELISSA E. ZUKOWSKI AND ANDREW BELUS

BACKGROUND

Utilization of PAs and NPs, collectively known as advanced practice providers, is now commonplace in the ED. As EDs continue to experience overcrowding due to rising patient volumes, an aging population, and a worsening boarding crisis, it has become clear that a collaborative model is necessary. APPs are part of the staffing model in diverse settings, including urban, rural, community, and academic hospitals. Some EDs only utilize APPs to evaluate and treat patients with lower ESI scores, while other APPs may care for critically ill patients. The AMA, ACEP, ABEM, and other professional boards advocate for physician-led care for all ED patients, while recognizing the value brought to the medical team by APPs.

Scope of Practice

In its most basic form, physician supervision consists of delegating which healthcare tasks an APP may or may not perform. The first factor determining APP scope of practice is state laws and regulations, which vary widely. All 50 states currently require PAs to have a formal agreement with a supervising physician, while NPs can legally practice independently in many states. Conversely, regulations allow wide latitude in the procedures a supervising physician may delegate to a PA, while some procedures and interventions (ie, blood transfusion and lumbar puncture) are specifically forbidden for NPs in certain settings. Supervising physicians must be familiar with local regulations to effectively supervise APPs.

Beyond state level regulations, each hospital and practice group will have their own norms and policies that further guide the scope of practice for APPs. For example, a rural ED may employ an APP as the only provider on shift. The APP in this setting, who may only have access to a supervising physician via telephone, will likely have a broader scope of practice than an APP working alongside a physician in an urban center.

The educational background, training, and experience of the APP are also critical in determining their scope of practice. Pediatrics is an important example of a specialized population—FNPs, PNPs, and PAs are all able to see children following their training programs, while other APPs cannot. An APP's background and comfort with a specific patient population are an important factor to consider when determining the scope of practice. The last, and perhaps most important factor in determining the APP scope of practice, is the comfort level of the individual supervising physician who will be delegating the tasks in question.

Onboarding

Bringing an APP into the department requires a multidisciplinary team. Often, the most successful model for APP leadership includes a department administrator, a medical director, and a lead APP who each work collaboratively to ensure the success and strength of the program. Understanding the training and background of the onboarding APP is of utmost importance. Variations in training can be very broad and may dictate what initial credentials, training, and onsite onboarding are needed for one APP compared to another. Many EDs begin by gradually progressing in responsibility and acuity as an APP, new to emergency medicine, gains experience in their respective departments. Many EDs offer "Boot Camps" to introduce or refresh skills, reviewing common chief complaints and procedures. Initial credentialing may require a focused evaluation of supervised skills ("Initial Focused Professional Practice Evaluation") until that APP can be signed off to perform the skillset independently. Each of these processes makes for a stronger, more cohesive team, which is critical to successful integration of APPs into an ED.

Structure of Supervision

As with onboarding, the structure of APP supervision will appropriately vary between individual APPs. A new graduate will require much closer supervision than a seasoned provider. Case presentations and face-to-face evaluation of the patient before discharge may be warranted for new graduate APPs until both the APP and the supervising physician are comfortable with greater autonomy. Retrospective chart review can act as a bridge to more independent practice with experienced providers seeking direct supervision only on a case-by-case basis.

Many models of supervision exist in EDs that utilize APPs. This variability allows APPs to flex to meet the needs of a wide range of clinical scenarios. A model for APP staffing in a rural setting likely looks different than in an urban setting. A community ED may choose to use its APPs differently than an academic center, where a balance must be struck between faculty physicians, resident learners, and the APP team. The most common models utilize APPs in lower-acuity treatment spaces or in the main ED, working alongside a physician colleague.

More recently, APPs have become key team members in triage, where they have been highly successful in initiating care, including ordering initial labs and imaging. These models have been critical in improving overall ED throughput and reducing key ED metrics such as door-to-doc times and LWOT numbers.

Lastly, some EDs are utilizing their APP workforce on the back end of the ED. Many EDs that oversee observation units find that APPs function very effectively in these care areas. In addition, some departments have used APPs for continuity of care for boarding patients, recognizing the need for consistent care teams for these patients.

Whichever model is selected for an individual department, success will lie in teamwork and open communication between all groups—physicians, APPs, and nurses. A clearly defined supervisory model that promotes collaboration will ensure provider satisfaction and highly reliable patient care and safety.

PEARLS

- Be well-versed in your individual state's laws and regulations and your hospital's policies and bylaws as they pertain to the APP scope of practice.
- Understand the specific educational background, training, and experience of each APP who is joining your ED team.
- Ensure a strong, cohesive leadership team and an individualized onboarding plan for your new APPs.
- APP supervision should be consistent and collaborative to maximize APP and physician satisfaction. Remove barriers to collaboration, whether actual or perceived.

SUGGESTED READINGS

Chekijian SA, Elia TR, Monti JE, Temin ES. Integration of advanced practice providers in academic emergency departments: best practices and considerations. *AEM Educ Train.* 2018;2(suppl 1):S48-S55.

Clark A, Amanti C, Sheng AY. Supervision of advanced practice providers. *Emerg Med Clin.* 2020;38(2):353-361.

344

WHAT TO DO WITH SO MANY? STRATEGIES FOR REDUCING EMERGENCY DEPARTMENT OVERCROWDING

JONATHAN SCOTT LOWRY

ED overcrowding has gone from an occasional, cyclic issue hospitals face to a pandemic level dealt with daily in nearly every ED across the country and much of the world. Although it is easy to blame COVID-19 for this problem, it was only the catalyst to our current situation. The short-term fix on "what to do with so many patients" is fairly straightforward. The long-term fix is more complicated. The most popular short-term fix is finding alternative care sites within the department. Hallway beds, chairs, double-rooming patients with curtains to separate them, treating patients in the lobby, or even adding portable tents in the parking lot are frequent flexes a department may implement to cram more patients into their overcrowded ED. What is the problem here? We are just adding patients to the department, not getting them out, like overfilling a balloon. If we don't let the air out, the balloon will burst. To use a classier medical analogy: "You can't cure constipation by adding more colon." ED overcrowding is a symptom of a larger problem; the fix requires hospital and system-wide change. Treating patients in hallways and chairs, the lobby, and tents in the parking lot are temporary fixes. Each of these alternative care spaces brings inherent dangers for the patients, providers, and the hospital itself. Sick patients cannot be treated adequately in a chair, most exams cannot be completed in the hallway, and patients cannot be properly monitored in a tent in the parking lot. Choosing the right patient for each site also becomes problematic when you have sicker patients waiting, not just "walking well."

Even before 2019, we had statistics from departments across the country showing patient arrival and acuity per hour with enough detail to allow comments at director courses like "We know how many patients will arrive; we know their chief complaints; we just don't know their names yet." This quote has stuck in my mind since an ACEP ED Directors Academy course before COVID-19. Many departments have this granular data, and most EMRs are able to spit it out with the click of a mouse. We can use these data to anticipate the incoming needs for our departments and adjust our staffing to match. In a perfect system, matching our workforce to our incoming needs should result in zero wait times and empty lobbies. Yet, our lobbies are overflowing, and our wait times are exceeding the length of our shifts. We have patients dying in waiting rooms across the country while waiting to be seen. Bottlenecked patient flow disrupts the correlation of patient influx and department census. Staffing to influxes no longer works when the patients do not leave the department. You have to staff to match the census and take care of the patients *still* in the department.

When anticipating surges, validated tools, such as the NEDOCS score, can be very useful in showing the status of the department and identifying triggers to activate contingencies like opening those aforementioned alternative care sites and expediting discharges upstairs. Having a specific score set as a trigger to switch to survival mode can be very helpful for both staff buy-in and administrative support. The issue here becomes sticking to the plan each time the score reaches this trigger point without inciting "alarm fatigue." The threshold to activate your alternative plans needs to be low enough that you have time to get things in motion before the situation gets worse. There also needs to be a *lower* number or a set of requirements that triggers the deactivation of the flex plan. If the activation and deactivation numbers are too close, you will yo-yo back and forth too quickly, setting yourself up for alarm fatigue and failure.

One validated solution, published throughout the literature, involves the use of inpatient hallway beds. When admitted patients are moved upstairs into inpatient hallways to await rooming, they are bedded faster than waiting in the ED for the same room. Building a NEDOCS score as a trigger to open inpatient hallway beds would be a great pop-off valve for acute surges in the ED that may prevent the need for more drastic measures.

Creating a clear plan to deal with your patient's surge is critical to managing the bolus when it inevitably comes. Fixing an overcrowded system is complicated; it requires a high level of hospital administration to manage. The only way to fix ED overcrowding is to fix the whole hospital system's throughput. You have to get existing patients out of the ED to see new ones and clear the waiting room—circling back to that colon metaphor, the solution to constipation isn't building a bigger colon. ED boarding compounds every aspect of ED overcrowding. Without high-level administrative support, system changes cannot take place, and smaller efforts on the departmental side will realistically just be band-aids—band-aids that, of course, you will receive after waiting 12 hours to be seen.

PEARLS

- Alternative care sites can help see more patients in a full ED.
- Matching staffing to patient flow is efficient until the ED is saturated.
- ED census measures, such as NEDOCS, can help set triggers for when to activate surge policies.
- ED overcrowding is a symptom of a larger problem; the fix requires hospital and even system-wide change.

Suggested Readings

Hernandez N, John D, Mitchell J. A reimagined discharge lounge as a way to an efficient discharge process. *BMJ Qual Improv Rep.* 2014;3(1):u204930.w2080.

Janke AT, Melnick ER, Venkatesh AK. Hospital occupancy and emergency department boarding during the COVID-19 pandemic. *JAMA Netw Open.* 2022;5(9):e2233964.

Laam LA, Wary AA, Strony RS, Fitzpatrick MH, Kraus CK. Quantifying the impact of patient boarding on emergency department length of stay: all admitted patients are negatively affected by boarding. *J Am Coll Emerg Open.* 2021;2:e12401.

Stead LG, Jain A, Decker WW. Emergency department over-crowding: a global perspective. *Int J Emerg Med.* 2009;2:133-134.

345

IT'S NOT MY FAULT! HOSPITAL ISSUES LEADING TO ED BOARDING AND HOW TO FIX THEM

JONATHAN SCOTT LOWRY

Bottlenecks and delays in ED throughput come from sources internal and external to the ED. Internal issues are the first to be blamed in every system: slow doctors with excessive workups (it *is* my fault?), increased doctor-to-disposition times (it *really* is?), resource overutilization, and slow room/bed turnover. Internal issues are easy to point fingers at; however, time and time again, they have been shown to be almost irrelevant in systems with ED overcrowding (It's *not* my fault! Phew!). External issues, such as radiology turnaround times, lab delays, consult response times, and boarding, account for the vast majority of ED-specific delays. Every delay adds to ED length of stay, and the perpetual influx of patients worsens overcrowding further. ED boarding compounds these issues by forcing the department to see and treat the same number of patients, even though we already know they are coming in, through a significantly reduced number of beds. This leads to only the sickest patients coming back to open rooms, requiring admission, clogging yet another bed, and decreasing the number of rooms available to see patients. In this way, ED boarding increases ED boarding in a continual positive feedback loop. Queuing theory describes the dramatic consequences of removing beds, just like reducing a teller at a bank, or a register at a retail store. It forces providers to seek out and develop alternative care spaces to treat patients.

While the internal and external issues noted above are additive to the problem, ED boarding is multiplicative. The most effective measure we can take to decrease ED overcrowding is to reduce or remove ED boarding. Keeping ED rooms open allows the department to evaluate and treat additional patients. The rest of the issues now become your problems, and barriers to efficiency can be addressed within the ED. Without fixing the boarding problem, the other issues are moot. When a 60-bed ED has 45 boarders, slow radiology turnaround times and long waits for consults feel like they are absolutely destroying the department's efficiency; if you were functioning with all 60 beds, the impact would be significantly minimized.

ED boarding is a multisystem problem that begins with bed availability on the inpatient side. Hospital census versus capacity is comparable to ED boarding. If the hospital has all of its beds open and staffed, ED boarding is limited until the hospital approaches capacity. Most systems have been shown to start backing up at 85% inpatient capacity. Incoming inpatient admissions are as predictable as ED patient arrivals, with statistics to tabulate patient arrivals from each source to inpatient floors. We may not know names, but we know how many and what diagnoses we will admit. Staffing beds to this anticipated number should be the starting point. Beyond that, with the predictable number of incoming admissions, the fix to hospital overcrowding is discharge—with a focus on decreased hospital length of stay. Barriers to hospital discharge become the next logical target. Within the hospital, rapid consult service response times, early physical and occupational therapy evaluations, pharmacy medicine reconciliation, and after-care planning all facilitate earlier hospital discharge. Creation of time goals or deadlines and actionable plans for these services helps to eliminate barriers to discharge.

Safe discharge with case management and pharmacy medication reconciliation is argued by some internists to be *the* major delay in inpatient discharges. Case management and environmental services should be overstaffed. Using the queuing theory, they should be upstaffed until they have 10% to 15% downtime per shift to avoid bottlenecks. Other delays are external to the hospital, such as limited bed availability at skilled nursing facilities. This can be difficult to address without the hospital system acquiring such facilities.

Another target for increasing hospital throughput to decrease boarding and overcrowding is consult response times. Every patient in the ED should be admitted or discharged in less than 4 hours. Consultants often request imaging, which may require labs for contrast or negative pregnancy test, often done in series rather than parallel. If a consult is going to take more than an hour, consider admission for evaluation and workup. One argument against admitting for consults is that bylaws for most hospitals state consults in the ED should be seen in hours, whereas a consult on the floor must be seen in days. Because of potential delay upstairs, the admitting team may request the ED team to have the patient seen by the consultant before admission. Consultants may be busy in the OR or in clinic seeing patients. So the consult is put off until after the OR case or after the clinic is over. This further delays disposition and ties up a room pending consultation before admission (or an inpatient discharge!). These hours waiting for consults dramatically increase the length of stay, hold up the bed, and decrease patient satisfaction (direct negative correlation with the length of stay and ED wait time). Tracking consult response times and actually holding departments accountable for following the hospital bylaws is the only way to decrease this delay. Adding ancillary staff like APPs to assist in consults is one cost-effective response.

The high level of change that will be needed to fix ED boarding will require buy-in and support from administration at the top of the food chain of your system. It will take a village, not just our own shop.

PEARLS

- Bottlenecks and delays in ED throughput come from sources internal and external to the ED.
- ED boarding is a multisystem problem that begins with bed availability on the inpatient side.
- You have to fix ED boarding before other internal changes will be effective.
- Real change to fix ED overcrowding requires changes at the hospital level.

Suggested Readings

Fomundam S, Herrmann JW. *A Survey of Queuing Theory Applications in Healthcare*. Institute for Systems Research Technical Reports; 2007. http://hdl.handle.net/1903/7222

Kelen G, Peterson S, Pronovost P. In the name of patient safety, let's burden the emergency department more. *Ann Emerg Med*. 2016;67(6):737-740.

Patel P, Combs M, Vinson DR. Reduction of admit wait times: the effect of a leadership-based program. *Acad Emerg Med*. 2014;21:266-273.

346

YOUR DEPOSITION

KEVIN M. KLAUER

What we do not understand will not only be anxiety provoking but can result in self-victimization from the "law" of unintended consequences. Your deposition is a prime example. A deposition is defined by Black's Law Dictionary as "A witnesses out of court testimony that is reduced to writing for later use in court or for discovery purposes."

What is importantly *not* part of that definition is "This is the doctor's day in court." The misapprehension that this is your day in court is perhaps the greatest and most dangerous misunderstanding that physicians have of the legal process.

Your deposition will be scheduled early in the course of a medical-legal case. The deposition is the cornerstone of the discovery phase. Many decisions will be made based on your deposition performance, which may even include dismissing the claim(s) against you. However, if the plaintiff's attorney has done their homework, dismissal is very unlikely, as the goal of the deposition isn't to "find facts" but rather to find facts that support specific arguments and theories of allegation.

Generally speaking, there are several goals of a deposition: testing existing theories/allegations, identifying new theories, sizing you up, and setting the trap.

Prior to pursuing a case, the plaintiff's attorney will secure experts to review the case and provide an opinion regarding whether or not the care fell below the standard of care, what aspects of the care were substandard, and whether they are defensible. These experts will provide the basis for the claim and the allegations against you. However, these theories and allegations must be tested. Does the defendant have a plausible explanation? Are there additional facts that would undermine their theories? These and other questions are answered through the deposition process.

To a large extent, depositions are fishing expeditions. Such fishing expeditions may yield new facts, new insights, and even new theories/allegations to pursue. That is why, when being deposed by a plaintiff's attorney, it is your day to be as quiet as possible and is not "your day in court." Make them do the work. Do not fall victim to the well-intentioned urge to explain yourself in the hopes of convincing them that their allegations are wrong. The more you say, the more is transcribed, and the more you will be accountable for at a future date, in particular, at trial. In other words, if they want to fish for facts to use against you, don't throw the fish in their boat. Make them work for it.

Much of the discovery phase of a lawsuit is determining strategy. Another very important aspect is to determine what kind of witness you will make. Are you credible? Will the jury like you? Are you overtly nervous? Can you defend your actions and the care you provided? These and many other questions will be answered in your deposition. As a matter of fact, they are likely to audio or video your deposition for this exact purpose. If you are a good witness, this will play well for you. If you aren't, this is more opportunity and leverage for the plaintiff's attorney to pursue higher settlement demands.

Perhaps, the most challenging part of the deposition is maintaining consistency of your message. This can be mentally taxing. The last thing you want is the plaintiff's attorney using your own words to discredit you. It is bad enough that they can secure expert witnesses to weaken your case, but it is devastating when the defendant aids them in this crusade. As previously noted, the plaintiff's attorney has theories, and they intend to prove them at your expense. They are likely to ask you the same question or similar questions multiple times. Don't lose your focus. This is a game of cat and mouse, and they will try to shape your testimony as a trap to be used against you.

The trap is a product of mental confusion. If they ask you a question enough times or in enough different ways, you are likely to contradict yourself. You will be asked a similar or identical question at trial, and such self-incriminating statements will be recited in front of the jury. No one will know what trickery occurred to extract that particular response from you; it will simply appear that on the day of your deposition, you said one thing, and in the courtroom, you said another. So, be smart, be consistent, and be quiet. The less said in a deposition, the better.

Preparation for your deposition is critical. Mock depositions to prepare for anticipated lines of questioning are essential. Your defense counsel can assist with crafting your messages and getting you comfortable with the process. Plan on a long day. You should be well rested and well fed. Although it seems like a fine line, you're being deposed, not interrogated. If you want a break for any reason, just ask for one. Dress in business attire, be respectful, be truthful, and maintain good eye contact. If you don't understand a question, don't answer it until it is clarified.

PEARLS

- The purpose of the deposition is fact-finding but not to discover the truth.
- Consistent application of carefully reasoned responses to difficult questions is critical to protecting yourself.
- Approach this like an important exam: study, get plenty of rest, and eat a good meal in advance.
- If you don't remember, simply respond, "I don't remember."
- If at all possible, be cordial, positive, engaging, and maintain eye contact.

Suggested Readings

Bal BS. An introduction to medical malpractice in the United States. *Clin Orthop Relat Res.* 2009;467(2):339-347.

Carrier ER, Reschovsky JD, Mello MM, et al. Physicians' fears of malpractice lawsuits are not assuaged by tort reforms. *Health Aff.* 2010;29:91585-91592.

Kessler DP. Evaluating the medical malpractice system and options for reform. *J Econ Persp.* 2011;25(2):93-110.

Struve CT. Malpractice crisis: improving the medical malpractice litigation process. *Health Aff.* 2004;23:433-441.

Weinstock MB, Klauer KM, Henry GL. *Bouncebacks! Medical.* Anadem Publishing; 2007.

347

SAY WHAT? HOW TO MAXIMIZE THE TRANSFER OF CARE WITH YOUR EMS PROVIDERS

JOHN BROWN AND JEFF COVITZ

INTRODUCTION

One of the most neglected areas of critical patient care in emergency medicine involves the fostering of the strong connection needed between prehospital providers (your EMS crews) and ED personnel. This chapter will focus on improving three critical time intervals in the trajectory of care for patients who transition from the 911 system to your ED.

BEFORE PATIENT ARRIVAL

Many EDs provide direct medical oversight (online medical control) for EMS provider agencies in their jurisdiction. Communication systems often involve a remote (off-site) connection between providers and a qualified emergency physician by radio or cell phone on a recorded line. It is important to understand what the purpose of the EMS provider's call is: help with treatment, destination triage, managing the risk in an "against medical advice" patient disposition, or termination of resuscitation efforts. Remember that "lights and sirens" transport of a patient in the latter two situations involves inherent risks to the patient, the providers, the public, and sometimes, to the family. Be sure that provider-to-physician communication is clear on the reason for the consultation and ask the provider to "Lead with the Headline."

WHEN THE PATIENT ARRIVES IN THE ED

Consider the following scenario from a critically ill patient delivered by your EMS providers:

As the paramedics wheel the patient into the resuscitation room, you notice a supraglottic airway in place, and the patient is attached to the EMS cardiac monitor, but you can barely make out a rhythm . . . paced? The paramedics and firefighters wheeling in the patient are drenched in sweat.

You shout above the cacophony of voices in the room:

"I'll take a report!"

You are half listening to the paramedic, something about PEA to v-fib to brady to paced, and feeling for a radial pulse while one of the nurses is removing the prehospital defib pads and replacing them. The paramedic shouts something,

"Hey! . . . . pacer . . . ! Being paced!"

You ignore it as the ED's cardiac monitor connects to the patient. You feel no femoral pulse and note wide, complex PEA on the monitor.

"He doesn't have a pulse." You shout, *"Begin CPR."*

You are annoyed that EMS brought in a patient without recognizing that he does not have a pulse. The paramedic is still speaking, but you disregard him, disconnecting the supraglottic airway to intubate the patient. A nurse abruptly closes a curtain, effectively shutting out the team of paramedics and firefighters from the room.

After the difficult airway is secured, followed by several more interventions by you and your ED staff, you pronounce:

"Time of death, 16:40."

Emergency physicians need to appreciate the emotional (and physical) investment paramedics and EMTs place in a high-acuity EMS call. They exert tremendous physical and emotional energy to bring the patient to you with a pulse and blood pressure. It is critical to have a single point of contact on the hospital team side, with the receiving physician using closed-loop communication techniques to ensure that critical information is received and understood. Unless an immediate life threat is detected, the cessation or removal of field-provided therapeutic interventions is unwarranted and may produce direct harm.

Develop a culture of open communication; it is critical to encourage direct contact between EMS providers and ED physicians. Patients have a reasonable expectation that the prehospital-to-hospital handoff should be as seamless as possible—that everything the EMS crew knows, the ED staff knows, allowing the ED physician to build upon everything the EMS crew has accomplished.

After the EMS Crew Has Left the ED

While following the guidelines listed so far in this chapter will help you minimize gaps in communication or concerns you might have over patient care, there still may be a need to follow up with EMS providers or their organizations after their departure from your ED. Your EMS 911 dispatch center can contact the relevant EMS supervisor and request additional patient care information from the treating EMS providers. They can also report a concern you might have with the patient's care. If your EMS system has moved to an electronic, cloud-based data system, you can obtain read-only access to prehospital care records. Concerns over patient care you might have cannot be reviewed and converted to action for improvement unless you take the time to report them in the same respectful, professional, and timely manner that you appreciate yourself when receiving feedback on your own patient care skills.

PEARLS

- If you're providing online medical oversight remotely to your EMS providers, be sure they "paint" an adequate picture of the case for you.
- Don't remove life-sustaining equipment from a patient brought to you by EMS (eg, pacemaker) unless you are sure that either they are harming the patient or that you are completely ready to provide a substitute.
- Identify yourself as the responsible person to take the report from the EMS provider and use closed-loop communication techniques.
- Develop a culture of open communication with your EMS providers so they are comfortable approaching you with concerns and prioritize interacting with them when they bring a patient to your ED.
- Contact your EMS dispatch center and the on-duty EMS supervisor for critical information lost in the transfer of care or to assist with a critical concern about care rendered to an EMS patient.

Suggested Readings

Ragger K, Hiebler-Ragger M, Herzog G, Kapfhammer HP, Unterrainer HF. Sense of coherence is linked to post-traumatic growth after critical incidents in Austrian ambulance personnel. *BMC Psychiatry.* 2019;19:89.

Watanabe BL, Patterson GS, Kempema JM, Magallanes O, Brown LH. Is use of warning lights and sirens associated with increased risk of ambulance crashes? A contemporary analysis using national EMS Information System (NEMSIS) data. *Ann Emerg Med.* 2019;74(1): 101-109. https://www.sciencedirect.com/science/article/pii/S0196064418313258

Wood K, Crouch R, Rowland E, Pope C. Clinical handovers between prehospital and hospital staff: literature review. *Emerg Med J.* 2015;32:577-581. https://emj.bmj.com/content/32/7/577.info

348

I'm Out of Here! Pitfalls in the AMA Process

Christina Sajak

As emergency physicians, we hope that all patients presenting for care in our departments agree with our recommended diagnostic and therapeutic interventions. In fact, working collaboratively with patients has become so important to us that shared decision-making has become the norm. Nonetheless, despite our best efforts, we have all found ourselves in situations in which patients decline our recommended care and opt to leave the department—otherwise known as leaving *AMA*. In fact, this is estimated to occur in 1% to 2% of all ED discharges. This can occur for a variety of reasons: disagreement on the diagnosis or plan, inconvenience, cost or insurance barriers, social responsibilities, fear or denial, frustration, or conflict, to name a few. We all know that a patient walking in those double doors labeled "Emergency" triggers the requirement for a medical screening examination and stabilization. Likewise, before patients walk back out of those doors against the advice of a medical provider or refuse particular aspects of care while still a patient, certain basic requirements must be fulfilled.

An important, sometimes forgotten, first step of the AMA process is simply ascertaining why the patient is declining the care. In instances where fear or denial may be contributing to a patient's refusal, a more in-depth bedside conversation that may or may not involve the patient's support system may lead the patient to change their mind. In some cases, social work or case management can be particularly helpful when outside social responsibilities are identified as interfering with a patient's ability to proceed with the recommended care.

In an effort to understand a patient's reasoning, the EM physician must also begin the process of assessing capacity. It is essential not only to assess but also to document that a patient declining care has decision-making capacity. Such an assessment includes the patient's ability to (1) understand the information, including diagnosis and risk-benefit; (2) appreciate the information; (3) demonstrate appropriate reasoning; and (4) state a clear expression of a choice. If, for any reason, the patient is felt not to have capacity, the AMA process cannot continue.

Next, the emergency medicine provider should have a full discussion with the patient about indications for the recommended care, as well as potential benefits of receiving the care. This discussion should also include the potential risks of foregoing or delaying the recommended care. Patients should be given the opportunity to ask any questions that arise, which may also help the physician determine the level of understanding of the patient. It is important to discuss any alternative tests or therapies that the patient may be agreeable to, often referred to as the "next best option." For example, a patient with an infection who declines admission for IV antibiotics should be offered appropriate oral antibiotics upon leaving AMA. Due to the importance and complexity of these conversations, they are best had in a quiet area with the provider near eye level to patient, and with a nurse or other staff member there to witness.

When the AMA process occurs because a patient wants to leave the hospital, there are additional considerations for the EM physician. All patients who leave the department AMA should be encouraged to return at any time to continue their care. They should all receive or have the opportunity to receive discharge instructions, including connection to follow-up care, return precautions, and any necessary prescriptions or appropriate assistive devices, such as splints and boots.

Many departments and hospitals also have specific forms to document a patient declining recommended intervention or leaving AMS. When possible, these should be correctly completed and witnessed not only for documentation purposes but walking through the forms can also help ensure that all critical steps have been completed. Occasionally, the patient will decline to sign these forms. It is important to note that this does not affect the AMA process but should be reflected in the physician's documentation.

Documentation surrounding AMA interactions is crucial. In addition to noting that the patient has capacity, it is important to include the patient's reasoning for declining or leaving, steps the care team took to try to facilitate the patient receiving appropriate care, consideration of the "next best option," as well as the risk-benefit conversation and discharge instruction conversation, if applicable. In the age of the electronic medical record, many emergency medicine physicians have taken to developing a personal smart phrase surrounding AMA, which can help to keep documentation factual and thorough. Whenever smart phrases are used, the physician should make the necessary effort to edit and individualize the phrase to the specific encounter. In addition, having the phrase reviewed by your department's legal or risk management team before implementation is recommended.

PEARLS

- AMA applies not only to discharge but also to individual components of care, such as testing, procedures, and therapeutics.
- Identifying a patient's reasoning for declining care may reveal opportunities to remove barriers to care and prevent the AMA process.
- If a patient does not have capacity, the AMA process cannot continue.
- When possible, hospital-specific AMA forms should be completed and conversations witnessed by another health care professional.

- Patients declining recommended interventions must be given the highest level of care that is acceptable to them, as well as appropriate prescriptions, discharge, and follow-up information.

SUGGESTED READINGS

Alfandre DJ. "I'm going home": discharges against medical advice. *Mayo Clin Proc*. 2009;84(3):255-260. PMID: 19252113.

Magauran BG Jr. Risk management for the emergency physician: competency and decision-making capacity, informed consent, and refusal of care against medical advice. *Emerg Med Clin North Am*. 2009;27(4):605-614-viii.

349

I'VE BEEN SERVED! WHAT DO I DO NOW?

CHRISTINA SAJAK AND GREGORY JASANI

According to the American Medical Association, over 50% of emergency medicine physicians report having been sued at least once during their careers. This means that, unfortunately, you are more likely than not to be involved with the U.S. justice system sometime over the course of your practice. While potentially unavoidable, understanding the basis of a malpractice suit can help you navigate the process (and potentially avoid being named in the first place!).

There are four tenets that form the basis of malpractice claims in this country. A malpractice claim must prove that

1) A professional duty was owed to the patient.
2) There was a breach of such duty.
3) An injury resulted from the breach.
4) Damages (financial and/or emotional) resulted as a result of the injury.

Obviously, for emergency medicine physicians, a professional duty is owed to any patient who walks through the doors of the ED due to EMTALA. For the second tenet, breach of duty, most plaintiffs will invoke "standard of care" to argue that the physician breached their professional duty. The third and fourth tenets tend to be dependent on the case and claim but often center around delayed or missed diagnosis and the subsequent harm. Often, the plaintiff and attorney team will claim that the bad outcome of a patient was otherwise avoidable.

The process of a malpractice suit begins before the physician is ever notified. A plaintiff goes to a legal team with their complaint, and the plaintiff then requests a medical record request. Plaintiff attorneys will then have the medical records reviewed by experts who comment on whether or not standard of care was met. Plaintiff attorneys will have as many medical experts review the case as needed, until they find an expert whose opinion is favorable to them. If the attorney believes they have an opportunity for success, they will file a claim or suit. Filing must be done within the statute of limitations, which varies by state, and can be time stamped from the date of occurrence OR the time of discovery of injury.

If the abovementioned conditions are met, the physician will receive formal notification and be "served papers," which can occur at inopportune times, including while on shift. The most important first step is to reach out to your institution's risk management/legal department as well as your malpractice carrier. They will be instrumental in guiding you through the discovery process, which can last months to years, depending on the case. Discovery phase includes deposition, which is a recorded interview completed under oath, and can be prolonged over several days. Following discovery, the case may go to arbitration or be settled; in fact, some health insurance plan agreements contain language that requires malpractice cases to go to arbitration rather than trial. If arbitration remains unsuccessful in resolving the case, it will go to trial.

If you find yourself on the receiving end of a lawsuit, utilize your resources. In most cases, your institution's legal and risk management departments will reach out to you to help you with the process, but you should never hesitate to contact them with questions or concerns. Many institutions now have practicing physicians as part of the risk management team. They will work with you to prepare you for the next step in the process. You should never engage with the plaintiff's attorney or participate in legal activities without first talking with your own legal team. In addition, be aware that any reading or preparation you do for a case is discoverable. Similarly, you should never retroactively alter a patient's chart after learning of a lawsuit. That is also discoverable and will make it harder to defend that care you provided.

Being named in a malpractice suit is every physician's nightmare, but unfortunately, it will happen to many of us during our careers. The best defense against a case going to trial is to continue to practice quality, evidence-based medicine and to document that care appropriately. However, if it does happen, engage with the legal experts at your institution to help you prepare as well as you can. With proper preparation, the chances of having a verdict reached against you are incredibly small. According to a recent retrospective review of ED and urgent care malpractice cases, on average, two-thirds of all claims were dropped, withdrawn, or dismissed. Another 20% of claims were settled for well below malpractice policy limits, and the vast majority (~90%) of the cases that went to trial had verdicts for the defendants.

Despite knowing that more than half of us will end up being named in a lawsuit during the course of our careers, it can be an isolating and anxiety-provoking experience. Many report difficulties in their professional and personal lives in the time following a formal notification, which can last to the end of the claim or even longer. Take time for yourself, seek assistance when needed, and know you are not alone. You and the work you do are important! Familiarize yourself with the legal process, use your resources, and continue to provide excellent patient care and the chances of a judgment against you are very small!

PEARLS

- Malpractice claims actually begin well before the physician is notified.
- Statute of limitations varies by state.

- Immediately after receiving formal notification, contact your risk management department and malpractice carrier.
- Any reading you do "to prepare" for the case/deposition/trial is considered discoverable.
- Most cases never go to trial, but those that do almost always go in favor of you!
- While being named in a malpractice case may feel isolating, you are never alone.

Suggested Readings

Bookman K, Zane RD. Surviving a medical malpractice lawsuit. *Emerg Med Clin North Am*. 2020;38(2):539-548.

Wong KE, Parikh PD, Miller KC, Zonfrillo MR. Emergency department and urgent care medical malpractice claims 2001-15. *West J Emerg Med*. 2021;22(2):333-338. PMID: 33856320.

350

See No Evil: Mandatory Reporting Obligations

Gregory Jasani and Rachel Wiltjer

Mandatory reporting laws are present in all 50 U.S. states. Consequences of failure to report are variable, ranging from fines to jail time to professional consequences. The laws are intended to protect either (1) a specific person (generally a "vulnerable person") or (2) the general population. The breadth of occurrences requiring reporting is state dependent, so be aware of local requirements. Laws can be mandatory or permissive; permissive reporting protects clinicians from consequences for good faith reporting of certain situations. This highlights the distinction of moral versus legal responsibility and introduces the possibility for bias in reporting.

A common area of mandatory reporting that speaks to public safety relates to impaired driving. The range of conditions that require reporting is broad, with some states having very specific wording and others more general. Seizures are the most commonly cited condition, but some states also include dementia, syncope, and alcohol usage. The AMA has published a policy statement supporting mandatory reporting of these impairments, noting an ethical obligation to patient and public safety. ACEP has taken a more moderate approach, advising caution against reporting based solely on diagnosis. ACEP also advocates for physician protection when reporting in good faith out of concern for patient or public safety.

Mandatory reporting laws regarding reportable diseases exist with public safety in mind. The most obvious of these include communicable diseases such as tuberculosis, HIV, other STDs, and COVID, but many states or municipalities include diseases such as anthrax, arboviruses, and various other resistant or invasive pathogens. This list varies based on the location but is generally accessible on health department websites. Reporting may be carried out by the laboratory department, so be aware of physician responsibilities at your institution.

Child abuse and neglect is probably the most well-known situation requiring mandatory reporting. All 50 states have some legislation dictating this requirement; circumstances for reporting, time frame in which reporting is required, and intake of reports vary by location. In some institutions, assistance (social work or other specialty services) may be available for report filing. Because it's a time-consuming process requiring information not pertinent to the patient's medical care, familiarity with the process can increase efficiency for the independently reporting emergency physician. Like child abuse and neglect, all U.S. states (although not all territories) require reporting of abuse and neglect of older or vulnerable adults. The definition of vulnerable adult is variable but generally includes cognitive deficits, developmental delay, and/or physical disabilities.

State law varies on reporting of perinatal substance abuse. Currently, 20 states require physicians to report pregnant mothers using illicit substances, classifying this as child abuse. Four additional states require reporting if the physician reasonably expects the substance use is associated with child maltreatment.

IPV may trigger mandatory reporting. This has fomented ethical debate out of concern that patients may avoid care if they fear reporting, viewing the hospital as unsafe. Older studies have documented that as many as 40% of victims of IPV do not support mandatory reporting. Therefore, it is important to discuss reporting with the patient to encourage understanding. It is worth being aware of nuance in reporting IPV, including whether it is mandated or permissive. Use discretion if reporting is protected, but not mandated to support victims.

Mandatory reporting of sexual assault raises similar ethical and safety concerns. In many areas, statutory offenses are classified under child abuse reporting, separate from sexual assault. Other situations may fall under IPV reporting. Several states that do not have reporting laws specific to sexual assault still require reporting of injuries (accidental and/or nonaccidental depending on the jurisdiction). California, Massachusetts, and Rhode Island have mandatory reporting of rape separate from other reportable situations.

Various traumatic injuries require reporting, generally directly to law enforcement. Specifics vary by location but often include injuries involving a weapon or interpersonal violence. All states require animal bite reporting to animal control, the department of health, or law enforcement to ensure the animal will be observed for signs of rabies.

Physicians are legally obligated to inform third-party individuals of threats of harm to their health. The Tarasoff rule, named after the Supreme Court case establishing the precedent, requires physicians to warn individuals if a patient makes credible threats against them. Patients expressing homicidal ideations toward a person must be held until the nature of the threat is assessed. It is generally advisable to inform law enforcement in addition to the individual.

In all states, concerns that a physician is impaired due to alcohol or drug dependency must be reported. The AMA defines the impaired physician as one who is unable to fulfill professional and personal responsibilities because of psychiatric illness, alcoholism, or drug addiction. Approximately 8% to 12% of physicians will develop an addiction during their careers, with anesthesia and emergency medicine physicians at particularly high risk. Any good faith concern that a colleague is impaired must be reported; physicians can report without fear of retaliation. Reports should be made to the state medical society or licensing board, which works with the physician to identify and treat substance or psychiatric illness before punitive action. Success rates have been shown to be high with proper support.

Engaging colleagues to help with mandatory reporting can ease our burden. Social workers may fill out the pertinent forms for suspected abuse; nurses can report animal bites to animal control. If delegating, it is important to touch base to ensure that the tasks are completed, since, as a physician, it is ultimately your responsibility.

PEARLS

- Mandatory reporting laws are meant for protection: of an individual or the general population.
- Organizations such as ACEP advocate for physician protection when reporting in good faith out of concern for patient or public safety.
- Know the applicable laws where you practice.
- Know that you are protected from retaliation for reports made in good faith.
- Know local mechanisms for reporting common mandated events.
- Use your resources to try to decrease your time commitment to reporting.

Suggested Readings

American College of Emergency Physicians. Domestic family violence policy statement. 2019. https://www.acep.org/patient-care/policy-statements/domestic-family-violence/

Geiderman JM, Marco CA. Mandatory and permissive reporting laws: obligations, challenges, moral dilemmas, and opportunities. *JACEP Open*. 2020;1:38-45.

Gupta M. Mandatory reporting laws and the emergency physician. *Ann Emerg Med*. 2007; 49(3):369-376.

351

Material Injury: Simple Steps to Preserve Forensic Evidence

Janet Carroll and Elizabeth Karagosian

Healthcare forensics represents the intersection of the medical and criminal justice systems. When a patient presents with injuries resulting from crime or violence, in addition to providing medical care, healthcare professionals should consider the patient's forensic needs. Carefully documented event histories and injury identification, or lack thereof, are critical forensic components. Knowledge about forensic evidence collection and the medical forensic options for different patient populations is essential to providing comprehensive patient care.

State/Jurisdictional Considerations

Specific guidelines regarding forensic evidence collection and time frames vary by state/jurisdiction, each having their own mandatory reporting requirements in relation to minors, vulnerable adults, gunshot wounds, stabbings, and "serious bodily injuries."

General Evidence Collection Principles

- If your facility utilizes forensic nurses, consider consultation as guided by hospital policy.
- Every patient deserves a comprehensive medical forensic evaluation, regardless of their ability to recall the event.
- The patient can decline any and all aspects of evidence collection, history-taking, examination, and photography.
- History-taking should be done privately with the patient. Ask questions in a nonleading manner, such as "What occurred that led to your emergency visit today?" to avoid influencing the patient's response.
- Offer a complete head-to-toe skin assessment, making sure to fully undress and examine the patient, documenting any injuries, wounds, and areas of tenderness.
- Before evidence collection, avoid nonemergent measures that would remove DNA evidence, such as washing/bathing, wound care, mouth care, oral intake, and placing a Foley. If the patient must void, instruct the patient to avoid wiping.
- When substances such as saliva, ejaculate, or blood are suspected on dry, nonmucosal surfaces, such as the skin or external anogenital areas, collect specimens using Q-tip swabs moistened with sterile water (avoid saline as it may interfere with forensic crime lab analysis). When obtaining specimens, simultaneously and "gently" roll two swabs on the skin. Applying too much pressure when swabbing will obtain a disproportionate amount of the patient's DNA.
- Change gloves between every piece of evidence collection to avoid cross-contamination.
- Swab all bite marks for saliva, regardless of time line.
- Dry evidence before packaging to avoid molding/degrading of DNA on specimens.
- Use paper, not plastic bags, to collect clothing. If you need bags or other evidence containers, ask law enforcement to provide them.
- Sharp objects should be placed in containers that allow for drying and minimize the risk of injury.
- Handle objects sparingly, using gloved fingers or covered forceps to avoid marking specimens.
- Do not cut clothing through any holes or rips to preserve defects resulting from assault.
- If the patient presents in clothing worn during the assault, collect and package each piece separately.
- If there is concern that the patient was drugged, follow state/jurisdictional guidelines for urine and/or blood collection. If urine is collected, the "dirty" urine should be placed on ice to reduce drug metabolism.
- With pediatric deaths concerning for abuse/neglect, the patient's body should not be left alone with the family/caregivers. A staff member should be assigned to document patient contact, for example, kissing and crying onto the patient. In some instances, the family/caregiver will not be allowed to touch the patient until a medical examiner is consulted.

Chain of Custody

- Maintain chain of custody until all evidence is transferred to law enforcement or into hospital storage, if allowed by your jurisdiction and hospital policy, complying with chain of custody standards. A chain of custody form is required when evidence is transferred, indicating the item, date and time of transfer, and signature of each person releasing/accepting the evidence.

Forensic Photography

- Obtain consent or follow hospital policy for those patients unable to consent.
- Photographs become part of the medical record, should only be released to law enforcement under jurisdictional protocol, and may require patient consent.
- Each injury/wound should have three photographs:
  1) A long shot includes the adjacent joints for location identification purposes.
  2) A close-up shot
  3) A close-up of a measuring tool or standardized object
- Whether or not photographs are taken, a body map diagram should be utilized to document the injury location.
- If photographs are taken, consider utilizing a photolog to reference descriptions of traumatic findings on a body map diagram.
- Consider follow-up photography to capture the progression of newly and/or previously visible injuries.

Strangulation

- Perform a detailed event history and comprehensive physical assessment, including a complete neurologic examination, given the high risk of morbidity and mortality.
- Utilize a "nonfatal strangulation documentation tool" for history taking and physical assessment.
- Note that a lack of identifiable injury does not rule out strangulation.

Suspect Exams

- Complete only under a search warrant, court order, or at the request of the patient.
- Law enforcement must remain present during the evaluation for staff safety.
- Only collect the items listed on the search warrant/court order, or, if the patient consents, according to jurisdictional guidelines.

Documentation Pearls

- Determine event time and location for time frame and jurisdictional needs.
- Only ask open-ended, nonleading questions.
- Capture patient history in quotes whenever possible.
- Use observations to objectively document the patient's emotional state.
- Do not use the terms "alleged," "allegation," or "alleges."
- Do not date bruises.
- Do not document the "entrance" or "exit" description for gunshot wounds.
- Do not draw unfounded conclusions; document what you see, hear, and do.

PEARLS

- Follow your state/jurisdictional protocols specific to medical forensic evaluations, patient options, and mandatory reporting requirements.
- Be objective, comprehensive, and as detailed as possible when documenting event histories and exam findings. The medical record is evidentiary material.
- Limited event recall or lack of physical evidence and/or exam findings does not rule out an assault.
- Avoid activities that could degrade the evidence.
- Observe proper packaging techniques.

Suggested Readings

American College of Emergency Physicians (ACEP), ed. *Evaluation and Management of the Sexually Assaulted or Sexually Abused Patient*. 2nd ed. 2013.
International Association of Forensic Nurses. *Non-Fatal Strangulation Documentation Toolkit*. 2016.
National Institute of Justice. *National Best Practices for Sexual Assault Kits: A Multidisciplinary Approach*. Chapter 2. U.S. Department of Justice; 2017.
Stark MM. *Clinical Forensic Medicine: A Physicians Guide*. 4th ed. Springer; 2020.

352

Caring for the Intimate Partner Violence Victim

Victoria J. Martin

IPV is frighteningly common, affecting millions of people in the United States every year. According to the CDC, approximately 41% of women and 26% of men report IPV at some point in their lifetime. IPV encompasses a number of behaviors, including physical violence, sexual violence, stalking, and psychological aggression. Many people affected by IPV experience injury, death, chronic medical problems, mental health problems, substance use disorders, legal entanglements, and missed work as a result of the violence. US crime reports show that one-fifth of all homicides, and over half of homicides where the victim is female, are carried out by a current or past intimate partner. IPV affects all people, but marginalized groups such as sexual and gender minority youth and people from racial and ethnic minority groups are at higher risk. The vast majority of victims are women.

Make the Diagnosis

Victims of IPV present for healthcare twice as frequently as they report to police. All patients should be screened for IPV, and there are a number of screening tools available. Elements of the history and patient encounter that should raise suspicion for IPV include a partner who is verbally abusive, controlling, or won't leave the room; inconsistent explanation for injuries; missed appointments; delayed presentation of injuries; late initiation of prenatal care; multiple abortions; frequent ED or urgent care visits; inappropriate affect; and reluctance to be examined. Injuries concerning IPV include, but are not limited to, any injury that is not well explained; multiple injuries in various stages of healing; central injuries (head, neck, face, and thorax); injuries of the teeth or genitals; broken fingernails; bite marks; burns; ligature marks; bruising on the neck, which could be a result of strangulation; and defensive wounds on the forearms. Abdominal injuries in pregnant patients, STIs, and unintended pregnancies may also be indicators of IPV.

Provide Medical Care and Emotional Support

Address any traumatic injuries and perform a thorough trauma evaluation as needed. Provide a forensic exam when indicated, preferably utilizing an experienced forensic examiner (ie, SANE or equivalent). Offer empathy and support, and take care to use neutral, nonjudgmental language—"I am so sorry this is happening to you." Validate the victim; acknowledge how difficult it must be for them to disclose the information—"This is not your fault." and "You don't deserve to be treated this way." Do not pressure them to leave the relationship; they may not be ready to take action at the time of your visit. Instead, focus on moving them forward on the continuum of precontemplation, contemplation, determination, and action while recognizing that for many patients, the journey is not linear. Protect the patient's privacy and confidentiality.

Assess Safety

Assess for safety and create a safety plan. There is a free, validated danger assessment tool at https://www.dangerassessment.org/DATools.aspx, which can help identify risk factors for lethality and more severe violence. It is critical to put a safety plan in place, using local resources, including an IPV hotline or advocate. The plan should include a signal to children or neighbors to call 911, a place to go, and an emergency kit with important documents, keys, and money. Victims should be counseled that, in times of escalating conflict, they should avoid rooms that contain weapons and hard surfaces. Over time, abusive episodes tend to escalate in severity and frequency.

Engage Support Services

Providers should refer victims to counseling while being careful not to provide written materials that may be discovered by the abuser. If the abuser is present at a visit, they should not be confronted and care should be taken to ensure that the abuser is not able to view sensitive notes in the medical record. When a victim attempts to leave an abuser, the violence often escalates. Providers should not encourage victims to leave but should support them and provide resources when they decide to leave on their own.

Document Appropriately

Careful documentation can be critical when legal issues arise. Note specifics, including the time, date, and nature of the abuse. Include patient quotes where appropriate. Be sure that all documentation is secure so that the abuser cannot gain access to the notes. The victim may request that information regarding IPV not be documented for fear that their abuser will discover it. Photographs (with consent) and drawings of injuries, as well as the involvement of a forensic examiner, can be helpful, especially when an evidence collection kit ("rape kit") is needed. Choose your language carefully. Don't use words like "claims" or "denies" that may be interpreted as implying you don't believe the patient; instead, use more neutral, straightforward language such as "states" or "reports." Know your state laws to determine when mandatory reporting is required: This is commonly abuse involving children, the older adults, persons with disability, and injuries resulting from a weapon that require reporting. Be aware that child maltreatment often coexists with IPV. In some states, knowledge of IPV mandates reporting to child protective services. In situations where a report must be made or when the provider determines it should be made, it may be advantageous for the victim to make the report themselves to indicate to child protective services that they are able to provide a safe environment for the children. Remember that health care providers are mandatory reporters.

PEARLS

- Make the diagnosis through screening and awareness of red flags in the history, exam, and patient interaction.
- Empathy and validation are paramount in your patient interaction.
- Assess the immediate risk and establish a safety plan.
- Know your local resources and engage in support services.
- Document appropriately; refer and arrange follow-up.
- Know your regional mandatory reporting obligations.

SUGGESTED READINGS

Centers for Disease Control and Prevention. Intimate Partner Violence. https://www.cdc.gov/violenceprevention/intimatepartnerviolence/index.html

Choo EK, Houry DE. Managing intimate partner violence in the emergency department. *Ann Emerg Med.* 2015;65(4):447-451.e1.

Liebschutz, JM, Rothman, EF. Intimate-partner violence—what physicians can do. *N Engl J Med.* 2012;367:2071-2073.

National Domestic Violence Hotline. www.thehotline.org/. 1-800-799-SAFE (7233). Futures without violence. https://www.futureswithoutviolence.org/

NCADV. Learn More. https://ncadv.org/learn-more/resources

OASH, US Department of Health & Human Services. Resources by State on Violence Against Women. https://www.womenshealth.gov/relationships-and-safety/get-help/state-resources

353

IDENTIFYING VICTIMS OF HUMAN TRAFFICKING

JANET CARROLL AND ELISHA PAUL DEKONING

HT is increasingly prevalent in our society, and victims are being identified in health care with increasing frequency. The United Nations defines HT as the "recruitment, transfer, harboring, or receipt of persons by means of threat or use of force or other forms of coercion, abduction, fraud, deception, the abuse of power, or a position of vulnerability to achieve the consent of a person, having control over another person, for the purpose of exploitation" (UNODC, Global Report on Trafficking in Persons 2020). Coercion can be used to achieve consent; thus, consent does not mean it is not trafficking. HT includes sex trafficking, forced labor, and domestic servitude. Commercial sex under 18 years is considered trafficking by law. HT permeates every societal demographic and geographic region. Very rarely is a patient "rescued" in the ED, but trafficked individuals are likely to interact with the health care system while being trafficked, giving health care workers a unique opportunity to provide resources and potentially connect victims to agencies that can eventually put them on a path to freedom.

Recognizing the Trafficked Patient

It is unlikely that a trafficked individual will openly admit their situation; they may be afraid, their captor/handler may accompany them to their health care encounter, or they may not realize that help is available and "freedom" is possible. No single finding is pathognomonic of HT, but history and examination clues exist that, taken in sum, may suggest that a patient is being trafficked. Trafficked patients frequently present with another individual, often identified as a significant other/spouse, aunt/uncle, or employer, who seeks to provide all details of the patient's history and to whom the patient may appear unusually deferential. If separated (which can be challenging), inconsistencies may appear in the patient's story. The patient may seem reluctant or circumspect, and they may lack personal identification. Clues from the history include multiple sexual partners, numerous unwanted pregnancies, and fragmented or delayed medical care. They may have an unusual attachment to their cell phone (their link to their handler) and may be unaware of what city/state they are in.

Clues on physical examination include signs of physical neglect, poor eye contact, evasiveness, defiance/anger, confusion, fear, submissiveness, and/or hypervigilance. Labor trafficking may be suggested by injuries from an industrial accident without appropriate protective gear; dizziness, headaches, or confusion from head injury; chronic complaints from poor work conditions; or evidence of untreated injuries. Clues of sex trafficking include bruises, bite marks, burns, branding, or tattoos; substance abuse; multiple or frequent pregnancies, repeated abortions or miscarriages, or complications from attempted abortions; and pelvic complaints such as persistent or inadequately treated STIs, genital or rectal trauma, or impacted foreign bodies on vaginal examination. In general, examination findings inconsistent with the patient's story should raise concern.

How (and How Not) to Respond

Using a trauma-informed care approach, the provider should remain nonjudgmental and nonbiased. The patient may come across as difficult, uninterested, or uncooperative due to fear, vulnerability, sleep, and/or food deprivation, or they may be impaired by drugs or alcohol. These behaviors may be part of the patient's coping or survival skills. Provide a sense of calm and safety, build trust, actively listen, and keep the patient informed of what to expect and who will be involved in their care. Empower patient decision-making, offer support, and fully inform them of any mandatory reporting requirements.

All patients should be screened for HT privately, but achieving this privacy can be difficult: remember, the handler is intelligent, controlling, and/or threatening enough to control another human. With this in mind, common excuses such as needing a radiologic test or urine sample should be used only if appropriate to the chief complaint. Use a hospital-provided interpreter if one is needed; do not use the person who accompanied them to the ED. Documentation should include specific details, quotes, and pictures as appropriate, but take care to secure the note so the trafficker cannot gain access (see Chapter 352). Screening questions should highlight why you are asking and what resources you have, for example, "We have patients who experience HT in our community and we have resources that may help." While several screening tools are available (eg, "RAFT" tool or the "Adult Human Trafficking Screening Tool and Guide" by the National HT Training and Technical Assistance Center), it is best to develop and follow facility-specific protocols.

If you have identified a victim of HT,

1) Involve social work and forensic nursing, if available.
2) Call the local crisis center advocate for confidential support and safety planning.
3) Alert security/law enforcement if safety issues are present.
4) If the patient is ready to leave the situation, consider admission for safety and any psychiatric or medical needs. Assist with residential trafficking facility referral forms (eg, Sheltered Alliance Rapid Referral), facilitate reporting to law enforcement, and provide follow-up referrals.
5) If there is not a mandatory reporting requirement and the patient is not prepared to leave their situation, support them with nonjudgmental and nonbiased care. If safe, provide written information including the National HT Hotline number, local resource brochures, and residential trafficking facility options and offer follow-up appointments (social work, substance use, psychiatry, medical) as appropriate.

PEARLS

- History and/or physical examination clues may suggest a patient is being trafficked.
- Obtain the history from the patient privately.
- Your job is not to "rescue" the patient; the adult patient has the right to decline care and return to the trafficking situation.
- Consider admitting patients who indicate they are ready to be "free."
- Understand your legal reporting obligations.
- National HT Hotline: Text BEFREE to 233733 or call 1-888-373-7888.

Suggested Readings

Catholic Health Initiatives online course. HT and the role of the health provider. Accessed February 15, 2024. https://www.catholichealthinitiatives.org/addressing-human-trafficking-course/story_html5.html

Children's Healthcare of Atlanta. *Human trafficking: guidelines for healthcare providers*. Accessed February 15, 2024. https://www.choa.org/medical-professionals/referrals-and-transfers/directory-of-services/child-protection-resources/institute-on-healthcare-and-human-trafficking

Chisolm-Straker M, Singer E, Strong D, et al. Validation of a screening tool for labor and sex trafficking among emergency department patients. *J Am Coll Emerg Physicians Open*. 2021;2(5):e12558.

Greenbaum J. A short screening tool to identify victims of child sex trafficking in the health care setting. *Pediatr Emerg Care*. 2018;34(1):33-37.

Human Trafficking Guidebook. Accessed February 15, 2024. https://www.massmed.org/Patient-Care/Health-Topics/Violence-Intervention-and-Prevention/Human-Trafficking-(pdf)/

National Human Trafficking Resource Center, Polaris Project. *Comprehensive Human Trafficking Assessment*. Accessed February 15, 2024. https://humantraffickinghotline.org/en/resources/comprehensive-human-trafficking-assessment-tool

Additional Resources

National Human Trafficking Hotline. Accessed February 15, 2024. https://humantraffickinghotline.org/en/resources/comprehensive-human-trafficking-assessment-tool
National Trafficking Sheltered Alliance for residential referrals. https://shelteredalliance.org/
Polaris Project. www.PolarisProject.org
Trauma-Informed Care Implementation Resource Center. https://www.traumainformedcare.chcs.org/
UNODC, Global Report on Trafficking in Persons 2020. United Nations publication, Sales No. E.20.IV.3

354

Pearls for the Safer Sign-Out

Brent King

Transitions of care between providers are inevitable in modern medical practice. Such transitions (also called "handoffs" or "sign-outs") are especially common in emergency medicine as emergency physicians usually work shifts, and patients may not have completed their care before the end of a provider's shift. In these cases, responsibility for the patient will be transferred to a new provider. Transitioning the patient's care from one provider to another can be among the most potentially dangerous periods in the care process. During a transition, important information can be miscommunicated or forgotten and critical tasks may not be performed, leaving the patient vulnerable to medical error and the provider at risk for litigation.

Several authors and organizations have created approaches to this problem. These methods have in common a structured and standardized method of transitioning care. Often, these take the form of a checklist characterized by an easy-to-recall mnemonic, which helps the provider remember all of the critical points. Some examples include the "I-PASS" or "I-PASS the BATON" tool and the "SBAR" tool, but there are many locally developed tools available, as well. A good handoff tool should have four characteristics: (1) it should be tailored to the specific clinical situation and context. Transitioning a patient's care from the ED to the intensive care unit may be different than transitioning their care to a new ED provider. Likewise, transitioning the care of a patient who has undergone an extensive workup is different than transitioning the care of a patient with a relatively straightforward problem or one who is early in their evaluation. (2) It should be structured so that each handoff is conducted in a consistent manner, with the information being conveyed in the same order. (3) It should include all of the critical information necessary for the next provider to effectively manage the patient. (4) It should allow for two-way communication between providers so that questions can be answered and concerns addressed before the new provider, assuming care of the patient.

The author's ED structures the transition process as follows:

- Identify the patient including age, gender, preferred pronouns, and any significant others who are with the patient, especially if the patient is a child or otherwise requires the assistance of another person in daily life.
- State the patient's current status in the ED, usually, "active"—still under the care of the ED—or "admitted"—care has been transitioned to an inpatient provider, but the patient has yet to leave the ED, or prepared for discharge.
- State the overall clinical status of the patient. The author's institution uses three categories: "stable," "watcher," and "critical." Stable patients require only routine care and monitoring. Those designated as "watchers" require additional attention, usually because they have the potential to become unstable but they may also have behavioral issues that could become problematic. Patients designated as "critical" require intensive monitoring and frequent reevaluation.
- Describe the history of the patient's present illness and their pertinent past medical history.
- Describe the patient's ED course from arrival to the present.
- Describe significant positive and negative test results.
- Describe any consultations obtained, the results of these consultations, and state whether any consultants have yet to see the patient.
- Describe significant social factors such as whether the patient will need a ride back to their home and shelter placement.
- Summarize what tasks need to be accomplished for the patient, which of those the off-going provider(s) will do before departure and which the oncoming provider(s) have agreed to do.
- Close the loop by ensuring that everyone agrees to the duties assigned in the prior step and that any questions are answered. Ideally, the oncoming provider will summarize the information received to ensure that they understand the situation.

Throughout the process of transitioning care between providers, two-way communication is crucial, and providers should pause frequently to allow for questions and to check for understanding.

PEARLS

- The risks associated with transitions in care can be reduced by using an organized and structured system.
- A tool or checklist can help ensure that all of the elements important to a safe and effective patient handoff are included and that information is transferred effectively.
- Two-way communication is a critical part of a good care transition process. Questions should be encouraged.
- The oncoming and off-going providers should clarify who will take responsibility for any unfinished tasks.
- The oncoming provider should briefly summarize their understanding of the patient's situation to ensure that the information has been communicated correctly.

Suggested Readings

Ehlers P, Seidel M, Schachers S, et al. Prospective observational multisite study of handover in the emergency department: theory versus practice. *West J Emerg Med*. 2021;22:401-409.

Kwok ESH, Clapham G, White S, et al. Development and implementation of a standardized emergency department inter-shift handover tool to improve physician communication. *BMJ Open Qual*.2020;9:e000780.

Norman S, DiCicco F, Simpson J. Emergency Room Safer Transfer of Patients (ER-STOP): a quality improvement initiative at a community-based hospital to improve the safety of emergency room patient handovers. *BMJ Open*. 2018;8:e019553.

Turner JS, Courtney RD, Sarmieto E, et al. Frequency of safety-net errors in the emergency department: effect of patient handoffs. *Am J Emerg Med*. 2021;42:188-191.

355

Collaborating With Difficult Consultants

Nikki Cali

Emergency medicine physicians speak with consultants in nearly every department of the hospital, consulting specialty services for a variety of reasons including management recommendations, procedural assistance, and facilitation of follow-up for safe discharges. It is important to recognize what consultants are available at your institution since this varies greatly between academic, community, and freestanding EDs. Consultant availability also varies based on time of day, so be aware of the differences between consultation during business hours versus consultation in the middle of the night.

It is imperative to put in the appropriate work before, during, and after consultation to achieve effective and efficient care for patients. Clearly expressed, closed-loop communication is at the center of this process and will help you avoid common errors when collaborating with your next consultant on shift.

Before Calling the Consultant

Know the purpose of your call. Have a clear question or actionable item for the consultant. Be able to provide basic information about the patient—name, MRN, location—and pertinent exam findings, imaging, or lab results that are available and/or pending.

Contact the appropriate service or provider on call. Be sure to follow the correct chain of command for contact as well. As simple as it sounds, it can be detrimental to the effectiveness of your consultation and delay disposition if you are waiting to hear from a provider who is not on call and has never received your message. Check with your department's unit secretary or daily call schedule to save yourself time and efficiency on the front end of your consultation.

Consider if the consultation will change patient management or outcomes. This is an important consideration when working overnight and will help build rapport with consultants, especially in the community setting, when many of them are not in the house. Importantly, when consultation changes management or outcomes in a time-sensitive manner, do not hesitate to place the consultations at any time of day or night.

Update your patients. If your patient has a diagnosis that warrants a specialty consultation, please notify them. It is unsettling for a patient to find out about a new diagnosis, treatment options, or admission plan while meeting the consultant for the first time. This can place our consultants in a precarious position when trying to establish a new patient relationship. As the ED physician, it is our responsibility to maintain cohesive care for our patients and keep them informed about their workup.

DURING THE CONSULTATION

Lead with the punchline. Catch your consultant's attention. They do not want to be bogged down by erroneous details of the patient's past medical history at the start of the consultation. State clearly the reason for the consultation and request.

Advocate for your patient. Assuming you put in the work before calling the consultant, have a clear question or actionable item. Be able to support your concerns on behalf of the patient.

Remain calm. This is where consultations have the potential to become derailed. Maintain a calm, nonconfrontational demeanor when having a conversation with a consultant. Communication is often misconstrued when using platforms such as secured messaging apps or even over the phone. Face-to-face communication remains the gold standard when possible. If the consultant is not understanding your question or request through secured messaging, propose escalation to a phone call. If there is a misunderstanding on the phone and it is within reason, ask the consultant to come to the ED to discuss the patient in person. Many consultations require physical evaluation of the patient, so the consultant can let you know what they think after they see the patient.

Summarize all actionable items and the outcome of the consultation. Establish what steps will be taken by both parties and when contact should be made again. Establish certain "if/then" scenarios when applicable to help eliminate any delays in disposition.

AFTER THE CONVERSATION WITH THE CONSULTANT

Document the conversation in the medical record. Document the medical decision-making of the conversation and include a time stamp, who you spoke with, and the outcome of your consultation.

Perform actionable items. This can range from ordering new studies, gathering supplies, or placing the patient in a specific examination room. Be sure to uphold your responsibilities during the consultation as it will not go unnoticed.

Follow-up with the consultant. Although this is important from a medicolegal perspective, it is also necessary for quality patient care. Make sure the consultant completes their actionable items, whether that includes coming to see the patient, writing a note, or placing admission orders. If there is a delay that may harm the patient or impede flow, do not hesitate to reengage with the consultant.

Update the patient care team. Consultations can change patient care plans, and the entire team should be updated accordingly. Was the nurse notified of additional labs or imaging? Is the patient NPO? Keeping the patient and their care team informed helps expedite additional workup recommended by the consultant, leading to a more efficient disposition.

PEARLS

- Know the purpose of your consultation. Have a clear question or actionable item before calling the consultant.
- Lead with the punch line. If the consultant wants more details, the consultant will ask for more details.
- Advocate for the patient while maintaining a calm, nonconfrontational demeanor.
- Summarize the result of the consultation and the next steps that will be taken by both parties.
- Document the time and medical decision-making of your consultation in the medical record.

Suggested Readings

Ackery AD, Adams JW, Brooks SC, Detsky AS. How to give a consultation and how to get a consultation. *CJEM*. 2011;13(4):289-291. PMID: 21722561.

Chan T, Bakewell F, Orlich D, Sherbino J. Conflict prevention, conflict mitigation, and manifestations of conflict during emergency department consultations. *Acad Emerg Med*. 2014;21(3):308-313. PMID: 24628756.

Kessler CS, Tadisina KK, Saks M, et al. The 5Cs of consultation: training medical students to communicate effectively in the emergency department. *J Emerg Med*. 2015;49(5):713-721.

356

Caring for the Inpatient Boarder

Nicholas D. Poole and Jennifer V. Pope

Boarding admitted patients in the ED is not a novel phenomenon, but it has become a more glaring issue in the wake of increasing ED visits and hospital capacity constraints. Adverse effects resulting from the practice of boarding inpatients in the ED include delays in the evaluation of new ED patients, ED overcrowding, increased costs, prolonged lengths of stay, and, most importantly, increased medical errors and patient mortality. The purpose of this chapter is not to offer systemic solutions to inpatient boarding in the ED but rather to describe best practices to manage this situation. Best practices include coordination with inpatient nursing, physicians, and administration to reduce harm, decrease burnout, and achieve the best outcomes for patients.

ED and Inpatient Nurses

Floor-level boarders require different resources than ED patients, including initiation of home medications, releasing standing orders for scheduled medications, and many other aspects of inpatient care that can be challenging for ED nurses, especially when they are simultaneously caring for acute ED patients. A multipronged approach toward nursing care for boarders is recommended, including cohorting boarding patients, floating floor nurses to the ED to care for these patients, and implementing inpatient nurse leadership rounding. The goal is to effectively create an inpatient-style area within the ED. Nurses who are familiar with inpatient care, and who are supported by inpatient nursing leadership, increase patient and nursing satisfaction and decrease strain on ED nursing. Inpatient nurse-leader rounding can help improve patient satisfaction by reassuring patients they are getting high-quality care even in an alternative setting. It also helps connect inpatient nurse leadership with the ED staff and encourages a team approach to tackling boarding and decompressing the ED.

THE ED PHYSICIAN, THE HOSPITALISTS, AND ADJUSTED WORKFLOW

Once a patient has been admitted, hospitals should have clear guidelines (ideally a policy) regarding who "owns" that patient. In the case of floor-level admissions, the hospitalist is often responsible for patient care, regardless of location, including boarding in the ED. This clear delineation of responsibility is important for patient safety and for nursing-physician communication. Although inpatient boarders are often not seen until later in the day, there are multiple benefits to rounding on these patients earlier. First, the boarding patient often feels overlooked and frustrated with the delay in getting an inpatient bed. Early rounding and clear communication of the goals of the day allow them to feel engaged by their team and to understand who is caring for them. Second, early rounding on patients allows for prompt discharging, resulting in the opening of ED space. It also allows for early detection of a change in patient status requiring changes in level of care. While the boarding patient is admitted and under the care of the hospitalist, the ED physician still needs to be aware of the patient and any acute changes to the patient's condition. The oncoming ED team should receive sign-out from the outgoing team in both verbal and standardized electronic format. While the nurses caring for the patient will primarily be communicating with the hospitalist team, nurses should be aware of clear triggers, such as unstable vital signs and acute changes in mental status, which would require them to involve the ED physician.

The care of ICU boarders represents a unique challenge as they require high level of attention from both nurse and physician teams. Like other boarders, ICU nurses should be floated to the ED to care for ICU boarding patients. Multiple models exist as to physician responsibility for the critical care patient in the ED, including the critical care team remotely caring for the patient, the ED team caring for the patient until they are transferred to the ICU, and hybrid models with special critical care areas of the ED devoted to high-acuity patients. In as many settings as possible, teams devoted solely to critical patients should be used. Most importantly, hospitals should have clear guidelines about who is primarily responsible for these patients once they have admission orders to ensure patient safety and to allow for clear nurse-physician communication.

PEARLS

- ED boarding of admitted patients is a prevalent phenomenon in nearly every ED in the country and is likely to increase with rising ED visits and continued hospital capacity constraints. To optimize care for these patients, it is important to consider these best practice pearls:
- Nursing responses should include floating floor and ICU nurses to the ED, cohorting boarding patients, and inpatient nurse-leader rounding. These actions

optimize safety, improve patient and nurse satisfaction, and allow for a team approach.
- Hospitals should have clear guidelines regarding physician ownership of floor-level boarding patients.
- Hospitalists and consultants should round early on ED boarders to help with prompt disposition, to recognize potential changes in level of care, and to improve patient satisfaction.
- The ED physicians should ensure clear verbal and standardized electronic handoff of ED boarders and establish triggers for nurses to involve the ED team.
- Hospitals should have guidelines regarding physician ownership of ICU boarding patients, which may involve shared management models.

Suggested Readings

Bornemann-Shepherd M, Le-Lazar J, Flynn Makic MB, DeVine D, McDevitt K, Paul M. Caring for inpatient boarders in the emergency department: improving safety and patient and staff satisfaction. *J Emerg Nurs*. 2015;41(1):23-29.

Janke AT, Melnick ER, Venkatesh AK. Hospital occupancy and emergency department boarding during the COVID-19 pandemic. *JAMA Netw Open*. 2022;5(9):e2233964.

Jayaprakash N, Pflaum-Carlson J, Gardner-Gray J, et al. Critical care delivery solutions in the emergency department: evolving models in caring for ICU boarders. *Ann Emerg Med*. 2020;76(6):709-716.

Shah S. *7 ways to solve the ED boarding challenge*. Emergency Physicians Monthly. October 31, 2018. https://epmonthly.com/article/7-ways-to-solve-the-ed-boarding-challenge/

Sun BC, Hsia RY, Weiss RE, et al. Effect of emergency department crowding on outcomes of admitted patients. *Ann Emerg Med*. 2013;61(6):605-611.e6.

SECTION XXVIII
PAIN MANAGEMENT

357

Ketamine for Procedural Sedation and Pain Management in the Emergency Department

R. Gentry Wilkerson

Many ED encounters are due to acute painful conditions. After recognizing that opioids administered in and prescribed from the ED contributed to the development of the opioid epidemic, alternative pain management strategies were sought. Ketamine has been established to be a safe and effective analgesic when administered appropriately in the ED.

How It Works

Ketamine, a portmanteau of ketone and amine, is an arylcycloalkylamine with chiral chemical structure that plays a role in the physiologic effects encountered with administration. Previously, ketamine was only available as a racemic mixture but now comes in both the S(+) and R(−) forms. It is the S(+) stereoisomer that is primarily responsible for the analgesic effect of ketamine having a 4-fold greater potency than the R(−) stereoisomer and 2-fold the potency of the racemic mixture. The S(+) stereoisomer has also been shown to be effective in the treatment of major depressive disorder and reduces the incidence of suicidal ideation.

The primary mechanism of action of ketamine is as a noncompetitive antagonist of the NMDA receptor, similar to the related but much more PCP. NMDA receptors have a central role in the development of chronic pain. Continuous activation of the NMDA receptors leads to increased responsiveness of spinal cord neurons and development of the central sensitization of chronic pain. Ketamine also provides direct analgesic effect through agonism at the mu-, delta-, and kappa-opioid receptors. Potentiation of mu-opioid receptor–mediated signaling by ketamine results in a lower dose of opioids required to have the same clinical effect. There is evidence that interactions at AMPA receptors, cannabinoid systems, mTOR signal pathway, cholinergic system, monoaminergic system, and sigma-1 receptors contribute to ketamine's clinical effects.

Extensive first-pass metabolism of ketamine leads to limited bioavailability with oral (~17%) and rectal (~25%) administration. Intranasal use of ketamine has as much as 50% bioavailability. Intramuscular administration has very high (93%) bioavailability. The distribution half-life is 7 to 11 minutes, and it rapidly crosses the blood-brain barrier. It is metabolized predominately by the liver where it undergoes N–dealkylation by cytochrome P450 3A4 primarily to form norketamine. Norketamine is a less potent metabolite that gets hydroxylated and excreted in bile and urine.

In addition to analgesia, the clinical effects of ketamine include sedation, bronchodilation, and sympathetic stimulation. Some of the effects are dose dependent. At higher doses, ketamine results in a state of dissociation where the patient has an altered level of consciousness with feelings of detachment, altered perception of visual and auditory stimuli, and amnesia. Lower or subdissociative doses of ketamine can be used for its analgesic properties. There is no consensus on the optimal dose of subdissociative ketamine. Most studies use an IV dose of 0.1 to 0.6 mg/kg. Psychomimetic symptoms, with both positive and negative symptoms of psychosis, can be seen with both bolus dosing and continuous infusions of ketamine. Ketamine should be avoided in patients with schizophrenia as it may exacerbate this condition.

How It's Used—Procedural Sedation

Ketamine is frequently used to provide sedation along with analgesia during acute painful procedures in the ED. It may be used as a single agent or in combination with another medication such as propofol, fentanyl, or a benzodiazepine. A combination of ketamine and propofol, commonly referred to as "ketofol," is safe and effective for procedural sedation and analgesia, although it is unclear that its use is associated with improved clinical outcomes compared to monotherapy with only ketamine. Ketamine allows the patient to maintain protective airway reflexes, although it has been associated with the development of idiosyncratic laryngospasm in less than 1% of patients.

During procedural sedation, the goal is to achieve full dissociation. This usually requires a bolus dose of at least 1 mg/kg IV or 4 mg/kg intramuscularly. These doses can be repeated as the clinical effect begins to wear off. For procedures known to have a long duration, the bolus dose can be followed by a continuous infusion of 10 to 20 mcg/kg/min. Emergence reactions complicate up to 30% of procedural sedations with ketamine in adults. The rate is lower in children (<10%). These are psychomimetic episodes of restlessness, agitation, dysphoria or euphoria, nightmares, or hallucinations. Benzodiazepines may be given before the procedure to reduce the risk of developing an emergence reaction or they may be given once an emergence reaction has occurred. It is unclear if placing a patient who has received ketamine into a low-stimulation environment is effective in decreasing the incidence of emergence reactions. Hypersalivation is frequently seen with ketamine administration, but it is rarely of clinical significance and does not require pretreatment with atropine or glycopyrrolate. Ketamine may be preferred in patients with hypotension as it is associated with elevations in blood pressure.

Ketamine is a safe and effective medication for procedural sedation. It should be used in a monitored setting by clinicians who are knowledgeable in the medication, its side effects, and in airway management. Patients can be discharged when their pain is controlled, vital signs are normal, mental status and physical function have returned to normal, and a reliable person who can provide support is present.

How It's Used—Analgesia

Ketamine can be used at subdissociative doses as an analgesic to treat severe traumatic and nontraumatic pain. It can be used as an adjunct when sufficient pain relief is not achieved with opioids. It can also be used as the initial drug of choice for patients in whom opioids may not be appropriate. Conditions where ketamine has been effectively used include renal colic, sickle cell disease, pancreatitis, and acute traumatic injuries. It is unclear if there is an analgesic ceiling whereby additional ketamine will provide no further pain relief. Recent data suggest that very low doses such as 0.15 mg/kg IV given as a bolus may be just as effective as higher doses with a better safety profile. Ketamine is also effective for treatment of severe pain when given as a continuous infusion at a rate of 0.15 to 0.3 mg/kg/h.

Oral administration of ketamine has been used for acute pain management although the racemic drug is only available as an IV formulation. The bioavailability of oral administration is low and has substantial variation among individuals making appropriate dosing difficult. Other methods of administration reported include intranasal and intramuscular. Appropriate dosing, while not standardized, for these other routes of administration include oral 0.5 mg/kg, intranasal 1 mg/kg, and intramuscular 0.5 to 1 mg/kg.

PEARLS

- Ketamine's antagonism at the NMDA receptor is the primary mechanism for its clinical effect.
- An analgesic ceiling for ketamine may exist with no benefit seen beyond doses of 0.15 mg/kg IV.
- Higher, dissociative doses of ketamine used for procedural sedation may be associated with development of psychotomimetic effects such as agitation, nightmares, and hallucinations.
- Other adverse events associated with ketamine use include development of emergence reactions, hypersalivation, and laryngospasm.
- Ketamine may be given as monotherapy or in combination with other medications intended to augment the analgesic effect or decrease the rate of certain complications.

Suggested Readings

Balzer N, McLeod SL, Walsh C, Grewal K. Low-dose ketamine for acute pain control in the emergency department: a systematic review and meta-analysis. *Acad Emerg Med.* 2021; 28(4):444-454.

Beaudrie-Nunn AN, Wieruszewski ED, Woods EJ, Bellolio F, Mara KC, Canterbury EA. Efficacy of analgesic and sub-dissociative dose ketamine for acute pain in the emergency department. *Am J Emerg Med.* 2023;70:133-139.

Corwell BN, Motov SM, Davis NL, Kim HK. Novel uses of ketamine in the emergency department. *Expert Opin Drug Saf.* 2022;21(8):1009-1025.

Riccardi A, Guarino M, Serra S, et al. Narrative review: low-dose ketamine for pain management. *J Clin Med.* 2023;12(9):3256.

Strayer RJ, Shy BD. Best practice during procedural sedation with ketamine. *Am J Emerg Med.* 2017;35(2):315-316.

Pitfalls in Ultrasound-Guided Nerve Blocks

Jose Acosta and Arun Nagdev

Ultrasound-Guided Nerve Blocks (UNGBs) are becoming integrated into emergency care of the acutely injured patients. Overreliance on opioid-based monomodal therapy has deleterious downstream effects, and emergency physicians have begun to incorporate a multimodal pain management pathway using UGNBs in combination with pharmacologic therapies (eg, ketamine, nonsteroidal anti-inflammatory drugs, acetaminophen, gabapentanoids, topical creams/patches). This chapter will review common errors with the performance of UGNBs outside the OR.

Pitfall 1: Failure to Aspirate Before Injecting Anesthetic

Intravascular injection of anesthetic medication during UGNBs is the most common cause of LAST. LAST is characterized by central nervous system and cardiac changes that occur within seconds to 30 minutes after injection of a local anesthetic. It has a spectrum of severity that ranges from perioral numbness, tachycardia, and hypertension to seizures, coma, respiratory and cardiac arrest. To reduce the possibility of LAST, we recommend to always aspirate first to ensure placement of the needle tip outside of the intravascular space and to then slowly inject small aliquots of anesthetic (3-5 mL). If anechoic fluid is not clearly seen after injection of anesthetic, intravascular placement should be suspected, and the procedure should be halted.

Pitfall 2: Inappropriate Anesthetic Dosing

LAST is a worrisome, albeit rare complication of UGNBs. Along with always ensuring that anesthetic is not deposited into the intravascular space, we recommend to always use a weight-based dosing calculator before every block to ensure that dosing of anesthetic is kept under maximum recommended levels. Clinicians should be aware that patients with advanced age and renal, cardiac, and hepatic dysfunction will have a reduced maximum dose. It is imperative to have intralipid treatment with clear instructions for administration available and easily accessible in the event that LAST is suspected.

Pitfall 3: Failure to Select the Appropriate Needle

The needle bevel/tip is the angular tip that facilitates entrance into tissue. There are different types of bevels: A-bevel, B-bevel, C-bevel, which are classified by the angle of the bevel. Classically, an A-bevel has a 12° to 15° angled tip while the B-bevel has an 18° to 20° angle and the C-bevel has a 25° to 30° angle. The steeper the angle of the tip (C-bevel) implies a blunt needle and should be used, if possible, for UGNBs. If a C-bevel needle is not readily available in your department, a 20- to 22-gauge Quincke spinal needle may be used as an alternative. Blunt needles are believed to offer several advantages over sharp, long (cutting) bevel needles: reduced risk of intraneural or intrafascicular peripheral nerve injury, reduced risk of intravascular injection, and greater sense of resistance to applied pressure, which better allows the user to perceive different tissue planes. We recommend speaking with your anesthesia colleagues and using similar block needles as those used daily in the OR to ensure consistency for all clinicians at your institution.

Pitfall 4: Allowing the Needle Tip to Be in Close Proximity to the Nerve

For the core group of blocks in the ED (eg, femoral nerve, erector spinae, serratus anterior, interscalene brachial plexus, supraclavicular brachial plexus, transverse abdominal plane), we recommend targeting the fascial plane for anesthetic deposition. These planes are the potential space between the two layers of fascia from surrounding muscles which contain nerves and vessels. This "stay away" approach is believed to lower the risk of intraneural injury by preventing inadvertent direct trauma to nerve fascicles by the block needle. Normal saline can be injected to ensure the correct fascial plane has been opened (hydrodissection) as well as improve needle tip visualization (hydrolocalization). After clear visualization of the needle tip and appropriate fascial plane spread, the anesthetic can be administered in gentle aliquots.

Pitfall 5: Not Using Color Doppler (Overreliance on B-Mode Imaging)

After clear nerve bundle visualization with B-mode imaging, we recommend using color Doppler to ensure the lack of vasculature in the projected pathway of the needle. Also, in proximal nerve roots such as the interscalene brachial plexus, nerve bundles are commonly anechoic and can be easily confused with vasculature. Clinicians performing UGNBs should be comfortable with performing color Doppler evaluation (and adjusting the pulse repetition frequency to optimize the elimination of artifacts) in addition to using standard gray-scale, B-mode ultrasound imaging. We recommend evaluating both the nerve bundle as well as the planned path of the needle so that inadvertent puncture is prevented.

Summary

UGNBs are a skill that all emergency medicine physicians should possess to optimally treat pain in the ED. They are a part of the multimodal approach to pain and can be safely and easily performed at bedside. Awareness of the common pitfalls in UGNBs will help prevent iatrogenic injury and other complications.

PEARLS

- Always use a weight-based calculator to determine the maximum dose.
- Use a blunt tip needle to prevent peripheral nerve injury.
- Stay away from the nerve and open fascial planes with saline first.
- Use color Doppler to prevent vascular puncture.
- Aspirate before injecting small aliquots of anesthetic.

Suggested Readings

Bloc S, Ecoffey C, Dhonneur G. Controlling needle tip progression during ultrasound-guided regional anesthesia using the hydrolocalization technique. *Reg Anesth Pain Med*. 2008; 33(4):382-383. PMID: 18675754.

Chin KJ, Versyck B, Elsharkawy H, et al. Anatomical basis of fascial plane blocks. *Reg Anesth Pain Med*. 2021;46(7):581-599. PMID: 34145071.

Hahn C, Nagdev A. Color Doppler ultrasound-guided supraclavicular brachial plexus block to prevent vascular injection. *West J Emerg Med.* 2014;15(6):703-705. PMID: 25247047.

Heavner JE, Racz GB, Jenigiri B, Lehman T, Day MR. Sharp versus blunt needle: a comparative study of penetration of internal structures and bleeding in dogs. *Pain Pract.* 2003; 3(3):226-231. PMID: 17147672.

Mahajan A, Derian A. Local anesthetic toxicity. [Updated October 3, 2022]. In: *StatPearls* [Internet]. StatPearls Publishing; 2022. https://www.ncbi.nlm.nih.gov/books/NBK499964;

Sites B, Antonakakis JG. Ultrasound guidance in regional anesthesia: state of the art review through challenging clinical scenarios. *Local Reg Anesth.* 2009;2:1-14.

359

TRAMA-DON'T: REASONS TO AVOID USING TRAMADOL

JACK MCGEACHY

Throughout the history of medicine, there have been analgesics that are perceived to be a safe and effective middle ground between nonopioids and full-agonist opioids. These can be considered "compromise opioids" because they are often prescribed to patients with pain who are not considered to require full agonists but who may report that nonopioid analgesics such as acetaminophen and NSAIDs are ineffective. An example is codeine (3-methylmorphine), a prodrug with little analgesic effect that must be converted to morphine to provide analgesia. It was considered a safe alternative to morphine with a wide therapeutic index and low risk of respiratory depression. Since 2011, multiple agencies, including the World Health Organization, the FDA, and the European Medicines Agency, have removed codeine from recommendations or placed warnings on its use after recognizing safety concerns with the drug. Another example of a "compromise opioid" is propoxyphene, which was introduced into the United States in 1957. After initial widespread adoption, it was recognized that its analgesic effects were minimal and that it carried higher risks than originally believed. Its major metabolite is nor-dextropropoxyphene, which is excreted by the kidneys. Accumulation of nor-dextropropoxyphene can lead to depression of the cardiac, respiratory, and central nervous systems. Ever since its introduction in 1995, the synthetic opioid tramadol has become the most widely prescribed "compromise opioid." According to the US Agency for Healthcare Research and Quality, more than 5 million people in the United States were prescribed tramadol in 2019.

"Compromise opioids" are a problematic category of drugs. The main issue is that it is impossible to create a nonaddictive opioid. Regardless of an opioid's strength, there is the potential for misuse due to the intrinsic euphoric effects. Moreover, stereotypical side effects of opioids are a class effect and all opioids have the potential to cause some degree of sedation, pruritus, nausea, constipation, confusion, and respiratory depression, among others. For tramadol, there are a multitude of additional possible side effects due to its interaction with receptors other than opioid receptors.

Misconceptions About Tramadol

Many of the misconceptions surrounding tramadol involve its mechanism of action, safety, abuse potential, or prescribing regulations. Many clinicians seem to believe that tramadol is either not an opioid or such a weak opioid that the risk of abuse is negligible. Tramadol is a mu-opioid receptor agonist, albeit a weak one. It is currently a schedule IV-controlled substance, although many have advocated for a move to schedule II consistent with other opioid medications. Schedule IV drugs have fewer regulations placed on their prescriptions. Schedule IV drugs can be prescribed over the phone and refilled, whereas schedule II drugs must be prescribed using paper or transmitted electronically and refills are not permitted. The ease with which tramadol can be prescribed increases the likelihood that clinicians will choose this medication over other opioids subject to stricter regulations.

Tramadol itself may be a weak opioid agonist, but the CYP2D6 enzyme converts tramadol in the liver to *o*-desmethyl tramadol, a drug with much stronger mu-agonism. People with CYP2D6 gain of function mutations (ie, "super-metabolizers") experience more intense euphoria. Rates of CYP2D6 super-metabolizers vary according to population group. It is rare that a prescriber of tramadol has any knowledge of the patient's CYP2D6 status and, thus, has no idea of the potency of this medication.

The second misconception is a failure of the prescriber to appreciate the pharmacodynamics of tramadol, notably its actions on systems beyond mu-opioid receptors. Tramadol is also a serotonin and norepinephrine reuptake inhibitor. It has muscarinic and anticholinergic properties. Additionally, it is a GABA-A inhibitor and a serotonin 5-HT2C antagonist. All of these additional actions contribute to its side effect profile.

Tramadol's actions can create intolerable neuropsychiatric side effects and delirium. Increased serotonergic activity can precipitate serotonin syndrome in patients taking other serotonergic drugs. Tramadol prolongs the QTc interval, which can trigger torsades de pointes. Finally, GABA-A inhibition can lower the seizure threshold. Because of these risks, the FDA advises that patients who are 17 years of age and older take no more than 400 mg of tramadol daily. This daily limit is decreased to 200 mg in patients with a creatinine clearance less than 30 mL/min and 300 mg in patients older than 75. Patients with cirrhosis should not take more than 50 mg every 12 hours. Tramadol has a "black box warning" for use in children under 12 years of age.

Lastly, tramadol is not a very effective analgesic. A 2017 Cochrane review found low to very low-quality evidence that tramadol provided better relief of neuropathic pain than placebo. However, 60% of patients experienced side effects and 20% stopped the drug due to these side effects. For patients with osteoarthritis, a 2019 Cochrane review found no benefit for tramadol when compared to NSAIDs. Similar to the 2017 review, 66% of the tramadol group experienced side effects and the drop out rate was 19%. Tramadol has also been associated with a higher mortality rate than NSAIDs used for osteoarthritis.

A World Without Tramadol

Most patients who are prescribed tramadol have moderate to severe pain and likely have not had adequate analgesia with the use of acetaminophen or NSAIDs. In this case, a short course of opioids may be warranted. Rather than trying to avoid opioids by prescribing a "compromise opioid," an appropriate mu-opioid receptor agonist should be prescribed. As mentioned previously, there are full mu-opioid receptor agonists such as codeine and propoxyphene that are problematic and should be avoided if not already withdrawn from the market (propoxyphene). Oral morphine is an excellent choice when given 5 to 10 mg every 6 hours. It produces less euphoria than oxycodone or hydromorphone but provides similar analgesia.

Unfortunately, to accurately dose this quantity requires the oral solution (10 mg or 20 mg per 5 mL), which is frequently out-of-stock in US pharmacies. Morphine tablets are small and difficult to divide accurately. Hydrocodone is equianalgesic to oral morphine, meaning that 1 mg of hydrocodone equals 1 mg of morphine. It is widely available and similar to morphine, it produces less euphoric reinforcement. The only drawback is that instant-release hydrocodone is only available compounded with acetaminophen, which can be contraindicated in some patients and increases the risk of accidental acetaminophen overdose.

In summary, when considering a prescription of tramadol for your patient with pain, just trama-don't!

PEARLS

- Tramadol is a weak mu-opioid receptor agonist; however, some patients with CYP2D6 gain of function mutations convert tramadol to the active metabolite, *o*-desmethyl tramadol.
- Tramadol is also a serotonin and norepinephrine reuptake inhibitor, a GABA-A inhibitor, and a serotonin 5-HT2C antagonist with muscarinic and anticholinergic properties.
- Tramadol is associated with multiple side effects, leading to its having a "black box" warning for use in children under 12 years of age.
- Tramadol is not a very effective analgesic.

Suggested Readings

Duehmke RM, Derry S, Wiffen PJ, Bell RF, Aldington D, Moore RA. Tramadol for neuropathic pain in adults. *Cochrane Database Syst Rev*. 2017;6(6):CD003726.

Mullins PM, Mazer-Amirshahi M, Pourmand A, Perrone J, Nelson LS, Pines JM. Tramadol use in United States Emergency Departments 2007–2018. *J Emerg Med*. 2022;62(5):668-674.

Toupin April K, Bisaillon J, Welch V, et al. Tramadol for osteoarthritis. *Cochrane Database Syst Rev*. 2019;5(5):CD005522.

Zeng C, Dubreuil M, LaRochelle MR, et al. Association of tramadol with all-cause mortality among patients with osteoarthritis. *JAMA*. 2019;321(10):969-982.

360

NSAIDs in Older Adults

Andrew K. Chang and Emma R. Furlano

NSAIDs are used to treat both acute and chronic pain. They are one of the most frequently used analgesics in the ED with ibuprofen being the third most commonly administered medication. Over-the-counter agents include ibuprofen, naproxen, and aspirin, while prescription medications include celecoxib.

The mechanism of action for NSAIDs involves the inhibition of prostaglandin synthesis, specifically the step in which the enzyme cyclooxygenase (COX) metabolizes arachidonic acid to form prostaglandin. COX-1 is an isoform found in platelets and is expressed throughout the body. The isoform COX-2 is induced in endothelial cells by laminar or mechanical stress, causing an inflammatory response including warmth, pain, erythema, and swelling. Nonselective NSAIDs, such as ibuprofen and naproxen, inhibit both COX-1 and COX-2, whereas selective NSAIDs (eg, celecoxib) inhibit COX-2 only. Aspirin is a nonselective agent that when given at lower doses (60-150 mg/d) causes acetylation of COX-1, which results in decreased platelet synthesis of thromboxane A_2 but does not cause decreased production of prostacyclin by the vascular cell wall. Higher daily doses of aspirin result in decreased prostacyclin production.

NSAIDs have important adverse effects in various organ systems, and these are often exacerbated in older adults due to multiple physiologic changes that can affect NSAID pharmacokinetics. Gastric motility and renal clearance decrease with aging, which can lead to reduced elimination of NSAIDs as most NSAIDs undergo hepatic metabolism and are then renally cleared. NSAIDs can promote fluid retention and increase the risk of heart failure, in addition to causing hypertension. Several COX-2 inhibitors have been withdrawn from the market due to thrombotic events, though celecoxib is still available and has a more favorable GI safety profile than nonselective NSAIDs. NSAIDs may increase the risk of GI bleeding up to 4-fold. The AGS recommends avoiding chronic use of NSAIDs unless other alternatives are not effective, and that a PPI should be added when NSAIDs are used chronically. NSAIDs should also be taken with food to decrease the risk of GI upset. Neurologic manifestations of NSAIDs in therapeutic dosing can cause headache, drowsiness, and dizziness along with rare drug-induced aseptic meningitis. These symptoms could potentially lead to increased likelihood of falls in the geriatric population. NSAIDs affect the renal system and can cause sodium retention, nephrotic syndrome, interstitial nephritis, and renal papillary necrosis. The risk of developing these side effects increases with age. Most of these effects can be reversible, but renal papillary necrosis may result in the need for hemodialysis. Acute tubulointerstitial nephritis can occur with short-term NSAID use and result in elevation of BUN in older adults though these typically normalize with discontinuation of the NSAID.

Adverse effects of NSAIDs have become even more important in older adults (age 65 and older), whose population has grown rapidly since 2010. Indeed, those aged 80 years and older represent the fastest-growing segment in the United States, with a growth rate twice that for people aged 65 years and older and almost 4 times that for the total population.

The importance of NSAID-induced adverse effects is demonstrated by their inclusion in the AGS Beers Criteria for potentially inappropriate medication use in older adults. This list compiles medications potentially to avoid or consider with caution because they may present an unfavorable balance of benefits and harms to older adults. The list, updated in 2023, recommends avoiding use of indomethacin and ketorolac. It also recommends avoiding chronic use of other NSAIDs (eg, naproxen, ibuprofen) unless other alternatives are ineffective, and recommends avoiding short-term scheduled use in combination with oral or parenteral corticosteroids, anticoagulants, or antiplatelet agents unless other alternatives are ineffective. Older patients often have multiple medical comorbidities and take medications that may have drug-drug interactions with NSAIDs. Examples include the disruption of the protective cardiovascular effects of aspirin and decreased renal clearance of methotrexate.

Given the potential adverse effects of NSAIDs and drug-drug interactions in older adults, alternative medications should be initiated if possible. Acetaminophen is typically a first-line choice for analgesia and fever in older adults. It may be administered orally and rectally, as well as intravenously, though some hospitals have restricted intravenous use due to cost. Although acetaminophen inhibits COX pathways, it has minimal peripheral anti-inflammatory properties while having strong central nervous system antipyretic and analgesic effects. If opioids are determined to be the most appropriate treatment for an older adult, they should be started at the lowest effective dose and for as short a duration as possible. A stool softener should be co-prescribed with opioids. Adjunctive therapies, such as peripheral femoral nerve block for acute hip fractures, may also lessen the need for analgesics with potentially harmful adverse effects.

Topical treatments for pain, including topical NSAIDs (eg, diclofenac gel), are reasonable alternatives to oral NSAIDs for localized pain control since they have decreased systemic absorption. Topical products may have decreased efficacy in older adults due to changes in skin with aging that affect absorption. Other topical agents include lidocaine cream and menthol salicylate.

Despite their potential downsides, NSAIDs are important analgesics used to treat older patients in the ED. Single and short-term (ie, 3-5 days) use is likely safe in older adults though alternatives should be considered whenever possible.

PEARLS

- Although NSAIDs can cause GI, renal, and cardiovascular adverse effects in older adults, a single dose or short-term use is generally safe in the ED population.
- When NSAIDs are used in older adults, naproxen and ibuprofen are preferred. Indomethacin and ketorolac should be avoided.
- Given the increased risk for adverse events, consider alternatives to NSAIDs, such as acetaminophen, in the appropriate clinical context.
- Medication lists should be examined in older adults since NSAIDs can cause multiple drug-drug interactions.

Suggesting Readings

By the 2023 American Geriatrics Society Beers Criteria® Update Expert Panel. American Geriatrics Society 2023 updated AGS Beers Criteria® for potentially inappropriate medication use in older adults. *J Am Geriatr Soc*. 2023;71(7):2052-2081.

Ribeiro H, Rodrigues I, Napoleão L, et al. Non-steroidal anti-inflammatory drugs (NSAIDs), pain and aging: adjusting prescription to patient features. *Biomed Pharmacother*. 2022; 150:112958.

Wongrakpanich S, Wongrakpanich A, Melhado K, Rangaswami J. A comprehensive review of non-steroidal anti-inflammatory drug use in the elderly. *Aging Dis*. 2018;9(1):143-150.

361

DOSE YOUR OPIOIDS CORRECTLY

T. ANDREW WINDSOR AND MEGHIN MOYNIHAN

The first decision to make when prescribing an opioid is whether it is even necessary in the first place. Opioids should not be considered first-line therapy for conditions such as osteoarthritis, migraine headaches, or chronic atraumatic low back pain. Opioids often provide no further analgesia than with what is provided by acetaminophen or NSAIDs as monotherapy or in combination. Opioids may be indicated for certain conditions causing moderate to severe pain, especially if other alternatives are contraindicated or have been proven ineffective.

When used, opioids should ideally be given at the lowest effective dose and as part of multi-modal therapy that also includes nonopioid treatment. Unfortunately, there is no "one-size-fits-all" approach to opioid dosing. Patients who chronically take opioids or have a history of opioid use disorder may have increased drug tolerance and require higher dosing to achieve the same level of analgesia as an opioid-naive patient. Similarly, clinical factors such as patient's age, weight, comorbidities, and other concomitant medications may also require dosing adjustment of the prescribed opioid for safety or efficacy.

CHOOSING AN OPIOID

Assuming that an opioid is necessary and appropriate, the next choice is to decide between oral and parenteral options. Factors including the severity of pain, the desired speed of onset of analgesia, and the duration of action play into this decision. Oral opioids can be effective for a wide variety of ED complaints and may be appropriate if the patient has normal gastrointestinal absorption and does not have a contraindication to taking medicine by mouth. Most oral opioids undergo first-pass metabolism, which leads to an onset of effect of about 30 to 45 minutes. There are negligible differences in efficacy at equianalgesic dosing (**Table 361.1**). When treating acute pain with an oral opioid in the ED or at discharge, immediate-release formulations should be used rather than extended-release or long-acting opioids.

Unlike oral agents, opioids given IV will have a rapid onset of action, usually within about 5 minutes. Intramuscular injection is usually not recommended due to unpredictable absorption rates. There is no true "minimum" amount of time required between additional dosing of an IV opioid if the desired level of analgesia has not been achieved; however, peak plasma levels and respiratory depression can be delayed beyond the onset of action. Peak plasma concentrations for an IV opioid given as a bolus tend to occur within about 20 minutes, although the peak physiologic effects (eg, miosis, respiratory depression) can occur as much as an hour later for morphine. Additional doses administered within this time have the potential to stack and lead to an overdose if the patient is not appropriately monitored. It is prudent to reassess pain control and side effects every 15 to 30 minutes for the first hour to decide if additional doses are warranted rather than allowing the patient to remain in significant pain for 2 to 3 hours if they tolerated the first dose.

TABLE 361.1 SAMPLE STARTING AND EQUIANALGESIC DOSES OF COMMON OPIOIDS

Opioid	PO (Starting)	IV (Starting)	Duration	PO (Equianalgesic)	IV (Equianalgesic)
Fentanyl	N/A	0.25-1 mcg/kg	0.5-1 h	N/A	0.15 mg (150 mcg)
Hydromorphone	1-2 mg	0.015 mg/kg	4-5 h	5 mg	2 mg
Morphine	10-15 mg	0.05-0.1 mg/kg	3-6 h	25 mg	10 mg
Oxycodone	5-10 mg	N/A	4-6 h	20 mg	N/A
Hydrocodone	5-10 mg	N/A	4-6 h	25 mg	N/A
Oxymorphone	10-20 mg	N/A	4-6 h	10 mg	N/A
Tramadol	25-50 mg	N/A	4-6 h	120 mg	N/A
Codeine	30-60 mg	N/A	4-6 h	200 mg	N/A

IV, intravenous; N/A, not available; PO, by mouth.

Please consult the manufacturer's full prescribing information and institutional protocols for individual medication guidance.

PITFALLS

A common pitfall when administering opioids is underdosing, thereby undertreating pain. Does your computer system pre-populate morphine 4 mg IV, regardless of the patient's characteristics? The reason might be more practical than anything evidence based. Many hospitals now stock single-use, preloaded syringes to avoid dosing errors or diversion. These often come in 2, 4, 8, or 10 mg/mL syringes. It may not be possible to stock all these concentrations in the ED, so if 5 mg of morphine was ordered and only the 4 mg syringes were stocked, it would require two syringes and nursing protocols generally require "wasting" or disposing of the unused 3 mg. Repeat that for thousands of patients annually, and that's a lot of waste. However, be aware that the "standard" dose may be ineffective for your patient. A reasonable approach for a generally healthy patient is to consider a weight-based starting dose (e.g., 0.1 mg/kg IV morphine or equianalgesic equivalent) although a single dose may not provide adequate analgesia.

Members of socioeconomically marginalized groups, those with substance use disorders, patients with chronically relapsing painful diseases such as SCD, or those with cancer-related pain are also at risk of undertreatment. Unconscious (or conscious) bias can play as much a part in this phenomenon as a lack of understanding of the specific underlying disease process. For example, a patient with SCD suffering a VOC may experience severe, debilitating pain without any of the outward distress or vital sign abnormalities one might see in a patient who underwent trauma. Many have had to contend with their condition since childhood and are very familiar with effective doses or have a high tolerance due to chronic medications. If a clinician rarely treats this condition, it may feel odd to have a patient state that they require 4 mg of hydromorphone IV, for example. However, the use of aggressive analgesia has been shown to reduce hospitalization rates with VOC. If utilization of such high doses is unverifiable and the clinician is not confident of the need, the key is to follow the principle of frequent (every 15-30 minutes) reassessment and to continue treating.

Assessing for increased risk of opioid-related harm or adverse effects, specifically respiratory/CNS depression, should be done before prescribing any opioids for home. Key populations to consider include patients 65 years old or older, those with obstructive sleep apnea, patients already taking other CNS depressants, and those with hepatic or renal insufficiency. If opioids are deemed necessary, consider dose reductions, cautious counseling, or close monitoring in these at-risk populations. Morphine and codeine should specifically be avoided in those with renal impairment (CrCl <30 mL/min) due to the accumulation of their active metabolites. Other agents should start at 25% to 50% of their usual doses. The same reductions should be made with any agent used in patients with hepatic impairment.

PEARLS

- Oral opioids can be useful for a variety of ED complaints, and most have similar efficacy at equianalgesic dosing.
- Weight-based dosing of IV opioids is more likely to be effective than using "standard" empiric doses.
- Be aware of potential biases that could affect appropriate treatment of pain in marginalized or vulnerable populations.
- Avoid morphine and codeine in patients with renal impairment due to accumulation of active metabolites.
- Reassess your patient within the first 15-30 minutes to determine if your initial chosen IV opioid dose was effective.

Suggested Readings

Chang AK, Bijur PE, Esses D, Barnaby DP, Baer J. Effect of a single dose of oral opioid and nonopioid analgesics on acute extremity pain in the emergency department: a randomized clinical trial. *JAMA.* 2017;318(17):1661-1667.

Coluzzi F, Caputi FF, Billeci D, et al. Safe use of opioids in chronic kidney disease and hemodialysis patients: tips and tricks for non-pain specialists. *Ther Clin Risk Manag.* 2020; 16:821-837.

Jones CM, McAninch JK. Emergency department visits and overdose deaths from combined use of opioids and benzodiazepines. *Am J Prev Med.* 2015;49:493-501.

Roth JV. Opioid-induced respiratory depression: is hydromorphone safer than morphine? *Anesth Analg.* 2021;132(4):e60.

362

Awesome Analgesic Adjuncts

Adam Barnathan and Samuel Harris

In many cases, treating pain should be considered an emergency. Opioids are often used as a first-line treatment for pain; however, they should be used thoughtfully. The risk of opioid use disorder increases with the duration and dose that is used. There are a multitude of procedural techniques and nonopioid medications that can be used to reduce or replace opioid utilization altogether. A few of the often-underutilized techniques for mitigating musculoskeletal pain in the ED require using your procedural skills. These include nerve blocks, intra-articular blocks, hematoma blocks, and trigger point injections.

PROCEDURAL ADJUNCTS FOR PAIN MANAGEMENT

The most common indication for a nerve block is to provide analgesia during the repair of a laceration. Anesthesia of the affected area allows for extensive cleaning of contaminated wounds, removal of foreign bodies, and of course the repair itself. Often nerve blocks are done on the digits, palms, or soles; however, an astute clinician could perform a nerve block for almost any surface on the body. Nerve blocks performed distant to the site of injury will not distort tissue prior to repair and thus can improve cosmetic outcomes in sensitive areas such as the vermilion border of the lips. They are also very useful in the setting of dental pain where a long-acting agent can be used to bridge a patient to the dentist or allow time for antibiotics to work.

Intra-articular injections can be used during reduction of shoulder or ankle dislocations, and they also provide effective although temporary relief for patients with osteoarthritis of the knees. Hematoma blocks, whereby local anesthetic is administered into a fracture space after aspiration of blood, provide sufficient analgesia for many uncomplicated extremity fractures requiring reduction and splinting. Trigger points have been described as discrete, hyperirritable nodules of skeletal muscle fascia. In some patients, trigger point injections are effective at providing myofascial pain relief through needle stimulation and treatment with anesthetics, steroids, or botulinum toxin. These are most effective when used for an appropriate indication and with proper patient selection. There is some limited evidence that trigger point injections result in improved analgesia, decreased length of stay in the ED, and decreased opioid utilization.

There are many benefits to the use of these techniques. They are safe and easy to do especially when using ultrasound guidance. They provide great pain control and can prevent undesirable side effects of opioids. These techniques also use less local anesthetic, limiting the risk of toxicity, especially in the pediatric population. Additionally, they often save time, cost, and resources by limiting the use of procedural sedation. If appropriately documented, many of these are also billable procedures. If used as a first-line treatment and adequate analgesia is not obtained, escalation of analgesia can occur with pharmacologic interventions or, when appropriate, procedural sedation.

PHARMACOLOGIC ADJUNCTS FOR PAIN MANAGEMENT

There are multiple pharmacologic options that can be employed to assist with pain management. Over-the-counter analgesics such as NSAIDs and acetaminophen provide excellent analgesia for many painful conditions if taken appropriately. They can be used as a solitary agent to avoid the use of opioids. Even in more painful conditions, these medications can be opioid sparing. Although safe for most patients, acetaminophen should not be used in patients with severe liver disease. Similarly, NSAIDs are generally safe but all have a risk of cardiovascular and gastrointestinal complications.

LET gel is a topical anesthetic that is frequently utilized for pediatric laceration repair, but it can be used for patients of all ages. At times, it may not provide complete analgesia but will at least reduce the pain and amount of subsequently injected local anesthetic. It can also be used topically at the site of a nerve block, such as prior to a painful digital block. It can take 45 minutes to take full effect, and thus should be applied early. To ensure continued contact with the skin, cover the LET gel with a transparent adhesive film dressing.

Ketamine is an effective analgesic when given at sub-dissociative intravenous doses of 0.1 to 0.6 mg/kg. This may be particularly useful when treating an opioid-tolerant patient. It also has the added benefit of being safe in those with borderline hemodynamics. Benzodiazepines are frequently coadministered to reduce the likelihood of an emergence reaction.

Pain management for patients presenting with headaches can be challenging. There are numerous underlying causes for headaches and patient-specific factors so that there is no one-size-fits-all approach. A multimodal approach to headaches may include medications such as NSAIDs, acetaminophen, antipsychotics, antihistamines, antiemetics, caffeine, triptans, antiepileptics, steroids, magnesium, and fluids.

Psychosocial Adjuncts for Pain Management

An invaluable component of treating patients with acute and chronic pain is as simple as having a conversation. The use of anticipatory guidance to set expectations regarding the timeline and treatment options for pain can improve outcomes and minimize risk. Patients should be educated regarding the side effects of agents and alternatives should be discussed. A holistic approach should be taken to encourage nonpharmacologic options and address the psychological aspect of pain. These interventions can include ice, heat, compression, elevation, massage, exercise, physical therapy, breathing techniques, or even therapy. The cumulative benefit of patient education and engagement in their own treatment cannot be understated.

Conclusion

A multimodal approach to pain is essential in today's climate. Patients deserve effective pain management while the clinicians caring for these patients need to maintain judicious prescribing to avoid opioid overutilization. Utilization of all the tools and techniques available will help to achieve this delicate balance.

PEARLS

- A multimodal approach to pain control in the ED leads to improved analgesia, increased patient satisfaction, and decreases the likelihood that a patient will develop opioid dependence.
- Opioid pain medications should be prescribed for no greater than 3 days based on evidence showing dependency is more likely with increased dosage and duration.
- Counseling patients regarding the expectations of pain control, risk of dependence, and addiction has been shown to lower rates of opioid use and improve patient satisfaction.
- Managing the anxiety related to pain by utilizing therapeutic touch, breathing techniques, and nonpharmacologic modalities (ice, compression, stretching, etc) should not be underestimated. This should be part of the anticipatory guidance provided to all patients with pain upon discharge.
- We are at the frontline of this deadly opioid epidemic and managing pain is a skill that must be trained in order to be the most prepared provider in the room.

Suggested Readings

Dowell D, Ragan KR, Jones CM, Baldwin GT, Chou R. CDC clinical practice guideline for prescribing opioids for pain—United States, 2022. *MMWR Recomm Rep*. 2022;71(3):1-95.

Motov S, Rockoff B, Cohen V, et al. Intravenous subdissociative-dose ketamine versus morphine for analgesia in the emergency department: a randomized controlled trial. *Ann Emerg Med*. 2015;66(3):222-229.e1.

Skelly AC, Chou R, Dettori JR, et al. *Noninvasive Nonpharmacological Treatment for Chronic Pain: A Systematic Review Update*. Agency for Healthcare Research and Quality (US); 2020.

363

Time Matters! Effective Pain Management in Your Sickle Cell Patient

Annie Rominger

Sickle cell disease (SCD) is one of the most common inherited diseases in the United States with approximately 100,000 people living with this condition. SCD primarily affects Black individuals (1 out of every 365 births) and some Hispanics (1 out of every 16,300 births). The most common complication of this disease is an acute pain crisis, which is an episode of severe pain from a vaso-occlusive ischemic event lasting hours to days. Patients with SCD typically have home medications to treat pain and present to the ED when their outpatient treatment is ineffective in controlling their pain.

There are an estimated 135,000 ED visits in the United States per year for acute pain crises in patients with SCD. Unfortunately, these patients have faced barriers to receiving adequate pain control in the acute setting. The barriers include availability of appropriate analgesics in the ED, physician concern about opioid misuse, variability in treatment care, physician bias, and systemic racism. In pediatric patients with SCD with an acute pain crisis, caregivers reported that ED physicians rejected patient's and caregiver's attempts to advocate for their own needs and discounted the severity of the patient's pain. They also reported racism contributing to inadequate pain control for the patient.

In 2020, the ASH updated the SCD pain management guidelines. The focus of these guidelines in the acute setting include time to analgesics, frequent reassessments, individualized opioid dosing, and the use of other nonopioid pharmacologic therapies. ASH recommends assessment and analgesic administration within 1 hour of ED arrival in patients with SCD presenting with an acute pain crisis and pain reassessment every 30 to 60 minutes. In a busy ED, it may be difficult to evaluate the patient, insert an IV catheter, and give an appropriate analgesic within 1 hour. Therefore, patients should be given a subcutaneous injection or IN administration of opioids if insertion of an IV is delayed. IN fentanyl has been shown to be a feasible alternative to IV morphine to treat pain in both adult and pediatric patients with SCD with a VOC. A study by Assad et al in 2023 showed patients given IN fentanyl had a 17.25% reduction in mean pain scores, which was not statistically different than the 17.15% seen in those who received IV morphine. There were decreased readmission rates, increased ED discharge rates, and decreased time to administration without significant differences in side-effect profiles. In summary, give opioid pain medication early and consider subcutaneous or IN administration if there are delays to IV insertion.

The ASH guidelines also recommend individualized, patient-tailored pain management plans. This takes into consideration each patient's baseline opioid therapy and medications that have been previously effective. These care plans should be developed with SCD physicians and imbedded into the patient's medical record. A recent study in a pediatric ED showed that after the implementation of individualized care plans, the time to first opioid administration decreased by almost 100 minutes. Patient preference should be taken into consideration and part of a shared decision-making process. If an individualized care plan has not been developed for a patient, standardized ED order sets are effective in decreasing pain and admission rates in patients with VOC. One study showed a 67% reduction rate of hospital admissions following the implementation of a standardized order set for patients with VOC. A set treatment plan and shared decision-making address many of the reported barriers encountered by patients with SCD seeking ED care for an acute pain crisis.

ASH recommends the use of NSAIDs and other nonopioid pharmacologic therapies when treating patients with SCD with a VOC in the acute setting. The panel recommends a 5- to 7-day course of NSAIDs in addition to opioids for acute pain management of VOC. However, this should not be administered in patients with certain other comorbidities, including peptic ulcer disease, renal dysfunction, or those on anticoagulation therapy. ASH recommends against steroids for the treatment of VOC. In fact, recent literature has demonstrated that exposure to steroids increases the risk of developing a severe VOC. ASH does recommend subanesthetic (analgesic) dose ketamine for pain that is refractory to opioid treatment (dose: 0.1-0.3 mg/kg/h). Regional anesthesia should be considered for localized pain that is refractory to traditional pain control.

The ASH panel did not make any specific recommendations for IV fluids because there are limited data to support or refute its use. Patients with SCD may have underlying renal or cardiac dysfunction and IV fluids may worsen these conditions. The panel did acknowledge that the risk of harm from IV fluids is higher in adults than children since they have more comorbid conditions. Therefore, the use of IV fluids should be considered on an individualized basis.

In summary, there are many patients with SCD who present to US EDs for an acute pain crisis, and often, they require additional analgesia. In 2020, the ASH developed guidelines for the treatment of patients with SCD presenting with acute pain, which focus on early analgesic treatment with frequent reassessments, tailored care plans, and optimal use of nonopioid pharmacologic agents.

PEARLS

- Barriers to pain control are physician bias, apprehension about opioid use, variability in treatment plans, racism.
- Assessment and opioid administered should occur within 1 hour of arrival.
- Pain reassessment should occur every 30 to 60 minutes.

- Individualized pain care plans are recommended but standardized care plans are effective if no individualized care plan exists.
- Nonopioid pharmacologic treatments can be effective in opioid refractory pain.

SUGGESTED READINGS

Assad O, Zamora R, Brown K, et al. IF IM in a crisis: intranasal fentanyl versus intravenous morphine in adult vaso-occlusive crisis. *Am J Emerg Med*. 2023;64:86-89.

Brandow AM, Carroll CP, Creary S, et al. American Society of Hematology 2020 guidelines for sickle cell disease: management of acute and chronic pain. *Blood Adv*. 2020;4(12):2656-2701.

Lapite A, Lavina I, Goel S, et al. A qualitative systematic review of pediatric patient and caregiver perspectives on pain management for vaso-occlusive episodes in the emergency department. *Pediatr Emerg Care*. 2023;39(3):162-166.

Tanabe P, Bosworth HB, Crawford RD, et al. Time to pain relief: a randomized controlled trial in the emergency department during vaso-occlusive episodes in sickle cell disease. *Eur J Haematol*. 2023;110(5):518-526.

Wachnik AA, Welch-Coltrane JL, Adams MCB, et al. A standardized emergency department order set decreases admission rates in in-patient length of stay for adult patients with sickle cell disease. *Pain Med*. 2022;23(12):2050-2060.

364

EFFECTIVE STRATEGIES FOR THE TREATMENT OF PATIENTS WITH OPIOID DEPENDENCY

KATHY LESAINT AND CURTIS GEIER

The ongoing opioid epidemic in the United States continues to cause overdose deaths and related morbidity and mortality. It is now generally accepted that all physicians, regardless of medical specialty, can make a significant impact on the treatment of a patient with OUD. Because EDs are often the first point of contact for individuals experiencing opioid overdose or seeking treatment for OUD, ED physicians can play a key role in providing timely and effective care for these patients. Professional organizations such as the American College of Emergency Physicians advocate for ongoing focused quality efforts for improving treatment for patients with OUD.

HARM REDUCTION FOR PATIENTS WITH OUD

The principle of harm reduction is a key component in caring for patients with OUD. Harm reduction utilizes strategies to reduce the negative consequences associated with the use of opioids. The goal is to encourage individuals to be as healthy as possible by "meeting them where they are." In other words, physicians should promote health for all patients who use substances, whether or not they are ready for initiation of medications for treatment.

Recently, some harm reduction initiatives that have gained traction in the ED arena include reducing stigma education, naloxone distribution, motivational interviewing, screening and treatment for comorbidities (eg, HIV, hepatitis C, skin and soft tissue infections), and referral to community harm reduction programs. Some EDs offer provision of safer use kits, which may include clean needles, pipes, syringes, and fentanyl test strips. Implementation of such interventions requires planning, executive leadership support, and creating a dialogue of culture change.

MEDICATIONS FOR OUD

For patients who are ready to initiate medications for treatment, three medications are approved by the FDA for the treatment of OUD: naltrexone, buprenorphine, and methadone. Naltrexone is a long-acting opioid receptor antagonist that inhibits the effects of opioid agonists. It is administered as a daily oral dose or as a once-monthly intramuscular injection. Given its high potential to cause precipitated withdrawal, naltrexone is rarely initiated in the ED setting.

Buprenorphine and methadone are more frequently initiated in the ED. Buprenorphine is a partial agonist at the mu-opioid receptor and offers a better safety profile than methadone. Buprenorphine binds to the opioid receptor with a high affinity, and subsequent administration or use of full opioid agonists has limited effect. It also has a ceiling effect in which it is able to quell withdrawal symptoms, but carries a low risk of respiratory depression at maximal dosage. Methadone is a full opioid receptor agonist. While it is an effective therapeutic consideration, it carries a larger risk of central nervous and respiratory depression than buprenorphine. Patient preference should be considered when initiating either buprenorphine or methadone.

TREATMENT OF OPIOID WITHDRAWAL

Physiologic findings of opioid withdrawal include restlessness, nausea, vomiting, diarrhea, piloerection, diaphoresis, yawning, mydriasis, and mild autonomic hyperactivity. Psychological effects include pain, anxiety, stress intolerance, irritability, and drug cravings. Although opioid withdrawal is very uncomfortable, it is rarely life-threatening. The most widely used tool to assess opioid withdrawal severity is the COWS, which measures 11 signs and symptoms of opioid withdrawal.

The degree of dependence, and thus the severity of opioid withdrawal, is directly related to the intensity (eg, dose, duration, continuity) of exposure. In general, spontaneous withdrawal typically occurs 8 to 12 hours after last use of a short-acting opioid and 16 to 24 hours after use of a long-acting opioid. Precipitated withdrawal, on the other hand, develops abruptly after the administration of an opioid antagonist or a partial agonist with tighter binding affinity. Massive catecholamine release during precipitated withdrawal has been reported to cause autonomic instability and cardiovascular complications.

Medications such as clonidine, loperamide, metoclopramide, and ondansetron can also be used to counter autonomic hyperactivity and/or vomiting and diarrhea associated with withdrawal. These adjunctive medications can help alleviate some withdrawal discomfort but are not adequate for long-term treatment of OUD. The consensus in the ED is to use buprenorphine or methadone to treat opioid withdrawal and as a bridge to long-term treatment. At this time, there is no definitive or "gold-standard" approach to ED dosing strategies for buprenorphine or methadone, and guidelines for optimal dosing vary.

Before initiating buprenorphine or methadone, a patient with OUD must be in opioid withdrawal. A concern with initiating buprenorphine is the risk of causing precipitated withdrawal. Therefore, patients who choose to be started on buprenorphine should have a COWS score of at least 8 to 13. Additionally, there is no consensus on the optimal initial and maximal dosages of buprenorphine though 8 to 16 mg and 32 to 48 mg, respectively, are reasonable. For patients who do not yet have a COWS of at least 8 but request buprenorphine for the treatment of OUD, an unobserved induction protocol (ie, prescription given for home initiation) or microdosing (ie, use of small doses of buprenorphine titrated up over 5-7 days) is an alternative approach. These methods have not been extensively studied in the ED patient population.

Methadone, on the other hand, may be a better option for patients who are not in sufficient withdrawal for the initiation of buprenorphine. Methadone initiation from the ED should only occur if patients are able to follow up at an opioid treatment program (methadone clinic) within 72 hours for continuation of treatment. It is reasonable to initiate methadone in the ED at 30 mg.

REGULATORY AND LEGAL ISSUES

There are no legal requirements to provide follow-up for patients, although appropriate outpatient linkage is key to sustaining treatment and reduction of morbidity from substance use. While the patient is in the ED, current US regulations permit physicians to utilize any medication for the treatment of opioid withdrawal symptoms, including buprenorphine and methadone. Additionally, regulations allow for patients who are already stabilized on buprenorphine or methadone to be continued on their outpatient dose while in the ED.

A DATA-Waiver registration is no longer required to treat patients with buprenorphine for OUD. Methadone can be initiated and administered in the ED for up to 72 hours while follow-up is arranged, but methadone for the treatment of OUD cannot be legally prescribed from the ED. New federal and state guidelines may allow dispensing of buprenorphine and methadone from the ED, although widespread practice and operationalization have not yet occurred.

PEARLS

- Harm reduction strategies such as education about stigma and distribution of naloxone kits can help reshape the culture and improve care of patients with substance use disorders.
- Initiation of treatment for OUD from the ED is safe, efficacious, and encouraged by existing emergency medicine organizations.
- Buprenorphine may be initiated in the ED and prescribed by emergency medicine providers.
- Methadone may be initiated and continued for 72 hours, but may not be prescribed. Linkage to an opioid treatment program, or methadone clinic, should be arranged.

SUGGESTED READINGS

D'Onofrio G, O'Connor PG, Pantalon MV, et al. Emergency department-initiated buprenorphine/naloxone treatment for opioid dependence: a randomized clinical trial. *JAMA*. 2015;313(16):1636-1644.

Hatten BW, Cantrill SV, Dubin JS, et al. Clinical policy: critical issues related to opioids in adult patients presenting to the emergency department. *Ann Emerg Med*. 2020;76(3):e13-e39.

Herring AA, Perrone J, Nelson LS. Managing opioid withdrawal in the emergency department with buprenorphine. *Ann Emerg Med*. 2019;73(5):481-487.

Strayer RJ, Hawk K, Hayes BD, et al. Management of opioid use disorder in the emergency department: a white paper prepared for the American Academy of Emergency Medicine. *J Emerg Med*. 2020;58(3):522-546.

365

MANAGEMENT OF ACUTE PAIN IN PATIENTS ON BUPRENORPHINE

R. GENTRY WILKERSON

Buprenorphine, a partial agonist of the MOR, is one of three medications along with methadone and naltrexone approved by the FDA for the treatment of OUD. Since it was first approved in 2002, buprenorphine has increasingly been chosen to treat OUD due to similar effectiveness to methadone but with increasingly less stringent regulations regarding prescribing. Buprenorphine has high affinity but low intrinsic activity at the MOR and functions as an antagonist at the KOR. Buprenorphine has a ceiling effect for respiratory depression but continues to have a dose-dependent analgesic effect. Confusion exists among clinicians on the optimal approach to acute pain management in patients on buprenorphine.

MAXIMIZE NONPHARMACOLOGIC AND NONOPIOID STRATEGIES

Regardless of the severity of the acute painful condition, all attempts should be made to employ pain management strategies that involve nonpharmaceutical approaches and nonopioid medications. Nonpharmacologic interventions should be tailored to the etiology of the painful condition. For musculoskeletal sprains and strains, these strategies include temperature-based therapy with cold or warm packs, immobilization, and elevation of the affected extremity to reduce swelling, along with rest to prevent aggravation of the injury. Massage and physical therapy may be employed. Other examples of nonpharmacologic interventions include acupuncture/acupressure, hypnosis, and biofeedback.

For many types of minor to moderately painful conditions, the use of acetaminophen and NSAIDs has been shown to be as effective as opioids for analgesia. Acetaminophen, given at recommended doses, has an excellent safety profile and does not inhibit platelet function, which may be advantageous if operative intervention is indicated. Acetaminophen is available in oral, rectal, and intravenous formulations. Scheduled dosing as opposed to "as needed" dosing is endorsed by multiple organizations to reduce delays in administration and provide a more even analgesic effect. A portion of acetaminophen is metabolized by the liver to produce a toxic byproduct—NAPQI—that is then inactivated by conjugation with glutathione. Acetaminophen should not be used in patients with severe liver disease due to the depletion of glutathione stores. NSAIDs function as inhibitors of COX enzymes. Nonselective NSAIDs, including aspirin, ibuprofen, and naproxen, inhibit both isoforms of COXs, COX-1 and COX-2. Selective NSAIDs preferentially inhibit COX-2, which is found at sites of inflammation, more than COX-1, which is located on platelets, blood vessels, and the stomach. NSAIDs are available in oral, intramuscular, intravenous, and topical formulations. All NSAIDs carry FDA warnings regarding cardiovascular complications, including myocardial infarction and stroke, as well as gastrointestinal adverse events, including bleeding, ulceration, and perforation. It is recommended to use the lowest effective dose for the shortest possible duration.

Other nonopioid analgesics include gabapentanoids (eg, pregabalin and gabapentin), local anesthetic agents (eg, lidocaine, tetracaine, and benzocaine), glucocorticoids, and ketamine. Gabapentin and pregabalin are FDA-approved for the treatment of post-herpetic neuralgia. Pregabalin has additional indications for the treatment of diabetic peripheral neuropathy, fibromyalgia, and neuropathic pain due to spinal cord injury. Despite these relatively few approved indications, prescriptions for gabapentanoids have increased as clinicians seek nonopioid alternatives due to the epidemic of opioid misuse and overdose. Data on the effectiveness of gabapentanoids for various painful conditions demonstrate minimal benefit, if any. An increased risk of respiratory depression has been found with the coadministration of gabapentanoids and opioids. Lidocaine and other anesthetic agents can be used topically and transdermally to provide local anesthesia. These are excellent choices when the cause of an acute painful condition is localized to a specific area, such as a skin abscess or dental cavity. Intravenous administration of lidocaine has been used for conditions such as kidney stones, migraine headaches, back pain, and other painful conditions. The benefit of IV lidocaine is temporary, and the optimal dosing strategy is ill-defined. Dosing should employ ideal body weight with infusions of 1 to 5 mg/kg/h most commonly used. Caution should be used in patients with liver disease due to the metabolism of lidocaine by the CYP450 system. Detailed information on the use of ketamine can be found in Chapter 357.

CONTINUATION OF BUPRENORPHINE DURING ACUTE PAIN MANAGEMENT

Concerns exist that continuation of buprenorphine treatment may interfere with acute pain management due to the high affinity of buprenorphine for MORs competing for full-agonist opioid therapy. There is growing evidence that continuing buprenorphine results in better overall analgesia, although a definitive clinical trial is lacking. There are reports that for patients in whom buprenorphine was discontinued, increased doses of full-agonist opioids are required due to the total overall opioid deficit created. Most now recommend continuing the home dose of buprenorphine during treatment for an acute, painful event. For mild-to-moderate pain not adequately controlled with nonpharmacologic and nonopioid medications, the dose of buprenorphine can be increased up to 32 mg/d, divided into doses administered every 6 to 8 hours. If the patient receives buprenorphine via long-acting implants or depot injections, it would be challenging to increase the dose of buprenorphine, and other strategies should be employed.

USE OF FULL-AGONIST OPIOIDS

Full-agonist opioids such as oxycodone, morphine, hydromorphone, and fentanyl have a greater intrinsic analgesic effect than buprenorphine. The addition of short-acting opioids to the home regimen of buprenorphine should be considered for moderate-to-severe painful conditions or those unresponsive to all other modalities. Doses required are typically higher than those used for opioid-naïve patients. The use of full-agonist opioids likely increases the risk of relapse in patients with OUD. Ideally, the use of full-agonist opioids should be a shared decision with the patient who has been made aware of such risks. Additionally, the clinician managing the patient's medication for OUD should be made aware. The lowest dose for the shortest duration possible should be used. If needed for more than a few days, a tapering plan should be created to wean the patient from the full opioid agonist to prevent the development of opioid withdrawal symptoms.

PEARLS

- Buprenorphine has a ceiling effect, whereby increasing the dose of buprenorphine does not increase the risk of respiratory depression.
- Nonpharmacologic and nonopioid medications should be utilized to provide analgesia for all severities of pain in patients who are on OUD treatment with buprenorphine.
- There is increasing evidence that continuing home doses of buprenorphine lead to better outcomes during acute pain management.
- Increasing the dose of buprenorphine may be an effective pain control strategy as it has a dose-dependent analgesic effect.
- Full-agonist opioids can be utilized while continuing treatment with buprenorphine, but this carries a risk of relapse, and the decision to use this modality should be shared with the patient who has been informed of the risks, benefits, and alternatives.

SUGGESTED READINGS

Alford DP, Compton P, Samet JH. Acute pain management for patients receiving maintenance methadone or buprenorphine therapy [published correction appears in *Ann Intern Med.* 2006;144(6):460]. *Ann Intern Med.* 2006;144(2):127-134.

Buresh M, Ratner J, Zgierska A, Gordin V, Alvanzo A. Treating perioperative and acute pain in patients on buprenorphine: narrative literature review and practice recommendations. *J Gen Intern Med.* 2020;35(12):3635-3643.

Cooper R, Vanjani R, Trimbur MC. Acute pain management in patients treated with buprenorphine: a teachable moment. *JAMA Intern Med.* 2019;179(10):1415-1416.

Dowell D, Ragan KR, Jones CM, Baldwin GT, Chou R. CDC clinical practice guideline for prescribing opioids for pain—United States, 2022. *MMWR Recomm Rep.* 2022;71(3):1-95.

Warner NS, Warner MA, Cunningham JL, et al. A practical approach for the management of the mixed opioid agonist-antagonist buprenorphine during acute pain and surgery. *Mayo Clin Proc.* 2020;95(6):1253-1267.

INDEX

Note: Page numbers in *italics* denote figures; those followed by a "t" denote tables.

A

AAA (*see* Abdominal aortic aneurysm)
Abdominal aortic aneurysm (AAA), 451
Abdominal pain, 805–806
Abdominal trauma, 656–658
  FAST examination, 656–657
  in geriatric patients, 658
  mechanism of injury, imaging based on, 656–657
    blunt, 657, *657*
    penetrating, 657
  in pediatrics, 658
  in pregnant women, 658
ABG (*see* Arterial blood gases)
Abnormal ECG, 196
Abscess, 263–264
Acalculous cholecystitis, 219–220, 232, *233*
Accidental hypothermia, 325
Accidental hypothermic cardiac arrest
  physiology, signs, and symptoms, 325
  treatment/management, 326–327
Acclimatization, 308
ACE-inhibitor, angioedema
  adjunct medications, 397–398
  diagnosis of, 396
  early airway assessment and intervention, failure to perform, 398
  inappropriate discharge from the ED, 398
  treatment, 396, 396t
  types of, 395–396
ACEP Clinical Policy, 465
Acetaminophen, 362, 453
Acetaminophen toxicity, 215, 613–615
  acetylcysteine for, 615
  chronic ingestions, treatment for, 615
  NAC
    patients with liver failure, 614
    toxic level result after 8 hours, 614
  screening, 615
  symptoms and signs of, 613
  treatment for, 613
Acetylcysteine, 615
Acid-base disturbance, 275–277
Acidosis, 76–78
ACLS (*see* Advanced cardiovascular life support)
ACS (*see* Acute compartment syndrome)
ACS (*see* Acute coronary syndrome)
Activated charcoal, 637, 639, 648
Acute adrenal crisis, 289
Acute angle-closure glaucoma, 340, 342, 488

Acute anterior uveitis, 340–341
Acute asthma exacerbation, magnesium in, 600–601
  data, 600–601
  mechanism of action, 600
  patient selection, 601
Acute cardiogenic pulmonary edema, nitroglycerin in, 187–188
Acute cholangitis, 245–247
  biliary obstruction, causes of, 246t
Acute compartment syndrome (ACS), 445–447
Acute coronary syndrome (ACS), 372–373
  age differences, 136
  alcohol consumption and, 184
  atypical risk factors for, 182–185
  cancer and, 183
  chronic kidney disease and, 183
  health disparities, 136
  HIV and, 184–185
  older adults, 137–139
    interpretation of ECG, 138
    risk stratification, 138–139
    signs and symptoms, 137–138
  pregnancy and, 184
  race and ethnicity, 136
  rheumatologic disorders and, 183
  serial ECGs, 141–143, *143*
  sex differentiations, 135
  ST segment elevation, 144–147
  systemic infection and, 184
  transgender, 135–136
Acute disseminated encephalomyelitis (ADEM), 403–404
Acute diverticulitis, 209–210
  assessment, 210
  indications for CT and antibiotics, 210t
  management, 211
  risk factors for, 210t
Acute liver failure (ALF), 214–215
  acetaminophen toxicity and, 215
  diagnosis of, 215
  N-acetylcysteine and, 215–216
  right upper quadrant ultrasound, 215–216
  supportive care, 215–216
Acute mesenteric arterial occlusion, 203
Acute mesenteric ischemia (AMI)
  clinical presentation, 204
  diagnosis, 204
  etiologies, 203–204
  management, 204–205

949

Acute mountain sickness (AMS), 307
  acclimatization, 308
  descent, 308
  medications, 308
  pediatrics, 308
  prevention and treatment, 308, 309t
Acute nodular septal panniculitis, 268
Acute pain, 815, 945–947
  buprenorphine, 945–947
Acute pancreatitis (AP)
  hazards of imaging, 206
  imaging for management and prognosis, 206
  imaging in diagnosis, 205–206
  severe, antibiotics for, 217–218
Acute respiratory distress syndrome (ARDS)
  refractory hypoxemia in patients with, 113t
Acute retroviral syndrome (ARS), 411–412
Acute variceal hemorrhage
  consultation and disposition, 202
  presentation, 201
  stabilization, 201–202
  treatment, 202
Acute vestibular syndrome (AVS), 479
  postexposure, 479
  spontaneous, 479–480
AD (*see* Aortic dissection)
Ad26.COV2.S (Janssen/Johnson & Johnson), 881, 882t, 884
Adalimumab (Humira), 400
ADEM (*see* Acute disseminated encephalomyelitis)
Adjunctive therapies, 178
Adrenal crisis, 289, 290
Adrenal insufficiency
  adrenal crisis, workup in, 290
  management, 290
  patients at risk, 289
  signs and symptoms, 289
  when to suspect, 289–290
Advanced cardiovascular life support (ACLS), 326
Advanced practice providers (APPs), 893–895
  background, 893–894
  onboarding, 894
  scope of practice, 894
  structure of supervision, 894–895
AEF (*see* Aortoenteric fistula)
AGE (*see* Arterial gas embolism)
Agitation
  in ED
    antipsychotics used for, 552t
    droperidol for, 552
    management of, 549–550, 549t
    serotonin toxicity with, 628–629
Airborne transmission, 436–437
Air trapping, 107–108, *107*
Airway management
  acidosis, 76–78
  asthma, 73–75
    endotracheal intubation, 74–75
    non-invasive positive pressure ventilation, 74
  bag-valve mask (BVM) ventilation
    equipment, 61–62
    JAWS acronym, 62
    mask seal, 62
    ventilation, 62–63
  bougie-assisted cricothyroidotomy, 81–82
    contraindications, 82
    post cricothyrotomy, 83
    preparation, 82
    procedure, 82–83
  emergency airway management
    approach, 69–70
    SOAP ME mnemonic for, 68–69
  endotracheal intubation (ETI), 63–64
    asthma and, 73–75
    hemodynamic effects of, 64
    obesity and, 70–73, *72*
    pre-intubation resuscitation, 64–65
    risk for decompensation, 64
  obesity, 70–73
  pediatric, 761–763
  pregnancy
    conditions contributing to respiratory depression in, 84t
    gravid patient, preparation for establishing definitive airway for, 85t
    intubation, 84–86
  rapid sequence intubation
    paralysis, 67
    premedication, 66
    sedation, 66–67
  view, loss of
    first-pass options, 78–79
    rescue approaches, 79
    tools and anatomy to navigating, 78–79
    troubleshooting, 80
Airway pressure release ventilation (APRV), 109–110
Airway resistance, 100
Alcohol consumption, and acute coronary syndrome, 184
Alcoholic ketoacidosis, 298–299
Alcohol intoxication, 611
Alcohols, toxic, 616–617
  ethylene glycol, 616
    ingestion, treatment for, 617
  isopropyl, 617
  methanol, 616
    ingestion, treatment for, 617
Alcohol use disorder, and suicide, 541
Alcohol withdrawal, 612
Alcohol withdrawal syndrome (AWS), *98*
  advantages of phenobarbital for, 97
  dosing, 97–98
  traditional treatment, 96–97
  treated with phenobarbital, disposition for, 98–99
ALF (*see* Acute liver failure)
Allis technique, 754
Altered mental status, and beta-blockers toxicity, 637
AMA (*see* American Medical Association)
American Academy of Pediatrics, 559
American Burn Association, 666
American Heart Association, 674

American Medical Association (AMA), 904–907, 909
American Urological Association, 572
AMI (*see* Acute mesenteric ischemia)
Amiodarone, 167
  in cardiac arrest, 7
Amoxicillin, 371
Amphotericin B, 567
AMS (*see* Acute mountain sickness)
Analgesia, and sedation
  benzodiazepines, 95
  dexmedetomidine, 94–95
  fentanyl or hydromorphone (opioids), 94
  ketamine, 95
  post-intubation, 93–96
  propofol, 94
  Richmond Agitation-Sedation Scale, 96t
Anaphylaxis
  epinephrine in, 391–392
  second-line medications in, 393–395
Anastomotic leak, 236–237
Aneurysmal LV, 146
Angioedema
  ACE-inhibitor
    adjunct medications, 397–398
    diagnosis of, 396
    early airway assessment and intervention, failure to perform, 398
    inappropriate discharge from the ED, 398
    treatment, 396, 396t
    types of, 395–396
Angiotensin-converting enzyme 2 (ACE2) receptor, 870
Antibiotics
  for abscess, 263–264
  acute diverticulitis, 210t
  appendicitis, 199–200
  for chronic obstructive pulmonary disease, 424
  febrile neutropenia, 371
  necrotizing fasciitis, 256–257
  for severe acute pancreatitis, 217–218
Anti-CD20 mAbs, 399–400
Anticoagulants, 377t
  antithrombotic MOA/half-life, 376t
  DOACs and antiplatelet agents, 376–377
  and hemorrhage, 375
  reversal, 375–377
  warfarin reversal, 375–376
Antihistamines, 394, 396
Antiplatelet agents, 376–377, 680
Antiseizure medications, 484–486
Antithrombotic MOA/half-life, 376t
Anti-TNF mAbs, 400
Antivenom, 328–329
Antiviral therapy, 421t
Anxiety
  and chest pain, 139–141
  defined, 542
  in emergency department, 542–545
  management, 543–544
  signs and symptoms of, 542–543, 543t
  special population, 544–545
    disposition, 544–545

older patients, 544
pediatrics, 544
pregnancy, 544
Aorta injuries, IR for, 670
Aortic dissection (AD), 180
  complications, 181–182
  diagnosis, 181
  ED management, 181
  predictive value of historical and physical examination features for, 180t
Aortoenteric fistula (AEF), 238–240
AP (*see* Acute pancreatitis)
Apixaban, 680
Appendicitis, 771–773, 772t
  antibiotic treatment alone, 199–200
  antibiotic treatment not alone, 199
  complications, 773
  history, 771
  pediatrics, 200
  scoring systems, 771
  treatment, 200, 773
  workup—imaging, 771
  workup—labs, 771–773
APPs (*see* Advanced practice providers)
APRV (*see* Airway pressure release ventilation)
ARDS (*see* Acute respiratory distress syndrome)
Argatroban, 680
ARS (*see* Acute retroviral syndrome)
Arterial blood gases (ABG), 284–286
Arterial gas embolism (AGE), 315–316
Arthrocentesis, 457, 717–719
  complications and pitfalls, 718–719
  contraindications, 717
  indications, 717
  synovial fluid interpretation, 718
  technique, 717–718
Ascending cholangitis, 245
Ask-Tell-Ask approach, 889–890
Asphyxiation, 398
Asthma, 73–75, 793–795
  endotracheal intubation, 74–75
  magnesium in, 600–601
    data, 600–601
    mechanism of action, 600
    patient selection, 601
  non-invasive positive pressure ventilation, 74
Asthma exacerbation, 45
Atrial fibrillation
  rate control, 172
  rhythm control, 172–173
  in Wolff-Parkinson-White Syndrome, 174–176, *175*
Austere environment, lifesaving procedures, 748–749
  airway management, 748
  finger thoracostomy, 748–749
  hemorrhage control, 749
Auto-PEEP, 102, *102*
Autotrigger, 105
AVAPS (*see* Average volume-assured pressure support)
Avastin (*see* Bevacizumab)
Average volume-assured pressure support (AVAPS), 110

AVS (*see* Acute vestibular syndrome)
AWS (*see* Alcohol withdrawal syndrome)
Aztreonam, 371

B

B2 receptor antagonists, 398
Back pain, 776–778
 can't miss diagnoses, 777–778
 emergency, 450–451
 epidural abscess on, 443–444
 history and physical exam, 776
 MSK low back pain, 452–453
 muscle relaxers, 452–453
 opioids, 452–453
 steroids, 452–453
 workup, 777
Bacteria (*see also specific types*)
Bacterial meningitis, 488
Bag-valve mask (BVM) ventilation, 2, *71*, 79
 equipment, 61–62
 JAWS acronym, 62
 mask seal, 62
 ventilation, 62–63
Balanced transfusion, 681–682
Balloon tamponade, for UGIB, 736–738
 complications, 737–738
 contraindications, 736
 indications, 736
 technique, 736–737
 types, 736–737, *737*
Baloxavir (Xofluza), 422, 422t
BCVI (*see* Blunt cerebrovascular injury)
Benign syphilis, 433t
Benzodiazepines, 65, 95, 178, 716
 for alcohol withdrawal, 612
 avoiding, ICU boarder, 121
 generalized convulsive status epilepticus, 485
 for serotonin toxicity, 629
 for sympathomimetic toxidrome, 621, 631
Benzonatate, 644
Beovu (*see* Brolucizumab)
Beta-blockade, 168
Beta-blockers
 toxicity, 636–638
  glucagon for, 637
  management of, 637
 use of, 9
Beta-hemolytic streptococci, 841
Beta-lactam antibiotic allergies, 579
Bevacizumab (Avastin), 400
Bicarbonate therapy, 286–288
Bicarbonate therapy, TCA toxicity, 642
Bilevel positive airway pressure (BiPAP), 44–45, *44*, 74, 491
Biliary obstruction, 222
Biliary obstruction, causes of, 246t
Biliary POCUS, 225, *226–228*
 acalculous cholecystitis, 232, *233*
 emphysematous cholecystitis, 232, *233*
 gallbladder, *226–232*
 hyperechoic cholelithiasis, *226, 232*
 pathology, 225t
 pneumobilia, *234*
 point-of-care ultrasound test characteristics, 228t
 visualizing gallbladder, 228–229t
BiPAP (*see* Bilevel positive airway pressure)
Bite, 327–328
 clinical presentation, 328
 North American pit vipers, 328
 treatment, 328–329
Bivalirudin, 680
Bleeding dialysis fistula, 573–574
Blood-borne transmission, 437
Blood product transfusion, 33
Blood transfusion, 383–384
 avoiding, ICU boarder, 121
 cryoprecipitate, 385
 factors VIII, IX, 386
 packed red blood cells, 384, 384t
 plasma (frozen and liquid), 385
 platelets, 385
 risks and complications of, 384
 type, screen, and crossmatch, 384
 whole blood, 384
Blunt cerebrovascular injury (BCVI), 659–660
 CTA screening, 660
 Denver Screening Criteria, 659–660
 high-risk injury patterns associated with, 659, 660t
 signs and symptoms of, 659, 660t
Blunt trauma, 811
BNT162b2 (Pfizer-BioNTech), 881, 882t, 884
Boarding
 ED and inpatient nurses, 922–923
 ED physician/hospitalists/adjusted workflow, 923
 psychiatric patients, 554–555
  communication, 555
  consultation, 554
  defined, 554
  evaluation, 554
  home medications, 554–555
  reassessments, 555
  recommendations, 554
 ventilator management, 608–609
Bolus-dose vasopressors (*see* Push-dose pressor (PDP))
Bottom surgery, 564
Bougie, 79
Bougie-assisted cricothyroidotomy, 81–82
 contraindications, 82
 post cricothyrotomy, 83
 preparation, 82
 procedure, 82–83
Boyle's law, 314
Brachiocephalic trunk, 352
Bradykinin pathway, *397*
Breath, shortness of, 605–607
 cardiovascular, 605
 endocrine-metabolic, 605–606
 ENT, 605
 hematologic, 606
 musculoskeletal, 606
 neuromuscular, 606
 psychologic, 606–607
 toxins, 606

Breath stacking (*see* Air trapping)
Brolucizumab (Beovu), 400
Brugada syndrome, 147, 169
Bullous pemphigoid
  defined, 258–259, 259t
  follow-up, 260
  treatment, 259–260
Bupivacaine, 725
Buprenorphine, 546–547, 943, 945–947
  acute pain management, 946
  full-agonist opioids, 947
  maximize nonpharmacologic and nonopioid strategies, 945–946
Burns, major
  %TBSA estimation tools, 667–668, *668*
  ABCs of, 666–668
  airway, 666
  defined, 666
  fluid resuscitation, 667
  patient guidelines for, 666t
  Rule of Nines, *667*
  transfer, 668
BVM ventilation (*see* Bag-valve mask ventilation)

C

C1 esterase inhibitor concentrate, 397
CAD (*see* Cervical artery dissection)
CAGE-AID Questionnaire, 546, 546t
Calcaneus fractures, 697
Calcium, 33
  in cardiac arrest, 7
Calcium channel beta blockers, 58t
Calcium channel blockers toxicity, 636–638
  dihydropyridine agents, 636
  management of, 637
Canadian TIA score, 473, 474t
Canalith (canalolith) repositioning maneuver, 481, *482*
Cancer, and acute coronary syndrome, 183
Cannabinoid hyperemesis syndrome (CHS), 635
Capacity assessment, 556–558
  accommodations, 557–558
  components of, 556–557, 557t
    appreciation, 557
    expression, 557
    reasoning, 557
    understanding, 557
  drugs/alcohol intoxication, 558
  minors in ED, 558
Carbon monoxide toxicity, 625–627
  HBO role in, 626–627
  incidence/causes, 625–626
  initial ED management, 626
  pathophysiology, 626
  presentation, 626
Cardiac arrest (*see also* Sudden cardiac arrest)
  amiodarone in, 7
  calcium in, 7
  epinephrine in, 6
  lidocaine in, 7
  magnesium sulfate in, 7
  oxygenation, optimizing, 14–16
  postcardiac arrest, 16
  blood pressure goals, clinical trials of, 17
  guideline recommendations, 17
  refractory, 12–13
  sodium bicarbonate in, 6
  targeted temperature management in, 21
  vasopressin in, 7
  ventilation, optimizing, 14–16
Cardiac cath team, 18–19
Cardiac surgery, 801–804, *802, 803*
Cardiac tamponade, *39*, 156–157
  clinical presentation of, 38
  definitive management of, 40
  evaluation of, 38–40
  initial resuscitation of, 40
Cardiogenic pulmonary edema, acute, 187–188
Cardiogenic shock, 23, 24t
  defined, 41
  intravenous fluids, 42–43
  pharmacologic support for, 42
  refractory, 12
  temporary MCS, 43
Cardiology
  acute cardiogenic pulmonary edema
    nitroglycerin in, 187–188
  acute coronary syndrome
    age differences, 136
    alcohol consumption and, 184
    atypical risk factors for, 182–185
    cancer and, 183
    chronic kidney disease and, 183
    health disparities, 136
    HIV and, 184–185
    older adults, 137–139
    pregnancy and, 184
    race and ethnicity, 136
    rheumatologic disorders and, 183
    serial ECGs, 141–143, *143*
    sex differentiations, 135
    ST segment elevation, 144–147
    systemic infection and, 184
    transgender, 135–136
  anxiety, in with chest pain, 139–141
  aortic dissection, 180
    complications, 181–182
    diagnosis, 181
    ed management, 181
  atrial fibrillation
    rate control, 172
    rhythm control, 172–173
    in Wolff-Parkinson-White Syndrome, 174–176, *175*
  chest pain
    cardiac tamponade, 156–157
    esophageal rupture, 157
    non-ACS causes of, 155–157
    pulmonary embolism (PE), 156
    stress test for, 162–164
    TAD, 155–156
    tension pneumothorax, 156
  congenital heart disease, 158–159
  ECGs
    lead misplacement, 148–150
    serial, 141–143, *143*

Cardiology (*continued*)
  hypertensive emergencies, 177–179
  myocarditis masquerade
    clinical presentation, 191, 192t
    consensus based diagnostic and therapeutic algorithm, *194*
    diagnosis, 192–193
    prognosis, 193
    treatment, 193
  occlusion myocardial infarction, 161t
    echocardiography, 161
    OMI *vs.* NOMI paradigm, 160–161
    STEMI-NSTEMI paradigm, 160
  older adults, 137–139
    acute coronary syndrome
      interpretation of ECG, 138
      risk stratification, 138–139
      signs and symptoms, 137–138
  STEMI in RBBB, 151–153, *153*
  ST segment elevation
    aneurysmal LV, 146
    early repolarization, 145, *145*
    electrolytes, 144–145
    inflammation, 146
    LBBB and ventricular-paced rhythm, 145
    neurogenic, 147
    Osborn waves, 146–147
    sudden death, 147
    thrombotic occlusion, 146
    ventricular hypertrophy, 145, *146*
  syncope, 195–197, 197t
  transcutaneous pacing, 169–170
    complications, 171
    procedure, 170–171
  troponins, high-sensitivity, 153–155
  ventricular assist device (VAD), 189–191, *190*
  ventricular storm
    management of, 167–169
  ventricular tachycardia, 164–166
Cardiovascular syphilis, 433t
Cardioversion, 5
Care of minor burns, 855–857
  classification, 856
  initial management, 856
  minor burn criteria, 856
  wound care, 857
Carfentanyl, 623
CAR-T therapy
  -related cytokine release syndrome, 378
    assessment and management, 379, 379t
    diagnosis, 379
  -related ICANS, 378
    assessment and management, 380t
    diagnosis, 379
Catheter-associated urinary tract infection (CAUTI), 583–584
  bacteria, types of, 583
  contributing factors, 583
  sample collection, 583
  symptomatology, 583–584
  treatment, 583–584
Cauda equina syndrome, 450
Caustic ingestion, 221–222

CAUTI (*see* Catheter-associated urinary tract infection)
Cecal volvulus, 250
Ceftriaxone, 202, 578
Celecoxib, 932
Cellulitis, 261–263
Central retinal artery occlusion, 343
Central retinal vein occlusion, 344
Cerebral edema, 782
Cerebral venous sinus thrombosis (CVST), 468–470, 488
  clinical manifestations, 469t
  risk factors, 469t
Cerebral venous thrombosis (CVT), 488
Cerebrovascular injury, blunt, 659–660
  CTA screening, 660
  Denver Screening Criteria, 659–660
  high-risk injury patterns associated with, 659, 660t
  signs and symptoms of, 659, 660t
Certolizumab pegol (Cimzia), 400
Cervical artery dissection (CAD), 461–463
  clinical features of, 463t
  neurologic findings, patients with, 462–463
  vertebral artery dissection, 462
Cervical dilators, 515
Chance fracture, 711–712
CHD (*see* Congenital heart disease)
Chest pain (*see also* Acute coronary syndrome)
  anxiety and, 139–141
  non-ACS causes of, 155–157
    cardiac tamponade, 156–157
    esophageal rupture, 157
    pulmonary embolism (PE), 156
    tension pneumothorax, 156
    thoracic aortic dissection (TAD), 155–156
  stress test for, 162–164
Chest tube placement, 742–744
  complications, 743
  contraindications, 743
  setup, 743
  technique, 743–744
Chiasmal and retrochiasmal disorders, 344
Child abuse, 757–758, 909
Chlamydia trachomatis, 578
Chronic kidney (CKD), and acute coronary syndrome, 183
Chronic obstructive pulmonary disease (COPD), 45, 423–424
CHS (*see* Cannabinoid hyperemesis syndrome)
CICO situation, 70
Cimzia (*see* Certolizumab pegol)
Ciprofloxacin, 371
CKD (*see* Chronic kidney)
Clavulanic acid, 371
Clevidipine, 178, 178t, 472
Clindamycin, 371
Clinical practice
  advanced practice providers (APPs), 893–895
    background, 893–894
    onboarding, 894
    scope of practice, 894
    structure of supervision, 894–895

American Medical Association (AMA), 904–907, 909
  boarding inpatients, 922–924
    ED and inpatient nurses, 922–923
    ED physician/hospitalists/adjusted workflow, 923
  difficult consultants, 920–922
  discharge documentation, 891–893
  emergency department (ED)
    boarding, 898–899
    overcrowding, 896–897
  EMS provider, 902–903
  handoffs/sign-outs, 918–919
  human trafficking (HT), 915–917
    how to respond, 916–917
    trafficked patient, recognizing, 916
  intimate partner violence (IPV), 909, 913–915
    assess safety, 914
    document appropriately, 914–915
    engage support services, 914
    make the diagnosis, 913–914
    provide medical care and emotional support, 914
  mandatory reporting laws, 908–910
  material injury, 910–913
    chain of custody, 912
    documentation pearls, 912
    forensic photography, 912
    general evidence collection principles, 911
    state/jurisdictional considerations, 911
    strangulation, 912
    suspect exams, 912
  patient satisfaction, 887–888
  patient's death to family members, delivering bad news about, 889–890
  your deposition, 900–901
Coagulopathy, trauma-induced, 682
Cocaine, 622
Cognitive impairment, 137
Cold water immersion (CWI), 321
Coma, 296–297
Compartment syndrome, 687
Compliance and airway resistance, 100
Compromise opioid, 930, 931
Computed tomographic angiography (CTA), 464
Computed tomographic venography (CTV), 470
Computed tomography (CT)
  acute diverticulitis, 210t
  in acute pancreatitis, 205–206
  of face and neck, 347–348
  in inflammatory bowel disease, 208
  ovarian torsion, 502
  on pregnancy, 251–253
    fetal exposure, 252t
    utero induced deterministic radiation effects, 253t
Congenital heart disease (CHD), 158–159
Congestive heart failure (CHF), non-invasive positive pressure ventilation during, 45
Conjunctivitis, 332
Constipation, 789–790, 790t
Contact dermatitis, 262
Contact transmission, 436

Continuous positive airway pressure (CPAP), 44, *44*
Continuous renal replacement therapy (CRRT), 118, 119t
COPD (*see* Chronic obstructive pulmonary disease)
CO toxicity, 310–311
Coumadin, 679
COVID-19 pandemic, 791, 887, 896
  clinical presentation of, 865–866
  evaluation of, 866
  long COVID, 869–872
    future studies, 871–872
    management, 871
    pathophysiology, 870–871, *870*
    prevalence, 870
    symptoms, 871
  mechanical ventilation, 878–880, *880*
    adequate PEEP to prevent atelectrauma, 879
    assess and limit distending pressures, 879
    prevent aspiration, 880
    tidal volume, 879
  MIS-C, 867–869
    signs and symptoms of, 868, 868t
    timely diagnosis of, 868
  risk factors for, 866
  tests, 872–874
    early months of, 872
    RT-PCR false positives, 873–874
    sensitivity of RT-PCR, 873
  therapeutics, 877t
  vaccinations, 883–885
    anaphylaxis, 884
    children, 885
    GBS, 885
    myocarditis and pericarditis, 884–885
    pregnancy, complications of, 885
    VITT, 884
  vaccines, 881–883
COWS score, 546
CPAP (*see* Continuous positive airway pressure)
Cricothyrotomy, 79, 83, 748
Critical care
  alcohol withdrawal syndrome
    advantages of phenobarbital for, 97
    dosing, 97–98
    traditional treatment, 96–97
    treated with phenobarbital, disposition for, 98–99
  analgesia and sedation
    benzodiazepines, 95
    dexmedetomidine, 94–95
    fentanyl or hydromorphone (opioids), 94
    ketamine, 95
    post-intubation, 93–96
    propofol, 94
    Richmond Agitation-Sedation Scale, 96t
  end-of-life care
    in emergency department, 130–132
  extracorporeal membrane oxygenation
    application and main indications, 128–129
    in emergency department, 128–130
    exclusion criteria, 129

Critical care (*continued*)
   other indications, 129
   fluid boluses
      benefits and harms of, 114–115
      initial liberal *vs.* restrictive approach to fluid loading, 115
      volume responsiveness after initial fluid strategy, 115–116
   ICU boarder
      benzodiazepines, avoiding, 121
      DVT, avoiding, 122
      excess fluid administration, avoiding, 120–121
      high-dose opioid infusions, avoiding, 121
      nephrotoxic medications, avoiding, 121–122
      unnecessary blood transfusion, avoiding, 121
   implementing ED-initiated ECMO, 129–130
   initial vent settings, 89–93, *90*
   mechanical ventilation, 108–109
      airway pressure release ventilation, 109–110
      average volume-assured pressure support, 110
      pressure regulated volume control, 109
      pressure support ventilation, 109
      synchronized intermittent mandatory ventilation, 109
   push-dose pressor, 122–123
      human error, 124
      patient selection, 123–124
      systems-based protocols, 124
   refractory hypoxemia
      in intubated patient, 111–113
      in patients with ARDS, 113t
   renal replacement therapy
      access site, 118
      contraindications, 118
      in emergency department, 116–120
      indications, 117
      modes of, 118–119
      risks, 117
   ventilator-associated pneumonia, 125–127
      measures reducing risk of, 127t
   ventilator pressures
      auto-PEEP, 102, *102*
      compliance and airway resistance, 100
      inspiratory plateau pressure, 100–101, *101*
      monitoring, 99–103
      peak inspiratory pressure, 100–101, *101*
   ventilator waveforms, 103
      air trapping, 107–108, *107*
      autotrigger, 105
      double triggering, 106, *107*
      flow asynchrony, 106, *106*
      ineffective triggering, 105, *105*
      normal waveforms, 104, *104*
      patient-ventilator asynchrony, 105
CRITOE mnemonic, 686, 686t
Croup (laryngotracheitis), 764–765
CRRT (*see* Continuous renal replacement therapy)
CRS (*see* Cytokine release syndrome)
Cryoprecipitate, 385
Crystalloids, 682
C-SSRS, 541

CT (*see* Computed tomography)
CTA (*see* Computed tomographic angiography)
CTV (*see* Computed tomographic venography)
Cutaneous
   abscess, 263–264
   bullous pemphigoid
      defined, 258–259, 259t
      follow-up, 260
      treatment, 259–260
   cellulitis, 261–263
   hidradenitis suppurativa
      clinical presentation, 272–273
      ED management and definitive therapy, 273
      I&D, 273
   mpox virus, 265–267
   necrotizing fasciitis
      antibiotic therapy, 256–257
      classification, 255, 255t
      clinical presentation, 256, 256t
      diagnostic imaging, 257
      differential diagnosis, 256, 256t
      evaluation, 256, 257t
      HBO therapy, 257
      LRINEC Score, 257
      risk factors, 256
   pemphigus vulgaris
      defined, 258–259, 259t
      follow-up, 260
      treatment, 259–260
   staphylococcal toxic shock syndrome
      clinical presentation, 270–271
      diagnostic criteria, 271
      pathogenesis, 270
      treatment, 271
   systemic Illnesses
      DRESS, 268–269
      EN, 268
      LE, 268
      neonatal HSV, 267–268
   varicella-zoster virus (chickenpox), 265–267
CVST (*see* Cerebral venous sinus thrombosis)
CVT (*see* Cerebral venous thrombosis)
CWI (*see* Cold water immersion)
Cyanide toxicity, 310–311
CYP2D6 enzyme, 931
Cyproheptadine, for serotonin toxicity, 629
Cytokine release syndrome (CRS), 378
   assessment and management, 379, 379t
   diagnosis, 379

D

Dabigatran, 680
Dalton's law, 314
DBZD, substances of use, 624
DCS (*see* Decompression sickness)
Decompression sickness (DCS), 315–316
Decontamination, 58, 647–649
   activated charcoal, 648
   dermal, 649
   gastric lavage, 649
   GI, 647–648
   multidose activated charcoal, 648
   ocular, 649
   whole bowel irrigation, 648

Deep dive on decompression illness, 314–316
Deep Head Hanging maneuver, 481
Deep vein thrombosis (DVT), 122
Defibrillation, 4
  dual sequential, 10
  troubleshooting, 10
Defibrillator pads
  anterolateral placement of, *4*
  anteroposterior placement of, *4*
  cardioversion, 5
  defibrillation, 4
  placement of, 3–4
  transcutaneous pacing, 5
Delirium, 819–821, 826
  defined, 537
  dementia *vs.*, 537–539
  diagnosis of, 537–538
  etiologies of, 539t
  features of, 538t
  risk factors for, 537
Delta-9-THC, 633–634
Dementia, 822–823
  causes of, 537
  defined, 537
  delirium *vs.*, 537–539
  diagnosis of, 537–538
  etiologies of, 539t
  features of, 538t
  risk factors for, 537
Dental infections
  history and physical exam, 347
  imaging, 347–348
  management, 348
Dental trauma, 361
  bleeding, 363
  pain control, 362
  trauma, 362–363
Dermal decontamination, 649
Descent, 308
Dexmedetomidine, 94–95, 538
Dextrose, for salicylate poisoning, 619
Diabetic ketoacidosis (DKA), 277, 781–783
  children in, 782
  fluid choice, 278
  insulin management, 278–279, 278t
  management of, 782
  potassium supplementation, 279
  sodium bicarbonate, utilization of, 279
Dialysis, 638
Dialysis fistula hemorrhage, 573–574
Dialyzable toxins, 638–640
  lithium, 639
  metformin, 639–640
  salicylates, 639
Diazepam, 486t
Dietary supplements, 631
Difficult consultants, 920–922
Digital blocks, 842–843
Digoxin, 58t
DIHS (*see* Drug-induced hypersensitivity syndrome)
Dihydropyridine agents, 636
Dihydropyridine CCBs, 643
Dilated pupil, 340

Dilute vasopressor infusions, 30–31
Direct oral anticoagulants (DOACs), 376–377
Direct thrombin inhibitors, 680
Discharge documentation, 891–893
Dislodged trach, replacing, 354–356
Distributive shock, 23, 24t
Dix-Hallpike test, 480–484, *483*
Dizziness, 477–480
  acute vestibular syndromes, 479
    postexposure, 479
    spontaneous, 479–480
  episodic vestibular syndromes, 478
    spontaneous, 479
    triggered, 479
DKA (*see* Diabetic ketoacidosis)
DOACs (*see* Direct oral anticoagulants)
Dobutamine, 42
Dopamine, 42
DOPES mnemonic, 111, 111t
Double triggering, 106, *107*
DRESS syndrome, 268–269
Droperidol, 551–553
  for agitation, 552
    recommended dosing, 553t
  history of, 551
  policy statement on use of, 552
Droplet transmission, 436
Drowning, 317–319
Drug-induced hypersensitivity syndrome (DIHS), 268
Dry drowning, 317–319
  treatment strategies, 318t
Dual sequential defibrillation, 10
Dumping syndrome, 237
DVT (*see* Deep vein thrombosis)
Dyspnea, in pregnancy
  diagnosis, 507–508
  presentation, 508
  pulmonary embolism, 508
  treatment, 508

E

EAH (*see* Exercise-associated hyponatremia)
Ear injuries/lacerations, 849–851
Early anastomotic stricture, 237
Early repolarization, 145, *145*
ECG (*see* Echocardiography)
Echocardiography (ECG), 161, 641
  abnormal, 196
  features of limb lead reversal, *148–149*
  features of RA/RL reversal, *149*
  features of superior lead placement, 150, *150*
  lead misplacement, 148–150
  occlusion myocardial infarction and, 161
  in older adults, 138
  post-ROSC
    considerations, 48
    patterns, 47–48
    push for delayed, 48
    push for immediate, 48
  serial, 141–143, *143*
  with sinus tachycardia and low QRS voltage, *39*
  stratification, 18–19

Eclampsia, 503–504
ECLS (*see* Extracorporeal life support)
ECMO (*see* Extracorporeal membrane oxygenation)
Ectopic pregnancies, 514
ED (*see* Emergency department)
Edoxaban, 680
EGD (*see* Esophagogastroduodenoscopy)
Eikenella corrodens, 844
Electrical storm, 8–9
Electrocardiogram (ECG), during childhood, 778–781, *780*
Electrolytes, 144–145
Elimination of poisons, 58–59
Embolic occlusion, 203
Emergency airway management
  approach, 69–70
  SOAP ME mnemonic for, 68–69
Emergency department
  abscess incision and drainage, 837–838
  agitation
    antipsychotics used for, 552t
    droperidol for, 552
    management of, 549–550, 549t
  anxiety, 542–545
    defined, 542
    disposition, 544–545
    management, 543–544
    older patients, 544
    pediatrics, 544
    pregnancy, 544
    signs and symptoms of, 542–543, 543t
  boarding, 898–899
    communication, 555
    consultation, 554
    defined, 554
    evaluation, 554
    home medications, 554–555
    reassessments, 555
    recommendations, 554
  droperidol, 551–553
    for agitation, 552
    history of, 551
    policy statement on use of, 552
    recommended dosing, 553t
  medical clearance, 559–560
    screening tests, 560t
  minors in, 558
  nasopharyngoscopy, 731–733
    indications, 732
    patient assessment, 732
    patient preparation, 732
    procedural considerations, 732–733
    resources, 733
  overcrowding, 896–897
  paracentesis, 722–723
    complications, 723
    contraindications, 722
    indications, 722
    technique, 722–723
  pediatric procedural sedation, 766–768, 767t
  procedural sedation, 713–716
    patient assessment, 713–714
    pharmacologic selection, 714–716, 715t
    procedure setup, 714
  Psychiatric Emergency Services, 555
  pyelonephritis, 570–571
    antibiotic regimens for, 571
    error in ED management of, 570
  renal stone disease, 575–577
    antibiotics for, 576–577
    clinical presentation of, 575
    diagnosis of, 575–576
    disposition, 576–577
    medical management for, 576
  substance use disorders, 545–548
    CAGE-AID Questionnaire, 546, 546t
    harm reduction, 548
    intervention, 546–547
    National Institute on Drug Abuse Quick Screen, 546
    referral for treatment, 547–548
    screening, 546
    treatment algorithm for, *547*
  ventilator management, for boarded patient, 608–609
Emergency physicians, follow-up phone calls, 888
Empathy, 888
Emphysematous cholecystitis, 232, *233*
EMS provider, 902–903
EN (*see* Erythema nodosum)
Encephalitides, immune-mediated
  clinical presentation, 402
  diagnosis, 402–403
  disposition, 403
  management, 403
  pathophysiology, 402
  pediatric considerations, 403–404
Endocrine/metabolic physiology
  acid-base disturbance, 275–277
  adrenal insufficiency
    adrenal crisis, workup in, 290
    management, 290
    patients at risk, 289
    signs and symptoms, 289
    when to suspect, 289–290
  bicarbonate therapy, 286–288
  diabetic ketoacidosis (DKA), 277
    fluid choice, 278
    insulin management, 278–279
    potassium supplementation, 279
    sodium bicarbonate, utilization of, 279
  hyperglycemic hyperosmolar state, 281–284
  hyperkalemia, 300–303
  hyponatremia, 304–306
  inborn errors of metabolism
    classification, 291–292
    diagnosis/clinical presentation, 292
    treatment/management, 293
    workup, 292
  ketoacidosis
    alcoholic ketoacidosis, 298–299
    IEMs, 299–300
    salicylate ingestion, 299
    starvation ketoacidosis, 299
  myxedema coma, 296–297
  orthostatic hypotension, 280–281

thyroid storm, 293–294
  diagnosis, 294–295
  management, 295
  VBG wizardry, 284–285
    HCO_3^- of, 285
    lactate of, 285–286
    pCO_2 of, 285
    pH of, 285
End-of-life (EOL) care, 130–132
Endophthalmitis, 343
Endotracheal intubation (ETI), 2, 63–64
  asthma and, 73–75
  hemodynamic effects of, 64
  obesity and, 70–73, 72
  pre-intubation resuscitation, 64–65
  risk for decompensation, 64
  for salicylate poisoning, 619
Endovascular thrombectomy (EVT), 492–494
Envenomation, 327–329
Environmental
  accidental hypothermic cardiac arrest
    physiology, signs, and symptoms, 325
    treatment/management, 326–327
  acute mountain sickness (AMS), 307
    acclimatization, 308
    descent, 308
    medications, 308
    pediatrics, 308
    prevention and treatment, 308, 309t
  bite, 327–328
    clinical presentation, 328
    North American pit vipers, 328
    treatment, 328–329
  deep dive on decompression illness, 314–316
  dry drowning, 317–319
    treatment strategies, 318t
  exercise-associated hyponatremia
    identification and diagnosis, 312–313
    pathophysiology, 312
    treatment, 313–314
  HBOT mechanisms
    emergency-capable, 322–323
    frontiers, 323
    hyperbaric medicine, contacting, 324
    indications, 323–324
    other indications, 324
  heat stroke management, 319–322
  high-altitude cerebral edema, 307
    acclimatization, 308
    descent, 308
    medications, 308
    pediatrics, 308
    prevention and treatment, 308, 309t
  high-altitude pulmonary edema, 307–308
    acclimatization, 308
    descent, 308
    medications, 308
    pediatrics, 308
    prevention and treatment, 308, 309t
  smoke inhalation
    systemic toxins, 310–311
    thermal burns, 310
EOL care (see End-of-life care)
EPA (see Spinal epidural abscess)

EPAP (see Expiratory positive airway pressure)
Epidural abscess, 450–451
Epiglottitis, 333–335
Epinephrine, 42, 73–74, 396
  in anaphylaxis, 391–392
  in cardiac arrest, 6
Episodic vestibular syndrome (EVS), 478
  spontaneous, 479
  triggered, 479
Epistaxis
  initial measures, 345
  packing, 346
  persistent bleeding, 346
  reassessment, 345–346
Epley maneuver, 480–484, 483t
Erysipelas, 261
Erythema nodosum (EN), 268
Escherichia coli, 769
Esophageal obstruction, 221
Esophageal perforation
  clinical presentation, 212
  diagnosis, 213
  treatment, 213
Esophageal rupture, 157
Esophagogastroduodenoscopy (EGD)
  biliary obstruction, 222
  caustic ingestion, 221–222
  esophageal obstruction, 221
  foreign body ingestion, 221
  upper gastrointestinal bleeding, 222
Ethylene glycol, 616
  ingestion, treatment for, 617
ETI (see Endotracheal intubation)
Etomidate, 65, 66, 75, 716
EVS (see Episodic vestibular syndrome)
EVT (see Endovascular thrombectomy)
Exercise-associated hyponatremia (EAH)
  identification and diagnosis, 312–313
  pathophysiology, 312
  treatment, 313–314
Expiratory positive airway pressure (EPAP), 44–45, 44
Extracorporeal cardiopulmonary resuscitation, 11
Extracorporeal life support (ECLS), 326
Extracorporeal membrane oxygenation (ECMO), 11
  additional considerations, 13
  application and main indications, 128–129
  basic configuration, 11, 12
  in emergency department, 128–130
  exclusion criteria, 129
  implementing ED-initiated, 129–130
  indications in ED, 12–13
  other indications, 129
Extremity trauma
  hemostasis, 654
  IR for, 671
  vascular injury in, 654–655
    computed tomography angiogram (CTA), 655
    hard signs of, 654, 655t
    proximity wounds, 655
    soft signs of, 655, 655t
Eyelid lacerations, 846–849, *847*

F

Facial feminization surgery, 563
Facial trauma, 362
Factors IX, 386
Factors VIII, 386
Factor Xa inhibitors, 680
FAINT Score, 196
Faricimab (Vabysmo), 400
FBs (*see* Foreign bodies)
Febrile neutropenia, antibiotics for, 370–371
Febrile traveler, 429–432
   epidemiology, 429–430
   etiologies of fever, 431t
   history, 430
   incubation period, 429t
   physical exam/workup, 430–431
Feminizing procedures, 563
Femoral nerve/fascia iliaca compartment blocks, 725
Fentanyl, 94, 623, 716
FFP (*see* Fresh frozen plasma)
Fiber-optic scope, 79
Fingernail faux pas, 860–862, *860*
Finger thoracostomy, 728
Fistula, bleeding dialysis, 573–574
Flexor tenosynovitis, 458–460
Flow asynchrony, 106, *106*
Fluid administration, 26–27
   avoiding, ICU boarder, 120–121
Fluid boluses
   benefits and harms of, 114–115
   initial liberal *vs.* restrictive approach to fluid loading, 115
   volume responsiveness after initial fluid strategy, 115–116
Fluoroquinolone, 371, 582
Foley catheter, 733–735
   indications, 734
   insertion, 734
   risks of catheterization, 734
   troubleshooting, 734–735
Fomepizole, 617
Fondaparinux, 680
Foreign bodies (FBs)
   aspirated, 350–351
   choosing lure, 350
   complications, 351
   ingestion, 221
   seeing is believing, 349
   tools for removal, 350t
   wound, 858–859
Fosphenytoin, 486t
Fournier gangrene, 566–567
   classic presentation of, 566
   defined, 566
   diagnosis of, 567
   infection, sources of, 566
   management of, 567
Fraction of inspired oxygen (FiO_2), 91
Fractures
   calcaneus, 697
   chance, 711–712
   fragility, 807

   Jones', *688*, 689
   Maisonneuve, 692
      mechanism of injury, 692–693
      with proximal fibula fracture, *693*
      treatment of, 693–694
   pelvic
      bedsheet to stabilize, 662
      causes of, 661
      point-of-care ultrasound, 662, *662*
      RSI, 663
      treatment for, 661
   proximal fibula, 692–694, *693*
   proximal humerus, 708–710, *708–709*
   Pseudo-Jones, 688–689
   rib, hip/vertebral compression, 807–809, *809*
   scaphoid, 694–696
      Herbert classification of, 696, 696t
   scapula, 690–691
   stress, 689
   supracondylar, 685–687
      compartment syndrome, 687
      CRITOE mnemonic, 686, 686t
      extension-type, classification of, 686t
      types of, 685
   tibial plateau, 703–706, *704–705*
      diagnostic imaging for, 704–705
      Schatzker classification system of, 706, *706*
      treatment for, 705
Fragility fracture, 807
Fresh frozen plasma (FFP), 385, 398

G

GAS (*see* Gender affirming surgeries)
Gastric bypass
   evaluation and management, 236–237
   overall approach, 235–236
   Roux-en-Y gastric bypass, 236–237, *236*
   surgical procedure, 235
Gastric lavage, 649
Gastric volvulus, 250
Gastroenterology
   acalculous cholecystitis, 219–220
   acute cholangitis, 245–247
      biliary obstruction, causes of, 246t
   acute diverticulitis, 209–210
      assessment, 210
      indications for ct and antibiotics, 210t
      management, 211
      risk factors for, 210t
   acute liver failure, 214–215
      acetaminophen toxicity and, 215
      diagnosis of, 215
      N-acetylcysteine and, 215–216
      right upper quadrant ultrasound, 215–216
      supportive care, 215–216
   acute mesenteric ischemia
      clinical presentation, 204
      diagnosis, 204
      etiologies, 203–204
      management, 204–205
   acute pancreatitis
      hazards of imaging, 206
      imaging for management and prognosis, 206

INDEX

imaging in diagnosis, 205–206
acute variceal hemorrhage
  consultation and disposition, 202
  presentation, 201
  stabilization, 201–202
  treatment, 202
aortoenteric fistula, 238–240
appendicitis
  antibiotic treatment alone, 199–200
  antibiotic treatment not alone, 199
  pediatrics, 200
  treatment of choice, 200
biliary POCUS, 225, *226–228*
  acalculous cholecystitis, 232, *233*
  emphysematous cholecystitis, 232, *233*
  gallbladder, *226–232*
  hyperechoic cholelithiasis, *226, 232*
  pathology, 225t
  pneumobilia, *234*
  point-of-care ultrasound test characteristics, 228t
  visualizing gallbladder, 228–229t
CT on pregnancy, 251–253
  fetal exposure, 252t
  utero induced deterministic radiation effects, 253t
esophageal perforation
  clinical presentation, 212
  diagnosis, 213
  treatment, 213
esophagogastroduodenoscopy (EGD)
  biliary obstruction, 222
  caustic ingestion, 221–222
  esophageal obstruction, 221
  foreign body ingestion, 221
  upper gastrointestinal bleeding, 201, 222
gastric bypass
  evaluation and management, 236–237
  overall approach, 235–236
  Roux-en-Y gastric bypass, 236–237, *236*
  surgical procedure, 235
inflammatory bowel disease
  imaging, 207–208
jaundice, 247–249
PEG tubes, displaced, 223–224
perforated peptic ulcer, 240–241
  complications, 241
  diagnosis, 241
  management, 241–242
  presentation of, 241
  risk factors, 241
severe acute pancreatitis
  antibiotics for, 217–218
spontaneous bacterial peritonitis
  diagnosis, 243–244
  examination, 243
  pathogenesis, 243
  positive cultures in a discharged patient, 244
  treatment, 244
volvulus, 249–250
  cecal volvulus, 250
  gastric volvulus, 250
  pediatric volvulus, 250–251

sigmoid volvulus, 250
GCA (*see* Giant cell arteritis)
GCSE (*see* Generalized convulsive status epilepticus)
Gelfoam, 363
Gender affirming surgeries (GAS), 563–565
  feminizing procedures, 563
  general considerations, 564
  masculinizing procedures, 564
  transfeminine patient, 565
  transmasculine patient, 565
Generalized convulsive status epilepticus (GCSE), 485, 486t
Genitourinary
  catheter-associated urinary tract infection (CAUTI), 583–584
    bacteria, types of, 583
    contributing factors, 583
    sample collection, 583
    symptomatology, 583–584
    treatment, 583–584
  dialysis fistula hemorrhage, 573–574
  Fournier gangrene, 566–567
    classic presentation of, 566
    defined, 566
    diagnosis of, 567
    infection, sources of, 566
    management of, 567
  gender affirming surgeries (GAS), 563–565
    feminizing procedures, 563
    general considerations, 564
    masculinizing procedures, 564
    transfeminine patient, 565
    transmasculine patient, 565
  priapism, 571–572
    American Urological Association guidelines, 572
    defined, 571
    error in management of, 571–572
    etiology of, 572
    ischemic, 571
    nonischemic, 571
    treatment of, 572
    types of, 571
  prostatitis, 580–582
    ABP, 580
    antibiotic selection, 582
    asymptomatic inflammatory, 580
    CBP, 580
    classification of, 580
    CP/CPPS, 580
    diagnosis of, 580
    treatment of, 580, 581t
  pyelonephritis, 570–571
    antibiotic regimens for, 571
    error in ED management of, 570
  renal stone disease, 575–577
    antibiotics for, 576–577
    clinical presentation of, 575
    diagnosis of, 575–576
    disposition, 576–577
    medical management for, 576
  STI treatment guidelines, 577–579

Genitourinary (*continued*)
 beta-lactam antibiotic allergies, 579
 Chlamydia trachomatis, 578
 Mycoplasma genitalium, 578–579
 Neisseria gonorrhoeae, 578
 pelvic inflammatory disease, 578
 penicillin allergies, 579
 Trichomonas vaginalis, 578
 testicular torsion, 568–569
  evaluation of, 569
  symptoms of, 568
  treatment of, 569
Gentamicin, 371
Geriatric abuse, 812–814, 813t
Geriatric patients
 abdominal trauma, 658
 agitation, management of, 549–550
 anxiety, 544
 ED
  goals of, 824–825
  Guidelines, 826
  screening, 826–827
 medical clearance, 559–560
  screening tests, 560t
 suicidal risk assessment, 540–541
  psychiatric history, 540
  risk factors, 540
Geriatrics
 delirium, 819–821, 826
 dementia, 822–823
 geriatric abuse, 812–814, 813t
 geriatric ED patient, goals of, 824–825
  screening, 826–827
 older adults
  overdiagnosing and overtreating UTIs, 817–819
  pain medications and procedural sedation in, 815–817
 older adults, polypharmacy in, 832–834
 pelvic fragility fractures, 808
 perform mobility testing, 830–831
  functional mobility assessment tools, 831t
  mobility assessment, 830
  post-assessment interventions, 830–831
 rib, hip/vertebral compression fractures, 807–809, *809*
 safe discharge, 828–829
  ancillary services, 829
  clinical approach, 828
  high risk identification, 828
  medications, 828
  mentation, 828
  mobility, 829
  what matters, 829
 trauma, 810–812
Giant cell arteritis (GCA), 343, 488–489
GI decontamination, 647–648
Gingival bleeding, 363
Globe rupture, 672–673
 ED role in, 673
 examination for, 672
Glottic visualization, 762
Glucocorticoids, 394, 524

Grip technique, 71, *71*
Gufoni maneuver, 481
Guillain-Barré, 606

H

HACE (*see* High-altitude cerebral edema)
Haloperidol, 551–553
Hand hygiene, 436
Handoffs/sign-outs, 918–919
HAPE (*see* High-altitude pulmonary edema)
Hartmann, Alexis, 28
HBO therapy, 257
 in carbon monoxide toxicity, 626–627
 mechanisms
  emergency-capable, 322–323
  frontiers, 323
  hyperbaric medicine, contacting, 324
  indications, 323–324
  other indications, 324
Headache, 487–489
 acute angle-closure glaucoma, 488
 bacterial meningitis, 488
 carotid artery dissection, 488
 cerebral venous thrombosis/cerebral venous sinus thrombosis, 488
 giant cell arteritis, 488–489
 subarachnoid hemorrhage, 487–488, 489t
Head, ears, eyes, nose, and throat (HEENT)
 dental infections
  history and physical exam, 347
  imaging, 347–348
  management, 348
 dental trauma, 361
  bleeding, 363
  pain control, 362
  trauma, 362–363
 dislodged trach, replacing, 354–356
 epiglottitis, 333–335
 epistaxis
  initial measures, 345
  packing, 346
  persistent bleeding, 346
  reassessment, 345–346
 foreign bodies
  aspirated, 350–351
  choosing lure, 350
  complications, 351
  seeing is believing, 349
  tools for removal, 350t
 herpes zoster ophthalmicus
  presentation, 331–332
  treatment, 332
 lateral canthotomy with cantholysis, 356–357
  complications and follow-up, 358
  indications and contraindications, 357
  supplies and procedure, 357, *358*
 parapharyngeal abscess, 335–337
 POCUS pearls for the eye
  diagnostic findings, 365
  preparing to scan, 364
  scanning technique tips, 364
 post-tonsillectomy bleed

preparation and intervention, 359–360, 360t
risk factors and anatomic changes, 359
therapeutics, 360–361
red eye, 339
history, 340
ophthalmology, 340–341
physical examination, 340
retropharyngeal abscess, 335–337
tracheoinnominate fistula
acute management for ongoing hemorrhage, 353
anatomy, 352
diagnostics, 353
risk factors, 352
sentinel bleed and catastrophic hemorrhage, 352–353
tympanic membrane perforation, 337–339
vision loss
acute angle-closure glaucoma, 342
causes of, 342–344
central retinal artery occlusion, 343
central retinal vein occlusion, 344
chiasmal and retrochiasmal disorders, 344
differential diagnosis for, 342t
endophthalmitis, 343
giant cell arteritis, 343
keratitis, 343
optic neuritis, 344
retinal detachment, 343
uveitis, 343
vitreous hemorrhage, 343
Health disparities, 136
Heat stroke (HS), 319–322
HEENT (*see* Head, ears, eyes, nose, and throat)
Hematology/oncology
anticoagulants, 377t
antithrombotic MOA/half-life, 376t
DOACs and antiplatelet agents, 376–377
and hemorrhage, 375
warfarin reversal, 375–376
blood transfusion, 383–384
cryoprecipitate, 385
factors VIII, IX, 386
plasma (frozen and liquid), 385
platelets, 385
PRBCs, 384, 384t
risks and complications of, 384
type, screen, and crossmatch, 384
whole blood, 384
CAR-T-related cytokine release syndrome, 378
assessment and management, 379, 379t
diagnosis, 379
CAR-T-related ICANS, 378
assessment and management, 380t
diagnosis, 379
febrile neutropenia
antibiotics for, 370–371
hemolytic uremic syndrome, 368, 369t
leukemia
differential diagnosis, 388
epidemiology, 387
family discussion, 388
laboratory evaluation, 387–388
oncologic emergencies, 388
in pediatrics, 386–389
physical examination, 387
symptoms, 387
sickle cell attacks
acute coronary syndrome, 372–373
infection, 374
sequestration, 373–374
stroke, 373
thrombotic thrombocytopenic purpura, 367–368, 369t
transfusion-associated circulatory overload, 381–383
transfusion related acute lung injury, 381–383
Hematometra, 514
Hemodialysis, 639
for salicylate poisoning, 619–620
Hemolytic uremic syndrome (HUS), 368, 369t
Hemoperitoneum, 723
Hemoptysis, 588–590
causes of, 588–590, 589t
management of, 590
Hemorrhage
anticoagulants and, 375
dialysis fistula, 573–574
Hemostasis, 654
Herbal supplements, 631, 632t
Herpes zoster ophthalmicus (HZO)
presentation, 331–332
treatment, 332
HFNC (*see* High-flow nasal cannula)
HG (*see* Hyperemesis gravidarum)
HHS (*see* Hyperglycemic hyperosmolar state)
HiB vaccine, 333
Hidradenitis suppurativa (HS)
clinical presentation, 272–273
ED management and definitive therapy, 273
I&D, 273
HIET (*see* High-dose insulin therapy)
High-altitude cerebral edema (HACE), 307
acclimatization, 308
descent, 308
medications, 308
pediatrics, 308
prevention and treatment, 308, 309t
High-altitude pulmonary edema (HAPE), 307–308
acclimatization, 308
descent, 308
medications, 308
pediatrics, 308
prevention and treatment, 308, 309t
High-dose insulin therapy, 645–646
adverse effects, 646
dosing protocols, 646
High-dose opioid infusions, 121
Highest quality CPR, 1–3
components of, 1
ETCO2 monitoring, 2
real-time feedback monitoring, 2
High-flow nasal cannula (HFNC), 44–46, *44*, *46*, 74, 591–592
High-pressure injection injuries, 698–699, *699*

Hill-Sachs defect, 707–708
HINTS examination, 475–477
Hip dislocation, 753–756
  diagnostic tests, 754
  physical examination, 753–754
  positioning and technique, 755t
  procedural sedation, 754
  reduction technique, 754, 756
HIV, and acute coronary syndrome, 184–185
HIV PEP (*see* HIV post-exposure prophylaxis)
HIV post-exposure prophylaxis (HIV PEP), 413–415
  exposures associated, with, 413–414
  importance of, 415
  initiation, 414–415
  regimens, 414t
HOTT acronym, 674
HS (*see* Heat stroke)
HS (*see* Hidradenitis suppurativa)
HSV (*see* Neonatal herpes simplex virus)
HT (*see* Human trafficking)
Human trafficking (HT), 915–917
  how to respond, 916–917
  trafficked patient, recognizing, 916
Humira (*see* Adalimumab)
Hunter criteria, serotonin toxicity, 629
HUS (*see* Hemolytic uremic syndrome)
Hydralazine, 178
Hydromorphone (opioids), 94
Hyperacute (gonococcal) conjunctivitis, 341
Hyperangulated blades, 79
Hyperbaric oxygen therapy, 311
Hyperechoic cholelithiasis, *226*, *232*
Hyperemesis gravidarum (HG), 523–525
  disposition, 525
  ED evaluation, 523–524
  management, 524
Hyperglycemic hyperosmolar state (HHS), 281–284
Hyperkalemia, 300–303, 303t
Hypertensive emergencies, 177–179
Hypertensive urgency, 179
Hyperthermia, 622
Hyperthyroidism, 605
Hypoglycemia, 605
  in alcohol intoxication, 611
Hyponatremia, 304–306
  classifications and symptoms, 305t
  treatment approaches by etiology, 306t
Hypotension, 392
  in alcohol intoxication, 611
Hypothermia, 146–147
  in alcohol intoxication, 611
Hypothermia After Cardiac Arrest With Nonshockable Rhythm trial, 21
Hypothermia, therapeutic, 20
Hypothyroidism, 605
Hypovolemia, 603
Hypovolemic shock, 23, 24t
Hypoxemia, 591–592
Hysterectomy, 564
HZO (*see* Herpes zoster ophthalmicus)

I

IBD (*see* Inflammatory bowel disease)
ICAD (*see* Internal carotid artery dissection)
ICANS, 378
  assessment and management, 380t
  diagnosis, 379
ICH (*see* Intracerebral hemorrhage)
IEMs (*see* Inborn errors of metabolism)
IHD (*see* Intermittent hemodialysis)
Immune-based therapy toxicities
  anti-CD20 mAbs, 399–400
  anti-TNF mAbs, 400
  VEGF mAbs, 400
Immune dysfunction, 867
Immune-mediated encephalitides, 401–402
  clinical presentation, 402
  diagnosis, 402–403
  disposition, 403
  management, 403
  pathophysiology, 402
  pediatric considerations, 403–404
Immunology
  ACE-inhibitor angioedema
    adjunct medications, 397–398
    diagnosis of, 396
    early airway assessment and intervention, failure to perform, 398
    inappropriate discharge from the ED, 398
    treatment, 396, 396t
    types of, 395–396
  anaphylaxis
    epinephrine in, 391–392
    second-line medications in, 393–395
  immune-based therapy toxicities
    anti-CD20 mAbs, 399–400
    anti-TNF mAbs, 400
    VEGF mAbs, 400
  immune-mediated encephalitides, 401–402
    clinical presentation, 402
    diagnosis, 402–403
    disposition, 403
    management, 403
    pathophysiology, 402
    pediatric considerations, 403–404
  liver transplantation, 407–408
    assessing recipient, 408–409
    pediatrics, 409–410
    significance of timing, 408t
  lung transplantation
    infection and malignancy, 405
    initial impression, 405
    management, 406–407
    mechanical complications, 406
    rejection, 406
Inborn errors of metabolism (IEMs)
  classification, 291–292
  diagnosis/clinical presentation, 292
  ketoacidosis, 299–300
  treatment/management, 293
  workup, 292
Inclusion (chlamydial) conjunctivitis, 341
Induction induced sympatholysis, 64
Ineffective triggering, 105, *105*

Infection, 374, 515, 848, 855 (*see specific types*)
Infectious disease
  acute retroviral syndrome (ARS), 411–412
  chronic obstructive pulmonary disease, 423–424
  febrile traveler, 429–432
    epidemiology, 429–430
    etiologies of fever, 431t
    history, 430
    incubation period, 429t
    physical exam/workup, 430–431
  HIV post-exposure prophylaxis, 413–415
    exposures associated, with, 413–414
    importance of, 415
    initiation, 414–415
    regimens, 414t
  influenza treatment, 421–423
  meningitis, 418–420
    diagnostic testing, 419
    physical examination, 419
    treatment, 419–420
  mpox, 425–426
  osteomyelitis, 427–428
    diagnosis, 427t
    finding consistent, with, 428t
  sepsis, 438–441
    source control in, 439–441
    studies, 438–439
    surviving sepsis campaign and SEP-1, 438
  source control, 439–441
    anatomy, 441t
    defined, 440
    needs, 440
    timing, 440
  spread, preventing, 436–437
    airborne transmission, 436–437
    blood-borne transmission, 437
    contact transmission, 436
    droplet transmission, 436
    isolation precautions, 436–437
  syphilis, 432–435
    diagnostic testing, 432, 434
    stages, 433t, 434t
    treatment for, 434–435
    treatment regimens, 434t
  toxic shock syndrome (TSS), 416–418
    diagnosis, 417
    management, 417
    presentation, 416–417
Infectious flexor tenosynovitis, 458–460
Inflammation, 146
Inflammatory bowel disease (IBD) imaging, 207–208
Infliximab (Remicade), 400
Influenza treatment, 421–423, 422t
Initial vent settings, 89–93, *90*
Innominate artery, 352
Inspiratory flow rate, 91
Inspiratory plateau pressure (P$_{plat}$), 90–91, 100–101, *101*
Inspiratory positive airway pressure (IPAP), 44
Intensive care unit (ICU) boarder
  benzodiazepines, avoiding, 121
  DVT, avoiding, 122
  excess fluid administration, avoiding, 120–121
  high-dose opioid infusions, avoiding, 121
  nephrotoxic medications, avoiding, 121–122
  unnecessary blood transfusion, avoiding, 121
Intermittent hemodialysis (IHD), 118, 119t
Internal carotid artery dissection (ICAD), 488
Intimate partner violence (IPV), 909, 913–915
  assess safety, 914
  document appropriately, 914–915
  engage support services, 914
  make the diagnosis, 913–914
  provide medical care and emotional support, 914
Intracerebral hemorrhage (ICH), 471–472
  BP management, in, 471t
Intracranial pressure, 497–499
Intraocular pressure, 340
Intravenous fluids, 42–43
Intubation, 46
  optimization, 51
IPAP (*see* Inspiratory positive airway pressure)
IPV (*see* Intimate partner violence)
Iritis, 332
Ischemic priapism, 571
  treatment of, 572
Ischemic stroke, 466–467
Isoniazid, 58t
Isopropyl alcohol toxicity, 617
IV liothyronine (T3), 297

J

Jaundice, 247–249
  defined, 247
  toxins and, 248
  with unconjugated hyperbilirubinemia, 248
Jones' fractures, *688*, 689
JYNNEOS vaccine, 426

K

Kallikrein inhibitors, 397
Kanavel signs, 459
Keratitis, 343
Ketamine, 65, 66, 67, 75, 95, 716, 925–927, 939
  administration, 927
  analgesia, 926–927
  extensive first-pass metabolism, 925–926
  primary mechanism, 925
  procedural sedation, 926
Ketoacidosis
  alcoholic ketoacidosis, 298–299
  IEMs, 299–300
  salicylate ingestion, 299
  starvation ketoacidosis, 299
Ketofol, 926
Kidney injuries, IR for, 670
Kidney stones, 575–577
  antibiotics for, 576–577
  clinical presentation of, 575
  diagnosis of, 575–576
  disposition, 576–577
  medical management for, 576

Knee pain, 454–456
  examination, 455
  history of, 454–455
  workup and imaging, 455
Kratom, 624
Kyphosis, 606

L

Labetalol, 178t, 472
Lacerations, 835
Lacosamide, 486t
LAST (*see* Local anesthetic systemic toxicity)
Last known well time (LKWT), 492–494
Latent syphilis, 433t, 434t
Lateral canthotomy with cantholysis, 356–357
  complications and follow-up, 358
  indications and contraindications, 357
  supplies and procedure, 357, *358*
Left bundle branch block (LBBB)/
    ventricular-paced rhythm, 145
Leukemia
  differential diagnosis, 388
  epidemiology, 387
  family discussion, 388
  laboratory evaluation, 387–388
  oncologic emergencies, 388
  in pediatrics, 386–389
  physical examination, 387
  symptoms, 387
Levetiracetam, 486t
Levofloxacin, 582
Lidocaine, 168, 725
  in cardiac arrest, 7
Limp, 774–775
  infection, 774
  inflammation, 775
  injury, 774–775
  neoplastic, 775
  structural, 775
Linton-Nachlas tube (LNT), 736, *737*
Lipodermatosclerosis, 261
Lisfranc injury, 700–701, *702*
Lithium toxicity, 639
Liver injuries, IR for, 670
Liver transplantation, 407–408
  assessing recipient, 408–409
  pediatrics, 409–410
  significance of timing, 408t
LKWT (*see* Last known well time)
LNT (*see* Linton-Nachlas tube)
Local anesthetic systemic toxicity (LAST), 928
Long COVID, 869–872
  future studies, 871–872
  management, 871
  pathophysiology, 870–871, *870*
  prevalence, 870
  symptoms, 871
Lorazepam, 486t
Lower extremity blocks, 725
LP (*see* Lumbar puncture)
LRINEC Score, 257
Lumbar puncture (LP), 719–721
  antibiotics administration, 720
  consent and contraindications, 719–720
  imaging, 720
  midazolam, 720
  patient positioning, 720–721
  post-LP pain, 721
  sterility, 720
Lung transplantation
  infection and malignancy, 405
  initial impression, 405
  management, 406–407
  mechanical complications, 406
  rejection, 406
Lupus erythematosus (LE), 268
Lutz sign, 259

M

Macklin effect, 597
Magnesium sulfate, in cardiac arrest, 7
Magnetic resonance imaging (MRI)
  acute pancreatitis, 205–206
  inflammatory bowel disease, 208
  spinal epidural abscess, 444
  for subarachnoid hemorrhage, 464
Magnetic resonance venography (MTV), 470
Maisonneuve fracture, 692
  mechanism of injury, 692–693
  with proximal fibula fracture, *693*
  treatment of, 693–694
Major burns
  ABCs of, 666–668
  airway, 666
  defined, 666
  fluid resuscitation, 667
  patient guidelines for, 666t
  Rule of Nines, *667*
  %TBSA estimation tools, 667–668, *668*
  transfer, 668
Mammalian bite wounds, 845
Mandatory reporting laws, 908–910
Manual left uterine displacement, 2
Marginal ulceration, 237
Marijuana, 633–635
  acute toxicity, 634
  cannabinoid hyperemesis syndrome
      (CHS), 635
  diagnostic testing, 634–635
  management, 634–635
  pharmacokinetics/pharmacodynamics, 634
  THC, 633–634
  urine drug screening, 635
Masculinizing procedures, 564
MASH approach, 112, 112t
Massive transfusion (MT), 32–33
Mastectomy, 564
MAT (*see* Medical-assisted therapy)
Material injury, 910–913
  chain of custody, 912
  documentation pearls, 912
  forensic photography, 912
  general evidence collection principles, 911
  state/jurisdictional considerations, 911
  strangulation, 912
  suspect exams, 912
MC (*see* Myxedema coma)
McMahon score, 449

MCS, temporary, 43
Mechanical ventilation, 108–109
　airway pressure release ventilation, 109–110
　average volume-assured pressure support, 110
　pressure regulated volume control, 109
　pressure support ventilation, 109
　for salicylate poisoning, 619
　synchronized intermittent mandatory ventilation, 109
Mediastinal emphysema
　(see Pneumomediastinum)
Medical-assisted therapy (MAT), 546, *547*
Medical clearance, 559–560
　screening tests, 560t
Medication-assisted abortions, 513
Meningitis, 418–420
　diagnostic testing, 419
　physical examination, 419
　treatment, 419–420
Mesenteric venous thrombosis, 204
Metformin, 639–640
Methadone, 943
Methanol, 616
　ingestion, treatment for, 617
Metoclopramide, 524
Metoidioplasty, 564
Metronidazole, 578
MG (*see* Myasthenia gravis)
MI (*see* Myocardial infraction)
Midazolam, 65, 486t, 716, 720
Milrinone, 42
Minnesota tube, 736, *737*
MIS-C, 867–869
Misoprostol toxicity, 515
Monomorphic ventricular arrhythmias, 9
Motor vehicle crash (MVC), 516–517
　additional considerations, 517
　airway and breathing, 516
　circulation, 516
　disability and fetal considerations, 516–517
　ED evaluation, 516
　secondary survey, 517
Mpox virus, 265–267, 425–426
MRI (*see* Magnetic resonance imaging)
mRNA-1273 (Moderna), 881, 882t, 884
MSK low back pain, 452–453
MT (*see* Massive transfusion)
MTV (*see* Magnetic resonance venography)
Multidose activated charcoal, 648
Multimorbidity, 138
Muscle relaxers, 452–453
Musculoskeletal (nontrauma)
　acute compartment syndrome (ACS), 445–447
　back pain
　　emergency, 450–451
　　epidural abscess on, 443–444
　　MSK low back pain, 452–453
　　muscle relaxers, 452–453
　　opioids, 452–453
　　steroids, 452–453
　infectious flexor tenosynovitis, 458–460
　knee pain, 454–456
　　examination, 455
　　history of, 454–455
　　workup and imaging, 455
　rhabdomyolysis, 447–449
　septic joint, 456–457
　spinal epidural abscess, 443–445
MVC (*see* Motor vehicle crash)
Myasthenia gravis (MG), 490–492
　drugs to avoid, 491
Myasthenia gravis, 606
Mycoplasma genitalium, 578–579
Myocardial infraction (MI), 146
Myocarditis masquerade
　clinical presentation, 191, 192t
　consensus based diagnostic and therapeutic algorithm, *194*
　diagnosis, 192–193
　prognosis, 193
　treatment, 193
Myxedema coma (MC), 296–297

N

NAC (*see* N-acetylcysteine)
N-acetylcysteine (NAC), 215–216
Naloxone, 57
　for opioid use disorder, 548
Naltrexone, 943
Nasopharyngoscopy, in ED, 731–733
　indications, 732
　patient assessment, 732
　patient preparation, 732
　procedural considerations, 732–733
　resources, 733
National Institute on Drug Abuse Quick Screen, 546
NCCTH (*see* Noncontrast CT head)
Neck injuries, 651–653
　computed tomography angiogram (CTA), 652–653
　hard signs of, 652t
　management of, 652
　no-zone approach, 651
　soft signs of, 652t
　superficial/deep, 652
　zones of neck, 651, 651t
Necrotizing fasciitis (NF)
　antibiotic therapy, 256–257
　classification, 255, 255t
　clinical presentation, 256, 256t
　diagnostic imaging, 257
　differential diagnosis, 256, 256t
　evaluation, 256, 257t
　HBO therapy, 257
　LRINEC Score, 257
　risk factors, 256
Necrotizing soft-tissue infection (NSTI)
　(*see* Necrotizing fasciitis (NF))
Needle bevel/tip, 928
Needle cricothyrotomy, 79
Needle decompression, 727–728
　bougie, 728
　finger thoracostomy, 728
　landmarks, 727–728
　ultrasound, 728
Neisseria gonorrhoeae, 578
Neonatal herpes simplex virus (HSV), 267–268

Neonatal resuscitation, 759–761
  advanced resuscitation, 760–761
  basic resuscitation, 759–760
  warming the baby, 760
Nephrotoxic medications avoiding, ICU boarder, 121–122
Nerve blocks, ultrasound-guided regional, 724–726
  femoral nerve/fascia iliaca compartment blocks, 725
  lower extremity blocks, 725
  potential benefits, 724–725
  risks and complications, 726
  technique, 725–726
  upper extremity blocks, 725
Neurogenic, 147
Neurology
  antiseizure medications, 484–486
  cerebral venous sinus thrombosis (CVST), 468–470
    clinical manifestations, 469t
    risk factors, 469t
  cervical artery dissection (CAD), 461–463
    clinical features of, 463t
    neurologic findings, patients with, 462–463
    vertebral artery dissection, 462
  Dix-Hallpike and Epley maneuvers, 480–484
  dizziness, 477–480
    AVS, 479–480
    EVS, 478–479
  headache, 487–489
    acute angle-closure glaucoma, 488
    bacterial meningitis, 488
    CAD, 488
    CVT/CVST, 488
    GCA, 488–489
    subarachnoid hemorrhage, 487–488, 489t
  HINTS examination, 475–477
  intracerebral hemorrhage (ICH), 471–472
    BP management, in, 471t
  ischemic stroke, 466–467
  myasthenic, 490–492
  psychogenic nonepileptiform seizures (PNES), 495–496
    diagnosis, 495–496, 495t
    generalized, 495
    treatment, 496
  subarachnoid hemorrhage (SAH), 464–465
  transient ischemic attack (TIA), 473–475
    Canadian, score, 474t
  traumatic brain injury (TBI), 497–499
    intracranial pressure, 497–499
  wake-up stroke, 492–494
    evaluation, 492–493
    evidence, 493
    searching, 493–494
Neurosyphilis, 433t, 434t
Neurotoxicity, 57–58
Neutropenic fever, 370
NF (see Necrotizing fasciitis)
Nicardipine, 177, 178t, 471–472
NIH COVID-19 Treatment Guidelines, 875
Nikolsky sign, 259

NIPPV/NPPV (see Non-invasive positive pressure ventilation)
Nirmatrelvir/ritonavir (Paxlovid), 875
NMB agents, 72
NMDA receptor, 925
Noncontrast CT head (NCCTH), 492
Nondihydropyridine CCBs, 643
Non-invasive positive pressure ventilation (NIPPV/NPPV), 44–46, 44, 74, 77
Nonischemic priapism, 571
  treatment of, 572
Nonocclusive mesenteric ischemia, 203–204
Non-ST-elevation myocardial infarction (NSTEMI), 141, 160, 161t
Nonsteroidal anti-inflammatory medications (NSAIDs), 362, 453, 932–934
  importance of, 933–934
  mechanism of, 933
Norepinephrine, 17, 42, 65
Normal saline, administration of, 28–29
North American pit vipers, 328
Novavax (see NVX-CoV2373 (Novavax))
NSAIDs (see Nonsteroidal anti-inflammatory medications)
NSTEMI (see Non-ST-elevation myocardial infarction)
NVX-CoV2373 (Novavax), 881, 882t, 884

O

Obesity, 70–73
Obstetrics/gynecology
  eclampsia, 503–504
  hyperemesis gravidarum, 523–525
    disposition, 525
    ED evaluation, 523–524
    management, 524
  motor vehicle crash (MVC), 516–517
    additional considerations, 517
    airway and breathing, 516
    circulation, 516
    disability and fetal considerations, 516–517
    ED evaluation, 516
    secondary survey, 517
  ovarian torsion, 501–502
    bedside examination, 501–502
    CT, 502
    ultrasound, 502
  pelvic examination of, 518–519
    accuracy and interexaminer reliability, 518–519
    patient consideration, 518
    STI testing, 519
    warranted, 519
  perimortem cesarean delivery (PMCD), 505–507
  peripartum cardiomyopathy, 509–513
    lab and diagnostic comparison of, 510t
    pharmacologic management, 511–512t
  postabortion complications, 513–515
    evaluation of, 514–515
    self-managed abortions of, 515
  pregnancy, dyspnea in, 507–509
    diagnosis, 507–508

PE, risk of, 508
  presentation, 508
  treatment, 508
 sexual assault survivor, 520–522
  diagnostic evaluation, 520–521
  discharge instructions, 522
  documentation pitfalls, 521
  examination, 520
  laws and protocols, 521
  postexposure prophylaxis, 521, 522t
  stabilization and evaluation, 520
  trauma, 521
Obstruction, 80
Obstructive lung disease, 89–90
Obstructive shock, 23, 24t
Occlusion myocardial infarction (OMI), 161t
 echocardiography, 161
 STEMI-NSTEMI paradigm, 160
 vs. NOMI paradigm, 160–161
Ocrelizumab (Ocrevus), 399
Ocrevus (*see* Ocrelizumab (Ocrevus))
Octreotide, 202
Ocular decontamination, 649
OESIL Score, 196
OH (*see* Orthostatic hypotension)
Older adults, 136, 137–139
 acute coronary syndrome
  interpretation of ECG, 138
  risk stratification, 138–139
  signs and symptoms, 137–138
 overdiagnosing and overtreating UTIs, 817–819
  interpreting the results, 818
  symptoms and signs of, 818
  test, 817–818
 pain medications and procedural sedation in, 815–817
 polypharmacy in, 832–834
  geriatric patients, prescribing best practices for, 833
  pharmacokinetics, 832–833
OM (*see* Otitis media)
OMI (*see* Occlusion myocardial infarction)
Opiates, 58t
Opioids, 623, 643–644, 935–937, 936t
 for back pain, 452–453
Opioid use disorder (OUD), 942–944 (*see also* Substance use disorders)
 abstinence-based therapy, 546
 harm reduction, 548, 942–943
 medications, 943
 referral for treatment, 547–548
 regulatory and legal issues, 944
 treatment, 943–944
 treatment algorithm for, *547*
Optic nerve, 365
Optic neuritis, 344
Orthopedics
 calcaneus fractures, 697
 chance fracture, 711–712
 high-pressure injection injuries, 698–699, *699*
 Jones' fractures, *688*, 689
 Lisfranc injury, 700–701, *702*

Maisonneuve fracture, 692
 mechanism of injury, 692–693
 with proximal fibula fracture, *693*
 treatment of, 693–694
proximal fibula fracture, 692–694, *693*
pseudo-Jones fractures, 688–689
scaphoid fracture, 694–696
 Herbert classification of, 696, 696t
scapula fracture, 690–691
shoulder dislocation, 707–710
 glenolabral pathology, 707–708
 Hill-Sachs defect, 707–708
 proximal humerus fractures, 708–710, *708–709*
 special populations, 710
stress fractures, 689
supracondylar fractures, 685–687
 compartment syndrome, 687
 CRITOE mnemonic, 686, 686t
 extension-type, classification of, 686t
 types of, 685
tibial plateau fracture, 703–706, *704–705*
 diagnostic imaging for, 704–705
 Schatzker classification system of, 706, *706*
 treatment for, 705
zone 1 tuberosity avulsion fractures, 688–689
zone 2 metaphysis/diaphysis, 689
zone 3 proximal diaphysis, 689
Orthostatic hypotension (OH), 280–281
Osborn waves, 146–147
Oseltamivir (Tamiflu), 422, 422t
Osteomyelitis, 427–428
 diagnosis, 427t
 finding consistent, with, 428t
Otitis media (OM), 337–339
OUD (*see* Opioid use disorder)
Ovarian torsion, 501–502
 bedside examination, 501–502
 CT, 502
 ultrasound, 502
Overdrive pacing, 170
Oxygenation, optimizing, 14–16

P

Packed red blood cells (pRBCs), 384, 384t, 681–683
PAILS mnemonic, 146
Pain management
 buprenorphine, 945–947
  acute pain management, 946
  full-agonist opioids, 947
  maximize nonpharmacologic and nonopioid strategies, 945–946
 ketamine, 925–927
  administration, 927
  analgesia, 926–927
  extensive first-pass metabolism, 925–926
  primary mechanism, 925
  procedural sedation, 926
 nonsteroidal anti-inflammatory medications (NSAIDs), 932–934
  importance of, 933–934
  mechanism of, 933
 opioids, 935–937, 936t

Pain management (*continued*)
opioid use disorder (OUD), 942–944
  harm reduction, 942–943
  medications, 943
  regulatory and legal issues, 944
  treatment, 943–944
pharmacologic adjuncts, 938–939
procedural adjuncts, 938
psychosocial adjuncts, 939
sickle cell disease (SCD), 940–941
tramadol, 930–932
  misconceptions, 931
  world without, 931–932
ultrasound-Guided Nerve Blocks (UNGBs), 928–929
PALS program, 783–786
algorithms, 784, 785t
pediatric assessment, 784, *784*
systematic approach, 784
Pancreas, injuries, IR for, 671
Pantoprazole, 202
Parapharyngeal abscess, 335–337
Paracentesis, in emergency department, 722–723
complications, 723
contraindications, 722
indications, 722
technique, 722–723
Paralysis, 67
Parapharyngeal abscess, 335–337
Pasteurella multocida, 844
Patient-centered care, 888
Patient experience, 887–888
Patients, communication with, 887–888
Patient satisfaction, 887–888
Patient's death to family members, delivering bad news about, 889–890
Patient-ventilator asynchrony, 105
Paxlovid (*see* Nirmatrelvir/ritonavir (Paxlovid))
PDP (*see* Push-dose pressor)
PE (*see* Pulmonary embolism)
Peak inspiratory pressure (PIP), 100–101, *101*
Pediatric myocarditis, mishaps in, 791–793
diagnostic studies, 792
management, 792–793
patient assessment, 791
Pediatrics
abdominal trauma, 658
acute mountain sickness, 308
agitation, management of, 549–550
airway, 761–763
anxiety, 544
appendicitis, 200, 771–773, 772t
  complications, 773
  history, 771
  scoring systems, 771
  treatment, 773
  workup—imaging, 771
  workup—labs, 771–773
asthma, 793–795
back pain, 776–778
  can't miss diagnoses, 777–778
  history and physical exam, 776
  workup, 777
blunt cerebrovascular injury (BCVI), 659–660

CTA screening, 660
Denver Screening Criteria, 659–660
high-risk injury patterns associated with, 659, 660t
signs and symptoms of, 659, 660t
cardiac surgery, 801–804, *802, 803*
child abuse, 757–758
constipation, 789–790, 790t
croup (laryngotracheitis), 764–765
diabetic ketoacidosis (DKI), 781–783
electrocardiogram (ECG), during childhood, 778–781, *780*
emergency department (ED)
pediatric procedural sedation, 766–768, 767t
high-altitude cerebral edema, 308
high-altitude pulmonary edema, 308
immune-mediated encephalitides, 403–404
indications and contraindications for TcP in, 171
injuries, IR for, 671
leukemia in, 386–389
limp, 774–775
infection, 774
inflammation, 775
injury, 774–775
neoplastic, 775
paralysis, 775
structural, 775
liver transplantation, 409–410
medical clearance, 559–560
screening tests, 560t
neonatal resuscitation, 759–761
advanced resuscitation, 760–761
basic resuscitation, 759–760
warming the baby, 760
PALS program, 783–786
algorithms, 784, 785t
pediatric assessment, 784, *784*
systematic approach, 784
pediatric myocarditis, mishaps in, 791–793
diagnostic studies, 792
management, 792–793
patient assessment, 791
resuscitative endovascular balloon occlusion of aorta in, 37
spinal motion restriction, 664–665
status epilepticus, 798–801
initial management and first-line therapy, 799, 799t
refractory status and additional diagnostic workup, management of, 800
second-line therapy, 799–800
special considerations, 800
suicidal risk assessment, 540–541
psychiatric history, 540
risk factors, 540
trauma, 796–798, 797t
urinary tract infection (UTI), 768–770
risk factors, 768–769
young infants, 786–788
clinical signs and symptoms, 786
historical guidelines, 787
PCT, 787
and age, 787

practical considerations and confounders, 787–788
2021 AAP guidelines, 787
Pediatric volvulus, 250–251
PEEP (*see* Positive end-expiratory pressure)
PEG tubes, displaced, 223–224
Pelvic examination, 518–519
  accuracy and interexaminer reliability, 518–519
  patient consideration, 518
  STI testing, 519
  warranted, 519
Pelvic fractures
  bedsheet to stabilize, 662
  causes of, 661
  point-of-care ultrasound, 662, *662*
  RSI, 663
  treatment for, 661
Pelvic fragility fractures, 808
Pelvic inflammatory disease (PID), 578
Pelvis injuries, IR for, 670
Pemphigus vulgaris
  defined, 258–259, 259t
  follow-up, 260
  treatment, 259–260
Penetrating abdominal injury, IR for, 671
Penicillin, 434t, 435
Penicillin allergies, 579
Peptic ulcer disease (PUD) (*see* Perforated peptic ulcer)
Peramivir (Rapivab), 422, 422t
PERC rule, 585
Perforated peptic ulcer, 240–241
  complications, 241
  diagnosis, 241
  management, 241–242
  presentation of, 241
  risk factors, 241
Perform mobility testing, 830–831
  functional mobility assessment tools, 831t
  mobility assessment, 830
  post-assessment interventions, 830–831
Pericardial effusion, 677–678
  diagnostic consideration, 677
  drain, 677–678
  procedure, 678
Pericarditis, 146
Perimortem cesarean delivery (PMCD), 505–507
Peripartum cardiomyopathy (PPCM), 509–513
  lab and diagnostic comparison of, 510t
  pharmacologic management, 511–512t
Peripheral pressor
  dilute concentration of, 30–31
  evaluating infusion site, 31
  risks of administration, 30
  selection of IV site for, 30
PH (*see* Pulmonary hypertension)
Phalloplasty, 564
Phenibut, 624
Phenobarbital
  for alcohol withdrawal, 612
  for alcohol withdrawal syndrome, 97
  disposition for, 98–99
  dosing, 97–98

Physostigmine, 631, 642
PID (*see* Pelvic inflammatory disease)
PIP (*see* Peak inspiratory pressure)
Pit vipers, 328
Plantar puncture wound pearls/pitfalls, 839–841
Plasma, 33
Plasma (frozen and liquid) transfusion, 385
Platelets transfusion, 385
PMCD (*see* Perimortem cesarean delivery)
PNES (*see* Psychogenic nonepileptiform seizures)
Pneumobilia, *234*
Pneumomediastinum, 597–599
  diagnosis of, 598
  management of, 599
  pathophysiology of, 597–598
  secondary, 598
  signs and symptoms of, 598
  spontaneous, 597–598
  tension, 598
POCUS pearls for eye
  diagnostic findings, 365
  preparing to scan, 364
  scanning technique tips, 364
Poison Control Center, 59
Poisoning
  airway and breathing, 57
  circulation, 57
  decontamination, 58
  enhanced elimination, 58–59
  evaluation of, 54–57
  neurotoxicity, 57–58
  poison control consultation, 59
  toxidromes, 55–56t
  toxin-dependent stabilization, 58t
Polymorphic ventricular arrhythmias, 9
Popliteal sciatic blocks, 725
Positive end-expiratory pressure (PEEP), 44, 91, 92t
Postabortion, complications, 513–515
  evaluation of, 514–515
  self-managed abortions of, 515
Postcardiac arrest, 16
  blood pressure goals, clinical trials of, 17
  guideline recommendations, 17
Post–cardiac arrest syndrome, 14
Post-COVID-19 syndrome, 869
Posterior acoustic shadowing, 229, *231*
Posterior vitreous detachment, 365
Post-tonsillectomy bleed
  preparation and intervention, 359–360, 360t
  risk factors and anatomic changes, 359
  therapeutics, 360–361
PPCM (*see* Peripartum cardiomyopathy)
PPIs (*see* Proton pump inhibitors)
pRBCs (*see* Packed red blood cells)
Pregnancy
  and acute coronary syndrome, 184
  anxiety, 544
  computed tomography on
    fetal exposure, 252t
    utero induced deterministic radiation effects, 253t

Pregnancy (*continued*)
conditions contributing to respiratory depression in, 84t
dyspnea in, 507–509
diagnosis, 507–508
PE, risk of, 508
presentation, 508
treatment, 508
gravid patient, preparation for establishing definitive airway for, 85t
intubation, 84–86
Pregnant women, abdominal trauma, 658
Pre-intubation resuscitation, 64–65
Premedication, 66
Preoxygenation, 46, 71
Pressure regulated volume control (PRVC), 109
Pressure support ventilation (PSV), 109
Priapism, 571–572
American Urological Association guidelines, 572
defined, 571
error in management of, 571–572
etiology of, 572
ischemic, 571
nonischemic, 571
treatment of, 572
types of, 571
Primary hypoxemic respiratory failure, 45–46
Primary syphilis, 433t, 434t
Procainamide, 168
Procedural sedation, 713–716
patient assessment, 713–714
pharmacologic selection, 714–716, 715t
procedure setup, 714
Procedures/skills
arthrocentesis, 717–719
complications and pitfalls, 718–719
contraindications, 717
indications, 717
synovial fluid interpretation, 718
technique, 717–718
austere environment, lifesaving, 748–749
airway management, 748
finger thoracostomy, 748–749
hemorrhage control, 749
balloon tamponade, for UGIB, 736–738
complications, 737–738
contraindications, 736
indications, 736
technique, 736–737
types, 736–737, *737*
chest tube placement, 742–744
complications, 743
contraindications, 743
setup, 743
technique, 743–744
Foley catheter insertion, 733–735
indications, 734
risks of catheterization, 734
troubleshooting, 734–735
hip dislocation, 753–756
diagnostic tests, 754
physical examination, 753–754
positioning and technique, 755t
procedural sedation, 754
reduction technique, 754, 756
lumbar puncture (LP), 719–721
antibiotics administration, 720
consent and contraindications, 719–720
imaging, 720
midazolam, 720
patient positioning, 720–721
post-LP pain, 721
sterility, 720
nasopharyngoscopy, in ED, 731–733
indications, 732
patient assessment, 732
patient preparation, 732
procedural considerations, 732–733
resources, 733
needle decompression, 727–728
bougie, 728
finger thoracostomy, 728
landmarks, 727–728
ultrasound, 728
paracentesis, 722–723
complications, 723
contraindications, 722
indications, 722
technique, 722–723
sedation, 713–716
patient assessment, 713–714
pharmacologic selection, 714–716, 715t
procedure setup, 714
shunt systems, 750–752
failure, causes of, 751
failure, workup of, 751–752
tap, 752
splinting, 738–739
general procedure, 738–739
indications, 740–741t
special considerations, 739
type, 740–741t
ultrasound for line confirmation, 729–730
placement guide, 729–730
postplacement confirmation, 730
postprocedural complications, 730
ultrasound-guided regional nerve blocks, 724–726
femoral nerve/fascia iliaca compartment blocks, 725
lower extremity blocks, 725
potential benefits, 724–725
risks and complications, 726
technique, 725–726
upper extremity blocks, 725
US-guided IV placement, pitfalls in, 745–747
procedural mechanics, 746–747, *746*
procedural preparation, 745–746
procedural success, 747
target vein selection, 745
Prolonged QT syndromes, 169
Promethazine, 524
Prophylactic antibiotics, 844–846, 845t
Propofol, 66, 67, 94, 716
Prostatitis, 580–582
ABP, 580

antibiotic selection, 582
asymptomatic inflammatory, 580
CBP, 580
classification of, 580
CP/CPPS, 580
diagnosis of, 580
treatment of, 580, 581t
Proton pump inhibitors (PPIs), 202
Proximal fibula fracture, 692–694, *693*
Proximal humerus fractures, 708–710, *708–709*
PRVC (*see* Pressure regulated volume control)
Pseudo-Jones fractures, 688–689
Pseudomonas aeruginosa, 841, 845
PSV (*see* Pressure support ventilation)
Psychiatric patients, boarding, 554–555
  communication, 555
  consultation, 554
  defined, 554
  evaluation, 554
  home medications, 554–555
  reassessments, 555
  recommendations, 554
Psychogenic nonepileptiform seizures (PNES), 495–496
  diagnosis, 495–496, 495t
  generalized, 495
  treatment, 496
Psychology
  agitation
    antipsychotics used for, 552t
    droperidol for, 552
    management of, 549–550, 549t
  anxiety, 542–545
    defined, 542
    disposition, 544–545
    management, 543–544
    older patients, 544
    pediatrics, 544
    pregnancy, 544
    signs and symptoms of, 542–543, 543t
  boarding, psychiatric patients
    communication, 555
    consultation, 554
    defined, 554
    evaluation, 554
    home medications, 554–555
    reassessments, 555
    recommendations, 554
  dementia *vs.* delirium, 537–539
    defined, 537
    diagnosis of, 537–538
    etiologies of, 539t
    features of, 538t
    risk factors for, 537
  droperidol, 551–553
    for agitation, 552
    history of, 551
    policy statement on use of, 552
    recommended dosing, 553t
  medical clearance, 559–560
    screening tests, 560t
  substance use disorders, 545–548
    CAGE-AID Questionnaire, 546, 546t
    harm reduction, 548
    intervention, 546–547
    National Institute on Drug Abuse Quick Screen, 546
    referral for treatment, 547–548
    screening, 546
    treatment algorithm for, *547*
  suicide risk assessment, 540–541
    and alcohol use disorder, 541
    psychiatric history, 540
    risk factors, 540
    support tools, 541
pUF, 119, 119t
Pulmonary embolism (PE)
  acute, management of, 53
  dyspnea in pregnancy, 508
  extracorporeal membrane oxygenation in, 12
  stratification of, 52–53
  thrombolysis, 53
  thrombolytic therapy, 53
Pulmonary embolism, 156, 585–587
  classifications of, 593–594, *594*
  D-dimer, 586
  decision-making algorithm for, *596*
  diagnosis of, 585
  high pretest probability of, 586
  low pretest probability of, 585–586
  moderate pretest probability of, 586
  PERC rule, 585
  prevalence of, 586
  risk stratification algorithm, *587*
  Wells score, 585
Pulmonary hypertension (PH), 602–604
  classification of, 50t
  continue medications in ED, 51
  intubation optimization, 51
  pathophysiology of, 602–603
  resuscitate RV to avoiding deterioration, 50–51
  and RV failure, 49–50
  volume overload consequences, 603–604
  WHO classification, 602t
Pupillary constriction, 340
Pupillary reactivity, 340
Pupillary reflex, 365
Push-dose pressor (PDP), 122–123
  human error, 124
  patient selection, 123–124
  systems-based protocols, 124
Pyelonephritis, 570–571
  antibiotic regimens for, 571
  error in ED management of, 570

Q
QRS interval, 641

R
Race and ethnicity, 136
Rapid sequence intubation (RSI), 86
  paralysis, 67
  premedication, 66
  sedation, 66–67
Rapid ultrasound for shock and hypotension (RUSH), 25, *26*

Rapivab (*see* Peramivir (Rapivab))
Rate control, atrial fibrillation, 172
REBOA (*see* Resuscitative endovascular balloon occlusion of aorta)
Red eye, 339
  history, 340
  ophthalmology, 340–341
  physical examination, 340
Refractory cardiac arrest, extracorporeal membrane oxygenation in, 12–13
Refractory cardiogenic shock, extracorporeal membrane oxygenation in, 12
Refractory hypoxemia
  in intubated patient, 111–113
  in patients with ARDS, 113t
Regional anesthesia, 816
Relenza (*see* Zanamivir (Relenza))
Remdesivir, 875
Remicade (*see* Infliximab (Remicade))
Renal replacement therapy (RRT)
  access site, 118
  contraindications, 118
  in emergency department, 116–120
  indications, 117
  modes of, 118–119
  risks, 117
Renal stone disease, 575–577
  antibiotics for, 576–577
  clinical presentation of, 575
  diagnosis of, 575–576
  disposition, 576–577
  medical management for, 576
Respiratory failure with refractory hypoxia, 13
Respiratory rate, 91
Resuscitation (*see also* Cardiac arrest; Echocardiography)
  cardiac tamponade, 38–41
  cardiogenic shock, 41–43
  defibrillator pads, 3–5
  extracorporeal membrane oxygenation (ECMO), 11–13
  highest quality CPR, 1–3
  high-flow nasal cannula, 44–46
  massive transfusion, 32–34
  non-invasive positive pressure ventilation, 44–46
  normal saline administration, 28–29
  oxygenation, optimizing, 14–16
  peripheral pressors, 30–31
  poisoning, 54–59
  pulmonary embolism, 52–54
  pulmonary hypertension, 49–51
  REBOA placement, 36–37
  resuscitative thoracotomy, 34–35
  shock
    cardiogenic, 23, 24t
    defined, 22
    distributive, 23, 24t
    fluid management, 26–27
    hypovolemic, 23, 24t
    obstructive, 23, 24t
    rapid ultrasound for shock and hypotension (RUSH), 25, *26*
  sonography in hypotension and cardiac arrest, 26, *26*
  TEE, 27
  targeted temperature management (TTM)
    guidelines for use of, 21
    pathophysiologic rationale and targeted outcomes of, 20
  ventilation, optimizing, 14–16
  ventricular fibrillation (VF), 8–10
  ventricular tachycardia (VT), 8–10
Resuscitative endovascular balloon occlusion of aorta (REBOA), 35
  in pediatric patients, 37
  zones and appropriate placement, 36–37
Resuscitative thoracotomy (RT), 34–35, 675
Retained products of conception (RPOC), 514
Retinal detachment, 343, 365
Retrobulbar hematoma, 365
Retrochiasmal disorder, 344
Retropharyngeal abscess, 335–337
Return of spontaneous circulation (ROSC), 2, 14–15, *15*
  post-ROSC ECG
    considerations, 48
    patterns, 47–48
    push for delayed, 48
    push for immediate, 48
Rhabdomyolysis, 447–449
Rheumatologic disorders/acute coronary syndrome, 183
Rhythm control, atrial fibrillation, 172–173
Rib, hip/vertebral compression fractures, 807–809, *809*
Richmond Agitation-Sedation Scale, 96t
Right bundle branch block (RBBB), ST-elevation myocardial infarction in, 151–153, *153*
Rituxan (*see* Rituximab (Rituxan))
Rituximab (Rituxan), 399
Rivaroxaban, 680
Road rash, 853–855
  anesthesia, 854
  assessment, 854
  cosmetics, 854–855
  dressings, 854
  scrub, 854
Rocuronium, 67, 75
Ropivacaine, 725–726
ROSC (*see* Return of spontaneous circulation)
ROSE Risk Score for syncope, 196
RPOC (*see* Retained products of conception)
RRT (*see* Renal replacement therapy)
RSI (*see* Rapid sequence intubation)
RT (*see* Resuscitative thoracotomy)
RT-PCR
  false positives, 873–874
  pharmacologic management matters in, 875–876
  sensitivity of, 873
  testing, 874
Rule of Nines, *667*
Rumack-Matthew nomogram, 614
RUSH (*see* Rapid ultrasound for shock and hypotension)

S

Safe discharge, 828–829
  ancillary services, 829
  clinical approach, 829
  high risk identification, 828
  medications, 828
  mentation, 828
  mobility, 829
  what matters, 829
SAFE-T, 541
SAH (see Subarachnoid hemorrhage)
SALAD technique, 80
Salicylate ingestion, 299
Salicylate poisoning, 618–620
  AC for, 619
  dextrose, 619
  endotracheal intubation, 619
  hemodialysis, 619–620
  mechanical ventilation, 619
  mixed respiratory alkalosis with metabolic acidosis, 618
  overdose history, 618
  serum and urinary alkalinization, 619
  serum salicylate concentration for, 618
  treatment decisions, 619
Salicylates, 639
Salicylate toxicity, 644
Salpingo-oophorectomy, 564
SARS-CoV-2 (see COVID-19 pandemic)
SBP (see Spontaneous bacterial peritonitis)
SBT (see Sengstaken-Blakemore tube)
SBT (see Short Blessed Test)
Scalpel-finger-bougie technique, 72
Scalp wounds, 862–864
Scaphoid fracture, 694–696
  Herbert classification of, 696, 696t
Scapula fracture, 690–691
SCD (see Sickle cell disease)
Scleritis, 341
Sclerosing panniculitis, 261
Scoliosis, 606
Screening labs, 559–560
Scrotoplasty, 564
SCUBA diving, 314
SCUF (see Slow continuous ultrafiltration)
Secondary insults, 498–499
Secondary pneumomediastinum, 598
Secondary syphilis, 433t, 434t
Sedation, 66–67
Seizures, 641
Self-managed abortions of, 515
Sengstaken-Blakemore tube (SBT), 736, 737
Sentinel injuries, 757
Sepsis, 438–441
  source control in, 439–441
  studies, 438–439
  surviving sepsis campaign and SEP-1, 438
Septic arthritis, 456
Septic joint, 456–457
Sequestration, 373–374
Serotonin antagonists, 524
Serotonin toxicity, 628–629
  diagnosis of, 629
  Hunter criteria, 629
  treatment of, 629
  xenobiotics, 628t
Serum ethanol level, 559–560
Sexual assault survivor, 520–522
  diagnostic evaluation, 520–521
  discharge instructions, 522
  documentation pitfalls, 521
  examination, 520
  laws and protocols, 521
  postexposure prophylaxis, 521, 522t
  stabilization and evaluation, 520
  trauma, 521
Sexually transmitted infections (STIs)
  treatment guidelines, 577–579
    beta-lactam antibiotic allergies, 579
    Chlamydia trachomatis, 578
    Mycoplasma genitalium, 578–579
    Neisseria gonorrhoeae, 578
    pelvic inflammatory disease, 578
    penicillin allergies, 579
    Trichomonas vaginalis, 578
SGA placement, 2, 79
SHoC (see Sonography in hypotension and cardiac arrest)
Shock
  cardiogenic, 23, 24t
  defined, 22
  distributive, 23, 24t
  fluid management, 26–27
  hypovolemic, 23, 24t
  obstructive, 23, 24t
  rapid ultrasound for shock and hypotension (RUSH), 25, 26
  sonography in hypotension and cardiac arrest, 26, 26
  TEE, 27
Short Blessed Test (SBT), 826
Shortness of breath, 605–607
  cardiovascular, 605
  endocrine-metabolic, 605–606
  ENT, 605
  hematologic, 606
  musculoskeletal, 606
  neuromuscular, 606
  psychologic, 606–607
  toxins, 606
Shoulder dislocation, 707–710
  glenolabral pathology, 707–708
  Hill-Sachs defect, 707–708
  proximal humerus fractures, 708–710, 708–709
  special populations, 710
Shunt systems, 750–752
  failure
    causes of, 751
    workup of, 751–752
  tap, 752
Sickle cell attack
  acute coronary syndrome, 372–373
  infection, 374
  sequestration, 373–374
  stroke, 373
Sickle cell disease (SCD), 940–941

Sigmoid volvulus, 250
Signs of life, defined, 674
SIMV (*see* Synchronized intermittent mandatory ventilation)
Sinus bradycardia, *302*
Slit-lamp examination, 340
Slow continuous ultrafiltration (SCUF), 119, 119t
Small bowel obstruction, 237
Smoke inhalation
　systemic toxins, 310–311
　thermal burns, 310
SOAP ME mnemonic, 68
Sodium bicarbonate, in cardiac arrest, 6
Sodium-channel blockers, 58t
Sonography in hypotension and cardiac arrest (SHoC), 26, *26*
Source control, 439–441
　anatomy of infections requiring, 441t
　defined, 440
　needs, 440
　timing, 440
Spinal epidural abscess (EPA), 443–445
Spinal epidural metastasis, 451
Spinal immobilization, 664–665
　defined, 664
Spinal motion restriction, 664–665
　goal of, 664
Spleen injuries, IR for, 670
Splinting, 738–739
　general procedure, 738–739
　indications, 740–741t
　special considerations, 739
　type, 740–741t
Spontaneous bacterial peritonitis (SBP)
　diagnosis, 243–244
　examination, 243
　pathogenesis, 243
　positive cultures in a discharged patient, 244
　treatment, 244
Spontaneous pneumomediastinum, 597–598
Spontaneous polymorphic ventricular arrhythmias, 9
Spread of infection, preventing, 436–437
　isolation precautions, 436–437
　　airborne transmission, 436–437
　　blood-borne transmission, 437
　　contact transmission, 436
　　droplet transmission, 436
Staphylococcal toxic shock syndrome (STSS)
　clinical presentation, 270–271
　diagnostic criteria, 271
　pathogenesis, 270
　treatment, 271
Staphylococcus aureus, 838, 841, 844
Starvation ketoacidosis, 299
Stasis dermatitis, 261
Status epilepticus, 798–801
　initial management and first-line therapy, 799, 799t
　refractory status and additional diagnostic workup, management of, 800
　second-line therapy, 799–800
　special considerations, 800

"Stay away" approach, 929
ST-elevation myocardial infarction (STEMI), 141, 160
　in RBBB, 151–153, *152*
STEMI (*see* ST-elevation myocardial infarction)
Steroids, 396, 452–453
STIs (*see* Sexually transmitted infections)
Streptococcus pyogenes, 844
Stress fractures, 689
Stress testing, 162–164
Stridor, 764
Stroke, 373 (*see also* Wake-up stroke)
ST segment elevation
　aneurysmal LV, 146
　early repolarization, 145, *145*
　electrolytes, 144–145
　inflammation, 146
　LBBB and ventricular-paced rhythm, 145
　neurogenic, 147
　Osborn waves, 146–147
　sudden death, 147
　thrombotic occlusion, 146
　ventricular hypertrophy, 145, *146*
STSS (*see* Staphylococcal toxic shock syndrome)
Subarachnoid hemorrhage (SAH), 464–465, 487–488, 489t
Submassive PE, thrombolytic therapy, 593–595
Substances of use, 623–624
　carfentanyl, 623
　DBZD, 624
　fentanyl, 623
　kratom, 624
　opioids, 623
　phenibut, 624
　THC, 623–624
　xylazine, 623
Substance use disorders
　in emergency department, 545–548
　　CAGE-AID Questionnaire, 546, 546t
　　harm reduction, 548
　　intervention, 546–547
　　National Institute on Drug Abuse Quick Screen, 546
　　referral for treatment, 547–548
　　screening, 546
　　treatment algorithm for, *547*
Succinylcholine, 67, 75
Suction, 79
Sudden cardiac arrest, cardiac cath team following, 18
　ECG stratification, 18–19
　guideline recommendations, 19
Sudden death, 147
Suicide
　and alcohol use disorder, 541
　risk assessment, 540–541
　　psychiatric history, 540
　　risk factors, 540
　　support tools, 541
Suicide Prevention Resource Center ED Guide, 541
Sulfonylureas, 644
Supine roll test, 481, *483*

Supplements, 630–631
  dietary, 631
  herbal, 631, 632t
Supracondylar fractures, 685–687
  compartment syndrome, 687
  CRITOE mnemonic, 686, 686t
  extension-type, classification of, 686t
  types of, 685
Surgical abortions, 513–514
Surgical cricothyroidotomy, 82
Surgicel, 363
Surviving Sepsis Campaign guideline, 30
Sustained low-efficiency dialysis, 119, 119t
Sutures, 835–836
Sympathomimetic toxidrome, 620–622
  benzodiazepines for, 621
  patient management, 622
  signs and symptoms of, 621
Synchronized intermittent mandatory ventilation (SIMV), 109
Syncope, 195–197, 197t
Syphilis, 432–435
  diagnostic testing, 432, 434
  stages, 433t, 434t
  treatment for, 434–435
  treatment regimens, 434t
Systemic Illnesses
  DRESS, 268–269
  EN, 268
  LE, 268
  neonatal HSV, 267–268
Systemic infection and acute coronary syndrome, 184
Systemic toxins, 310–311

T

TACO (*see* Transfusion-associated circulatory overload)
TAD (*see* Thoracic aortic dissection)
Tamiflu (*see* Oseltamivir (Tamiflu))
Targeted Normothermia After Out-of-Hospital Cardiac Arrest, 21
Targeted temperature management (TTM)
  guidelines for use of, 21
  pathophysiologic rationale and targeted outcomes of, 20
TBI (*see* Traumatic brain injury)
TCA (*see* Traumatic cardiac arrest)
TcP (*see* Transcutaneous pacing)
TdP, 9
TEE, 27
TEG, 33, 680
Tendon/nerve injuries, 851–853
  appropriately splint and immobilize, 852
  assess neurovascular status, 852
  consultation and referral, 852–853
  copiously irrigate the wound, 851
  documentation, 853
  ensure patient education and follow-up, 852
  mechanisms of, 851
  perform functional testing, 852
  properly examine the wound, 852
Tension pneumomediastinum, 598

Tension pneumothorax, 156
Terminal QRS distortion, 145
Tertiary syphilis, 433t, 434t
Testicular torsion, 568–569
  evaluation of, 569
  symptoms of, 568
  treatment of, 569
Tetanus treatment recommendations, 845t
THC, 623–624, 633–634
Therapeutic hypothermia, 20
Thermal burns, 310
Thoracic
  acute asthma exacerbation, magnesium in, 600–601
    data, 600–601
    mechanism of action, 600
    patient selection, 601
  hemoptysis, 588–590
    causes of, 588–590, 589t
    management of, 590
  high-flow nasal cannula (HFNC), 591–592
  pneumomediastinum, 597–599
    diagnosis of, 598
    management of, 599
    pathophysiology of, 597–598
    secondary, 598
    signs and symptoms of, 598
    spontaneous, 597–598
    tension, 598
  pulmonary embolism (PE), 585–587
    D-dimer, 586
    diagnosis of, 585
    high pretest probability of, 586
    low pretest probability of, 585–586
    moderate pretest probability of, 586
    PERC rule, 585
    prevalence of, 586
    risk stratification algorithm, *587*
    Wells score, 585
  pulmonary hypertension (PH), 602–604
    pathophysiology of, 602–603
    volume overload consequences, 603–604
    WHO classification, 602t
  shortness of breath, 605–607
    cardiovascular, 605
    endocrine-metabolic, 605–606
    ENT, 605
    hematologic, 606
    musculoskeletal, 606
    neuromuscular, 606
    psychologic, 606–607
    toxins, 606
  submassive PE
    thrombolytic therapy for, 593–595
  ventilator management, for boarded ED patient, 608–609
Thoracic aortic dissection (TAD), 155–156
Thoracotomy
  ED, 675
    pathologies to address in, 676t
Thrombolysis, 53
Thrombolytic therapy, 53, 593–595
Thrombotic occlusion, 146, 203

Thrombotic thrombocytopenic purpura (TTP), 367–368, 369t
Thyroid storm, 293–294
  diagnosis, 294–295
  management, 295
  signs and symptoms, 294t
TIA (*see* Transient ischemic attack)
Tibial plateau fracture, 703–706, *704–705*
  diagnostic imaging for, 704–705
  Schatzker classification system of, 706, *706*
  treatment for, 705
TIC (*see* Trauma-informed care)
Tidal volume (V$_t$), 89–90
TIFs (*see* Tracheoinnominate fistulas)
Tissue-type plasminogen activator (tPA), 492–494
TMT joint injury, 700–701, *702*
Tobramycin, 371
Top surgery, 564
Torsades de pointes, 551
Torticollis, 335–337
Toxic alcohols, 616–617
Toxicity
  immune-based therapy
    anti-CD20 mAbs, 399–400
    anti-TNF mAbs, 400
    VEGF mAbs, 400
Toxicology
  acetaminophen toxicity, 613–615
    acetylcysteine for, 615
    chronic ingestions, treatment for, 615
    patients with liver failure, NAC, 614
    screening, 615
    symptoms and signs of, 613
    toxic level result after 8 hours, NAC, 614
    treatment for, 613
  alcohol intoxication, 611
  alcohols, toxic, 616–617
    ethylene glycol, 616
    isopropyl, 617
    methanol, 616
  alcohol withdrawal, 612
  beta-blockers toxicity, 636–638
    glucagon for, 637
    management of, 637
  calcium channel blockers toxicity, 636–638
    dihydropyridine agents, 636
    management of, 637
  carbon monoxide toxicity, 625–627
    HBO role in, 626–627
    incidence/causes, 625–626
    initial ED management, 626
    pathophysiology, 626
    presentation, 626
  decontamination, 647–649
    activated charcoal, 648
    dermal, 649
    gastric lavage, 649
    GI, 647–648
    multidose activated charcoal, 648
    ocular, 649
    whole bowel irrigation, 648
  dialyzable toxins, 638–640
    lithium, 639
    metformin, 639–640
    salicylates, 639
  high-dose insulin therapy, 645–646
    adverse effects, 646
    dosing protocols, 646
  marijuana, 633–635
    acute toxicity, 634
    cannabinoid hyperemesis syndrome (CHS), 635
    diagnostic testing, 634–635
    management, 634–635
    pharmacokinetics/pharmacodynamics, 634
    THC, 633–634
    urine drug screening, 635
  salicylate poisoning, 618–620
    AC for, 619
    dextrose, 619
    endotracheal intubation, 619
    hemodialysis, 619–620
    mechanical ventilation, 619
    mixed respiratory alkalosis with metabolic acidosis, 618
    overdose history, 618
    serum and urinary alkalinization, 619
    serum salicylate concentration for, 618
    treatment decisions, 619
  substances of use, 623–624
    carfentanyl, 623
    DBZD, 624
    fentanyl, 623
    kratom, 624
    opioids, 623
    phenibut, 624
    THC, 623–624
    xylazine, 623
  supplements, 630–631
    dietary, 631
    herbal, 631, 632t
  sympathomimetic toxidrome, 620–622
    benzodiazepines for, 621
    patient management, 622
    signs and symptoms of, 621
  TCA toxicity, 640–642
    bicarbonate therapy, 642
    ECG, 641
    features of, 641
    GI decontamination, 641
    physostigmine, 642
    QRS interval, 641
    seizures, 641
Toxic shock syndrome (TSS), 416–418
  diagnosis, 417
  management, 417
  presentation, 416–417
Toxidromes, 55–56t
Toxin-dependent stabilization, 58t
tPA (*see* Tissue-type plasminogen activator)
Tracheoinnominate fistulas (TIFs)
  acute management for ongoing hemorrhage, 353
  anatomy, 352
  diagnostics, 353
  risk factors, 352
  sentinel bleed and catastrophic hemorrhage, 352–353
Tracheostomy, 354–356

TRALI (*see* Transfusion related acute lung injury)
Tramadol, 833, 930–932
　misconceptions, 931
　world without, 931–932
Tranexamic acid (TXA), 33, 397, 680
Transcutaneous pacing (TcP), 169–170
　complications, 171
　procedure, 170–171
Transcutaneous pacing, 5
Transfeminine patient, gender affirming surgeries, 565
Transfusion-associated circulatory overload (TACO), 381–383
Transfusion related acute lung injury (TRALI), 381–383
Transgender, 135–136
Transient ischemic attack (TIA), 473–475
Transmasculine patient, gender affirming surgeries, 565
Trauma, 796–798, 810–812
　abdominal trauma, 656–658
　　blunt trauma, 657, *657*
　　FAST examination, 656–657
　　in geriatric patients, 658
　　mechanism of injury, imaging based on, 656–657
　　in pediatrics, 658, 797t
　　penetrating trauma, 657
　　in pregnant women, 658
　balanced transfusion, 681–682
　blunt cerebrovascular injury (BCVI), 659–660
　　CTA screening, 660
　　Denver Screening Criteria, 659–660
　　high-risk injury patterns associated with, 659, 660t
　　signs and symptoms of, 659, 660t
　cardiac arrest, 674–676
　　checklist for, 675t
　　ED thoracotomy, 675, 676t
　　emerging technologies, 675–676
　　hypovolemia, 674
　　oxygenation, 674–675
　　REBOA, 675–676
　　reversible causes of, 674
　　signs of life, 674
　　tamponade, 675
　　tension pneumothorax, 675
　crystalloids, 682
　globe rupture, 672–673
　　ED role in, 673
　　examination for, 672
　major burns
　　%TBSA estimation tools, 667–668, *668*
　　ABCs of, 666–668
　　airway, 666
　　defined, 666
　　fluid resuscitation, 667
　　patient guidelines for, 666t
　　Rule of Nines, *667*
　　transfer, 668
　neck, 651–653
　　computed tomography angiogram (CTA), 652–653
　　hard signs of, 652t
　　management of, 652
　　no-zone approach, 651
　　soft signs of, 652t
　　superficial/deep, 652
　　zones of, 651, 651t
　OR *vs.* IR, 669–671
　　aorta, 670
　　extremities, 671
　　kidney, 670
　　liver, 670
　　pancreas, 671
　　pediatric injuries, 671
　　pelvis, 670
　　penetrating abdominal injury, 671
　　spleen, 670
　　vascular, 671
　pelvic fractures
　　bedsheet to stabilize, 662
　　causes of, 661
　　point-of-care ultrasound, 662, *662*
　　RSI, 663
　　treatment for, 661
　pericardial effusion, 677–678
　　diagnostic consideration, 677
　　drain, 677–678
　　procedure, 678
　PRBCs, 681–683
　spinal immobilization, 664–665
　spinal motion restriction, 664–665
　trauma-induced coagulopathy, 682
　vascular injury, 654–655
　　computed tomography angiogram (CTA), 655
　　hard signs of, 654, 655t
　　proximity wounds, 655
　　soft signs of, 655, 655t
　whole blood, 682
Trauma-induced coagulopathy, 682
Trauma-informed care (TIC), 550
Traumatic brain injury (TBI), 497–499
　intracranial pressure, 497–499
　　secondary insults, 498–499
Traumatic cardiac arrest (TCA), 674–676
　checklist for, 675t
　ED thoracotomy, 675
　　pathologies to address in, 676t
　emerging technologies, 675–676
　REBOA, 675–676
　reversible causes of, 674
　　hypovolemia, 674
　　oxygenation, 674–675
　　tamponade, 675
　　tension pneumothorax, 675
　signs of life, 674
　toxicity, 640–642, 643
　　bicarbonate therapy, 642
　　ECG, 641
　　features of, 641
　　GI decontamination, 641
　　physostigmine, 642
　　QRS interval, 641
　　seizures, 641

Triage-TiTrATE-Test approach, 478, *478*
Trichomonas vaginalis, 578
Trichomoniasis, 578
Troponins, high-sensitivity, 153–155
TSS (*see* Toxic shock syndrome)
TTM (*see* Targeted temperature management)
TTP (*see* Thrombotic thrombocytopenic purpura)
TXA (*see* Tranexamic acid)
Tympanic membrane perforation, 337–339

U

UDS, 559–560
UGIB (*see* Upper gastrointestinal bleeding)
Ultrasound, 502
  for line confirmation, 729–730
    placement guide, 729–730
    postplacement confirmation, 730
    postprocedural complications, 730
  right upper quadrant, 215–216
Ultrasound-guided arthrocentesis, 718
Ultrasound-Guided Nerve Blocks (UNGBs), 928–929
Ultrasound-guided regional nerve blocks, 724–726
  femoral nerve/fascia iliaca compartment blocks, 725
  lower extremity blocks, 725
  potential benefits, 724–725
  risks and complications, 726
  technique, 725–726
  upper extremity blocks, 725
UNGBs (*see* Ultrasound-Guided Nerve Blocks)
Unstable angina, 141
Unstable bradycardia, 170
Upper extremity blocks, 725
Upper gastrointestinal bleeding (UGIB), 201, 222
Urinary tract infection (UTI), 768–770
  catheter-associated, 583–584
    bacteria, types of, 583
    contributing factors, 583
    sample collection, 583
    symptomatology, 583–584
    treatment, 583–584
  pyelonephritis, 570–571
    antibiotic regimens for, 571
    error in ED management of, 570
  risk factors, 768–769
U.S. Agency for Healthcare Research and Quality, 729
US-guided IV placement, pitfalls in, 745–747
  procedural mechanics, 746–747, *746*
  procedural preparation, 745–746
  procedural success, 747
  target vein selection, 745
Uterine artery embolization, 514
Uterine atony management, 514
Uterine perforation, 514
UTI (*see* Urinary tract infection)
Uveitis, 343

V

Vabysmo (*see* Faricimab (Vabysmo))
Vaccination mpox, 426
Vaccinations, 883–885
  anaphylaxis, 884
  children, 885
  GBS, 885
  myocarditis and pericarditis, 884–885
  pregnancy, complications of, 885
  VITT, 884
VAD (*see* Ventricular assist device)
VAD (*see* Vertebral artery dissection)
Valproic acid, 486t
The Van Beek Criteria, 861
Vancomycin, 371, 567
VAP (*see* Ventilator-associated pneumonia)
Varicella-zoster virus (chickenpox), 265–267
Vascular injury, 654–655
  computed tomography angiogram (CTA), 655
  hard signs of, 654, 655t
  IR for, 671
  proximity wounds, 655
  soft signs of, 655, 655t
Vaso-occlusive episode (VOE), 372–373
Vasopressin, 65
  in cardiac arrest, 7
Vasopressor, peripheral (*see* Peripheral pressor)
VBG (*see* Venous blood gas)
VEGF mAbs, 400
Veno-arterial extracorporeal membrane oxygenation, 11–12, *12*
Venous blood gas (VBG), 284–285
  HCO_3^- of, 285
  lactate of, 285–286
  pCO_2 of, 285
  pH of, 285
Venous thromboembolism (VTE), 585
  pulmonary embolism (PE), 585–587
    D-dimer, 586
    diagnosis of, 585
    high pretest probability of, 586
    low pretest probability of, 585–586
    moderate pretest probability of, 586
    PERC rule, 585
    prevalence of, 586
    risk stratification algorithm, *587*
    Wells score, 585
Veno-venous extracorporeal membrane oxygenation, 11–12, *12*
Ventilation optimizing, 14–16
Ventilation-induced lung injury (VILI), 102
Ventilator-associated pneumonia (VAP), 125–127
  defined, 125
  measures reducing risk of, 127t
Ventilator pressures
  auto-PEEP, 102, *102*
  compliance and airway resistance, 100
  inspiratory plateau pressure, 100–101, *101*
  monitoring, 99–103
  peak inspiratory pressure, 100–101, *101*
Ventilator waveforms, 103
  air trapping, 107–108, *107*
  autotrigger, 105
  double triggering, 106, *107*
  flow asynchrony, 106, *106*
  ineffective triggering, 105, *105*
  normal waveforms, 104, *104*

patient-ventilator asynchrony, 105
Ventricular assist device (VAD), 189–191, *190*
Ventricular fibrillation (VF), 8–10
Ventricular hypertrophy, 145, *146*
Ventricular-paced rhythm, 145
Ventricular storm (VS), management of, 167–169, *168*
Ventricular tachycardia (VT), 8–10, 164–166
Verbal de-escalation, 549–550, 549t
Vertebral artery dissection (VAD), 488
VF (*see* Ventricular fibrillation)
View, loss of
 first-pass options, 78–79
 rescue approaches, 79
 tools and anatomy to navigating, 78–79
 troubleshooting, 80
VILI (*see* Ventilation-induced lung injury)
Visceral leishmaniasis (VL), 79
Vision loss
 acute angle-closure glaucoma, 342
 causes of, 342–344
 central retinal artery occlusion, 343
 central retinal vein occlusion, 344
 chiasmal and retrochiasmal disorders, 344
 differential diagnosis for, 342t
 endophthalmitis, 343
 giant cell arteritis, 343
 keratitis, 343
 optic neuritis, 344
 retinal detachment, 343
 uveitis, 343
 vitreous hemorrhage, 343
Visual acuity, 340
Vitamin K antagonists, 679
Vitreous hemorrhage, 343, 365
VOE (*see* Vaso-occlusive episode)
Volkmann contracture, 687
Volume depletion, 280–281
Volvulus, 249–250
 cecal volvulus, 250
 gastric volvulus, 250
 pediatric volvulus, 250–251
 sigmoid volvulus, 250
VT (*see* Ventricular tachycardia)
VTE (*see* Venous thromboembolism)
Vulnerable adult, definition of, 909

W

Wake-up stroke, 492–494
 evaluation, 492–493
 evidence, 493
 searching, 493–494
Warfarin, 679
Warfarin reversal, 375–376
WCT (*see* Wide complex tachycardia)
WE (*see* Wernicke encephalopathy)
Wells score, 585
Wernicke encephalopathy (WE), 611
Whole blood, 682
Whole blood transfusion, 384
Whole bowel irrigation, 648

Wide-complex tachycardia (WCT), 57
 differential diagnosis of, *165*
Wolff-Parkinson-White Syndrome, 174–176, *175*
World Health Organization, 256, 869, 930
Wound care
 abscess incision and drainage, ED, 837–838
 care of minor burns, 855–857
  classification, 856
  initial management, 856
  minor burn criteria, 856
  wound care, 857
 digital blocks, 842–843
 ear injuries/lacerations, 849–851
 eyelid lacerations, 846–849, *847*
 fingernail faux pas, 860–862, *860*
 foreign body, wound, 858–859
 plantar puncture wound pearls/pitfalls, 839–841
 prophylactic antibiotics, 844–846, 845t
 road rash, 853–855
  anesthesia, 854
  assessment, 854
  cosmetics, 854–855
  dressings, 854
  scrub, 854
 scalp wounds, 862–864
 sutures, 835–836
 tendon/nerve injuries, 851–853
  appropriately splint and immobilize, 852
  assess neurovascular status, 852
  consultation and referral, 852–853
  copiously irrigate the wound, 851
  documentation, 853
  ensure patient education and follow-up, 852
  mechanisms of, 851
  perform functional testing, 852
  properly examine the wound, 852
WPW syndrome, 174

X

Xenobiotics, 628t, 643
Xofluza (*see* Baloxavir (Xofluza))
Xylazine, 623

Y

Yacovino maneuver, 481
Young infants, 786–788
 clinical signs and symptoms, 786
 historical guidelines, 787
 PCT, 787
  and age, 787
  practical considerations and confounders, 787–788
 2021 AAP guidelines, 787
Your deposition, 900–901

Z

Zanamivir (Relenza), 422, 422t
Zone 1 tuberosity avulsion fractures, 688–689
Zone 2 metaphysis/diaphysis, 689
Zone 3 proximal diaphysis, 689